Wiro J. Niessen   Max A. Viergever (Eds.)

Medical Image Computing and Computer-Assisted Intervention – MICCAI 2001

4th International Conference
Utrecht, The Netherlands, October 14-17, 2001
Proceedings

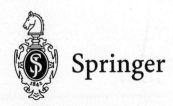

Springer

Series Editors

Gerhard Goos, Karlsruhe University, Germany
Juris Hartmanis, Cornell University, NY, USA
Jan van Leeuwen, Utrecht University, The Netherlands

Volume Editors

Wiro J. Niessen
Max A. Viergever
University Medical Center Utrecht, Image Sciences Institute
Heidelberglaan 100, 3584 CX Utrecht, The Netherlands
E-mail: {wiro/max}@isi.uu.nl

Cataloging-in-Publication Data applied for

Die Deutsche Bibliothek - CIP-Einheitsaufnahme

Medical image computing and computer assisted intervention : 4th
international conference ; proceedings / MICCAI 2001, Utrecht, The
Netherlands, October 14 - 17, 2001. Wiro J. Niessen ; Max A. Viergever
(ed.). - Berlin ; Heidelberg ; New York ; Barcelona ; Hong Kong ; London ;
Milan ; Paris ; Tokyo : Springer, 2001
 (Lecture notes in computer science ; Vol. 2208)
 ISBN 3-540-42697-3

CR Subject Classification (1998): I.5, I.4, I.3.5-8, I.2.9-10, J.3

ISSN 0302-9743
ISBN 3-540-42697-3 Springer-Verlag Berlin Heidelberg New York

Springer-Verlag Berlin Heidelberg New York
a member of BertelsmannSpringer Science+Business Media GmbH

http://www.springer.de

© Springer-Verlag Berlin Heidelberg 2001
Printed in Germany

Typesetting: Camera-ready by author, date conversion by Boller Mediendesign
Printed on acid-free paper   SPIN 10840779   06/3142   5 4 3 2 1 0

Preface

In the four years of its existence, MICCAI has developed into the premier annual conference on medical image computing and computer-assisted intervention. The single-track conference has an interdisciplinary character, bringing together researchers from both the natural sciences and various medical disciplines. It provides the international forum for developments concerning all aspects of medical image processing and visualization, image-guided and computer-aided techniques, and robot technology in medicine.

The strong interest in MICCAI is confirmed by the large number of submissions we received this year, which by far surpassed our expectations. The arrival of the shipload of papers just before the deadlines (one in the European and the other in the American time zone) was a particularly enjoyable experience, as was the whole procedure of preparing the scientific programme. Both the quantity and quality of the submissions allowed us to compose a volume of high quality papers, which we are sure will contribute to the further development of this exciting field of research.

As for the hard numbers, in total 338 submissions were received. Next to full papers, short communications were solicited for works in progress, hardware prototypes, and clinical case studies. Long papers were reviewed by three or four reviewers and short papers by two or three reviewers. The final selection of papers was carried out by the Programme Board. Out of the 246 long papers, 36 were accepted for oral presentation and 100 as full posters. An additional 75 of the long papers, and 47 out of 92 short papers were accepted as short posters. We are indebted to the the Scientific Review Committee and the Programme Board for their timely and high-quality reviews. The entire review procedure was carried out electronically. We are very grateful for the dedicated work performed by Shirley Baert and Josien Pluim in setting up and maintaining the web based review system, which made our task substantially easier.

We are very pleased to welcome delegates attending MICCAI 2001 in Utrecht. It is a small and friendly city with a beautiful centre and nice atmosphere, even if it rains (which it usually does in October). We hope that the conference proves to be both scientifically and socially an enjoyable and stimulating experience. For researchers who are unable to attend, we hope that the proceedings provide a valuable record of the scientific programme and we look forward to meeting you at the next MICCAI, which will be held in Tokyo, Japan, in 2002.

August 2001   Wiro J. Niessen and Max A. Viergever

Conference Organizing Committee

Fourth International Conference on
Medical Image Computing and Computer-Assisted Intervention
Utrecht, The Netherlands
14-17 October 2001

General Chair

Max A. Viergever   University Medical Center Utrecht,
                                    The Netherlands

Co-chairs

Takeyoshi Dohi   University of Tokyo, Japan
Michael W. Vannier   University of Iowa, USA

Programme Chair

Wiro J. Niessen   University Medical Center Utrecht,
                                    The Netherlands

Programme Board

Nicholas Ayache   INRIA, Sophia Antipolis, France
James S. Duncan   Yale University, New Haven, USA
David J. Hawkes   King's College London, UK
Ron Kikinis   Harvard Medical School, Boston, USA
J. B. Antoine Maintz (tutorials) Utrecht University, The Netherlands
Lutz.-P. Nolte   University of Bern, Switzerland
Kenneth Salisbury   Stanford University, USA
Jun-Ichiro Toriwaki   University of Nagoya, Japan
Dirk Vandermeulen   Catholic University Leuven, Belgium

Conference Managers

Sandra Boeijink   University Medical Center Utrecht,
Caroline Hop   The Netherlands

Local Organizing Committee

Margo Agterberg
Shirley Baert
Gerard van Hoorn
Marjan Marinissen
Josien Pluim
Luuk Spreeuwers
Koen Vincken   University Medical Center Utrecht,
Theo van Walsum   The Netherlands

Scientific Review Committee

John Adler	Stanford University Medical Center, USA
Amir Amini	Washington University, St. Louis, USA
Ludwig Auer	ISM, Salzburg, Austria
Shirley Baert	University Medical Center Utrecht, The Netherlands
Christian Barillot	IRISA, Rennes, France
Jan Blankensteijn	University Medical Center Utrecht, The Netherlands
Leendert Blankevoort	Academic Medical Center Amsterdam, The Netherlands
Michael Brady	University of Oxford, UK
Michael Braun	University of Technology, Sydney, Australia
Ivo Broeders	University Medical Center Utrecht, The Netherlands
Elizabeth Bullitt	University of North Carolina, Chapel Hill, USA
Aurelio Campilho	University of Porto, Portugal
Philippe Cinquin	University of Grenoble, France
Kevin Cleary	Georgetown University Medical Center Washington DC, USA
Jean Louis Coatrieux	INSERM, Rennes, France
Alan Colchester	University of Kent at Canterbury, UK
Louis Collins	Montreal Neurological Institute, Canada
Christos Davatzikos	Johns Hopkins University, Baltimore, USA
Brian Davies	Imperial College, London, UK
Takeyoshi Dohi	University of Tokyo, Japan
Kunio Doi	University of Chicago, USA
Norberto Ezquerra	Georgia Institute of Technology, Atlanta, USA
Aaron Fenster	J.P. Robarts Research Institute, London, Canada
Michael Fitzpatrick	Vanderbilt University, Nashville, USA
Robert Galloway	Vanderbilt University, Nashville, USA
James Gee	University of Pennsylvania, Philadelphia, USA
Guido Gerig	University of North Carolina, Chapel Hill, USA
Frans Gerritsen	Philips Medical Systems, Best, The Netherlands
Maryellen Giger	University of Chicago, USA
Michael Goris	Stanford University Medical Center, USA
Eric Grimson	Massachusetts Institute of Technology, Cambridge, USA
Alok Gupta	Siemens Corporate Research, Princeton, USA
Marco Gutierrez	University of Sao Paulo, Brasil
Pierre Hellier	INRIA, Rennes, France
Marcel van Herk	The Netherlands Cancer Institute, The Netherlands

Derek Hill	King's College London, UK
Karl Heinz Höhne	University of Hamburg, Germany
Xoji Ikuta	Nagoya University, Japan
Branislav Jaramaz	UPMC Shadyside Hospital, Pittsburgh, USA
Ferenc Jolesz	Harvard Medical School, Boston, USA
Leo Joskowicz	Hebrew University of Jerusalem, Israel
Nico Karssemeijer	University Hospital Nijmegen, The Netherlands
Christoph Kaufmann	National Capital Area Medical Simulation Center, Bethesda, USA
Erwin Keeve	Research Center Caesar, Bonn, Germany
Burt Klos	Catharina Hospital, Eindhoven, The Netherlands
Stephane Lavallée	PRAXIM, La Tronche, France
Boudewijn Lelieveldt	Leiden University Medical Center, The Netherlands
Heinz Lemke	Technical University Berlin, Germany
Murray Loew	George Washington University, Washington DC, USA
Anthony Maeder	Queensland University of Technology, Brisbane, Australia
Isabelle Magnin	INSA de Lyon CREATIS, France
Sherif Makram-Ebeid	Philips Research PRF, Paris, France
Armando Manduca	Mayo Clinic, Rochester, USA
Jean-Francois Mangin	Service Hospitalier Frederic Joliot, Orsay, France
Calvin Maurer Jr.	Stanford University, USA
Tim McInerney	Ryerson University, Toronto, Canada
Chuck Meyer	University of Michigan, Ann Arbor, USA
Michael Miga	Vanderbilt University, Nashville, USA
Ralph Mösges	University of Cologne, Germany
Sandy Napel	Stanford University, USA
Mads Nielsen	IT University of Copenhagen, Denmark
Robert Nishikawa	University of Chicago, USA
Allison Noble	University of Oxford, UK
Herke-Jan Noordmans	University Medical Center Utrecht, The Netherlands
Wieslaw Nowinski	Kent Ridge Digital Labs, Singapore
Silvia Olabarriaga	Federal University of Rio Grande do Sul, Brasil
Charles Pelizzari	University of Chicago, USA
Franjo Pernuš	University of Ljubljana, Slovenia
Terry Peters	University of Western Ontario, London, Canada
Stephen Pizer	University of North Carolina, Chapel Hill, USA

Frans Vos	Delft University of Technology, The Netherlands
Albert Vossepoel	Delft University of Technology, The Netherlands
Theo van Walsum	University Medical Center Utrecht, The Netherlands
Simon Warfield	Brigham and Women's Hospital, Boston, USA
Juergen Weese	Philips Hamburg, Germany
Harrie Weinans	University of Rotterdam, The Netherlands
Sandy Wells	Harvard Medical School, Boston, USA
Guang-Zhong Yang	Imperial College, London, UK
Alistair Young	University of Auckland, New Zealand
Alex Zijdenbos	Montreal Neurological Institute, Canada
Karel Zuiderveld	Vital Images, Plymouth, USA

MICCAI Board

Nicholas Ayache   INRIA, Sophia Antipolis, France
Alan C. F. Colchester   University of Kent at Canterbury, UK
Anthony M. DiGioia   UPMC Shadyside Hospital, Pittsburgh, USA
Takeyoshi Dohi   University of Tokyo, Japan
James Duncan   Yale University, New Haven, USA
Karl Heinz Höhne   University of Hamburg, Germany
Ron Kikinis   Harvard Medical School, Boston, USA
Stephen M. Pizer   University of North Carolina, Chapel Hill, USA
Richard A. Robb   Mayo Clinic, Rochester, USA
Russell H. Taylor   Johns Hopkins University, Baltimore, USA
Jocelyne Troccaz   University of Grenoble, France
Max A. Viergever   University Medical Center Utrecht,
                           The Netherlands

Table of Contents

Oral Sessions

Image-Guided Surgery I

Shape Analysis

Segmentation I

Quantitative Image Analysis I

Segmentation II

Image-Guided Surgery II

Registration II

Quantitative Image Analysis II

Posters

Medical Robotics and Devices I

Image-Guided Surgery I

Simulation, Planning, and Modelling I

Segmentation I

Registration I

Poster Session II

Medical Robotics and Devices II

Computer-Aided Diagnosis

Visualization and Augmented Reality

Registration II

Quantitative Image Analysis

Poster Session III

Time Series Analysis

Registration III

Simulation, Planning, and Modelling II

Segmentation III

Image-Guided Surgery II

Short Posters

Image-Guided Surgery I

Simulation, Planning and Modelling I

Registration I

Segmentation and Shape Analysis I

Visualization and Augmented Reality I

Quantitative Image Analysis I

Time Series Analysis I

Image-Guided Surgery II

Simulation, Planning, and Modelling II

Registration II

Segmentation and Shape Analysis II

Medical Robotics and Devices I

Time Series Analysis II

Simulation, Planning, and Modelling III

Registration III

Segmentation and Shape Analysis III

Computer-Aided Diagnosis

Visualization and Augmented Reality II

Medical Robotics and Devices II

A Method for Tracking the Camera Motion of Real Endoscope by Epipolar Geometry Analysis and Virtual Endoscopy System

Kensaku Mori[1,2], Daisuke Deguchi[2], Jun-ichi Hasegawa[3], Yasuhito Suenaga[2], Jun-ichiro Toriwaki[2], Hirotsugu Takabatake[4], and Hiroshi Natori[5]

[1] Image Guidance Laboratory, Department of Neurosurgery, Stanford University,
[2] Graduate School of Engineering, Nagoya University, Furo-cho, Chikusa-ku, Nagoya
464-8603, Japan
{ddeguchi,mori,toriwaki,suenaga}@nuie.nagoyap-u.ac.jp
[3] School of Computer and Cognitive Sciences, Chukyo University, Toyota, Japan
[4] Minami-ichijyo Hospital, Sapporo, Japan
[5] School of Medicine. Sapporo Medical University, Sapporo, Japan

Abstract. This paper describes a method for tracking the camera motion of a real endoscope by epipolar geometry analysis and image-based registration. In an endoscope navigation system, which provides navigation information to a medical doctor during an endoscopic examination, tracking the camera motion of the endoscopic camera is one of the fundamental functions. With a flexible endoscope, it is hard to directly sense the position of the camera, since we cannot attach a positional sensor at the tip of the endoscope. The proposed method consists of three parts: (1) calculation of corresponding point-pairs of two time-adjacent frames, (2) coarse estimation of the camera motion by solving the epipolar equation, and (3) fine estimation by executing image-based registration between real and virtual endoscopic views. In the method, virtual endoscopic views are obtained from X-ray CT images of real endoscopic images of the same patient. To evaluate the method, we applied it a real endoscopic video camera and X-ray CT images. The experimental results showed that the method could track the motion of the camera satisfactorily.

1 Introduction

An endoscope is a tool for observing the inside of a human body. A medical doctor inserts an endoscope inside a patient for diagnosis. The endoscope is controlled by only watching a TV monitor. Accordingly, it is hard to know the precise current location of the endoscopic camera. If it were possible to track the camera motion of an endoscope and display the current location to a medical doctor during an endoscopic examination in real time, this would be help the medical doctor greatly.

Virtual endoscope systems (VESs) are now widely used as systems that visualize the inside of the human body based on 3-D medical images in the medical

W. Niessen and M. Viergever (Eds.): MICCAI 2001, LNCS 2208, pp. 1–8, 2001.

field [1]. The user of a VES can fly through inside an organ or perform some quantitative measurements. The user can also create an examination path for a biopsy. The VES visualizes not only information about the target organ's wall but also information beyond the target organ by employing a translucent display technique. If we could fuse real and virtual endoscopes in the examination room, we could help medical doctors more easily operate endoscopes. Endoscope navigation systems, which provide navigation information to medical doctors during endoscopic examinations, should have two fundamental functions: (a) tracking of the camera motion of the endoscope and (b) presentation of the navigation information.

There are two types of endoscopes, i.e., rigid endoscopes and flexible endoscopes. It is difficult to acquire the tip position of a flexible endoscope by using an external positional sensor, since the body of the flexible endoscope can be bent into any form. Attaching a sensor at the tip is also hard due to space limitations.

Several research groups have already reported methods of registering real and virtual endoscopic images by using image-based registration techniques [2,3]. Bricault et al. [2] performed a frontier-work on the registration of real and virtual endoscopic images. They used branching structure information of the bronchi. This registration was statically performed. Unfortunately, they did not consider the continuous tracking of the camera motion. Our group also reported a method for the continuous tracking of the camera motion by using optical flow analysis and image-based registration [5]. We detected only the forward and backward motion of the endoscope from optical flow patterns. The image-based registration was performed as the precise estimation of the endoscope's position. The main problem of this previous methods was that it could not estimate the camera motion correctly around areas where there were no feature structures such as a branching structure. For example, the previous method could not detect the rotational motion inside a tube when we could not see branching structures.

This paper describes a method for tracking the camera motion of a flexible endoscope by using epipolar geometry analysis and image-based registration between real endoscopic (RE) and virtual endoscopic (VE) views enabling us to track the camera motion continuously. In Section 2, we briefly explain the epipolar geometry analysis, which is a fundamental theory of this paper. We describe the details of the proposed method in Section 3. Experimental results and discussions are shown in Section 4.

2   Recovering the Camera Motion

2.1   Epipolar Geometry

The proposed method directly estimates the camera motion by using the epipolar geometry [6]. The epipolar geometry defines the relationship of cameras located at two different positions. Figure 1 is an illustration that explains the relationship of two position-varied cameras. Let $\mathbf{X}$ be a point located in a 3-D space, and $\mathbf{C}$

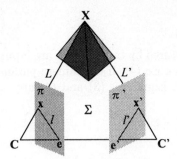

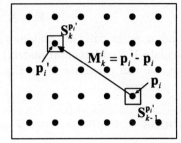

Fig.1 Epipolar geometry.   **Fig.2** Finding a corresponding point-pair.

and $\mathbf{C}'$ the locations of the two cameras. The plane Σ is a plane defined by $\mathbf{C}$, $\mathbf{C}'$, and $\mathbf{X}$. $\mathbf{x}$ and $\mathbf{x}'$ are projected points of $\mathbf{X}$ on the image planes π and π'. Any point located on the line $\mathbf{L}$ should always be projected to the same point $\mathbf{x}$. The line $\mathbf{l}'$ is a projected line of $\mathbf{L}$ on the image plane π' defined by the camera $\mathbf{C}'$. $\mathbf{L}'$ and $\mathbf{l}$ are defined in the same way. The lines $\mathbf{l}$ and $\mathbf{l}'$ are called "epipolar lines". It is obvious that the epipolar lines pass the points $\mathbf{e}$ and $\mathbf{e}'$, called "epipoles", on each projection plane. The epipoles show the relationship between the two viewpoints $\mathbf{C}$ and $\mathbf{C}'$.

2.2   Epipolar Equation

Let us assume that the initial camera position $\tilde{\mathbf{x}}$ moves to $\tilde{\mathbf{x}}'$ by the rotational motion $\mathbf{R}$ and the translational motion $\mathbf{T}$. In this case, the relationship between $\tilde{\mathbf{x}}$ and $\tilde{\mathbf{x}}'$ is expressed by the following equation.

$$\lambda' \tilde{\mathbf{x}}' = \lambda R \tilde{\mathbf{x}} + \eta \mathbf{T}, \tag{1}$$

where λ and η are constants. Figure 2 shows the relation of each vector in Eq. (1). Since $\lambda' \tilde{\mathbf{x}}'$, $\lambda R \tilde{\mathbf{x}}$, and $\eta \mathbf{T}$ exist in the same plane, the following equation should be satisfied.

$$\tilde{\mathbf{x}}' \cdot (\mathbf{T} \times R \tilde{\mathbf{x}}) = 0, \tag{2}$$

where $\cdot$ and $\times$ mean the inner product and the cross product, respectively. Equation (2) can be rewritten as Eq.(3) by using $\mathbf{T} \times R\tilde{x} = [\mathbf{T}]_\times R\tilde{\mathbf{x}}$, $\mathbf{E} = [\mathbf{T}]_\times R$, and $[\mathbf{T}]_\times = \begin{pmatrix} 0 & -T_3 & T_2 \\ T_3 & 0 & -T_1 \\ -T_2 & T_1 & 0 \end{pmatrix}$.

$$\tilde{\mathbf{x}}'^T \mathbf{E} \tilde{\mathbf{x}} = 0. \tag{3}$$

$\mathbf{E}$ is called the "Essential matrix". When we denote $\mathbf{A}$ as the camera parameter matrix defined by the focal length, the unit length of each axis, the center position of an image, and the angle of each axis, Eq. (3) is rewritten by using $\tilde{\mathbf{m}} = \mathbf{A}\tilde{\mathbf{x}}$ and $\tilde{\mathbf{m}}' = \mathbf{A}\tilde{\mathbf{x}}'$ as

$$\tilde{\mathbf{m}}'^T \mathbf{F} \tilde{\mathbf{m}} = 0. \tag{4}$$

Here

$$E = A^T FA. \tag{5}$$

If corresponding point-pairs of two views captured by two cameras are inputted, we can calculate F (fundamental matrix) from Eq (4). If the camera parameter A is known, we can calculate E by Eq. (5). Equations (3) and (4) are called "epipolar equations".

3   Methods

3.1   Preparation

Coordinate System in Tracking The goal of tracking the camera motion is to obtain a sequence of viewing parameters of the real endoscope that is represented in the CT coordinate system. Each viewing parameter is represented as $Q = (P, w)$ here. $P = (x, y, z)$ is the camera position of the endoscope, and $w = (\alpha, \beta, \gamma)$ represents the camera orientation. The final goal of the tracking is to find a Q able to generate a virtual endoscopic view that is similar to the current frame of the real endoscopic video for each frame.

Rendering of VE Images The proposed method uses VE images for tracking. Accordingly, VE views are obtained by rendering the shape of the target organ and setting the viewpoint inside the organ with the perspective projection. In the tracking, a lot of views should be rendered. Since the surface rendering can be accelerated with conventional PC-based graphics boards, we employ the surface rendering method to render VE views.

In a real endoscope, the light power decreases with the square of the distance from the light source. The VES can simulate this effect. Although all organs have complex reflection properties, we ignore these properties except for diffuse reflection properties when rendering for simplification purpose. All lighting parameters are manually adjusted so that the VE views are close to the real views. Lens system distortion is also ignored at present.

3.2   Processing Overview

The inputs of the system are a real endoscopic video and an X-ray CT image of the same patient. The method consists of two processing steps: (a) direct camera motion estimation by solving an epipolar equation and (b) image-based registration between RE and VE images. In the former step, we calculate corresponding point-pairs from two time-adjacent images. The rotation and the translation motion of the real endoscopic camera are found by substituting the coordinates of these point-pairs into the epipolar equation. Then we perform the image based registration [4]. The observation parameter of the VES, which generates the most similar VE view to the current frame of the real endoscopic video, is obtained here by generating VE views while changing the observation parameter. The search area of this process is limited to within the area around the motion computed by the direct estimation process.

3.3   Processing Procedure

Calculation of Corresponding Point-Pairs We calculate pairs of two corresponding points on two time-adjacent real endoscopic images, $\mathbf{R}_{k-1}$ and $\mathbf{R}_k$. $\mathbf{R}_{k-1}$ and $\mathbf{R}_k$ are the previous frame and the current frame of the real endoscopic video, respectively. The sampled points are defined on $\mathbf{R}_{k-1}$ as shown in Fig. 1. We define a small subimage $\mathbf{S}_{k-1}^{\mathrm{P}i}$ for each sample point i on $\mathbf{R}_{k-1}$. The center point $\mathbf{p}_i$ of $\mathbf{S}_{k-1}^{\mathrm{P}i}$ is located at the same position as sample point i. The size of $\mathbf{S}_{k-1}^{\mathrm{P}i}$ is given beforehand. We search for a subimage $\mathbf{S}_k^{\mathrm{P}'i}$ that is similar to $\mathbf{S}_k^{\mathrm{P}i}$. The center point of $\mathbf{S}_k^{\mathrm{P}'i}$ is noted as $\mathbf{p}'_i$, which can be found as the position that maximizes the correlation between subimages $\mathbf{S}_{k-1}^{\mathrm{P}i}$ and $\mathbf{S}_k^{\mathrm{P}'i}$. We consider the two points $\mathbf{p}_i$ and $\mathbf{p}'_i$ as a pair of corresponding points.

Calculation of the Fundamental Matrix This process calculates a fundamental matrix $\mathbf{F}$ from the point-pairs obtained in the previous step. Let $(u_i v_i)^T$ and $(u'_i v'_i)^T$ be $(u_i v_i) = \mathbf{A}u_i$ and $(u'_i v'_i) = \mathbf{A}u'_i$. We use $(u_i\ v_i\ 1)^T$ and $(u'_i\ v'_i\ 1)^T$ as $\tilde{\mathbf{m}}$ and $\tilde{\mathbf{m}}'$ in Eq. (4) for the corresponding point-pair i. When we describe $\mathbf{F} = \begin{pmatrix} f_{11}\ f_{12}\ f_{13} \\ f_{21}\ f_{22}\ f_{23} \\ f_{31}\ f_{32}\ f_{33} \end{pmatrix}$, Eq. (4) can be rewritten as

$$\left(uu'\ vu'\ u'\ uv'\ vv'\ v'\ u\ v\ 1 \right) \mathbf{f} = 0, \tag{6}$$

where $\mathbf{f} = \left(f_{11}\ f_{12}\ f_{13}\ f_{21}\ f_{22}\ f_{23}\ f_{31}\ f_{32}\ f_{33} \right)^T$. To find $\mathbf{F}$, eight point-pairs are required at least. For n point-pairs, the above equation can be expressed as

$$\mathbf{Uf} = \begin{pmatrix} u_1 u'_1\ v_1 u'_1\ u'_1\ u_1 v'_1\ v_1 v'_1\ v'_1\ u_1\ v_1\ 1 \\ \vdots \qquad\qquad\qquad\qquad\qquad \vdots \\ u_n u'_n\ v_n u'_n\ u'_n\ u_n v'_n\ v_n v'_n\ v'_n\ u_n\ v_n\ 1 \end{pmatrix} \mathbf{f} = \mathbf{0}. \tag{7}$$

The fundamental matrix $\mathbf{F}$ is calculated by solving Eq. (7).

Calculation of the Translation and the Rotation Motion This process computes the translation and the rotation motions from the obtained $\mathbf{F}$. We can obtain $\mathbf{T}$ and $\mathbf{R}$ by solving the following equations sequentially.

$$\mathbf{E}^T \mathbf{T} = 0 \tag{8}$$

$$\mathbf{R}\mathbf{E}^T = [\mathbf{T}]_\times^T \tag{9}$$

Image Based Registration This process finds the observation parameter that generates the VE view that is the most similar to $\mathbf{R}_k$. Let $\mathbf{V}(\mathbf{Q})$ be the VE view rendered by using the observation parameter $\mathbf{Q}$. The search process is performed by the following maximization process,

$$\max_{\mathbf{Q}} E\left(\mathbf{R}_k, \mathbf{V}(\mathbf{Q}) \right). \tag{10}$$

6   K. Mori et al.

Table 1. Tracking results

| Video Clip | Number of frames | Number of successful frames | |
		Previous method	Proposed method
(a)	543	375	487
(b)	100	8	73
(c)	299	173	247
(d)	320	51	190

$E(\mathbf{A}, \mathbf{B})$ is a function for measuring the similarity between two images $\mathbf{A}$ and $\mathbf{B}$. We use the correlation of the two images as E. The operation (10) is executed by employing Powell's method. We set the rotational motion of the initial parameter of the search as $\mathbf{R}$ acquired by Eq. (9). The direction specified by $\mathbf{T}$ is used for eliminating the search area of the translation motion.

4   Experimental Results and Discussion

We implemented the proposed method on a conventional Microsoft Windows-based PC machine (CPU: Pentium III 1GHz, Main memory: 1Gbyte, Graphics board: nVidia GeForce2 GTS). A bronchoscopic video and a chest X-ray CT image of the same patient were used for evaluating the performance of the proposed method. All of the processes were executed as off-line jobs due to the processing speed. The endoscopic video was recorded onto a digital video tape in an examination room and the images were captured frame by frame. Each frame of the video was converted from a color image into a gray-scale image. The real endoscope was performed under a conventional protocol. The specifications of the CT image were: 512x512x180 image size, 5mm thickness, and 1mm reconstruction pitch. A set of triangle patches was generated to render VE views from the bronchus region extracted from the CT image by the method in [1].

We evaluated the performance of the proposed method by counting the number of frames tracked correctly. The authors (including engineering and medical doctors) evaluated the results by observing real and virtual endoscopic images, since it is hard to obtain the real 3-D position of a bronchoscope camera. Table 1 shows the results of the evaluation. This table also includes results obtained by a previous method [5]. About 500 frames were successfully tracked. We can see improvements in the tracking, especially in frames where some specific structures cannot be seen.

Figure 3 shows results of camera motion tracking. The left side figures of each column are sequences of real endoscopic images. The corresponding virtual bronchoscopic images are displayed on the right side. These virtual images were generated by rendering VE views at estimated viewpoints. The results show that the method could track the real endoscope camera motion satisfactorily. In the case of video clip (a) where tracheal tumor can be observed, both the previous method and the proposed method can be seen to have worked well.

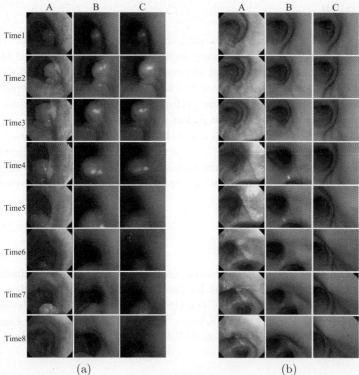

(a)   (b)

Fig.3 Results of camera motion tracking. The images in column A are real endoscopic images, those in B results obtained by the proposed method, and those in C were results obtained by a previous method [5].

From the scene where the tumor disappears from the views by due to endoscope movements, the proposed method can be seen to have continued its successful tracking, while the previous method failed. In video clip (b), the endoscope passes through an area where there are few feature structures. The proposed method can be seen to have performed the tracking correctly, while the previous method failed in tracking at Time3 and could no longer perform estimation, for the rest of the frames.

The processing time for one frame was also significantly reduced from fifteen second of the previous method to six seconds for the proposed one. This was because the result obtained by the direct estimation process eliminated the search area of the image-based registration process. Generally speaking, the image-based registration process is a time-consuming task, since we should generate a lot of virtual views to obtain an optimal parameter.

5   Conclusion

This paper described a method for tracking the camera motion of a real endoscope by using a camera motion recovery technique and an image-based registration technique. The translation and the rotational motion were directly estimated from corresponding point-pairs of two images by solving an epipolar equation. Then, precise estimation was performed by comparing VE and RE images. The experimental results showed that the method can track the camera motion in scenes where we cannot see feature structures in endoscopic views. Future work includes: (a) evaluation with a large number of cases, (b) development of a precise validation method, (c) improvement of the procedure for finding corresponding point-pairs by employing sub-pixel matching, and (d) reduction of the processing time.

Acknowledgement

The authors thank our colleagues for their useful suggestions and discussions. Parts of this research were supported by the Grant-In-Aid for Scientific Research from the Ministry of Education, the Grant-In-Aid for Scientific Research from Japan Society for Promotion of Science, and the Grant-In-Aid for Cancer Research from the Ministry of Health and Welfare of Japanese Government.

References

1. K. Mori, J. Hasegawa, J. Toriwaki, et al., Automated extraction and visualization of bronchus from 3-D CT images of Lung, In N.Ayache, (ed.) Computer Vision, Virtual reality and Robotics in Medicine, Lecture Notes in Computer Science, Vol. 905, pp.542-548, Springer-Verlag, Berlin Heidelberg New York, 1995
2. I. Bricault G. Ferretti, P. Cinquin, Registration Real and CT-Derived Virtual Bronchoscopic Images to Assist Transbronchial Biopsy, IEEE Trans. on Medical Imaging, 17, 5, pp.703-714, 1998
3. A.J. Sherbondy, A.P. Kiraly, A.L. Austin, et al., Virtual bronchoscopic approach for combining 3D CT and endoscopic video, Processing of SPIE Vol.3978, pp.104-115, 2000
4. A. Roche, G. Malandain, N. Ayache, S. Prima, Toward a Better Comprehension of Similarity Measures Used in Medical Image Registration, Lecture Notes Computer Science, 1679 (Proc. of MICCAI'99), pp.555-566, 1999
5. K.Mori, Y.Suenaga, J.Toriwaki, et al., Tracking of camera motion of real endoscope by using the Virtual Endoscope System, Proc. of CARS2000, pp.85-90, 2000
6. Gang Xu, Zhengyou Zhang, Epipolar Geometry in Stereo, Motion and Object Recognition, Kluwer Academic Publishers, Sept 1996

Real-Time Visual Tracking of the Surgeon's Face for Laparoscopic Surgery

Atsushi Nishikawa[1], Toshinori Hosoi[1], Kengo Koara[1], Daiji Negoro[1],
Ayae Hikita[1], Shuichi Asano[1], Fumio Miyazaki[1], Mitsugu Sekimoto[2],
Yasuhiro Miyake[2], Masayoshi Yasui[2], and Morito Monden[2]

[1] Department of Systems and Human Science,
Graduate School of Engineering Science, Osaka University
1-3 Machikaneyama-cho, Toyonaka City, Osaka 560-8531, Japan
[2] Department of Surgery and Clinical Oncology,
Osaka University Graduate School of Medicine
2-2 Yamadaoka, Suita City, Osaka 565-0871, Japan

Abstract. We have developed an image-based human-machine interface
that tracks the surgeon's face robustly in real-time(30Hz) and does not
require to use any body-contacted sensing devices. Based on this face
tracker we have developed a new robotic laparoscope positioning system
for solo surgery. Our system completely frees the surgeon's hands and
feet from the laparoscope guiding task. To evaluate the performance of
the proposed system and its applicability to clinical use, an *in vivo* experiment was carried out in which a surgeon used the system to perform
a laparoscopic cholecystectomy on a pig.

1 Introduction

In current laparoscopic surgery, a camera assistant usually holds the laparoscope
for the surgeon and positions the scope according to the surgeon's instructions.
This method of operation is frustrating and inefficient for the surgeon because
commands are often interpreted and executed erroneously by the assistant. The
views may be suboptimal and unstable because the scope is sometimes aimed
incorrectly and vibrates due to the assistant hand trembling. The introduction
of robotic technologies –development of robotic laparoscope positioning systems
to replace the human assistant– is a major step towards the solution of this
problem and the user(surgeon)-friendly design of human-machine interface that
controls the laparoscope positioner plays an important role in this step.

Almost all the laparoscope positioning systems proposed so far only have
the human-machine interface requiring the use of the surgeon's hand and/or
foot such as instrument-mounted buttons/joystick, foot pedal and the like[1,2,3].
This type of interface, however, seems to be sometimes uneasy to use because the
surgeon already uses his/her hands/feet to control a variety of surgical tools. To
solve this problem, several researchers have tried to introduce "voice" controller
interface based on the use of advanced voice recognition systems[4,5,6]. It seems
an effective approach because the verbal instructions are natural for human and

W. Niessen and M. Viergever (Eds.): MICCAI 2001, LNCS 2208, pp. 9–16, 2001.

the use of neither hands nor feet is required in controlling the laparoscope. However, it has originally some limitations such as reduced accuracy in positioning, long reaction time and erratic movements in a noisy environment. We believe that the surgeon's head controllable laparoscope is the best solution because nonverbal instructions such as facial gestures are more intuitive and faster than verbal instructions(typically voice commands) and have the potential ability to represent not only the direction of scope motion but also the motion degrees such as velocity so that the laparoscope positioning accuracy may be improved. Several laparoscope manipulators with the head controller interface have been developed[7,8,9]. Such systems, however, require not only head movements but also simultaneous control of a foot/knee switch. Furthermore, the surgeon must wear a head-mounted sensing devices such as headband and gyro sensor, which are stressful for surgeon.

We have developed an image-based human-machine interface that tracks the surgeon's face robustly in real-time(30Hz) and does not require to use any body-contacted sensing devices. Based on this face tracker we have developed a new robotic laparoscope positioning system for solo surgery. Our system completely frees the surgeon's hands and feet from the laparoscope guiding task.

2   Real-Time Face Tracking

In operation, the laparoscopic surgeon usually stands in front of the TV monitor on which the scope image is displayed and gazes at a surgical point of interest on the screen. Therefore, if a surveillance camera is placed just over the TV monitor, the surgeon's face can be observed almost all the time. However, as the surgeon wears a gown, a cap and a mask, almost all the face features such as mouth, nose, and hair do not appear in the surveillance image. We at first turn our attention to the surgeon's irises. The main reason is the following: in our case, not only it is ensured that both left and right irises always appear in the image but also it is easier to detect them than in the general case of face image processing.

2.1   Iris-Based Method

Basically the iris has a low intensity and a circular shape. Thus we do not use color image but gray-value one. The surgeon's face image is taken by a CCD camera and its intensity information is digitized into the memory of the host computer through a video capturing device at a frequency of 30Hz. The video capturing process is done in parallel to the following image processing so that the surgeon's irises are also detected and tracked at a rate of 30Hz. The outline of our algorithm for detecting the surgeon's irises and an example of the detection process are respectively shown in Fig. 1 and Fig. 2.

First of all, based on the previous frame information two rectangle-shaped windows(respectively for tracking the left/right irises) are set on the image. The following processes run only within the rectangles and not the whole image. The

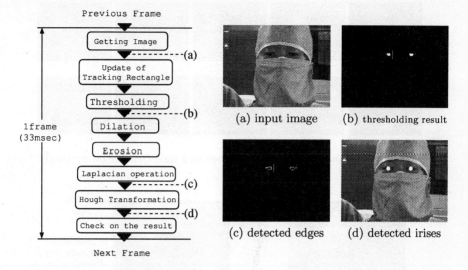

Fig. 1. Iris detection algorithm

Fig. 2. An example of iris detection process

widow images are thresholded at a level, driving lower intensity pixels to 1 and higher ones to zero. For example, see Fig. 2(a)(original) and (b) (result). (in the latter figure, the white region indicates the extracted low-intensity pixels and the rectangle indicates the tracking window.) The gaps are then bridged through dilation-erosion process. After that, the resulting image is convolved with the Laplacian edge operator so that the edge image is yielded such as Fig. 2(c). Finally the Hough transformation technique is used to detect circular shapes as the surgeon's irises. This result is shown in Fig. 2(d). The circular region detected by the Hough technique are overlaid on the original image. Fig. 3 shows ten images taken from a tracking sequence. In addition to the tracking rectangles, the estimates of the surgeon's irises are marked with circular boundaries.

2.2 Marker-Based Method

The iris-based method requires "careful" selection of the thresholding/Hough transformation parameters according to illumination conditions or individual variations in visible size of irises(a part of them is occluded by the eyelid). To cope with this problem, as the alternative, we also developed a marker-based method for face tracking. The marker we use is black(for non-color image processing) and made of low-reflectance materials, and has a long-narrow rectangle shape. It is attached on the surgical cap in advance (see Fig. 3). The flow of marker-based tracking process is the following: (1) the black region is at first extracted by simple thresholding, (2) the conventional labeling algorithm is executed on the thresholded image so that the maximal region is selected as the marker region,

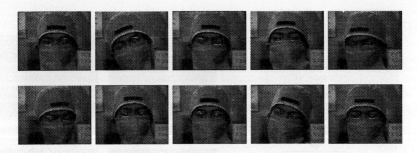

Fig. 3. Real-time tracking of the surgeon's face (iris-based method)

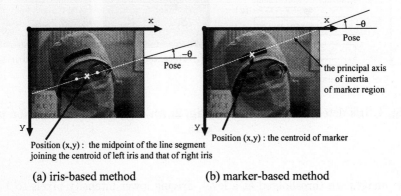

(a) iris-based method   (b) marker-based method

Fig. 4. Estimating the position and the pose of the surgeon's face

(3) the centroid of the marker and its principal axis of inertia are calculated for robust and rapid tracking at the next frame. The marker-based face tracker can also work at a frequency of 30Hz.

2.3   Estimation of the Position and the Pose of the Surgeon's Face

We have already assumed that a CCD camera can be placed just over the TV monitor on which the laparoscope image is displayed. In standard laparoscopic surgery such as laparoscopic cholecystectomy, we can also assume *distance-constant* and *fronto-parallel* interaction, i.e., that the surgeon's face remains almost parallel to the TV monitor screen and the distance between the surgeon and the screen is almost constant during the whole interaction time. In this case, the position and the pose of the surgeon's face can be easily estimated in real-time from the result of the image processing described above (see Fig. 4). Notice that during such kind of interaction the face DOF(degrees of freedom) are reduced from six to three –namely, a translation 2 dimensional vector (x, y) and a rotation θ in the face plane.

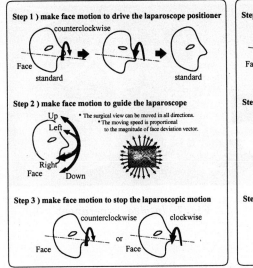

(a) Face motions for maintaining the point of interest in the image center

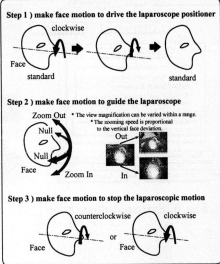

(b) Face motions for providing the required target magnification

Fig. 5. Positioning the laparoscope by making face motion

3   Application to Laparoscopic Surgery

The proposed method was applied to laparoscopic cholecystectomy on a pig.

3.1   Face Gestures

At first, we worked out a method for positioning the laparoscope only by face motion. It consists of the following three steps (see Fig. 5).

1. *Make face motion to drive the laparoscope positioner*
   In this step, the following three consecutive face motions are required. (1) put the position and pose of the face in standard, (2) roll the face counterclockwise/clockwise, (3) return the face "precisely" to the standard position/pose. The counterclockwise rotation is selected when the surgeon wants to guide the laparoscope for maintaining the surgical point of interest in the center of the video frame, while the clockwise motion is made when he/she wants to guide it for providing the required target magnification. Notice that the surgeon cannot make these consecutive motions unconsciously.
2. *Make face motion to guide the laparoscope*
   Once coming into the step, as shown in Fig. 5, the face motion is represented as a vector from the standard position, and the direction and the magnitude of the vector are respectively transformed into the direction and the velocity of the laparoscopic motion, according to the surgeon's requirement.

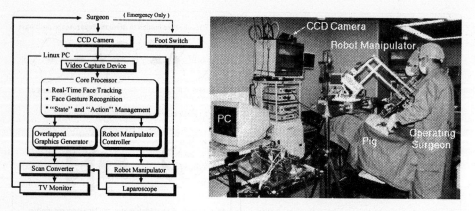

Fig. 6. System configuration   **Fig. 7.** *In vivo* experiment

3. *Make face motion to stop the laparoscopic motion*
   In this final step, all the surgeon has to do is to roll the face. Note that this
   action is very easy to make.

Notice that these gestures can be recognized based on the time sequence of the
estimated position and pose of the surgeon's face.

3.2 Face Tracker-Based Laparoscope Positioning System

Based on the face tracker and the gesture recognizer, we have developed a novel
robotic laparoscope positioning system for solo surgery. The system configuration is shown in Fig. 6. Our laparoscope positioning system mainly consists of a
CCD camera, a video capture board, a general PC(Intel Pentium III, 600MHz,
OS: Linux), a robot manipulator that holds a laparoscope, a scan converter for
superimposing some graphics on the scope image, and a foot switch (in an emergency only). The core system in the PC can detect and track the surgeon's face
features(either left/right irises or a marker) in real-time(30Hz) from a sequence
of video images taken through the CCD camera and estimates the position and
the pose of the surgeon's face from the image processing result and then recognizes the face gestures. According to the motion recognition result, the control
command is sent to the laparoscope manipulator.

3.3 Laparoscopic Cholecystectomy on a Pig

To evaluate the applicability of our system to clinical use, an *in vivo* experiment
was carried out in which a surgeon used the system to perform a laparoscopic
cholecystectomy on a pig (see Fig. 7). Instead of human camera assistant, the
system was applied to all of the procedure after trocar insertion. As a result, the
whole operative procedure was successfully and safely completed with our system. No one used the emergency foot switch for shutting down the system. The

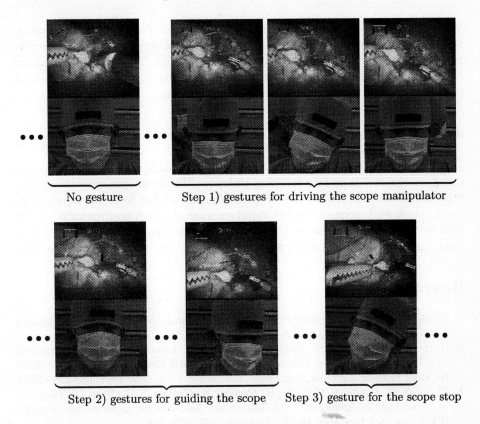

No gesture   Step 1) gestures for driving the scope manipulator

Step 2) gestures for guiding the scope   Step 3) gesture for the scope stop

Fig. 8. A scene in the *in vivo* laparoscopic cholecystectomy experiment

number of the lens cleaning was also zero. The operating time from trocar insertion till the removal of the gallbladder inclusive was about 44 minutes. In this experiment, no case has been found in which the robot obstructed the surgeon's work and neither particular incidents nor technical problems had occurred. Fig. 8 shows a scene of the surgeon's facial motions in the experiment(upper part: the scope image which the surgeon looked at, lower part: the surgeon's face image from the surveillance camera, each pair was taken at the same time).

The number of times in operation that the surgeon made face motions to the system to drive the laparoscope manipulator(i.e., step 1 of Fig. 5) was 97 times, which was broken down into 40 times for maintaining the point of interest in the image center, 50 times for providing the required target magnification, and 7 times for being not recognized by the system. No case was found in which the system mistook any other motion such as unintentional action of the operating surgeon and/or another surgeon who looked at the experiment. (e.g., see Fig. 8. In the 2nd-4th images, a surgeon was walking behind the operating surgeon.) The number of times that the surgeon made face gestures to stop the laparoscope motion (step 3 of Fig. 5) was 90 times and these were all recognized completely.

We got many positive comments such as fast reaction time, high positioning accuracy, and easy and intuitive camera guidance(for step 2 of Fig. 5), from the surgeons who performed or looked at the experiment. The operating surgeon, however, also made a negative comment that after the experiment he felt a little fatigue in the cervix from a lot of rolling face motions.

4   Conclusion

We have developed a new robotic laparoscope positioning system for solo surgery based on the real-time face tracking technique. In an *in vivo* experiment, our system succeeded in freeing the surgeon's hands and feet from the laparoscope guiding task while achieving safety, rapid reaction, and high positioning accuracy. Now we are studying a new method for guiding the laparoscope with the aim of reducing not only mental stress but also "physical" one such as cervical fatigue.

References

1. Sackier, J.M., Wang, Y.: Robotically Assisted Laparoscopic Surgery. From Concept to Development. Surg Endosc **8** (1) (Jan 1994) 63–66
2. Hurteau, R., DeSantis, S., Begin, E., Gagner, M.: Laparoscopic Surgery Assisted by a Robotic Cameraman: Concept and Experimental Results. In: Proc. 1994 IEEE Int Conf Robotic Automat, San Diego, California, USA, May 1994, pp. 2286–2289
3. Taylor, R.H., Funda, J., Eldridge, B., Gomory, S., Gruben, K., LaRose, D., Talamini, M., Kavoussi. L, Anderson, J.: A Telerobotic Assistant for Laparoscopic Surgery. IEEE Eng Med Biol Mag **14** (3) (May-Jun 1995) 279–288
4. Allaf, M.E., Jackman, S.V., Schulam, P.G., Cadeddu, J.A., Lee, B.R., Moore, R.G., Kavoussi, L.R.: Laparoscopic Visual Field. Voice vs Foot Pedal Interfaces for Control of the AESOP Robot. Surg Endosc **12** (12) (Dec 1998) 1415–1418
5. Buess, G.F., Arezzo, A., Schurr, M.O., Ulmer, F., Fisher, H., Gumb, L., Testa, T., Nobman, C.: A New Remote-Controlled Endoscope Positioning System for Endoscopic Solo Surgery. the FIPS Endoarm. Surg Endosc **14** (4) (Apr 2000) 395–399
6. Munoz, V.F., Vara-Thorbeck, C., DeGabriel, J.G., Lozano, J.F., Sanchez-Badajoz, E., Garcia-Cerezo, A., Toscano, R., Jimenez-Garrido, A.: A Medical Robotic Assistant for Minimally Invasive Surgery. In: Proc. 2000 IEEE Int Conf Robotic Automat, San Francisco, California, USA, Apr 2000, pp. 2901–2906
7. Finlay, P.A., Ornstein, M.H.: Controlling the Movement of a Surgical Laparoscope. EndoSista, with Four Degrees of Freedom, Operates in Concert with Surgeon's Intuitive Head Motions. IEEE Eng Med Biol Mag **14** (3) (May-Jun 1995) 289–291
8. Dowler, N.J., Holland, S.R.J.: The Evolutionary Design of an Endoscopic Telemanipulator. IEEE Robotic Automat Mag **3** (4) (Dec 1996) 38–45
9. Kobayashi, E., Masamune, K., Sakuma, I., Dohi, T., Hashimoto, D.: A New Safe Laparoscopic Manipulator System with a Five-Bar Linkage Mechanism and an Optical Zoom. Comput Aided Surg **4** (4) (1999) 182–192

Computer-Based Periaxial Rotation Measurement for Aligning Fractured Femur Fragments: Method and Preliminary Results

Ofer Ron[1], Leo Joskowicz[1], Ariel Simkin[2], and Charles Milgrom[2]

[1] School of Computer Science and Engineering
The Hebrew University of Jerusalem, Jerusalem 91904 Israel.
[2] Dept. of Orthopaedic Surgery, Hadassah Univ. Hospital, Jerusalem, Israel.
josko@cs.huji.ac.il

Abstract. We describe a new computer-based method for periaxial rotation measurement of healthy and fractured femurs during closed femoral fracture reduction surgery from CT. The method provides a comparative quantitative measure to align the distal and proximal femur fragments based on periaxial rotation. We define periaxial rotation in terms of patient-specific bone features and describe an algorithm for automatically extracting these features from the CT. The algorthm extracts condyle landmarks and neck axis of the healthy bone, determines its periaxial rotation, and extrapolates this data, assuming mirror symmetry between the healthy and the fractured bone, to measure periaxial rotation between the fractured fragments. Unlike existing techniques, our method requires minimal user intervention. We applied the method to a patient data set and simulated a reduction based on the anteversion measurements with satisfactory results.

1 Introduction

Reducing the surgeon cumulative radiation exposure and improving the positioning accuracy are key issues in computer-assisted orthopaedic surgery. We have developed FRACAS, a computer-integrated system for closed long bone fracture reduction [5]. The system replaces uncorrelated static fluoroscopic images with a virtual reality display of 3D bone models created from preoperative CT and tracked intraoperatively in real time.

An important issue in closed medullary nailing is correctly aligning for periaxial rotation the distal and proximal fragments of the fractured femur during surgery. Precise alignment is necessary to ensure correct postoperative functionality. Currently, the surgeon performs the alignment by making a qualitative assessment of the fragments position on uncorrelated intraoperative fluoroscopic images, comparing them with preoperative X-rays of the healthy bone, and manipulating the bone fragments in an attempt to achieve a symmetric result. This procedure is lengthy, error-prone, and highly dependent on the surgeon, resulting in a non-negligible percentage of suboptimal outcomes.

W. Niessen and M. Viergever (Eds.): MICCAI 2001, LNCS 2208, pp. 17–23, 2001.
© Springer-Verlag Berlin Heidelberg 2001

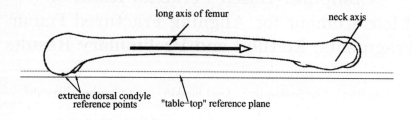

Fig. 1. *Definition of periaxial rotation*

We have developed a new modeling and visualization software tool for assisting surgeons in correctly aligning for periaxial rotation the distal and proximal fragments of the fractured femur during closed femoral fracture reduction surgery. The modeling module allows surgeons to preoperatively build surface models from CT data of the fractured and the healthy bone, identify and derive relevant anatomical data from these models, and define comparative periaxial rotation measurement with minimal user intervention. The visualization module presents two three-dimensional views (frontal and lateral) of the proximal and distal fragment models, a cross section of the femoral shaft of both fragments close to the fracture location, and their anatomical axes whose relative positions are updated in real time from position data obtained from an optical tracking device. The measure of their periaxial rotation is displayed and updated, providing a comparative patient-specific quantitative measurement to evaluate the quality of the alignment. The surgeon utilizes the views and the periaxial rotation value to bring the bone fractures into alignment without further use of fluoroscopy.

In this paper, we describe the computer-based method for periaxial rotation measurement of healthy and fractured femurs. We define periaxial rotation in terms of patient-specific bone features and describe an algorithm for automatically extracting these features from the CT. Periaxial rotation is the angle between the axis of the femoral neck and the "table top" reference plane, which is the plane passing through the extreme dorsal points of the medial and lateral condyles and parallel to the main axis of the femur (Figure 1). By spatially relating the proximal and distal fragments, this definition allows the extension of periaxial rotation measurements to the fractured femur, which could not be obtained with existing methods. The algorithm extracts condyle landmarks and neck axis of the healthy bone, determines its periaxial rotation, and extrapolates this data, assuming mirror symmetry between the healthy and the fractured bone, to measure periaxial rotation between the fractured distal and proximal fragments. In contrast with existing techniques, our method requires minimal user intervention in the modeling and measurement process.

2   Previous Work

Periaxial rotation measurement is closely related to anteversion measurement. Most previous research addresses the problem of establishing methods for accurately measuring anteversion using X-rays, CT scans, and computer reconstructed models. The main difficulty is that the measure of femoral anteversion is not uniquely defined, and there are discrepancies as to what is best way to measure femoral anteversion. Consequently, most of the efforts have been focused on creating new measurement protocols using CT scans or X-Rays.

Hoftstatter et al [4] describe a system to assist surgeons in femoral fracture reduction and periaxial rotation correction based on fluoroscopic images. Periaxial rotation is defined from manually selected landmarks in AP and lateral fluoroscopic images and is updated in real time during the procedure. The long axis of the healthy femur and fractured femur are identified independently, so they do not account for the arching of the femur. The drawbacks of this method are the manual landmark selection and the inaccurate fragment axes definition.

Egund and Palmer [1] describe a method which consists of acquiring several CT slices at selected locations, manually extracting geometric features from those slices, defining a reference plane and a plane though the femur head from the features, and measuring anteversion as the angle between the plane normals. Herman and Egund [3] propose to measure anteversion from three CT slices and from fluoroscopic images of the whole femur at precise predetermined viewpoints. The method requires significant manual user intervention. Herman and Egund [2] determine that the femur positioning on CT slices does influence the femoral anteversion measurement, and conclude that a full 3D reconstruction of the bone from the CT scans is necessary to compensate for non standard bone positioning.

Comparison studies of alternative methods of measuring femoral anteversion with radiographic methods have also been conducted. Murphy [7] compares four different definitions of anteversion measurement and conclude that the "table top" method for locating the condylar plane (which we refer to as the table top plane), is the simplest, most reproducible, and is most similar to the clinical method of measurement. Sugano [8] compares various definitions and measurement procedures based on different data for anteversion. They provide a precise statistical evaluation of each of the methods by comparing their results to an anteversion value (termed "true anteversion") measured by positioning a 3D model reconstructed from CT slices of the femur in a position close to the the classical clinical method of measuring anteversion manually. They conclude that most methods either overestimate or underestimate the average and standard deviation of the method utilizing the full 3D reconstruction.

In contrast with previous approaches, our work aims at providing a comparative measure of femur anteversion before and after the fracture, rather than attempting to find an absolute measure of anteversion or periaxial rotation only applicable to healthy femurs. We believe that this relative measure is the most useful one for restoring function and improving surgical outcomes. The emphasis is on precise and robust automatic location of geometric features in the bone models.

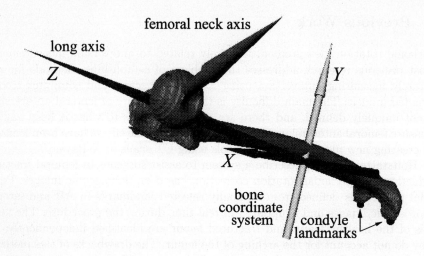

Fig. 2. *Healthy femur feature extraction*

3 Our Method

The inputs are three surface bone models (triangular surface meshes) of the healthy femur and the distal and proximal fragments of the fractured femur. The models can be readily obtained from CT data using standard segmentation and surface construction techniques, [5]. The output is a set of relevant geometric features (femur main axes, condyle landmarks, femur head and neck axis) and a measure of periaxial rotation.

The method consists of three steps. First, we extract the geometric features of the healthy femur and compute from them its periaxial rotation (Figure 2). Next, we extract the geometric features of the fractured femur proximal and distal fragments (Figure 3) by using the healthy femur features as reference (Figure 4). Finally, we use this information for accurate alignment of proximal and distal fragments during surgery. We briefly describe each step next.

The periaxial rotation value for the healthy bone is obtained in two steps (Figures 2 and 3). First, we compute the principal axes of the healthy femur, and the proximal and distal fragments of the fractured femur using the Principal Axis Transformation (PAX) technique [9]. PAX computes the three major orthogonal axes of mass distribution of a solid object. The principal axis is the one with the highest mass distribution (largest eigenvalue). We then manually orient the axes according to a preferred orientation, which can be chosen arbitrarily. This establishes a reference frame for the location of the model vertices and geometric features. Correct orientation of the principal axes is crucial to the correctness of the computations, and thus has to be set by the user. Orientations are defined for bones whose condyles are touching the table (healthy bone and distal fragment), or whose lesser trochanter is touching the table (proximal fragment). The long axis (Z) is parallel to the table top and oriented toward the femur head, away

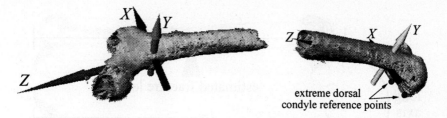

Fig. 3. *Features of proximal (left) and distal (right) fragments*

from the condyles. The second axis parallel to the table top (X) is always oriented in the opposite direction from the femoral head. The axis orthogonal to the table top (Y) is always oriented upwards. This axes orientation defines a right (left) axis system for the right (left) leg bones, and embodies our assumption that the left and right femurs of a normal patient are approximately mirror-symmetric about the YZ plane. We use this new coordinate system with its origin at the centroid of the model for all subsequent computations.

Second, we extract the relevant geometric features from the healthy bone: the two extreme dorsal condyle points and the axis passing through the femur's neck. The extreme dorsal condyle points are the lowest points with respect to the Y axis which lie on opposite sides of the YZ plane. The femoral neck axis is the principal axis found by PAX on the region upwards of the lesser trochanter (femur head and neck). Model vertices in this region are found by "cutting" the femur twice above the fracture twice with a plane parallel to the XY plane. Finally, we compute the periaxial rotation from the condyle landmarks and the femur neck axis as the angle between the plane normal and the femur neck axis.

The relevant geometric features of the fractured femur fragments are extracted in an identical manner. The condyle landmarks and long axis are extracted for the distal fragment, and the femoral neck axis for the proximal. We approximate the location of the fracture on the healthy bone by assuming mirror symmetry between healthy and fractured bone, splitting the healthy bone model at that location, and calculating the principal axes for the interpolated distal fragment (Figure 4). We calculate the rigid transformation that takes the interpolated distal fragment coordinate system to the real distal fragment coordinate system. We then transform the femoral long axis of the healthy femur to the distal fragment coordinate system (as given by PAX) using this transformation, defining it as the interpolated long axis of the fractured femur. We then define the "table top" reference plane for the distal fragment as the plane containing the distal fragment condyle landmarks and parallel to the interpolated long axis.

The periaxial rotation value is computed and updated in real time during surgery by using the known location of the proximal and distal fragments in world coordinates to relate the table top plane defined for the distal fragment to the neck axis of the proximal fragment. The periaxial rotation value is computed for any spatial configuration of the fragments as their relative positions change.

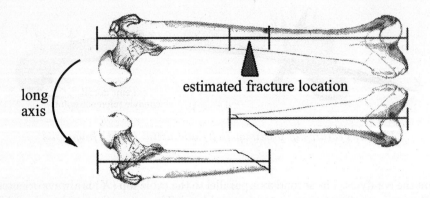

Fig. 4. *Fracture extrapolation on healthy bone*

The advantages of our method are several. First, no additional images are required. The bone models are the same models used for navigation during surgery, which are derived from the preoperative CT scan. Second, no manual CT slice selection is required. The method automatically identifies the slices belonging to regions of interest where geometric features will be extracted. Third, the feature extraction on both the healthy and the fractured femur is fully automatic, which ensures robustness, reproducibility, and accuracy. Fourth, the method is position scan independent. The computation of the periaxial rotation is independent of the scanning position of both femurs, since feature extraction is relative and coordinate transformations for matching them are computed explicitly.

4   Experimental Results

The main difficulty in designing experiments to validate our approach is that there is no "golden standard" for determining the correct absolute value of the periaxial rotation. Instead, we designed experiments to determine the usefulness of the method in fracture reduction. We have obtained scans of several actual fracture cases and dry femurs and have performed periaxial rotation measurements on them. When only one dry femur is available, we create a mirror image and "break" it to obtain distal and proximal fragments.

To determine the effectiveness of the method, we have performed the following in-vitro experiment using a whole dry femur and a physical fracture simulator device [6]. First, we CT scan the femur and construct a surface model of it. Then, we break the femur into two fragments, CT scan both fragments, and construct reflected models of them. We extract the geometric features and compute periaxial rotation on the three models as described above. We then a attach an optical tracking instrument to each fragment, register each to its model using contact-based registration techniques [10], and cover both fragments with a cloth, so that they can be manipulated but not seen. We perform fragment alignment using the visualization software and the periaxial rotation information only. Once the alignment has been performed according to the software, we compare it with the actual physical position of the bone fragments and ask a surgeon to determine if the discrepancy is acceptable. While the comparison is only qualitative, the initial results are encouraging.

We are planning on carrying the first in-vivo test in the near future. We will use the traditional fluoroscopic validation method to qualitatively evaluate if the periaxial rotation measurement combined with the visualization method reduces the reduction time and provides satisfactory results.

References

1. Egund N., Palmer J., 1984, "Femoral Anatomy Described in Cylindrical Coordinates Using Computed Tomography". *Acta Radiologica Diagnosis*, vol. 25, pg. 209-215.
2. Hermann K.L., Egund N., 1997, "CT Measurement of Anteversion in the Femoral Neck: The Influence of Femur Positioning".*Acta Radiologica*, vol 38,pg. 527-532.
3. Hermann K.L., Egund N., 1998, "Measuring Anteversion in the Femoral Neck from Routine Radiographs".*Acta Radiologica*, vol 39,pg. 410-415.
4. Hofstatter, R., Slomczykowski, M., Krettek, C., et al. 2000, "Computer-Assisted Fluoroscopy-based reduction of femoral fractures and antetorsion correction", *J. of Computer-Aided Surgery*, Vol 5(5).
5. Joskowicz, L., Milgrom, C., Simkin, A., Tockus, L., Yaniv, Z., 1999, "FRACAS: A System for Computer-Aided Image-Guided Long Bone Fracture", Journal of Computer-Aided Surgery, Vol 3(6), May.
6. Joskowicz, L., Milgrom, C., and Simkin, A., 2000, "Simulator and Distal Targeting Device for In-Vitro Experimentation and Training in Computer-Aided Closed Medullary Nailing", Proc. 14th Int. Congress on Computer-Assisted Radiology and Surgery, CARS'2000, Lemke et. al. eds, Elsevier, pp 969-975.
7. Murphy, S., Simon S., Kijewski, P., et al., 1987, "Femoral Anteversion". *The Journal of Bone and Joint Surgery, Inc.*, vol 69-A, pg. 1169-1176.
8. Sugano N., , Noble, P., and Kamaric, E., 1998, "A Comparison of Alternative Methods of Measuring Femoral Anteversion".*Journal of Computed Assisted Tomography*, vol 22(4), pg. 610-614.
9. Tsao J., Chiodo, C., Williamson, D., Wilson, M., and Kikinis, R., 1998, "Computer-Assisted Quantification of Periaxial Bone Rotation from X-Ray CT".*Journal of Computed Assisted Tomography*, vol. 22(4), pg. 615-620.
10. Yaniv, Z., Sadowsky, O., and Joskowicz, L., 2000, "In-Vitro Accuracy Study of Contact and Image-Based Registration: Materials, Methods, and Experimental Results", Proc. 14th Int. Congress on Computer-Assisted Radiology and Surgery, CARS'2000, Lemke et. al. eds, Elsevier, pp. 141-146.

Acknowledgement

This research was supported in part by a grant from the Israel Ministry of Industry and Trade for the IZMEL Consortium on Image-Guided Therapy. We thank Ofri Sadowski and Ziv Yaniv for their help in formulating the ideas presented in this paper.

Shape versus Size: Improved Understanding of the Morphology of Brain Structures

[1,2]Guido Gerig, [1]Martin Styner, [3]Martha E. Shenton, [2]Jeffrey A. Lieberman

[1]Department of Computer Science, UNC, Chapel Hill, NC 27599, USA
[2]Department of Psychiatry, UNC, Chapel Hill, NC 27599, USA
[3]Department of Psychiatry, VAMC-Brockton, Harvard Medical School, Boston, USA
gerig@cs.unc.edu, martin_styner@ieee.org

Abstract. Standard practice in quantitative structural neuroimaging is a segmentation into brain tissue, subcortical structures, fluid space and lesions followed by volume calculations of gross structures. On the other hand, it is evident that object characterization by size does only capture one of multiple aspects of a full structural characterization. Desirable parameters are local and global parameters like length, elongation, bending, width, complexity, bumpiness and many more. In neuroimaging research there is increasing evidence that shape analysis of brain structures provides new information which is not available by conventional volumetric measurements. This motivates development of novel morphometric analysis techniques answering clinical research questions which have been asked for a long time but which remained unanswered due to the lack of appropriate measurement tools. Challenges are the choice of biologically meaningful shape representations, robustness to noise and small perturbations, and the ability to capture the shape properties of populations that represent natural biological shape variation. This paper describes experiments with two different shape representation schemes, a fine-scale, global surface characterization using spherical harmonics, and a coarsely sampled medial representation (3D skeleton). Driving applications are the detection of group differences of amhygdala-hippocampal shapes in schizophrenia and the analysis of ventricular shape similarity in a mono/dizygotic twin study. The results clearly demonstrate that shape captures information on structural similarity or difference which is not accessible by volume analysis. Improved global and local structure characterization as proposed herein might help to explain pathological changes in neurodevelopment/neurodegeneration in terms of their biological meaning.

1. Introduction

In-vivo imaging studies of brain structures have provided valuable information about the nature of neuropsychiatric disorders including neurodegenerative diseases and/or disorders of abnormal neurodevelopment. Deformities in brain structure in Alzheimer's and Huntington's disease are believed to be due the effects of the disease process in adulthood after a period of normal neurodevelopment, while diseases like Autism and Fragile X syndrome are thought to involve abnormal neurodevelopment which give rise to the symptoms of the illness. Schizophrenia, on the other hand, is

W. Niessen and M. Viergever (Eds.): MICCAI 2001, LNCS 2208, pp. 24–32, 2001.

often subject to conflicting hypotheses about the cause and temporal evolution of the neuropathologic features of the disorder. Structural imaging studies so far have most often focused on volumetric assessment of brain structures, for example full brain or hemispheric gray and white matter, ventricular volume and hippocampus. Increasing evidence for structural changes in small subregions and parts of structures drive development of new structure analysis techniques. Wang [Wang 2000] found that while hippocampal volume did not discriminate schizophrenia groups from control groups, shape measurements did provide a distinct group separation. The paper further discusses that summary comparisons of whole structures ignores the possibility of detecting regional differences. Csernansky [Csernansky et al., 1998] suggests that a full characterization of neuroanatomical abnormalities will increase our understanding of etiology, pathogenesis, and pathophysiology of schizophrenia. Results show that the analysis of hippocampal shape discriminates schizophrenia and control subjects with greater power than volumetry [see also Haller et al., 1996,1997]. [Suddath et al., 1990] found smaller anterior hippocampi in affected vs. unaffected MZ twins. All these studies advocate new morphometry techniques to study shape rather than gross volume and to provide quantitative measures that are not only statistical significant but also neuroanatomically relevant and intuitive.

2. Shape Modeling

Surface-based shape representation: We applied a technique for surface parametrization that uses expansion into a series of spherical harmonics (SPHARM) [Brechbuehler, 1995, Szekely et al., 1996, Kelemen, 1999]. The development parallels the seminal work of Cootes & Taylor [Cootes et al., 1995] on active shape models but is based on a parametric object description (inspired by Staib and Duncan [Staib, 1996]) rather than a point distribution model. SPHARM is a global parametrization method, i.e. small local changes can affect all parameters. It allows simple alignment of structures and gives a good initial point-to-point correspondence.
Medially-based surface shape representation: As an alternative to surface-based global shape representation, the UNC research group is working on a 3D skeletal representation with coarse to fine sampling (Pizer, 1999, Yushkevich, 2001, Styner, 2000, 2001). The medial shape representation provides locality of width and bending on a hierarchy of scales. Parameters derived from the medial representation are more intuitive than Fourier coefficients and will help to develop shape descriptions expressed in natural language terms.

3. Applications in Neuroimaging

The following subsections describe applications of surface-based and medially-based shape representation methods in two clinical studies.

3.1 Statistical Analysis of Amygdala-Hippocampal Asymmetry in Schizophrenia

We studied the asymmetry of the hippocampal complex for a group of 15 controls and 15 schizophrenics (collaboration with M. E. Shenton, Harvard). Asymmetry was assessed by segmentation using deformable models (Kelemen, 1999), by flipping one object across the midsagittal plane, by aligning the reference and the mirrored object using the coordinates of the first ellipsoid, and by calculating the MSD between the two surfaces (Fig.1).

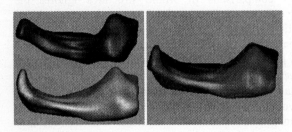

Fig. 1. Analysis of amygdala-hippocampal left/right asymmetry. The left hippocampal complex is mirrored, aligned and overlaid (right) to calculate the mean square distance between surfaces.

As shape difference measures can be largely influenced by object size differences, we normalized all the objects by volume. The statistical analysis can be based on the single features L/R volume asymmetry or L/R shape difference, but also by combining both values (Table 1, Fig.2). Similarly to published results [Csernansky et al., 1998], we found that the volume asymmetry expressed by $(|L-R|)/(L+R)$ did not discriminate the groups well if we consider classification (70%), although the group difference was significant (P<0.0032). Using both shape and volume in a composite analysis (Fig. 2 right) results in a correct classification of 13 out of 15 for both groups and thus in an overall classification rate of 87%. We used a support vector machine (SVM) method (Vapnik, 1998). Unbiased classification performance was obtained by leave-one-out tests.

	Volume	Shape	Volume & Shape
	rel. L-R diff.	MSD surfaces	
Student t-test	F=10.4, P<0.0032	F=5.0, P<0.0335	F=11.19, P<0.0024
Classification	70%	73%	87% (SVM)

Table 1. Statistics of left/right asymmetry analysis of the amygdala-hippocampal complex for volume and shape characterization. Classification is poor and not much better than a guess for volume and shape only, whereas the combined analysis shows a significantly improved classification rate despite of the small numbers of 15 controls and 15 schizophrenics.

3.2 Similarity of Lateral Ventricles in Mono-/Dizygotic Twin Study

The study of identical (monzygotic, MZ) and nonidentical twins (dizygotic, DZ) provides an excellent opportunity to study similarities and differences of the morphology with respect to a genetic effect. Moreover, discordant twins, i.e. one subject affected by illness and the related subject healthy, allow further insight into the genetic factor of illness [Suddath, 1990]. We have access to an MRI twin study of

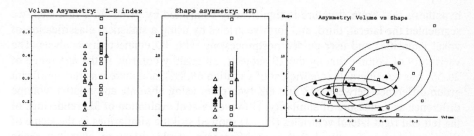

Fig. 2. Statistics of volume, shape and volume&shape lateralization of the amygdala-hippocampal complex in schizophrenia. The left figure shows the statistics of the volume asymmetry index (|R-L|/(R+L)) for the control and schizophrenics groups. The middle figure illustrates the shape difference (mean square difference between corresponding surface points, MSD) for both groups after volume normalization of each structure. The figure to the right shows a combined analysis of volume and shape asymmetry, illustrated as a two-dimensional feature space. Controls and schizophrenics are marked by dark triangles and open squares, respectively, with overlay of quartile ellipsoids.

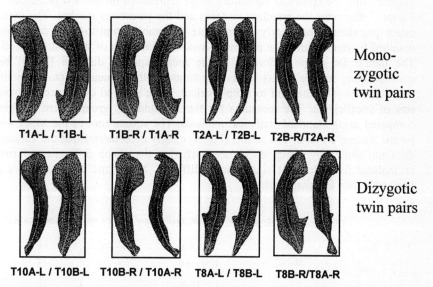

Fig. 3. Illustration of aligned and normalized surfaces of left and right ventricles of MZ (upper row) and DZ (lower row) twin pairs. The parametrization is overlaid as a surface mesh. The color major meridian lines show the stable point-to-point correspondences between surfaces. Visually, shapes of MZ twins are more similar than shapes of DZ twins. Please not that all the shapes are normalized by volume.

10 twin pairs, all healthy controls, to study volume and shape of brain structures. Image data is part of a research of D. Weinberger at NIHM and is published in [Bartley, 1997]. We were interested in the shape variability of the lateral ventricles as ventricular changes are often found to be a marker for disease, e.g. in schizophrenia. We tested the hypothesis that ventricles of MZ twin pairs are more similar than ventricles of non-identical twin pairs and of unrelated pairs, to corroborate the

hypothesis that brain structure is significantly controlled by genes. In a first step, we segmented the lateral, third, and forth ventricles by using a statistical classification of voxel intensities and user-guided postprocessing with 3D connectivity analysis. The variability of volume among the 20 subjects, all healthy controls in the age range of 26-35, was considerable (coefficient of variation 68.8%), and there was no significant group difference between MZ and DZ twin pairs using absolute and relative volume difference as a measure of similarity. However, visual evaluation of 3D renderings of the left and right lateral ventricles (Fig. 3) showed striking similarities in the shape of these structures. To avoid that size differences would dilute or alter the shape measurements, the size of all structures was normalized by volume. We then applied two shape representation methods, surface representation based on spherical harmonics [Kelemen, 1999] and 3D medial mesh representation presented in [Pizer, 1999, Styner, 2000,2001].

Shape analysis using surface representation
The binary segmentations of the left and right ventricles were parametrized and aligned using the spherical harmonics shape representation method [Kelemen, 1999]. Figure 3 illustrates the resulting surfaces and the parameter meshes. The overlaid of major meridian lines clearly demonstrate the stable point-to-point correspondence obtained by normalizing the parameter space to the poles of the first order ellipsoid. The metric for shape difference is the mean squared distance (MSD) between corresponding surface points. Given the nature of the expansion into harmonics, we can use Parseval's theorem to simply calculate the squared differences between two sets of coefficients. The measures for the MZ and DZ groups were analyzed and compared using standard statistical methods. The square root of the MSD was used for the student's t-tests. The results (Fig. 4) clearly demonstrate that the volume index does not show any group differences, whereas the shape difference of structures normalized for volume is significantly different. MZ shape pairs are more similar (p<0.012) than DZ shape pairs.

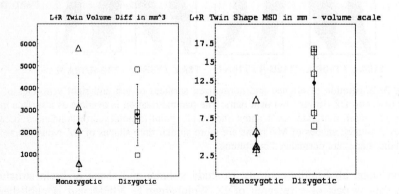

Fig 4. The volume difference index ({R-L|/(R+L)) of the ventricles of MZ and DZ twin pairs is nonsignificant (p < 0.75). The shape difference (√MSD) after volume normalization (right) results in a significantly lower shape difference for MZ than for DZ (p < 0.012).

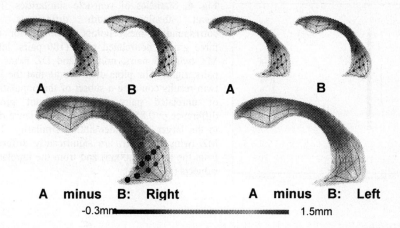

Fig. 5. Shape comparison of ventricles based on medial representations. Right and left lateral ventricles of paired twins A and B are shown in the upper row. The larger figures at the bottom row represent the medial mesh with width (radius) difference at corresponding mesh points. The size and color of the disks indicate local differences between twin A and B in the range of minus 0.3mm till 1.5mm.

Shape analysis using medial mesh representation

The structures aligned and normalized using the spherical harmonics as described above were processed by deformation of a sampled medial model [Styner and Gerig, 2000,2001]. The mesh of a shape model, derived from a population of ventricular shapes, was deformed to optimally match the new binary structures. The deformation results in a point-to-point correspondence of the discrete set of mesh points (Fig. 5). At each mesh node, we know the position in space and the local width (radius). We used both features independently to test whether the width itself without considering any mesh deformation, or the mesh deformation without considering any width changes, was more significant to find group differences between MZ and DZ twins. Figure 5 and Table 2 demonstrate that the group difference of the width measure alone is highly significant ($p<0.0065$) to tell that ventricular shapes in MZ twin pairs are more similar than in DZ pairs. We also tested a third group, which are all the unrelated pairs in our study of 20 subjects (Figure 6). The statistical tests show that the DZ distribution seems to be part of the unrelated pairs distribution. This result is plausible since non-identical twins have the same age and in our study the same gender, which explains the smaller variance of the DZ distribution. The same tests have bee applied to the second feature, the mean absolute distance (MAD) between the mesh node positions. This feature would significantly respond to mesh deformations, e.g. bending, disregarding any local width changes. The results were less significant ($p<0.035/0.011$, Table 2) but present additional shape information. Combined measures using a larger set of local features are currently studies. The interesting shape analysis results have to be compared with the volume analysis presented in the previous section, which was not significant at all, suggesting that shape analysis reveals new information not accessible by simple volume analysis.

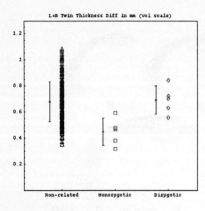

Fig. 6. Statistics of ventricle similarities. The mean absolute width differences at corresponding mesh points is shown for the three groups nonrelated pairs (180 pairs, left), MZ twins (5 pairs, middle) and DZ twins (5 pairs, right). The plots demonstrate that the DZ twin results could be a subset of the population of unrelated pairs (non significant group difference p<0.8562), with smaller variance due to the larger age/gender/sibling similarity. The MZ twins, however, are significantly different from the DZ (p<0.0065) and from the unrelated subjects (p<0.0009).

4. Discussion

This paper clearly demonstrates that shape features provide new information about group differences which is not provided by volume or size only. These results were expected since we intuitively know that structural differences between objects are only poorly defined by volumetric measurements. On the other hand, standard practice in neuroimaging analysis is still volumetry, measuring the brain volume or the volume of subcortical structures and ventricles. We will further extend our new methodology and apply the measurements to data from large clinical studies, in particular to the study of schizophrenia, the enlargment of ventricles in premature infants, to hippocampal measurements in epilepsy, and to autism and Fragile-X studies.

Width similarity		
	DZ	unrelated
MZ	0.0065	0.0009
DZ		0.8562
Location similarity		
	DZ	unrelated
MZ	0.0356	0.0110
DZ		0.6699

Table 2. Shape similarity of left and right ventricles between MZ/DZ/unrelated pairs using the sampled medial mesh representation. The table shows the p-values for testing mean differences of the width similarity measure (mean absolute radius differences, top) and location similarity measure (mean absolute position difference, bottom).

The comparison of the surface and the medial shape representation with respect to their power of finding group differences clearly demonstrates that the medial representation shows improved significance even using only part of the local shape information, here the width at a discrete set of corresponding mesh points. This is equivalent to flattening the mesh and looking only at the width parameter at the sampling points. The mesh deformation itself, independent of the width, can be described as a bending or straightening of figures. In our ventricle study, this measurement was less significant but still below a p-value of 5%. We plan to combine both, width and position, to further improve the discrimination power. A most significant advantage of a sampled medial representation versus a Fourier surface description is the locality of shape information [Yushkevich, 2001], as we can ask for group differences of a part of the mesh only or even at single mesh elements. In epilepsy and schizophrenia, e.g., several groups found significant shape differences using global parametrization or a large set of features. However, such analysis does not give any answer to where and what the pathological differences would be. We will apply our framework to hippocampal and ventricular analysis in studies where group differences were already found, and will test the possibilities for locality and type of shape change given by our new methods.

Acknowledgements:

We acknowledge D. Weinberger and W. Douglas, NIMH Neuroscience at St. Elizabeth, Washington for providing the twin datasets. We are further thankful to S. Pizer, T. Fletcher and S. Joshi, UNC Computer Science, for providing the m-rep tools for deformable medial meshes.

Bibliography

Bartley, A.J., Douglas, W.J., and Weinberger, D.R., Genetic variability of human brain size and cortical gyral patterns, Brain (1997), 120, 257-269.

Brechbuehler, Ch, Gerig, G. and Kuebler, O. "Parametrization of closed surfaces for 3D shape description", Comp. Vision and Image Underst. (CVIU), Vol. 61, No. 2, pp. 154-170, 1995

Cootes T.F. et al. (1995) Active Shape Models - Their Training and Application, Computer Vision and Image Understanding, 61(1), pp. 31-59.

Csernansky, J., Joshi, S., Wang, L., Haller, J., Gado, M., Miller, J., Grenander, U., and Miller, M., *Hippocampal morphometry in schizophrenia via high dimensional brain mapping*, Proc. Natl. Acad. Sci. USA, 95:11406-11411, Sept. 1998

Haller, J., Christensen, G. E., Joshi, S.C, Newcomer, J. W., Miller, M. I., Csernansky, J. G., Vannier, M. W., Hipppocampal MR imaging morphometry by means of general pattern matching, Radiology, Vol. 199, pp. 787-791, 1996.

Haller,J., Banerjee, A., Christensen, G. E, Joshi, S.C.,Miller, M.I., Vannier, M.W., J. Csernansky, G., "Three-Dimensional Hipocampal Volumetry by High Dimensional Transformation of a neuroanatomical Atlas,", Radiology, Vol. 202, pp. 504-510, 1997.

Kelemen, A., Szekely, G. and Gerig, G. (1999) Elastic Model-Based Segmentation of 3D Neuroradiological Data Sets, *IEEE Transactions On Medical Imaging*, 18, 828-839.

Pizer, S.M., Fritsch, D.S., Yushkevich, P.A., Johnson, V.E., and Chaney, E.L., Segmentation, Registration, and Measurement of Shape Variation via Image Object Shape, IEEE TMI 18(10):851-865, Oct. 1999

Shenton ME, Wible CG, McCarley RW. (1997) MRI studies in schizophrenia, In: Krishnan KRR, Doraiswamy PM (Eds.), Brain Imaging in clinical Psychiatry. Marcel Dekker, Inc. pp. 297-380.

Staib L.H. and Duncan J.S. (1996) Model-based Deformable Surface Finding for Medical Images, IEEE Trans. Med. Imaging, 15(5), pp. 1-12.

Styner, M. and Gerig, G., Hybrid boundary-medial shape description for biologically variable shapes, Proc. IEEE Workshop on Mathematical Methods in Biomedical Image Analysis (MMBIA), pp. 235-242, June 2000

Styner, M. and Gerig, G., Medial models incorporating object variability for 3D shape analysis, to be published in Proc. of IPMI 2001, Springer Verlag, June 2001

Suddath, R.L., Christison, G.W., Torrey, E.F., Casanova, M.F., and Weinberger, D.R., Anatomical abnormalities in the brains of monozygotic twins discordant for schizophrenia. [Published erratum in New England Journal of Medicine, 322:1616, 1990.], New England Journal of Medicine, 322:789-794, 1990.

Székely, G, A Kelemen, C Brechbühler, G Gerig (1996). Segmentation of 2-D and 3-D objects from MRI volume data using constrained elastic deformations of flexible Fourier contour and surface models. *Medical Image Analysis* 1(1): 19-34.

Vapnik, Statistical Learning Theory, 1998

Wang, L., Sarang, C.J., Miller, M.I., Grenander, U., and Csernansky, J.G., Statistical Analysis of Hippocampal Asymmetry, in press, NeuroImage. to appear 2001.

Yushkevich, P., Pizer, S.M., Joshi, S., and Marron, J.S., Intuitive, Localized Analysis of Shape Variability, to be published in Proc. IPMI 2001, Springer Verlag, June 2001

Hippocampal Shape Analysis Using Medial Surfaces

Sylvain Bouix[1], Jens C. Pruessner[2], Donald L. Collins[2], and Kaleem Siddiqi[1]

[1] Centre for Intelligent Machines & School of Computer Science
[2] McConnell Brain Imaging Centre, Montreal Neurological Institute
McGill University, Montreal, Canada

Abstract. Within the medial temporal lobe, significant attention has been paid to the analysis of the hippocampus (HC) in MR images because of its intimate connection to memory, emotion and learning. Volume changes in the HC have been recorded in conjunction with Alzheimer's disease, post-traumatic stress disorder and depression. Recent studies have also found a significant reduction in HC volume that is related to gender; it is found in men but not women. In this paper we demonstrate a shape analysis of the HC and employ it to investigate gender differences in normal subjects. For each subject we extract the dominant medial sheet of the HC, find the plane defined by its two principal eigen vectors and then express the medial surface radius as a height function over this plane. This allows us to statistically quantify the relationship between several independent variables and local object width.

1   Introduction

In studies employing hippocampus (HC) and amygdala (AG) segmentation based on magnetic resonance (MR) imaging, varying degrees of volume loss in conjunction with Alzheimer's disease, depression and post-traumatic stress disorder have been observed. The precise nature of this loss and its connection to variables such as age and gender remains somewhat controversial, pointing to the need for better quantitative models of 3D shape to be used in this context. With respect to structures such as the HC, a good candidate is the medial surface. The most prominent medial surface sheet can be used to register individual data sets, following which more precise comparisons can be made [13].

Medial models have been successfully used in medical image analysis in a number of contexts, e.g., see [7,4] for some recent applications. Applying these methods in 3D presents a challenge because only a small class of computationally reliable algorithms exist. One such class relies on pruning strategies for 3D Voronoi diagrams [1,6]. This has recently been used in conjunction with a boundary description to provide a characteristic model for 3D shape analysis [13]. An important idea is the use of a medial primitive [8] to describe the most prominent medial sheet and provide an intrinsic frame of reference by which different data sets can be registered.

W. Niessen and M. Viergever (Eds.): MICCAI 2001, LNCS 2208, pp. 33–40, 2001.

In this paper we adopt a similar strategy, but use a novel algorithm we have developed for computing medial surfaces. Our main goal is to apply this methodology to a data set for which volume loss in relation to gender and age has been previously investigated [9]. The main idea is to extract the dominant medial sheet of the HC for each subject, find the plane defined by its two principal eigen vectors and then express the medial surface radius as a height function over this plane. This in turn allows us to statistically examine the relationship of independent variables with local object width.

2   Divergence Based Medial Surfaces

In this section we review the algorithm for computing medial surfaces [11,2].

2.1   The Hamilton Jacobi Formulation

Consider the grassfire flow

$$\frac{\partial S}{\partial t} = \mathcal{N} \tag{1}$$

acting on a closed 3D surface S, such that each point on its boundary is moving with unit speed in the direction of the inward normal $\mathcal{N}$. In physics, such equations are typically solved by looking at the evolution of the phase space of an equivalent Hamiltonian system. Let D be the Euclidean distance function to the initial surface S_0. The magnitude of its gradient, $\|\nabla D\|$, is identical to 1 in its smooth regime. The associated Hamiltonian system is given by:

$$\dot{\mathbf{p}} = (0, 0, 0), \qquad \dot{\mathbf{q}} = -(D_x, D_y, D_z). \tag{2}$$

Hamiltonian systems are conservative and hence the vector field $\dot{\mathbf{q}}$ is divergence free. However, this property does not hold at singularities of $\dot{\mathbf{q}}$, which coincide with medial surface points. We use the divergence theorem to measure the net outward flux of $\dot{\mathbf{q}}$ through a surface

$$\int_v \mathrm{div}(\dot{\mathbf{q}})\mathrm{d}v \equiv \int_S < \dot{\mathbf{q}}, \mathcal{N} > \mathrm{d}s. \tag{3}$$

In the limit as the volume enclosed by the surface shrinks to zero we obtain a numerical approximation to the divergence which is used to guide a thinning process in a cubic lattice, while taking care to preserve the object's topology.

2.2   Preserving Homotopy

A point is a *simple* point if its removal does not change the topology of the object. Hence in 3D, its removal must not disconnect the object, create a hole, or create a cavity. Malandain *et al.* have introduced a topological classification of a point x in a cubic lattice by computing two numbers [5]: i) C^*: the number of 26-connected components 26-adjacent to x in $O \cap N_{26}^*$, and ii) $\bar{C}$: the number of 6-connected components 6-adjacent to x in $\bar{O} \cap N_{18}$. Further, they have shown that if $C^* = 1$ and $\bar{C} = 1$, the point is *simple*, and hence removable.

The basic strategy now is to guide the thinning of the object by the total outward flux measure computed over a very small neighborhood. Points with the most negative outward flux are the strongest medial surface points. The process is stopped when all surviving points are not simple, or have a total outward flux below some chosen (negative) value, or both. Unfortunately the result is not guaranteed to be a thin set, i.e., one without an interior.

This last constraint can be satisfied by defining an appropriate notion of an endpoint in a cubic lattice. In $\mathcal{R}^3$, if there exists a plane that passes through a point p such that the intersection of the plane with the object includes an open curve which ends at p, then p is an end point of a 3D curve, or is on the rim or corner of a 3D surface. This criterion can be discretized easily to 26-connected digital objects by examining 9 digital planes in the 26-neighborhood of p [10]. The thinning process proceeds as before, but the threshold criterion for removal is applied only to endpoints.

2.3 Segmenting the Medial Surface

The medial surface can now be segmented using the classification of [5]. Specifically, the numbers C^* and $\bar{C}$ can be used to classify curve points, surface points, border points and junction points. However, junction points can be misclassified as surface points when certain special configurations of voxels occur. These cases have to be dealt with using a new definition for simple surfaces [5].

Let x be a surface point ($\bar{C} = 2$ and $C^* = 1$). Let B_x and C_x be the two connected components of $\bar{O} \cap N_{18}$ 6-adjacent to x. Two surface points x and y are in an equivalence relation if there exists a 26-path $x_0, x_1, ..., x_i, ..., x_n$ with $x_0 = x$ and $x_n = y$ such that for $i \in [0, ..., n-1]$, $(B_{x_i} \cap B_{x_{i+1}} \neq \emptyset$ and $C_{x_i} \cap C_{x_{i+1}} \neq \emptyset)$ or $(B_{x_i} \cap C_{x_{i+1}} \neq \emptyset$ and $C_{x_i} \cap B_{x_{i+1}} \neq \emptyset)$. A *simple surface* is defined as any equivalence class of this equivalence relation.

We use this definition in our framework to find all the different simple surfaces comprising the medial surface of an object. The first unmarked surface point on the medial surface is found and used as a "source" to build its corresponding simple surface using a depth first search strategy. The next simple surface is built from the next unmarked point and so on, until all medial surface points are marked.

3 Hippocampal Data

In a previously published analysis [9], the left and right HC and AG were manually segmented from T1-weighted MR images (three dimensional spoiled gradient echo acquisition with sagittal volume excitation; repetition time 18, echo time 10, flip angle 30 degrees) from 80 normal healthy subjects. These subjects included 39 healthy men and 41 healthy women in the age range of 18 to 42 years (mean age 25.4 +/- 5.6 years). The MRI data for each subject was first corrected for

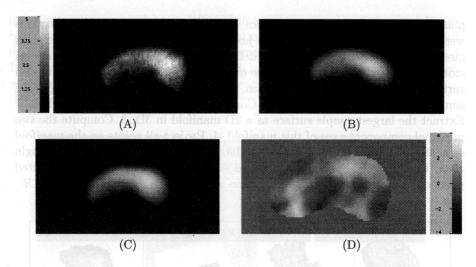

(A)   (B)

(C)   (D)

Fig. 3. Horizontal section of medial surface radius function, anterior at the right, posterior at the left and medial at the top of image. (A) Radius function projected onto a 2D sheet for one subject. The grey bar (left side) indicates a radius of 0 to 5 mm. (B) Average radius function for left female hippocampus. This image is created by computing the average, on a pixel-by-pixel basis, of the radius function of the left HC for the 41 women in the study. One can see that on average the head of the HC (right side, image B) is approximately 10mm thick from top to bottom and that the tail (left side) gradually decreases in thickness. (C) Average radius for right female hippocampus. There appears to be a difference between the left and right sides. In order to localize statistically significant differences, a pairwise age corrected t-statistic image was computed for right-left (D). High intensity areas indicate regions where the right side is larger than the left.

gender and age on the right hemisphere than on the left; the resulting t-values are higher in the right hemisphere. Adjacent regions of positive and negative t-values indicate possible local translation. Evidence for this effect at the head and tail of the right hemisphere HC indicate a rotation of female HC with respect to the male HC, with womens' HC head moving laterally and the tail moving medially. However, the difference in magnitude between the two regions suggests differences in the size of the medial anterior section of the HC between males and females. We note that the recent study in [13] reports that the right HC is on average thicker than the left, although the connection to gender was not examined.

Second, Fig. 5 shows the individual age regression maps for the 4 groups. The intensity of the image is directly proportional to the magnitude (and sign) of the regression of the medial surface radius function with age and thus reveals information about the effect of age on the location of shape differences. The

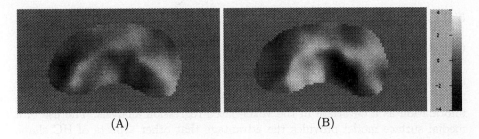

(A)   (B)

Fig. 4. Regression of gender, correcting for age, left (A) and right (B) hemi
spheres. The grey bar indicates a range of t-values from -4.0 to 4.0.

most apparent result is that the regressions are stronger in men than in women,
and stronger on the right side in both sexes. We can see positive correlations in
the medial anterior region of (A), suggesting a thickening of the alveus with age
in females. In males, there is a significant decrease in the anterior and posterior
regions, corresponding to the uncal recess and the inferior horn of the lateral
ventricles. These results confirm those found in our previous study [9].

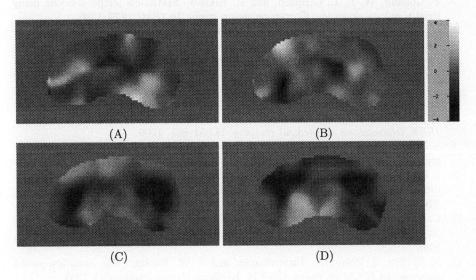

(A)   (B)

(C)   (D)

Fig. 5. Regression of age for women left (A) and right (B) hemispheres; and men
left (C) and right (D). The grey bar indicates t-values from -4.0 to 4.0.

5   Conclusions

Our experiments indicate that association with HC shape is stronger in men. This confirms our previous results which showed a stronger (negative) correlation of volume with age in men than in women. Future studies need to address the association between shape and volume more precisely, possibly by adding volume information as a covariate in the voxel-based regression analysis. The use of a medial surface model provides the advantage that other aspects of HC shape (such as boundary curvature) can also be incorporated as a height function, allowing for further quantitative analysis.

References

1. D. Attali, G. S. di Baja, and E. Thiel. Skeleton simplification through non-significant branch removal. *Image Processing and Communications*, pages 63–72, 1997.
2. S. Bouix and K. Siddiqi. Divergence-based medial surfaces. In *ECCV'2000*, pages 603–618, Dublin, Ireland, June 2000.
3. D. L. Collins, P. Neelin, T. M. Peters, and A. C. Evans. Automatic 3d inter-subject registration of mr volumetric data in standardized talairach space. *Journal of Computer Assisted Tomography*, 18:192–205, 1994.
4. P. Golland, W. E. L. Grimson, and R. Kikinis. Statistical shape analysis using fixed topology skeletons: Corpus callosum study. In *IPMI'1999*, 1999.
5. G. Malandain, G. Bertrand, and N. Ayache. Topological segmentation of discrete surfaces. *International Journal of Computer Vision*, 10(2):183–197, 1993.
6. M. Näf, O. Kübler, R. Kikinis, M. E. Shenton, and G. Székely. Characterization and recognition of 3d organ shape in medical image analysis using skeletonization. In *IEEE Workshop on Mathematical Methods in Biomedical Image Analysis*, 1996.
7. S. M. Pizer, D. S. Fritsch, P. Yuskhevich, V. Johnson, and E. Chaney. Segmentation, registration and measurement of shape variation via image object shape. *IEEE Transactions on Medical Imaging*, 18:851–865, 1999.
8. S. M. Pizer, A. Thall, and D. T. Chen. M-reps: A new object representation for graphics. *ACM Transactions on Graphics (submitted)*, 1999.
9. J. C. Pruessner, D. L. Collins, M. Pruessner, and A. C. Evans. Age and gender predict volume decline in the anterior and posterior hippocampus in early adulthood. *The Journal of Neuroscience*, To appear, 2001.
10. C. Pudney. Distance-ordered homotopic thinning: A skeletonization algorithm for 3d digital images. *Computer Vision and Image Understanding*, 72(3):404–413, 1998.
11. K. Siddiqi, S. Bouix, A. Tannenbaum, and S. W. Zucker. The hamilton-jacobi skeleton. In *ICCV'99*, pages 828–834, Kerkyra, Greece, September 1999.
12. J. G. Sled, A. P. Zijdenbos, and A. C. Evans. A non-parametric method for automatic correction of intensity non-uniformity in mri data. *IEEE Transactions On Medical Imaging*, 17(1):87–97, 1998.
13. M. Styner and G. Gerig. Medial models incorporating object variability for 3d shape analysis. In *IPMI'2001*, pages 502–516, 2001.
14. K. J. Worsley, J. B. Poline, and A. C. Evans. Characterizing the response of pet and fmri data using multivariate linear models. *NeuroImage*, 6:305–319, 1998.

Detecting Spatially Consistent Structural Differences in Alzheimer's and Fronto Temporal Dementia Using Deformation Morphometry

C. Studholme[1], V. Cardenas[1], N. Schuff[1], H. Rosen[2], B. Miller[2], and M. Weiner[1]

[1] Dept. Radiology, U.C.S.F., VAMC (114), 4150 Clement Street, San Francisco.
[2] Memory and Aging Center,Dept. Neurology, U.C.S.F., San Francisco
cs1@itsa.ucsf.edu

Abstract. Atrophy is known to occur at specific sites around the brain in both Alzheimer's disease (AD) and Fronto-Temporal Lobe Dementia (FTLD), inducing characteristic shape changes in brain anatomy. In this paper we employ an entropy driven fine lattice free form registration algorithm to investigate whole brain structural changes induced by these diseases relative to normal anatomy, using deformation morphometry. We focus on Alzheimer's disease (AD) and two common sub groups of FTLD: the frontal lobe variant (FTD) and semantic dementia (SD). The shape of each subject group was characterized at each point in the reference anatomy by the distribution of the determinant of the Jacobian of the transformation mapping the subject to a common reference anatomy. Statistical measures were then applied to locate points where voxel level differences in the Jacobian occur between a control group and each of the disease groups, indicating spatially consistent shape differences induced by a particular disease. Spatial maps of the statistical differences showed very different structural characteristics in each disease. AD was characterized by relative contractions in regions of the hippocampus and the parietal lobe and expansions of the ventricular CSF spaces. FTD was characterized by patterns of contraction in the frontal lobe. SD was characterized by large contractions in the temporal lobe, hippocampus and expansion of the ventricular CSF spaces.

1 Introduction

Alzheimer's disease (AD) and fronto-temporal lobe dementia (FTLD) are two forms of dementia with distinctly different etiologies but with clinical symptoms that are often difficult to distinguish. Therefore, improvements in the differential diagnosis between AD and FTLD are desirable for better staging of patients in drug trials and treatment planning. Computational shape analysis of structural MRI data that identifies anatomical changes in the brain has the potential to aid a differential diagnosis. Partially driven by the development of more accurate anatomical registration techniques, the field has expanded rapidly over

W. Niessen and M. Viergever (Eds.): MICCAI 2001, LNCS 2208, pp. 41–48, 2001.

the last few years. Much of the early work concentrated on specific anatomical regions such as the corpus callosum [7] which has remained an active area of methodological development [20]. Region based analysis techniques can rely on the identification and mapping of points on a specific anatomical boundary for statistical shape analysis [4,14] and has been used to analyze regional shape variation such as in the hippocampus in AD [6]. Whole brain approaches have concentrated on the analysis of the volume transformation describing the non rigid mapping between subjects and a reference anatomy [1,27]. A recent study of schizophrenia [10] analyzed low resolution 3D deformation fields and detected effects of disease without a-priori assumptions. Related techniques, such as voxel morphometry [2], which examine local changes in the regional density of particular tissue types, have detected significantly different structural patterns in degenerative diseases [22].

In this work we focus on purely deformation based morphometry relying on accurate registration to provide spatial transformations describing the subtle differences in brain shape. Specifically, we have used a high dimensional (many parameter) non-rigid free-form registration technique to map subject brains to a common reference space and then analysed the Jacobian of this transformation to look for characteristic differences in shape. We have used a voxel level Jacobian analysis to search for only those points of change which are both spatially and diagnostically consistent across the different groups.

2   Method

2.1   Inter-subject Registration

Quantification and comparison of shape differences in brain anatomy is dependent on the ability to find corresponding anatomical points in images of two different human brains. This is a fundamental problem stemming from the inherent variability of human brain anatomy, particularly in the cortex [3]. The field of non-rigid inter-subject brain mapping or atlas matching is extensive and beyond the scope of this paper. We have chosen to use a voxel based algorithm which provides fully automated registration estimates on a large range of data, primarily because the number of data-sets being examined precludes the use of perhaps more accurate methodology requiring some form of manual tracing or segmentation. Specifically we have made use of a voxel level free form deformation algorithm driven by normalised [24] mutual information [28,18] between the two MRI scans,

$$C(M_1; M_2) = \frac{H(M_1) + H(M_2)}{H(M_1, M_2)}, \tag{1}$$

where $H(M_1)$ and $H(M_2)$ are the marginal entropies of the reference $m_1 \in M_1$ and subject $m_2 \in M_2$ MRI values occurring in the volume of overlap of points in the reference and test subject MRI volumes, related by transformation $\mathbf{T}_{12}$. $H(M_1, M_2)$ is the joint entropy of the co-occurrence of the values in the two scans within this overlap. This provides spatial transformation estimates robust to tissue intensity changes which may arrise in degenerative diseases. This is a refinement of earlier registration methodology employed for tissue deformation [21] estimation and relative geometric imaging distortion [25] correction. For this application we have developed the algorithm and its implementation to provide a finer (2.4mm) B-Spline lattice estimate of the mapping between different brain anatomy. Further details of the registration algorithm used here are given in [23].

2.2   Shape Comparison

Choice of Reference Atlas: There are a number of approaches to constructing a common reference anatomy as a target for spatial normalisation. Because we are primarily concerned with accurate normalisation of different subject groups, rather than in the ability to report results in a standard anatomical coordinate system, we have chosen to use a single subject reference MRI as opposed to an averaged and blurred MRI, thus retaining the finest anatomical structures for registration. In earlier work [23] we examined the use of our non-rigid registration methodology in mapping different subject groups to old and young anatomical atlases. This demonstrated that the consistency of spatial normalization of older, younger or atrophied brains improved when the reference atlas was roughly age-matched. To age match our AD and FTLD subjects, we have chosen an older control subject (in this case a 72 year old female) as the reference space for the measurements.

Clinical Hypothesis for Shape Differences in AD and FTLD: Alzheimer's disease accelerates the loss of large projection neurons in the hippocampus [26] which may precede and is more severe than neuron loss in association cortex. MRI studies of AD [16,13] show generalized brain tissue loss, reduction in GM (particularly in the parietal lobes), ventricular enlargement, and changes in T2 signal intensity. Focal atrophy of the hippocampus occurs in normal aging [11], and to a greater extent in AD [12]. The rate of lateral ventricle enlargement (measured longitudinally), highly correlates with impaired cognition but shows variable overlap with controls [5].

In general, FTLD patients exhibit greater atrophy of anterior brain regions than AD and healthy elderly, while regions of the medial temporal lobe appears to be spared in FTLD [9]. FTLD, like AD, shows hippocampal atrophy [8], suggesting that sole hippocampal volume measurements may not be helpful to differentiate between FTLD and AD. Kaufer *et al.* [15] found a smaller anterior corpus callosum and enlarged pericallosal CSF spaces in FTLD when compared with AD. MRI also demonstrated cases with predominant temporal lobe atrophy and predominant frontal lobe atrophy in FTLD [19] supporting the existence of the temporal and frontal variants of FTLD.

Based on these previous findings, we hypothesized that our shape analysis between FTLD and AD would reveal 1) greater frontal lobe atrophy in FTLD, 2) greater anterior temporal lobe atrophy in FTLD, 3) atrophy of anterior corpus callosum and hypertrophy of pericallosal CSF spaces in FTLD, and 4) parietal lobe gray matter atrophy in AD.

Comparing Shape in Each Group: Following registration estimation, we have a B-Spline model of the transformation $(x_S, y_S, z_S) = T_{RS}(x_R, y_R, z_R)$ mapping between the reference anatomy and each subject. This global transformation consists of a rigid component describing the patient positioning, and the remaining non-rigid components describing the global and local shape differences between each subject and the reference anatomy. To examine the shape differences only we take the approach of Davatzikos [7] and Machado [17] and examine the differential properties of the spatially normalising transformation through the Jacobian matrix,

$$\mathbf{J}_{RS}(x_R, y_R, z_R) = \begin{bmatrix} \frac{\partial x_S}{\partial x_R} & \frac{\partial x_S}{\partial y_R} & \frac{\partial x_S}{\partial z_R} \\ \frac{\partial y_S}{\partial x_R} & \frac{\partial y_S}{\partial y_R} & \frac{\partial y_S}{\partial z_R} \\ \frac{\partial z_S}{\partial x_R} & \frac{\partial z_S}{\partial y_R} & \frac{\partial z_S}{\partial z_R} \end{bmatrix} \tag{2}$$

of the volume transformation, between reference and subject coordinates. This matrix describes the point-wise volume change in each axis when mapping points from the reference anatomy to each subject. Large values of components indicate expansions of anatomy, while small values indicate contractions. In our methodology, the partial derivatives making up the Jacobian are evaluated analytically from the B-Spline deformation model. For the work presented in this paper we have only considered the determinant of this Jacobian $J_{RS}(x_R, y_R, z_R) = |\mathbf{J}_{RS}(x_R, y_R, z_R)|$, which is a scalar summarizing the point-wise volume change. To analyze shape statistically we first consider a single group of subject MRIs mapped to a reference MRI. At each reference coordinate $\mathbf{x}_R$ there will be a set of Jacobian values,

$$\mathcal{J}_{RG}(\mathbf{x}_R) = \{J_{R1}(\mathbf{x}_R), J_{R2}(\mathbf{x}_R) \ldots J_{RN}(\mathbf{x}_R)\}, \tag{3}$$

where N is the number of subjects in the group. For a given location, this set of values will provide an estimate of the distribution in the point-wise volume at that point across the group of subjects, relative to the chosen reference anatomy. For points within the gray matter of the cortex for example, this volume measure will be primarily determined by the thickness of the cortex, relative to the thickness of the cortex at that point in the reference anatomy. Globally the average Jacobian over the brain volume for each subject will describe the relative size of each subject brain relative to the target anatomy. To remove the influence of brain size from the analysis we have chosen to scale each Jacobian value by the average Jacobian of the subject. To detect differences in shape of the distributions for AD $\mathcal{J}_{RA}(\mathbf{x})$, SD $\mathcal{J}_{RS}(\mathbf{x})$ and FTD $\mathcal{J}_{RF}(\mathbf{x})$ from the control group $\mathcal{J}_{RC}(\mathbf{x})$ at each point, we have used the effect size as employed by Davatzikos et al. [7] and Machado et al. [17], defined between the AD and control group as:

$$\mathcal{E}_{CA}(\mathbf{x}_R) = \frac{\mu_{RA}(\mathbf{x}_R) - \mu_{RC}(\mathbf{x}_R)}{\sigma_{C \cup A}(\mathbf{x}_R)}, \tag{4}$$

where $\mu_{RA}(\mathbf{x}_R)$ is the mean Jacobian determinant in the Alzheimer's group and $\mu_{RC}(\mathbf{x}_R)$ is the mean Jacobian determinant in the control group at location $\mathbf{x}_R$ in the reference anatomy. The standard deviation $\sigma_{C \cup A}(\mathbf{x}_R)$ is derived from the combined set of Jacobian values in the control and AD group.

Subject Imaging Data: For this study 40 Controls (17 Female, 23 Male), 31 AD (13 Female, 18 Male), 12 SD (2 Female, 10 Male), 14 FTD (3 Female, 11 Male) were imaged. All images were acquired using the same 3D gradient echo T1 weighted anatomical MPRAGE sequence (TR=10ms,TE=4ms). The images were reconstructed with a coronal slice plane at a voxel size of $1mm \times 1mm \times 1.5mm$. Overall, dementia severity as measured by a standard minimental state examination (MMSE) test was similar in the patient groups (Control= 29 ± 0.6), AD = 22 ± 5, AD=24 ± 3, FTD = 24 ± 6; with 30 representing cognitive normal and 0 severe dementia conditions).

3   Results

Figure 1 shows the spatial distribution of the effect size of the Jacobian of each disease group relative to the control group overlaid onto the average control MRI, where cyan-blue indicates expansion and yellow-red is contraction of regions control subjects to disease subjects. In AD, the most prominent differences with respect to controls were contractions in the hippocampus and temporal and parietal lobe without large changes in frontal lobe. In addition, AD patients had substantially increased temporal and lateral ventricular spaces compared to controls. In FTD, the most prominent contractions when compared to controls appeared in the anterior aspects of the putamen and frontal lobe regions, while hippocampus and temporal and parietal lobes were spared. In SD, the most prominent differences from controls were bilateral expansions of the anterior temporal horn of the ventricles, accompanied by contractions in the adjacent temporal lobe regions, including hippocampus and amygdala.

4   Discussion

In this work we have implemented a fully automated whole brain shape analysis technique based on an entropy driven fine-lattice volume registration algorithm and applied it to identify characteristic abnormal brain structure associated with three common forms of dementia: AD, FTD and SD. Cognitive and neurobehavioral studies have indicated differences between FTLD and normal controls, and between FTLD and AD. In addition, a handful of cognitive studies have begun to identify important differences between the sub-types of FTLD, such as early impairments of executive functions in FTD and profound semantic memory breakdown in SD. Our results further support this work indicating that differences between these dementia syndromes are associated with characteristic structural changes. One important observation was that consistent spatial shape differences were detected between the patient groups that had very similar levels of dementia severity as measured by MMSE. This implies that the spatial pattern of structural abnormality reflects primarily the regional distribution of pathology as opposed to being simply associated with dementia severity. Therefore, the different spatial patterns of shape deformation could aid a differential diagnosis between these different types of dementia.

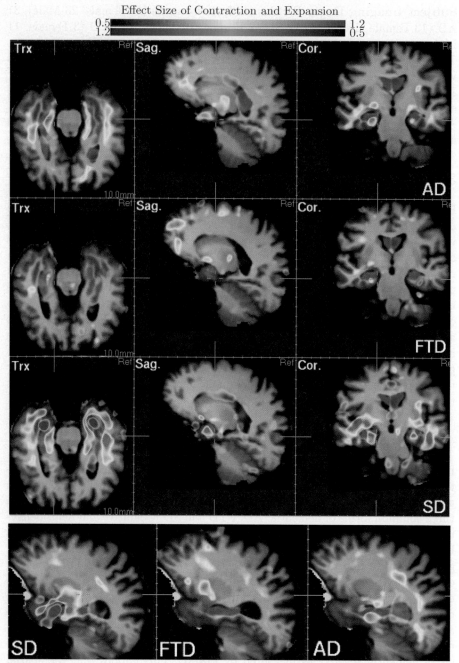

Fig. 1. Transaxial, sagittal and coronal slices through the averaged spatially normalised control group MRI (N=40) with colour overlay of the thresholded effect size of relative contraction (yellow-red) or expansion (cyan-blue) of tissue from the normal control group to the three disease groups. Top row shows AD, second from top FTD, third from top SD and the lower row shows a second set of sagittal slices through another plane illustrating further differences in the frontal and parietal lobe shape.

Overall, the groups of AD and SD subjects were older than the group of FTD subjects, and age-related atrophy is well established. FTLD subjects are generally younger than AD subjects, making age-matching difficult. A map of structural changes due to normal aging would assist in ruling out confounding effects of age. There are many other routes to extend and improve our initial analysis, looking, for example, at the individual components, rather than simply the determinant of the Jacobian, which could provide directional information about shape differences. Methods of statistically combining shape measurements from different locations will help to improve the statistical power of this analysis [20]. Additionally, other non-parametric statistical measures may well assist in comparing shape characteristics arising from unknown sub-groups within the clinically defined diagnoses.

Acknowledgments This work was funded by a NIH grants P01 AG12435, P01 AA11493 and R01 AG10897. The authors wish to thank D. Truran for helping select and prepare the atlas data, Dr B. Jagust for access to imaging data, Dr L. Rogers for advice on the statistical analysis and Dr J. Gee and Dr D. Pettey for discussions on the Jacobian shape analysis.

References

1. J. Ashburner and K.J. Friston. Nonlinear spatial normalization using basis functions. *Neuroimage*, 7(4):254–266, 1997.
2. J. Ashburner and K.J. Friston. Voxel-based morphometry-The methods. *Neuroimage*, 11:805–821, 2000.
3. A.J. Bartley, D.W. Jones, and D.R. Weinberge. Genetic variability of human brain size and cortical gyral patterns. *Brain*, pages 257–269, 1997.
4. F.L. Bookstein. Landmark methods for forms without landmarks: Morphometrics of group differences in outline shape. *Medical Image Analysis*, 1(3):225–243, 1997.
5. C. De Carli, J.V. Haby, J.A. Gilette D. Teichberg, S. Rapoport, and M.B. Schapiro. Longitudinal changes in lateral ventricular volume in patients with dementia of the alzheimer type. *Neurology*, 42:2029–2036, 1992.
6. J.G. Csernansky, L. Wang, S. Joshi J.P. Miller M. Gado D. Kido D. McKeel, J.C. Morris, and MI. Miller. Early DAT is distinguished from aging by high-dimensional mapping of the hippocampus. *Neurology*, 55(11):1636–1643, 2000.
7. C. Davatzikos, M. Vaillant, S.M. Resnick, J.L. Prince, S. Letovsky, and R.N. Bryan. A computerised approach for morphological analysis of the corpus callosum. *Journal of Computer Assisted Tomography*, 20(1):88–97, 1996.
8. R. Duara, W. Barker, and C.A. Luis. Frontotemporal dementia and alzheimer's disease: differential diagnosis. *Dement Geriatr Cogn Disord*, 10(1):37–42, 1999.
9. G.B. Frisoni, A. Beltramello, C. Geroldi, C. Weiss, A. Bianchetti, and M. Trabucchi. Brain atrophy in frontotemporal dementia. *J Neurol Neurosurg Psychiatry*, 61:157–165, 1996.
10. C. Gaser, H.P. Voltz, S. Kiebel, S. Riehemann, and H. Sauer. Detecting structural changes in whole brain based on nonlinear deformations- application to schizophrenia research. *Neuroimage*, 10:107–113, 1999.
11. J. Golomb, A. Kluger, and M.J. de Leon. Hippocampal formation size in normal human aging: a correlate of delayed secondary memory performance. *Learning and Memory*, 1:45–54, 1994.

12. C.R. Jack, C.R. Petersen, P.C. O'Brien, and E.G. Tangalos. MR-based hippocampal volumetry in the diagnosis of alzheimer's disease. *Neurology*, 42:183–188, 1992.
13. T.L. Jernigan, D.P. Salmonand N. Butters, and J. Hesselink. Cerebral structure on MRI, part II: specific changes in Alzheimer's and Huntington's diseases. *Biol Psychaitry*, 29:68–81, 1991.
14. S. Joshi. *Large Deformation Diffeomorphisms and Gaussian Random Fields for Statistical Characterization of Brain Sub-Manifolds*. PhD thesis, Washington Univ., 1997.
15. D.I. Kaufer, B.L. Miller, L. Itti, L.A. Fairbanks, J. Li, J. Fishman, J. Kushi, and J.L. Cummings. Midline cerebral morphometry distinguishes frontotemporal dementia and alzheimer's disease. *Neurology*, 48:978–985, 1997.
16. J.S. Luxenberg, J.V. Haxby, H. Creasey, M. Sundaram, and S.I. Rapoport. Rate of ventricular enlargement in dementia of the alzheimer type correlates with rate of neuropsychological deterioration. *Neurology*, 37:1135–1140, 1987.
17. A.M.C. Machado, J.C. Gee, and M.F.M. Campos. Atlas warping for brain morphometry. In *Proceedings of Medical Imaging 1998*, pages 642–651. SPIE Press, 1998. San Diego, California.
18. F. Maes, A. Collignon, D. Vandermeulen, G. Marchal, and P. Suetens. Multimodality image registration by maximisation of mutual information. *IEEE Transactions on Medical Images*, 16(2):187–198, 1997.
19. R.J. Perry and J.R. Hodges. Differentiating frontal and temporal variant frontotemporal dementia from alzheimer's disease. *Neurology*, 54:2277–2284, 2000.
20. D.J. Pettey and J.C. Gee. Using a linear diagnostic function and non-rigid registration to search for morphological differences between poluations: An example involving the male and female corpus callosum. In *Proceedings SPIE Medical Imaging*, volume 4322, page In Press, 2001.
21. D. Ruckert, C. Hayes, C. Studholme, M. Leach, and D.J. Hawkes. Non-rigid registration of breast MR images using mutual information. In W. M. Wells, A. Colchester, and S. Delp, editors, *Proceedings of MICCAI*, pages 1144–1152, 1998. Cambridge, MA, USA.
22. A.R.B. Serge, B Rombouts, F. Barkhof, M.P. Witter, and P. Scheltens. Unbiased whole-brain analysis of gray matter loss in alzheimer's disease. *Neuroscience Letters*, 285:231–233, 2000.
23. C. Studholme, V. Cardenas, and M. Weiner. Multi scale image and multi scale deformation of brain anatomy for building average brain atlases. In *Proceedings SPIE Medical Imaging*, volume 4322, page In Press, 2001.
24. C. Studholme, D.L.G. Hill, and D.J. Hawkes. An overlap invariant entropy measure of 3D medical image alignment. *Pattern Recognition*, 32(1):71–86, 1999.
25. C. Studholme, E. Novotny, R. Stokking, J.S. Duncan, I.G. Zubal, and D. Spencer. Alignment of functional data acquired before and after intra-cranial electrode implantation using non-rigid MRI registration. In *Proceedings of ISMRM 2000, Denver, Col., USA.*, page 585, 2000.
26. R.D. Terry, A. Peck, R. DeTeresa, R. Schechter, and D. Horoupian. Some morphometric aspects of the brain in senile dementia of the alzheimer type. *Annals of Neurology*, 10:184–192, 1981.
27. P. Thompson, R. Woods, M. Mega, and A. Toga. Mathematical/Computational challenges in creating deformable and probabilistic atlases of the human brain. *Human Brain Mapping*, 9:81–92, 2000.
28. W.M. Wells, P. Viola, H. Atsumi, S. Nakajima, and R. Kikinis. Multi-modal volume registration by maximisation of mutual information. *Medical Image Analysis*, 1(1):35–51, 1996.

Quantifying Small Changes in Brain Ventricular Volume Using Non-rigid Registration

Mark Holden, Julia A. Schnabel, and Derek L.G. Hill

Computational Imaging Science Group, Division of Radiological Sciences and Medical Engineering, Guy's, King's and St. Thomas' School of Medicine, Guy's Hospital, King's College London, UK
{mark.holden,julia.schnabel,derek.hill}@kcl.ac.uk

Abstract. Non-rigid registration can automatically quantify small changes in volume of anatomical structures over time by means of segmentation propagation. Here we use a non-rigid registration algorithm based on optimising normalised mutual information to quantify small changes in brain ventricular volume in MR images of a group of five patients treated with growth hormone replacement therapy and a control group of six volunteers. The lateral ventricles are segmented from each subject image by registering the brainweb image [1] which has this structure delineated. The mean (standard deviation) volume change measurements are 1.09cc (0.73cc) for the patient group and 0.08cc (0.62cc) for the volunteer group, this difference is statistically significant at the 1% level. We validate our volume change measurements by comparing them to previously published results obtained by visual inspection of difference images, and demonstrate high rank correlation coefficient ($\rho = 0.7$, n=11).

1 Introduction

Non-rigid registration algorithms have recently been used for quantifying change in volume of structures over time, and for quantifying differences between members of a cohort. One approach is to delineate a structure of interest from one image, and use the deformation field calculated by non-rigid registration of that image to a second image to delineate the same structure in the second image [2]. This approach is sometimes called segmentation propagation [3, 4], and is illustrated in Figure 1. Most non-rigid registration algorithms are very sensitive to differences in intensities between images, or to shading artefacts. Non-rigid algorithms that optimise an information theoretic similarity measure such as normalised mutual information are less likely to be sensitive to these effects.

Here we apply the non-rigid registration algorithm devised by Rueckert [5] to study a group of five adult patients being treated with growth hormone replacement therapy, and a group of six volunteers. This group was previously studied using rigid body registration and visual assessment of difference images [6], and that study determined that the greatest change in the patient images was a reduction in the volume of the lateral ventricles. We demonstrate that the non-rigid registration algorithm is able to quantify small changes in volume with

W. Niessen and M. Viergever (Eds.): MICCAI 2001, LNCS 2208, pp. 49–56, 2001.
© Springer-Verlag Berlin Heidelberg 2001

high precision, and also validate the results it produces by comparing them to a visual assessment score previously obtained for the same subjects.

The novelty of this work is the use of segmentation propagation to quantify very small changes in clinical serial MR images, and the comparison of these measurements with results of a blinded visual assessment of difference images for the same subjects. We use a generic atlas and therefore do not require subject-specific segmentation. In related work, the ability of the same algorithm to recover large deformations was validated using a biomechanical model [7].

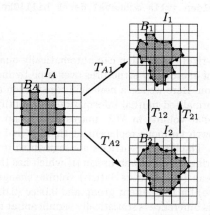

Fig. 1. Principle of segmentation propagation. I_A represents the atlas image with a segmented structure, B_A, defined by a connected set of boundary points at voxel locations, shown as dots and lines. I_1 and I_2 represent the baseline and repeat images of the patient. Non-rigid registration of I_A to I_1 and I_2 produces the transformations T_{A1} and T_{A2}. Registration of I_1 and I_2 produces the transformations T_{12} and T_{21}. Image I_A is transformed by T_{A1} and T_{A2} into the space of I_1 and I_2 which results in propagated structures B_1 and B_2. Because a transformation results generally in translations of boundary points by a non-integer number of voxels, the transformed set of boundary points does not, in general, coincide with the voxel locations of I_1 and I_2.

1.1   Review of Brainweb Simulated Normal Brain Image

The brainweb image is available from the McConnell brain imaging centre, Montreal Neurological Institute. It was created by first registering 27 (1mm isotropic voxels) T_1 weighted gradient echo scans of a normal volunteer [1]. These registered images were then corrected for RF inhomogeneity and intensity averaged to produce a high SNR image. This image was then classified into five tissue types: white matter, grey matter, CSF, fat, background; first automatically using a clustering algorithm and then by expert manual editing [1].

1.2 Review of Rueckert's Non-rigid Registration Algorithm

The non-rigid registration algorithm [5] we use here was designed for the registration of dynamic contrast enhanced MR breast images acquired only a few minutes apart. The algorithm uses a free-form deformation (FFD) to model local deformation. The FFD is constructed from a 3D tensor product of B-splines, and deformation is achieved by translating control points while optimising a cost function consisting of two terms: a measure of image similarity (normalised mutual information), and a regularization term (weighted by λ) that penalises high bending energy deformations. B-splines have compact support so moving one control point only affects the spline coefficients in a local neighbourhood and efficiently models local deformations. The degree of smoothness can be controlled by adjusting the control point spacing. Because B-splines are inherently smooth the deformation energy is typically low, hence, here we ignore the regularization term (i.e. $\lambda = 0$). The algorithm's optimisation involves translating the control points in steps along the direction of maximum gradient until either the magnitude of the gradient of the cost function is less than or equal to a threshold (Epsilon, set to zero here) or pre-specified number of iterations is exceeded. Then the step size is decreased by a factor of two and the process continues.

2 Materials and Methods

Clinical Data and Atlas

The clinical growth hormone dataset consists of three serial T_1 weighted MR scans of six volunteers and five growth hormone deficient patients with an inter-scan interval of three months. To estimate measurement precision we also acquired three MR scans of another volunteer with the same MR sequence as the patients, but with an inter-scan interval of less than five minutes. Our atlas (registration source image) is based on the brainweb normal brain image without added noise [1] – see review in section 1.1. To reduce image resampling error during affine registration this was interpolated with a Hanning windowed sinc kernel (radius 6 zero crossings) from $1 \times 1 \times 1$mm to the same voxel dimension as the clinical data, $1 \times 1 \times 1.8$mm. We use the brainweb supplied CSF classification to define the lateral ventricles, as illustrated in Figure 2. To facilitate the measurement of volume (change) this ventricular segmentation was converted to a binary mask image (background voxels = 0, ventricular voxels = 1000).

Registration and Volume Measurement Strategy

Registration was performed as a two stage process. First global motion and gross differences in head size were compensated for by the affine (12 degrees of freedom) registration algorithm devised by Studholme [8]. Because of large differences in orientation between the atlas image and the subject images, starting estimates within approximately 5mm and 5 degrees were interactively provided prior to affine registration. Secondly, local deformation was calculated using Rueckert's

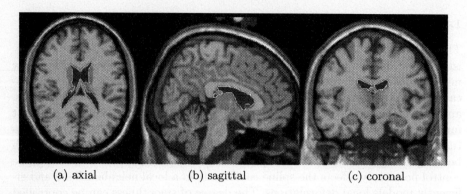

(a) axial   (b) sagittal   (c) coronal

Fig. 2. Atlas brain image ($1 \times 1 \times 1$ mm voxels) with accurate ventricular seg-mentation – outlined in white. Brainweb images supplied by McGill university, Montreal [1].

algorithm [5] (reviewed in section 1.2), first with a coarse grid (10mm control point spacing) then with a fine grid (5mm control point spacing). The full brain image was used for the coarse grid registration. For the fine grid registration, a region of interest (ROI) was defined surrounding the ventricles using the ventric-ular outline from the coarse grid registration solution dilated by 7mm to include a boundary layer at least one control point thick around the ROI, see Figure 3(a). Only voxels in this region were used for the fine grid registration, substan-tially reducing the execution time. For one patient with elongated ventricles, the dilation was increased as shown in Figure 3(b). To reduce the algorithm's

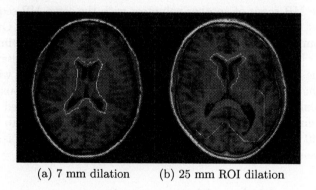

(a) 7 mm dilation   (b) 25 mm ROI dilation

Fig. 3. (a) Example of the atlas ventricles dilated by 7 mm and mapped to the space of a patient image. (b) Extra dilation (25 mm) for the patient with elongated ventricles to compensate for the larger deformation.

sensitivity to noise, especially at the fine control point spacing, the images were low-pass filtered with a Gaussian ($\sigma = 0.5$ voxels).

Ventricular volume (change) was measured by transforming, using linear interpolation, the ventricular binary mask into the space of the subject images using the deformation field calculated by non-rigid registration. Linear interpolation allowed the partial volume of the transformed boundary voxels to be calculated to sub-voxel accuracy, as illustrated in Figure 4. The volume of the mask in the transformed space was calculated by summing the voxel intensities and dividing by 1000 to give an estimate with a rounding error $\leq 0.05\%$.

(a)   (b)   (c)

Fig. 4. Schematic 1D diagram illustrating volume estimation by linear interpolation of a binary image. Shown in (a) is a voxel of unit intensity with neighbours of zero intensity. Translating one edge by 0.5 voxels increases the volume by 50%, shown as a dark grey region in (b). The neighbouring voxel is interpolated with an intensity of half a unit (c). Hence the measured volume will be 1 voxel in (a) and 1.5 voxels in (c).

3   Results

The measured ventricular volume for the three consecutive volunteer scans was 26.58cc, 26.49cc, 26.50cc which gave a measurement precision of $\sigma = 0.05$cc for the three consecutive scans.

The mean ventricular volume and volume change for the growth hormone study subjects at the 0, 3 and 6 months timepoints is shown in Table 1. Over six months there was a mean 1.2cc (5.5%) decrease in ventricular volume for the patient group compared to a 0.18cc (1.1%) increase for the controls. To test whether the volume change measurements for the two groups differed significantly, the Wilcoxon rank sum test (Matlab, Mathworks Inc, Natick, MA, USA) was used with the null hypothesis that there was no difference between the groups. This gave $p = 0.013$ (5% significance) for the 0 and 3 month scans and $p = 0.001$ (1% significance) for the 0 and 6 month scans. The p-values for both pairs of timepoints was $p = 0.0016$, which compares with $p = 0.0001$ found in our previous study involving qualitative ranking of difference images using a seven point scale [6]. To further compare the volume change measurements with those from the previously published study, we calculated the rank correlation coefficient (ρ), this gave $\rho = 0.76$ for zero to three months, $\rho = 0.72$ for zero to 6 months, and $\rho = 0.67$ overall. The ρ values indicate a significant correlation with the previously published visually assessment results at the 5% level, see [9] for $n = 11$. Figure 5 shows graphically the ventricular volume and volume change at the 0, 3 and 6 month timepoints for each of the eleven subjects.

Table 1. Mean (std) measured ventricular volume (cc) for patients and volunteers.

Mean (stdev) ventricular volume (cc)			
	timepoint		
group	0 months	3 months	6 months
patients	21.96 (6.16)	20.98 (6.66)	20.76 (6.73)
volunteers	16.08 (7.70)	16.06 (7.90)	16.27 (7.69)
Mean (stdev) of ventricular volume change (cc)			
	timepoints		
group	0 to 3 months	0 to 6 months	overall
patients	-0.98 (0.76)	-1.20 (0.76)	-1.09 (0.73)
volunteers	-0.02 (0.81)	0.18 (0.42)	0.08 (0.62)

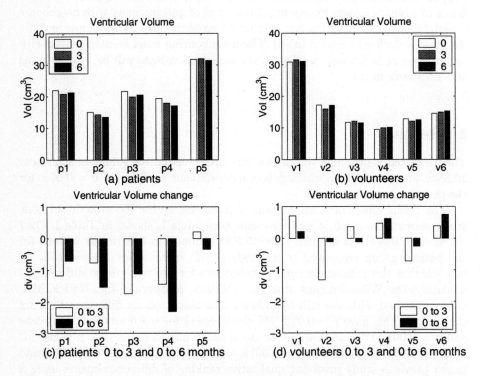

Fig. 5. Ventricular volume for the 11 subjects in the clinical growth hormone study. (a) and (b) refer to the measured ventricular volume for the 6 volunteers and 5 growth hormone patients at the three timepoints respectively. (c) and (d) refer to the change in ventricular volume from 0 to 3 months and from 0 to 6 months for growth hormone patients and volunteers respectively.

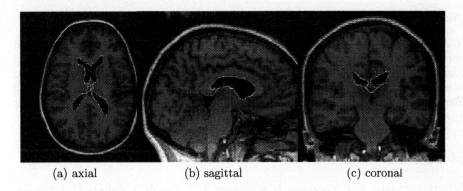

(a) axial   (b) sagittal   (c) coronal

Fig. 6. Example of segmentation propagation for patient 1. The boundary of the propagated ventricles is shown outlined in white.

4   Discussion and Conclusions

A key strength of Rueckert's non-rigid registration algorithm [5] is that it uses the mutual information (NMI) similarity measure whereas other non-rigid algorithms [10, 11] are based on intensity differences. Mutual information has the capability of registering images with non-linearly related voxel intensities. As a result, accurate registration of images that are derived from different scanners and images that are not corrected for intensity inhomogeneity is possible. So a generic brain atlas can be used without needing to acquire and segment extra volunteer images, as was required in previous work (e.g.[3]).

In this paper we have demonstrated that this approach is precise when applied to consecutive scans of a single subject ($\sigma < 0.05$cc) and that small changes of brain ventricular volume ($\approx$ 1cc) can be quantified by segmentation propagation using the Rueckert non-rigid registration algorithm. This is the first time that a non-rigid registration algorithm based on optimisation of mutual information has been shown to detect volume changes of this magnitude. These measurements are sufficiently accurate to significantly ($p \approx 0.01$) determine ventricular volume change for a group of five growth hormone patients compared to a group of six normal subjects. We have been able to validate the algorithm by demonstrating high correlation ($\rho \approx 0.7$, $n = 11$) between these results and those previously reported from ranking of differences images after rigid registration of the same images [6].

Although our results indicate high precision for one volunteer, and the set of measurements correlate with the previously published ones, the error appears to be larger than this precision value would suggest for individual cases. In particular, the measurements for volunteers v2 and v5, see Figure 5, indicate volume decreases of up to 1cc. Such decreases are inconsistent with the previous published results and implausible biologically and are most likely to be the result of registration error. Further improvements to the method of registration would probably reduce these errors.

Acknowledgements

We are grateful for Philips Medical Systems EasyVision advanced development for funding this work, to Daniel Rueckert for the use of his software, and to our colleagues in the Computational Imaging Science Group, led by Prof. David Hawkes, where the work was carried out. We are also grateful to the McConnell Brain Imaging Centre (BIC) Montreal Neurological Institute for the use of their brainweb simulated MR image.

References

[1] D. L. Collins, A. P. Zijdenbos, V. Kollokian, J. G. Sled, N. J. Kabani, C. J. Holmes, A. C. Evans: Design and construction of a realistic digital brain phantom. IEEE Trans on Medical Imaging **17** (1998) 463–468

[2] Bajcsy, R., Kovacic, S.: Multiresolution elastic matching. Computer Vision, Graphics and Image Processing **46** (1989) 1–21

[3] B. M. Dawant, S. L. Hartmann, J. P. Thirion, F. Maes, D. Vandermeulen, P. Demaerel: Automatic 3-D segmentation of internal structures of the head in MR images using a combination of similarity and free-form transformations: Part I, methodology and validation on normal subjects. IEEE Trans on Medical Imaging **18** (1999) 909–916

[4] G. Calmon, N. Roberts: Automatic measurement of changes in brain volume on consecutive 3D MR images by segmentation propagation. Magnetic Resonance Imaging **18** (2000) 439–453

[5] D. Rueckert, L. I. Sonoda, C. Hayes, D. L. G. Hill, M. O. Leach, D. J. Hawkes: Non-rigid registration using free-form deformations: Application to breast MR Images. IEEE Trans on Medical Imaging **18** (1999) 712–721

[6] E. R. E. Denton, M. Holden, E. Christ, J. M. Jarosz, D. Russell-Jones, J. Goodey, T. C. S. Cox, D. L. G. Hill: The identification of cerebral volume changes in treated growth hormone deficient patients using serial 3-D MR image processing. Journal of Computer Assisted Tomography **24** (2000) 139–145

[7] Schnabel, J.A., Tanner, C., Smith, A.C., Leach, M.O., Hayes, C., Degenhard, A., Hose, R., Hill, D.L.G., Hawkes, D.J.: Validation of non-rigid registration using Finite Element Methods. In: Proc. 17th Int. IPMI 2001 Conf. Vol LNCS 2082, Springer Verlag (2001) 344–357

[8] C. Studholme, D. L. G. Hill, D. J. Hawkes: Automated three-dimensional registration of magnetic resonance and positron emission tomography brain images by multiresolution optimization of voxel similarity measures. Medical Physics **24** (1997) 25–35

[9] M. Bland: An introduction to medical statistics. Oxford Medical Publications (1995) ISBN: 0-19-262428-8.

[10] G. E. Christensen, R. D. Rabbitt and M. I. Miller: Deformable templates using large deformation kinematics. IEEE Trans on Image Processing **5** (1996) 1435–1447

[11] J.-P. Thirion: Image matching as a diffusion process: an analogy with Maxwell's demons. Medical Image Analysis **2** (1998) 243–260

An Efficient Method for Constructing Optimal Statistical Shape Models

Rhodri H. Davies[1], Tim F. Cootes[1], John C. Waterton[2], and Chris J. Taylor[1]

[1] Division of Imaging Science, Stopford Building, Oxford Road, University of
Manchester, Manchester, M13 9PT, UK.
rhodri.h.davies@stud.man.ac.uk
[2] Enabling Science & Technology, AstraZeneca, Alderley Park, Macclesfield,
Cheshire, SK10 4TG, UK.

Abstract. Statistical shape models show considerable promise as a basis for segmenting and interpreting images. A major drawback of the approach is the need to establish a dense correspondence across a training set of segmented shapes. By posing the problem as one of minimising the *description length* of the model, we develop an efficient method that *automatically* defines a correspondence across a set of shapes. As the correspondence does not use an explicit ordering constraint, it generalises to 3D shapes. Results are given for several different training sets of 2D boundaries, showing the automatic method constructs better models than ones built by hand.

1 Introduction

Statistical models of shape show considerable promise as a basis for segmenting and interpreting images [4]. The basic idea is to establish, from a training set, the pattern of 'legal' variation in the shapes and spatial relationships of structures in a given class of images. Statistical analysis is used to give an efficient parameterisation of this variability, providing a compact representation of shape and allowing shape constraints to be applied effectively during image interpretation [5]. One of the main drawbacks of the approach is, however, the need - during training - to establish dense correspondence between shape boundaries over a reasonably large set of example images. It is important to establish the 'correct' correspondence, otherwise an inefficient parameterisation of shape can result, leading to difficulty in defining shape constraints. In practice, correspondence has often been established using manually defined 'landmarks'; this is both time-consuming and subjective. The problems are exacerbated when the approach is applied to 3D images.

Several previous attempts have been made to automate model building [1, 2, 3, 9, 10, 11, 12, 14, 16, 18] . The problem of establishing dense correspondence over a set of training boundaries can be posed as that of defining a parameterisation for each of the training shapes, leading to implicit correspondence between equivalently parameterised points. Different arbitrary parameterisations of the training boundaries have been proposed [1, 12] , but do not address the issue of

W. Niessen and M. Viergever (Eds.): MICCAI 2001, LNCS 2208, pp. 57–65, 2001.

optimality. Shape 'features' (e.g. regions of high curvature) have been used to establish point correspondences, [2, 11, 18] but, although this approach corresponds with human intuition, it is still not clear that it is in any sense optimal. A third approach, and that followed in this paper, is to treat finding the correct parameterisation of the training shape boundaries as an explicit optimisation problem.

The optimisation approach has been described by several authors [3, 6, 9, 14, 16]. The basic idea is to find the parameterisation of the training set that yields, in some sense, the 'best' model. We have previously described a minimum description length criterion that describes a set of shapes as efficiently as possible [6]. We showed that, by optimising the parameterisation of each shape, we could produce models that were superior to those built by hand. The optimisation scheme was, however, inefficient and took many hours to converge. In this paper, we describe a more efficient method and also consider the pose transformation for each shape. As the method applies only an implicit ordering constraint, it can be used on 3D shapes.

2   Statistical Shape Models

A statistical shape model is built from a training set of aligned example shapes. Each shape, Ψ_i $(i = 1 \ldots n_s)$, can (without loss of generality) be represented by a set of n points sampled along the boundary. These points are sampled according to the parameterisation, Φ_i of the shape. By concatenating the coordinates of its sample points into a $2n$-dimensional vector, $\mathbf{x}$ (where n is the number of points sampled on each shape), and using principal component analysis, each shape vector can be explained by a linear model of the form

$$\mathbf{x} = \bar{\mathbf{x}} + \mathbf{Pb} \tag{1}$$

where $\bar{\mathbf{x}}$ is the mean shape vector, the columns of $\mathbf{P}$ describe a set of orthogonal modes of shape variation and $\mathbf{b}$ is a vector of shape parameters. New examples of the class of shapes can be generated by choosing values of $\mathbf{b}$ within the range found in the training set. This approach can be extended easily to deal with continuous boundary functions [14], but for clarity we limit our discussion here to the discrete case.

The utility of the linear model of shape shown in (1) depends on the appropriateness of the set of boundary parameterisations $\{\Phi_i\}$ that are chosen. An inappropriate choice can result in the need for a large set of modes (and corresponding shape parameters) to approximate the training shapes to a given accuracy and may lead to 'legal' values of $\mathbf{b}$ generating 'illegal' shape instances. For example, consider two models generated from a set of 17 hand outlines. Model A uses a set of parameterisations of the outlines that cause 'natural' landmarks such as the tips of the fingers to correspond. Model B uses one such correspondence but then uses a simple path length parameterisation to position the other sample points. The variance of the three most significant modes of models A and B are (2.13, 1.16, 0.61) and (4.39, 1.56, 1.08) respectively. This suggests that model A is more compact than model B. All the example shapes generated by model A using values of **b** within the range found in the training set are 'legal' examples of hands, whilst model B generates implausible examples - this is illustrated in Fig. 1 .

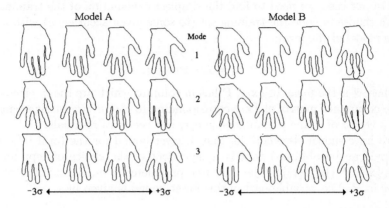

Fig. 1. The first three modes of variation ($\pm 3\sigma$) of models A and B

The set of parameterisations used for model A were obtained by marking the 'natural' landmarks manually on each training example, then using simple path length parameterisation to sample a fixed number of equally spaced points between them. This manual mark-up is a time-consuming and subjective process. In principle, the modelling approach extends to 3D, but in practice, manual landmarking becomes impractical. We aim to overcome these problems by building shape models *automatically*.

3   Automatic Model Building

We wish to optimise the parameterisations $\{\Phi_i\}$ of each shape in our training set $\{\Psi_i\}$. Since we wish to obtain a compact model with good generalisation ability we define the 'best' model as that which can account for the observations (the training shapes) in as simple a way as possible.

The configuration space of $\{\Phi_i\}$ is highly non-linear and has many local minima. Although stochastic optimisation techniques such as simulated annealing [13] and genetic algorithms [7] search for a truly *global* minima, they take many hours to converge. We overcome this problem by optimising $\{\Phi_i\}$ using a *multiresolution* approach. This allows a local optimisation method to be used at each resolution. We have used the Nelder-Mead simplex algorithm to produce the results in section 4.

3.1   An Information Theoretic Objective Function

To select a suitable objective function we must state the desirable properties of a statistical shape model. Ideally, we would like a model that is general (it can represent any instance of the object - not just those seen in the training set), specific (it can only represent valid instances of the object) and compact (it can represent the variation with as few parameters as possible). We therefore choose to follow the principle of Occam's razor : the simplest explanation generalises best. In our case, we need to find the simplest explanation of the training set.

We choose to code the training set (to some given accuracy δ) with a linear shape model of the form:

$$\mathbf{x}_i = \bar{\mathbf{x}} + \mathbf{P}\mathbf{b}_i + \mathbf{r}_i \qquad (2)$$

where $\bar{\mathbf{x}}$ is the mean of $\{\mathbf{x}_i\}$, $\mathbf{P}$ has m columns which are the m eigenvectors of the covariance matrix of $\{\mathbf{x}_i\}$ corresponding to the m largest eigenvalues λ_j, $\mathbf{b}_i$ is a vector of shape parameters, and $\mathbf{r}_i$ is a vector of residuals.

We have shown elsewhere [6] that a lower bound for the total information required can be obtained that is independent of the choice of representation of $(\bar{\mathbf{x}}, \{\mathbf{x}_i\}, \mathbf{P}, \{\mathbf{b}_i\}, \{\mathbf{r}_i\})$. The only free parameter is m, the number of shape modes in $\mathbf{P}$. The variable part of this lower bound is given by

$$F(m) = (n_p + n_s) \sum_{j=1}^{m} \log(\lambda_j) + [n_p(n_s - 1) - (n_p + n_s)]m \log(\lambda_{\mathbf{r}}) \qquad (3)$$

where n_s is the number of shapes, $n_p = 2n$, twice the number of sample points on each shape and $\lambda_{\mathbf{r}} = \frac{1}{n_p} \sum_{j=m+1}^{n_p} \lambda_j$.

The first term is analogous to the determinant of the covariance of $\{\mathbf{x}_i\}$ used by Kotcheff and Taylor [14] and favours a model with much variation described by a small number of modes. The second term penalises a large number of modes and/or large residuals. The optimal trade-off between describing systematic variability using the model versus describing each shape individually can be determined by varying m exhaustively between zero and an upper bound on m given by $\lambda_m > 12\alpha\lambda_{\mathbf{r}}/(2\pi e)$, where $\alpha = (\frac{n_p n_s}{n_p(n_s-1)-m(n_p-n_s)})$.

F_{min}, the minimum of F with respect to m can be used to asses the quality of a given model.

3.2   Multiresolution Parameterisation

Our training data are a set of shapes $\{\Psi_i\}$ represented parametrically as curves: $\Psi_i(t), (0 \leq t \leq 1)$. We can manipulate the correspondences of the shapes by reparameterising these curves:

$$\Psi_i(t) \rightarrow \Psi_i(t'), \;\; t' = \Phi_i(t), \;\; \text{where } \{\Phi_i : [0, 1] \rightarrow [0, 1]\} \qquad (4)$$

We select n corresponding uniformly sampled points from the reparameterised shapes. The method described in this section is applicable to both open and closed curves; for clarity, we will limit our discussion to the closed case.

Each $\Phi_i(t)$ must be a homeomorphic mapping of the interval [0,1]. We use a piecewise-linear approximation of each parameterisation $\Phi_i(t)$ by specifying a set of n_c *control points*, on each shape and linearly interpolating between them. The configuration space is therefore (sn_c)-dimensional. This search space is generally too large for a direct optimisation scheme to converge rapidly and reliably. We overcome this by using the following multiresolution approach:

- We begin with one control point, p_{1i}, on each shape. This point is allowed to assume any value in the range $[0,1]$. We use linear interpolation to sample $n/2$ points between $[0,p_{1i}]$ and $[p_{1i},1]$, see figure (2a). We find the values of $\{p_{1i}\}$ that minimise F_{min}. Once these values are found, they are fixed and recorded.
- We place two additional control points p_{2i} and p_{3i} between 0 and p_{1i} and between p_{1i} and 1 respectively. We equally space $n/4$ points in the intervals $[0,p_{2i}]$, $[p_{2i},p_{1i}]$, $[p_{1i},p_{3i}]$ and $[p_{3i},1]$ (see figure (2b)). We fix and record the optimal positions of $\{p_{2i}\}$ and $\{p_{3i}\}$.
- We continue adding additional control points in a similar fashion between the fixed control points $\{p_i\}$ until the parameterisation is suitably defined. See figures (2c) and (2d).

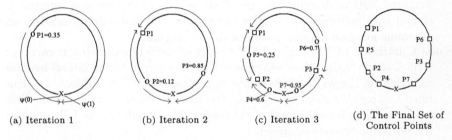

(a) Iteration 1   (b) Iteration 2   (c) Iteration 3   (d) The Final Set of Control Points

Fig. 2. A Demonstration of Parameterising a Circle. The 'X' represents the origin, the circles represent the current (flexible) control points and the squares represent the fixed control points. At each iteration, the current control points are allowed to move between the endpoints of the arrow.

At each iteration, the position of each control point is initialised as halfway along its allowed range - the equivalent of an arc-length parameterisation. As we have not used an explicit ordering constraint, the method may be used on shapes in 3D (see [6] for details).

3.3   Dealing with Pose Transformations

The pose of each shape affects the value of F_{min}. We therefore need to optimise the four parameters that allow a rigid transformation of each shape: translations d_x, d_y, scaling s and rotation θ. We have found that adding an additional $4n_s$ dimensions to each iteration significantly slows the optimisation and introduces many additional false minima. Better results can be achieved by performing a procrustes analysis [8] of the reparameterised shapes inside the objective function, before calculating the value of F_{min}.

4   Results

We tested our method on four different sets of object outlines. The algorithm was run for four iterations, giving 16 control points per shape. We compare the results to models built by equally-spacing points along the boundary and hand-built models, produced by identifying a set of 'natural' landmarks on each shape.

Our training sets consisted of manual-segmentations taken from:

Hand Outlines 17 images of a hand.

Rat Kidney 15 transverse, multislice T2-weighted magnetic resonance images (MRI) of rat kidneys. The repetition time was (TR) 2 sec; echo time (TE) 20 msec and slice thickness 1 mm. 41 contiguous transverse slices were acquired with a 64×64mm field of view and a $256 \times 256 \times 41$ image matrix. A single slice - containing most evidence of the collecting apparatus - was chosen from each image and the right kidney segmented.

Stroke Model 23 images collected from a previous study where permanent focal cerebral ischaemia was induced in rats [19]. For this study, only data from saline-treated animals were used. The experiment used in vivo multislice T2-weighted MRI as described in [19]. A single transverse slice was segmented, chosen with reference to an atlas of anatomy [15] and corresponded to an anatomic location 6.3 mm posterior to the bregma.

Knee Cartilage 15 T1-weighted MR images of the femoral articular cartilage [17]. A single sagital slice was chosen from the centre of the lateral femoral condyles. As the width of the femur varies from subject to subject, we identified comparable slices by selecting the slices halfway between (1) the first evidence of the lateral aspect of the meniscal horn and (2) the full extent of the posterior cruciate ligament.

In figure 3, we show qualitative results by displaying the variation captured by the first three modes of each model (the first three elements of **b** varied by $\pm 2\sigma$). We also give quantitative results in table 1, tabulating the value of F_{Min}, the total variance, and variance explained by each mode for each of the models.

The qualitative results in figure 3 show that the shapes generated within the allowed range of **b** are all plausible. The quantitative results in table 1 show that our method produces models that are significantly more compact than either the models built by hand or those obtained using equally-spaced points.

To test the generalisation ability of the models, we performed leave-one-out tests on each model described in table 1. In figure 4, we report the results on the hand outlines although the same trends appear in all datasets. As can be seen from the figure, the optimised model performs significantly better than both the manual and arc-length parameterised models for the entire range of included modes, suggesting better generalisation ability.

5   Conclusions

We have described an efficient method for automatically defining a set of dense correspondences to build statistical shape models. Results show that the models

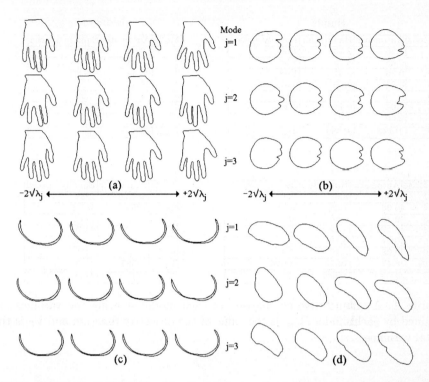

Fig. 3. The first three modes ($j = 1, j = 2, j = 3$) of variation ($\pm2\sigma$)of the models automatically generated from (a)hand outlines, (b)kidneys, (c) knee cartilage and (d)Stroke Model.

produced by our method are more compact and general than models built by hand - the current gold standard.

Our method finds an isomorphic mapping between each of a set of shape contours and the mean. Since it does not use an explicit ordering constraint, it generalises to higher-dimensional spaces. By starting our optimisation from equally-spaced points, the worst model the method can possibly produce is a procrustes-aligned, arc-length parameterisation.

Regular Principal Component Analysis can not capture non-linear variations (e.g caused by a sub-part rotating in the plane) with a single mode - this affects the generalisation ability, specificity and compactness of such linear models. The method described in this paper overcomes this by allowing points to 'slide' along the parameterisation to compensate for the non-linear movement - this allows the variation to be explained by a single mode.

We are currently experimenting with more continuous representations of the parameterisation using the cumulative distribution defined by a set of basis functions. We intend to generalise the principle so that it can be used to reparameterise the sphere and hence surfaces rendered from 3D images.

Hands

Mode	Automatic	Hand Built	Equally-spaced
1	1.20	2.13	4.39
2	0.68	1.16	1.56
3	0.39	0.61	1.08
4	0.21	0.50	0.67
5	0.08	0.15	0.36
6	0.04	0.14	0.26
V_T	2.69	5.04	8.72
F_{min}	31477	41563	45272

Kidneys

Mode	Automatic	Equally Spaced
1	128.2	306.19
2	53.98	197.18
3	33.65	109.86
4	28.57	70.20
5	14.50	41.98
6	8.55	23.63
V_T	284.48	802.72
F_{min}	4722	5485

Knee Cartilage

Mode	Automatic	Hand Built	Equally-spaced
1	6.90	8.03	8.07
2	0.68	1.29	1.36
3	0.32	0.66	0.69
4	0.17	0.22	0.23
5	0.11	0.17	0.18
6	0.08	0.10	0.11
V_T	8.47	10.73	11.24
F_{min}	25133	35969	37941

Stroke Model

Mode	Automatic	Equally Spaced
1	684.29	1389
2	306.62	581.7
3	59.47	174.5
4	54.65	88.70
5	36.59	40.51
6	27.15	34.9
V_T	12385	23135
F_{min}	3412	4752

Table 1. A quantitative comparison of each model showing the variance explained by each mode. F_{min} is the value of the objective function and V_T is the total variance.

Acknowledgements

Tim Cootes is funded under an EPSRC advanced fellowship grant. Rhodri Davies would like to thank the BBSRC and Astrazeneca pharmaceuticals, Alderely Park, Macclesfield, UK for their financial support.

References

[1] Baumberg, A. and D. Hogg, Learning Flexible Models from Image Sequences, in *European Conference on Computer Vision, ECCV'94*. p. 299-308.

[2] Benayoun, A., N. Ayache, and I. Cohen. Adaptive meshes and nonrigid motion computation. in *International Conference on Pattern Recognition. ICPR'94*

[3] Bookstein, F.L., Landmark methods for forms without landmarks: morphometrics of group differences in outline shape. *Medical Image Analysis*, 1997. 1(3): p. 225-243.

[4] Cootes, T., A. Hill, C. Taylor, and J. Haslam, The use of Active shape models for locating structures in medical images. *Image and Vision Computing*, 1994. 12: p. 355-366.

[5] Cootes, T., C. Taylor, D. Cooper and J. Graham, Active shape models - their training and application. *Computer Vision and Image Understanding*, 1995. 61: p. 38-59.

[6] Davies, Rh. H, T. Cootes and C. J. Taylor, A Minimum Description Length Approach to Statistical Shape Modelling, in *Information processing in medical imaging, IPMI'01*, (to appear)

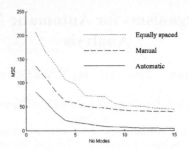

Fig. 4. Leave one out tests. The plot shows the number of modes used against the mean squared approximation error

[7] Goldberg, D.E., *Genetic Algorithms in Search, Optimisation and Machine Learning.* 1989: Addison Wesley.

[8] Goodall, C., Procrustes Methods in the Statistical Analysis of Shape. *Journal of the Royal Statistical Society B*, 1991. 53(2): p. 285-339.

[9] Hill, A. and C. Taylor. Automatic landmark generation for point distribution models. in *British Machine Vision Conference. BMVC'94.*

[10] Hill, A. and C.J. Taylor, A framework for automatic landmark identification using a new method of non-rigid correspondence. *IEEE Transactions on Pattern Analysis and Machine Intelligence, PAMI*, April, 2000.

[11] Kambhamettu, C. and D.B. Goldof, Point Correspondence Recovery in Non-rigid Motion, in *CVPR'92.* p. 222-227.

[12] Kelemen, A., G. Szekely, and G. Gerig, Elastic model-based segmentation of 3-D neuroradiological data sets. *IEEE trans. medical imaging*, 1999. 18(10): p. 828-839.

[13] Kirkpatrick, S., C. Gelatt, and M. Vecchi, Optimization by Simulated Annealing. *Science*, 1983. 220: p. 671-680.

[14] Kotcheff, A.C.W. and C.J. Taylor, Automatic Construction of Eigenshape Models by Direct Optimisation. *Medical Image Analysis*, 1998. 2: p. 303-314.

[15] G. Paxinos and C. Watson. *The rat brain in streotactic coordinates.* Academic Press, San Diego 1986

[16] Rangarajan, A., H. Chui and F. L. Bookstein,The Softassign Procrustes Matching Algorithm, in *IPMI'97.* p. 29-42.

[17] Solloway, S., Taylor, C.J., Hutchinson, C.E., Waterton, J.C., Quantification of Articular Cartilage from MR images using active shape models, in *Proceedings of the 4th European Conference on Computer Vision, ECCV' 96*, pp. 400-412.

[18] Wang, Y., B. S. Peterson, and L. H. Staib. Shape-based 3D surface correspondence using geodesics and local geometry. *CVPR 2000*, v. 2: p. 644-51.

[19] Waterton J. C. , B. J. Middleton, R. Pickford, C. P. Allott, D. Checkley and R. A. Keith, Reduced animal use in efficacy testing in disease models with use of sequential experimental designs. Developments in Animal and Veterinary Sciences, 31: Progress in the Reduction, Refinement and Replacement of Animal Experimentation, 737-745 (2000)

Deformable Organisms for Automatic Medical Image Analysis

Ghassan Hamarneh[1,2], Tim McInerney[3,2], and Demetri Terzopoulos[4,2]

[1] Dept. of Signals and Systems, Chalmers University of Technology, Göteborg 41296, Sweden
ghassan@s2.chalmers.se, www.s2.chalmers.se
[2] Dept. of Computer Science, University of Toronto, Toronto M5S 3H5, Canada
{ghassan,tim,dt}@cs.toronto.edu, www.cs.toronto.edu
[3] School of Computer Science, Ryerson University, Toronto M5B 2K3, Canada
tmcinern@scs.ryerson.ca, www.scs.ryerson.ca
[4] Courant Institute, New York University, New York NY 10003, USA
dt@cs.nyu.edu, www.mrl.nyu.edu

Abstract. We introduce a new paradigm for automatic medical image analysis that adopts concepts from the field of Artificial Life. Our approach prescribes deformable organisms, autonomous agents whose objective is the segmentation and analysis of anatomical structures in medical images. A deformable organism is structured as a 'muscle'-actuated 'body' whose behavior is controlled by a 'brain' that is capable of making both reactive and deliberate decisions. This intelligent deformable model possesses an 'awareness' of the segmentation process, which emerges from a conflux of perceived sensory data, an internal mental state, memorized knowledge, and a cognitive plan. We develop a class of deformable organisms using a medial representation of body morphology that facilitates a variety of controlled local deformations at multiple spatial scales. Specifically, we demonstrate a deformable 'worm' organism that can overcome noise, incomplete edges, considerable anatomical variation, and occlusion in order to segment and label the corpus callosum in 2D mid-sagittal MR images of the brain.

1 Introduction

The automatic segmentation and labeling of anatomical structures in medical images is a persistent problem that continues to defy solution. There is consensus within the medical image analysis research community that the development of general-purpose automatic segmentation algorithms will require not only powerful bottom-up, data-driven processes, but also equally powerful top-down, knowledge-driven processes within a robust decision-making framework that operates across multiple levels of abstraction [2]. Deformable models, one of the most actively researched model-based segmentation techniques [5], feature a potent bottom-up component founded in estimation theory, optimization, and physics-based dynamical systems, but their top-down processes have traditionally relied on interactive initialization and guidance by knowledgeable users. Attempts to fully automate deformable model segmentation methods have so far been less than successful at coping with the enormous variation in anatomical structures of interest, the significant variability of image data, the need for intelligent initialization conditions, etc.

W. Niessen and M. Viergever (Eds.): MICCAI 2001, LNCS 2208, pp. 66-76, 2001.
© Springer-Verlag Berlin Heidelberg 2001

The time has come to shift our attention to what promises to be a critical element in any viable, highly automated solution: the decision-making framework itself. Existing decision-making strategies for deformable models are inflexible and do not operate at an appropriate level of abstraction. Hierarchically organized models, which shift their focus from structures associated with stable image features to those associated with less stable features, are a step in the right direction [4,9]. However, high-level contextual knowledge remains largely ineffective because it is intertwined much too tightly with the low-level optimization-based mechanisms. It is difficult to obtain intelligent, global (i.e., over the whole image) model behavior throughout the segmentation process from such mechanisms. In essence, current deformable models have no explicit awareness of where they (or their parts) are in the image or what their objectives are at any time during the optimization process.

It is our contention that we must revisit ideas for incorporating knowledge that were explored in earlier systems (e.g., [14]), and develop new algorithms that focus on top-down reasoning strategies which may best leverage the powerful bottom-up feature detection and integration abilities of deformable models and other modern model-based medical image analysis techniques. We further contend that a layered architecture is appropriate, where the high-level reasoning layer has knowledge about and control over the low-level model (or models) at all times. The reasoning layer should apply an active, explicit search strategy that first looks for the most stable image features before proceeding to less stable image features, and so on. It should utilize contextual knowledge to resolve regions where there is a deficiency of image feature information.

To achieve these goals, we introduce a new paradigm for automatic medical image analysis that adopts concepts from the emerging field of Artificial Life. In particular, we develop *deformable organisms*, autonomous agents whose objective is the segmentation and analysis of anatomical structures in medical images. A deformable organism is structured as a 'muscle'-actuated 'body' whose behavior is controlled by a 'brain' that is capable of making both reactive and deliberate decisions. This intelligent deformable model possesses a non-trivial 'awareness' of the segmentation process, which emerges from a conflux of perceived sensory data, an internal mental state, memorized knowledge, and a cognitive plan. By constructing deformable organisms in a layered fashion, we are able to separate the knowledge-driven model-fitting control functionality from the data-driven, local image feature integration functionality, exploiting both for maximal effectiveness.

1.1 Artificial Life Modeling

The Artificial Life (ALife) modeling approach has been applied successfully to produce realistic computer graphics models of plants and animals [13]. Artificial animals are relevant to deformable organisms. Autonomous agents known as "artificial fishes" [12] serve to illustrate the key functional components of artificial animals: bodies that comprise muscle actuators, sensory organs (eyes, etc.) and, most importantly, brains consisting of motor, perception, behavior, learning and cognition centers. Controllers in the motor center coordinate muscle actions to carry out specific motor functions, such as locomotion and sensor actuation. The perception center employs attention mechanisms to interpret sensory information about the dynamic environment. The behavior center realizes an adaptive sensorimotor system through a repertoire of behavior routines that couple perception to action in meaningful ways. The learning center in the brain enables the artificial animal to learn motor control and behavior through practice and sensory reinforcement. The cognition center enables it to think.

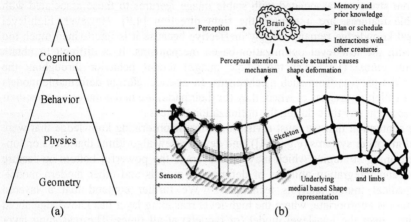

Fig. 1. (a) The ALife modeling pyramid (adapted from [12]). (b) A deformable organism: The brain issues 'muscle' actuation and perceptual attention commands. The organism deforms and senses image features, whose characteristics are conveyed to its brain. The brain makes decisions based on sensory input, memorized information and prior knowledge, and a pre-stored plan, which may involve interaction with other organisms.

To manage their complexity, artificial animal models are best organized hierarchically, such that each successive modeling layer augments the more primitive functionalities of lower layers. At the base of the modeling hierarchy (see Fig 1a), a geometric modeling layer represents the morphology and appearance of the animal. Next, a physical modeling layer incorporates biomechanical principles to constrain the geometry and simulate biological tissues. Further up the hierarchy is a motor control layer that motivates internal muscle actuators in order to synthesize lifelike locomotion. Behavioral and perceptual modeling layers cooperate to support a reactive behavioral repertoire. At the apex of the modeling pyramid is a cognitive modeling layer, which simulates the deliberative behavior of higher animals, governs what an animal knows about itself and its world, how that knowledge is acquired and represented, and how automated reasoning and planning processes can exploit knowledge to achieve high-level goals.

1.2   An Artificial Life Modeling Paradigm for Medical Image Analysis

Viewed in the context of the artificial life modeling hierarchy (Fig. 1a), current *automatic* deformable model-based approaches to medical image analysis include geometric and physical modeling layers only (in interactive deformable models, such as snakes, the human operator is relied upon to provide suitable behavioral level and cognitive level support). At the physical level, deformable models interpret image data by simulating dynamics or minimizing energy terms, but the models themselves do not monitor or control this optimization process except in a most primitive way. At the geometric level, aside from a few notable exceptions [11], deformable models are not generally designed with intuitive, multi-scale, multi-location deformation 'handles'. Their inability to perform global deformations, such as bending, and other global motions such as sliding and backing up makes it difficult to develop reasoning or planning strategies for these models at the correct level of abstraction [5].

In more sophisticated deformable models, prior information is used to constrain shape and appearance, as well as the statistical variation of these quantities [1,10]; however, these models have no explicit awareness of where they are and, consequently, the effectiveness of these constraints is dependent upon model starting conditions. The lack of awareness also prevents the models from knowing when to trust the image feature information and ignore the constraint information and vice versa. The constraint information is therefore applied arbitrarily. Furthermore, because there is no active, explicit search for stable image features, the models are prone to latching onto incorrect features [1] simply due to their proximity and local decision-making. Once this latching occurs, the lack of control of the fitting procedure prevents the model from correcting the misstep. The result is that the local decisions that are made do not add up to intelligent global behavior.

To overcome the aforementioned deficiencies while retaining the core strengths of the deformable model approach, we add high-level controller layers (a 'brain') on top of the geometric and physical (or deformation) layers to produce an autonomous deformable organism (Fig. 1b). The intelligent activation of these lower layers allows the organism to control the fitting/optimization procedure. The layered architecture approach allows the deformable organism to make deformation decisions at the correct level of abstraction.

The perception system of the deformable organism comprises a set of sensors that provide information. Any type of sensors can be incorporated, from edge strength and edge direction detectors to snake 'feelers'. Sensors can be focused or trained for specific image features and image feature variation in a task-specific way; hence, the organism can disregard sensory information superfluous to its current behavioral needs.

Explicit feature search requires powerful, flexible and intuitive model deformation control. We achieve this with a set of 'motor' (i.e. deformation) controllers, which are parameterized procedures dedicated to carrying out a complex deformation function, such as successively bending a portion of the organism over some range of angles or stretching part of the organism forward some distance.

The organism is 'self-aware' (i.e. knows where it and its parts are and what it is seeking) and therefore it effectively utilizes global contextual knowledge. The organism begins by searching for the most stable anatomical features in the image before proceeding to less stable features. Once stable features are found and labeled, the organism uses neighboring information and prior knowledge to determine the object boundary in regions known to provide little or no feature information.

Because the organism carries out active, explicit searches for object features, it is not satisfied with the nearest matching feature but looks further within a region to find the best match, thus avoiding local minimum solutions. Furthermore, by carrying out explicit searches for features we ensure correct correspondence between the model and the data. If a feature cannot be found, the organism flags the situation. Subsequently, if multiple plans exist, another plan could potentially be selected and the search for the missing feature postponed until further information is available.

2   A Deformable Organism for 2D MR Brain Image Analysis

To demonstrate the potential of our framework for medical image analysis, we have developed a deformable "worm" organism that can overcome noise, incomplete edges, considerable anatomical variation, and occlusion in order to segment and label the corpus callosum (CC) in 2D mid-sagittal MR images of the brain. We will now describe in detail the layered architecture for this particular deformable organism.

2.1   Geometric Representation

As its name suggests, the deformable worm organism is based on a medial representation of body morphology [3] that facilitates a variety of controlled local deformations at multiple spatial scales. In this shape representation scheme, the CC anatomical structure is described with four shape profiles derived from the primary medial axis of the CC boundary contour. The medial profiles describe the geometry of the structure in a natural way and provide general, intuitive, and independent shape measures. These profiles are: a length profile $L\langle m\rangle$, an orientation profile $O\langle m\rangle$, a left (with respect to the medial axis) thickness profile $T^l\langle m\rangle$, and a right thickness profile $T^r\langle m\rangle$ where $m = 1, 2, ..., N$ and N is the number of medial nodes. The length profile represents the distances between consecutive pairs of medial nodes, and the orientation profile represents the angles of the edges connecting the pairs of nodes. The thickness profiles represent the distances between medial nodes and their corresponding boundary points (Fig. 2, Fig. 3)[1].

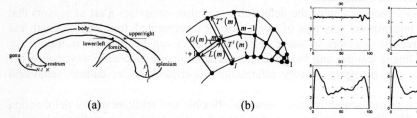

(a)   (b)

Fig. 2. (a) CC anatomical feature labels overlaying a reconstruction of the CC using the medial shape profiles shown in Fig. 3. (b) Diagram of shape representation.

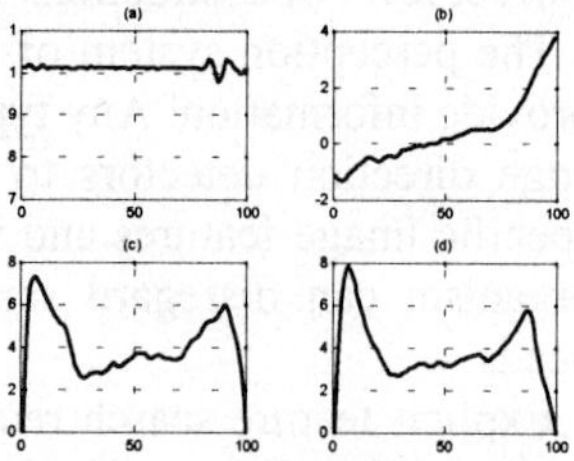

Fig. 3. Example medial shape profiles: (a) length, (b) orientation, (c) left and (d) right thickness profiles.

2.2   Motor System

Shape Deformation Actuators. In addition to affine transformation abilities (translate, rotate, scale), we control organism deformation by defining deformation

---

[1] Currently we construct medial profiles only from the primary medial axis and have not considered secondary axes. This may prevent the CC worm organism from accurately representing highly asymmetrical (with respect to the primary axis) parts of some corpora callosa. We also realize that our medial shape representation needs improvement near the end caps. We are currently exploring these issues, as well as issues related to the extension of our model to 3D, and we intend to make full use of the considerable body of work of Pizer *et al* [6,7,8] on these topics.

actuators in terms of the medial shape profiles (Fig. 4). Controlled stretch (or compress), bend, and bulge (or squash) deformations are implemented as deformation operators acting on the length, orientation, or thickness profiles, respectively. Furthermore, by utilizing a hierarchical (multiscale) and regional principal component analysis to capture the shape variation statistics in a training set [3], we can keep the deformations consistent with prior knowledge of possible shape variations. Whereas general, statistically-derived shape models produce global shape variation modes only [1,10], we are able to produce spatially-localized feasible deformations at desired scales, thus supporting our goal of intelligent deformation planning.

Several operators of varying types, amplitudes, scales, and locations can be applied to any of the length, orientation, and thickness shape profiles (Fig. 5a-d). Similarly, multiple statistical shape variation modes can be activated, with each mode acting at a specified amplitude, location and scale of the shape profiles (Fig. 5e-h). In general, operator- and statistics-based deformations can be combined (Fig. 5i) and expressed as

$$p_d = \bar{p}_d + \sum_l \sum_s \left(M_{dls} w_{dls} + \sum_t \alpha_{dlst} k_{dlst} \right) \tag{1}$$

where p is a shape profile, d is a deformation type (stretch, bend, left/right bulge), i.e. $p_d(m) : \{L(m), O(m), T^l(m), T^r(m)\}$, $\bar{p}$ is the average shape profile, k is an operator profile (with unity amplitude), l and s are the location and scale of the deformation, t is the operator type (e.g. Gaussian, triangular, flat, bell, or cusp), α is the operator amplitude, the columns of M are the variation modes for a specific d, l, and s, and w contains variation mode weights. Details can be found in [3].

Deformation (Motor) Controllers. The organism's low-level motor actuators are controlled by motor controllers. These parameterized procedures carry out complex deformation functions such as sweeping over a range of rigid transformation parameters, sweeping over a range of stretch/bend/thickness amplitudes at a certain location and scale, bending at increasing scales, moving a bulge on the boundary etc. Other high-level deformation capabilities include, for example, smoothing the medial/left/right boundaries, interpolating a missing part of the thickness profile, moving the medial axis to a position midway between the left and right boundaries, and re-sampling the model by including more medial and boundary nodes.

2.3 Perception System

Different parts of the organism are dynamically assigned sensing capabilities and thus act as sensory organs (SOs) or receptors. The locations of the SOs are typically confined to the organism's body (on-board SOs) such as at its medial or boundary nodes, at curves or segments connecting different nodes. In our implementation, the SOs are made sensitive to different stimuli such as image intensity, image gradient magnitude and direction, a non-linearly diffused version of the image, an edge detected (using Canny's edge detector) image, or even the result of a Hough transform. In general, a wide variety of image processing/analysis techniques can be applied to the original image.

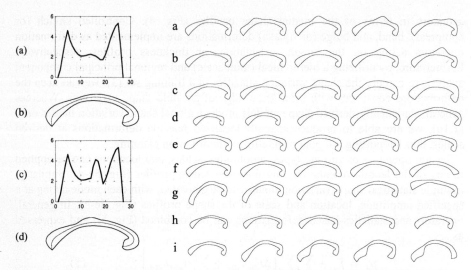

Fig. 4. Introducing a bulge on the upper boundary of the CC by applying a deform-ation operator on the upper thickness profile, $T^r(m)$. (a) $T^r(m)$ before and (c) after applying the operator. (b) The reconstructed shape before and (d) after the operator.

Fig. 5. Examples of controlled deformations: (a)-(c) Operator-based bulge deformation at varying locations/amplitudes/scales. (d) Operator-based stretching with varying amplitudes over entire CC. (e)-(g) Statistics-based bending of left end, right end, and left half of CC. (h) Statistics-based bulge of the left and right thickness over entire CC. (i) From left to right: (1) mean shape, (2) statistics-based bending of left half, followed by (3) locally increasing lower thickness using operator, followed by (4) applying operator-based stretch and (5) adding operator based bend to right side of CC.

2.4   Behavioral/Cognitive System

The organism's cognitive center combines sensory information, memorized information, and instructions from a pre-stored segmentation plan to carry out active, explicit searches for object features by activating 'behavior' routines. Behavior routines are designed based on available organism motor skills, perception capabilities, and available anatomical landmarks. For example, the routines implemented for the CC worm organism include: find-top-of-head, find-upper-boundary-of-CC, find-genu, find-rostrum, find-splenium, latch-to-upper-boundary, latch-to-lower-boundary, find-fornix, thicken-right-side, thicken-left-side, back-up. The behavior routines subsequently activate the deformation controllers to complete a stage in the plan and bring the organism closer to its intention of object segmentation.

The segmentation plan provides a means for human experts to incorporate global contextual knowledge. It contains instructions on how best to achieve a correct segmentation by optimally prioritizing behaviors. If we know, for example, that the corner-shaped rostrum of the CC is always very clearly defined in an MRI image, then the find-rostrum behavior should be given a very high priority. Adhering to the segmentation plan and defining it at a behavioral level affords the organism with an awareness of the segmentation process. This enables it to make effective use of prior shape knowledge – it is applied only in anatomical regions of the target object where there is a high level of noise or known gaps in the object boundary edges, etc. In the next section we describe the segmentation plan for the CC organism to illustrate this ability to harness global contextual knowledge.

3 Results

When a CC deformable worm organism is released into a 2D sagittal MRI brain image, it engages in different 'behaviors' as it progresses towards its goal. Since the upper boundary (Fig. 2a) of the CC is very well defined and can be easily located with respect to the top of the head, the cognitive center of the CC organism activates behaviors to first locate the top of the head and then move downwards (through the gray and white matter) in the image space to locate the upper boundary (Fig. 6.1-5). Next, the organism bends to latch to the upper boundary and activates a find-genu routine, causing the CC organism to stretch and grow along this boundary towards the genu (Fig. 6.6-7). Once the genu is located, the find-splenium routine is activated and the organism stretches and grows in the opposite direction (Fig. 6.11). The genu and splenium are easily detected by looking for a sudden change in direction of the upper boundary towards the middle of the head.

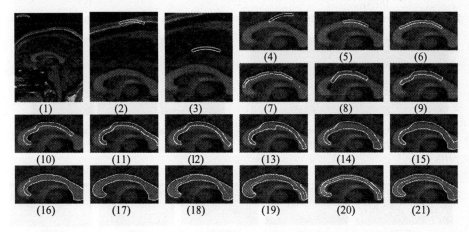

Fig. 6. Intelligent CC organism progressing through a sequence of behaviors to segment the CC

Once the genu is found, the organism knows that the lower boundary opposite to the genu is well defined so it backs up and latches to the lower boundary (Fig. 6.8). It then activates the find-rostrum behavior that tracks the lower boundary until it reaches the distinctive rostrum (Fig. 6.8-10). At the splenium end of the CC, the organism backs up and finds the center of a circle that approximates the splenium end cap (Fig. 6.12). The lower boundary is then progressively tracked from the rostrum to the splenium while maintaining parallelism with the organism's medial axis in order to avoid latching to the potentially occluding fornix (Fig. 6.13-14). However, the lower boundary may still dip towards the fornix, so a successive step is performed to locate where, if at all, the fornix occludes the CC, by activating the find-fornix routine (making use of edge strength along the lower boundary, its parallelism to the medial axis, and statistical thickness values). Thus, prior knowledge is applied only when and where required. If the fornix does indeed occlude the CC, any detected dip in the organism's boundary is repaired by interpolating neighboring thickness values. The thickness of the upper boundary is then adjusted to latch on to the corresponding boundary in the image (Fig. 6.15-17). At this point the CC organism has almost reached its goal; however, the medial axis is not in the middle of the CC organism (Fig. 6.18), hence the medial axis is re-parameterized by positioning the medial nodes halfway between the boundary nodes (Fig. 6.19-20). Finally the lower and upper boundaries are re-located again to obtain the final segmentation result (Fig. 6.21).

In addition, Fig. 7 demonstrates the detection and repairing of the fornix. Fig. 8 demonstrates the organism's self-awareness. Fig. 9 shows other segmentation results and several validated examples are also shown in Fig. 10.

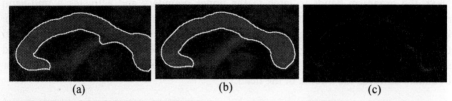

(a)   (b)   (c)

Fig. 7. (a) Before and (b) after detecting and repairing the fornix dip. (c) The gradient magnitude.

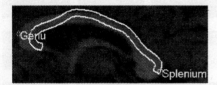   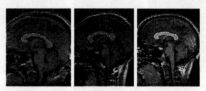

Fig. 8. The CC organism's self-awareness makes it capable of identifying landmark parts.   **Fig. 9.** Example segmentation results.

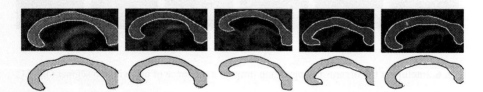

Fig. 10. Example segmentation results (top), also shown (in black) over manually segmented (gray) CC (bottom).

4   Conclusions

Robust, automatic medical image analysis requires the incorporation and intelligent utilization of global contextual knowledge. We have introduced a new paradigm for medical image analysis that applies concepts from artificial life modeling to meet this requirement. By architecting a deformable model-based framework in a layered fashion, we are able to separate the 'global' model-fitting control functionality from the local feature integration functionality. This separation allows us to define a model-fitting controller or 'brain' in terms of the high-level anatomical features of an object rather than low-level image features. The layered-architecture approach also provides the brain layer with precise control over the lower-level model deformation layer. The result is an intelligent organism that is continuously aware of the progress of the segmentation, allowing it to effectively apply prior knowledge of the target object. We have demonstrated the potential of this approach by constructing a Corpus Callosum "worm" organism and releasing it into MRI brain images in order to segment and label the CC.

Several interesting aspects of our approach are currently in consideration for further exploration. These include extending our model to 3D, designing a motion tracking plan and releasing an organism into time-varying image 'environments' (i.e. 4D images), exploring the use of multiple plans and plan selection schemes, and exploring the application of learning algorithms, such as genetic algorithms, to assist human experts in the generation of optimal plans. Another potentially important research direction is the use of multiple organisms that intercommunicate contextual image information (i.e. are 'aware' of one another).

Acknowledgements

GH was funded in part by the Visual Information Technology (VISIT) program, Swedish Foundation for Strategic Research (SSF). Dr. Martha Shenton of the Harvard Medical School generously provided the MRI data.

References

1. Cootes, T., Beeston, C., Edwards, G., Taylor, C.: A Unified Framework for Atlas Matching using Active Appearance Models. Image Processing in Medical. Imaging (1999) 322-333.
2. Duncan, J., Ayache, N.: Medical Image Analysis: Progress Over Two Decades and the Challenges Ahead. IEEE Trans. PAMI 22(1) (2000) 85 -106.
3. Hamarneh, G., McInerney, T.: Controlled Shape Deformations via Medial Profiles. Vision Interface (2001) 252-258.
4. McInerney, T., Kikinis, R.: An Object-based Volumetric Deformable Atlas for the Improved Localization of Neuroanatomy in MR Images. MICCAI (1998) 861-869.
5. McInerney, T., Terzopoulos, D.: Deformable Models in Medical Image Analysis: A Survey. Medical Image Analysis 1(2) (1996) 91-108.
6. Pizer, S., Fletcher, P., Fridman, Y., Fritsch D., Gash, A., Glotzer, J., Joshi, S., Thall A., Tracton, G., Yushkevich, P., Chaney, E.: Deformable M-Reps for 3D Medical Image Segmentation. Submitted to Medical Image Analysis (2000).
7. Pizer, S., Fritsch, D., Low, K., Furst, J.: 2D & 3D Figural Models of Anatomic Objects from Medical Images. Mathematical Morphology and Its Applications to Image Processing, Kluwer Computational Imaging and Vision Series, H.J.A.M. Heijmans, J.B.T.M. Roerdink, Eds. Amsterdam, (1998) 139-150.
8. Pizer, S., Fritsch, D.: Segmentation, Registration, and Measurement of Shape Variation via Image Object Shape. IEEE Transactions on Medical Imaging 18(10) (1999) 851-865.
9. Shen, D., Davatzikos, C.: An Adaptive-Focus Deformable Model Using Statistical and Geometric Information. IEEE Trans. PAMI 22(8) (2000) 906 -913.

10. Szekely, G., Kelemen, A., Brechbuehler C., Gerig, G.: Segmentation of 3D Objects From MRI Volume Data Using Constrained Elastic Deformations of Flexible Fourier Surface Models. Medical Image Analysis 1(1) (1996) 19-34.
11. Terzopoulos, D., Metaxas, D.: Dynamic 3D Models with Local and Global Deformations: Deformable Superquadrics. IEEE Trans. PAMI 13(7) (1991) 703-714.
12. Terzopoulos, D., Tu, X., Grzeszczuk, R.: Artificial Fishes: Autonomous Locomotion, Perception, Behavior, and Learning in a Simulated Physical World. Artificial Life 1(4) (1994)
13. Terzopoulos,D.:Artificial Life for Computer Graphics.Commun. ACM 42(8) (1999)32-42.
14. Tsotsos, J.K., Mylopoulos, J., Covvey, H.D., Zucker, S.W.: A Framework for Visual Motion Understanding. IEEE Trans. PAMI 2(6) (1980) 563-573.

Automatic Construction of 3D Statistical Deformation Models Using Non-rigid Registration

D. Rueckert[1], A.F. Frangi[2,3], and J.A. Schnabel[4]

[1] Visual Information Processing, Department of Computing, Imperial College, London, UK
dr@doc.ic.ac.uk, http://www.doc.ic.ac.uk/~/dr
[2] Grupo de Tecnologia de las Comunicaciones, Departamento de Ingenieria Electronica y Comunicaciones, Universidad de Zaragoza, Spain
[3] Image Sciences Institute, University Medical Center Utrecht (UMC), Utrecht, NL
[4] Computational Imaging Science Group, Guy's Hospital, King's College London, UK

Abstract. In this paper we introduce the concept of statistical deformation models (SDM) which allow the construction of average models of the anatomy and their variability. SDMs are built by performing a statistical analysis of the deformations required to map anatomical features in one subject into the corresponding features in another subject. The concept of SDMs is similar to active shape models (ASM) which capture statistical information about shapes across a population but offers several new advantages over ASMs: Firstly, SDMs can be constructed directly from images such as MR or CT without the need for segmentation which is usually a prerequisite for the construction of active shape models. Instead a non-rigid registration algorithm is used to compute the deformations required to establish correspondences between the reference subject and the subjects in the population class under investigation. Secondly, SDMs allow the construction of an atlas of the average anatomy as well as its variability across a population of subjects. Finally, SDMs take the 3D nature of the underlying anatomy into account by analysing dense 3D deformation fields rather than only the 2D surface shape of anatomical structures. We demonstrate the applicability of this new framework to MR images of the brain and show results for the construction of anatomical models from 25 different subjects.

1 Introduction

The significant inter-subject variability of anatomy and function makes the interpretation of medical images a very challenging task. Atlas-based approaches address this problem by defining a common reference space. Mapping data sets into this common reference space not only accounts for anatomical and functional variations of individual subjects, it also offers a powerful framework to facilitate comparison of anatomy and function over time, between subjects, between groups of subjects and across sites. Consequently, a number of different elastic [1] and fluid [2,3] warping techniques have been developed for this purpose. A recent review of different non-rigid registration techniques can be found in [4]. Traditional medical atlases contain information about anatomy and function from a single individual focusing primarily on the human brain

W. Niessen and M. Viergever (Eds.): MICCAI 2001, LNCS 2208, pp. 77–84, 2001.

[5]. Even though the individuals selected for these atlases may be considered normal, they may represent an extremum of a normal distribution. To address this problem, researchers have developed various probabilistic and statistical approaches which include information from a group of subjects making them more representative of the population under investigation [6,7,8].

Statistical models of shape variability [9] or Active Shape Models (ASM) have been successfully applied to perform various image analysis tasks in 2D and 3D images. In building those statistical models, a set of segmentations of the shape of interest is required as well as a set of landmarks that can be unambiguously defined in each sample shape. An extension of ASMs are the so-called Active Appearance Models (AAM) [10] which have been used for atlas matching. This model incorporates not only information about the spatial distribution of landmarks but also about the intensity distribution at the landmarks. In a different approach Wang et al. [11] suggested to use statistical shape information as priors for a non-rigid registration. A fundamental problem when building these models is the fact that it requires the determination of point correspondences between the different shapes. The manual identification of such correspondences is a time consuming and tedious task. This is particularly true in 3D where the amount of landmarks required to describe the shape accurately increases dramatically compared to 2D applications.

In a recent paper [12] we have described an automated way of establishing correspondences between different shapes via a non-rigid registration algorithm [13]. In this paper we present a natural extension of our previous approach in which we perform statistical analysis directly on the deformation fields required to match different anatomies. We use the term statistical deformation models (SDM) to describe this framework since it allows the construction of average models of the anatomy and their statistical variability across a population of subjects.

2 Method

Traditionally, landmarks are anatomically characteristic points which can be uniquely identified across a set of individuals. The goal of inter-subject registration is to find the optimal transformation $T_i : x \mapsto x'$ which maps any point x in the anatomy of the reference subject S_r into its corresponding point x' in the anatomy of any other subject S_i in the population class. Assuming a one-to-one correspondence of anatomical structures across subjects, the registration of images between different subjects yields a dense set of so-called *pseudo-landmarks*. In our new framework we perform a principal component analysis (PCA) on these pseudo-landmarks which is equivalent to performing a PCA on the deformation fields required to map the anatomy of one subject into the anatomy of another subject. In the following we will describe our new framework in more detail.

2.1 Non-rigid Registration

In practice, the anatomical variability between subjects cannot be sufficiently explained by an affine transformation which only accounts for differences due to position, orientation and size of the anatomy. To capture the anatomical variability, it will be necessary to employ non-rigid transformations such as elastic or fluid transformations. We are using a non-rigid registration algorithm which has been previously applied successfully to a number of different registration tasks [13,14]. This algorithm uses a combined transformation $\mathbf{T}$ which consists of a global transformation and a local transformation:

$$\mathbf{T}(\mathbf{x}) = \mathbf{T}_{global}(\mathbf{x}) + \mathbf{T}_{local}(\mathbf{x}) \tag{1}$$

The global transformation describes the overall differences between the two subjects and is represented by an affine transformation. The local transformation describes any local deformation required to match the anatomies of the subjects. We have chosen a free-form deformation (FFD) model based on B-splines which is a powerful tool for modelling 3D deformable objects. The basic idea of FFDs is to deform an object by manipulating an underlying mesh of control points. The resulting deformation controls the shape of the 3D object and can be written as the 3D tensor product of the familiar 1D cubic B-splines,

$$\mathbf{T}_{local}(\mathbf{x}) = \sum_{l=0}^{3} \sum_{m=0}^{3} \sum_{n=0}^{3} B_l(u) B_m(v) B_n(w) \mathbf{c}_{i+l,j+m,k+n} \tag{2}$$

where $\mathbf{c}$ denotes the control points which parameterise the transformation. The optimal transformation is found by minimising a cost function associated with the global transformation parameters as well as the local transformation parameters. The cost function comprises two competing goals: The first term represents the cost associated with the voxel-based similarity measure, in this case normalised mutual information [15], while the second term corresponds to a regularization term which constrains the transformation to be smooth [13].

The resulting transformation $\mathbf{T}$ maps each point in the anatomy of the reference subject S_r to the corresponding point in the anatomy of subject S. Since the transformation $\mathbf{T}$ is a sum (rather than a concatenation) of a global and local transformation, we need to remove any dependency of the local transformation on the global transformation (which is a result of the different position, orientation and size of each subject's anatomy):

$$\mathbf{x} + \mathbf{d}(\mathbf{x}) = \mathbf{T}_{global}^{-1}(\mathbf{T}_{global}(\mathbf{x}) + \mathbf{T}_{local}(\mathbf{x})) \tag{3}$$

Thus, the deformation $\mathbf{d}$ describes the anatomical variability across the population class in the coordinate system of the reference subject.

2.2 Construction of Statistical Deformation Models

The concept of statistical deformation models (SDMs) is closely related to the idea of ASMs. The key difference is that we apply a principal component analysis (PCA) to the deformation fields required to map one anatomy to another anatomy rather than to corresponding points: Suppose that we have n deformation fields described as vectors $\mathbf{d}_i$. These deformation fields are the result of the non-rigid registration algorithm described in the previous section and map the anatomy of the reference subject S_r into the anatomy of the other individuals S_i in the population class under investigation. Each deformation field d_i can be expressed as a concatenation of m 3-D vectors which describe the deformation at each voxel in the image of the reference subject. The goal of SDMs is to approximate the distribution of d using a parameterised linear model of the form

$$d = \hat{d} + \Phi b \tag{4}$$

where $\hat{d}$ is the average deformation field for all n subjects,

$$\hat{d} = \frac{1}{n} \sum_{i=1}^{n} d_i \tag{5}$$

and b is the model parameter vector. The columns of the matrix Φ are formed by the principal components of the covariance matrix S:

$$S = \frac{1}{n-1} \sum_{i=1}^{n} (d_i - \hat{d})(d_i - \hat{d})^T \tag{6}$$

From this, we can calculate the principal modes of variation of the deformation field as the eigenvectors ϕ_i and corresponding eigenvalues λ_i (sorted so that $\lambda_i \geq \lambda_{i+1}$) of S.

2.3   Interpretation of Statistical Deformation Models

A common problem encountered during the construction of a model of the average anatomy is the choice of the reference subject to which all other subjects are registered. Even though the reference subject selected may be considered normal, it may represent an extremum of a normal distribution. Assuming a perfect registration, the registration will align the anatomy of each subject with the anatomy of the reference subject. Thus, the average model will be constructed in the coordinate system of the reference subject. To remove any bias of the average model towards a particular anatomy, we can construct the average model of the anatomy in its *natural coordinate system*. This natural coordinate system is the coordinate system which requires the least residual deformation to explain the anatomical variability across all individuals. Based on a point x in the space of the reference subject we can find the corresponding point x' in its natural coordinates by applying the average deformation vector $\hat{d}$:

$$x' = x + \hat{d}(x) \tag{7}$$

Within this natural coordinate system we can now study the anatomical variability of the population class under investigation. Recall that in eq. (4) the vector b provides a parameterisation of the deformations in terms of its principal modes. Varying the parameter vector b will generate different instances of the deformation field. By applying these deformation fields to the average anatomy we can generate instances of the class of anatomy under analysis. Under the assumption that the cloud of deformation vectors at each point follows a multi-dimensional Gaussian distribution, the variance of the i-th parameter, b_i, across the population is given by eigenvalue λ_i. By applying limits to the variation of b_i, for instance $|b_i| \leq \pm 3\sqrt{\lambda_i}$, it can be ensured that a generated anatomy is similar to the anatomies in the training class.

Registration	L. nucleus caudate	R. nucleus caudate
Affine	48.86%	41.35%
Non-rigid (20 mm)	62.56%	58.98%
Non-rigid (10 mm)	75.01%	74.75%
Non-rigid (5 mm)	86.73%	85.65%

Table 1. Average overlap between the left and right nucleus caudate of the reference subject after registration with all other individuals.

3   Results

To demonstrate our approach we have used 25 brain MR images from different subjects with schizophrenia to construct a statistical deformation model of the brain. All images were acquired at the Department of Psychiatry of the University Medical Center Utrecht using a 3D FFE sequence (TE = 4.6 ms, TR = 30 ms, flip angle = 30°) on a 1.5 T MR imaging system (Philips Gyroscan ACS-NT). These images have a voxel size of $1 \times 1 \times 1.2$ mm^3 and $200 \times 200 \times 160$ voxels. Out of the 25 subjects we have randomly selected one individual which was used as the reference subject. We have then registered each of the remaining 24 individuals to this reference subject. For the non-rigid registration we have used control point spacings of 20 mm, 10 mm and finally 5 mm [13,14]. In order to assess the quality of the inter-subject registration, we have calculated the overlap between a manually segmented deep structure in the brain, the nucleus caudate, after affine and non-rigid registration. The results summarised in Table 1 show that after non-rigid registration the average overlap between the nucleus caudate of the reference subject and those of the remaining 24 individuals is more than 85%. Given the small size of the nucleus caudate this indicates a very good registration.

The first step of the construction of statistical deformation models is to build a model of the average anatomy of all subjects after non-rigid registration. The resulting *atlas* constructed in the coordinate system of the reference subject is shown in the top row of Figure 1 in form of an average intensity image[1]. In the second step we have removed any bias of the atlas towards the reference subject by applying the average deformation $\hat{d}$ to the atlas. The resulting atlas in its *natural coordinate system* is shown in the bottom row of Figure 1. In this example we can clearly see that the average reproduces the large ventricular system of the subject chosen as reference subject. Removing any bias of the atlas towards the reference subject yields an average model in which the ventricular system is significantly smaller.

The final step of the construction of statistical deformation models is the calculation of the principal modes of variation of the deformation field which give an indication of the anatomical variability across the population under investigation. We can generate the modes of variation by varying the shape parameter b_i and applying the resulting deformation field to the atlas. An example of the first three modes of variation is shown in Figure 2. Note, that in contrast to AAMs [10], our model does not incorporate any statistical information about intensities so that the intensities of the atlas are not affected

---

[1] Animated versions of Figure 1 and 2 are available at http://www.doc.ic.ac.uk/~dr/MICCAI01.

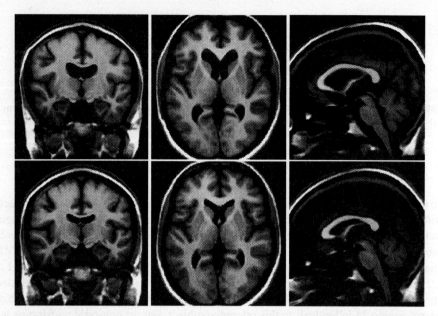

Fig. 1. The top row shows a coronal, axial and sagittal view of the average brain atlas of 25 different subjects constructed in the space of the reference subject. The bottom row shows the coronal, axial and sagittal view of the average brain atlas of 25 different subjects constructed in natural atlas coordinates. This coordinate system is obtained by applying the average deformation $\hat{d}$ to the coordinate system of the reference subject.

by the modes of variation. The total number of modes of variation corresponds to the number of individuals in the population class excluding the reference subject. In our example we have 24 different modes of variation of which the first 10 modes explain more than 70% of the cumulative anatomical variability while the first 18 modes explain more than 90% of this variability.

The interpretation of the modes of variation is difficult since they are not only the result of the variability of a single anatomical structure but the result of the variability of a large number of different anatomical structures as well as their inter-relationship. The interpretation is further complicated by the fact that a dense deformation field requires performing a PCA on a very high dimensional space ($200 \times 200 \times 160 = 6.4$ million deformation vectors). However, we can significantly reduce the dimensionality by performing the PCA directly on the control points of the FFD ($40 \times 40 \times 32 = 51200$ control points). This provides a very compact representation of deformation fields using B-spline basis functions. In future experiments we are planning to use a larger number of subjects to allow a robust statistical analysis of the deformation fields.

4   Discussion and Conclusions

In this paper we have presented a new method for the automatic construction of statistical deformation models (SDM). These models can be used to build an atlas of the

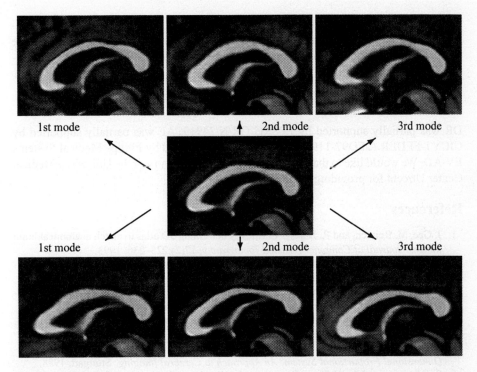

Fig. 2. Instances of the statistical deformation model showing the corpus callosum: Each image has been generated by varying the first three modes of variation between $-3\sqrt{\lambda_i}$ (top row) and $+3\sqrt{\lambda_i}$ (bottom row). The middle row corresponds to the average model.

average anatomy as well as its variability. This is achieved by performing a principal component analysis of the deformations required to map the anatomy of a reference subject to all other subjects in the population. A similar statistical analysis of deformation fields has been proposed by Gee et al. [7]. The key difference to the work by Gee et al. is the fact that our approach exploits the compact parameterization of the deformation fields by the B-spline representation. Our method can also be used for the construction of "stable" anatomical models which are not dependent on the choice of the reference subject. A related approach has been pursued by Guimond et al. [8]. Their approach also uses average deformations to construct an atlas of the shape and intensity. The advantage of the framework presented in this paper stems from the fact that the proposed framework allows not only to construct an atlas of the average anatomy but also a model of the principal modes of variation of this anatomy. This may be used to compare the morphometrics of an individual with those of a group or across different groups of individuals.

In practice inter-subject registration is a very challenging task and will lead to registration errors. In previous experiments we have found that our algorithm yields a registration accuracy between 1 and 2 mm when comparing different anatomical landmarks across individuals. This compares to an intra-observer variability between 0.2 and 0.9

mm for the localisation of anatomical landmarks. We are currently investigating the effect of registration errors on the statistical analysis of the deformation fields in more detail. We are also aiming to incorporate knowledge about landmarks into the registration algorithm.

Acknowledgements

DR was partially supported by EPSRC GR/N/24919. AF was partially supported by CICYT-FEDER (2FD97-1197-C02-01). JAS is supported by Philips Medical Systems EV-AD. We would like to thank the Department of Psychiatry of the University Medical Center Utrecht for providing the data.

References

1. J. Gee, M. Reivich, and R. Bajcsy. Elastically deforming 3D atlas to match anatomical brain images. *Journal of Computer Assisted Tomography*, 17(2):225–236, 1993.
2. G. E. Christensen, R. D. Rabbitt, and M. I. Miller. Deformable templates using large deformation kinematics. *IEEE Transactions on Image Processing*, 5(10):1435–1447, 1996.
3. M. Bro-Nielsen and C. Gramkow. Fast fluid registration of medical images. In *Proc. Visualization in Biomedical Computing (VBC'96)*, pages 267–276, 1996.
4. D. Rueckert. Non-rigid registration: Techniques and applications. In D. J. Hawkes, D. L. G. Hill, and J. Hajnal, editors, *Medical Image Registration*. CRC Press, 2001.
5. J. Talairach and P. Tournoux. *Co-Planar Stereotactic Atlas of the Human Brain: 3-Dimensional Proportional System: An Approach to Cerebral Imaging*. Stuttgart, 1988.
6. P. Thompson and A. W. Toga. Detection, visualization and animation of abnormal anatomic structure with a deformable probabilistic atlas based on random vector field transformations. *Medical Image Analysis*, 1(4):271–294, 1997.
7. J. C. Gee and R. K. Bajcsy. Elastic Matching: Continuum Mechnanical and Probabilistic Analysis. In A. W. Toga, editor, *Brain Warping*, pages 183-197. Academic Press, 1999.
8. A. Guimond, J. Meunier, and J.-P. Thirion. Average brain models. *Computer Vision and Image Understanding*, 77:192–210, 2000.
9. T. F. Cootes, C. J. Taylor, D. H. Cooper, and J. Graham. Active Shape Models - their training and application. *Computer Vision and Image Understanding*, 61(1):38–59, 1995.
10. T. F. Cootes, C. Beeston, G. J. Edwards, and C. J. Taylor. A unified framework for atlas matching using active appearance models. In *Proc. Information Processing in Medical Imaging (IPMI'99)*, pages 322–333, 1999.
11. Y. Wang and L. H. Staib. Elastic model based non-rigid registration incorporating statistical shape information. In *Proc. MICCAI '98*, pages 1162–1173, 1998.
12. A. F. Frangi, D. Rueckert, J. A. Schnabel, and W. J. Niessen. Automatic 3D ASM construction via atlas-based landmarking and volumetric elastic registration. In *Proc. Information Processing in Medical Imaging: (IPMI'01)*, pages 78–91, 2001.
13. D. Rueckert, L. I. Sonoda, C. Hayes, D. L. G. Hill, M. O. Leach, and D. J. Hawkes. Non-rigid registration using free-form deformations: Application to breast MR images. *IEEE Transactions on Medical Imaging*, 18(8):712–721, 1999.
14. J. A. Schnabel, D. Rueckert, M. Quist, J. M. Blackall, A. D. Castellano Smith, T. Hartkens, G. P. Penney, W. A. Hall, H. Liu, C. L. Truwit, F. A. Gerritsen, D. L. G. Hill and D. J. Hawkes. A Generic Framework for Non-Rigid Registration Based on Non-Uniform Multi-Level Free-Form Deformations. In *Proc. MICCAI '01*, 2001. In press.
15. C. Studholme, D. L. G. Hill, and D. J. Hawkes. An overlap invariant entropy measure of 3D medical image alignment. *Pattern Recognition*, 32(1):71–86, 1998.

A Learning Method for Automated Polyp Detection

S.B. Göktürk[1], C. Tomasi[1], B. Acar[2], D. Paik[2], C. Beaulieu[2], S. Napel[2]

[1] Robotics Lab., Computer Science Department, Stanford University
[2] Three Dimensional Imaging Lab., Department of Radiology, Stanford University
{gokturkb,tomasi,bacar}@Stanford.edu
{paik,cfb,snapel}@s-word.Stanford.edu

Abstract. Adenomatous polyps in the colon have a high probability of developing into subsequent colorectal carcinoma, the second leading cause of cancer deaths in United States. In this paper, we propose a new method for computer-aided diagnosis of polyps. Initial work with shape detection has shown high sensitivity for polyp detection, but at a cost of too many false positive detections. We present a statistical approach that uses support vector machines to distinguish the differentiating characteristics of polyps and healthy tissue, and subsequently uses this information for the classification of the new cases. One of the main contributions of the paper is a new 3-D pattern analysis approach, which combines the information from many random images to generate reliable signatures of the shapes. At 80% polyp detection rate, the proposed system reduces the false positive rate by 80% compared to previous work.

1 Introduction

Colon cancer is the second leading cause of cancer deaths in the United States. American adults have 1/20 chance of developing and 1/40 chance of dying from this disease [1]. Previous research has shown that adenomatous polyps, particularly those larger than 1 cm in diameter, have a high probability of developing into subsequent colorectal carcinoma [2]. Detection and removal of small polyps can totally eliminate the disease. Unfortunately, colon cancer is most often discovered after the patient develops symptoms, and by then, the likelihood of a cure has diminished substantially. Therefore, a cost-effective and patient-comfortable screening procedure is desirable in order to diagnose the disease in an earlier stage.

Optical colonoscopy is considered the definitive diagnostic test as it affords direct visualization and the opportunity for biopsy or removal of suspicious lesion [3]. This method involves an optical probe being inserted into the colon in order to examine the interior. An alternative, non-invasive method has recently been proposed: Computed tomography colonography (CTC) or virtual colonscopy is a technique that combines axial spiral CT data acquisition of the air-filled and cleansed colon with 3-dimensional imaging software to create endoscopic images of the colonic surface [4]. The initial clinical results are quite promising, yet the technique is still impractical due, in part, to the extensive amount of radiologist time involved in the process, which typically requires viewing over 300 512 by 512 images per patient study. In

W. Niessen and M. Viergever (Eds.): MICCAI 2001, LNCS 2208, pp. 85-93, 2001.
© Springer-Verlag Berlin Heidelberg 2001

order to help the radiologist be more time efficient and accurate, an automated screening method for computer-aided diagnosis of polyps is necessary.

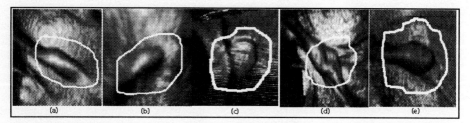

Fig. 1. (a),(b),(c) are polyps, (d) is a normal thickened fold (e) is retained stool.

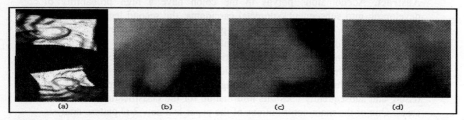

Fig. 2. (a) Two different 3-D views of a polyp. (b-d) Perpendicular images through the same polyp.

Automated polyp detection is a very recently growing area of research. The problem of identifying colonic polyps is very challenging because they come in various sizes and shapes, and because thickened folds and retained stool may mimic their shape and density. Figure 1 demonstrates the appearance of polyps and other tissue as they appear in a virtual colonoscopy study.

Initial studies concerning automated polyp detection have started from the intuitive observation that the shape of a polyp is similar to a hemisphere. In [5], Summers *et al.* computes the minimum, maximum, mean and Gaussian curvatures at all points on the colon wall. Following discrimination of polypoid shapes by their principal minimum and maximum curvatures, more restrictive criteria are applied in order to eliminate non-spherical shapes.

In [6], Paik *et al.* introduced a method based on the concept that normals to the colon surface will intersect with neighboring normals depending on the local curvature features of the colon. The method detects the polyps by giving the shapes a score based on the number of intersecting normal vectors. In [7], Yoshida *et al.* use curvedness to distinguish polyps from healthy tissue.

In [8], Göktürk and Tomasi designed a method based on the observation that the bounding surfaces of polyps are usually not exact spheres, but are often complex surfaces composed by small, approximately spherical patches. In this method, a sphere is fit locally to the isodensity surface passing through every CT voxel in the wall region. Densely populated nearby sphere centers are considered as polyp candidates.

Due to the large number of false positive detections, all of the methods mentioned above can be considered more as polyp *candidate* detectors than polyp detectors. This paper presents a statistical method to differentiate between polyps and normal tissue.

The input to the system is a set of small candidate volumes, which may or may not contain polypoid shapes. This set can be computed by one of the methods just discussed. Our novel volume processing technique generates shape-signatures for each candidate volume. The signatures are then fed to a support vector machine (SVM) classifier for the final diagnosis of the volume.

The paper is organized as follows: Section 2 explains both the volume processing and support vector classifier in detail. Section 3 describes the experimental setup and discusses our preliminary results. Section 4 gives some conclusions and possible directions for future work.

2 Our Method

Many radiologists prefer to view colon CT images through three perpendicular image planes aligned with the transaxial, sagittal, and coronal anotomical directions[4]. Figure 2 shows a polyp in 3-D and 3 perpendicular views through it in 2-D. These perpendicular planes capture substantial information about the shape, yet they are incomplete by themselves. A more accurate signature of the volume can be obtained by collecting statistics over several *triples* of mutually orthogonal planes, oriented along other than the anatomical directions. We use a histogram of several geometric attributes obtained from many triples of perpendicular random images as a feature-vector to represent the shape.

Computing shape features on triples of planes, rather than on individual planes, captures 3D shape aspects more completely. Taking histograms of these features over several random triples makes the resulting signatures invariant to rotations and translations. More details on our signatures are given sections 2.1 and 2.2. Support-vector machines, described in section 2.3, are then trained with signatures computed from an initial set, and are subsequently used to classify new volumes into polyps and normal tissues.

2.1 Image Processing

Each candidate volume is sliced with several triples of perpendicular planes. A polyp may not occupy the resulting images entirely. As a consequence, images are segmented, so as to disregard tissues surrounding the putative polyp. This segmentation process is described in section 2.1.1. Shape and intensity features are then computed in the resulting sub-windows, as discussed in section 2.1.2.

2.1.1 Segmentation
The size of the critical region varies depending on the size and the shape of the suspicious lesion. Here, we aim to discover the best square window that would capture the essentials of the shape. Figure 3 depicts the critical window for different shapes.

A window is considered good when it contains a shape that is approximately circular and has a small radius. Because elongated folds are common in the colon, it was found to be useful to also explicitly rule out elongated regions. To find an optimal window size *w*, an image is first binarized, and the following target function is computed for each window of size *w* and centered in the middle of the image:

$$f(w) = a_1 r + e_{circle} - a_2 e_{line} \tag{1}$$

Here, *r* is the radius of the circle that best fits the edges in the binarized image, e_{circle} is the residue to the best fitting circle, e_{line} is the residue to the best fitting line, and a_1 and a_2 are constants. Details of the fitting are described in the next section. The value of *w* that yields the smallest *f(w)* is chosen as the best window size.

2.1.2 Image Features

Image features should capture representative information about the candidate shape. Primitive shapes such as circle, quadric curve, and line (figure 4. d,e,f) are fit to the largest connected edge component, *i.e.* boundary of the shape.

A random slice of a sphere is a circle. Thus, fitting circles is a means of measuring the sphericity of the 3-D shape. When doing so, the residuals at each pixel on the boundary are first weighted with a Gaussian located at the image center, and shown in image 4(c). The purpose of these weights is to give more importance to boundary points of the shape than to those of the surrounding colon wall. The weighted residuals are then added together, and the least square solution gives the optimum circle. The residual to the least square solution is recorded as well.

Similarly, the residual to the optimum fitting line gives information on the flatness of the surface. Quadratic curves include any second order equation system of two variables. By fitting a quadratic curve to the boundary of the image, the ellipsoidal structure of the shape can be measured, thereby helping to capture similarity to a pedunculated polyp.

In order to extract information on higher order frequency characteristics of the boundary, 3rd order moment invariants are computed as well [9]. Specifically, given the coordinates of points on the plane, a *(p,q)*th moment and the third order moment invariant M are given by,

$$m_{pq} = \sum_{i=1}^{N} (x_i - x_0)^p .(y_i - y_0)^q \text{ and } M = (m_{30} + m_{12})^2 + (m_{03} + m_{21})^2$$

In addition to these shape features, intensity features are extracted from the tissue part of the image. The colon tissue is first separated away from the interior of the colon (air) by intensity thresholding. The mean and the standard deviation of the remaining intensity values are recorded as intensity measurements in the feature vector.

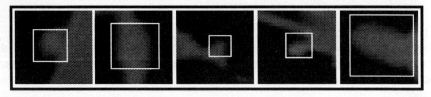

Fig. 3. 2-D images of five different suspicious lesions, with the size of the critical region varying from image to image.

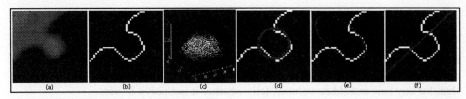

Fig. 4. (a) Sample image. (b) Edges. (c) Gaussian mask to weight the edge points on the image. (d) The circle fitted to the weighted edge points. (e) The quadratic fitted to the weighted edge points. (f) The line fitted to the edge points.

All the attributes mentioned so far are calculated for each random triple of images. The three images in each triple are sorted in the order of increasing radius of curvature, and the features above are listed into a vector in this order. This vector represents the signature of the shape, relative to that particular triple of perpendicular planes.

2.2 Vector Quantization

The features computed from each triple of perpendicular planes depend on the position and orientation of that particular triple. However, if histograms of feature distributions are computed from sufficiently many triples with random positions and orientations, the histograms themselves are essentially invariant to position and orientation. Explicit histograms, on the other hand, are out of the question, since the high dimension of the underlying feature space would imply prohibitive amounts of storage. A more efficient solution, proposed here, represents a histogram by first computing the representatives for the main clusters of features over a large collection of vectors. New feature vectors are then assigned to these clusters, rather than to fixed bins. This method is called *vector quantization* and is described in more detail in [10].

Let X_{ij} be the n-vector obtained from the jth random triple of perpendicular planes extracted from the ith shape. Having obtained X_{ij}'s from all of the shapes, the k-means algorithm [10] is used to compute vector clusters. Let X be the matrix each column of which contains one particular X_{ij}. The cluster centers are initialized to be the principal component directions of X. Subsequent iterations of the k-means algorithm then alternately reassign vectors to clusters and recompute cluster centers, resulting eventually into the optimum cluster centers B_i.

When forming feature histograms, the simplest strategy would be to have each vector increment a counter for the nearest cluster center. This method, however, is overly sensitive to the particular choice of clusters. We adopted a more robust solution, in which each feature vector partitions a unit vote into fractions that are inversely proportional to the vector's distances to all cluster centers. The histograms thus obtained, one per candidate volume, are the shape signatures used for classification as described in the next section.

2.3 Support Vector Machines

A classifier learning algorithm takes a *training set* as input and produces a *classifier* as its output. In our problem, a training set is a collection of candidate volumes that a radiologist has individually labeled as polyps or non-polyps. A classifier is a function that, for any new candidate volume, tells whether it is a polyp or not.

Mathematically, a classifier can also be viewed as a *hypersurface* in feature space, that separates polyps from non-polyps. Support vector machines (SVM) [11] implicitly transform the given feature vectors x into new vectors $\phi(x)$ in a space with more dimensions, such that the hypersurface that separates the x, becomes a *hyperplane* in the space of $\phi(x)$'s. This mapping from x to $\phi(x)$ is used implicitly in that only inner products of the form $K(x_i, x_j) = \phi(x_i)^T \phi(x_j)$ need ever to be computed, rather than the high dimensional vectors $\phi(x)$ themselves. In these so-called *kernels*, the subscripts i,j refer to vectors in the training set. In the classification process, only the vectors that are very close to the separating hypersurface need to be considered when computing kernels. These vectors are called the *support vectors*. Suppose that vector x_i in the training set is given (by the radiologist) a label $y_i = 1$ if it is a polyp and $y_i = -1$ if it is not. Then the optimal classifier has the form:

$$f(x) = sign\left(\sum_{SV's} \alpha_i y_i K(x_i, x) + b \right) \qquad \text{(A)}$$

Where SV denotes the set of support vectors, and the constants α_i and b are computed by the classifier-learning algorithm. See [11] for details. Computing the coefficients α_i, b is a relatively expensive (but well understood) procedure, but needs to be performed only once, on the training set. During volume classification, only the very simple expression (A) needs to be computed.

SVMs minimize the structural risk, given as the probability of misclassifying previously unseen data. In addition, SVMs pack all the relevant information in the training set into a small number of support vectors and use only these vectors to classify new data. This makes support vectors very appropriate for polyp recognition. More generally, using a learning method, rather than hand-crafting classification heuristics, exploits all of the information in the training set optimally, and eliminates the guess work from the task of defining appropriate discrimination criteria.

3 Experiments

We used a data set consisting of small candidate volumes from the CT scans of subjects enrolled in our CT colonography study comprising of 47 known colonic polyps and 250 other regions containing tissue from healthy mucosal surface. These healthy tissues were all false positives obtained in previous work [6,8], and essentially look quite like the true positive polyps. All the polyps were bigger than 5 mm in their principal radius. 150 random triples of perpendicular images were extracted from each candidate shape. A 30-vector was obtained for each triple, and 32 clusters were used in k-means clustering, resulting into a 32-vector signature per candidate shape.

Figure 5 shows examples of two polyps and one thickened, yet normal fold along with their corresponding signatures.

Linear, polynomial and exponential radial basis functions [11] were used as kernel functions in different experiments with support vector machine classifiers. To test for each candidate shape, the classifier was first trained with all the other shapes and then

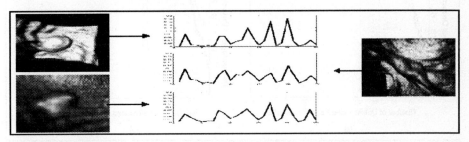

Fig. 5. Two polyps (left) and a very similarly shaped fold structure (right). As expected, the signatures are very similar, yet distinguishable.

used to test the shape. This cross-validation scheme was repeated for each candidate shape in the data set. Table 1 summarizes the results obtained from different kernel functions. The main objective of this work is to be able to achieve an accuracy of 80 or more with a minimum number of false positives (FPs). In previous work, comparable accuracy was obtained with about 100 FPs per colon for polyps of size 5mm or greater, and our approach is shown to be able to reduce the false positive rate by 80%, which inherently reduces the radiologist's interpretation time by the same amount.

A more quantitative analysis of the experiments can be achieved by replacing the zero-crossing ("sign") in expression (A), with a level crossing. As the level is decreased, more true polyps are detected, but at a cost of more false positives. The percentage of true polyp detections versus false positive detections is given in Fig.6(a).

Finally, we have analyzed the response of the system to different sizes of polyps. In previous studies, it has been shown that, polyps less than 1 cm in size are rarely malignant, with an incidence of carcinoma of only 1% [12]. However, the incidence of carcinoma increases to 37% in polyps greater than 2 cm in size [12]. Therefore, it is of critical importance to remove adenomatous polyps as small as 1 cm to impact the mortality of this disease. In figure 6(b), we illustrate the corresponding performance curves for polyps of size greater than 1 cm and smaller than 1 cm separately. The worse performance on smaller polyps can be explained by two reasons: First, folds in the human colon look similar to smaller polyps. Second and mainly, the resolution of current CT technology (voxel size is about .7 x .7 x 3.5 mm) is not high enough to capture shape descriptors for small objects. The results for bigger sized polyps were obtained using a 10-big-polyp training set. Since our methods rely on previous statistics, a bigger training set will improve the sensitivity of the system.

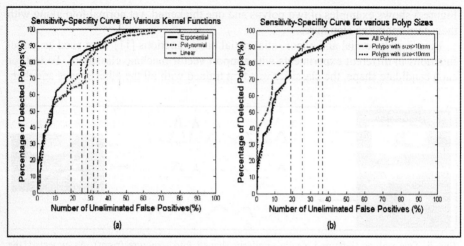

Fig. 6. Sensitivity vs. number of false positive detections. (a) Comparison between various kernel types. (b) Comparison between various polyp sizes.

Table 1. Improvements obtained by different kernel functions.

	Linear Kernel	Polynomial Kernel	Exponential Kernel
FP rate for 80% polyp detection	28.51	24.89	18.87
FP rate for 90% polyp detection	38.15	31.32	33.33
FP rate for 100% polyp detection	67.07	69.88	57.03

4 Conclusions and Future Work

Virtual colonoscopy is a promising new medical imaging technique to evaluate the human colon for precancerous polyps. Due to the large amount of radiologist time involved in reviewing hundreds of images in a search for small lesions, computer aided diagnosis is necessary to make the approach efficient and cost-effective. Previous automated detection methods had a high sensitivity for polyp detection, but relied on human observations to differentiate polyps from normal folds or retained fecal material. To be more accurate, we need a method that is capable of differentiating polyps from other normal healthy structures in the colon. In this study, we proposed a learning approach that yields a good polyp detection rate with a reasonable number of false positives, thereby showing the feasibility of computer-based screening. One of the main contributions of the paper is the new 3-D pattern analysis approach, which combines the information from many random images to generate reliable shape signatures. We also show that the use of support vector machines is capable of distinguishing implicitly the differentiating characteristics of polyps and healthy tissue, thus improving classification rates.

There are many directions for future investigation. First, we would like to analyze support vectors to observe the differentiating characteristics of polyps and healthy tissue. These observations might give valuable feedback in designing new features for the system. In addition, while the results reported in this paper are promising, more extensive case studies need to be carried out, and more comprehensive statistics must be collected. Finally, studies integrating these computer aided detection schemes with radiologist readers will be used to measure potential improvements in sensitivity and efficiency compared with unassisted radiologist interpretation.

References

[1] Wingo P.J., Cancer Statistics, *Ca Cancer Journal Clin*, 1995; 45:8-30.
[2] Thoeni R.F., Laufer I. "Polyps and cancer," *Textbook of Gastrointestinal Radiology*, Philadelphia: W.B. Saunders, 1994; 1160.
[3] Winawer S.J., Zauber A.G., Ho M.N., O'Brien M.J., Gottlieb L.S., Sternberg S.S., Waye J.D., et. al. "Prevention of colorectal cancer by colonoscopic polypectomy," The national polyp study workgroup, *N Engl J Med.* 1993; 329:1977-1981.
[4] Dachman A.H., Kuniyoshi J.K., Boyle C.M., Samara Y., Hoffman K.R., Rubin D.T., Hanan I., " Interactive CT colonography with three-dimensional problem solving for detection of colonic polyps," *American Journal of Roentgenology*, 1998; 171:989-995.
[5] Summers R.M., Beaulieu C.F., Pusanik L.M., Malley J.D., Jeffrey R.B., Glazer D.I., Napel S., "Automated polyp detector for CT colonography: feasibility study," *Radiology* ,216(1)284-90, 2000.
[6] Paik D.S., Beaulieu C.F., Jeffrey R.B., Jr., Karadi C.A., Napel S., "Detection of Polyps in CT Colonography: A Comparison of a Computer-Aided Detection Algorithm to 3D Visualization Methods," *Radiological Society of North America 85th Scientific Sessions*, Chicago, November 1999.
[7] H. Yoshida, Y. Masutani, P.M. MacEneaney, K. Doi, Y. Kim, A.H. Dachman, "Detection of colonic polyps in CT colonography based on geometric features," *Radiology*, vol. 217(SS), pp. 582-582, November 2000.
[8] Göktürk S.B., Tomasi C., "A graph method for the conservative detection of polyps in the colon," *2nd International Symposium on Virtual Colonoscopy*, Boston , October 2000.
[9] Hu M.K., "Visual pattern recognition by moment invariants," *IRE transactions on information theory*, vol. IT-8, pp 179-187, 1962.
[10] A.Gersho and R.M. Gray, *Vector Quantization and Signal Compression*, Kluwer Academic Press, 1992.
[11] Vapnik V., *Statistical Learning Theory*, New York, 1998.
[12] Hermanek P., "Dysplasia-carcinoma sequence, types of adenomas and early colo-rectal carcinoma," *European Journal of Surgery* , 1987, 13:141-3.

A CAD System for 3D Locating of Lesions in Mammogram

Yasuyo Kita[1], Eriko Tohno[2], Ralph P. Highnam[3], and Michael Brady[4]

[1] National Institute of Advanced Industrial Science and Technology,
1-1-1 Umezono,Tsukuba 305-8568, Japan
y.kita@aist.go.jp
[2] University of Tsukuba, 1-1-1 Tennodai, Tsukuba 305-8575, Japan
etohno@md.tsukuba.ac.jp
[3] Mirada Solutions, Mill street, Oxford OX2 0JK, UK
rph@mirada-solutions.com
[4] University of Oxford, Oxford OX1 3PJ, UK
jmb@robots.ox.ac.uk

Abstract. A CAD system for estimating the 3D (three dimensional) positions of lesions found in two mammographic views is described. The system is an extension of our previous method which finds corresponding 2D positions in different mammographic views by simulating breast compression [1] . In this paper, we first explain the principles and process flow of the system. The correctness of the 3D position calculated by the system is examined using breast lesions, which are found both in mammograms and in MRI data. Results from experiments show that the CAD system has clinical promise.

1 Introduction

Mammography (breast x-ray) is currently by far the best trade-off between specificity/sensitivity and cost to detect breast cancer in its early stages. As a result, screening programmes have been established in a number of countries, including the UK, Netherlands, Sweden, and Australia. Currently, screening programmes are being established in France, Germany, and Japan. There has been a considerable amount of previous work on CAD (Computer-Aided Diagnosis) systems for mammograms[2]. Most aim to detect lesions (including tumours) in images. Hardly any yield 3D (three dimensional) information, for example the 3D position and volume of lesions, which is important information for the ensuing diagnosis and treatment.

Obtaining 3D information about breast lesions from mammograms has not been accorded a great deal of attention, because breast compression (primarily to reduce x-ray dosage), which almost always varies markedly between the cranio-caudal (CC) and mediolateral oblique (MLO) views, involves a complicated relationship between the 2D positions of a point in the two images and its actual 3D position in the uncompressed breast. Although other modalities, most notably MRI, nuclear medicine and ultrasound, can be used to get the

W. Niessen and M. Viergever (Eds.): MICCAI 2001, LNCS 2208, pp. 94–102, 2001.
© Springer-Verlag Berlin Heidelberg 2001

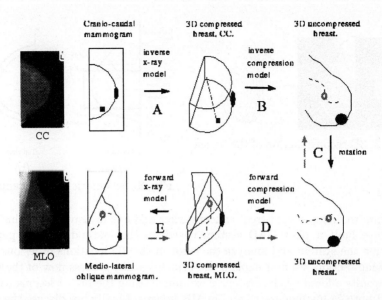

Fig. 1. Strategy for determining 3D position from two mammographic views.

required 3D information, some of the most important early indicators of cancer, e.g. calcifications, can only be observed in mammograms. It turns out that the 3D distribution of such early signs is clinically significant [3][4]. Nevertheless, few clinical studies consider how a lesion appears in an x-ray image based on the projective principle[5],[6].

It has recently been proposed that acquiring two views of the breast, medio-lateral oblique (MLO) and cranio-caudal (CC), greatly improves sensitivity and specificity. If a lesion is seen in both images, then, theoretically at least, its 3D position should be determined based on the principles of stereo vision. However, as we noted above, the breast compression in the CC and MLO differ quite markedly. As a result, the epipolar geometry, that is the determination of the straight line in one of the images that corresponds (ie the locus of candidate matches) to a point in the other image is deformed into a curve. Hence, the correspondence problem for lesions is not at all intuitive and becomes a difficult task. Kita, Highnam and Brady[1] proposed the first method to estimate curved epipolar lines by developing a simulation of breast deformation into stereo camera geometry. Using such curved epipolar lines, we can not only determine correspondences, but can estimate the 3D location of a lesion within the uncompressed breast. Using this information together with a quantitative measure obtained from calibrated image brightness, Yam et al. [3] showed how to match each microcalcification in the cluster between the two views and reconstructs the cluster in 3D. However, the correctness and accuracy of the 3D location obtained from the epipolar curves has not to date been investigated thoroughly.

The 3D position of a lesion in a mammogram, provided by our method, presents the radiologist with new, clinically significant, information that enables

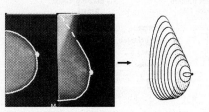

Fig. 2. 3D reconstruction of the breast

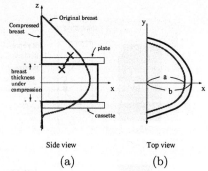

Side view   Top view

(a)   (b)

Fig. 3. Schematic breast compression

her/him to diagnose and treat cancer earlier and less invasively. For this reason, we have built a pilot CAD system based on the method. In this paper, we describe the system and analyze the error in the 3D locations of lesions. In the following section, we first explain the principles and process flow of the system. The results offered by the system is examined using the breast lesions which are found both in mammograms and in MR images. Finally, we discuss the current capabilities of this system at the present and what problems should be solved in the future.

2   CAD System for 3D Locating of Lesions in Mammogram

2.1   Principle

When a mammogram is performed, the breast is compressed between the film-screen cassette and compression plate in the direction of the x-ray source: "head to toe" for the CC view and "over the shoulder diagonally to the hip" for the MLO view. Figure 1 shows an overview of the system. Further detail is given in [1]. First, suppose that a point in one image is pointed at by a radiologist. The method calculates the epipolar curve, that is the locus of possible corresponding positions of the point in the other image by simulating the five steps of the process, A: back projection → B: uncompression → C: rotation → D: compression → E: projection as shown by the solid arrows. Next, the corresponding position is searched for along the epipolar curve. Once the correspondence is found along the curve, the corresponding 3D position in the uncompressed breast can be determined by back-tracking the movement of the point during the simulation as shown with the dashed arrows.

We define the canonical shape of the uncompressed breast as follows. According to established guidelines for taking mammograms [5], the breast is pulled gently away from the chest wall before compression so that all tissues can be seen without any folding. We define the breast shape when it satisfies this condition as the canonical shape, since it is close to the intrinsic shape of the breast without the effect of gravity. From the observation that the outlines of CC and MLO

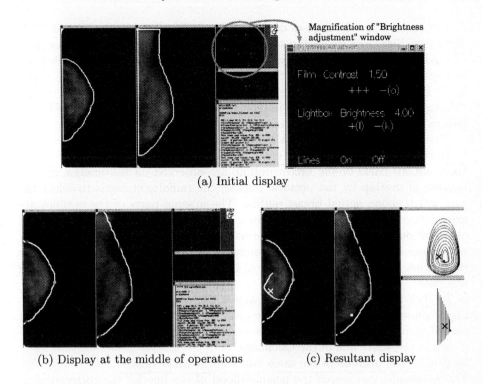

(a) Initial display

(b) Display at the middle of operations   (c) Resultant display

Fig. 4. Interface of the proposed system

images are, respectively, close in shape to the horizontal and vertical contours of the breast in this canonical state, the canonical shape can be reconstructed automatically from the outlines, as shown in Fig. 2.

The simulation of breast deformation caused by compression and uncompression is realized by the model proposed in [1], which calculates the position of any point of the breast under compression from its original position in the canonical state, and vice versa, as shown in Fig. 3a. Although in the previous paper [1], the distance from the nipple to the chest wall was assumed to be fixed during the compression, we observed that in practice the change in the distance caused by compression can be significant. Therefore, we have improved the compression model so that it can take account of the expansion of the horizontal cross section. The expansion rate, which is b/a in Fig. 3b, depends on the individual and the strength of compression. In comparison with the 3D breast shape of the corresponding MRI data, we currently select 1.1 as the average rate and use this value for all the experiments in this paper.

2.2   Operation

The data necessary as inputs to the system are the CC and MLO images of the same breast, as well as the angular separation between the CC and MLO directions, and the thicknesses of the compressed breast in the CC and MLO directions. Figure 4a shows the screen at the start. The left two windows show CC and MLO images respectively. Their brightness and contrast can be changed by clicking "+" and "-" in the "Brightness adjustment" window on the upper right. Beneath this window, the user can always see what to do next in the "Messages" window. White lines in the images are the outlines of possible breast regions which are automatically extracted[7].

The operation required of the radiologist is as follows:

1) To click edge points of breast outlines and the nipple positions.

Since not all parts of the breast outline are observed on the images, mainly because of overlap by the pectoral muscle, the radiologist needs to select the part which shows actual breast outline. The missing parts of the outlines are extrapolated by simple extension from the tangent to the adjoining part of the observed outline. As a result, the breast outlines are fixed as shown by the white lines in Fig.4b. The six gray points on the lines are points clicked by the radiologist. The 3D canonical shape of the breast is reconstructed from these two lines.

2) To click the position of a lesion in any of CC/MLO images.

Fig.4c shows an example in which the position illustrated by the white point in the MLO image was clicked. Within a second, the epipolar curve is displayed as shown in the white line in the CC image.

3) To click the position of the same lesion in the other image.

The radiologist can search the neighborhood of the line for the corresponding point. In the example shown in Fig. 4c, the position illustrated by the white cross was clicked. In one second, the estimated 3D position of the lesion is displayed in the right-hand two windows and marked with crosses in the top and side views of the 3D canonical shape.

If there is more than one lesion in the images, as is quite often the case, the radiologist can successively input the next lesion and can repeat steps 2) and 3). Although we show the images here in black-and-white, the windows are actually displayed using color marks.

3   Experiment

In general, it is difficult even for radiologists to determine accurate correspondences between the CC and MLO images. However, radiologists can determine some correspondences with confidence, based largely on the similarity of the intensity patterns in the two images. We have gathered five lesions for which correspondences between the CC and MLO images were known, and in such a way that the lesion is also observed in MRI data. We then applied our method to the lesions.

Regarding the prediction of the correspondence in the other image, the minimum distances from the correct position to the resultant epipolar curve are measured and listed in Table 1. The second column, CC→MLO is the case where the radiologist inputs the lesion in the CC image first, and then the sys-

Table 1   Minimum distance between the correct position and the resultant epipolar curve measured in pixels (0.3mm) in 600 × 800 images.

No.	CC→MLO	MLO→CC
1	24.3	2.0
2	2.4	0.6
3	22.5	18.3
4	2.1	1.8
5	80.0	37.5

Table 2   Relative 3D position of lesions to the nipple: Euclidean distance(x, y, z)(mm)(refer the 3D coordinates in Fig. 3)

No.	A: CC→MLO	B: MLO→CC	C: MRI	C-(A+B)/2
1	39.3(-5.6, -14.8, 36.0)	38.2(-9.3, -14.1, 34.3)	43.0(-37.5, -3.7, 20.7)	4.3(-30.1, 10.8, -14.4)
2	44.3(-27.3, 18.6, -29.5)	43.5(-27.8, 18.2, -28.1)	55.7(-51.3, 15.0, -15.5)	11.8(-23.8, -3.4, 13.3)
3	31.6(-26.9, 12.2, 11.1)	27.1(-24.0, 9.5, 8.3)	33.6(-31.7, 10.4, -4.2)	4.2(-6.3, -0.45, -13.9)
4	71.6(-51.7, 40.9, 27.9)	67.5(-44.1, 42.2, 28.9)	73.6(-72.4, 6.5, -11.8)	4.0(-24.5, -35.1, -40.2)
5	68.2(-16.6, 34.5, 56.2)	88.8(-29.5, 34.0, 76.5)	73.3 (-59.7, 23.0, 35.7)	-5.2(-36.7, -11.3, -30.7)

tem predicts the position in the MLO image, and vice versa for MLO→CC in the third column. As shown in the table, apart from case 5, the system gives good predictions which are less than 7.5 mm (25 pixels).

Fig. 5a and b show the best (No.2 in Table 1 & 2)and the worst (No.5) results respectively. The left-hand figures show the results obtained by the proposed system, while the right-hand ones are the side and top MIP (Maximum Intensity Projection) images obtained from MR images and the 3D breast shape reconstructed from the outlines in the MIP images. Since the MR images are taken with the breast pendulous while the subject lies on her front, the 3D breast shape from MRI data is elongated by gravity in the direction from the chest wall to the nipple, that is, in the x direction in the 3D coordinates of the system (see Fig. 3). Therefore, the canonical shape of the system should be close to a suitably reduced shape of the 3D breast in the MRI in the x direction. From this stand point, in case No.5, the nipple position in the 3D breast reconstructed from the mammogram looks unnaturally low as the canonical shape. The reason why this occured seems to be that the breast was not pulled away sufficiently from the chest wall before compression for the MLO image and was compressed under the condition that the breast is elongated downward (the negative z direction of the 3D coordinates) by gravity. We infer that this causes the epipolar curve to be transformed downwards from the actual corresponding position in the MLO image. If the guideline for taking mammograms was adhered to properly when taking the MLO image, the nipple position could be further up while the outline is not so different from the current state. We simulated this case by intentionally giving a higher position for the nipple on the MLO outline as shown in Fig.6. As one can see, the epipolar curve gets closer to the actual correspondence.

The 3D positions of lesions found in the MR images are marked by a cross in both the MIP images and in the reconstructed 3D shape. Table 2 shows the distances and relative positions of lesions to the nipple. The second, third and fourth columns are respectively the results obtained by the system with the first

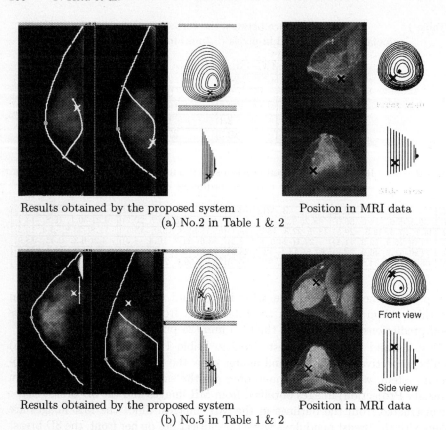

Results obtained by the proposed system   Position in MRI data
(a) No.2 in Table 1 & 2

Results obtained by the proposed system   Position in MRI data
(b) No.5 in Table 1 & 2

Fig. 5. Experimental results

input in the CC image and the second input of the corresponding position in the
MLO image, the results obtained by the system with the inputs in the reverse
order, and the values obtained from the MRI data. The fifth column shows the
difference between the MRI result and the average of the results by the proposed
system. On No.1, No.2 and No.3, the differences are under 15 mm apart from
the values of the x coordinates. One reason for the large difference in the x
coordinates is because the breast is elongated in the x direction in the MRI data
as noted above. Concerning cases No.4 and No5, their breasts are relatively large
so that their breasts have a "hanging bell" shape in the MRI data. The distance
of the nipple from the chest wall changes from about 75mm in their canonical
shape to about 90 mm in the 3D shape of the MRI data. These observations
show that the deformation from the canonical shape assumed for the breast
shape in the MRI data is too large to be ignored in these cases. Therefore, in
these two cases, comparison of the 3D coordinates appears nonsensical. This is
supported by the fact that the difference in Euclidean distances, which should
not be changed much by the effect of the deformation, is fairly small, less than

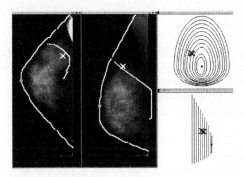

Fig. 6. Effect of the movement of the nipple

about 10mm, for all five data sets. From these observations, we conclude that the proposed system can estimate the 3D position in the canonical shape to about 10 mm error.

4   Conclusion

In this paper, we have described a developing CAD system for estimating the 3D positions of breast lesions found in two mammographic views. This is the first demonstration of a CAD system which enables the radiologist to obtain 3D information from a conventional pair of CC-MLO mammograms. Since some lesions are observed only in mammograms, this has considerable clinical significance.

From the experimental results, particularly the comparison with the 3D information provided by MRI data, the following two conclusions emerge. First, it is a necessary condition for applying this system that the breast is pulled gently away from the chest wall before the compression necessary for mammography, that is, in accordance with the established guidelines for taking mammograms. Since the effects of gravity on the soft, and sometimes heavy, breat tissue tends to prevent radiographers from adhering strictly to this condition, careful mammogram image formation is required, especially for MLO images. Second, we have concluded tentatively that the system achieves about 10mm errors in estimating the 3D locations of lesions. In order to assert this with greater certainty, however, we need more understanding of the breast deformation between the breast shape during MR image formation and its relationship to the canonical shape used in the system. This study is also important for the fusion of multi-modal data of the breast.

Acknowledgements

This research was partially supported by the Specific International Joint Research programme of AIST.

References

1. Y. Kita, R. P. Highnam and J. M. Brady: "Correspondence between different view breast X-rays using a simulation of breast deformation", In *Proc. of Computer Vision and Pattern Recognition '98*, pp. 700–707, 1998.
2. K. Doi, M. L. Giger, R. M. Nishikawa et al: "Recent progress in development of Computer-Aided Diagnostic(CAD) schemes", *Med Imag Tech*, Vol. 13, No. 6, pp. 822–835, 1995.
3. M. Yam, M. Brady, R. Highnam, C. Behrenbruch, R. English, and Y. Kita: "Three-dimensional reconstruction of microcalcification clusters from two mammographic views", *IEEE Trans. Medical Imaging*, vol. 20 no. 6, pp. 479–489, 2001.
4. W. J. H. Veldkamp, N. Karssemeijer, and J.H.C.L. Hendriks: "Automated classification of clustered microcalcifications into malignant and benign types", *Medical Physics*, vol. 27 no. 11, 2000.
5. E. Roebuck: *"Clinical radiology of the breast"*, Heinemann medical books, Oxford, 1990.
6. R. Novak: *"The transformation of the female breast during compression at mammography with special reference to the importance for localization of a lesion"*, ACTA radiologica supplement 371 Stockholm, 1989.
7. R. P. Highnam and J. M. Brady: *"Mammographic image processing"*, Kluwer Academic Publishing, 1999.

Analysis of Pulmonary Nodule Evolutions Using a Sequence of Three-Dimensional Thoracic CT Images

Y. Kawata[1], N. Niki[1], H. Ohmatsu[2], M. Kusumoto[3], R. Kakinuma[2],
K. Mori[4], H. Nishiyama[5], K. Eguchi[6], M. Kaneko[3], N. Moriyama[3]

[1]Dept. of Optical Science, Univ. of Tokushima,
{kawata, niki}@opt.tokushima-u.ac.jp
[2]National Cancer Center East,
[3]National Cancer Center, [4]Tochigi Cancer Center,
[5]The Social Health Medical Center, [6]National Shikoku Cancer Center

Abstract. This paper presents a method to analyze volume evolutions of pulmonary nodules for discrimination between malignant and benign nodules. Our method consists of four steps; (1) The 3-D rigid registration of the two successive 3-D thoracic CT images, (2) the 3-D affine registration of the two successive region-of-interest (ROI) images, (3) non-rigid registration between local volumetric ROIs, and (4) analysis of the local displacement field between successive temporal images In preliminary study, the method was applied to the successive 3-D thoracic images of two pulmonary lesions including a metastasis malignant case and a inflammatory benign to quantify the evolving process in the pulmonary nodules and surrounding structure. The time intervals between successive 3-D thoracic images for the benign and malignant cases were 150 and 30 days, respectively. From the display of the displacement fields and the contrasted image by the vector field operator based on the Jacobian, it was observed that the benign case reduced in the volume and the surrounding structure was involved into the nodule in the evolution process. It was also observed that the malignant case expanded in the volume. These experimental results indicate that our method is a promising tool to quantify how the lesions evolve their volume and surrounding structures.

1. Introduction

Physicians often wish to compare a sequence of thoracic CT images of the same patient and to analyze dynamical characteristic of pulmonary nodules. Computerized differentiation between the thoracic CT image sequences may assist physicians to detect abnormalities and to characterize interval changes in the known lung lesions. Though the correspondence between slice images of the nodule over time is interactively performed, the promising results for evaluating the likelihood of malignancy have been presented by using the sequence of thoracic CT images. Swensen et al [1] presented a technique based on differential enhancement of pulmonary nodules after the intravenous administration of iodinated contrast material to evaluate the likelihood of malignancy. Other group also demonstrated that the nodule enhancement was an indicator of malignancy based on the succession of

W. Niessen and M. Viergever (Eds.): MICCAI 2001, LNCS 2208, pp. 103-110, 2001.
© Springer-Verlag Berlin Heidelberg 2001

thoracic CT images [2]. Yankeleviz et al. presented a technique to evaluate nodule growth based on sequential thin-section CT images [3]. In their technique the nodule growth was assessed by comparison the image from the initial scan including the maximal area with the image form the repeat scan including the maximal area. This comparison was done by displaying the two image sets side by side. However, the thoracic CT images are not usually reproducible in terms of patient positioning, inspiration, and cardiac pulsation. The complexity of the lung deformation makes the analysis of sequential thoracic CT images difficult. In comparison with the existing approaches of deformation analysis of brain and heart diseases, few works have been done to address the problem of tracking interval changes in thoracic CT image sequences [4]. Fan and Chen [5] presented an approach to estimate volumetric lung warping and registration from 3-D CT images obtained at different stages of breathing. Their warping model was governed by a model derived from continuum mechanics and a 3-D optical flow.

The purpose of this study is to aid differential diagnosis of lung lesions through quantitative analysis of interval changes of the 3-D pulmonary nodule with respect to the internal structure of the nodule, the nodule margin characteristics, and the relationship between surroundings and the nodule. In this paper, we present an approach to analyze the displacement field of thoracic CT image sequences combining with 3-D rigid and affine registration, non-rigid registration, and vector field analysis. We apply our method to sequences of 3-D thoracic images with lesions to evaluate interval changes of 3-D pulmonary nodules.

2. Methods

2.1 Overview

The method consists of four steps; 1) The 3-D rigid registration of the two successive 3-D thoracic CT images., 2) the 3-D affine registration of the two successive region-of-interest (ROI) images extracted from two registered 3-D thoracic CT images, 3) non-rigid registration between local volumetric ROIs, 4) analysis of the local displacement field between successive temporal images. For the first step, we computed a rigid transformation between two successive 3-D thoracic CT images I_1 and I_2. We then resampled the image I_2 into I_2' to superpose I_2 to I_1 roughly. To avoid complexity of the whole lung deformation caused by a combination of body movement, heartbeats, and respiration, we interactively selected and extracted a local ROI image including a nodule of interest from the registered 3-D thoracic CT image. The ROI image was a cubic region (128x128x128 voxels). For both I_1 and I_2' the same location of the nodule center was interactively determined and the cubic region centering on this location was extracted. The ROI images extracted from I_1 and I_2' are denoted as F_1 and F_2, respectively. We then computed an affine transformation between two ROI images, F_1 and F_2, and we resampled image F_2 into F_2' to superpose to F_1. In our experiments we always resample the data into isotropic volumes before processing them. As previously ascertained by other researches [6],[7], the mutual information confirms to be a successful measure of goodness of fit for registration of images. Studholme presented that mutual information is not

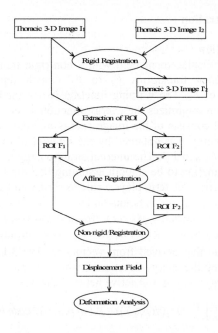

Fig. 1. Block diagram of the method.

independent of the overlap between two images and suggested the use of the normalized mutual information as a measure of image alignment [8]. We used the normalized mutual information as a voxel similarity measure. Next, we computed the non-rigid displacement between F_1 and F_2' using a warping function which maps F_1 to F_2'. The warping function is a displacement field represented by a 3-D array of displacement vectors. To design the warping function, we used the active net model proposed by Sakaue [9] for the extraction of a texture region. The active net model is a two-dimensional (2-D) elastic network model with is a 2-D extension of Snakes proposed by Kass [10]. This model deforms the net to wrap a target region minimizing the internal strain energy of the net and the image energy that attracts the net toward features such as edge of the target region. Witkin et al. formulated multidimensional matching and registration problems as the minimization of an energy measure that integrates a similarity term and a smoothness term of the deformation field [11]. Following their idea, the active net model also might be applied to estimate the non-rigid displacement by replacing the image energy with the integral of the density difference between the image sequences. In this study, we extended the active net into 3-D, which is called 3-D active net to estimate a volume displacement field between F_1 and F_2'. After computing the local displacement field between successive ROI images, we analyzed the displacement filed using the vector field operator based on the Jacobian operator [13].

2.2 Non-rigid Registration

2.2.1 Warping Function

We compute the 3-D displacement field with a non-rigid transformation based on a warping function which transforms F_1 to F_2' which represents as the affine transformation result of F_2. The warping function is designed by introducing a 3-D active net model which minimizes the energy functional and deforms elastically [9]. The energy functional consists of the image energy and the internal strain energy of the net. The image energy was obtained by the integral of the density difference of each voxels between F_1 and F_2'. The internal strain energy of the 3-D net constrains the non-rigid transformation to be smooth assuming that the local displacement field of the nodules is smooth. This term plays a role to shrink and smooth the 3-D net. By using three parameters, p, q, and r, points on the 3-D nets for 3-D images F_1 and F_2' are defined by $\mathbf{w}(p,q,r) = (x(p,q,r), y(p,q,r), z(p,q,r))$ and $\mathbf{v}(p,q,r) = (X(p,q,r), Y(p,q,r), Z(p,q,r))$ $(0 \le p \le 1, 0 \le q \le 1, 0 \le r \le 1)$, respectively. The warping function is given by a 3-D displacement field that derived from vectors $\mathbf{w}$. The 3-D displacement field is obtained by minimizing the energy functional, while the position of each vector $\mathbf{v}$ is fixed. The image energy term of 3-D active net is defined as

$$S(\mathbf{w}) = \int_0^1 \int_0^1 \int_0^1 (F'_2(\mathbf{v}(p,q,r)) - F_1(\mathbf{w}(p,q,r)))^2 \, dpdqdr \tag{1}$$

The internal strain energy of the 3-D active net is given by

$$R(\mathbf{w}) = \int_0^1 \int_0^1 \int_0^1 \frac{\alpha}{2}\left[\left(\frac{\partial \mathbf{w}}{\partial p}\right)^2 + \left(\frac{\partial \mathbf{w}}{\partial q}\right)^2 + \left(\frac{\partial \mathbf{w}}{\partial r}\right)^2\right] + \\ \frac{\beta}{2}\left[\left(\frac{\partial^2 \mathbf{w}}{\partial p^2}\right)^2 + \left(\frac{\partial^2 \mathbf{w}}{\partial q^2}\right)^2 + \left(\frac{\partial^2 \mathbf{w}}{\partial r^2}\right)^2 + 2\left(\frac{\partial^2 \mathbf{w}}{\partial p \, \partial q}\right)^2 + 2\left(\frac{\partial^2 \mathbf{w}}{\partial q \, \partial r}\right)^2 + 2\left(\frac{\partial^2 \mathbf{w}}{\partial r \, \partial p}\right)^2\right] dpdqdr$$

$$\tag{2}$$

where α and β are weighting parameters to control the first and the second terms. The first term results in the force to shrink the 3-D net. The second term makes the 3-D net shape smooth. Associated with the smoothness of the transformation R, the following energy functional of the 3-D active net is obtained.

$$J(\mathbf{w}) = \int_0^1 \int_0^1 \int_0^1 (F'_2(\mathbf{v}(p,q,r)) - F_1(\mathbf{w}(p,q,r)))^2 \\ + \frac{\alpha}{2}\left[\left(\frac{\partial \mathbf{w}}{\partial p}\right)^2 + \left(\frac{\partial \mathbf{w}}{\partial q}\right)^2 + \left(\frac{\partial \mathbf{w}}{\partial r}\right)^2\right] \\ + \frac{\beta}{2}\left[\left(\frac{\partial^2 \mathbf{w}}{\partial p^2}\right)^2 + \left(\frac{\partial^2 \mathbf{w}}{\partial q^2}\right)^2 + \left(\frac{\partial^2 \mathbf{w}}{\partial r^2}\right)^2 + 2\left(\frac{\partial^2 \mathbf{w}}{\partial p \, \partial q}\right)^2 + 2\left(\frac{\partial^2 \mathbf{w}}{\partial q \, \partial r}\right)^2 + 2\left(\frac{\partial^2 \mathbf{w}}{\partial r \, \partial p}\right)^2\right] dpdqdr \tag{3}$$

2.2.2 Implementation

As a practical computation, the 3-D net is approximated by a $n \times m \times l$ mesh;

$$\mathbf{w}(p,q,r) = \mathbf{w}(i\Delta n, j\Delta m, k\Delta l) = (x_{i,j,k}, y_{i,j,k}, z_{i,j,k}), \ 0 \le i \le n, 0 \le j \le m, 0 \le k \le l \quad (4)$$

where $\Delta n = 1/n, \ \Delta m = 1/m$, and $\Delta l = 1/l$. The grid points are placed on the cubic mesh. Each grid of 3-D net has 26-neighbors. The first term in Eq. (2) results in the force to shrink the boundary of the 3-D net. To prevent the boundary gird from shrinking, we fixed the position of the boundary nod of the 3-D net. We used an iterative technique [9] to obtain the 3-D active net that minimizing the energy functional in Eq. (3). The ROI images that we intend to match often contain vessels or bronchi with smaller diameter size than that of the nodule of interest. Therefore, we incorporated a hierarchical multiresolution approach in which the resolution of the mesh is increased, along with the image resolution in a coarse to fine manner.

2.3 Vector Field Operator

We characterize the obtained displacement field by using a vector field operator that transforms a 3-D vector field into 3-D scalar image. The value of each voxel in the scalar image varies with respect to the nodule evolution. Some vector field operators of the displacement field have been proposed. Thirion et al. proposed vector field operations based on the divergence and the norm of the displacement field [12]. Rey et al. pointed out that values obtained by their operators were hardly interpreted in terms of physical meanings and proposed another operator based on the Jacobian of the warping function that was derived from the displacement field [13]. They also demonstrated that the vector field operator based on the Jacobian provides a measure of evolution of a small volume. In this study, we adopt the Jacobian operator proposed by Rey. Let the value of the Jacobian operator at the point P be J. When $J > 1$, the evolution at the point P is considered as a local expansion and when $J < 1$, the evolution at the point P is considered as a local shrinking. When $J = 1$, no variation of volume at the point P is observed. The computation of the first derivatives in the Jacobian of the warping function was performed by using the recursive filtering proposed by Derich [14].

3. Results and Discussion

Thin-section CT images were obtained by the helical CT scanner (Toshiba TCT900S Superhelix) under the following conditions; beam width: 2mm, table speed: 2mm/sec, tube voltage; 120kV, tube current: 250mA. For the scan duration, patients held their breath at full inspiration. Per patient, about 60 slices at 1mm intervals were obtained to observe the whole nodule region and its surroundings. The range of pixel size in each square slice of 512 pixels was between 0.3x0.3 mm^2 and 0.4x0.4 mm^2. The 3-D thoracic image was reconstructed by a linear interpolation technique to make each voxel isotropic.

We present the application results of our method to two sets of successive 3-D thoracic CT images A and B. The data set A contains sequential 3-D thoracic CT

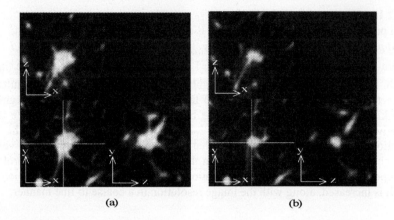

Fig. 2. ROI images of the benign nodule. (a) ROI image C_0 measured at T_0. (b) ROI image C_1 measured at T_1. Cross-sections for the xy-plane, yz-plane, xz-plane are shown.

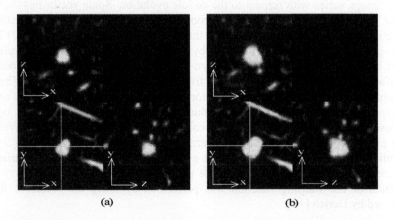

Fig.3. ROI images of the malignant nodule. (a) ROI image D_0 measured at T_2. (b) ROI image D_1 measured at T_3. Cross-sections for the xy-plane, yz-plane, xz-plane are shown.

images A_0 and A_1 of a patient with a benign nodule. These images A_0 and A_1 measured at different time T_0 and T_1, respectively. The period between T_0 and T_1 was 150 days. The data set B contains sequential 3-D thoracic CT images B_0 and B_1 of a patient with a malignant nodule. These images B_0 and B_1 measured at different time T_2 and T_3, respectively. The period between T_2 and T_3 was 30 days.

Figs. 2 and 3 show ROI images of benign (A_0 and A_1) and malignant (B_0 and B_1) It is observed that the benign nodule reduces its volume over time and the malignant nodule expands its volume over time.

We computed the displacement fields between two consecutive ROI images by using the non-rigid registration. Fig.4 shows the deformed grids of the benign and malignant nodules. It can be observed that the effect of a shrinking and an expansion of the grids for benign and malignant nodules evolutions. Fig.5 shows application

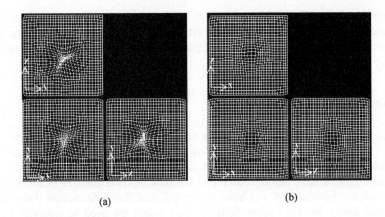

(a)   (b)

Fig. 4. 3-D Displacement fields. (a) Benign nodule. (b) Malignant nodule. Cross-sections of 3-D displacement field for the xy-plane, yz-plane, xz-plane are shown.

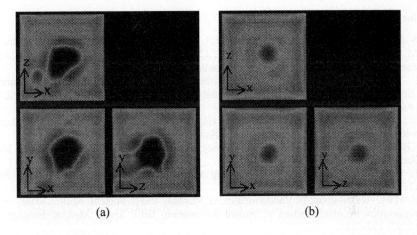

(a)   (b)

Fig.5. Applications of the vector field operator based on the Jacobian. (a) Benign nodule. (b) Malignant nodule. Cross-sections of 3-D displacement field for the xy-plane, yz-plane, xz-plane are shown.

results of the vector field operator based on the Jacobian. The more contrasted areas demonstrate the shrinking or the growing regions of nodules. From the display of the displacement fields and the contrasted image by the Jacobian operator, it is observed that the benign case reduces in the volume and the surrounding structure is involved into the nodule in the evolution process. It is also observed that the malignant case expands in the volume without deform the surrounding structure.

The application results of our method to the sequence of 3-D thoracic images demonstrate that the time interval changes of lesions can be made visible. Additionally, the experimental results shows that the displacement field computed by our method might be used to quantify how the lesions evolve their volume and surrounding structures by using the vector field operator based on the Jacobian. Real pulmonary nodules have a complex evolving process types such as tissue deformation, tissue displacement into other tissues, and combination of them. Still, the quantitative analysis of the displacement field of consecutive nodule images could aid physician diagnosis of indeterminate pulmonary lesions using only the static 3-D thoracic image.

4. Conclusion

We have presented a volumetric analysis method in evolving processes of pulmonary nodules by combining with 3-D rigid and affine registration, non-rigid registration, and vector field analysis. The application results of our method to the sequence of 3-D thoracic images have demonstrated that the time interval changes of lesions can be made visible. Additionally we have presented that the deformation field and the contrasted image by the vector field operator might be used to quantify how the lesions evolve their volume and surrounding structures. To analyze the capabilities of our method, we are collecting successive 3-D thoracic CT images from appropriate clinical cases.

References

1. S. J. Swensen, R. L. Morin, B. A. Schueler, L. R. Brown, D. A. Cortese, P. C. Pairolero, W. M. Brutinel : Solitary pulmonary nodule: CT evaluation of enhancement with iodinated contrast material - A preliminary report. Radiology, **182**, (1992)   343-347
2. K. Yamashita, S. Matsunobe, T. Tsuda, T. Nemoto, K. Matsumoto, H. Miki, J. Konishi, : Solitary pulmonary nodule: Preliminary study of evaluation with incremental dynamic CT. Radiology, **194**, (1995) 399-405
3. D. F. Yankelevitz, R. Gupta, B. Zhao, C. I. Henschke : Small pulmonary nodules: Evaluation with repeat CT – Preliminary experience. Radiology, **212**, (1999) 561-566
4. J. B. A. Maintz and M. A. Viergever: A survey of medical image registration. Medical Image Analysis, **2**, (1998) 1-36
5. L. Fan, C. W. Chen: 3D warping and registration from lung images. Proc. SPIE, **3660**, (1999) 459-470
6. F. Maes, A. Collignon, D. Vandermeulen, G. Marchal, and P. Suetens: Multimodality image registration by maximization of mutual information. IEEE Trans. Medical Imaging, **16**, (1997) 187-198
7. P. Viola, W. M. Wells III : Alignment by maximization of mutual information. Int. J. Computer Vision, **24**, (1997) 137-154
8. C. Studholme, D. L. G. Hill and D. J. Hawkes: An overlap invariant entropy measure of 3D medical image alignment. Pattern Recognition, **32**, (1998) 71-86
9. K. Sakaue and K. Yamamoto : Active net model and its application to region extraction. Journal of the Institute of Television Engineering, **45**, (1991) 1155-1163
10. M. Kass, A. Witkin and D. Terzopulos : Snakes: Active contour models. International Journal of Computer Vision, **1**, (1988) 321-331
11. A. Witkin, D. Terzopoulos, A.M. Kass : Signal matching through scale space, International Journal of Computer Vision, **1**, (1987), 133-144.
12. J.-P. Thirion and G. Calmon: Deformation analysis to detect and quantify active lesions in three-dimensional medical image sequences. IEEE Trans. Medical Imaging, **18**, (1999) 429-441
13. D. Rey, G. Subsol, H. Delingette, and N. Ayache : Automatic detection and segmentation of evolving processes in 3D medical images: Application to multiple sclerosis. Proc. Information Processing in Medical Imaging, IPMI'99, (1999) 154-167
14. R. Deriche : Recursively implementing the gaussian and its derivatives. INRIA Research Report, **1893**, (1993)

Intensity-Based Non-rigid Registration Using Adaptive Multilevel Free-Form Deformation with an Incompressibility Constraint

Torsten Rohlfing and Calvin R. Maurer, Jr.

Image Guidance Laboratories, Department of Neurosurgery, Stanford University
Medical Center, 300 Pasteur Drive, Room S-012, Stanford, CA 94305-5327, USA
{torsten.rohlfing,calvin.maurer}@igl.stanford.edu

Abstract. A major problem with non-rigid image registration techniques in many applications is their tendency to reduce the volume of contrast-enhancing structures [10]. Contrast enhancement is an intensity inconsistency, which is precisely what intensity-based registration algorithms are designed to minimize. Therefore, contrast-enhanced structures typically shrink substantially during registration, which affects the use of the resulting transformation for volumetric analysis, image subtraction, and multispectral classification. A common approach to address this problem is to constrain the deformation. In this paper we present a novel incompressibility constraint approach that is based on the Jacobian determinant of the deformation and can be computed rapidly. We apply our intensity-based non-rigid registration algorithm with this incompressibility constraint to two clinical applications (MR mammography, CT-DSA) and demonstrate that it produces high-quality deformations (as judged by visual assessment) while preserving the volume of contrast-enhanced structures.

1 Introduction

Non-rigid image registration algorithms [1,5,7] based on free-form deformations [3] have recently been shown to be a valuable tool in various medical image processing applications. However, a major problem with existing algorithms is that when they are applied to pre- and post-contrast image pairs, they produce transformations that substantially shrink the volume of contrast-enhancing structures. Tanner et al. [10] observed this for contrast-enhanced breast lesions and we have observed this for contrast-enhanced vessels in CT-DSA. This problem severely affects the usefulness of the resulting transformation for volumetric analysis, image subtraction, and multispectral classification.

To address this problem, an additional "energy" term is typically added to the intensity-based similarity measure to constrain the deformation to be smooth. Some authors use a mechanically motivated energy term that constrains the "bending energy" of the deformation [7]. A different approach uses "coupled" control points of the deformation to make the contrast-enhanced lesion locally

W. Niessen and M. Viergever (Eds.): MICCAI 2001, LNCS 2208, pp. 111–119, 2001.

rigid [10]. This approach of course requires identification of these structures prior to or during registration. Also, it prevents deformation of these structures even in cases where they have actually deformed.

In this paper, we present a novel incompressibility (local volume preservation) constraint based on the Jacobian determinant of the deformation. Soft tissue in the human body is generally incompressible. By penalizing deviations of the local Jacobian determinant of the deformation from unity, this knowledge can be incorporated into the registration process. The Jacobian has been used for analyzing non-rigid transformations [2,10]. This paper, as far as we are aware, is the first report of the use of this mathematical tool to enforce tissue incompressibility during the registration. We also introduce a locally adaptive deformation refinement and present some modifications to the implementation details of existing non-rigid registration algorithms. Both improvements lead to a substantial increase in computational efficiency.

We apply our intensity-based non-rigid registration algorithm using constrained adaptive multilevel free-form deformations to sample MR mammography and CT-DSA images and demonstrate that it produces high quality deformations while preserving the volume of contrast-enhanced structures.

2   Methods

General Registration Algorithm. Our rigid registration algorithm is based on an independent implementation [5,6] of a technique for rigid and affine registration described in Ref. [8]. It uses "normalized mutual information" (NMI) as the similarity measure [9]. In the first step, this method is employed directly for finding an initial rigid transformation to capture the global displacement of both images. The rigid transformation is then used as the initial estimate for the non-rigid registration. The non-rigid algorithm is an independent and modified implementation of a technique presented by Rueckert et al. [7]. It uses the same NMI similarity measure as the rigid registration. However, a different optimization technique (modified steepest-ascent line search [5]) is used to address the problem of the high dimensionality of the search space in the non-rigid case. In addition to the NMI similarity measure E_{NMI}, our technique incorporates an additional penalty term E_{Jacobian} to constrain the deformation of the coordinate space. A user-defined weighting factor ω controls the relative influence of E_{NMI} and E_{Jacobian}, combining both into the overall cost function E_{Total} as follows:

$$E_{\mathrm{Total}} = (1 - \omega)E_{\mathrm{NMI}} + \omega E_{\mathrm{Jacobian}}. \tag{1}$$

A description of the term E_{Jacobian} and its computation are provided below.

B-Spline Deformation. The non-rigid registration algorithm determines the set of parameters of a deformation **T** that optimizes the cost function in Eq. 1. **T** is defined on a uniformly spaced grid Φ of control points $\phi_{i,j,k}$, where $-1 \leq i < n_x - 1$, $-1 \leq j < n_y - 1$, and $-1 \leq k < n_z - 1$. Control points with i, j, or k equal to either 0 or $n_x - 3$ ($n_y - 3$ and $n_z - 3$ for j and k) are located on the edge of the image data. The spacings between the control points in x-,

y-, and z-directions are denoted by δ_x, δ_y, and δ_z, respectively. For any location (x, y, z), the deformation at these coordinates is computed from the positions of the surrounding $4 \times 4 \times 4$ neighborhood of control points:

$$\mathbf{T}(x, y, z) = \sum_{l=0}^{3} \sum_{m=0}^{3} \sum_{n=0}^{3} B_l(u) B_m(v) B_n(w) \phi_{i+l, j+m, k+n}. \tag{2}$$

Here, i, j, and k denote the index of the control point cell containing (x, y, z), and u, v, and w are the relative positions of (x, y, z) in the three dimensions. The functions B_0 through B_3 are the approximating third-order spline polynomials as described by Ref. [3].

The degrees of freedom of a B-spline based transformation are the coordinates of the control points $\phi_{i,j,k}$. In comparison to previous algorithms, ours does not consider these vectors to be offsets from the original control point positions with initial displacements of 0. Instead, we use them as absolute positions and initialize them as

$$\phi_{i,j,k}^{(0)} := (i\delta_x, j\delta_y, k\delta_z). \tag{3}$$

Thus, the actual coordinate transformation is $(x, y, z) \mapsto \mathbf{T}(x, y, z)$ rather than $(x, y, z) \mapsto (x, y, z) + \mathbf{T}(x, y, z)$. This makes application of the actual deformation computationally more efficient for two reasons: First of all, it immediately reduces the number of required real-value additions per transformed coordinate by 3. More importantly, $\mathbf{T}$ is linear with respect to the $\phi_{i,j,k}$. Therefore, an initial rigid transformation A can be incorporated by applying it to the control point positions ϕ:

$$(A \circ \mathbf{T})(x, y, z) = \sum_{l=0}^{3} \sum_{m=0}^{3} \sum_{n=0}^{3} B_l(u) B_m(v) B_n(w) (A\phi_{i+l, j+m, k+n}). \tag{4}$$

As a consequence, the computational cost for every transformed vector is reduced by the cost of a vector-matrix multiplication plus another vector addition. By implicitly applying the rigid transformation *after* the deformation, we ensure that this is mathematically equivalent to explicitly applying A (because computation of i, j, k, u, v, and w remains independent of A).

Deformation Constraint. The design of our deformation constraint is motivated by the observation that most tissues in the human body are incompressible. In a small neighborhood of the point (x, y, z), the local compression or expansion caused by the deformation $\mathbf{T}$ can be calculated by means of the Jacobian determinant:

$$J_{\mathbf{T}}(x, y, z) = \det \begin{pmatrix} \frac{\partial}{\partial x} \mathbf{T}_x(x, y, z) & \frac{\partial}{\partial y} \mathbf{T}_x(x, y, z) & \frac{\partial}{\partial z} \mathbf{T}_x(x, y, z) \\ \frac{\partial}{\partial x} \mathbf{T}_y(x, y, z) & \frac{\partial}{\partial y} \mathbf{T}_y(x, y, z) & \frac{\partial}{\partial z} \mathbf{T}_y(x, y, z) \\ \frac{\partial}{\partial x} \mathbf{T}_z(x, y, z) & \frac{\partial}{\partial y} \mathbf{T}_z(x, y, z) & \frac{\partial}{\partial z} \mathbf{T}_z(x, y, z) \end{pmatrix}. \tag{5}$$

The value of $J_{\mathbf{T}}(x, y, z)$ is equal to 1 if the deformation at (x, y, z) is incompressible, greater than 1 if there is local expansion, and less than 1 if there is compression. Since the 3-D spline is the tensor product of independent 1-D functions, its derivative with respect to x can easily be computed as follows:

$$\frac{\partial}{\partial x} \mathbf{T}_x(x, y, z) = \frac{1}{\delta_x} \sum_{l=0}^{3} \sum_{m=0}^{3} \sum_{n=0}^{3} \left(\frac{d}{du} B_l(u)\right) B_m(v) B_n(w) \phi_{i+l, j+m, k+n}. \quad (6)$$

The remaining derivatives are obvious. Computation of the entries of $J_\mathbf{T}$ is in fact very similar to computing $\mathbf{T}$ itself. Depending on the position in the matrix, the spline polynomial B in the respective dimension is simply replaced by its derivative. Using the above definition of $J_\mathbf{T}$, the incompressibility constraint penalty is defined as the normalized sum of the absolute logarithm of the local scaling divided by the global one:

$$E_{\text{Jacobian}} = \frac{1}{N_\Phi} \sum_{i,j,k} \left|\log(J_\mathbf{T}(\phi_{i,j,k}^{(0)})/S)\right|, \quad (7)$$

where $S = s_x s_y s_z$ is the total scaling of the initial affine (rigid plus anisotropic scaling) transformation A and s_x, s_y, and s_z are the scale factors in each dimension. This term penalizes deviations of $J_\mathbf{T}/S$ from 1, i.e., it penalizes local tissue expansion and compression. The motivation for using the log of the scaling ratio is to equally penalize a local scaling by cS and by S/c and thus achieve equal weighting of local expansion and compression. The penalty term is furthermore normalized by dividing by the number N_Φ of control points. This is necessary as during the application of a multilevel strategy the number of control points and therefore the number of addends in 7 increases by a factor of 8 per level.

Two properties of the penalty term E_{Jacobian} should be noted. First, the penalty term does not penalize rigid transformations with anisotropic scaling. Second, as $J_\mathbf{T}$ is evaluated only at the control points, the spline coefficients B as well as their derivatives take on particularly simple forms. For this reason, E_{Jacobian} can be computed very efficiently, which is important to keep execution time reasonable. The same is true for the discrete approximation to the derivatives of E_{Jacobian} with respect to the coordinates of any control point. For finite difference approximation to this derivative, a small offset ϵ is added to and subtracted from the respective parameter. E_{Jacobian} is then re-evaluated, yielding E_{Jacobian}^+ and E_{Jacobian}^-. As all addends in 7 outside a $4 \times 4 \times 4$ neighborhood of the affected control point are constant, they cancel out when $\Delta E_{\text{Jacobian}} = \frac{E_{\text{Jacobian}}^+ - E_{\text{Jacobian}}^-}{2\epsilon}$ is calculated. Computation can thus be restricted to the interior of the local neighborhood region.

Multilevel B-Splines. An arbitrary B-spline deformation can be refined to an identical deformation with the control point spacing in every dimension divided by 2. In the 1-D case, the transformed control point positions ϕ_i' of the refined grid can be computed from the coarse control points ϕ_i:

$$\phi_{2i+1}' = \frac{1}{2}(\phi_i + \phi_{i+1}) \text{ and } \phi_{2i}' = \frac{1}{8}(\phi_{i-1} + \phi_{i+1} + 6\phi_i). \quad (8)$$

This can be generalized to 3-D by applying the tensor product. For 2-D, the resulting explicit assignments are given in Ref. [3]; for 3-D they can be found in

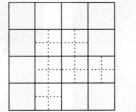 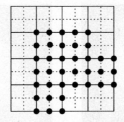

Fig. 1. Local (*left*) and global (*right*) refinement of the control point grid. Active control points are marked by • in the right picture.

Refs. [4,5]. However, it is sufficiently efficient and considerably more convenient to compute the tensor product on-the-fly using 8 rather than by applying the closed forms.

Grid Refinement and Fixed Control Points. Refinement of the control point grid by a factor of 2 per dimension increases the number of control points by roughly a factor of 8. The leads to a dramatic increase in computation time. However, not everywhere in the deformed image is the refined grid actually helpful. One approach is to refine the grid only in areas where small deformations could not be modeled otherwise (Fig. 1, left). However, for B-spline deformations it is difficult to preserve consistency at the transition from refined to unrefined grid cells.

We have therefore chosen an alternative approach that unites the power of multilevel deformations with the computational efficiency of locally refined control point grids. In fact, the deformation is globally refined. However, control points where there is insufficient local intensity variation (information) to meaningfully estimate finer deformation (e.g., control points in the image background) are fixed to their current positions. This means that their coordinates are no longer considered degrees of freedom of the deformation. Thus, they can be excluded from gradient computation and optimization. The only penalty still arising from the global refinement is the increased amount of memory required to store the locations of all control points in the refined grid. Computational efficiency is not affected by this as computation of the deformation is independent of the number of control points. In fact, as the globally refined grid is more regular than a locally refined one, the globally refined deformation can potentially be computed more efficiently than one defined on a locally refined grid.

Local Entropy. In order to determine which control points are fixed and which are considered variable, a local entropy criterion is applied. For each control point $\phi_{i,j,k}$, the entropy $H_{i,j,k}^R$ of the reference image data is computed over the region $D_{i,j,k}$ that is influenced by its position:

$$H_{i,j,k}^R = \frac{1}{|D_{i,j,k}|} \sum_{\mathbf{x} \in D_{i,j,k}} p(r(\mathbf{x})) \log p(r(\mathbf{x})). \tag{9}$$

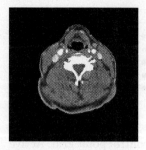 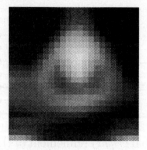 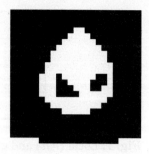

Fig. 2. Illustrative example of local entropy criterion. *Left:* Original CT image. *Center:* Local entropy in $4 \times 4 \times 4$ neighborhoods of the B-spline control points. *Right:* Binary image where feature voxels represent neighborhoods where local entropy is greater than 50% of the maximum. Control points where local entropy is less than 50% of the maximum (background voxels in the binary image) are fixed to their current positions.

Here, $r(\mathbf{x})$ are the voxels in $D_{i,j,k}$ and $p(r)$ is the probability of the respective grey value computed over all voxels in $D_{i,j,k}$. In addition, this local entropy is also computed for the corresponding region in the model image under the current deformation. Then, the maximum entropy over all control points is determined separately for the reference and the model image. Using these limits, a control point is fixed if and only if the local entropies associated with it are less than 50% of the respective maximum in the reference and model image. An example of this process is illustrated in Fig. 2. By considering the local entropies from both reference and model, it is ensured that the deformation remains active even in areas where one of the images has little structure as long as there is sufficient information in the other one.

3   Results

We applied the algorithm presented in this paper to two CT-DSA (head-and-neck and abdomen) and one MR mammography image data sets. Both types of study involve acquiring images before and after contrast injection. We registered each pair of images using rigid registration, unconstrained deformation, and deformation with the incompressibility constraint, and then computed subtraction images (post- minus pre-contrast). Figure 3 illustrates the results achieved using our technique in a subtraction image from one of the MR mammography data sets. The deformation algorithm started with a 40 mm control point spacing that was refined to 20 mm and then to 10 mm.

There is considerable artifact in the subtraction images obtained with rigid registration due to tissue deformation not captured by the rigid transformation. The unconstrained and the constrained non-rigid registrations produced subtraction images with substantially reduced motion artifact. Both non-rigid registration subtraction images visually appeared virtually identical, except that

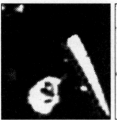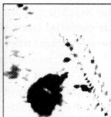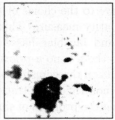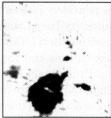

Fig. 3. *From left to right:* Original breast MR image (post contrast), subtraction image (post- minus pre-contrast) after rigid registration, after unconstrained deformation, and after deformation with the incompressibility constraint. The subtraction images are displayed with an inverse gray scale to produce a clear presentation in print. [Image data provided by Michael Jacobs and David Bluemke, The Johns Hopkins University School of Medicine, Baltimore, MD.]

contrast-enhanced structures (vessels in CT-DSA, tumor in MR mammography) visibly shrank in the unconstrained deformation subtraction images, but not in those obtained with constrained deformation. The shrinkage was quantified in the MR mammography study.

Volume Preservation. In the MR mammography image data set, the contrast-enhanced tumor was segmented (by region growing) in the stack of subtraction images used to generate the slices in Fig. 3. This allowed for the volumetric analysis of the different results. We found that after rigid registration the tumor occupied a volume of 4.46 ml. After unconstrained deformation, the tumor volume shrank by 27% to 3.25 ml. After deformation using the incompressibility constraint with a weight of 5×10^{-2}, the tumor volume remained virtually unchanged at 4.45 ml while still achieving the same visual artifact reduction. Using Jacobian weights of 10^{-3} and 10^{-2}, the tumor volume shrank only slightly to 4.31 ml. This reduction of 3% is within the estimated accuracy of the volume computation.

Computational Efficiency. Adaptive fixing of grid control points has two beneficial effects on the computation time. First, fixed parameters need not be considered for gradient estimation, thus directly reducing the computation time per optimization step. Also, the effective dimension of the search space is reduced, which decreases the number of optimization steps required to find the final solution. For typical image data, we experienced the fraction of fixed parameters to be somewhere between 30% and 60% depending on the ratio of object and background voxels. This lead to an observed reduction of computation time by at least 50%.

4 Discussion

We have presented a non-rigid registration algorithm with a novel incompressibility constraint. The Jacobian-based penalty term is effective and efficient. It is relatively insensitive to the choice of the weighting factor with respect to the intensity-based similarity measure. This is essential since the two terms in our cost function (NMI and Jacobian-based penalty term) are fundamentally different entities and thus there is no a-priori "correct" weighting.

Preliminary results on three image data sets suggest that incorporation of this constraint improves non-rigid registration of pre- and post-contrast images by substantially reducing the problem of shrinkage of contrast-enhanced structures. The energy term as well as its discrete derivative is easy to implement and can be computed rapidly. In fact, almost no performance penalty is experienced when using the Jacobian-based constraint. Our algorithm also incorporates locally adaptive multilevel refinement, which improves computational efficiency of the non-rigid registration.

5   Acknowledgments

The authors began this research in the Department of Neurological Surgery, University of Rochester, Rochester, NY. They gratefully acknowledge support for this work provided by the Ronald L. Bittner Endowed Fund in Biomedical Research. The authors thank Michael Jacobs and David Bluemke of The Johns Hopkins University School of Medicine, Baltimore, MD, for providing the image data shown in Figure 3.

References

1. ERE Denton, LI Sonoda, D Rueckert, DLG Hill, et al. Comparison and evaluation of rigid, affine, and nonrigid registration of breast MR images. *J Comput Assist Tomogr*, 23(5):800–805, 1999.
2. T Hartkens, D Hill, C Maurer, Jr, A Martin, et al. Quantifying the intraoperative brain deformation using interventional MR imaging. *Proc Int Soc Magn Reson Medicine*, 8:51, 2000.
3. S Lee, G Wolberg, SY Shin. Scattered data interpolation with multilevel B-splines. *IEEE Trans Visualization Comput Graphics*, 3(3):228–244, 1997.
4. T Rohlfing. *Multimodale Datenfusion für die bildgesteuerte Neurochirurgie und Strahlentherapie*. PhD thesis, Technische Universät Berlin, 2000.
5. T Rohlfing, CR Maurer, Jr, WG O'Dell, J Zhong. Modeling liver motion and deformation during the respiratory cycle using intensity-based free-form registration of gated MR images. In *Medical Imaging: Visualization, Display, and Image-Guided Procedures*, volume 4319. Proceedings of SPIE, 2001. (In press.)
6. T Rohlfing, JB West, J Beier, T Liebig, et al. Registration of functional and anatomical MRI: Accuracy assessment and application in navigated neurosurgery. *Comput Aided Surg*, 5(6):414–425, 2000.
7. D Rueckert, LI Sonoda, C Hayes, DLG Hill, et al. Nonrigid registration using free-form deformations: Application to breast MR images. *IEEE Trans Med Imaging*, 18(8):712–721, 1999.
8. C Studholme, DLG Hill, DJ Hawkes. Automated three-dimensional registration of magnetic resonance and positron emission tomography brain images by multiresolution optimization of voxel similarity measures. *Med Phys*, 24(1):25–35, 1997.

9. C Studholme, DLG Hill, DJ Hawkes. An overlap invariant entropy measure of 3D medical image alignment. *Pattern Recognit*, 33(1):71–86, 1999.

10. C Tanner, JA Schnabel, D Chung, MJ Clarkson, et al. Volume and shape preservation of enhancing lesions when applying non-rigid registration to a time series of contrast enhancing MR breast images. In *MICCAI 2000*, pages 327–337.

Mass Preserving Mappings and Image Registration

Steven Haker[1], Allen Tannenbaum[2], and Ron Kikinis[1]

[1] Department of Radiology, Surgical Planning Laboratory
Brigham and Women's Hospital, Boston, MA 02115
haker@bwh.harvard.edu
[2] Departments of Electrical and Computer and Biomedical Engineering
Georgia Institute of Technology, Atlanta, GA 30332-0250

Abstract. Image registration is the process of establishing a common geometric reference frame between two or more data sets from the same or different imaging modalities possibly taken at different times. In the context of medical imaging and in particular image guided therapy, the registration problem consists of finding automated methods that align multiple data sets with each other and with the patient. In this paper we propose a method of mass preserving elastic registration based on the Monge–Kantorovich problem of optimal mass transport.

1 Introduction

In this paper, we propose a method for image warping and elastic registration based on the classical problem of optimal mass transport. The mass transport problem was first formulated by Gaspar Monge in 1781, and concerned finding the optimal way, in the sense of minimal transportation cost, of moving a pile of soil from one site to another. This problem was given a modern formulation in the work of Kantorovich [15], and so is now known as the *Monge–Kantorovich problem*. This type of problem has appeared in econometrics, fluid dynamics, automatic control, transportation, statistical physics, shape optimization, expert systems, and meteorology [20].

The registration problem, i.e. the problem of of establishing a common geometric reference frame between two or more data sets, is one of the great challenges in medical imaging. Registration has a substantial recent literature devoted to it, with numerous approaches effective in varying situations. These range from optical flow to computational fluid dynamics [5] to various types of warping methodologies. See [17] for a review of the methods as well as an extensive set of references. See also [21] for a number of recent papers on the subject in the area of brain registration, and [14], [7] and [16] for representative examples of optical flow and elastic deformation model approaches.

The method we introduce in this paper is designed for elastic registration, and is based on an optimization problem built around the L^2 Monge–Kantorovich distance taken as a similarity measure. The constraint that we put on the transformations considered is that they obey a mass preservation property. We will

W. Niessen and M. Viergever (Eds.): MICCAI 2001, LNCS 2208, pp. 120–127, 2001.

assume that a rigid (non-elastic) registration process has already been applied before applying our scheme. For another application of such mass preserving mappings, see [11].

Our method has a number of distinguishing characteristics. It is parameter free. It utilizes all of the grayscale data in both images, and places the two images on equal footing. It is thus symmetrical, the optimal mapping from image A to image B being the inverse of the optimal mapping from B to A. It does not require that landmarks be specified. The minimizer of the distance functional involved is unique; there are no other local minimizers. Finally, it is specifically designed to take into account changes in density that result from changes in area or volume.

We believe that this type of elastic warping methodology is quite natural in the medical context where density can be a key measure of similarity, e.g., when registering the proton density based imagery provided by MR. It also occurs in functional imaging, where one may want to compare the degree of activity in various features deforming over time, and obtain a corresponding elastic registration map. A special case of this problem occurs in any application where volume or area preserving mappings are considered.

2   Formulation of the Problem

We now give a modern formulation of the Monge–Kantorovich problem. We assume we are given, *a priori*, two subdomains Ω_0 and Ω_1 of $\mathbf{R}^d$, with smooth boundaries, and a pair of positive density functions, μ_0 and μ_1, defined on Ω_0 and Ω_1 respectively. We assume $\int_{\Omega_0} \mu_0 = \int_{\Omega_1} \mu_1$ so that the same total mass is associated with Ω_0 and Ω_1. We consider diffeomorphisms $\tilde{u}$ from Ω_0 to Ω_1 which map one density to the other in the sense that

$$\mu_0 = |D\tilde{u}| \, \mu_1 \circ \tilde{u}, \tag{1}$$

which we will call the *mass preservation* (MP) property, and write $\tilde{u} \in MP$. Equation (1) is called the *Jacobian equation*. Here $|D\tilde{u}|$ denotes the determinant of the Jacobian map $D\tilde{u}$, and $\circ$ denotes composition of functions. In particular, Equation (1) implies that if a small region in Ω_0 is mapped to a larger region in Ω_1, then there must be a corresponding decrease in density in order for the mass to be preserved.

There may be many such mappings, and we want to pick out an optimal one in some sense. Accordingly, we define the squared L^2 Monge–Kantorovich distance as follows:

$$d_2^2(\mu_0, \mu_1) = \inf_{\tilde{u} \, \in \, MP} \int \|\tilde{u}(x) - x\|^2 \mu_0(x) \, dx. \tag{2}$$

An *optimal MP map* is a map which minimizes this integral while satisfying the constraint (1). The Monge–Kantorovich functional (2) is seen to place a penalty on the distance the map $\tilde{u}$ moves each bit of material, weighted by the material's mass. A fundamental theoretical result [4,10], is that there is a unique optimal $\tilde{u} \in MP$ transporting μ_0 to μ_1, and that this $\tilde{u}$ is characterized as the gradient of a convex function w, i.e., $\tilde{u} = \nabla w$. This theory translates into a practical advantage, since it means that there are no non-global minima to stall our solution process.

3   Computing the Transport Map

There have been a number of algorithms considered for computing an optimal transport map. For example, methods have been proposed based on linear programming [20], and on Lagrangian mechanics closely related to ideas from the study of fluid dynamics [3]. An interesting geometric method has been formulated by Cullen and Purser [6].

Let $u : \Omega_0 \rightarrow \Omega_1$ be an initial mapping with the mass preserving (MP) property. Inspired by [4,9], we consider the family of MP mappings of the form $\tilde{u} = u \circ s^{-1}$ as s varies over MP mappings from Ω_0 to itself, and try find an s which yields a $\tilde{u}$ without any curl, that is, such that $\tilde{u} = \nabla w$. Once such an s is found, we will have the Monge–Kantorovich mapping $\tilde{u}$. We will also have $u = \tilde{u} \circ s = (\nabla w) \circ s$, known as the *polar factorization* of u with respect to μ_0 [4].

3.1   Removing the Curl

Our method assumes that we have found and initial MP mapping u. This can be done for general domains using a method of Moser [18,8], or for simpler domains using a type of histogram specification; see [13]. Once an initial MP u is found, we need to apply the process which will remove its curl. It is easy to show that the composition of two mass preserving (MP) mappings is an MP mapping, and the inverse of an MP mapping is an MP mapping. Thus, since u is an MP mapping, we have that $\tilde{u} = u \circ s^{-1}$ is an MP mapping if

$$\mu_0 = |Ds| \, \mu_0 \circ s. \tag{3}$$

In particular, when μ_0 is constant, this equation requires that s be area or volume preserving.

Next, we will assume that s is a function of time, and determine what s_t should be to decrease the L^2 Monge–Kantorovich functional. This will give us an evolution equation for s and in turn an equation for $\tilde{u}_t$ as well, the latter being the most important for implementation. By differentiating $\tilde{u} \circ s = u$ with respect to time, we find

$$\tilde{u}_t = -D\tilde{u} \, s_t \circ s^{-1}, \tag{4}$$

while differentiating (3) with respect to time yields $\text{div}(\mu_0 \, s_t \circ s^{-1}) = 0$, from which we see that s_t and $\tilde{u}_t$ should have the following forms:

$$s_t = \left(\frac{1}{\mu_0}\zeta\right) \circ s, \quad \tilde{u}_t = -\frac{1}{\mu_0}D\tilde{u}\,\zeta, \tag{5}$$

for some vector field ζ on Ω_0, with $\mathrm{div}(\zeta) = 0$ and $\langle \zeta, n \rangle = 0$ on $\partial\Omega_0$. Here n denotes the normal to the boundary of Ω_0. This last condition ensures that s remains a mapping from Ω_0 to itself, by preventing the flow of s, given by $s_t = \left(\frac{1}{\mu_0}\zeta\right) \circ s$, from crossing the boundary of Ω_0. This also means that the range of $\tilde{u} = u \circ s^{-1}$ is always $u(\Omega_0) = \Omega_1$.

Consider now the problem of minimizing the Monge–Kantorovich functional:

$$M = \int \|\tilde{u}(x) - x\|^2 \mu_0(x) \, dx. \tag{6}$$

Taking the derivative with respect to time, and using the Helmholtz decomposition $\tilde{u} = \nabla w + \chi$ with $\mathrm{div}(\chi) = 0$, we find from (5) that

$$-\frac{1}{2} M_t = \int \langle \tilde{u}, \zeta \rangle = \int \langle \chi, \zeta \rangle. \tag{7}$$

Thus, in order to decrease M, we can take $\zeta = \chi$ with corresponding formulas (5) for s_t and $\tilde{u}_t$, provided that we have $\mathrm{div}(\chi) = 0$ and $\langle \chi, n \rangle = 0$ on $\partial\Omega_0$. Thus it remains to show that we can decompose $\tilde{u}$ as $\tilde{u} = \nabla w + \chi$ for such a χ.

3.2 Gradient Descent: $\mathbf{R}^d$

We let w be a solution of the Neumann-type boundary problem

$$\Delta w = \mathrm{div}(\tilde{u}), \quad \langle \nabla w, n \rangle = \langle \tilde{u}, n \rangle \text{ on } \partial\Omega_0, \tag{8}$$

and set $\chi = \tilde{u} - \nabla w$. It is then easily seen that χ satisfies the necessary requirements.

Thus, by (5), we have the following evolution equation for $\tilde{u}$:

$$\tilde{u}_t = -\frac{1}{\mu_0} D\tilde{u} \left(\tilde{u} - \nabla \Delta^{-1} \mathrm{div}(\tilde{u}) \right). \tag{9}$$

This is a first order non-local scheme for $\tilde{u}_t$ if we count Δ^{-1} as minus 2 derivatives. Note that this flow is consistent with respect to the Monge–Kantorovich theory in the following sense. If $\tilde{u}$ is optimal, then it is given as $\tilde{u} = \nabla w$, in which case $\tilde{u} - \nabla\Delta^{-1}\mathrm{div}(\tilde{u}) = \nabla w - \nabla\Delta^{-1}\mathrm{div}(\nabla w) = 0$ so that by (9), $\tilde{u}_t = 0$.

3.3 Gradient Descent: $\mathbf{R}^2$

The situation is somewhat simpler in the $\mathbf{R}^2$ case, due to the fact that a divergence free vector field χ can in general be written as $\chi = \nabla^\perp h$ for some scalar function h, where $\perp$ represents rotation by 90 deg, so that $\nabla^\perp h = (-h_y, h_x)$. In this case, we solve Laplace's equation with a Dirichlet boundary condition, and derive the evolution equation

$$\tilde{u}_t = \frac{1}{\mu_0} D\tilde{u} \nabla^\perp \Delta^{-1} \mathrm{div}(\tilde{u}^\perp). \tag{10}$$

3.4   Defining the Warping Map

Typically in elastic registration, one wants to see an explicit warping which smoothly deforms one image into the other. This can easily be done using the solution of the Monge–Kantorovich problem. Thus, we assume now that we have applied our gradient descent process as described above and that it has converged to the Monge–Kantorovich optimal mapping $\tilde{u}^*$. It is shown in [3] that the flow $X(x,t)$ defined by

$$X(x,t) = x + t\,(\tilde{u}^*(x) - x) \tag{11}$$

is the solution to a closely related minimization problem in fluid mechanics and provides appropriate justification for using (11) to define our continuous warping map X between the densities μ_0 and μ_1.

4   Implementation and Examples

We note that even though our non-local method requires that the Laplacian be inverted during each iteration, the problem has been set up specifically to allow for the use of standard fast numerical solvers which use FFT-type methods and operate on rectangular grids [19]. In practice, we found that the standard upwinding scheme was helpful for stability. For a local method in the 2D case, see [13].

We illustrate our methods with a pair of examples. In Figures 1 and 2 we show a brain deformation sequence. Two three dimensional MR data sets, acquired at the Brigham and Women's hospital, were used. The first data set was pre-operative, the second was acquired during surgery, after craniotomy and opening of the dura. Both were sub-sampled to 128x128x64 voxels and pre-processed to remove the skull. The Monge–Kantorvich mapping was found using the evolution equation (9) with intensity values as densities. This process took four hours on a single processor Sun Ultra 10. The warp function (11) together with (1) for the intensities were used to find the continuous deformation through time. The first image shows a planar axial slice, while subsequent images show 2D orthogonal projections of the 3D surfaces which constitute the path of the original slice.

The second example shows an application of our method to surface warping. We have used a colon surface here, but the method can be applied to any surface, such as that of the brain. Figure 3 shows a tubular portion of the colon surface obtained from a CT scan. We cut this tubular surface end to end and flattened it into the plane using a conformal mapping technique [12], as shown in Figure 4. It is well known that a surface of non-zero Gaussian curvature can not be flattened by any means without some distortion. The conformal mapping is an attempt to preserve the appearance of the surface through the preservation of angles. However, in some applications it is desirable to be able to preserve areas instead of angles, so that the sizes of surface structures are accurately represented in the plane. The Monge-Kantorovich approach allows us to find such an area-correct flattening. Specifically, once we have conformally flattened the surface, we define a density μ_0 to be the Jacobian of the inverse of the flattening map,

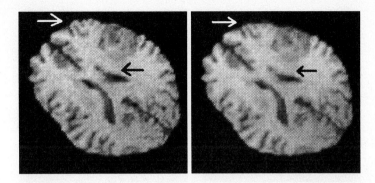

Fig. 1. Brain Warping: $t = 0.00$ (left), $t = 0.33$ (right). The $t = 0.0$ image was given, the $t = 0.33$ derived. The arrows indicate the regions of greatest deformation.

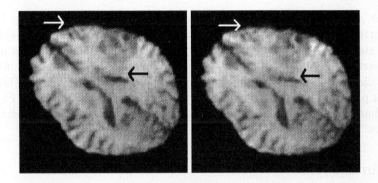

Fig. 2. Brain Warping: $t = 0.67$ (left), $t = 1.00$ (right). Both images were derived, the final $t = 1.00$ image to agree with the target volume according to (1). The arrows indicate the regions of greatest deformation.

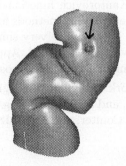

Fig. 3. Original Colon Surface. This portion of colon surface was extracted from CT data. The arrow indicates a phantom polyp. A shading scheme which highlights regions of high Gaussian curvature has been used.

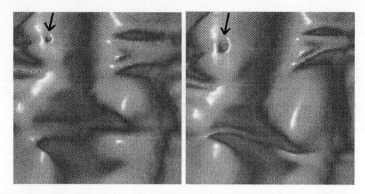

Fig. 4. Conformal (left) and Area Corrected (right) Flattenings. The arrows indicate the phantom polyp. The shading scheme is the same as in Figure 3. Note that the polyp appears in its true size in the area corrected mapping.

and set μ_1 to a constant. The Monge-Kantorovich optimal mapping is then area-correcting by (1). The resulting map took just a few minutes to calculate and is shown in Figure 4. Although corrected for area, surface structures are still clearly discernible. The curl-free nature of the Monge–Kantorovich mapping avoids distortion effects often associated with area preserving maps. There is a circular phantom polyp visible in the upper left corner of the images in Figure 4. Note that it is substantially larger in the area-corrected mapping, reflecting its true size.

5   Conclusions

In this paper, we presented a natural method for image registration based on the classical problem of optimal mass transportation. Although applied here to the Monge–Kantorovich problem, the method used to enforce the mass preservation constraint is general and has other applications. For example, any weighted linear combination of the Monge–Kantorovich functional and a standard L^2 energy functional can be used. Gradient descent methods for computing an optimal map in such cases can be derived in a manner very similar to that described above for the pure Monge–Kantorovich functional [1]. Applications of these techniques include brain surface flattening and virtual colonoscopy as described in [2,12].

Acknowledgments: This work was funded through NIH Grants PO1 CA67165, R01 RR11747, P41 RR13218, and an NIH training grant, as well as grants from AFOSR, ARO, MURI, NSF, Coulter, and NSF-LIS.

References

1. S. Angenent, S. Haker, A. Tannenbaum, and R. Kikinis, "On area preserving maps of minimal distortion," in *System Theory: Modeling, Analysis, and Control*, edited by T. Djaferis and I. Schick, Kluwer, Holland, 1999, pp. 275-287.

2. S. Angenent, S. Haker, A. Tannenbaum, and R. Kikinis, "Laplace-Beltrami operator and brain surface flattening," *IEEE Trans. on Medical Imaging* **18** (1999), pp. 700-711.

3. J.-D. Benamou and Y. Brenier, "A computational fluid mechanics solution to the Monge–Kantorovich mass transfer problem," *Numerische Mathematik* **84** (2000), pp. 375-393.

4. Y. Brenier, "Polar factorization and monotone rearrangement of vector-valued functions," *Com. Pure Appl. Math.* **64** (1991), pp. 375-417.

5. G. E. Christensen, R. D. Rabbit, and M. I. Miller, "Deformable templates using large deformation kinematics," *IEEE Trans. of Medical Imag.* **5** (1996) pp. 1435-1447.

6. M. Cullen and R. Purser, "An extended Lagrangian theory of semigeostrophic frontogenesis," *J. Atmos. Sci.* **41** (1984), pp. 1477-1497.

7. C. Davatzikos, "Spatial transformation and registration of brain images using elastically deformable models," *Comp. Vis. and Image Understanding* **66** (1997), pp. 207-222.

8. B. Dacorogna and J. Moser, "On a partial differential equation involving the Jacobian determinant," *Ann. Inst. H. Poincaré Anal. Non Linéaire*, **7** (1990), pp. 1-26.

9. W. Gangbo, "An elementary proof of the polar factorization of vector-valued functions," *Arch. Rational Mechanics Anal.* **128** (1994), pp. 381-399.

10. W. Gangbo and R. McCann, "The geometry of optimal transportation," *Acta Math.* **177** (1996), pp. 113-161.

11. A. F. Goldszal, C. Davatzikos, D. L. Pham, M. X. H. Yan, R. N. Bryan, and S. M. Resnick, "An image processing protocol for qualitative and quantitative volumetric analysis of brain images", *J. Comp. Assist. Tomogr.*, **22** (1998) pp. 827-837.

12. S. Haker, S. Angenent, A. Tannenbaum, and R. Kikinis, "Nondistorting flattening maps and the 3D visualization of colon CT images," *IEEE Trans. of Medical Imag.*, July 2000.

13. S. Haker and A. Tannenbaum, "Optimal transport and image registration," submitted to *IEEE Trans. Image Processing*, January 2001.

14. N. Hata, A. Nabavi, S. Warfield, W. Wells, R. Kikinis and F. Jolesz, "A volumetric optical flow method for measurement of brain deformation from intraoperative magnetic resonance images," *Proc. Second International Conference on Medical Image Computing and Computer-assisted Interventions* (1999), pp. 928-935.

15. L. V. Kantorovich, "On a problem of Monge," *Uspekhi Mat. Nauk.* **3** (1948), pp. 225-226.

16. H. Lester, S. R. Arridge, K. M. Jansons, L. Lemieux, J. V. Hajnal and A. Oatridge, "Non-linear registration with the variable viscosity fluid algorithm," *Information Processing in Medical Imaging* (1999), pp. 238-251.

17. J. B. A. Maintz and M. A. Viergever, "A survey of medical image registration," *Medical Image Analysis* **2** (1998), pp. 1-36.

18. J. Moser, "On the volume elements on a manifold," *Trans. Amer. Math. Soc.* **120** (1965), pp. 286-294.

19. W. Press, S. Teukolsky, W. Vetterling and B. Flannery, *Numerical Recipes in C: The Art of Scientific Computing*, 2nd Edition, Cambridge University Press, Cambridge U.K., 1992.

20. S. Rachev and L. Rüschendorf, *Mass Transportation Problems*, Volumes I and II, Probability and Its Applications, Springer, New York, 1998.

21. A. Toga, *Brain Warping*, Academic Press, San Diego, 1999.

Inverse Finite Element Characterization
of Soft Tissues

M. Kauer[1], V. Vuskovic[2], J. Dual[1], G. Szekely[3], and M. Bajka[4]

[1] Centre of Mechanics, ETH Zurich, 8092 Zurich, Switzerland
`martin.kauer@imes.mavt.ethz.ch`
[2] Institute of Robotics, ETH Zurich, 8092 Zurich, Switzerland
[3] Computer Vision Group, ETH Zurich, 8092 Zurich, Switzerland
[4] Department of Gynaecology, University Hospital, 8091 Zurich, Switzerland

Abstract. In this work a tissue aspiration method for the *in-vivo* determination of biological soft tissue material parameters is presented. An explicit axisymmetric finite element simulation of the aspiration experiment is used together with a Levenberg-Marquardt algorithm to estimate the material model parameters in an inverse parameter determination process. Soft biological tissue is modelled as a viscoelastic, non-linear, nearly incompressible, isotropic continuum. Viscoelasticity is accounted for by a quasi-linear formulation. The aspiration method is validated experimentally with a synthetic material. *In-vivo* (intra-operatively during surgical interventions) and *ex-vivo* experiments were performed on human uteri.

1 Introduction

Precise biomechanical characterization of soft tissues has recently attracted much attention in medical image analysis and visualization. Tissue elasticity can deliver valuable diagnostic information. Procedures as palpation have been used for centuries in medical diagnosis. On the other hand, current computer-assisted systems for medical diagnosis, therapy and training are increasingly relying on the availability of procedures allowing a realistic quantitative prediction of the mechanical behaviour of soft tissues.

Surgical navigation, as stereotaxy for limited access brain surgery [1] or image guided orthopaedic navigation [2] often relies on pre-operative images, which have to be aligned with the actual anatomy of the patient during operation. While efficient and precise algorithms have been developed for rigid registration [3], these can only be applied if organ deformation between the radiological data acquisition and the intervention can be excluded. Several studies underline the importance of duly considering elastic tissue deformation in neurosurgery [4] or even in orthopaedic applications [5].

Another area, where soft tissue modelling plays an important role is the development of virtual reality based simulators for surgery training. In addition to several academic research projects in the field of laparoscopic [6,7,8], arthroscopic

W. Niessen and M. Viergever (Eds.): MICCAI 2001, LNCS 2208, pp. 128–136, 2001.

[9] or eye surgery [10] simulators, e.g., a large number of commercial products is already available on the market.

The performance of the simulation in both application areas critically depends on the availability of appropriate methods for calculating soft tissue deformation. Besides highly simplified physically inspired models for laparoscopic training [6,7,11] or interpolative algorithms for landmark-based non-rigid matching [12], several attempts have been published to apply methods based on continuum mechanics. Finite element based simulation of soft tissue deformation has been applied both in surgical simulators [13,14] and elastic image registration especially in neurosurgical applications [15].

While the applied methods sometimes even allow fully volumetric modelling with non-linear effects [14], even the most sophisticated simulation algorithms are of limited use without precise information about the elastic properties of living tissue. Unfortunately, only very limited quantitative data are available about the biomechanical properties of soft tissues, especially for the *in-vivo* characterization of human organs. This is primarily due to the extreme technical and ethical demands on such experiments. In many cases direct access to the internal organs is necessary, which cannot be achieved during the usual surgical procedures without significantly disturbing or prolonging the intervention.

Most traditional methods of material testing like tensile experiments or compression techniques cannot be performed under such circumstances. Indentation methods have been used successfully for *in-vivo* experiments both on the skin [16] and on internal organs during surgery [17]. The resulting tissue deformation is sometimes measured by imaging techniques like ultrasound [18] or MR [19]. Surgical instruments have also been equipped with force-sensing capabilities allowing elasticity measurements [17,20]. These techniques have, however, disturbing drawbacks: they are restricted to one-dimensional testing, they lack well-defined boundary conditions during the experiment and often fail to address the viscoelastic properties of the tissue. MR elastography, allowing to spatially map and quantify small displacements caused by propagating harmonic mechanical waves [21] opened the way for volumetric non-invasive imaging of elastic properties in non-homogeneous organs. The resulting very small displacements (usually 1 mm or less) and the frequency range used do not allow, however, to predict the tissue behaviour in the range of the strains and strain rates observed during surgical interventions.

With the tissue aspiration method presented here we address the following targets: we generate well defined mechanical boundary conditions during the experiment, we are able to induce relatively large tissue deformations (depending on the maximum aspiration pressure) and the time dependent resolution of the deformation allows us to describe the viscoelastic properties of the tissue at a time scale relevant for actual surgical procedures.

2   Methods

2.1   Aspiration Experiment

In this work the experimental data used to characterize the soft tissues is acquired with a tissue aspiration experiment. The tissue aspiration instrument used is shown in Fig. 1. It was developed at the Institute of Robotics at the ETH Zurich. In the tissue aspiration experiment the aspiration tube is put against the target tissue and a weak vacuum is generated in the tube by connecting the aspiration tube to a low-pressure reservoir. A small mirror, placed next to the aspiration hole at the bottom of the tube, reflects the side-view of the aspirated tissue towards the video camera placed on top of the instrument. An optic fibre connected to a light source illuminates the tissue surface. The video camera grabs the images of the aspirated tissue with a frequency of approximately 25 Hz. The aspiration pressure is measured simultaneously with a pressure sensor. Only the profile of the aspirated tissue, represented by the outermost contour of the surface, is used to characterize the deformation. We assume that the experiment

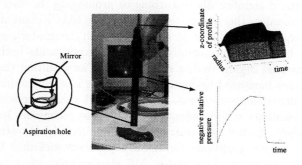

Fig. 1. Tissue Aspiration Experiment

occurs under axisymmetric conditions. Since tissues are in general anisotropic, the condition of axisymmetry will never be met exactly in the experiments. The resulting pressure and profile histories are the two data sets used to evaluate the aspiration experiments. With the profile data of the undeformed tissue a finite element model of the tissue surface is generated. The pressure data is applied to the surface of the finite element model as a surface load in order to simulate the aspiration experiment.

2.2   Soft Tissue Models

The soft tissue material models constitute a very important part of the simulation of the aspiration experiment. Due to their high water content soft biological tissues can be approximated as nearly incompressible materials. The following form of the strain energy function depending on the reduced invariants J_1, J_2, J_3 of the right Cauchy-Green deformation tensor $\mathbf{C}$ was used in an explicit displacement-pressure finite element formulation [21]

$$\bar{W} = \sum_{i=1}^{N} \mu_i (J_1 - 3)^i + \frac{1}{2}\kappa(J_3 - 1)^2. \tag{1}$$

The μ_i [N/m^2] are material parameters and κ [N/m^2] is the bulk modulus of the material. The degree of non-linearity of this constitutive equation can be determined with the parameter N. By setting $N = 1$ a nearly incompressible neo-Hookean material formulation results. The synthetic material employed in the experimental validation of the aspiration method and the human uteri are modelled with the strain energy function according to Eq. (1).

The viscoelastic material properties are modelled with a quasi-linear approach. The second Piola-Kirchhoff stresses $\mathbf{S}(t + \Delta t)$ at time $t + \Delta t$ in the material are additively composed of a purely elastic part $\mathbf{S}^e$ and a part incorporating the history dependence of the stresses

$$\mathbf{S}(t + \Delta t) = \mathbf{S}^e(\mathbf{C}(\mathbf{x}, t + \Delta t)) + \int_0^{t+\Delta t} \sum_{i=0}^{N_d} (c_i e^{-(t+\Delta t - s)/\tau_i} \frac{\partial}{\partial s} \mathbf{S}_{dev}^e(\mathbf{C}(\mathbf{x}, s))) ds \tag{2}$$

$$\mathbf{S}_{dev}^e = 2\partial(\sum_{i=1}^{N} \mu_i(J_1 - 3)^i / \partial \mathbf{C}), \qquad \mathbf{S}^e = 2\partial \bar{W}(J_1, J_2, J_3)/\partial \mathbf{C}. \tag{3}$$

The spectrum of $N_d + 1$ relaxation times τ_i with corresponding weighting factors c_i in Eq. (2) is used to model the viscoelastic material properties. Depending on the degree N of the strain energy function from Eq. (1) and on the number $N_d + 1$ of relaxation times used in the spectrum approximation of Eq. (2) the following material constants are determined by fitting the simulation of the aspiration experiment to the real aspiration experiment: $\mu_i, i = 1 \ldots N$ and $c_i, i = 1 \ldots N_d$. These parameters are grouped in the parameter vector $\mathbf{p}$. The bulk modulus κ of the material and the different relaxation times τ_i are not included in the parameter determination but set constant.

2.3   Inverse Finite Element Parameter Estimation

The employed material law represents the basis of the inverse parameter estimation. The material law is chosen according to *a priori* knowledge of the mechanical properties of the target tissue. The determination of the parameters contained in the chosen material law is then done by comparing the experimental and the simulated tissue profiles (Fig. 2). The quality of the match of the simulated data and the experimental data is measured by the objective function $o(\mathbf{p})$, which consists of the squared differences between simulated and experimentally determined profile data. The optimization algorithm searches for an optimal set of material parameters in order to minimize the objective function

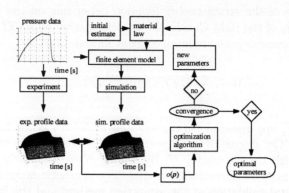

Fig. 2. Flow chart for parameter estimation algorithm

$o(\mathbf{p})$. The parameters corresponding to the computed minimum of the objective function are assumed to represent the real tissue parameters. From the many available algorithms for the optimization of the parameter vector $\mathbf{p}$ we chose the Levenberg-Marquardt method, which has already been shown to work well in finite strain applications [22],[23].

3   Results

3.1   Experimental Validation of the Method

An experimental validation of the aspiration method was performed on a synthetic material by predicting the behaviour in a tensile test with parameters obtained from the aspiration tests. Silgel, a very soft gel-like material, proved to be an ideal material to test the aspiration method. In tensile tests the neo-Hookean material formulation showed to adequately model the silgel material. The following four relaxations times are used to model the viscoelastic properties relevant for the stretch rates in the aspiration and the tensile experiments $\tau_0 = 0.036$ [s], $\tau_1 = 0.36$ [s], $\tau_2 = 3.6$ [s], $\tau_3 = 36$ [s]. The largest relaxation time $\tau_3 = 36$ [s] was determined by optimization from an aspiration experiment. The other relaxation times were equally distributed to obtain a good spectrum approximation. The values obtained for the different material model parameters from the aspiration experiment were then used to simulate tensile experiments. In Fig. 3 the force-elongation curves predicted by these simulations are compared to the corresponding experimentally determined force-elongation curves for different stretch rates. A good agreement between the predicted and the measured data is observed. A good material characterization with the aspiration technique was also possible by using only estimated values for the relaxation times τ_i.

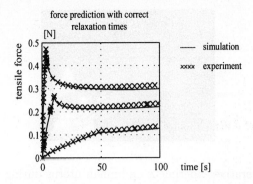

Fig. 3. Comparison of predicted force-elongation curves and experimentally determined data

3.2   In-Vivo Measurements on Human Uterus

The tissue aspiration technique was for the first time applied *in-vivo* on human tissue. In collaboration with the Department of Gynaecology of the University Hospital in Zurich intra-operative measurements on the human uterus were performed. From the continuum-mechanical point of view the uterus represents a very complex tissue. The uterus is a complex multilayered structure with strongly anisotropic properties. On the other hand it is of great advantage for us that the *hysterectomy* (removal of the uterus) is a quite frequently performed surgical intervention and we therefore have the chance to perform measurements on the organ before and after it is excerpted. In some of the cases the excerpted uteri show pathological changes. Three aspiration experiments are performed at different positions before the uterus is removed, then three measurements at the same locations on the removed uterus. The three positions are a ventral and a dorsal position and a position close to the fundus of the uterus. Due to the short duration of 20 seconds of the aspiration experiments the obtained material data is only valid for simulations within this time frame. Since we do not have any data regarding the viscoelastic relaxation times of the human uterus we use the following spectrum of relaxation times for our quasi-linear viscoelastic model $\tau_0 = 0.1$ [s], $\tau_1 = 1.0$ [s], $\tau_2 = 10.0$ [s]. The observed, strongly viscoelastic properties of the uterus would certainly require the inclusion of larger relaxation times in the material model but a robust determination of their weighting factors c_i calls for experiments of long duration which are not possible under *in-vivo* conditions. Tensile experiments performed by Yamada [24] on uteri of rabbits indicate a nearly linear stress-elongation behaviour of the uteri in tensile experiments up to extension ratios of 40%. We therefore assume that the human uterus mechanically behaves similar and use the following strain energy function to model the human uterus

$$\bar{W} = \mu_1(J_1 - 3) + \mu_2(J_1 - 3)^2 + \frac{1}{2}\kappa(J_3 - 1)^2. \tag{4}$$

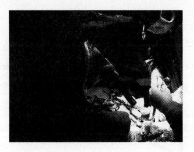

Fig. 4. Intra-operative experiment on human uterus during a hysterectomy

κ is set to $\kappa = 10^7$ [N/m^2]. Up to now *in-vivo* and *ex-vivo* measurements on six uteri were performed. These six measurements led to five data sets which

	location of performed aspiration experiment	μ_1 [Pa]	μ_2 [Pa]	c_0 []	c_1 []	c_2 []
uterus 3 in-vivo	ventral	1239	829	1.4	7.1	4.7
	dorsal	3044	1879	2.9	3.3	1.6
	fundus	3477	3580	0.5	5.0	1.8
uterus 3 ex-vivo	ventral	894	1306	1.7	3.4	1.9
	dorsal	708	3525	16.0	0.1	0.8
	fundus	754	2914	16.8	1.5	1.6

Table 1. Parameters for the polynomial material law obtained from the in-vivo and ex-vivo aspiration experiments performed on uterus 3

could be evaluated with the inverse parameter estimation algorithm, one data set showed too large a noise component. Stress-stretch curves simulated with the parameters gained from the aspiration experiments are shown in Fig. 5, the corresponding material parameters estimated for uterus 3 are given in Table 1. The time involved for one measurement is approximately one day where all the time needed for the preparatory work, e.g. for getting the patients' consent and having the aspiration instrument sterilized, is not counted here.

4   Discussion

The presented soft tissue aspiration method allows to determine the parameters of mechanical models for soft tissues under *in-vivo* conditions. An experimental validation of the aspiration method with a synthetic material showed that very good predictions of the material behaviour can be made also for states of deformation different from the one in the aspiration experiment. For the first time the aspiration method was employed intra-operatively under *in-vivo* conditions

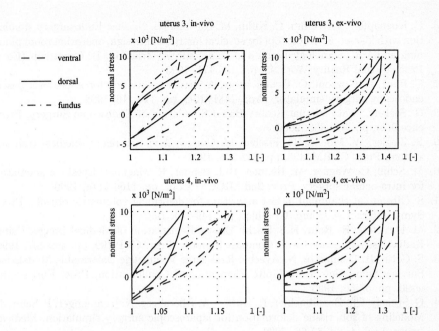

Fig. 5. Stress-stretch curves predicted with data from aspiration experiments on uterus 3 and uterus 4 at a stretch rate of ±0.02 [1/s]

on human uteri. A pronounced decrease in the uterine tissue stiffness was visible between the *in-vivo* and the *ex-vivo* measurements. The intersample variation of the tissue stiffness of all measurements seemed to be slightly higher than the stiffness variation observed on the single uteri. The maximum differences in stiffness observed in all performed measurements on the uteri were approximately equal in the *in-vivo* and the *ex-vivo* measurements. A statistical interpretation of the mechanical properties of the uterus does not seem appropriate due to the relatively small number of experiments performed.

References

1. H.F. Reinhardt: CT-guided real-time stereotaxy, Acta Neurochir. Suppl. (Wien) 46, pp. 107-8, 1989
2. A.M. Di Gioia, B. Jaramaz (Eds.): Medical Robotics and Computer-Assisted Orthopaedic Surgery, Operative Techniques in Orthopaedics 10(1), 2000
3. J.B.A. Mainz, M.A. Viergever: A survey of medical image registration, Med. Image Analysis 2(1) pp. 1-36, 1998
4. D.L.G. Hill, C.R. Maurer, R.J. Maciunas, J. A. Barwise, J.M. Fitzpatrick, M.Y. Wang: Measurement of Intraoperative Brain Surface Deformation under a Craniotomy, Neurosurgery, 43(2) pp. 514-526, 1998
5. J.A. Little, D.L.G. Hill, D.J. Hawkes: Deformations Incorporating Rigid Structures, Comp. Vision Image Underst. 66(2), pp. 223-232, 1997

6. U. Kuenapfel, H. Krumm, C. Kuhn, M. Huebner, B. Neisius: Endosurgery simulation with kismet, a flexible tool for surgical instrument design, operation room planning and VR technology based abdominal surgery training, B. Groettrup (Ed.), Proc. Virtual Reality World95, pp. 165-171, 1995
7. C. Baur, D. Guzzoni, O. Georg: Virgy, A virtual reality and force feedback based endoscopy surgery simulator, Proc. MMVR98, pp. 110-116, 1998
8. G. Szekely, et.al.: Virtual Reality-Based Simulation of Endoscopic Surgery, Presence 9(3), pp. 310-333, 2000
9. R. Ziegler, W. Mueller, G. Fischer, M. Goebel: A virtual reality medical training system, Proc. CVRMed95, pp. 282-286, 1995
10. M. Schill, C. Wagner, M. Hennen, H-J. Bender, R. Maenner: Eyesi - a simulator for intra-ocular surgery, Proc. 2nd MICCAI Conf, pp. 1166-1174, 1999
11. S. Gibson: 3d chainmail, a fast algorithm for deforming volumetric objects, Proc. Symp. Interactive Comp. Graphics, pp. 149-154, 1997
12. M. Fornefett, K. Rohr, H.S. Stiehl: Elastic Registration of Medical Images Using Radial Basis Functions with Compact Support, Proc. CVPR99, pp. 402-407, 1999
13. S. Cotin, H. Delingette, N. Ayache: Real-Time Volumetric Deformable Models for Surgery Simulation using Finite Elements and Condensation, Proc. Eurographics96, pp. 57-66, 1996
14. G. Szekely, Ch. Brechbuehler, R. Hutter, A. Rhomberg, N. Ironmonger, P. Schmid: Modeling of soft tissue deformation for laparoscopic surgery simulation, Medical Image Anal. 4, pp. 57-66, 2000
15. S.K. Kyriacou, D. Davatzikos: A Biomechanical Model of Soft Tissue Deformation with Applications to Non-rigid Registration of Brain Images with Tumor Pathology, Proc. MICCAI98, pp. 531-538, 1998
16. A.P. Pathak, M.B. Silver-Thorn, C.A. Thierfelder, T.E. Prieto: A rate-controlled indentor for in vivo analysis of residual limb tissues, IEEE Trans. Rehab. Eng. 6(1), pp. 12-20, 1998
17. F.J. Carter, T.G. Frank, P.J. Davies, D. McLean, A. Cuschieri: Biomechanical Testing of Intra-abdominal Soft Tissues, Med. Image Analysis, in press
18. J. Ophir, I. Cespedes, P. Ponnekanti, Y. Yazdi, X. Li: Elastography, a quantitative method for imaging the elasticity of biological tissues, Ultrasonic Imaging 13, pp. 111-134, 1991
19. J.B. Fowlkes et.al.: Magnetic resonance imaging techniques for detection of elasticity variation, Med. Phys 22(11), Pt. 1, pp. 1771-1778, 1995
20. R. Muthupillai, D.J. Lomas, P.J. Rossman, J.F.Greenleaf, A. Manduca, R.L. Ehman: Magnetic Resonance Elastography by Direct Visualization of Propagating Acoustic Strain Waves, Science 269, 99. 1854-1857, 1995
21. T. Sussman, K.J. Bathe: A Finite Element Formulation for Nonlinear Incompressible Elastic and Inelastic Analysis, Journal Computers & Structures, Vol. 26, pp. 357-409, 1987
22. S. K. Kyriacou, C. Schwab, J. D. Humphrey: Finite Element Analysis of Nonlinear Orthotropic Hyperelastic Membranes, Computational Mechanics, Vol. 18, pp. 269-278, 1996
23. M. J. Moulton, L. L. Creswell, R. L. Actis, K. W. Myers, M. W. Vannier, B. A. Szab, M. K. Pasque, An Inverse Approach to Determining Myocardial Material Properties, Journal of Biomechanics, Vol. 28, pp. 935-948, 1995
24. H. Yamada, Strength of Biological Materials, The William & Wilkins Company, Baltimore, 1970

A Microsurgery Simulation System

Joel Brown[1], Kevin Montgomery[2], Jean-Claude Latombe[1], and
Michael Stephanides[2]

[1] Computer Science Department, Stanford University
[2] Department of Surgery, Stanford University

Abstract. Computer systems for surgical planning and training are
poised to greatly impact the traditional versions of these tasks. These
systems provide an opportunity to learn surgical techniques with lower
costs and lower risks. We have developed a virtual environment for the
graphical visualization of complex surgical objects and real-time interaction with these objects using real surgical tools. An application for
microsurgical training, in which the user sutures together virtual blood
vessels, has been developed. This application demonstrates many facets
of our system, including deformable object simulation, tool interactions,
collision detection, and suture simulation. Here we present a broad outline of the system, which can be generalized for any anastomosis or other
procedures, and a detailed look at the components of the microsurgery
simulation.

1 Introduction

As computer power and graphics capabilities continue to increase, there is growing interest in surgical simulation as a technique to enhance surgeons' training.
Such training currently requires cadavers or laboratory animals. A computer
simulation option could reduce costs and allay ethical concerns, while possibly
decreasing training time and providing better feedback to the trainees. However, for surgical simulation to be useful it must be realistic with respect to
tissue deformation, tool interactions, visual rendering, and real-time response.
This paper describes a microsurgery training system based on novel computer
simulation techniques. The system allows a user to interact with models of deformable tissues using real surgical instruments mounted on trackers. It generates
a graphic rendering of the tissue deformations in real-time. Its key components
are new algorithms for fast and realistic simulation of tissue and suture, and for
detecting and processing contacts among rigid and deformable objects.

1.1 Related Work

Research on modeling soft-tissue deformation has increased dramatically in the
past few years, with focus on physically-based models for simulation. Terzopoulos and Waters [1] argue the advantages of using anatomy and physics rather
than just geometry for facial animation, and present a mass-spring model of

W. Niessen and M. Viergever (Eds.): MICCAI 2001, LNCS 2208, pp. 137–144, 2001.

facial tissue with muscle actuators. Joukhadar and Laugier [2] also use a mass-spring model with explicit integration techniques as the foundation of a general dynamic simulation system, and Baraff and Witkin [3] use masses and springs with implicit integration to simulate cloth. These mass-spring models are characterized by fast computation and simple implementation [10]. They can model in great geometric detail tissues that have nonlinear, non-homogeneous, and anisotropic visco-elastic properties.

Finite element models (FEMs) have been used in order to more rigorously capture biomechanical properties of human tissues. Works in [4,5] use FEMs to model facial tissue and predict surgery outcomes. The increased computational demands of finite elements are serious hurdles for real-time simulation. Numerical techniques, including pre-computation of key deformations, are proposed in [6,7] to significantly reduce computation. The endoscopic training tool of [8] describes a system which uses either mass-spring or FEM depending on the situation. The hybrid elastic approach of [11] combines aspects of both models in a simulation which allows deformation and cutting of tissues in real-time.

There are many other examples of mass-spring models and FEMs, as well as some alternate models, too numerous to cite them all here. The consensus is that FEMs can be very biomechanically accurate, but are not always appropriate for large deformations, or for real-time simulation of large geometries. Conversely, determining the proper parameters for mass-spring models can be very difficult, as can be determining proper placement of masses and springs to adequately model an object's volume. Surgical training simulation tends to rely more on visual realism than exact, patient-specific deformation (which may be more necessary in planning and predicting a specific patient's surgery, for example), and thus we have focused our research on mass-spring models, with an eye towards computation reduction for displaying complex virtual environments.

The need for suture simulation has been previously addressed in [12], and a performance study in [13] discusses the validity of using such a simulator to develop surgical skill, although it does not provide technical details of the actual simulation. More recently, [8] discusses many different aspects of suture simulation.

Interaction with virtual tools is another necessary component of any realistic simulator, and has attracted a fair amount of recent attention [9]. Surgical tools must not only be modeled accurately, but also pull, push, grasp, and cut other objects, often causing deformations by their actions. The first step of simulating such interactions is accurate collision detection, which has been studied extensively for rigid objects [16], although not nearly as much for deformable models. After detection, novel algorithms to handle collision response need to be developed to allow for a wide range of surgical actions [2].

1.2   Description of Microsurgery

Microsurgery is a well-established surgical field which involves the repair of approximately 1mm vessels and nerves under an operating microscope. It is a necessity in many reconstructive procedures, including the successful reattachment of severed digits. Using a forceps, the surgeon maneuvers a suture through the ends of two vessels, loops the suture around a second forceps, and pulls it tightly through itself to knot the vessels together. With several such stitches, the severed vessel can be repaired. Microsurgeons typically acquire their initial skills through months of practice in an animal lab, at which point they still require months of supervision in the operating room. Without practice, these skills can quickly degrade.

2   System Overview

Our software system includes a deformable object simulator, a tool simulator, and a collision detection module. A graphics display allows any number of objects to be rendered from a 3D virtual world onto the screen at 30 Hz or more. The user has complete control of the view, and may use stereo glasses for true binocular depth perception. The positions of the objects are read from the deformable object and tool simulators before each screen refresh.

Deformable object simulation is described in detail in the following two sections. Tool simulation synchronizes virtual surgical tools with real tools that are connected to external tracking devices. Virtual tools consist of one or more rigid parts modeled as triangulated surfaces. Their positions and orientations are controlled by the external devices at high update rates (typically 100 Hz), and other information from the devices may control relative rotations or translations of the parts that make up one tool. Interactions between tools and deformable objects, such as grabbing, poking, and cutting, are dependent on the collision detection module (Section 5).

The system also supports parallel processing using multithreading. Two separate threads of execution allow the simulation and collision detection to not conflict with the display. In this way, visual updates occur at a guaranteed rate while the simulation continues uninterrupted.

The setup for microsurgery includes two real surgical forceps instrumented to detect closure and attached to electromagnetic trackers (miniBIRD, Ascension Technology Corporation). The user's translation, rotation, opening, and closing of these forceps directly controls forceps models in the simulation. Using the forceps, models of blood vessels can be grabbed and deformed. A suture (needle and thread) can be manipulated to pierce through and realistically interact with the vessels and the forceps. Stereo glasses allow the necessary depth perception to complete the task. Figure 1a shows a user of the simulator.

3   Soft-Tissue Modeling

We represent the volumetric geometry of a deformable object by a 3D mesh M of n nodes N_i $(i = 1,...,n)$ connected by links L_{ij}, $i, j \in [1, n], i \neq j$. The nodes and links are grouped into triangles on the surface, for graphics purposes, but

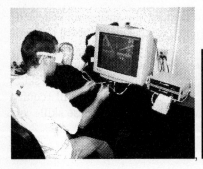 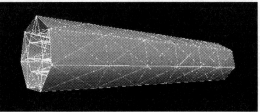

Fig. 1. (a) Setup for microsurgery (b) Shaded vessel shown with links

unrestricted below the surface. Each node maps to a specific point of the object, so that the displacements of the nodes describe the deformation of the object.

The viscoelastic properties of the object are described by additional data stored in the nodes and links of M. More precisely, a mass m_i and a damping coefficient c_i are associated with each node N_i, and a stiffness k_{ij} is associated with each deformable link L_{ij}. The internal force between N_i and N_j is $\boldsymbol{F}_{ij} = -k_{ij}\Delta_{ij}\boldsymbol{u}_{ij}$, where $\Delta_{ij} = l_{ij} - rl_{ij}$ is the current length of the link minus its resting length, and $\boldsymbol{u}_{ij}$ is the unit vector pointing from N_i toward N_j. The stiffness k_{ij} may be constant or a function of Δ_{ij}, and in both cases, $\boldsymbol{F}_{ij}$ is a function of only the coordinate vectors $\boldsymbol{x}_i$ and $\boldsymbol{x}_j$ of N_i and N_j. This representation makes it possible to describe objects that have nonlinear, non-homogeneous, and anisotropic properties.

At any instant of time t, the motion and deformation of M are described by a system of n second-order differential equations, each expressing the motion of a node N_i:

$$m_i\boldsymbol{a}_i + c_i\boldsymbol{v}_i + \sum_{j\in\sigma(i)} \boldsymbol{F}_{ij}(\boldsymbol{x}_i, \boldsymbol{x}_j) = m_i\boldsymbol{g} \qquad (1)$$

where $\boldsymbol{x}_i$ is the coordinate vector of N_i, $\boldsymbol{v}_i$ and $\boldsymbol{a}_i$ are its velocity and acceleration vectors, respectively, and $m_i\boldsymbol{g}$ is the gravitational force. $\sigma(i)$ denotes the set of the indices of the nodes in M connected by links to N_i. Some nodes may be fixed in space, or directly manipulated by surgical tools, in which case their positions are read from memory or computed from the positions of the tracking devices, rather than via (1).

To dynamically simulate the modeled tissue, we have implemented several numerical integration techniques to solve (1), including forward Euler, and second and fourth order Runge-Kutta solvers. These are all based on advancing the simulation by an amount of time Δt, and using the position, velocity, and force information for each node at time t to find positions and velocities at time $t + \Delta t$.

We have also developed a faster "quasi-static" algorithm, based upon the assumptions that the velocity of user-displaced nodes is small enough and damping large enough that the mesh achieves static equilibrium at each instant. These assumptions are reasonable for many human-body tissues and surgical operations on these tissues. Under these assumptions we can neglect dynamic inertial and damping forces, and compute the current shape of M by solving this system of equations:

$$\sum_{j \in \sigma(i)} F_{ij}(x_i, x_j) - m_i g = 0 \tag{2}$$

The reduced computation can be a significant savings in the many situations where the quasistatic assumptions are appropriate.

We let I be the set of indices of all variable nodes (those which are not fixed in space or directly grasped by the user), and let f_i be the total force acting on each variable node, $f_i = \sum_{j \in \sigma(i)} F_{ij} - m_i g$. An iterative algorithm for solving (2) at real-time animation rates is as follows:

1. Compute positions of user-displaced nodes from positions of tracking devices
2. Repeat until 1/30 sec. has elapsed:
   For every $i \in I$:
   (a) Update f_i based on (2): $f_i \leftarrow \sum_{j \in \sigma(i)} F_{ij} - m_i g$
   (b) Update x_i based on the force f_i: $x_i \leftarrow x_i + \alpha f_i$

Ideally, the value of α is chosen as large as possible such that the iteration converges, and the values f_i approach $\mathbf{0}$ before each redraw. This choice is typically determined by experimental trials. By performing rendering in a separate thread, the entire time interval is used for computing the equilibrium positions x_i of the nodes. By ordering the indices in I in a breadth-first manner starting at the user-displaced nodes, and proceeding along links in the mesh, forces converge faster. In addition, we can handle objects with many more nodes by limiting the deformation region to only those nodes within a certain distance of the user-displaced nodes, or by cutting off propagation when forces drop below a certain threshold.

The vessels in our simulation are modeled as double-hulled cylinders, with the inner and outer cylinders representing the thickness of the vessel. Each cylinder consists of several layers of nodes, with the layers evenly spaced, and each layer consists of several nodes evenly spaced around a circle. Each node is connected by deformable links to its neighbors within a layer and in neighboring layers. There are also connections between the inner and outer cylinders, which provide torsional stability, preventing the vessel from twisting around its long axis. The end layers of each vessel are fixed in space, representing the fact that the vessels are clamped down during surgery, and only a portion of their length can be manipulated. Figure 1b shows a smooth-shaded vessel and its underlying links.

As the user displaces individual nodes of the vessels, the quasi-static algorithm described above is used to calculate the deformation. Figures 2a and 2b show some examples of deforming the vessels with forceps.

4   Simulation of the Suture

The suture is deformable but not elastic, so the above deformation techniques based on mass-spring models are not applicable. Instead it should behave as a needle and thread, which can stretch minimally if at all, and has a free-form shape which is affected by gravity and direct contacts. To achieve realistic deformation, we model the suture as an articulated object: many short, linear links (edges) are connected together at nodes which act as spherical joints. The joints allow two degrees of rotational freedom, while the edges are rigid and short enough that the suture shape appears smooth. By keeping the angles between the first few edges fixed, we can model a rigid needle at one end of the suture.

To model the motion of the suture, constraint-based techniques are used. Any node of the suture may be constrained by another object in the system. For example, one node might be grasped by a forceps, and thus its position is constrained by the forceps. If the suture has pierced through a vessel, a node will be constrained by the position of the vessel. Finally, if the suture is draped over another object, nodes will be constrained by that object.

The motion is then calculated in a "follow-the-leader" manner as follows: a constrained node N_i is moved by the constraining object from $x_{i.old}$ to $x_{i.new}$. Its neighbor N_{i+1} then computes its new position $x_{i+1.new}$ as the point a distance d along the line from $x_{i.new}$ to $x_{i+1.old}$, where d is the (fixed) length of the edge connecting N_i and N_{i+1}. The same is done for node N_{i-1}. This motion is propagated up and down the suture to N_{i+1}, N_{i+2}, ... and N_{i-1}, N_{i-2}, ... until the next constrained node or one end of the suture is reached. For nodes between two constrained nodes N_i and N_j, the preceding algorithm will compute two preliminary results, propagating from N_i to N_j, and from N_j to N_i. These results are averaged to give the final position.

Certain constraints are designated as *soft*, such as where the suture is piercing a vessel or draped over another object, whereas the forceps grabbing the suture is a *hard* constraint. The distinction is that the suture can slide over and/or through a soft constraint, changing which node of the suture is constrained. It may be the case that two constraints move in opposing directions and cause the suture to stretch between them. In that case, the suture will slide through a soft constraint to decrease the stretch, but will break if between two hard constraints (in real surgery, it is not difficult to break the suture by pulling with both forceps in opposite directions). Additionally, if the suture is pierced through a vessel and is pulled on both ends, the suture will pull the vessel, causing it to deform as in Fig. 2c. Figure 2d shows the suture pulling together the two vessels.

5   Collisions and Interactions

Almost all object interactions depend at some level on collision detection [16]. Grabbing is achieved by finding nodes colliding with the tip of the grabbing object (e.g. forceps). Piercing the vessel requires finding a collision between the needle edges and a vessel face. Draping the suture around another object also involves edge to face collisions (Figures 2e and 2f show the suture around forceps and vessel), and draping it around itself requires edge to edge self-collisions. Other interactions modeled by the system (although not specifically in the microsurgery simulation) include prodding one object with another (face to face collisions), and cutting one object with another (edge to face collisions).

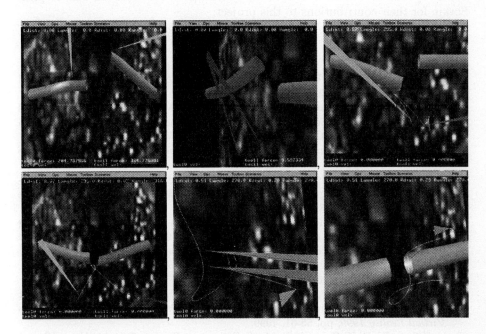

Fig. 2. (a)-(f): Scenarios for vessel, forceps, and suture interaction

The scheme we use for collision detection and distance computation is based on Quinlan's bounding sphere hierarchy [14]. This algorithm was extended by Sorkin [15] to allow for collisions between deforming objects by efficiently updating the bounding sphere hierarchies as these objects deform. We can comfortably find all collisions between forceps, vessels, and suture (including internal edge to edge collisions in the suture) at every redraw, without affecting the animation rate of the simulation.

6   Conclusions

By combining tool interactions, tissue deformation, collision detection, and high-resolution graphics, we have created a preliminary microsurgery simulation which has been exhibited to many plastic and reconstructive surgeons, and deemed realistic and potentially very useful. Our next step is experimental and clinical verification, by having surgeons who are learning the procedure use this tool, and assessing the quality of their virtual repairs through measurements such as angle and position of vessel piercing. We will then try to establish quantitatively how practicing with the simulator affects future quality of real vessel repairs.

Acknowledgements: This work was supported by NASA (NAS-NCC2-1010), NSF (IIS-99-07060-001), and NIH National Libraries of Medicine (NLM-3506). Special thanks also to Cynthia Bruyns, Frederic Mazzella and Stephen Sorkin for their contributions to this project.

References

1. D. Terzopoulos and K. Waters. Physically-Based Facial Modelling, Analysis, and Animation. *J. of Visualization and Computer Animation* Vol 1: 73-80, 1990.
2. A. Joukhadar and C. Laugier. Dynamic Simulation: Model, Basic Algorithms, and Optimization. In *Algorithms For Robotic Motion and Manipulation*, J. Laumond and M. Overmars (eds.), A.K. Peters Publisher, pp. 419-434, 1997.
3. D. Baraff and A. Witkin. Large Steps in Cloth Simulation. *ACM SIGGRAPH 98 Conference Proceedings*, pp. 43-52, 1998.
4. R. Koch, M. Gross, F. Carls, D. von Büren, G. Fankhauser, and Y. Parish, Simulating Facial Surgery Using Finite Element Models. *ACM SIGGRAPH 96 Conference Proceedings*, pp. 421-428, 1996.
5. S. Pieper, D. Laub, and J. Rosen. A Finite-Element Facial Model for Simulating Plastic Surgery. *Plastic and Reconstructive Surgery*, 96(5): 1100-1105, Oct 1995.
6. M. Bro-Nielsen and S. Cotin. Real-time Volumetric Deformable Models for Surgery Simulation using Finite Elements and Condensation. *Computer Graphics Forum*, 15(3): 57-66 (Eurographics '96), 1996.
7. J. Berkley, S. Weghorst, H. Gladstone, G. Raugi, D. Berg, and M. Ganter. Fast Finite Element Modeling for Surgical Simulation. *Proceedings of Medicine Meets Virtual Reality 1999*, pp. 55-61, 1999.
8. U. Kühnapfel, H. K. Çakmak, H. Maaß. Endoscopic Surgery Training Using Virtual Reality and Deformable Tissue Simulation. *Computers & Graphics*, Volume 24: 671-682, 2000.
9. C. Basdogan. Simulation of Instrument-Tissue Interactions and System Integration. *Medicine Meets Virtual Reality (MMVR2001)*, Newport Beach, CA, January 27, 2001, *http://eis.jpl.nasa.gov/~basdogan/Tutorials/MMVRTuto01.pdf*
10. S. Cotin, H. Delingette, and N. Ayache. Real-time Elastic Deformations of Soft Tissues for Surgery Simulation. *IEEE Transactions On Visualization and Computer Graphics*, 5(1): 62-73, January-March 1999.
11. S. Cotin, H. Delingette, and N. Ayache. A Hybrid Elastic Model Allowing Real-Time Cutting, Deformations and Force-Feedback for Surgery Training and Simulation. *The Visual Computer*, 16(8): 437-452, 2000.
12. H. Delingette. Towards Realistic Soft Tissue Modeling in Medical Simulation. *Proc. of the IEEE : Special Issue on Surgery Simulation*, pp. 512-523, April 1998.
13. R. O'Toole, R. Playter, T. Krummel, W. Blank, N. Cornelius, W. Roberts, W. Bell, and M. Raibert. Measuring and Developing Suturing Technique with a Virtual Reality Surgical Simulator. *J. of the American College of Surgeons*, 189(1): 114-127, July 1999.
14. S. Quinlan. Efficient Distance Computation Between Non-Convex Objects. *Proc. IEEE Int. Conf. On Robotics and Automation*, pp. 3324-3329, 1994.
15. S. Sorkin. *Distance Computing Between Deformable Objects*. Honors Thesis, Computer Sc. Dept., Stanford University, June 2000.
16. M. Lin and S. Gottschalk. Collision Detection Between Geometric Models: A Survey. *Proc. of IMA Conference on Mathematics of Surfaces*, pp. 37-56, 1998.

A Surgery Simulation Supporting Cuts and Finite Element Deformation

Han-Wen Nienhuys and A. Frank van der Stappen

Institute of Information and Computing Sciences, Utrecht University
PO Box 80089, 3508 TB Utrecht, The Netherlands
{hanwen,frankst}@cs.uu.nl

Abstract. Interactive surgery simulations have conflicting requirements of speed and accuracy. In this paper we show how to combine a relatively accurate deformation model—the Finite Element (FE) method—and interactive cutting without requiring expensive matrix updates or precomputation. Our approach uses an iterative algorithm for an interactive linear FE deformation simulation. The iterative process requires no global precomputation, so runtime changes of the mesh, i.e. cuts, can be simulated efficiently. Cuts are performed along faces of the mesh; this prevents growth of the mesh. We present a provably correct method for changing the mesh topology, and a satisfactory heuristic for determining along which faces to perform cuts. Nodes within the mesh are relocated to align the mesh with a virtual scalpel. This prevents a jagged surface appearance, but also generates degeneracies, which are removed afterwards.

1   Introduction

In a surgery simulator, surgeons can train surgical procedures on virtual patients. Such simulators offer a promise of reducing costs and risks when training surgeons. A training simulation can only replace training on live patients if it is realistic enough, and it can only reduce costs if it does not require big resources. Hence, the challenge in virtual surgery is to produce higher realism with as little computing resources as possible.

A full-fledged interactive surgery simulator consists of a core system that computes tissue response to surgical manipulations. It is supported by a display system for visual output and a force-feedback device for haptic output. The underlying problems in the core system, i.e. the soft tissue simulation, form the focus of our research.

A soft tissue simulation must provide convincingly accurate visual and haptic response to manipulations such as poking, pulling, cutting and cautering. We have chosen to simulate the elastic manipulations using the Finite Element Method (FEM). This method is based on a physical model of deformation, and solves the constitutive equations induced by that model. This makes the FEM potentially accurate from a physical point of view.

W. Niessen and M. Viergever (Eds.): MICCAI 2001, LNCS 2208, pp. 145–152, 2001.

We think that a physically accurate model will ultimately be preferable to ad-hoc heurististic models, such mass-spring models. Therefore we have chosen to use the simplest model available, static linear elasticity with linear geometry. Despite inaccuracies, we think that building a surgery simulation using this idealized model is a first step on the way to a physically accurate surgery simulation.

It has been suggested before that the FEM offers high fidelity tissue simulation. Bro-Nielsen [3], who first tried to use the FEM for surgery simulation, concluded that FEM is incompatible with cutting operations, because updating precomputed matrix inverses is too expensive for on-line operation. In our approach, we avoid these costly updates by using an iterative method that does not require global precomputed structures. To our best knowledge, this makes us the first to combine efficient cutting with an interactive FEM simulation [10].

Other prior work in deformation mostly uses heuristic models, such as Chain-Mail [11] or mass-spring models. These models are relatively straightforward to understand and implement, but they lack a rigorous physical basis. Recent advances have tried to incorporate aspects of the FEM into mass-spring models, blurring the distinction between these two approaches of soft-tissue simulation. For example, the hepatic surgery simulator project at INRIA uses uses a mass-spring model where the forces are inspired by linear and non-linear FEM, yielding what they call a tensor-mass model [5].

In the absence of cutting, full FEM implementation using matrix factorization have shown to be feasible. For example James and Pai [8] have produced interactive linear FEM simulations by removing internal nodes of the mesh. This is an algebraic procedure, and is more or less equivalent to precomputing a matrix inverse. Zhuang and Canny [12] achieve interactive non-linear deformation, also by matrix precomputations.

We combine the FEM for soft tissue simulation with algorithms for cutting. Since the deformation operates on a mesh, the cutting problem boils down to cutting in meshes. The basic problem with cutting in meshes is that one tetrahedron sliced with a blade does not yield two tetrahedra. The same holds for any other finite class of polygonal solids.

To accomodate cuts, the system has to contain routines that adapt the mesh to make cuts appear where a user performed them. Of course, this routine can only use a restricted set of shapes, e.g. tetrahedra. We have attempted to come up with an approach that does not significantly increases the size of the mesh. This is a desirable property, since the performance of the deformation simulation is directly proportional to the mesh size.

Earlier work solved cutting operations simplistically by removing those parts of the mesh that came in contact with a surgical tool [4]. In more recent work involving cuts, the basis is some deformable model defined on a tetrahedral mesh, with a subdivision scheme to accomodate cuts. Bielser was the first to demonstrate fully volumetric cuts, albeit with an expensive scheme [2] that was later refined [1]. Other efforts include a dynamic level-of-detail model [6] and other subdivision schemes [9]. A common characteristic of subdivision schemes is that they increase the mesh size, which degrades the performance of the simulation.

In this paper we discuss our FEM deformation scheme first. Then we discuss the cutting algorithm. We conclude with a discussion.

2 Finite Element Deformation

In the Finite Element Method (FEM), the material under scrutiny is subdivided in simple elements. If one assumes that these elements deform in a limited number of ways, then the behavior of the entire subdividision can be computed, yielding an equation that relates deformation and elastic force.

We have chosen a tetrahedral elements for the mesh. Such a mesh is the simplest mesh to allow arbitrary shapes to be constructed in 3D. In the linear elasticity model, the relation between displacements of the nodes in a tetrahedron τ and elastic force $\mathbf{f}_{v,\tau}$ exerted by that tetrahedron on a node v is linear. The total elastic force $\mathbf{f}_v$ on v then is the contribution from all tetrahedra incident with that node

$$\mathbf{f}_v = \sum_{\tau, \tau \ni v} \mathbf{f}_{v,\tau} \tag{1}$$

As can be seen, this quantity f_v depends only on displacements of nodes that are connected to v by an edge. Hence, we can calculate the elastic force locally for every node in the mesh.

The total deformation is determined by balancing all external forces with all elastic forces. In an equation, this is described as

$$f_{\text{external}G} = -K^G u^G. \tag{2}$$

In this equation $f_{\text{external}G}$ and u^G represent the total external force on and displacement of the tissue respectively. Both are vectors of dimension $3n$, where n is the number of nodes in the mesh. The matrix K^G combines all force-displacement relations in one big $3n \times 3n$-matrix called *global stiffness matrix*. In fact, every entry of the vector $K^G u^G$ is an elastic force that can be computed by Equation (1); in other words: $K^G u^G$ can be computed using only local information, i.e. without generating the matrix K^G itself.

This insight is the key to our solution method: we use an iterative method that only requires calculating $K^G v^G$ for some $3n$-vector v^G in every iteration. In our implementation, we have chosen the conjugate gradient algorithm [7], but any other algorithm of the Krylov-subspace type could also be used.

We have found the conjugate gradient algorithm to be efficient enough for interactive use. For larger models, the solution does not appear instanteneous, though: the solution process is noticeable, and appears as a quickly damping vibration of the object. Our simulation is static, so the relaxation time and vibration frequencies have no obvious relation with temporal behavior in reality. It is therefore not clear how much this will detriment the realism of a real simulation.

On a single 500 Mhz Xeon CPU we can manipulate a model of 7986 tetrahedra and 1729 nodes interactively. The relaxation process runs at approximately 50 iterations per second. In this mesh, the Lamé-material parameters are
$\lambda = \mu = 1$, which corresponds with Poisson ratio $\nu = 0.25$. For this material and
this model, we observed that this model generally requires between 70 and 200
iterations to reach convergence.

3   Cuts

Surgery can only be meaningfully simulated if there is support for changing the
tissue. We have taken the operation of cutting as a basic task to model. Cutting
in our FE simulation amounts to cutting in a tetrahedral meshes. The problem
with cutting in a tetrahedral mesh, is maintaining both tetrahedrality and making the cut appear where the user performed it. Most previous work proposed
subdivision methods to achieve this: every tetrahedron that is encountered during a cut is subdivided to accomodate the scalpel path. There are two inherent
problems with this approach: Firstly, the mesh will always grow more complex,
which brings down performance. Secondly, If the scalpel passes close by features
of the mesh, then unconditional subdivision leads to degeneracies, such as elongated or flattened tetrahedra. These degeneracies can cause numerical problems
in the simulation.

In an attempt to overcome these problems, we have taken the extreme opposite of subdivision: our cutting method does not perform any subdivision at all.
We achieve this by adapting the mesh locally so that there are always triangles
on the scalpel path, and performing the cut along those triangles. This procedure
can be subdivided into three subtasks, schematically shown in Figure 1.

- Selecting faces from mesh for dissecting and repositioning. We call this process *surface selection*.
- Repositioning nodes from the mesh so the selected faces are on the scalpel
  path. We call this process *node snapping*.
- Modifying the mesh to reflect the incision. We call this process *dissection*.

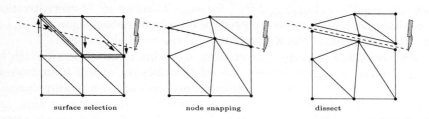

surface selection   node snapping   dissect

Fig. 1. Three steps in performing a cut, shown in 2D

Faces are selected on basis of edge-scalpel intersections: for each tetrahedron, we intersect the scalpel path with all edges of the tetrahedron. From every edge of the tetrahedron, we select the node closest to the intersection point. The set of nodes that is acquired in this way generally has three or less points, and represents a feature of the tetrahedron. The set of faces selected in this way is an approximation of the scalpel path: it is always close to the scalpel sweep, it is connected, and it generally does not branch.

Nodes are repositioned by projecting them orthogonally onto the scalpel path. For nodes that are on the boundary, this projection is done within the surface triangle containing the intersection. This minimizes the shape change caused by node repositioning.

Modifying the structure of the mesh is achieved by a flexible data structure. We have chosen a data-structure that closely mirrors a theoretical mesh description by means of simplicial complexes. This enabled us to construct verifiable algorithms to perform the modification.

Finally, the entire mesh has to be checked for connectivity: new loose components can be created by the cuts. To guarantee the existence of a solution, all new loose components must be fixed.

We have implemented this scheme, and succeeded in our goal: performing cuts without enlarging the mesh complexity. Figures 3 and 4 show the result for a single straight cut. The result of node snapping is clearly shown here. Figure 2 shows a large curved cut.

We also encountered a number of problems with this cutting scheme:

- A face is only selected when the scalpel crosses a tetrahedron completely. This means that there will be a lag between the cut instrumented by the user and the cut realized in the mesh.
- Node snapping cannot always be done without changing the external shape of the mesh: for instance, when the scalpel enters close to a corner of the mesh, that corner will move. In Figure 1, this happens with the upper left corner.
- Projecting nodes within the mesh can causes degeneracies: if four nodes of one tetrahedron are selected, node snapping will flatten that tetrahedron.

The last situation is relatively rare. It depends on the starting quality of the mesh, and the orientation of the scalpel path relative to the tetrahedralization. We found that the number of degeneracies were in the order of 5 % of the number of faces dissected for a typical cut in a Delauney tetrahedralization of a 8000 element cube.

However, when a degeneracy happens, it causes serious problems in the deformation routines, since a zero-volume tetrahedron respond to forces with infinite deformations. This prompted us to implement a routine that removes these degeneracies. After each cut, all tetrahedra of the mesh are scrutinized. Tetrahedra with low volumes or suspect aspect-ratios are classified according to their shape, and then an attempt is made to remove them. This search is repeated until there are no degeneracies left.

We observed that in most cases, the degeneracy removal is successful, and the number of tetrahedra only increases slightly due to the degeneracy removal, in the order of 1 %. Unfortunately, our current algorithm cannot repair all types of degeneracies.

4   Discussion

We have made a twofold contribution: first, we have described how to implement a static FEM analysis without requiring precomputation, thus enabling interactive cutting. We have obtained very satisfactory results, with deformations running at interactive rates for models with 2000 nodes.

Like all previous contributions in interactive surgery simulation, we assume a number of idealizations. We plan to refine our approach to deformation to obtain a more realistic simulation. At present, the simulation assumes the following:

- Force and deformation are proportional. This is the *linear material model*. Soft tissue has highly non-linear behavior: its resistance to stretching increases at higher stress levels.
- The deformation is assumed to be small. This is the *linear geometry approximation*. This assumption is valid when analyzing relatively stiff structures. Soft tissue is not stiff, which easily leads to big deformations.
- The simulation is static, i.e. only equilibrium situations are simulated, neglecting effects such as vibrations, inertia and viscosity.

Second, we have experimented with a cutting approach that does not increase the size of the mesh per se. We have had mixed success. On one hand, we learned that it was possible to execute this idea. On the other hand we found some serious drawbacks. There is an inherent lag between the scalpel and the realized cut. This effect may be alleviated by finely subdividing the mesh near the cut-area. However, this negates the original purpose of not increasing the mesh size. Second, we found that repositioning nodes within the mesh can easily generate degeneracies, which in turn have to be eliminated.

This experience prompts us to seek future work in cutting in a more flexible approach. In effect, other work unconditionally subdivides the mesh near the cut, while we unconditionally do not subdivide. In the future we will look at an approach that takes a middle road and retetrahedralizes the cut-area on demand, so that the mesh will be as fine as needed.

References

1. Daniel Bielser and Markus H. Gross. Interactive simulation of surgical cuts. In *Proc. Pacific Graphics 2000*, pages 116–125, Hong Kong, China, October 2000. IEEE Computer Society Press.
2. Daniel Bielser, Volker A. Maiwald, and Markus H. Gross. Interactive cuts through 3-dimensional soft tissue. In P. Brunet and R. Scopigno, editors, *Computer Graphics Forum (Eurographics '99)*, volume 18(3), pages 31–38, 1999.

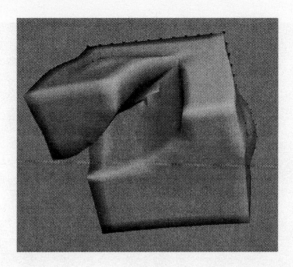

Fig. 2. A $12 \times 12 \times 12$ cube with a big cut. The material has Lamé-parameters $\lambda = \mu = 1$. The rear face of the cube is fixated.

3. Morten Bro-Nielsen. *Medical Image Registration and Surgery Simulation.* PhD thesis, Dept. Mathematical Modelling, Technical University of Denmark, 1997.
4. S. Cotin, H. Delingette, and N. Ayache. A hybrid elastic model allowing real-time cutting, deformations and force-feedback for surgery training and simulation. *The Visual Computer*, 16(8):437–452, 2000.
5. G. Picinbono and H. Delingette and N. Ayache. Non-linear and anisotropic elastic soft tissue models for medical simulation. In *ICRA2001: IEEE International Conference Robotics and Automation*, Seoul, Korea, May 2001.
6. Fabio Ganovelli, Paolo Cignoni, Claudio Montani, and Roberto Scopigno. A multiresolution model for soft objects supporting interactive cuts and lacerations. *Computer Graphics Forum*, 19(3):271–282, 2000.
7. Gene H. Golub and Charles F. Van Loan. *Matrix Computations.* John Hopkins University Press, Baltimore, Maryland, 1983.
8. Doug L. James and Dinesh K. Pai. Artdefo—accurate real time deformable objects. In *SIGGRAPH*, pages 65–72, 1999.
9. Andrew B. Mor and Takeo Kanade. Modifying soft tissue models: Progressive cutting with minimal new element creation. In *Medical Image Computing and Computer Assisted Intervention (MICCAI)*, number 1935 in Lecture Notes in Computer Science, pages 598–607. Springer-Verlag, 2000.
10. Han-Wen Nienhuys and A. Frank van der Stappen. Combining finite element deformation with cutting for surgery simulations. In A. de Sousa and J.C. Torres, editors, *EuroGraphics Short Presentations*, pages 43–52, 2000.
11. Markus A. Schill, Sarah F. F. Gibson, H.-J. Bender, and R. Männer. Biomechanical simulation of the vitreous humor in the eye using an enhanced chainmail algorithm. In *Medical Image Computing and Computer Assisted Intervention (MICCAI)*, pages 679–687, 1998.
12. Yan Zhuang and John Canny. Real-time global deformations. In *Algorithmic and Computational Robotics*, pages 97–107, Natick MA, 2001. A. K. Peters.

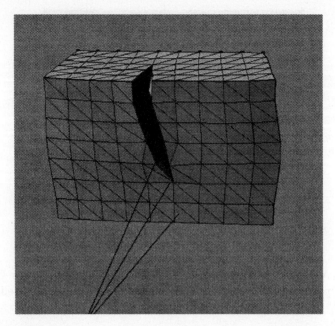

Fig. 3. A incision in a mesh with 480 nodes and 1890 tetrahedra, material parameters $\mu = \lambda = 1$. A dilating force is applied to the left and right. Edges are shown to demonstrate repositioning. The last scalpel movement and the next scalpel movement are indicated by the two partially penetrating triangles.

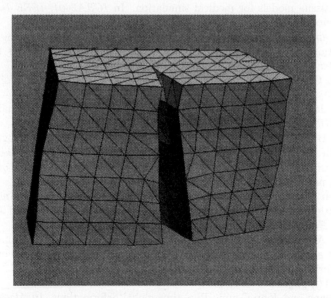

Fig. 4. The same incision, now completed.

Patient-Specific Simulation of Carotid Artery Stenting Using Computational Fluid Dynamics

Juan R. Cebral[1], Rainald Löhner[1], Orlando Soto[1],
Peter L. Choyke[2], and Peter J. Yim[2]

[1]School of Computational Sciences, George Mason University, 4400 University Drive,
M.S. 4C7, Fairfax, Virginia 22030, USA
{jcebral, lohner, soto}@gmu.edu
[2]Diagnostic Radiology Department, National Institutes of Health, Building 10, Room
1C660, Bethesda, Maryland 20892, USA
{pyim, pchoyke}@nih.gov

Abstract. An image-based computational methodology to predict the outcome of carotid artery stenting procedures is presented. Anatomically realistic models are reconstructed from contrast-enhanced magnetic resonance angiography images using deformable models. Physiologic flow conditions are obtained from phase-contrast magnetic resonance angiography data. Finite element flow calculations are obtained before and after modifying the anatomical models in order to simulate stenting procedures. The methodology was tested on image data from a patient with carotid artery stenosis. Significant changes in the blood flow through the common carotid and internal carotid artery were found after conducting a "virtual stenting" intervention. Pending experimental validation, this methodology may potentially be used to plan and optimize vascular stenting procedures on a patient-specific basis.

1 Introduction

Stroke is the leading cause of long-term disability and third cause of death after cancer and heart disease in the western world. Carotid artery atherosclerosis is a major cause of stroke. However, to date there is incomplete knowledge of the atherosclerotic disease, its associated risks, and the optimal medical therapy[1]. Carotid artery stenting is being actively explored as a less invasive alternative to the traditional carotid artery endarterectomy[2]. Complications of angioplasty and stenting include cerebral embolism associated with intravascular manipulation, hemodynamic compromise during balloon inflation, vessel dissection, early restenosis or occlusion and cerebral hyperperfusion and intracranial hemorrhage[3]. Restenosis after angioplasty and stenting remains a major problem limiting the efficacy of the procedure. Even though the mechanisms of in-stent restenosis are not fully understood, stent implantation changes the geometry of the vessel creating new regions of decreased and increased shear stress that might be related to the observed restenosis patterns[4,5,6]. The planning of a stenting procedure and the prevention of complications are done based on the experience of the operator and the long-term outcomes are still not established. Image-based computational hemodynamics is

W. Niessen and M. Viergever (Eds.): MICCAI 2001, LNCS 2208, pp. 153–160, 2001.
© Springer-Verlag Berlin Heidelberg 2001

154   J.R. Cebral et al.

increasingly been used to study genesis and progression of vascular disease[7,8], enhance image-based diagnosis[9] and plan surgical and interventional procedures[10,11].

The aim of this paper is to present a computational modeling methodology to predict the outcome of carotid artery stenting procedures. The basis of the method is the integration of computational fluid dynamics (CFD) and medical imaging techniques. Patient-specific anatomical information and physiological flow conditions are obtained from magnetic resonance angiography (MRA) data. First, a realistic model of the carotid bifurcation is constructed from 3D contrast-enhanced MRA images. The geometry of this model is then modified to simulate the introduction of a vascular stent. Blood flow calculations are then conducted using finite element methods and physiologic conditions derived from phase-contrast MRA flow measurements. Finally, the blood flows before and after the introduction of the stent are compared. It is anticipated that this methodology will enable accurate predictions of blood flow patterns after performing a stenting procedure. These predictions might potentially be used to design, plan and optimize stenting interventions for individual patients[11].

2 Methods

2.1 Magnetic Resonance Angiography Data

The anatomical information used to construct realistic 3D geometrical models of the carotid artery bifurcation was obtained from high-resolution 3D contrast-enhanced MRA images. These images were taken using an intra-venous injection of bolus of Gd-DTPA on a 1.5T GE scanner.

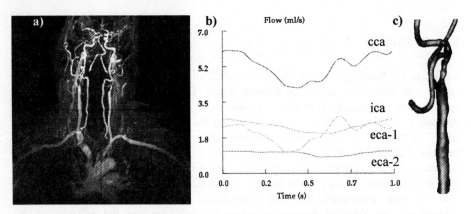

Fig. 1. MRA data: a) MIP rendering of contrast-enhanced MRA images; b) flow-rate curves obtained from phase-contrast MRA velocity measurements; c) model of the carotid bifurcation.

Blood flow velocity measurements were taken on 2D cross-sectional planes using gated cine phase-contrast MRA. Time-dependent flow curves were obtained by integration of the velocity profiles over the cross-sectional area of the carotid artery.

Flow curves above and below the bifurcation were used to impose physiologic flow boundary conditions. The maximum intensity projection (MIP) of the anatomical images of a patient with moderate carotid artery stenosis is shown in figure 1a. The flow curves obtained in the common carotid artery (CCA), the internal carotid artery (ICA) and the external carotid artery (ECA) are presented in figure 1b. The final anatomical model of the carotid bifurcation is shown in figure 1c.

2.2 Anatomical Model Construction

Accurate reconstruction of vessel anatomies from medical images is a challenging problem due to image artifacts, noise and limited resolution. However, many segmentation algorithms have been devised. We use a semi-automatic technique based on cylindrical deformable models[12]. With this approach each branch of the carotid artery is reconstructed independently. In this manner, problems associated to self-intersections or intersections with other close arteries or veins present in the images are avoided.

Once a surface triangulation was constructed for each arterial branch, a surface-merging algorithm[13] was used to obtain a watertight surface model of the carotid bifurcation. In the sequel, we refer to this model as the pre-operative model. This surface model was then used as a support surface to generate a volumetric finite element grid. Given a desired element size distribution, specified via background grids and sources, a new surface triangulation was generated using an advancing front technique[14]. Either linear or quadratic interpolation can be used to reposition points on the support surface. Topological constraints were used to avoid jumps between different arterial branches. The space inside the new triangulation was then filled with tetrahedral elements using a traditional advancing front grid generation method[15].

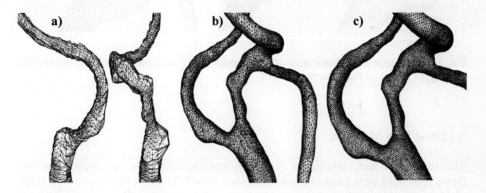

Fig. 2. Anatomical model before stenting: a) reconstructed arterial branches; b) merged model; c) surface of the finite element grid.

The element size was selected to yield approximately ten points across the smallest cross-section, resulting in roughly 0.5 million tetrahedral elements. The grid

J.R. Cebral et al.

generation process is illustrated in figure 2. The reconstructed arterial branches and the bifurcation model after merging are shown in figures 2a and 2b, respectively.

A rigid flow-through phantom of the carotid bifurcation under steady flow conditions as well as MRA data of normal human subjects have previously been used to validate the methodology[9]. These studies show that MRA data can be used to accurately model blood flow in the carotid artery.

The surface model of the carotid bifurcation was then modified to simulate the presence of the stent. A cylindrical surface representing the stent was first created along the axis or centerline of the ICA. The arterial centerline was automatically extracted from the previous finite element grid using a skeletonization procedure operating on tetrahedral meshes, devised for visualization of blood flows in realistic arterial models[16,17]. The final geometrical model was then obtained by merging the pre-operative and the stent models. In what follows, we refer to this model as the post-operative model. A new finite element grid was generated using the same element size distribution as in the pre-operative case. The geometry of the stent, the post-operative model, and the corresponding finite element grid are shown in figure 3a, 3b and 3c, respectively

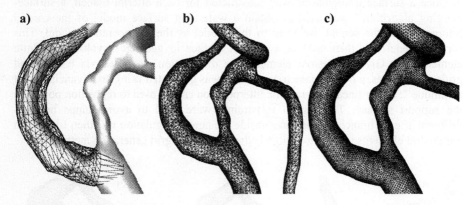

Fig. 3. Introduction of a virtual stent: a) stent geometry; b) anatomical model including after stenting; c) surface of the finite element grid.

2.3 Blood Flow Modeling

The time-dependent, non-linear Navier-Stokes equations for an incompressible, Newtonian fluid were used to model the blood flow[18]. The Newtonian approximation yields reasonable results in large arteries such as the carotids[19]. The vessel walls were assumed to be rigid, mainly due to a lack of pressure and elasticity information required to model compliant walls. However, it is known that atherosclerotic arteries tend to be stiffer than normal arteries; therefore this assumption is not entirely unjustified. In future studies we intend to gather all the necessary information to incorporate wall compliance, and conduct fluid-structure interaction calculations[9].

The fluid equations were solved using a fully implicit time discretization algorithm based on a stabilized fractional step method and linear finite element spatial discretizations[20]. Explicit time integration schemes, although very accurate, impose a limit on the maximum time-step size that can be used which is several orders of magnitude smaller than the period of the cardiac cycle. Thus, using such methods requires several thousands of time-steps per cardiac cycle. However, implicit schemes allow arbitrary time-step sizes, which are then selected in order to yield an accurate solution (e.g. 100 time-steps per heartbeat).

Physiologic flow boundary conditions are imposed using the flow curves derived from the phase-contrast MRA velocity measurements. At the boundaries where time-dependent flows are prescribed, a velocity profile is computed as the superposition of Womersley solutions[21] corresponding to different Fourier modes of the flow waveform[22].

3 Results

Two blood flow calculations were performed, corresponding to the pre- and post-operative models. In the pre-operative model, time-dependent flows were prescribed at the ICA and ECA's. Traction-free boundary conditions were used in the CCA, imposing a zero pressure (p=0), thus the computed pressures represent pressure drops relative to the entrance of the CCA. During this simulation, the pressure drop between the CCA and the ICA were stored. For the post-operative model, time-dependent flows were prescribed at the ECA's, zero pressure was imposed at the CCA and the time-dependent pressure drop calculated in the pre-operative model was imposed at the ICA. These boundary conditions assume that the flow in the ECA's and the pressure gradient in the ICA do not change significantly after the implantation of the stent. These assumptions, which may be reasonable for cases of moderate stenosis, enable the prediction of the new flow pattern and wall shear stress distribution after stenting. However, further testing and validation of these assumptions are required.

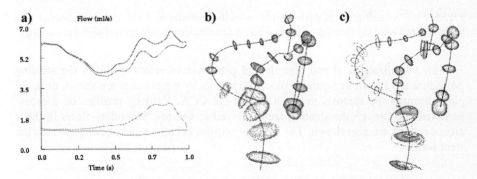

Fig. 4. a) Change in the flow rate curves through the CCA and ICA after implantation of the vascular stent; b) velocity contours before stenting; c) velocity contours after stenting.

Both flows through the CCA and the ICA change due to the introduction of the stent in the ICA. The stent size is approximately 3.7 cm in length and 2.8 mm in radius. The change in the time-dependent flow curves precipitated by the introduction of the stent is shown in figure 4a. Quantitatively, the flow through the CCA increases by 14 % at peak systole and by 4 % at end diastole. In the ICA the flow increases by 156 % at peak systole and 21 % at end diastole. Average flows during a cardiac cycle through the CCA and ICA change by 6 % and 63 %, respectively. Velocity contours at peak systole before and after stenting are plotted in a series of cuts normal to the arterial axis in figures 4b and 4c, respectively.

The change in the flow pattern and wall shear stress distribution is illustrated in figures 5. Figures 5a and 5b show velocity contours in a cut parallel to the arterial axis while figures 5c and 5d show the wall shear stress maps at peak systole. It is interesting to note much stronger secondary flows after stenting in the internal and common carotids due to the increased flow.

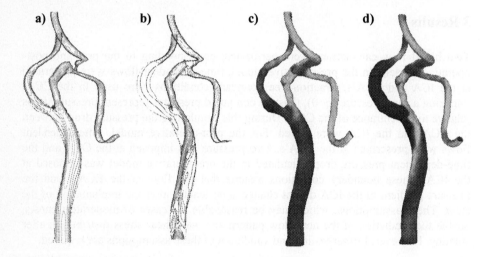

Fig. 5. Flow visualization at peak systole: velocity contours in a cut along the arterial axis before (a) and after (b) stenting; wall shear stress distributions before (c) and after (d) stenting.

Flow visualizations at end diastole and peak systole before and after the stenting procedure are shown in figure 6. Blood flow velocity magnitudes are shown on a cut plane through the stenosis in the ICA and the CCA. Velocity profiles on a cross-sectional cut through the stenosis are displayed as vectors. Secondary flows in these cross-sections are also shown. The velocity profiles become more skewed towards the stent walls.

4 Discussion

An image-based computational methodology to predict patient-specific blood flow in the carotid artery after a stenting procedure has been presented. Anatomical and physiologic data are obtained from MRA images and used to construct finite element models of the carotid artery hemodynamics.

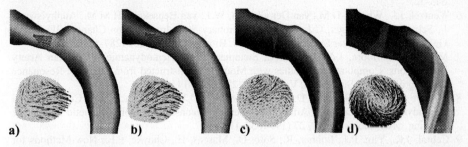

Fig. 6. Flow visualization showing velocity magnitudes, velocity profiles and secondary flows in the region of the stenosis: a) before stenting, end diastole; b) before stenting, peak systole; c) after stenting, end diastole; d) after stenting, peak systole.

Significant changes in the blood flow rates as well as average flows through both the common carotid and the internal carotid arteries were found after the introduction of a vascular stent into the internal carotid artery. The stenting procedure also changes significantly the flow pattern and the wall shear stress distribution. These predictions are particularly important in order to study complications of the stenting procedures such as restenosis, hyperperfusion syndrome and cerebral hemorrhage.

The significance of these results is that, pending experimental validation, the present methodology can be used to predict the outcome and therefore optimize carotid stenting procedures.

Limitations of the methodology include the assumption of rigid vessel walls, errors in the anatomical reconstruction and errors in the velocity measurements using MRA data. Even though the rigid wall assumption may be reasonable for stenotic arteries, wall compliance may play an important role in the development of restenosis at the ends of the stent. Future work will focus on quantification of these errors, validation studies using multi-modality image data, and verification of the post-operative boundary conditions.

References

1. Connors III, J.J.: The Nature of Cervical Carotid Stenosis. Techniques in Vascular and Interventional Radiology, 3(2) (2000) 62-64.
2. Vitek, J.J., Roubin, G.S., New, G., Al-Mubarek, N., Iyer, S.S.: Carotid Stenting. Techniques in Vascular and Interventional Radiology, 3(2) (2000) 75-85.
3. Meyers PM, Higashida RT, Phatouros C, Malek AM, Lempert TE, Dowd CF, Halbach VV: Cerebral Hyperperfusion Syndrome after Percutaneous transluminal Stenting of the Craniocervical Arteries. *Neurosurgery*, 47(2), (2000) 335-345.
4. Berger, S.A., Jou, L.D.: Flow in Stenotic Blood Vessels. Annual Review of Fluid Mechanics, 32 (2000) 347-82.

5. Jou, L.D., Saloner, D.: A Numerical Study of Magnetic Resonance Angiography Images for Pulsatile Flow in the Carotid Bifurcation. Medical Engineering and Physics, 20(9) (1998) 643-52.
6. Wentzel, J.J., Whelan, D.M., van Der Giessen, W.J., van Beusekom, H.M.M., Andhyiswara, I., Serruys, P.W., Slager, C.J., Kram, R.: Coronary Stent Implantation Changes 3D Vessel Geometry and 3D Shear Stress Distribution. J. Biomech., 33 (2000) 1287-1295.
7. Milner, J.S., Moore, J.A., Rutt, B.K., Steinman, D.A.: Hemodynamics of Human Artery Bifurcations: Computational Studies with Models Reconstructed from Magnetic Resonance Imaging of Normal Subjects. J. Vasc. Surg., 27 (1998) 143-156.
8. Moore, J.A., Steinman, D.A., Holdsworth, D.W.: Accuracy of Computational Hemodynamics in Complex Arterial Geometries Reconstructed from Magnetic Resonance Imaging. Ann. Biomed. Eng., 27 (1999) 32-41.
9. Cebral, J.R., Yim, P.J., Lohner, R., Soto, O., Marcos, H., Choyke, P.L.: New Methods for Computational Fluid Dynamics Modeling of Carotid Artery from Magnetic Resonance Angiography. Proc. SPIE Medical Imaging, 4321, paper No. 22 (2001).
10. Perktold, K., Hofer, M., Karner, G., Trubel, W., Schima, H.: Computer Simulation of Vascular Fluid Dynamics and Mass Transport: Optimal Design of Arterial Bypass Anastomoses. Proc. ECCOMAS 98, 2, John Wiley & Sons, (1998) 484-489.
11. Taylor, C.A., Draney, M.T., Ku, J.P., Parker, D., Steele, B.N., Wang, K., Zarins, C.K.: Predictive Medicine: Computational Techniques in Therapeutic Decision-Making. Computer Assisted Surgery 4 (1999) 231-247.
12. Yim, P.J., Cebral, J.R., Mullick, R., Choyke, P.L.: Vessel Surface Reconstruction with a Tubular Deformable Model. Submitted to IEEE Trans. Medical Imaging (2001).
13. Cebral, J.R., Löhner, R., Choyke, P.L., Yim, P.J.: Merging of Intersecting Triangulations for Finite Element Modeling. J. Biomech. (2001) in press.
14. Löhner, R.: Regridding Surface Triangulations. J. Comp. Phys., 126 (1996) 1-10.
15. Löhner, R.: Automatic Unstructured Grid Generators. Finite Elements in Analysis and Design, 25 (1997) 111-134.
16. Cebral, J.R., Löhner, R.: Flow Visualization On Unstructured Grids Using Geometrical Cuts, Vortex Detection and Shock Surfaces. AIAA-01-0915 (2001).
17. Cebral, J.R., Löhner, R.: Visualization of Blood Flow Computations in Realistic Anatomical Models Using Geometrical Surface Cuts. Submitted to IEEE Trans. Visualization and Computer Graphics (2001).
18. Taylor, C.A., Hughes, T.J.R., Zarins, C.K.: Finite Element Modeling of Blood Flow in Arteries. Comput. Methods Appl. Mech. Engrg. 158 (1998) 155-196.
19. Zhao, S.Z., Xu, X.Y., Hughes, A.D., Thom, S.A., Stanton, A.V., Ariff, B., Long, Q.: Blood Flow and Vessel Mechanics in a Physiologically Realistic Model of a Human Carotid Arterial Bifurcation. J. Biomech. 33 (2000) 975-984.
20. Soto, O., Löhner, R., Cebral, J.R., Codina, R.: A Time-Accurate Implicit Monolithic Finite Element Scheme for Incompressible Flow Problems. Proc. ECCOMAS CFD, Swansea, UK (2001) to appear.
21. Womersley, J.R.: Method for the Calculation of Velocity, Rate of Flow and Viscous Drag in Arteries When the Pressure gradient is Known. J. Physiol. 127 (1955) 553-563.
22. Cebral, J.R., Lohner, R., Burgess, J.E.: Computer Simulation of Cerebral Artery Clipping: Relevance to Aneurysm Neuro-Surgery Planning. Proc. ECCOMAS, Barcelona-Spain (2000).

Volume Rendering of Segmented Tubular Objects

Elizabeth Bullitt[1] and Stephen Aylward[2]

Departments of [1]Surgery, [1,2]Radiology, and [2]Computer Science, University of North Carolina, Chapel Hill, NC
bullitt@med.unc.edu, aylward@unc.edu

Abstract. This paper describes a new method of combining ray casting with segmented tubular objects, such as blood vessels, for purposes of clinically useful display. The method first projects segmented tubes using a modified z-buffer that additionally records information about the objects projected. A subsequent step selectively volume renders only through the object volumes recorded by the z-buffer. In common with traditional "block" volume rendering the actual image data is shown, of importance when the boundary of a segmented object is uncertain. Unlike traditional "block" volume rendering, the approach permits user manipulation of objects, operates rapidly, and provides depth information even for maximum intensity projection. Although our methods were developed for display of the intracerebral vasculature, the approach is applicable to volume rendering of tubular objects throughout the body.

1. Introduction

This paper describes a new method of combining volume rendering and segmentation that maximizes the strengths of each approach. The goal is to provide a method of three-dimensional (3D) visualization that will be useful to clinicians who need to understand complex vascular anatomy in 3D, who may or may not have access to specialized hardware, and who may be distrustful of automated segmentation methods that sharply define objects subsequently shown only by surface rendering.

From the clinical perspective, an ideal method of visualizing 3D volume data should include:

1) The ability to visualize "truth" (the actual image data as seen in high quality images),
2) The ability to view objects rapidly and interactively from any point of view,
3) The ability to interactively remove obscuring objects and/or to obtain relevant information about selected objects or groups of objects,
4) The ability to run the software on any platform/hardware so that surgical planning can be done on office machines or at home.

This paper describes an approach that combines segmentation with volume rendering in order to do all of the above. The basic methodology employs segmentation to define regions that are subsequently selectively volume rendered using a modified z-buffer. "Fuzzy margins" can be set so that desired amounts of the

W. Niessen and M. Viergever (Eds.): MICCAI 2001, LNCS 2208, pp. 161-168, 2001.
© Springer-Verlag Berlin Heidelberg 2001

actual image data are shown regardless of the boundary definitions provided by segmentation. No time is wasted casting rays through non-interesting space, so the implementation operates efficiently even without hardware optimization. Individual objects or groups of objects can be interactively selected, queried, and manipulated. Depth information is available even for maximum intensity projection (MIP), thus adding to the image information available for each image frame.

The methods described here were initially developed for visualization of the intracerebral vasculature as extracted from magnetic resonance angiograms (MRA) and as seen by maximum intensity projection (MIP). However, the approach is applicable to display of tubular objects extracted from any type of 3D image data and from any part of the body.

2. Methods

2.1 Image Acquisition and Image Segmentation

For this study, 12 patients underwent 3D, time of flight MRA in a Siemens 1.5 T Vision unit with a quadrature head coil and with magnetization transfer suppression. Images were acquired in the axial projection over a 7.6 cm volume, using 69 1 mm contiguous sections and an x and y spacing of 0.85 mm. An additional patient was studied by 3D digital subtraction angiography (3D-DSA). Siemens has given us a 3D volume representing this patient's right carotid circulation.

We have previously described and evaluated methods of segmenting vessels from 3D images [1], [2] and of providing directed graph descriptions of these segmented vessels [3], [4], [5]. The approach is applicable to any type of 3D data including MR, computed tomography, 3D-DSA, ultrasound, and confocal microscopy. In brief, each vessel must be provided an initial seed point. The program then automatically defines an image intensity ridge representing the vessel's 3D skeleton curve, with a subsequent automatic calculation of vessel width at each skeleton point. Graph description is performed largely automatically, employing both distance and image intensity measurements. We have tested the resultant vessel trees against digital subtraction angiographic data obtained from the same patient [3], [5], [6]. The output of the segmentation/tree definition program is a set of vessels, each of which is comprised of a set of 3D skeleton points with an associated width at each point, and with additional information available about the connectivity of each vessel.

2.2 Visualization

The visualization method consists of two steps: front projection of segmented objects using a modified z-buffer algorithm, and subsequent volume rendering so that a pixel's ray is processed only if that ray intersects a volume of interest. If more than one object projects to the same pixel, volume rendering is only performed for the object closest to the ray source. This approach provides an efficient means of volume rendering that does not waste time in processing empty space or in analyzing distant objects that project to the same pixel as a closer object.

For tubular objects such as blood vessels, the approach is simple. For segmented vessels, each vessel skeleton point is projected upon the viewplane. If more than one point projects to the same pixel, the point closest to the ray source is given priority.

Tubular objects are circular in cross section. Each 3D vessel point can therefore be viewed as a sphere whose projection will be circular (or close to circular) on the projection plane. Given the depth (Z) coordinate of each vessel skeleton point, knowledge of that point's radius, and knowledge of the viewing geometry, the radius of each projected point can be calculated on the viewplane. A fast Bressenham filled circle algorithm is used to calculate the associated viewplane pixels from which to back project rays. These rays are selectively cast only through the appropriate 3D object of interest, and only for the distance indicated by that object's radius. If another object has already been identified as projecting to a portion of a filled viewplane circle, the object closest to the ray source is given priority.

A byproduct of the approach is that each viewplane pixel of interest is automatically labeled with the identification number of the object projecting to it and with that object's relevant point identification number. Any subsequent "point and click" operation to interactively select an object can thus be processed rapidly without requiring a 3D search.

2.3   Evaluation

We have processed 12 patient MRA data sets and an additional patient studied by 3D digital subtraction angiography (3D-DSA) using the methods outlined above. Two patients were normal, two had base-of-the-brain tumors, one an aneurysym, one an intracerebral hemorrhage, and 7 an arteriovenous malformation (AVM). The intracerebral vasculature normally consists of three vascular trees: two carotid circulations and one vertebrobasilar circulation. All three intracerebral vascular trees were defined for all 12 patients who underwent MRA. Only one vessel tree was available for the patient who was studied by 3D-DSA.

Images were projected using perspective, MIP projection, a field of view of 20 degrees, and a large window of 500 x 500 pixels. The program allows interactive manipulation of the point of view as well as the ability to interactively select objects. All tests and evaluations were done on an 850 MHz, Pentium III laptop computer running Windows 2000.

Image quality was assessed by side-to-side comparison with the excellent quality, MIP volume renderings of the publically available Visualization Toolkit (VTK) [7]. For purposes of comparison, the viewing geometry was set identically in each window, and the volume of space given to VTK for volume rendering was the bounding box of the segmented vessels shown in the other window.

Volume rendering over large volumes, under perspective projection, and using large display windows is usually very slow without specialized hardware. For each of the 12 patients studied by MR (and for whom the full intracranial volume was thus available for analysis), we tested the time to render the vasculature 10 times into a 500 x 500 pixel display window.

3. Results

3.1 Image Quality

MRAs are noisy, and the quality of an image produced by volume rendering is often degraded by noise. An advantage of selective volume rendering through segmented objects is that little or no background noise is present. In addition, traditional methods of volume rendering may suffer from image obscuration when objects of interest and extraneous objects occupy the same block of space. Selective volume rendering does not have this limitation. Figure 1 shows a patient with an intracerebral hemorrhage. The vasculature adjacent to the hemorrhage cannot be visualized by traditional volume rendering, but is readily appreciated following vessel segmentation.

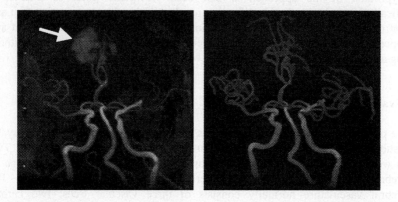

Fig. 1. Comparison of block volume rendering (left) with volume rendering using segmentation (right) in a patient with an intracerebral blood clot (arrow). The image at left is noisy and the pattern of the vasculature is obscured in the vicinity of the clot.

Another advantage of the proposed approach is that depth information is available on any individual view. This leads to images of higher quality and informational content. Figure 2 illustrates the depth information available by our approach. The patient shown is normal.

3.2 Image Manipulation

An advantage of segmented object display over traditional block volume rendering is that individual objects or groups of objects can be selected and manipulated by the user. Figure 3 shows a patient with an AVM whose vessels were extracted from a 3D-DSA. The number of vessels and the degree of projection overlap make it difficult to discern the feeding arteries. By using graph descriptions of segmented objects, a single mouseclick can hide a vessel subtree, thus allowing easier analysis of the vascular feeding pattern.

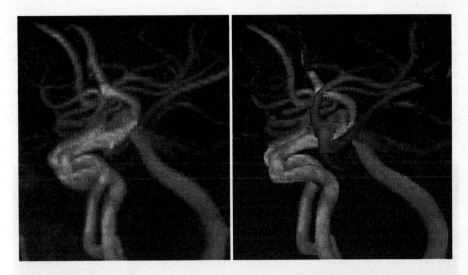

Fig. 2. Depth information from an individual MIP view. No depth information is available with traditional "block" volume rendering (left), and the resultant image is confusing. Useful depth information is available by the approach outlined in this report (right).

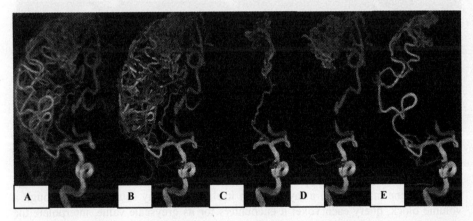

Fig. 3. Block volume rendering (A) and segmented vessel volume rendering (B) of a patient with an AVM defined by 3D-DSA. Our graph descriptions of segmented vessels permit hiding an entire vessel subtree with a single mouseclick. C-E illustrate how the arterial feeding patterns can be clarified when subtrees are selectively hidden.

A disadvantage of segmentation is that the definition of object boundaries may be uncertain or inaccurate. An advantage of combining volume rendering with segmentation is that the actual image data is shown in the region of interest. If the clinician is concerned that segmentation may be inaccurate, our approach allows arbitrary dilation of segmented boundary margins so that more of the actual image data can be seen. Figure 4 shows a patient with a mycotic aneurysm of the middle cerebral artery. Our segmentation did not show an aneurysm neck, and the question was raised whether a neck might actually be present. Figure 4 shows a selective volume rendering of the relevant vessels using a radius of 1.0, 2.0, and 2.5 times the length of each point's radius as determined by segmentation. No aneurysm neck is present, and the initial segmentation was correct. However, the fact that a clinician can check the segmentation against the actual image data is reassuring to the clinician and adds a significant safety factor if 3D volume visualizations are to be used for surgical planning.

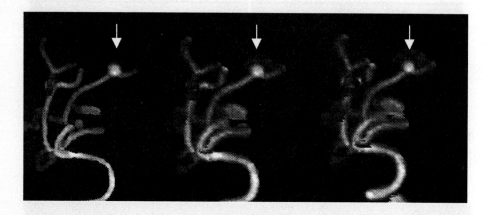

Fig. 4. Volume rendering using fuzzy segmentation boundaries. The patient has an aneurysm (arrow) and the question was whether an aneurysm neck might be present. From left to right, volume rendering is shown for 1.0, 2.0, and 2.5 times the radius at each vessel point.

3.3 Image Rendering Speed

Traditional methods of high quality volume rendering are slow because each pixel on the viewplane must define a ray between itself and the ray source, walk through a volume block, query each voxel it encounters for its greyscale value, interpolate the greyscale values of adjacent voxels, and then process each interpolated value. Under conditions of traditional "block" volume rendering, much time is wasted in processing voxels without useful informational content. The software algorithm described in this report is capable of fast, interactive volume rendering because it spends time casting rays only through structures of interest. Our approach allows interactive manipulation of object position/orientation on a laptop computer without specialized hardware, using a large display window of 500 x 500 pixels, under conditions of perspective projection, and displaying the entire intracranial vasculature.

Time tests for the 12 images analyzed under the difficult conditions listed above indicated a mean rendering time of better than 5 frames a second. More specifically, the mean time to render an image was slightly less than 0.2 seconds with a standard deviation of 0.1 seconds.

4. Discussion

This report describes a new method of visualizing segmented tubular objects using a modified z-buffer and selective ray-casting. The resultant visualizations allow direct display of image intensity values, the ability to manipulate/query objects interactively, high quality images, fast interaction time, depth information on individual frames, and the capacity to provide "fuzzy" segmented object boundaries so that the actual image data can be shown beyond segmented object margins if the accuracy of segmentation is in doubt.

Other investigators have also approached the issue of selective volume rendering using segmented objects. Like our own method, such approaches offer significant advantages over traditional "block" volume rendering. However, unlike the "shell" rendering approach of Grevera [8], our method does not require explicit construction of object surfaces, allows ray casting precisely through the confines of the objects of interest, and provides high-quality, interpolated images at even high magnification. Unlike the 3D spatial subdivision and labeling approach of Zuiderveld [9], our method avoids walking rays through empty space, allows arbitrary dilation of segmentation boundaries, and permits user-defined manipulation of connected groups of objects. We therefore believe that our approach provides a new and powerful visualization method likely to be useful to clinicians.

A disadvantage of the proposed methodology is that it is applicable only to tubular objects. We are currently exploring methods of extending the approach to segmented objects of any arbitrary configuration.

In addition to the vascular visualizations enabled by the proposed approach, we can also offer significant, hardware-independent increases in rendering speed. Image size appears to be increasing in parallel with hardware improvements. A more efficient software algorithm can take advantage of hardware optimizations and, regardless of the hardware available, should perform better than a less efficient approach. Moreover, a number of algorithms are available that speed orthographic projection. Our current program is implemented only for the more complex case of perspective projection; further speed improvements should be possible under orthographic visualizations. It should be noted, however, that the rendering speed improvements offered by our approach will be most marked when small objects are scattered over a wide volume of space. If the objects of interest consist only of closely apposed cubic blocks, our approach will operate no more quickly than traditional volume rendering methods, although the other advantages of our methodology will still apply.

Acknowledgments

Supported by R01CA67812 NIH-NCI, P01CA47982 NIH-NCI and Intel and Microsoft equipment awards. Algorithms for vessel segmentation and description have been licensed to Medtronic Corp. (Minn., Minn) and to R2 Technology (Los Altos, CA).

References

1. Aylward, S.R., Pizer, S.M., Bullitt, E., Eberly, D.: Intensity ridge and widths for 3D object segmentation and description IEEE WMMBIA IEEE 96TB100056 (1996) 131-138.
2. Aylward S.R., Bullitt E.: A comparison of methods for tubular object centerline extraction. (2001) Accepted IEEE-TMI .
3. Bullitt E., Aylward S., Liu A., Stone J., Mukherji S., Coffey C., Gerig G., Pizer S.M.: 3D graph description of the intracerebral vasculature from segmented MRA and tests of accuracy by comparison with x-ray angiograms. IPMI 99; Lecture Notes in Computer Science (1999) 1613:308-321.
4. Bullitt E., Aylward S., Bernard E., Gerig G.: Special Article. Computer-assisted visualization of arteriovenous malformations on the home pc (2001) Neurosurgery 48: 576-583.
5. Bullitt E., Aylward S., Smith K., Mukherji S., Jiroutek M., Muller K.: Symbolic Description of Intracerebral Vessels Segmented from MRA and Evaluation by Comparison with X-Ray Angiograms (2001) in press Medical Image Analysis.
6. Bullitt E., Liu A., Aylward S., Coffey C., Stone J., Mukherji S., Muller K., S, Pizer S.M.: Registration of 3D cerebral vessels with 2D digital angiograms: Clinical evaluation Academic Radiology (1999) 6:539-546.
7. Schroeder W., Martin K., Lorensen B.: The Visualization Toolkit. Prentice Hall, New Jersey (1998). Open source software is available at http://www.kitware.com/vtk.html.
8. Grevera G., Udupa J., Odhner D.:An order of magnitude faster isosurface rendering in software on a PC than using dedicated, general purpose rendering hardware. IEEE Transactions of Visualization and Computer Graphics (2000) 6:335-345.
9. Zuiderveld K.: Visualization of multimodality medical volume data using object-oriented methods. Thesis. Universiteit Utrecht, Utrecht. ISBN 90-393-0687-7 (1995).

Clinical Evaluation of an Automatic Path Tracker for Virtual Colonoscopy

Roel Truyen[1], Thomas Deschamps[2], and Laurent D. Cohen[3]

[1] Philips Medical Systems Nederland,
EasyVision Advanced Development
roel.truyen@philips.com
[2] Laboratoire d'Electronique Philips France,
thomas.deschamps@philips.com
[3] Laboratoire CEREMADE, Université Paris Dauphine, France,
laurent.cohen@ceremade.dauphine.fr

Abstract. Virtual colonoscopy is a minimally invasive technique allowing early detection of colorectal polyps. A path or centerline through the colon can be very useful to perform virtual endoscopy. Manual path tracking is a very time-consuming task and the resulting path depends a lot on the experience of the operator. This severely limits the applicability of the path-based visualization and inspection methods.

An automatic path tracker for virtual endoscopy was introduced in [3], based on previous work on minimal path extraction ([1]). First, we briefly recall the theory of the automatic path tracker, detailing how we adapt this method for virtual colonoscopy. We show the speed and robustness of this automatic path tracker by means of a multi-user study where we measured the total user time and the difference in results between users on 29 clinical cases.

1 Introduction

The physician's efficacy in virtual colonoscopy can be increased by using an automatic path tracking tool. This tool must be easy to learn and operate, fast and the result should be largely operator-independent. In that case, a less experienced technologist can track a path during a preprocessing step, reducing the time spent by the physician. We have used an automatic path tracker that was first presented for virtual endoscopy in [2]. Based on the theory of minimal paths [1], several improvements were brought in [3] to accelerate the computations.

In this paper we briefly recall the theory of minimal paths, then we detail how we apply the method of [1] to the particular case of colonoscopy, and finally we present a clinical evaluation of the path tracker. In section 2, we describe the method to automatically extract a path between user defined start and end points. In section 3, we detail how we applied the technique for path tracking in the CT colon. The results of a clinical multi-user validation are presented in section 4. A short conclusion summarizes the benefits of the automatic path tracker.

W. Niessen and M. Viergever (Eds.): MICCAI 2001, LNCS 2208, pp. 169–176, 2001.

2   Finding a Path in a 3D Tubular Structure

2.1   Path of Minimal Cost

We formulate the path construction as a minimal cost path search. As an example, see Fig. 1 where we want to extract a path in a vessel between two points. If we use the grey level itself as the local cost, the minimal cost path will follow the dark lumen of the vessel as much as possible.

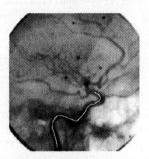

Fig. 1. Extracting a path on a digital subtracted angiography (DSA) image

In [1], the authors proposed to extract the minimal path by formulating a simplified snake energy model for the path C, without the second derivative term of the classical formulation of [5]:

$$E(C) = \int_{\Omega} \{w + P(C(s))\}ds = \int_{\Omega} \left\{ \tilde{P}(C(s)) \right\} ds \ . \tag{1}$$

where Ω is the domain of definition of C, s represents the arc-length parameter, and $w > 0$ is a regularization term which constrains the length and the curvature of C, as shown in [1]. The potential term P only depends on image grey-value information, and should be low at the image positions where the path should go.

First step is to compute the *minimal action map* $U(p)$, which is defined as the cost of the minimal cost path between a starting point p_0 and any point p:

$$U(p) = \inf_{p_0, p} \left\{ \int_{\Omega} \tilde{P}(C(s))ds \right\} \ . \tag{2}$$

It can be shown that U satisfies the *Eikonal* equation, that is also used in geometric optics to describe lightwave propagation.

$$\|\nabla U\| = \tilde{P} \ . \tag{3}$$

The minimal action map U computed according to the Eikonal equation (3) has a global minimum $U(p_0) = 0$ at the start point p_0.

In a second step, the minimal cost path is extracted by a simple gradient descent on the *minimal action map* $U(p)$ from the desired end point p_e back to the starting point p_0.

2.2   Fast Marching Algorithm

In order to discretize equation 3, authors in [3] based on previous work in [7] have proposed an iterative method to calculate the unknown u at each voxel (i, j, k) as:

$$
\begin{aligned}
(\max\{u - U_{i-1,j,k}, u - U_{i+1,j,k}, 0\})^2 + \\
(\max\{u - U_{i,j-1,k}, u - U_{i,j+1,k}, 0\})^2 + \\
(\max\{u - U_{i,j,k-1}, u - U_{i,j,k+1}, 0\})^2 = \tilde{P}'_{,j,k} .
\end{aligned}
\tag{4}
$$

giving the correct viscosity-solution u for $U_{i,j,k}$. This quadratic equation implies that the action U at (i, j, k) depends only on the 6-neighbors that have lower action values, and that the action can only grow when iterating.

Based on this observation, the *fast marching* technique introduces order in the selection of the voxels, and the Eikonal equation can be solved using a front propagation technique. Starting from the initial point p_0 with $U = 0$, this algorithm chooses at each iteration the voxel with minimum action value and solves equation (4) in its 6-neighborhood. This corresponds to a wavefront that expands with a speed inversely proportional to the local potential $\tilde{P}$. Wavefront expansion will stop when the desired end point p_e is reached.

To perform these operations efficiently with $O(N \log_2 N)$ complexity on a N voxel grid, the voxels are stored in a min-heap data structure (see details in [7]). It is shown in [3], that when we have reached the end point p_e, we have visited the necessary set of voxels for the path construction. Therefore, we can constrain the computations to this set of voxels, thus saving computation time.

3   Application to Virtual Colonoscopy

3.1   Problem Formulation

In virtual colonoscopy, we want to extract the colon centerline as a navigation guide for a virtual endoscopic camera. This centerline should stay in the colon lumen, pass through the center as much as possible, start and end at user defined points, and be smooth. User interaction can be reduced by automatically detecting the end point of the path.

3.2   Cost Function

In a CT colon scan, the contrast between the air-filled colon lumen and the surrounding tissue is very high, and the Houndsfield values $I(\mathbf{x})$ of both structures are very constant. Therefore, we can simply use a thresholding function as the potential in each voxel: $P(\mathbf{x}) = 0$ if $I(\mathbf{x}) < T$ and $P(\mathbf{x}) = C$ elsewhere.

The minimal cost path using this thresholded cost will be the path with minimal Euclidean length between the start and end point that still stays inside the colon.

3.3 Path Centering

If we use the cost function defined in section 3.2, the minimal path will not be centered. The effect near a turn in the structure is shown in Fig. 2-left (dashed line) and a virtual view in Fig. 2-middle. This is due to the fact that the Euclidean path length is minimized, and no cost benefit is given for centering.

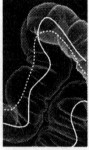
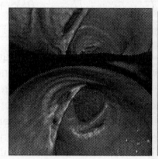
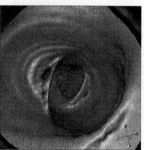

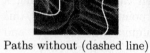
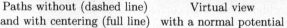

Paths without (dashed line)   Virtual view   Virtual view
and with centering (full line)   with a normal potential   with a centering potential

Fig. 2. Centering the path in the colon

In [3] a technique is detailed how to center paths in a tubular shape, using the front propagation method at each step. A short outline of the method:

1. The propagated front is used to obtain a segmentation of the colon, in a way similar to [6].
2. The distance $\mathcal{D}$ to the colon wall is calculated in every voxel using a front propagation with constant potential. This distance is used to define a new potential P' as $P'(\mathbf{x}) = A \, \exp(-B\mathcal{D})$ where the constants A and B are chosen according to the size of the colon.
3. Finally a minimal path search is done using the centering potential P'. The final centered path is shown in Fig. 2-left in full line its virtual view is shown in Fig. 2-right.

3.4 End Point Detection

The wavefront expansion will stop when a user defined point has been reached. However, in practical applications it is better to automatically detect the end-point of the path for the following reasons :

- it reduces user interaction and therefore saves time and creates a user-independent result;
- a less experienced user may put the end point in the wrong location;
- the colon is often obstructed by remaining fluid, stool or colon contractions.

It is possible to detect when the propagating wavefront expands outside the colon lumen by simply checking the potential value of the voxel added to the front. When this occurs, the entire colon lumen connected to the start point has been searched. The last voxel that was reached before expanding outside the colon lumen is the point that has the largest Euclidean distance (inside the colon) from the starting point, and is therefore chosen as automatic end point. The centering as explained in section 3.3 will be done between the starting point and the automatically detected end point.

3.5 Some Results

Some results of the path tracker are shown in Fig. 3. We can clearly see the complex tortuous shape of the colon, and the quality of the resulting path.

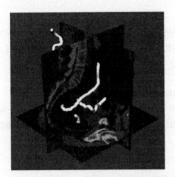 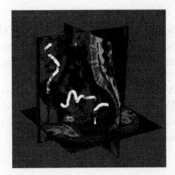

Fig. 3. Different views on a tracked path

4 Clinical Study

4.1 Goal

A multi-user clinical study was performed using a prototype based on EasyVision (Philips Medical Systems). The purpose was to measure the speed and user-dependence of the automatic path tracker. To this aim, the path tracking tool has been evaluated by 5 different operators :

- two physicians with manual path tracking experience ($P1$, $P2$);
- two operators with abdominal anatomy knowledge but no virtual colonoscopy practice ($M1$, $M2$);
- one reference operator (R) familiar with the automatic path tracking tool.

As a comparison the user R also manually defined a path twice on the same dataset.

4.2 Data

Spiral CT data (5 mm slice thickness, 3 mm reconstruction interval) from 15 patients were used, corresponding to a total of 29 scans. During the patient preparation phase the colon was emptied as much as possible, and distended by inflating room air. In most cases, both prone and supine scanning was done.

4.3 Measurements

Time For each user, the wall clock time was measured using an automatic logging mechanism. In general, path construction consisted of following steps :

1. load and inspect data
2. place starting point in the cecum
3. track + center path
4. check result and modify/continue tracking if necessary

The time necessary to perform steps 3 and 4 were measured and both user interaction time and calculation time were taken into account.

User-Dependence To measure the user-dependence of the path tracker, resulting paths P from different users were compared to the corresponding path R obtained by reference user in the following way :

1. **Warp path $P(i)$ and $R(j)$ to a common length parameter k**
   We want to locally stretch and compress paths $P(i)$ and $R(j)$ using warping functions $w_P(k)$ and $w_R(k)$. The goal is to obtain the optimal warping satisfying

   $$(w_P, w_R) = argmin_{w_1, w_2} \left(\sum_k \|P(w_1(k)) - R(w_2(k))\| \right) \qquad (5)$$

   where all points of P and R are addressed by the warping. This mapping is calculated using the Dynamic Time Warp algorithm ([8]).

2. **Calculate Euclidean distances d between corresponding points**
   After warping, the path distances d can be calculated as

   $$d_{P,R}(k) = \|P(w_P(k)) - R(w_R(k))\| \qquad (6)$$

   and are shown in Fig.4 as a function of the common path length k.

3. **Extract the common part**
   To exclude the effect of the exact start and end point, we only consider the common part of paths P and R, which is defined in Fig.4.

4. **Measure the similarity S between the paths**
   We propose to measure the similarity by using the percentage of the common path length k where the distance d is below a threshold t, written as $\mathcal{S}^t_{(P,R)}$.

The chosen measure for path similarity $\mathcal{S}^t_{(P,R)}$ is symmetrical, it is robust to a complete different choice in starting position, and it gives a more reliable result of similarity between paths than e.g. the maximum distance.

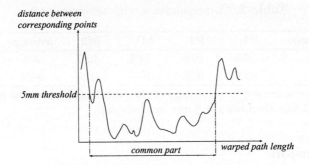

Fig. 4. The Euclidean difference between corresponding points plotted versus the warped path length k. The common part is defined as the longest possible stretch between two positions where the distance falls below the threshold of 5 mm.

Table 1. Timing results of the automatic path tracker.

time	P1	P2	M1	M2	R	average	manual
user time	2.8	4.6	5.3	4.5	2.0	3.6	30.0
calculation time	1.0	1.0	1.2	1.7	1.3	1.2	
total time	3.8	5.6	6.5	6.2	3.2	**4.8**	30.0

Time expressed in minutes per scan.

4.4   Results

Time The results of the time measurements are show in Table 1. The average time needed for path tracking is 4.8 minutes per scan, measuring both user interaction time and calculation time.

No significant differences (95% confidence level, student t-test) were found between the experienced physicians ($P1$ and $P2$) and the other users ($M1$, $M2$), excluding the reference user R. These results are in agreement with a previously published study [4], where an average of 4.5 minutes was measured on 27 cases. The timing for the manual case has no statistical meaning, but is merely given for comparison.

User-Dependence Table 2 summarizes the measurements of the path correspondence using the similarity measures S^2 (2 mm threshold) and S^5 (5 mm threshold) as defined in section 4.3.

On the average, an automatically defined path differs less than 5 mm from the reference over 94% of its length. Again, the results of the manual path tracking is given for comparison. Both manually tracked paths differed less than 5 mm over only 68% of their lengths.

Table 2. Correspondence with reference path.

correspondence	P1	P2	M1	M2	average	manual
$\mathcal{S}^2$	79%	89%	81%	92%	85%	20%
$\mathcal{S}^5$	89%	97%	93%	95%	**94%**	68%

Correspondence expressed in percentage of the path length where the reference path is closer than 2 mm (first row) or 5 mm (second row).

5   Conclusion

Automatic path tracking provides a fast and easy way to determine the colon centerline. The resulting path lies completely inside the colon, is as much centered as possible and is smooth.

The path tracker can be used by less experienced operators without significant differences in time or resulting centerline. This is an important result, since it allows to separate the path tracking task from the actual inspection task. The former task can be done as a preprocessing step by a different person since the results of the path tracker are largely operator-independent. Separating path tracking and inspection will increase the physician's efficacy, reduce the cost and allow a more widespread application of path-based navigation and visualization.

References

1. Cohen, L.D., Kimmel, R.: Global Minimum for Active Contour Models: A Minimal Path Approach. International Journal of Computer Vision. **24** (1997) 57–78
2. Deschamps, T., Cohen, L.D.: Automatic construction of minimal paths in 3D images for virtual endoscopy. Computer Assisted Radiology and Surgery, CARS'99, Paris. (1999)
3. Deschamps, T., Cohen, L.D.: Minimal Paths in 3D Images and Application to Virtual Endoscopy. European Conference on Computer Vision, ECCV'00, Dublin. (2000)
4. Rogalla P., Verdonck B., Truyen R., Hamm B.: Efficacy of automatic path tracking for virtual colonoscopy. RSNA 1999
5. Kass, M., Witkin, A., Terzopoulos, D.: Snakes: Active contour models. International Journal of Computer Vision. **4** (1988) 321–331
6. Malladi, R., Sethian, J.A.: A Real-Time Algorithm for Medical Shape Recovery. Proceedings of International Conference on Computer Vision. (1998) 304–310
7. Sethian J.A.: Level set methods: Evolving Interfaces in Computational Geometry, Fluid Mechanics, Computer Vision and Materials Sciences. Cambridge University Press (1999)
8. Rabiner, L. R., Rosenberg, A. E., and Levinson, S. E.: Considerations In Dynamic Time Warping Algorithms For Discrete Word Recognition IEEE Trans. On Acoustics, Speech and Signal Processing , vol. ASSP-26, No. 6, pp. 575-582, December 1978.

Evaluation of Diffusion Techniques for Improved Vessel Visualization and Quantification in Three-Dimensional Rotational Angiography

Erik Meijering[1], Wiro Niessen[1], Joachim Weickert[2], and Max Viergever[1]

[1] Image Sciences Institute, University Medical Center Utrecht,
Heidelberglaan 100, NL-3584 CX Utrecht, the Netherlands.
{erik,wiro,max}@isi.uu.nl
http://www.isi.uu.nl/
[2] Computer Vision, Graphics and Pattern Recognition Group,
Department of Mathematics and Computer Science,
University of Mannheim, D-68131 Mannheim, Germany.
Joachim.Weickert@uni-mannheim.de
http://www.cvgpr.uni-mannheim.de/weickert/

Abstract. Three-dimensional rotational angiography (3DRA) is a promising imaging technique which yields high-resolution isotropic 3D images of vascular structures. Raw 3DRA images, however, usually suffer from a high noise level and the presence of other artifacts. For accurate visualization and quantification of vascular anomalies, noise reduction is therefore highly desirable. In this paper we analyze the effects of several linear and nonlinear filtering techniques for that purpose. From the results of *in vitro* experiments we conclude that edge-enhancing anisotropic diffusion is very suitable for mentioned tasks. However, in view of the computational requirements of this technique, the regularized isotropic nonlinear diffusion scheme may be considered a useful alternative.

1 Introduction

Three-dimensional rotational angiography (3DRA) is a relatively new technique for imaging blood vessels in the human body [1,2,3,4,5]. Using a standard C-arm imaging system, this technique yields high-resolution isotropic 3D datasets reconstructed from 2D X-ray angiography images acquired during a 180-degree rotation of the X-ray source-detector combination following a single injection of contrast material. The vascular structures of interest can afterwards be studied from any desired angle by the use of 3D visualization techniques. The absence of overprojections and the high resolution of the resulting datasets make the technique also potentially interesting for quantitative studies.

However, visualization of raw 3DRA images is usually unacceptable, due to the high noise level and the presence of reconstruction artifacts and unwanted structures resulting from inhomogeneous surrounding tissue. In order to improve

W. Niessen and M. Viergever (Eds.): MICCAI 2001, LNCS 2208, pp. 177–185, 2001.

the quality of volume and surface renderings, some form of noise reduction must be applied to the raw data prior to visualization. Although application of noise reduction techniques may result in qualitatively better renderings, the effects of such techniques on the subsequent quantification of vessels and vascular anomalies based on those renderings have not yet been reported in the literature. Analysis of these effects is important, as particular techniques may increase the user-dependency of volume and surface renderings—which are generally based on one or more user-defined thresholds—and thus the reliability of quantitative measurements obtained from those renderings. In this paper we evaluate several linear and nonlinear diffusion filtering techniques for noise reduction by analyzing their effects on the quality of visualization and the accuracy of quantification of vascular anomalies in 3DRA images.

2   Diffusion Techniques

The noise reduction techniques considered in this study are uniform filtering, Gaussian filtering or linear diffusion, regularized isotropic nonlinear diffusion, and edge-enhancing anisotropic diffusion, which are briefly described next.

Uniform Filtering. The simplest and computationally cheapest approach to reduce noise in images is to average the grey-values of voxels in a cubic neighborhood around each voxel by means of separable uniform filtering (UF):

$$I(\mathbf{x}) = (I_0 * U_m)(\mathbf{x}), \qquad \mathbf{x} = (x, y, z) \in X, \tag{1}$$

where I_0 denotes the original 3D image, $X \subset \mathbb{R}^3$ is the image domain, and $U_m(\mathbf{x}) = u_m(x)u_m(y)u_m(z)$ denotes the 3D normalized uniform filter given by $u_m(\xi) = m^{-1}$ if $|\xi| \leq \frac{1}{2}m$, $m \in \mathbb{N}$ odd, and $u_m(\xi) = 0$ otherwise.

Gaussian Filtering. Another frequently used approach to image smoothing is Gaussian filtering (GF), also implemented by separable convolution:

$$I(\mathbf{x}) = (I_0 * G_\sigma)(\mathbf{x}), \qquad \mathbf{x} = (x, y, z) \in X, \tag{2}$$

with $G_\sigma(\mathbf{x}) = g_\sigma(x)g_\sigma(y)g_\sigma(z)$, and g_σ denoting the Gaussian with standard deviation σ. The process (2) constitutes the solution to the linear diffusion equation $\partial_t I(\mathbf{x}; t) = \nabla \cdot \nabla I(\mathbf{x}; t)$, with $\sigma = \sqrt{2t}$ and initial condition $I(\mathbf{x}; 0) = I_0(\mathbf{x})$.

Regularized Isotropic Nonlinear Diffusion. The first nonlinear technique included in this study is the regularized version of the Perona-Malik scheme [6]. This scheme (RPM) is obtained from the linear diffusion equation by including a gradient-dependent diffusivity:

$$\partial_t I(\mathbf{x}; t) = \nabla \cdot \left(D\big(\|\nabla I_\tau(\mathbf{x}; t)\|^2\big) \nabla I(\mathbf{x}; t) \right), \tag{3}$$

where the gradient is computed at scale $\sigma_n = \sqrt{2\tau}$, $\tau > 0$. In our study, we used [7] $D(\xi^2) = 1 - \exp\big(-3.31488/(\xi/\zeta)^8\big)$, where $\zeta > 0$ corresponds to the minimum contrast needed for structures in order to be preserved.

Edge-Enhancing Anisotropic Diffusion. The second nonlinear diffusion technique (EED) does not only take into account the contrast of an edge, but also its orientation. This is achieved by replacing the scalar-valued diffusivity in (3) by a diffusion tensor [7]:

$$\partial_t I(\mathbf{x}; t) = \nabla \cdot \Big(\mathbf{D}\big(\nabla I_\tau(\mathbf{x}; t)\big) \nabla I(\mathbf{x}; t) \Big), \tag{4}$$

where $\mathbf{D}$ is constructed from the system of orthonormal eigenvectors $\mathbf{v}_1 \| \nabla I(\mathbf{x}; \tau)$, $\mathbf{v}_2 \perp \nabla I(\mathbf{x}; \tau)$, $\mathbf{v}_3 \perp \nabla I(\mathbf{x}; \tau)$ and $\perp \mathbf{v}_2$, and corresponding eigenvectors $\lambda_1 = D\big(\|\nabla I(\mathbf{x}; \tau)\|^2\big)$ and $\lambda_2 = \lambda_3 = D(0) = 1$, with D as in RPM. With this choice of $\mathbf{D}$, smoothing along edges is preferred over smoothing across them.

3   Vascular Anomalies

Currently, 3DRA is used primarily for visualization and subsequent quantification of carotid stenosis and intracranial aneurysms [3,4,5]. We briefly discuss the measures used for quantification of these anomalies.

Carotid Stenosis. For the quantification of the degree of stenosis of the internal carotid artery (ICA) we used the North American Symptomatic Carotid Endarterectomy Trial (NASCET) measure and the common carotid measure (CC) [8], respectively defined as $D_{\text{NASCET}} = (1 - d_\text{S}/d_{\text{ICA}})$ and $D_{\text{CC}} = (1 - d_\text{S}/d_{\text{CCA}})$, with d_S, d_{ICA}, and d_{CCA} as in Fig. 1. Both measures involve measuring the luminal diameter at the point of maximum stenosis (d_S). The NASCET measure furthermore involves the diameter (d_{ICA}) of a visible portion of disease-free ICA distal to the stenosis, whereas the CC measure uses the diameter (d_{CCA}) of the visible disease-free distal common carotid artery (CCA).

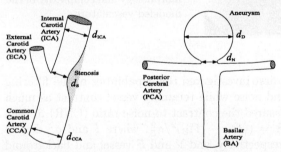

Fig. 1. Diameters involved in the different measures for quantification of internal carotid stenosis (**left**) and intracranial saccular aneurysms (**right**).

Intracranial Aneurysms. For quantification of intracranial aneurysms, several measures were considered. The first is the dome diameter (d_D, see Fig. 1), which has been shown to relate significantly to risk of rupture [9]. The second measure considered in this study is the diameter of the aneurysmal neck (d_N), which is important in selecting an appropriate clip in the case of surgical intervention or for predicting successful obliteration of the aneurysmal lumen in the case of endovascular treatment [10]. The ratio between diameters d_N and d_D of the aneurysm has also been suggested as a guideline in deciding between surgical or endovascular treatment [11].

4 Experiments and Results

The experiments were carried out on phantoms for which ground truth was available. In this section we describe the phantoms and image acquisition, the method of evaluation, and the results.

Phantoms and Image Acquisition. Images were obtained of a carotid anthropomorphic vascular phantom (CAVP) with an asymmetrical stenosis in the ICA, and an intracranial anthropomorphic vascular phantom (IAVP) with a berry aneurysm at the tip of the basilar artery (BA). The phantoms (R. G. Shelley Ltd., North York, Ontario) represent average dimensions of the corresponding vascular structures in the human body: $d_s = 1.68$mm, $d_{ICA} = 5.6$mm, $d_{CCA} = 8.0$mm, $d_N = 2.6$mm, and $d_D = 12.9$mm. Each of the phantoms was filled with contrast material (50% diluted Ultravist-300, Schering, Weesp) and an Integris V3000 C-arm imaging system (Philips Medical Systems, Best) was used to acquire 100 X-ray angiography images (resolution 512^2 pixels, 10 bits/pixel, see Fig. 2 for examples) during automatic rotation of the C-arm over 180 degrees lasting eight seconds. A modified filtered back-projection algorithm was then applied to generate 3DRA images at resolutions of 128^3 voxels of size 0.6^3mm^3 and 256^3 voxels of size 0.3^3mm^3, 16 bits/voxel.

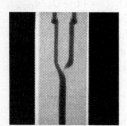 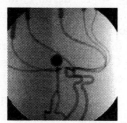

Fig. 2. Sample X-ray projection images taken from the rotational angiography runs of the CAVP (**left**) and the IAVP (**right**). The images give an impression of the morphology and complexity of the modeled vasculature.

Method of Evaluation. We first investigated the capabilities of the filtering techniques to reduce background noise while retaining vessel contrast as much as possible. To this end we measured the contrast-to-noise ratio (CNR) in each of the vessels of interest: CNR $= (\langle I \rangle_V - \langle I \rangle_B)^2 / \sigma_B^2$, where I and σ^2 denote image intensity and variance, respectively, and V and B vessel and background regions. For B, a fixed background region was selected in each of the images. The CNR was measured as a function of "evolution time", t. This variable is explicitly present in RPM and EED, and together with the temporal step-size Δt determines the number of iterations of the discretized differential equation to be carried out. For GF we have the relation $t = \sigma^2 / 2$. For UF we used the same relation, with σ the standard deviation of u_m, so that $t = m^2 / 24$, where m is a discrete variable for which we took values of $1, 3, 5, 7, 9$, and 11. To allow a direct comparison of the results of UF and GF, RPM, and EED, the measurements for the latter schemes were carried out at corresponding evolution times $t = 0.0$ (original), 0.375, 1.042, 2.042, 3.375, and 5.042. In all experiments, the additional parameters of RPM and EED were fixed to $\sigma_n = 0.5$ and $\zeta = 0.05$, which seemed to be appropriate values according to initial experiments.

Next, the effects of the techniques on quantification of the vascular anomalies were investigated. Therefore, the diameters d_s, d_{ICA}, d_{CCA}, d_N, and d_D were measured as a function of both t and the threshold parameter θ. For t we used the same values as in the CNR measurements. The parameter θ is used in practice to separate relevant (vascular) from non-relevant (noise and other) structures in the visualizations, on the base of which quantification takes place. In order to use acquisition independent values for θ, the images were "normalized" so as to make the average background intensity 0.0 and the average intensity within the vessels 1.0. Together with the ground-truth values, the results allowed for an assessment of both accuracy and robustness to threshold selection of quantitative measurements and their dependency on the filter strength.

Finally, we looked at the qualitative (visual) effects of the different noise reduction techniques. These concerned the apparent (not measured) dimensions of the vascular anomalies in 3D visualizations of the filtered 3DRA datasets and their dependency on the user-controlled threshold parameter, as well as the apparent smoothness of the vascular structures in these visualizations. To this end, both exo- and endovascular surface renderings were generated by using a standard Phong shading technique.

Results. Because of space limitations we have to confine ourselves here to showing only some of the results and to summarize the overall findings. Examples of CNR measurement results carried out in high-resolution 3DRAs of the CAVP and IAVP are given in Fig. 3. The results showed that the four schemes UF, GF, RPM, and EED reduce noise equally well in vessel segments with a relatively large luminal diameter (typically larger than 10 voxels). For segments with smaller diameters, the nonlinear filtering techniques (RPM and EED) outperformed the linear techniques (UF and GF) for larger evolution times.

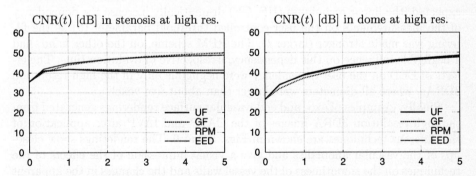

Fig. 3. Contrast-to-noise ratio (CNR) as a function of evolution time (t) for the four techniques (UF, GF, RPM, EED), measured in the stenosis (**left**) and dome (**right**) in the high-resolution 3DRA reconstruction of the CAVP and IAVP, respectively.

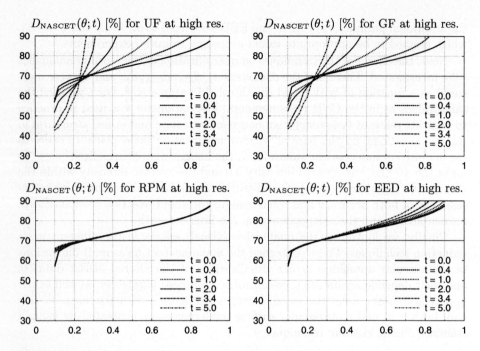

Fig. 4. Degree of stenosis (D_{NASCET}) as a function of the user-controlled threshold (θ) and evolution time (t) for the four techniques (UF, GF, RPM, EED), as measured in the high-resolution reconstruction of the CAVP. The true value is $D_{\text{NASCET}} = 70\%$.

Whereas the CNR measurements concerned the behavior of the techniques in the background and the interior of vessels, the diameter measurements revealed their performance at the transitions from background to vessel. Examples of the results of these experiments are given in Fig. 4. These results showed that, as expected, the linear techniques (UF, GF) dramatically increase the dependency of the measurements on the user-controlled threshold parameter (θ) as the filtering was made stronger (larger t). The RPM scheme, on the other hand, had a negligible influence on this dependency, irrespective of evolution time. The effects of EED on the user-dependency were negligible only in the high-resolution 3DRAs, where all diameters were larger than about five voxels.

Finally, examples of exo- and endovascular surface renderings generated from the high-resolution 3DRA images of the CAVP and IAVP after application of the different techniques are shown in Figs. 5 and 6. The renderings show close-ups of the vascular anomalies and give a visual impression of the effects of the techniques on the smoothness of the vessel walls and the changes in the apparent dimensions of the anomalies when varying the user-controlled threshold. The renderings support the findings of the quantification experiments: the linear techniques increased the user-dependency of the vascular dimensions, while the negative effects of RPM and EED were marginal. The smoothness of the vessel

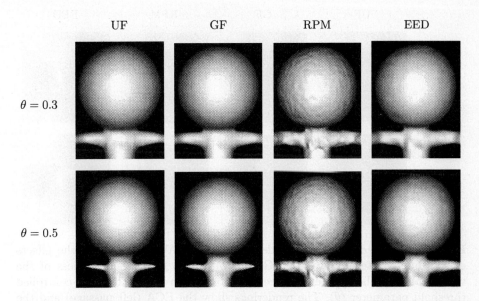

Fig. 5. Exovascular surface renderings of the IAVP illustrating the effects of the different techniques (UF, GF, RPM, EED) on the smoothness of the vessel walls and the apparent size of especially the neck of the aneurysm when varying the user-controlled threshold parameter (θ). The renderings show a close-up of the neck and the dome of the aneurysm, the BA and both PCAs, at $t = 2.042$.

walls, however, was considerably improved by EED, while most of the noise in these edge regions was retained by RPM.

5   Discussion and Conclusions

Overall, the results of our *in vitro* experiments suggest that for vessels with sufficiently large luminal diameter, EED is most suitable: the increase in the user-dependency of quantifications and visualizations is considerably less than with UF or GF, and it is better at reducing noise at the vessel walls than RPM. The sub-optimal performance of EED in vessel segments with very small luminal diameters is most probably due to the fact that the amount of blurring in the plane orthogonal to a local gradient is equal in all directions. We suspect that in order for EED to work adequately also in these cases, it is necessary to make a distinction between the directions corresponding to minimal and maximal curvature, which requires the use of second-order information (Hessian). Early experiments with curvature-based anisotropic diffusion schemes [12] have shown promising results, but more elaborate evaluations are required to determine the clinical implications. Other disadvantages of EED are its memory requirements and its relatively high computational cost. If these are decisive factors, RPM may be a reasonable alternative, for which more efficient algorithms exist [7].

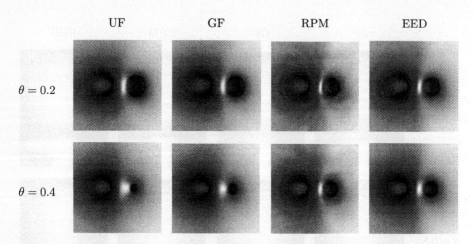

Fig. 6. Endovascular surface renderings of the CAVP illustrating the effects of the different techniques (UF, GF, RPM, EED) on the smoothness of the vessel walls and the apparent degree of stenosis when varying the user-controlled threshold parameter (θ). The renderings show the ECA (left passage) and the stenosis in the ICA (right passage), viewed from within the CCA, at $t = 2.042$.

References

1. R. Fahrig *et al.*, "Use of a C-arm system to generate true three-dimensional computed rotational angiograms: Preliminary *in vitro* and *in vivo* results", *Am. J. Neuroradiol.*, vol. 18, 1997, pp. 1507–1514.
2. B. A. Schueler *et al.*, "Three-dimensional vascular reconstruction with a clinical X-ray angiography system", *Acad. Radiol.*, vol. 4, 1997, pp. 693–699.
3. J. Moret *et al.*, "3D rotational angiography: Clinical value in endovascular treatment", *Medicamundi*, vol. 42, 1998, pp. 8–14.
4. R. Anxionnat *et al.*, "3D angiography: Clinical interest. First applications in interventional neuroradiology", *J. Neuroradiol.*, vol. 25, 1998, pp. 251–262.
5. Y. Trousset *et al.*, "A fully automated system for three-dimensional X-ray angiography", in *Computer Assisted Radiology and Surgery (CARS'99)*, Elsevier Science, Amsterdam, 1999, pp. 39–43.
6. F. Catté *et al.*, "Image selective smoothing and edge detection by nonlinear diffusion", *SIAM J. Num. Anal.*, vol. 29, 1992, pp. 182–193.
7. J. Weickert, *Anisotropic Diffusion in Image Processing*, B. G. Teubner, Stuttgart, Germany, 1998.
8. P. M. Rothwell *et al.*, "Equivalence of measurements of carotid stenosis. a comparison of three methods on 1001 angiograms", *Stroke*, vol. 25, 1994, pp. 2435–2439.
9. N. Yasui *et al.*, "Subarachnoid hemorrhage caused by previously diagnosed, previously unruptured intracranial aneurysms: A retrospective analysis of 25 cases", *Neurosurgery*, vol. 39, 1996, pp. 1096–1100.
10. A. Fernandez Zubillaga *et al.*, "Endovascular occlusion of intracranial aneurysms with electrically detachable coils: Correlation of aneurysm neck size and treatment results", *Am. J. Neuroradiol.*, vol. 15, 1994, pp. 815–820.

11. L. Parlea *et al.*, "An analysis of the geometry of saccular intracranial aneurysms", *Am. J. Neuroradiol.*, vol. 20, 1999, pp. 1079–1089.
12. K. Krissian *et al.*, "Directional anisotropic diffusion applied to segmentation of vessels in 3D images", in *Scale-Space Theory in Computer Vision*, vol. 1252 of *Lecture Notes in Computer Science*, Springer-Verlag, Berlin, 1997, pp. 345–348.

Eddy-Current Distortion Correction and Robust Tensor Estimation for MR Diffusion Imaging

J.-F. Mangin[1,3], C. Poupon[1,2,3,4], C. Clark[1,3], D. Le Bihan[1,3], and I. Bloch[2,3]

[1] Service Hospitalier Frédéric Joliot, CEA, 91401 Orsay, France
mangin@shfj.cea.fr, http://www-dsv.cea.fr/
[2] Département Signal et Images, CNRS URA 820, ENST, Paris
[3] Institut Fédératif de Recherche 49
[4] GE Medical Systems, Buc, France

Abstract. This paper presents a new procedure to estimate the diffusion tensor from a sequence of diffusion-weighted images. The first step of this procedure consists of the correction of the distortions usually induced by eddy-current related to the large diffusion-sensitizing gradients. This correction algorithm relies on the maximization of mutual information to estimate the three parameters of a geometric distortion model inferred from the acquisition principle. The second step of the procedure amounts to replacing the standard least squares based approach by the Geman-McLure M-estimator, in order to get rid of outlier related artefacts. Several experiments prove that the whole procedure highly improves the quality of the final diffusion maps.

1 Introduction

There is currently considerable interest in the use of MRI for imaging the apparent diffusion of water in brain tissues [13]. When anisotropy of the 3D diffusion process is of interest, for instance for fiber bundle tracking [18], a symmetric diffusion tensor D has to be calculated for each voxel from a series of diffusion-weighted volumes [3, 2]. Each such volume is acquired with a different applied diffusion-sensitizing gradient [21]. These gradients are applied in order to vary a symmetric matrix b (s/mm^2) that depends on the gradient direction, strength and timing [15]. The diffusion-sensitizing gradient affects the signal intensity of any given voxel in a manner that can be described by the linear equation:

$$\ln S(b) = \ln S(0) - D_{xx}b_{xx} - 2D_{xy}b_{xy} - 2D_{xz}b_{xz} - D_{yy}b_{yy} - 2D_{yz}b_{yz} - D_{zz}b_{zz}, \tag{1}$$

where S denotes the signal of the selected voxel. When a sufficient number of different b matrices is used, the diffusion tensor D can be estimated.

Such calculations are simple if each voxel in the different volumes represents the same point in the anatomy of the subject, but can be impractical if different volumes of the series are distorted relative to each other. Diffusion-weighted images, however, are often acquired using Echo-Planar Imaging (EPI), to reduce acquisition time. Unfortunatelly, this fast acquisition scheme is highly sensitive

W. Niessen and M. Viergever (Eds.): MICCAI 2001, LNCS 2208, pp. 186–194, 2001.

to eddy currents induced by the large diffusion gradients [8]. These eddy currents can cause significant distortions in the phase-encoding direction where the image bandwidth is quite low (see Fig. 1). Since the degree and nature of this artefact typically vary both with the strength and orientation of the diffusion-sensitizing gradient, distortions can dramatically change the direction of highest diffusion supposed to correspond to fiber direction.

The methods for reducing the effects of eddy currents may be divided into four categories. The first one simply consists of modifications of the gradient sequences [1]. This approach, however, seems unsufficient to get completely rid of artefacts. Other approaches are retrospective and can be considered as registration methods. Some of them which rely on MR physics require additional experimental data [11]. Others simply use a distortion geometric model inferred from the acquisition principle, which leads to estimate a few parameters using a standard similarity measure like cross-correlation [8, 6, 4]. The last kind of approaches stem from recent progress in the definition of robust similarity measures. To our knowledge, such approaches have only been applied in functional MRI to correct for distortions induced by susceptibility artefacts in EPI, using a free deformation model with a high number of parameters [12, 9]. In this paper we propose to estimate the few parameters of the distortion geometric model from the mutual information in order to achieve a robust correction. This approach largely improves previous ones. Simpler similarity measures, indeed, seem not sufficient to perfectly take into account the complex dependencies embedded in equation 1. Moreover, the fact that a priori knowledge on the deformation main effects allows us to estimate only three paramaters per slice highly simplifies the optimization process.

This paper proposes a second improvement of the standard calculation of the diffusion tensor D. The linearity of Eq. 1 usually leads to a least squares based regression method [2]. This approach, however, is not robust to the various kinds of noises that can be observed in diffusion-weighted data [5]. Non Gaussian noise can stem for instance from physiological motions (brain beat), subject motions or residual distortions. While careful acquisition schemes including cardiac gating and navigator echo may reduce some of these problems, some weaknesses of the tensor diffusion model lead to other regression problems: each voxel includes several water compartments endowed with different diffusion processes that are mixed up in the data [7]. Hence, in order to overcome the influence of outliers on the tensor estimation, we propose the use of a standard robust M-estimator [16]. A comparison of the behaviour of both regression methods in the presence of various levels of corrupted data prove the interest of the robust approach.

2   Distortion Correction

In the following, echo-planar diffusion-weighted images were acquired in the axial plane. Blocks of eight contiguous slices were acquired each 2.8mm thick. Seven blocks were acquired covering the entire brain corresponding to 56 slice locations. For each slice location 31 images were acquired; a T2-weighted image

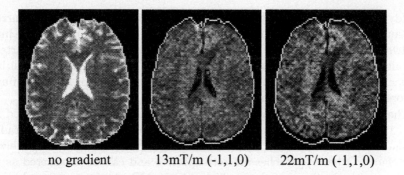

no gradient   13mT/m (-1,1,0)   22mT/m (-1,1,0)

Fig. 1. *Example of eddy-current related distortions (8mm in the worst case)*

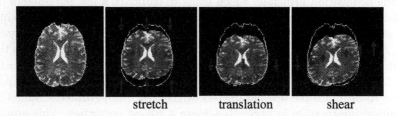

stretch   translation   shear

Fig. 2. *The simple geometric model of eddy-current related distortions*

with no diffusion sensitization followed by 5 diffusion sensitized sets (b values linearly incremented to a maximum value of $1000s/mm^2$) in each of 6 non-colinear directions. In order to improve the signal to noise ratio this was repeated 4 times, providing 124 images per slice location. The image resolution was 128 x 128, field of view $24cm \times 24cm$, $TE = 84.4ms$, $TR = 2.5s$

For each slice, all acquisitions are aligned with the first image of the series. For convenience we use the notation that the image is in the XY plane, and the phase-encoding direction lies along Y. Simple considerations about MR physics lead to the following distortion model [8]:

– A residual gradient in the slice-encoding direction Z produces uniform translation along Y;
– A residual gradient in the frequency-encoding direction X produces a shear parallel to Y (a translation linearly related to X);
– A residual gradient in the phase-encoding direction Y produces a uniform scaling in Y direction.

Hence, the geometric model (see Fig. 2) can be written for each column X as:

$$Y' = SY + T_0 + T_1X. \tag{2}$$

An additional global multiplicative correction by $\frac{1}{S}$ has to be applied to the slice intensities, which is done after estimation of (S, T_0, T_1).

To take into account the complex dependencies between the target image, which is a standard T2-weighted image, and the diffusion-weighted images, the

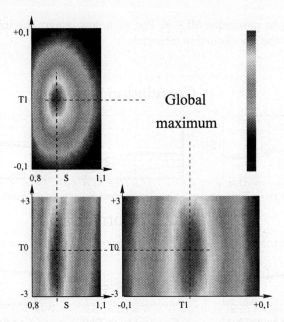

Fig. 3. *Orthogonal slices of the mutual information crossing at the global maximum.*

similarity measure used to estimate the optimal (S, T_0, T_1) is the mutual information (MI) [10, 14]. Since the two images to be aligned are 128x128 slices to be compared to the usual 3D situation, a Parzen window is used to get a robust estimation of the joint intensity distribution. This Parzen window is a truncated Gaussian kernel sufficient to smooth the joint histogram. This approach turned out to be crucial to prevent the maximization algorithm to be trapped in MI local maxima. Hence, estimation of $MI(S, T_0, T_1)$ consists of a linear resampling of the image to be aligned according to Eq. 2, followed by the application of the Parzen window to the joint histogram. Then MI can be computed from:

$$MI(S, T_0, T_1) = \sum_{i_t=0}^{M-1} \sum_{i_a=0}^{M-1} p(i_t, i_a) \log \frac{p(i_t, i_a)}{p(i_t)p(i_a)},$$

where M is the sampling of the joint probability distribution (in practice $M = 64$), i_t the intensity in the target image and i_a the intensity in the image to be aligned. The marginal probabilities $p(i_t)$ and $p(i_a)$ are computed by row and column summation.

Since 123 realignments have to be performed for each slice of the volume, a fast optimization scheme is required. Fortunately, the use of a Parzen window leads to a rather smooth MI landscape around the global maximum (see Fig. 3). In some cases, several maxima have been observed near the global one. In such situations, however, we could not claim that the global maximum was a better solution than the surrounding maxima. Hence, Powell algorithm has been used in the following to maximize MI [19]. For each new image, the initial position is (1,0,0), namely the no distortion situation.

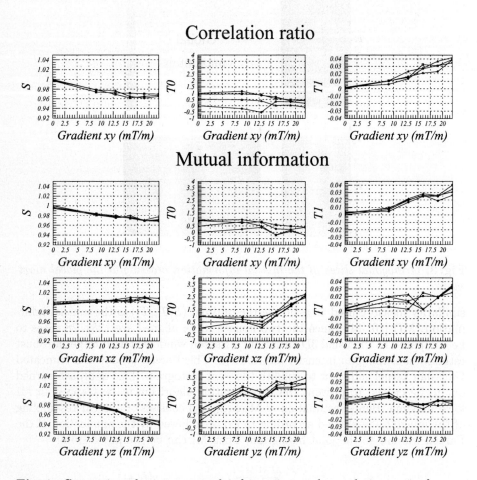

Fig. 4. *Comparison between mutual information and correlation ratio for one gradient direction: (1,1,0). Reproducibility of the correction process across the four repetitions in three gradient directions, (1,1,0), (1,0,1) and (0,1,1), with six different strengths.*

Thanks to the four repetitions embedded in our acquisition process, the accuracy and the robustness of the correction process can be evaluated. A first experiment consists of comparing the results obtained using mutual information with the results obtained using another similarity measure: the correlation ratio [20]. While both methods have given similar results, the variability across the four repetitions was higher for the correlation ratio (see Fig. 4). Hence, mutual information has been chosen as more adapted to diffusion-weighted images.

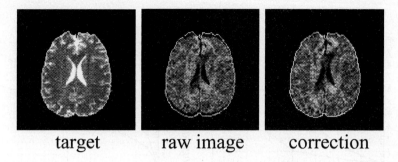

target   raw image   correction

Fig. 5. *Example of distortion correction*

In general, the correction was reproducible across the four repetitions (see Fig. 4). The largest variability was observed for the translation parameter T_0, which can be understood from the shape of MI landscape (see Fig. 3). MI isophotes, indeed, are rather cylindrical with a T0 oriented axis along which some local maxima can be observed. An interesting result is the fact that the highest variability is obtained for the three repetitions of the pure T2-weighted target (no sensitizing gradient) for which $S = 1$, $T_1 = 0$ but $T_0 \neq 0$. This observation tends to prove that eddy currents have long term trends that corrupt several consecutive acquisitions. Finally, the estimated distortions fit well with the physical interpretation mentioned above: The **xy** and **yz** gradients induce a scaling, the **xz** and **yz** gradients induce a global translation, and the **xy** and **xz** gradients induce a shearing.

3   Robust Tensor Estimation

Estimation of the diffusion tensor is done from linear equation 1. While tradition and ease of computation have made the least squares method the popular approach for this regression analysis [2], this method becomes unreliable if outliers are present in the data. Robust regression methods can be used in such situations [16]. The M-estimators are the more popular robust methods. These estimators minimize the sum of a symmetric, positive-definite function $\rho(\epsilon_i)$ of the residuals ϵ_i, with a unique minimum at $\epsilon_i = 0$. A residual is defined as the difference between the data point and the fitted value. For the least squares method $\rho(\epsilon_i) = \epsilon_i^2$. Several ρ functions have been proposed which reduce the influence of large residual values on the estimated fit. We have chosen one of the most popular ones, the Geman-McLure estimator $\rho(\epsilon_i) = \frac{\epsilon_i^2}{\epsilon_i^2 + C^2}$, where $C = 1.48 median_i \{\|\epsilon_i\|\}$. The M-estimate of the diffusion tensor is obtained by converting the minimization into an iterated weighted least squares problem. The initial guess is the solution of the standard least squares.

In order to compare the behaviour of both M-estimators, raw data have been corrupted with various levels of outliers (of course some actual outliers are also present in these data). For a given experiment, a percentage P of the 124 images is modified. For such images, an additional error e is added to each voxel. This

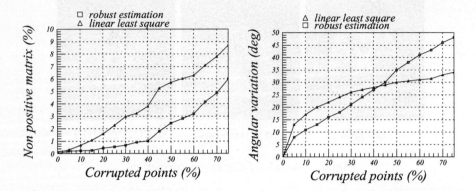

Fig. 6. *Influence of outliers on the number of non positive matrices and on the direction of highest diffusion.*

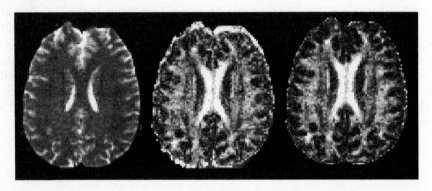

Fig. 7. Left: *raw T2-weighted image.* **Right:** *tensor fractional anisotropy [17] without and with distortion correction and robust regressor. Fractional anisotropy is a simple ratio which measures the variability between the diffusion tensor eigenvalues.*

error is sampled from a Gaussian distribution whose mean is the mean intensity inside the brain, and whose standard deviation is a tenth of the mean. Two measures allow us to assess the effect of these outliers. The first one is the number of non positive estimated tensors, which have no physical interpretation. Such situations may occur because no positivity constraint is embedded in the fitting process. The second measure is the mean angular variation between the direction of highest diffusion with and without outliers. This direction corresponds to the tensor eigenvector associated with the largest eigenvalue. The evolution of these measures relative to the percentage of outliers P is proposed in Fig. 6. The superiority of the Geman-McLure estimator is straightforward.

4   Conclusion

This paper has presented a robust procedure to estimate the diffusion tensor from a sequence of diffusion-weighted images. Further work, however, could still improve this procedure. For instance, a fitting method including a positivity constraint on the tensor eigenvalues should be designed. Furthermore, the issue of distortion correction in the presence of subject motions remains completely open, like in the case of functional MRI. Nevertheless, our new procedure already highly improves the quality of the diffusion map which is illustrated by anisotropy images in Fig. 7.

References

[1] A. L. Alexander, J. S. Tsuruda, and D. L. Parker. Elimination of eddy current artefacts in diffusion-weighted echo-planar images: the use of bipolar gradient. *Magn. Reson. Med.*, 38:1016–1021, 1997.

[2] P.J. Basser, J. Mattiello, and D. LeBihan. Estimation of the effective self-diffusion-tensor from the NMR spin echo. *J. of Magn. Reson., Series B*, 103:247–254, 1994.

[3] P.J. Basser, J. Mattiello, and D. LeBihan. Mr diffusion tensor spectroscopy and imaging. *Biophysical Journal*, 66:259–267, 1994.

[4] M. E. Bastin. Correction of eddy current-induced artefacts in diffusion tensor imaging using iterative cross-correlation. *Magn. Reson. Imag.*, 17:1011–1024, 1999.

[5] M.E. Bastin, P.A. Armitage, and I. Marshall. A theoretical study of the effect of experimental noise on the measurement of anisotropy in diffusion imaging. *Magnetic Resonance Imaging*, 16(7):773–785, 1998.

[6] F. Calamante, D.A. Porter, D.G. Gadian, and A. Connelly. Correction for eddy current induced B0 shifts in diffusion-weighted echo-planar imaging. *Magnetic Resonance in Medicine*, 41:95–102, 1999.

[7] C. A. Clark and D. LeBihan. Water diffusion compartmentation and anisotropy at high b values in the human brain. *Magn. Reson. Med.*, 44:852–859, 2000.

[8] J.C. Haselgrove and J.R. Moore. Correction for distorsion of echo-planar images used to calculate the apparent diffusion coefficient. *Magn. Reson. Med.*, 36, 1996.

[9] P. Hellier and C. Barillot. Multimodal non-rigid warping for correction of distortions in functional MRI. In *MICCAI, LNCS-1935*, pages 512–520, 2000.

[10] W. Wells III, P. Viola, H. Atsumi, S. Nakajima, and R. Kikinis. Multi-modal volume registration by maximization of mutual information. *MIA*, 1:35–51, 1996.

[11] P. Jezzard, A. Barnett, and C Pierpaoli. Characterization and correction for eddy current artefacts in echo planar diffusion imaging. *MRM*, 39:801–812, 1998.

[12] J. Kybic, P. Thévenaz, A. Nirkko, and M. Unser. Unwarping of EPI images. *IEEE Trans. Medical Imaging*, 19(2):80–93, 2000.

[13] D. Le Bihan, J.-F. Mangin, C. Poupon et al. Diffusion tensor imaging: concepts and applications. *Journal of Magnetic Resonance Imaging*, 13:534–546, 2001.

[14] F. Maes, A. Collignon, D. Vandermeulen, G. Marchal, and P. Suetens. Multi-modality image registration by maximisation of mutual information. *IEEE Trans. Medical Imaging*, 16(2):187–198, 1997.

[15] J. Mattiello, P. J. basser, and D. LeBihan. The b matrix in diffusion tensor echo-planar imaging. *Magn. Reson. Med.*, 37:292–300, 1997.

[16] P. Meer, D. Mintz, and A. Rosenfeld. Robust regression methods for computer vision: a review. *International Journal of Computer Vision*, 6(1):59–70, 1991.

[17] C. Pierpaoli and P. J. Basser. Toward a quantitative assessment of diffusion anisotropy. *Magn. Reson. Med.*, 36:893–906, 1996.

[18] C. Poupon, J.-F. Mangin, C. A. Clark, V. Frouin, D. LeBihan, and I. Bloch. Towards inference of the human brain connectivity from MR diffusion tensor data. *Medical Image Analysis*, 5:1–15, 2001.

[19] M. Powell. An efficient method for finding the minimum of a function of several variables without calculating derivatives. *The Computer Journal*, 7:155–162, 1964.

[20] A. Roche, G. Malandain, X. Pennec, and N. Ayache. The correlation ratio as a new similarity measure for multimodal image registration. In *MICCAI'98, MIT, USA, LNCS-1496, Springer Verlag*, pages 1115–1124, 1998.

[21] E.O. Stejskal and J.E. Tanner. Spin diffusion measurements: spin echoes in the presence of a time-dependent field gradient. *Journal of Chemical Physics*, 42(1):288–292, 1965.

Edge Preserving Regularization and Tracking for Diffusion Tensor Imaging

Klaus Hahn[1], Sergei Prigarin[2], and Benno Pütz[3]

[1] Institute of Biomathematics and Biometrics of the National Research Center for
Environment and Health — GSF — , Postfach 1129, D–85758 Neuherberg, Germany
`hahn@gsf.de`
[2] Institute of Computational Mathematics and Mathematical Geophysics,
Novosibirsk, Russia
`smp@osmf.sscc.ru`
[3] Max-Planck-Institute of Psychiatry, München, Germany
`puetz@mpipsykl.mpg.de`

Abstract. Two major problems in MR Diffusion Tensor Imaging, regularization and tracking are addressed. Regularization is performed on a variance homogenizing transformation of the tensor field via a nonlinear filter chain to preserve discontinuities. The suitability of the smoothing procedure is validated by Monte Carlo simulations. For tracking, the tensor field is diagonalized and a local bilinear interpolation of the corresponding direction field is performed. The track curves, which are not restricted to the measured grid, are modeled by following stepwise the interpolated directions. The presented methods are illustrated by applications to measured data.

1 Introduction

Diffusion Tensor Imaging, which can appreciably contribute to explore anatomical connectivity, recently became a main topic in human brain mapping. Two essential problems on the way to detect the flow of axon fibers are discussed in this paper: Improvement of the low signal to noise ratio in the tensor field via regularization and modeling of the axon bundle flow.

Regularization or, equivalently, smoothing including convenient priors is essential for the quantification of anisotropy and direction of the diffusion field as convenient measures are biased by low signal to noise ratio [1,2]. Smoothing can be performed on different levels of description for the direction field, e. g., on the diffusion weighted images of the measured signal [3], on the tensor field [4] or on the vector field of the main diffusion directions [5]. Our approach regularizes a variance homogenizing transformation of the tensor field, as the noise variance of the tensor field is strongly dependent on measuring parameters and the field amplitude. The signals in the tensor field show discontinuous patterns, due to tissue or organ dependent changes in the anisotropy of diffusion. Therefore, an edge preserving smoother which does not blur the field is applied. A validation of this smoothing method is performed by a Monte Carlo simulation

W. Niessen and M. Viergever (Eds.): MICCAI 2001, LNCS 2208, pp. 195–203, 2001.

via the Stejskal-Tanner equations [6]. Our smoothing procedure concerns the increase of signal to noise ratio on the measurement grid, so it concerns averaged properties of the actual axon flow. Tracking on the other hand is regarded as a way to model this flow below the grid scale. To achieve this, the smoothed tensor field is diagonalized and the direction field of the principal eigenvectors is further analyzed. For a given seed point in white matter, not necessarily on the grid, the track of axon fibers is modeled. To do this, the direction field is interpolated locally by a bilinear procedure, then the track is followed by differential equation discretization. The method is applied to real data and results concerning the corpus callosum region are presented. The diffusion tensor images were acquired on a 1.5 T clinical scanner (Signa Echospeed, GE) using a diffusion weighted EPI sequence with 6 non-collinear gradient orientations and 4 b-factors, b_{max}=880 s/mm^2. 24 contiguous slices with a spatial resolution of $1.875{\times}1.875{\times}3$ mm^3 were acquired.

2   Edge Preserving Regularization of the Diffusion Tensor Field

Our approach to regularization or smoothing is similar to that of Basser et al. [4], as we are essentially smoothing the tensor field [7]. However, in contrast to Basser et al., who use linear B-Spline approximation which gives blurring of the resulting fields, we use nonlinear filters which are edge preserving and homogenizing, as the measured fields show clear discontinuities and as the curvature of the direction field should be small [5]. This smoothing technique differs from that used by Parker et al [3], who use the "Perona Malik-variant" of the diffusion equation. We use a chain of three dimensional nonlinear Sigma filters, the "Aurich-chain" [8], which is easy to implement and has suitable numerical and statistical properties.

According to the exponential behavior of the Stejskal-Tanner equations [9,1,2],

$$F_I^b(\boldsymbol{x})/F^0(\boldsymbol{x}) = \exp(-b\hat{\boldsymbol{G}}_I^T * D(\boldsymbol{x}) * \hat{\boldsymbol{G}}_I) \tag{1}$$

where $D(\boldsymbol{x})$ is the spatial tensor field, $F_I^b(\boldsymbol{x}) = |Signal_I^b(\boldsymbol{x}) + n_{Re} + in_{Im}|$ with $n_{Re}, n_{Im} \in N(0,\sigma)$, $F^0(\boldsymbol{x})$ is the T_2-weighted field, $b > 0$ is the diffusion weighting parameter, and $\hat{\boldsymbol{G}}_I, I = 1,\dots,6$ are normalized gradient vectors. For high b-values the variance of the noise in the tensor field $D(\boldsymbol{x})$ depends strongly on the amplitude, see Fig. 1 for one dimensional simulated examples. Therefore, to achieve noise homogeneity, an important prior condition for smoothing by filters, filtering should not be performed on the coefficients D_{xx}, D_{xy}, etc. of the symmetric $D(\boldsymbol{x})$ matrix directly but on it's exponential, e. g. on $f = \exp(-bD_{xx}(\boldsymbol{x}))$.

The fields in Eq. (1) show discontinuities, which are due to voxel wise changes in diffusion anisotropy (caused, e. g., by tissue dependent anisotropy or by fiber crossing creating partial volume effects), see Fig. 2, Panel A. Therefore, nonlinear edge preserving filtering is applied. For every field f the "Aurich-chain" is formulated in three dimensions according to:

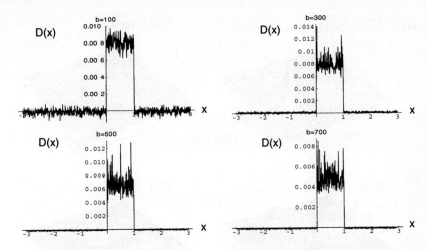

Fig. 1: A smooth tensor coefficient $D(x)$ for one space dimension is assumed as a step function. According to the Monte Carlo simulation described in text $\sigma = 0.03F^0$ complex Gaussian noise is added to the Signal and $D(x)$ is plotted for b=100, 300, 500, and $700\,\mathrm{s/mm^2}$. The variance depends strongly on b and on the amplitude of the field

$$
f(\boldsymbol{x})_{\mathrm{new}} = \sum_{\boldsymbol{y}\in\mathrm{Neighborhood}(\boldsymbol{x})} \exp\left(-\frac{(\boldsymbol{x}-\boldsymbol{y})^2}{2\sigma^2}\right) \exp\left(-\frac{(f(\boldsymbol{x})-f(\boldsymbol{y}))^2}{2\tau^2}\right) \frac{f(\boldsymbol{y})}{Norm}
$$

$$
= F_\sigma^\tau \circ f(\boldsymbol{x})
$$

$$
Norm = \sum_{\boldsymbol{y}\in\mathrm{Neighborhood}(\boldsymbol{x})} \exp\left(-\frac{(\boldsymbol{x}-\boldsymbol{y})^2}{2\sigma^2}\right) \exp\left(-\frac{(f(\boldsymbol{x})-f(\boldsymbol{y}))^2}{2\tau^2}\right) \qquad (2)
$$

$$
f(\boldsymbol{x})_{\mathrm{smooth}} = F_{\sigma*1.59*1.59}^{(\tau/3)/2} \circ F_{\sigma*1.59}^{\tau/3} \circ F_\sigma^\tau \circ f(\boldsymbol{x}) \quad ,
$$

where σ is the voxel width and τ is three times an estimate of the smallest step in the field f which should be preserved. A lower bound of this step is given by the standard deviation of the noise in f.

This algorithm is statistically robust with respect to noise details (deviations from independent Gaussian noise), numerically stable, and computationally fast, as tabulation methods can be used. See [10] for further details and for a review of recent edge preserving smoothers. In Fig. 2, Panel B, some tensor coefficients of the smoothed field are shown, three iterations in the chain gave a suitable flatness of the resulting field, which is equivalent to a low curvature in the direction field.

In addition, to demonstrate the quality of our filter method, a validation based on Monte Carlo simulation was performed. The smoothed three dimensional tensor data around the corpus callosum which are partially shown in Fig. 2, Panel B, were used as reference. By Eq. (1) they were corrupted with noise via the following steps: Assume F^0=1000 and derive via Eq. (1) $Signal_I^b(\boldsymbol{x})$, for b=100, 300, 500, and $700\,\mathrm{s/mm^2}$ and $\hat{\boldsymbol{G}}_1 = (1,0,0)$, $\hat{\boldsymbol{G}}_2 = (0,1,0)$, $\hat{\boldsymbol{G}}_3 = (0,0,1)$, $\hat{\boldsymbol{G}}_4 = (1/\sqrt{2},1/\sqrt{2},0)$, $\hat{\boldsymbol{G}}_5 = (1/\sqrt{2},0,1/\sqrt{2})$, and $\hat{\boldsymbol{G}}_6 = (0,1/\sqrt{2},1/\sqrt{2})$. These

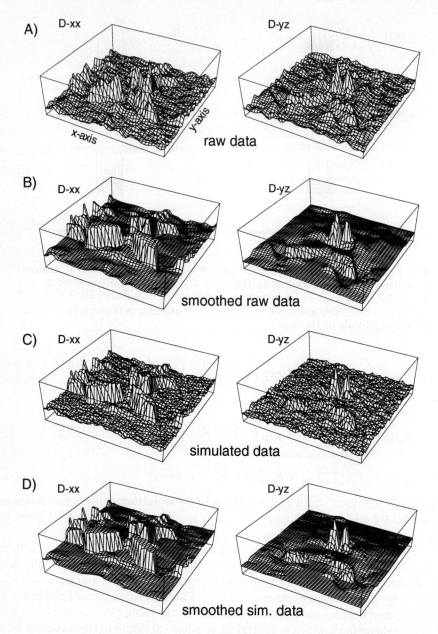

Fig. 2: In Panel A, axial slices of $D_{xx}(\boldsymbol{x})$ and $D_{yz}(\boldsymbol{x})$ for identical regions around the corpus callosum are shown for raw data. Panel B presents the corresponding smoothed fields. Panel C shows the noise corrupted fields of Panel B, see Monte Carlo simulation in text for details. Panel D demonstrates that the applied smoother indeed reproduces Panel B with high precision

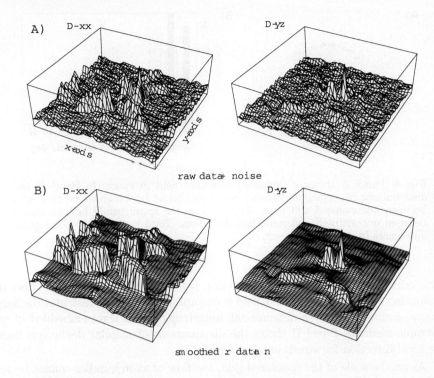

Fig. 3: Effect of the robust smoother on tensor coefficients (as in Fig. 2)

25 fields, including F^0, were then corrupted by complex Gaussian noise, $N(0, \sigma)$, with $\sigma=3\%$ of $F^0(x)$. The corresponding tensor field $D(x)$ was calculated at every space point via multivariate linear regression. This regression comprised all 24 linear equations corresponding to the logarithmic variant of Eq. (1) for the four b-values. Some coefficients of the resulting noisy tensor field $D(x)$ are shown in Fig. 2, Panel C. Smoothing of $D(x)$ was performed in the same way as for the raw data, using $b=400\,\mathrm{s/mm^2}$ in the exponential transformation, with results shown in Fig. 2, Panel D. The good agreement with the reference in Panel B demonstrates the suitability of the applied filter method. In a second test the raw data signals of Fig. 2, Panel A were additionally corrupted by adding the noise of Panel C, as shown in Fig. 3, Panel A. An application of the filter chain demonstrates the robustness of the method as seen in Fig. 3, Panel B.

3   Tracking

To derive the main diffusion directions of the axon bundles the smoothed tensor field, $D(x)$, was numerically diagonalized by singular value decomposition at every grid point x_i, resulting in three eigenvalues and eigenvectors (orientations modulo π) for every voxel. The field of eigenvectors corresponding to the largest

A)   B)

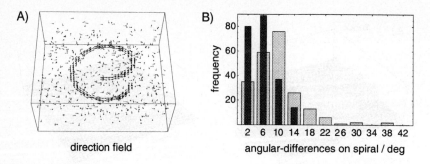

direction field   angular-differences on spiral / deg

Fig. 4: Panel A shows a simulated direction field in space. In Panel B the distributions of angular differences are given: broad bars correspond to angles between uncorrupted and noisy directions on the spiral, small bars to angles between uncorrupted and smoothed directions. Total frequencies versus angle differences in degrees are given.

eigenvalue, $\hat{e}(x_i)$, gives the main direction field. In Fig. 4 the positive effect of smoothing on the main direction field is exemplified. Panel A illustrates the field around a simulated three-dimensional, anisotropic spiral tract embedded in an isotropic medium. Panel B shows the distributions of angular deviations from the ideal direction for voxels on the spiral.

As on the scale of the measured grid, the flow of axon bundles cannot be resolved completely, the regularization deals with averaged quantities. Correspondingly, in regions of crossing or merging axon directions cancellation is possible, leading to partial volume voxels with artificially low anisotropy. To introduce the direction information into these voxels, a rotation algorithm was developed, which proceeds essentially in two steps:

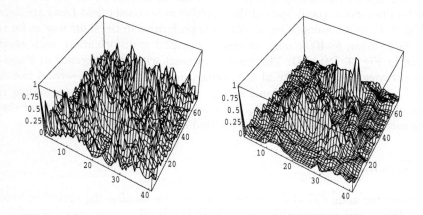

Fig. 5: The anisotropy coefficient $A_{\mathrm{major}} \in [0,1]$ for the axial region of Fig. 2; left: based on raw data, right: based on smoothed tensor field

1. According to the eigenvalues of the partial volume voxel, decide if the isotropy is two or three dimensional by the following procedure: Sort the eigenvalues in decreasing order and check if the first two or three eigenvalues are close (if the local tensor is disk shaped or spherical).
2. Then, two or three directions are mapped to this voxel by an algorithm which minimizes (modulo π) the mean angular deviation of a rotating vector to the main streams of directions in the neighborhood. In case of a two dimensional isotropy, the corresponding eigenvectors define the rotation plane of the vector, in case of three dimensions the rotation covers a sphere.

To model the direction of the axon bundles below the grid resolution, a local bilinear interpolation of the discrete direction field was performed, according to:

$$\hat{e}(x) = \sum_{x_i \in 8-\text{neighborhood}(x)} \hat{e}(x_i) \cdot \left|1 - \frac{|x - x_i|}{\Delta x}\right| \cdot \left|1 - \frac{|y - y_i|}{\Delta y}\right| \cdot \left|1 - \frac{|z - z_i|}{\Delta z}\right| ,$$

(3)

where $\Delta x, \Delta y$, and Δz are the grid lengths.

If a partial volume voxel which includes several directions is in the 8-neighborhood, that direction which is closest to those of the neighboring standard voxels is chosen. The standard voxels have a cigar shaped tensor and are chosen by an anisotropy coefficient above a certain threshold. Anisotropy coefficients are strongly biased by noise, a review of recent coefficients and a discussion of their noise dependence is given in [2]. The effect of the presented regularization on the coefficient

$$A_{\text{major}} = \frac{\lambda_1 - (\lambda_2 + \lambda_3)/2}{\lambda_1 + \lambda_2 + \lambda_3} \qquad \text{for sorted eigenvalues} \quad \lambda_1 \geq \lambda_2 \geq \lambda_3 \quad (4)$$

is shown in Fig. 5, where the anisotropy for the raw data is compared to those of the smoothed tensor field, the region presented is the same as in Fig. 2.

On the basis of this interpolated direction field, tracks of axon bundles can be calculated as follows:

1. Choose the seed point of the track and the initial orientation via the nearest standard voxel.
2. Align the neighboring directions according to the initial orientation and calculate the interpolated direction by Eq. (3).
3. Proceed with a fixed step length Δs in this direction.
4. If the anisotropy is above the threshold, use the new position as seed point, the direction of step 3 to determine the initial orientation for the next iteration, and continue with step 2.

For $\Delta s \to 0$, this procedure essentially approaches an initial value problem for differential equations [4], according to this in step 3 a Runge-Kutta procedure gives more stable results. In Fig. 6 the direction field of the smoothed tensors is shown for 5 axial slices around the corpus callosum for $A_{\text{major}}^{\text{smoothed data}} \geq 0.3$. Several calculated tracks in are included.

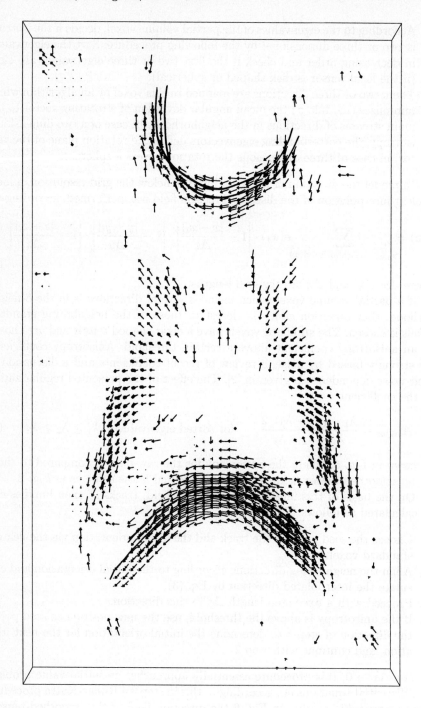

Fig. 6: The direction field around the corpus callosum as in Fig. 2 for 5 contiguous axial slices. Voxels for $A_{\mathrm{major}} > 0.3$, based on the smoothed tensor field, are shown. Several calculated tracks are included

4   Conclusion

Spatially smoothing the tensor field is equivalent to a homogenization of the directions of the eigenvectors and of the eigenvalues which are derived by diagonalization. Therefore smoothing has an important impact on anisotropy coefficients and on tracking. For anatomical and geometrical reasons, the tensor field shows discontinuous patterns. In the corpus callosum region, anatomy gives rise to abrupt changes in the anisotropy signal from one voxel to the next. Similarly, for crossing or merging fiber tracks, the finite grid resolution can produce voxel-wise changes in anisotropy or partial volume effects. Therefore, edge preserving smoothing is the method of choice to regularize diffusion signals or their tensor fields. The proposed tracking method was tested in model cases and by application to real data. Near the corpus callosum, where we found only standard voxels, reasonable results were achieved. Crossing and partial volume situations were up to now studied only by model simulations, more analyses are necessary to adapt the proposed method, which can handle only isolated, non-standard voxels, to realistic situations. The present tracking algorithm uses local information of the direction field only and proceeds in the frame of an initial value problem. To explore anatomical connectivity boundary value conditions which introduce anatomical knowledge about the starting and ending regions of the tracks should also be treatable. Furthermore, it seems to be experimentally evident that partial volume voxels with crossing tracks can also appear as groups or larger clusters in white matter [11]. For both reasons more global tracking methods than the present ones should additionally be applied. This could be achieved, e. g., by optimization methods of variational calculus which offer a flexible tool to combine global aspects with convenient priors.

Acknowledgment: We thank Dr. D. P. Auer for her kind interest and Dr. C. Gössl for providing us with the test example in Fig. 4. In addition, we would like to thank the referees for fruitful suggestions.

References

1. Pierpaoli C and Basser PJ. *Magn. Reson. Med.* **36** 893-906 (1996)
2. Skare S, Li TQ, Nordell B, and Ingvar M. *Magn. Reson. Imag.* **18** 659-669 (2000)
3. Parker GJM, Schnabel JA, Symms MR, et al. *J. Magn. Reson. Imag.* **11** 702-710 (2000)
4. Basser PJ, Pajevic S, Pierpaoli C, et al. *Magn. Reson. Med.* **44** 625-632 (2000)
5. Poupon C, Clark CA, Frouin V, et al. *NeuroImage* **12** 184-195 (2000)
6. Stejskal EO and Tanner JE. *J. Chem. Phys.* **42** 288-292 (1965)
7. Hahn K, Prigarin S, and Pütz B. *NeuroImage* **13** S142 (2001)
8. Aurich V and Weule J. Non-linear gaussian filters performing edge preserving diffusion. In *Proc. 17. DAGM-Symposium*, pages 538-545, Bielefeld, Springer (1995)
9. Henkelmann M. *Med. Phys.* **12** 232-233 (1985)
10. Winkler G, Aurich V, Hahn K, et al. *Pattern Recognition and Image Analysis* **9** 749-766 (1999)
11. Wiegell MR, Larsson HBW, and Wedeen VJ. *Radiology* **217** 897-903 (2000)

A Statistical Framework for Partial Volume Segmentation

Koen Van Leemput[1,2], Frederik Maes[1], Dirk Vandermeulen[1], and Paul Suetens[1]

[1] Katholieke Universiteit Leuven, Medical Image Computing, Radiology-ESAT,
UZ Gasthuisberg, Herestraat 49, B-3000 Leuven, Belgium
[2] Helsinki University of Technology, Laboratory of Biomedical Engineering,
P.O. Box 2200, FIN-02015 HUT, Finland
koen.vanleemput@hut.fi

Abstract. Accurate brain tissue segmentation by intensity-based voxel classification of MR images is complicated by partial volume (PV) voxels that contain a mixture of two or more tissue types. In this paper [1], we present a statistical framework for PV segmentation that combines and extends existing techniques. We think of a partial volumed image as a downsampled version of a fictive higher-resolution image that does not contain partial voluming, and we estimate the model parameters of this underlying image using an Expectation-Maximization algorithm. This leads to an iterative approach that interleaves a statistical classification of the image voxels using spatial information and an according update of the model parameters. We illustrate the performance of the method on simulated data and on 2-D slices of real MR images. We demonstrate that the use of appropriate spatial models not only improves the classification, but is often indispensable for robust parameter estimation as well.

1 Introduction

Previously we presented a fully automated model-based approach for intensity-based tissue classification of MR images of the brain [1]. The method uses an Expectation-Maximization (EM) algorithm [2] to iteratively estimate during classification the parameters of tissue-specific Gaussian intensity models, of a polynomial model for MR bias field correction, and of a Markov random field (MRF) prior that models spatial interactions between neighboring voxels. Prior knowledge about the expected distribution of the various tissue classes in the image is derived from a digital brain atlas that is co-registered with the image under study, which allows full automation of the method.

Whereas this technique assigns each voxel to a single tissue type, the limited spatial resolution of MR imaging and the complex shape of the tissue interfaces in the brain imply that a large part of the voxels in MR brain images are so-called partial volume (PV) voxels, i.e. voxels that contain not a single tissue, but

---

[1] This paper is a short version of a technical report KUL/ESAT/PSI/0102. Available:
http://bilbo.esat.kuleuven.ac.be

W. Niessen and M. Viergever (Eds.): MICCAI 2001, LNCS 2208, pp. 204–212, 2001.
© Springer-Verlag Berlin Heidelberg 2001

rather a mixture of two or more tissue types. In this paper, we therefore extend our approach by explicitly including a model for such PV voxels. We derive an EM algorithm for assessing the Maximum Likelihood (ML) parameters of the resulting image model, and demonstrate that this leads to a general PV segmentation framework that enables estimation of tissue-specific means and covariance matrices guided by spatial information, while classifying the image voxels at the same time.

2   Image Model

Let $L = \{l_j, j = 1, 2, \ldots, J\}$ be a label image with a total of J voxels, where $l_j \in \{1, 2, \ldots, K\}$, denotes the one of K non-mixed tissue types to which each voxel j belongs. These labels are assumed to be drawn according to some probability distribution $f(L \mid \Phi_L)$ with parameters Φ_L to be specified further that imposes certain spatial constraints. Suppose that a non-mixed intensity image $Y = \{y_j, j = 1, 2, \ldots, J\}$ is generated from L by drawing a sample from a probability distribution $f(Y \mid L, \Phi_Y)$ parameterized by Φ_Y. We assume that the intensity of each class k is normally distributed with mean μ_k and covariance Σ_k, such that $\Phi_Y = \{\mu_k, \Sigma_k, k = 1, 2, \ldots, K\}$ and $f(Y \mid L, \Phi_Y) = \prod_j f(y_j \mid l_j, \Phi_Y) = \prod_j G_{\Sigma_{l_j}}(y_j - \mu_{l_j})$ with $G_{\Sigma}(\cdot)$ the zero-mean normal distribution with covariance matrix Σ. With the exception of an explicit model for the MR bias field, which we assume here not to be present for the sake of simplicity, this was the image model used in our previous work [1].

Now an extra step is added, where Y is not directly observed, but downsampled by a factor M to yield a partial volumed MR image $\tilde{Y} = \{\tilde{y}_i, i=1, 2, \ldots I\}$ with only $I = J/M$ voxels. The observed intensity $\tilde{y}_i$ in voxel i of the downsampled image $\tilde{Y}$ is modeled as the sum of the intensities y_j of all the subvoxels in the original image Y that underlie i. In voxels where not all subvoxels belong to the same tissue type, this causes partial voluming. Let t_i be a vector that contains the relative amount of each class k, $k=1, 2, \ldots K$ in voxel i. A value of $t_{ik} = 1$ for some class k means that all the subvoxels underlying voxel i belong to class k, whereas a value of $t_{ik} = 0$ indicates that i does not contain class k at all. It can be shown that the observed intensity $\tilde{y}_i$ in a voxel is governed by a normal distribution that only depends on its mixing proportions t_i:

$$f(\tilde{y}_i \mid t_i, \Phi_Y) = G_{\tilde{\Sigma}(t_i)}(\tilde{y}_i - \tilde{\mu}(t_i)) \tag{1}$$

with $\tilde{\mu}(t_i) = M \cdot \sum_k t_{ik} \mu_k$ and $\tilde{\Sigma}(t_i) = M \cdot \sum_k t_{ik} \Sigma_k$.

This model is illustrated in figure 1 on a 2-D example for two classes and $M = 3^2$ subvoxels per voxel. Figure 1f also shows the normal distributions $f(\tilde{y}_i \mid t_i, \Phi_Y)$ for each mixture $t = (\alpha, 1-\alpha)$ with $\alpha \in \{0, 1/M, 2/M, \ldots, (M-1)/M, 1\}$, weighted by the number of times each mixture occurs in the image. Note that these mixture distributions do not all have the same weight, indicating that not all mixtures are equally likely. Summing the distributions of all non-pure mixtures yields a model for the intensity distribution of PV voxels.

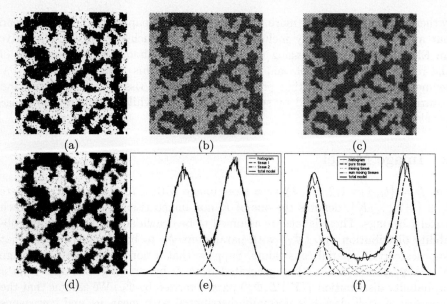

Fig. 1. PV image model: (a) label image L with 2 classes drawn according to some statistical model; (b) intensity image Y obtained from L assuming the intensity of each class to be normally distributed; (c) downsampled image $\tilde{Y}$ containing partial voluming; (d) tissue fraction $t_{i1} = 1 - t_{i2}$ in each voxel i of $\tilde{Y}$; (e) and (f): histograms of Y and $\tilde{Y}$ respectively and their underlying models.

3   Model Parameter Estimation

Given the observed data $\tilde{Y}$, the aim is to reconstruct the label image L or, more modestly, to estimate the tissue fractions t_i in each voxel. Before these issues can be addressed, the model parameters $\Phi = \{\Phi_Y, \Phi_L\}$ need to be estimated somehow from $\tilde{Y}$. In this paper, we estimate the parameters that maximize the likelihood of the data $f(\tilde{Y} \mid \Phi) = \sum_L f(\tilde{Y} \mid L, \Phi_Y) f(L \mid \Phi_L)$ with $f(\tilde{Y} \mid L, \Phi_Y) = \prod_i f(\tilde{y}_i \mid t_i, \Phi_Y)$ given by (1). To this end, we use an EM algorithm that iteratively maximizes the expected value of the log-likelihood $\log f(Y, L \mid \Phi)$ of the unknown data $\{Y, L\}$, where the expectation is based on the observed data $\tilde{Y}$ and the parameters $\Phi^{(m-1)}$ estimated in the previous iteration $(m-1)$ (see [3] for details):

Expectation step : find the function

$$Q(\Phi \mid \Phi^{(m-1)}) = E_{L,Y}[\log f(Y, L \mid \Phi) \mid \tilde{Y}, \Phi^{(m-1)}] \qquad (2)$$

Maximization step: find

$$\Phi^{(m)} = \arg\max_{\Phi} Q(\Phi \mid \Phi^{(m-1)})$$

Because $f(\boldsymbol{Y}, \boldsymbol{L} \mid \boldsymbol{\Phi}) = f(\boldsymbol{Y} \mid \boldsymbol{L}, \boldsymbol{\Phi}_Y).f(\boldsymbol{L} \mid \boldsymbol{\Phi}_L)$, the expectation function can be written as $Q(\boldsymbol{\Phi} \mid \boldsymbol{\Phi}^{(m-1)}) = Q_Y(\boldsymbol{\Phi}_Y \mid \boldsymbol{\Phi}^{(m-1)}) + Q_L(\boldsymbol{\Phi}_L \mid \boldsymbol{\Phi}^{(m-1)})$. Maximization of Q_Y yields closed-form expressions for estimating the class intensity parameters $\boldsymbol{\Phi}_Y$ that depend on the posterior probabilities $f(t_i \mid \tilde{\boldsymbol{Y}}, \boldsymbol{\Phi}^{(m-1)})$. These depend on the prior spatial model $f(\boldsymbol{L} \mid \boldsymbol{\Phi}_L)$, for which three different models were investigated [3]:

Model A: no spatial correlation Every mixing combination t has a spatially invariant prior probability π_t.

Model B: no spatial correlation and uniform prior Every mixing combination t has a spatially invariant prior probability π_t, that is the same for all non-pure t.

Model C: Markov random field The spatial distribution of labels l_j in L is governed by an Ising/Potts MRF whose parameters regulate how much of each tissue is present and how voxels of a particular tissue type are clustered.

For models A and B, $f(t_i \mid \tilde{\boldsymbol{Y}}, \boldsymbol{\Phi}^{(m-1)}) \propto f(\tilde{\boldsymbol{y}}_i \mid t_i, \boldsymbol{\Phi}_Y^{(m-1)}) \cdot \pi_t^{(m-1)}$ with the prior probabilities π_t estimated by maximization of $Q_L(\boldsymbol{\Phi}_L \mid \boldsymbol{\Phi}^{(m-1)})$. For model C, $f(t_i \mid \tilde{\boldsymbol{Y}}, \boldsymbol{\Phi}^{(m-1)})$ can not be calculated analytically. We therefore use the MCEM algorithm [4] to approximate the expectation over the labels $\boldsymbol{L}$ in (2) by sampling the distribution $f(\boldsymbol{L} \mid \tilde{\boldsymbol{Y}}, \boldsymbol{\Phi}^{(m-1)})$. The MRF parameters are calculated using the pseudo-likelihood approximation [5].

4 Results

The performance of the 3 spatial models was validated on simulated 2-D data generated with different parameter sets $\boldsymbol{\Phi}$ according to model C, i.e. with the underlying label image $\boldsymbol{L}$ modeled as an MRF sample. The three spatial models A, B and C were fitted to the data starting from the same randomized initial parameters. In all cases, the MRF model C resulted in more accurate classifications than model A and B [3]. Moreover, models A and B, which are entirely histogram-based, often failed to correctly estimate the underlying model parameters. In many cases the use of prior spatial knowledge as provided by model C showed indispensable for robust estimation of the model parameters.

Figure 2 shows an example with 2 classes and $M = 3^2$ subvoxels per voxel. Model A fits the histogram well, but the underlying model is not correctly estimated. Since there is no restriction on the weights π_t for the mixing proportions t, the algorithm has simply adjusted these to get a good histogram fit, thereby setting the prior probability for pure tissue to zero. With model B, all the mixing fractions corresponding to non-pure tissues are forced to have the same weight, resulting in the typical flat shape of the total intensity model for PV voxels that is commonly used in the literature [6,7,8,9]. However, the true mixing fractions in this example are not equal at all and therefore model B is condemned to fail. Only model C succeeds to retrieve the correct model parameters.

Figure 3 shows an example for 3 classes and $M = 2^2$ subvoxels per voxel. Because the intensity of voxels mixing the tissues with the lowest and highest

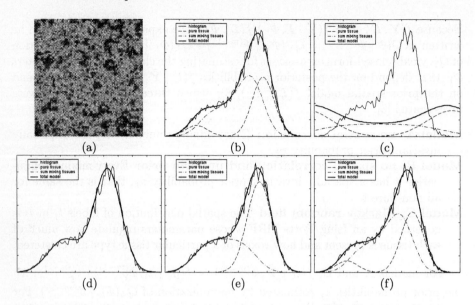

Fig. 2. Simulated data, two tissue types: (a) observed data $\tilde{Y}$; (b) histogram of $\tilde{Y}$ with the underlying model overlayed; (c) model initialization; (d,e,f): resulting histogram fit obtained with models A, B and C, respectively.

intensity is similar to the intensity of pure voxels of the tissue type with intermediate intensity, model A is severely underconstrained in this case and was therefore not considered. Model B and C fit the global histogram equally well, but only model C retrieves the correct model parameters, while model B yields incorrect parameters that are different with different initializations [3].

Our current implementation of the MRF of model C is only 2-D, implying that tissue boundaries are assumed to be orthogonal to the image slice. Figure 4a shows an axial slice of a high-resolution 1 mm isotropic T1-weighted image of the head through the central part of the brain where this assumption is more or less valid. Since different combinations of mixing tissues have overlapping intensities, model A was not considered. Comparing the results obtained with models B and C, it is clear that the MRF of model C reduces the noise in the segmentations considerably and forces partial volume voxels to lie on the border between the constituent tissues, in contrast to model B.

5   Discussion

Our statistical framework for PV segmentation is an extension of the methods of Choi *et al.* [10], Pham and Prince [11] and Nocera and Gee [12] when model C is used. Defining an MRF prior that imposes similar tissue combinations t_i over neighboring voxels, these approaches iteratively assign a mixing fraction t_i to each voxel and update the mean intensity of every pure tissue type. However,

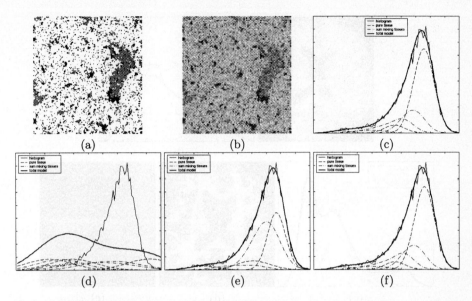

Fig. 3. Simulated data, three tissue types: (a) label image $\boldsymbol{L}$; (b) observed partial volumed image $\hat{\boldsymbol{Y}}$; (c) histogram of $\hat{\boldsymbol{Y}}$ with the true model overlayed; (d) model initialization; (e,f) histogram fit obtained with model B and C, respectively.

these methods assume that all tissues have the same diagonal covariance structure, which does not need to be the case in real MR data, and the estimation of this covariance is not addressed. Furthermore, the methods in [10,12] use an MRF that simply imposes similar $\boldsymbol{t}_i$ over neighboring voxels, which erroneously encourages voxels to contain equal amounts of every tissue type everywhere in the image, in combination with extreme values for the mean intensity of pure tissues [3]. In contrast, our method additionally estimates tissue-specific covariance matrices as well, and defines an MRF model on subvoxels rather than on the voxels directly, thereby naturally imposing homogeneous regions of pure tissues bordered by PV voxels.

Our method is also an extension of the PV techniques of Santago and Gage [8], Wu *et al.* [9], Laidlaw *et al.* [6] and Ruan *et al.* [7]. These methods estimate their parameters by fitting the model to the histogram, thereby discarding all spatial information, and assume that all mixing proportions are equally alike when two tissues mix in a voxel, similar to our model B. However, the assumption of equally probable mixing fractions lacks any basis, as can be seen from figures 1f and 2b. Our model A does not make any prior assumption about the mixing proportions at all, but this introduces so many degrees of freedom that the model fitting is severely underconstrained. However, in contrast to [6,7,8,9], our approach allows incorporating a prior spatial model to guide the model fitting, which allows the mixing proportions to be non-uniform without making the estimation problem underconstrained.

210   K. Van Leemput et al.

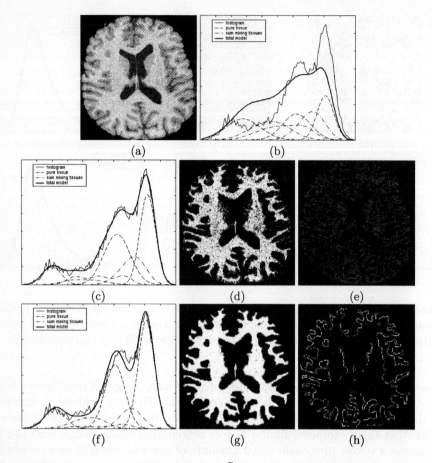

Fig. 4. 2-D MR image: (a) image data $\tilde{Y}$; (b) histogram with the model initialization overlayed; (c,d,e) resulting histogram fit, expected fraction of white matter and estimated probability for partial voluming between white and gray matter, obtained using model B; (f,g,h) idem, but using model C.

While there may be many parameter sets that provide a close histogram fit, what discriminates the true solution is that it provides a meaningful classification in the images in agreement with the spatial model. With model C, our method iteratively interleaves a statistical classification of the image voxels using spatial information and an according update of the model parameters. Our results demonstrate that the use of such spatial information during the model fitting is often required in order to obtain reliable results.

6   Conclusion

In this paper, we presented a statistical framework for PV segmentation that combines and extends existing techniques. A partial volumed image is considered a downsampled version of a fictive higher-resolution image that does not contain partial voluming, and the model parameters of this underlying image are estimated using an EM algorithm. This leads to an iterative approach that interleaves a statistical classification of the image voxels using spatial information and an according update of the model parameters. We have demonstrated on simulated data that the use of appropriate prior spatial models not only improves the classification, but is often indispensable for robust parameter estimation as well. Future work will focus on developing such models that accurately describe the shape of the brain.

Acknowledgments

This work was supported by the EC-funded BIOMED-2 program under Grant BMH4-CT96-0845 (BIOMORPH) and Grant BMH4- CT98-6048 (QAMRIC), and by the Research Fund KULeuven under Grant GOA/99/05 (VHS+). The work of K. Van Leemput was supported by a grant from the IWT, Belgium. F. Maes is a Postdoctoral Fellow of the FWO-Vlaanderen, Belgium. The work of D. Vandermeulen was supported in part by the F.W.O.-Vlaanderen under Grant 1.5.397.97.

References

1. K. Van Leemput, F. Maes, D. Vandermeulen, and P. Suetens. Automated model-based tissue classification of MR images of the brain. *IEEE Transactions on Medical Imaging*, 18(10):897–908, october 1999.
2. A. P. Dempster, N. M. Laird, and D. B. Rubin. Maximum likelihood from incomplete data via the EM algorithm. *Journal of the Royal Statistical Society*, 39:1–38, 1977.
3. K. Van Leemput, F. Maes, D. Vandermeulen, and P. Suetens. A statistical framework for partial volume segmentation. Technical Report KUL/ESAT/PSI/0102, K.U.Leuven, ESAT, Leuven, Belgium, April 2001. Available: http://bilbo.esat.kuleuven.ac.be.
4. G. C. G. Wei and M. Tanner. A monte carlo implementation of the EM algorithm and the poor man's data augmentation algorithm. *J. Amer. Stat. Assoc.*, 85:699–704, 1990.
5. J. Besag. Efficiency of pseudo-likelihood estimation for simple gaussian fields. *Biometrika*, 64:616–618, 1977.
6. D. H. Laidlaw, K. W. Fleischer, and A. H. Barr. Partial-volume bayesian classification of material mixtures in MR volume data using voxel histograms. *IEEE Transactions on Medical Imaging*, 17(1):74–86, february 1998.
7. S. Ruan, C. Jaggi, J. Xue, J. Fadili, and D. Bloyet. Brain tissue classification of magnetic resonance images using partial volume modeling. *IEEE Transactions on Medical Imaging*, 19(12):1179–1187, December 2000.
8. P. Santago and H.D. Gage. Quantification of MR brain images by mixture density and partial volume modeling. *IEEE Transactions on Medical Imaging*, 12(3):566–574, September 1993.

212   K. Van Leemput et al.

9. Z. Wu, H.-W. Chung, and F.W. Wehrli. A bayesian approach to subvoxel tissue classification in NMR microscopic images of trabecular bone. *MRM*, 31:302–308, 1994.

10. H. S. Choi, D. R. Haynor, and Y. Kim. Partial volume tissue classification of multichannel magnetic resonance images–a mixel model. *IEEE Transactions on Medical Imaging*, 10(3):395–407, september 1991.

11. D. L. Pham and J. L. Prince. Unsupervised partial volume estimation in single-channel image data. In *Proceedings of IEEE Workshop on Mathematical Methods in Biomedical Image Analysis – MMBIA'00*, pages 170–177, 2000.

12. L. Nocera and J. C. Gee. Robust partial volume tissue classification of cerebral MRI scans. In K. M. Hanson, editor, *Proceedings of SPIE Medical Imaging 1997: Image Processing*, volume 3034 of *SPIE Proceedings*, pages 312–322. Bellingham, WA:SPIE, 1997.

From Sinograms to Surfaces: A Direct Approach to the Segmentation of Tomographic Data

Vidya Elangovan and Ross T. Whitaker

School of Computing, University of Utah
Salt Lake City, UT, USA

Abstract. Under ideal circumstances the problem of tomographic reconstruction is well-posed, and measured data are sufficient to obtain accurate estimates of volume densities. In such cases segmentation and surface estimation from the *reconstructed volume* are justified. In other situations the reconstructed volumes are not suitable for subsequent segmentation. This can happen in the case of incomplete sinograms, noise in the measurement process, or misregistration of the views. This paper presents a direct approach to the segmentation of incomplete and noisy tomographic data. The strategy is to impose a fairly simple model on the data, and treat segmentation as a problem of estimating the *interface* between two substances of somewhat homogeneous density. The segmentation is achieved by simultaneously deforming a surface model and updating density parameters in order to achieve a best fit between the projected model and the input sinograms. The deformation is implemented with level-set surface models, calculated at the resolution of the input data. Several computational innovations make the approach feasible with state-of-the-art computers. The usefulness of the approach is demonstrated by reconstructing the shape of spiny dendrites from electron microscope tomographic data.

1 Introduction

Certain kinds of tomographic reconstruction problems are ill-posed due to incomplete sinogram data. Difficulties in reconstructing volumes from such data are aggravated by noise in the measurements and misalignments among projections. This paper addresses the problem of segmentation in the context of such difficult tomography problems in biology and medicine. The usual approach for segmentation (indeed, any kind of post processing) in such cases is to reconstruct the volume, as best as possible, from the measured data using standard techniques such as filtered backprojection. Segmentation is then performed based on the grey-scale properties of that volume. However, the ill-posed nature of the reconstruction problem tends to produce various kinds of grey-scale artifacts, which state-of-the-art segmentation techniques cannot overcome. This paper presents a *direct* approach to segmentation, which uses the information in the sinograms instead of working with the reconstructed volumes and their associated artifacts. This direct strategy alleviates the effects of noise and misregistration and provides surface models of objects directly from incomplete sinograms.

The application studied in this paper is electron microscope tomography (EMT). While this data serves to motivate and demonstrate the proposed method, the characteristics of EMT are not unique, and the principles developed in this paper are applicable

W. Niessen and M. Viergever (Eds.): MICCAI 2001, LNCS 2208, pp. 213–223, 2001.

to a variety of clinical and biological problems. EMT data, which deals with structures of very small dimensions (on the order of a few micrometers), has several inherent problems. First, there are technical limits to the projection angles from which data can be measured. These limits are due to the mechanical apparatus used to tilt the specimens and the tradeoff between the destructive effects of electron energy and the effective specimen thickness, which increases with tilt angle. Usually, the maximum tilt angle is restricted to about ±60–70 degrees. Figure 1 (a) shows an illustration of the geometry of this limited-angle scenario. The second problem with EMT data is the degree of electron scattering, which results in projection images (sinograms) that are noisy relative to many other modalities, e.g. X-ray CT. Finally, due to the flexible nature of biological objects and the imperfections in the tilting mechanism, the objects undergo some movements while being tilted. Manual alignment procedures used to account for this tend to produce small misregistration errors. The segmentation approach described in this paper works well despite these limitations in the data.

Typically EMT data sets are produced using some kind of a contrast-enhancing mechanism (a dye) that highlights regions of interest, e.g. the interior of a cell. Thus, an ideal measurement and reconstruction would present a volume with two distinct densities (or electron opacities); one for the undyed regions (the background) and another for the dyed region (the foreground, or object). In practice, the densities are not homogeneous for either the object or the background. However, to the extent that the inhomogeneities are random and small relative to the contrast between the object and the background, the problem can be posed as estimating the interface between the object and the surrounding tissue and the densities of those two materials.

Our strategy, therefore, is to estimate the interface between two relatively homogeneous materials directly from the sinogram data, by deforming a surface model so that its forward projection is a best fit to the input data. For this work, the "best fit" is the sinogram that minimizes the mean square difference to the input. Other statistically-based metrics can be easily incorporated into this formulation, but that subject is beyond the scope of this paper. The relationship between *surface shape* and the associated projections is nonlinear, and we therefore use an iterative approach that deforms a surface model to achieve incrementally better fits. This requires a surface representation, which is sufficiently expressive to capture complex shape while allowing incremental, local deformations. For this we use a level-set surface model, which is a volume with grey-scale values that change according to a partial differential equation that controls surface movements. We consider the densities of the object and background as unknowns and estimate them simultaneously with the surface fitting. Refer to figure1b for a schematic of the approach. We apply the proposed method to limited-angle, noisy, misregistered EMT data of a small section of a *spiny dendrite*. However, the basic assumptions of the approach are consistent with tomographic imaging modalities that are characterized by contrasting foreground and background, such as SPECT or PET.

The remainder of this paper is as follows. Section 2 gives a brief account of related work. Section 3 lays out the mathematical formulations of our segmentation strategy, the resulting surface deformation, the level-set evolution equations and the computational innovations that result in a fast and accurate implementation. Sections 4 and 5 give experimental results and conclusions.

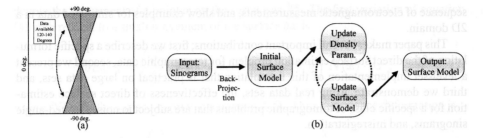

Fig. 1. (a) Illustration of limited-angle tomography, data missing in the shaded region (b) Schematic of the proposed method

2 Related Work

Several tomographic reconstruction methods are described in the literature [8], [13], and the method of choice depends on the quality of projection data. Filtered backprojection (FBP), the most widely used approach, works well in the case of the full-data reconstruction problem, where one is given *enough high-quality projections over 180 degree angular range*. Statistical, iterative approaches such as maximum-likelihood (ML) and maximum a posteriori (MAP) estimation have been proved to work well with *noisy* projection data, but generally rely on complete data sets. Some hybrid approaches [9], [12] have been specifically designed to deal with *limited-angle* tomography by "guessing" missing sinogram data via some extrapolation technique. A few researchers have proposed direct surface estimation using the projection data. For instance, Battle *et al.* [1], [2] use geometric deformable models for 3D tomographic reconstruction of objects of constant interior density in the context of SPECT imaging. They pose the inverse problem in a Bayesian framework and used a MAP estimate to compute the reconstruction of the shape of synthetic heart and lung phantoms represented as triangulated surface meshes. The fitting is accomplished by progressive surface refinement, but is limited in fidelity by the formulation and the surface representation. They demonstrate robustness to noise, but show results only for simulated data and do not study the effects of incomplete data.

The literature describes many examples of level-sets as curve and surface models for image segmentation [15], [10], [17], [3]. The authors have examined their usefulness for 3D segmentation of EMT *reconstructions* [19], the results of which are limited in quality due to reconstruction artifacts. Recently, several authors [4], [16] have proposed level-set formulations for finding piecewise smooth approximations to images in the context of segmentation. We assert that while level-sets are an interesting technology for modeling deformable surfaces, they are only as good as the data that drives their deformation—better results can be obtained by better formulations of the relationship between the models and the data.

Several authors have proposed solving *inverse problems* using level sets, with a more direct relationship between the data and the model. Santosa [14] lays out this basic strategy and demonstrates the idea on some small problems such as de-blurring 2D, binary images. Dorn *et al.* [5], [6] use this strategy to solve for permittivity using a

a stable fashion, and a variety of researchers have proposed computationally efficient algorithms. We use the sparse-field algorithm [18], which computes updates on a (relatively) small set of grid points, called the *active layer*, which is only one point wide, and can position level-set surface models to sub-voxel accuracy.[1] The curvature, κ, is computed as described in the literature [15], [17] using central differences on the discrete approximation to ϕ.

3.2 Initialization

The deformable model fitting approach requires an initial model, i.e. $\phi(x, t = 0)$. One reasonable way to obtain this is by thresholding the "best" information available prior to our solution, which is a volume reconstructed by filtered backprojection. In practice we do not require the initial model to be particularly close to the desired solution, and thus the threshold is not a critical parameter.

3.3 Estimation of Density Parameters

We consider the object and background to be homogeneous substances of *unknown* densities β_1 and β_0 respectively, and these density parameters affect the error term in equation (4). We update the estimate of the surface model iteratively, and at each iteration we reestimate the quantities β_1 and β_0 in such a way that the energy, E_{data} is minimized. Treating Ω as constant, equation (4) is quadratic in the density parameters. Thus, β_1 and β_0 are computed from the following linear system:

$$\frac{\partial E_{\text{data}}}{\partial \beta_0} = 0, \quad \frac{\partial E_{\text{data}}}{\partial \beta_1} = 0. \tag{11}$$

Variations in instrumentation can cause variations in the brightness levels of the images taken at different angles. In such cases we estimate sets of such parameters, i.e., $\beta_1(\theta_i)$ and $\beta_0(\theta_i)$ for $i = 1 \ldots M$.

3.4 Speed and Accuracy Considerations

Because we are combining the reconstruction problem (which is known to be time consuming) with the level-set deformation, our approach is computationally intensive. Specifically, computing $\hat{p}(r, s, \theta)$ is a major bottleneck. Computing this term involves re-computing the sinogram of our model as it moves. In the worst case, we would re-project the entire model every time the surface moves.

To address this computational concern, we have designed and implemented a method, that we call *incremental projection update* (IPU). Rather than fully recompute $\hat{p}$ at every iteration, we maintain a current running version of $\hat{p}$ and update it to reflect the changes in the model as it deforms. Changes in the model are computed only on a small

---

[1] The implementation in this paper is built on VISPACK, a C++ open-source software library for processing images, volumes and level-set surface models. The library is available at http://www.cs.utah.edu/ ∼ whitaker.

set of grid points in the volume, and therefore the update time is proportional to the area of the surface, rather than the size of the volume it encloses.

The IPU strategy works with the the sparse-field algorithm [18] as follows. At each iteration, the sparse-field algorithm updates only the active layer (one voxel wide) and modifies the set of active grid points as the surface moves. The incremental projection update strategy takes advantage of this to selectively update the model projection to reflect those changes. At each iteration, the amount of change in an active point's value determines the direction of motion of that particular surface point. This quantitative measure determines what portions of the projection $\hat{p}$ change (and by how much), and we can update it accordingly. Thus, the IPU maintains sub-voxel accuracy at a relatively low computational cost.

4   Experimental Results

In order to verify the correctness of the proposed method we first present results of digitally simulated slices (2D) for comparison against a ground truth, $f(x, y)$. The synthesized image is a homogeneous object on a homogeneous background. Projections of 128 samples each span 134 degrees (limited-angle) at two degree increments for a total of 67 views. To simulate misregistration errors, we randomly translate the image by plus/minus one pixel before taking the projections, and we corrupt each projection with additive, independent, Gaussian noise. Figure 2 shows the segmentation results for one simulated 2D slice. The input image (figure 2a) has three ellipses with two of them connected to each other. The incomplete, noisy, misaligned sinogram from this simulation (figure 2b) results in a rather poor backprojection (figure 2d). Figures 2c and 2f show the initial model and the final model after 150 iterations respectively overlaid on the input data. The initial model obtained from the backprojection is not a good estimate, it contains parts that do not belong to the object and it is missing some other pieces. The deformation process corrects these errors, and the final model captures all these connections and accurately estimates the contour corresponding to the input data. The final estimated sinogram, shown in figure 2e, demonstrates that the proposed method fills in the missing information in a reasonable way.

We also applied our algorithm to 3D EMT data obtained from a 3 MeV UHVEM. This 3D data set consists of 67 tilt series images, each corresponding to one view of the projection. Each tilt series image is of size 424x334. The volume reconstructed by FBP is of size 424x424x334. Figure 4a and 4b show the sinogram corresponding to a single slice of this data set and the estimate of the same sinogram created by the method. Figure 4e shows the surface estimate intersecting this slice overlaid on the backprojected slice. Some structures not seen in the backprojection are introduced in the final estimation, but the orientation of the structures introduced suggests that these structures were in the original object but were lost in the reconstruction artifacts during the backprojection. This hypothesis is consistent with the results of the simulated data. Also, the proposed method captures line-by-line brightness variations in the input sinogram (as explained in section 3.3). This suggests that the density estimation procedure is correct. Figure 5 shows the 3D initialization and the final 3D surface estimate. The figure also

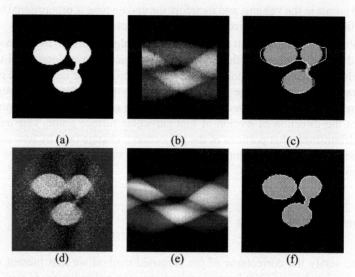

(a)   (b)   (c)

(d)   (e)   (f)

Fig. 2. Results of a 2D simulation: (a) Digitally simulated input image (b) limited-angle, noisy, misaligned sinogram created by projecting the input image (c) Initial model obtained by thresholding the backprojection (d) Backprojection showing artifacts (e) Sinogram estimated by the proposed method (f) Final model showing the correct segmentation of the input (Note: The initial and final contours are overlaid on the input data)

shows enlarged initial and final versions of a small section of the surface. The enlarged versions clearly illustrate the missing structures getting filled in.

Figure 3a shows a plot of the percentage error, relative to the RMS magnitude of the input sinogram, versus number of iterations. The error converges to a constant value within approximately 50 iterations for the simulated data, whereas it takes about 150 iterations for the real dendrite data. This is justified by the complexity of the real data compared to the simulated data. Also, the percentage error is lower for simulated data, which suggests the higher degree of noise and inhomogeneities in the EMT data. Figure 3b shows the convergence of the average value of the density parameter $\beta_1(\theta_i)$ for a single slice of the EMT dendrite data. The final surface estimate for the EMT dendrite data required 250 iterations, which took approximately 5 hours on a single processor of Silicon Graphics Onyx2 workstation.

5   Conclusions

We have demonstrated direct segmentation and surface modeling using sinograms for difficult tomography problems. Our results show that this approach is better than working with reconstructed volumes and their associated artifacts. In the particular case EMT dendrite data, the method appears superior to the current practice of hand segmentation, which requires more time and fails to capture the same level of detail.

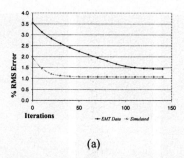 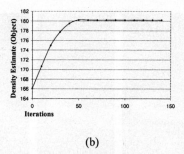

(a)   (b)

Fig. 3. Convergence plots: (a) Percentage error versus number of iterations for simulated and dendrite data. (b) The estimated object density parameter (average of $\beta_1(\theta_i)$ over all angles) for the EMT dendrite data versus the number of iterations

This work promises a number of interesting future directions. One direction is to extend the method to work for non homogeneous substances or multiple densities. In principle, one can modify the level-set equations to accommodate non-homogeneous density functions, that could also be estimated simultaneously with the surface estimate. Also, one could have several, interacting surface models, each one enclosing a different substance. Another direction is to apply the approach to other kinds of tomography, which have the similar problems. For example, a limited-angle problem occurs in cardiac CT imaging, where the carriage containing X-ray emitters and detectors can only travel part of the way through the full angular range before significant heart motion occurs. Finally, preliminary results show that the method can reconstruct surface shapes even in the extreme case of very few projections. This suggests that the approach could have applications in angiography and fluoroscopy.

6   Acknowledgments

This work is supported by the National Science Foundation under grants 0089915 and 9982273, the Office of Naval Research under grant N00014-01-10033, and the National Library of Medicine *Insight* project. The authors thank the National Center for Microscopy and Imaging Research (NCMIR) at San Diego for providing the EMT spiny dendrite data and Gordon Kindlmann for his valuable suggestions and volume analysis tools.

References

1. Battle, X.L., Cunningham, G.S., Hanson, K.M. (ed.): 3D tomographic reconstruction using geometrical models. Proc. SPIE Medical Imaging: Image Processing **3034** (1997) 346–357
2. Battle, X.L., Bizais, Y.J., Le Rest, C., Turzo, A., Hanson, K.M. (ed.): Tomographic reconstruction using free-form deformation models. Proc. SPIE Medical Imaging: Image Processing **3661** (1999) 356–367

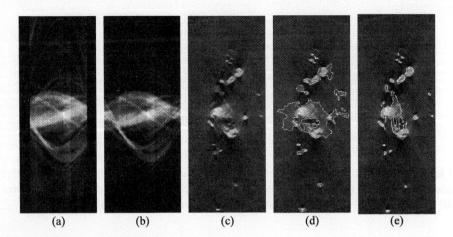

(a)   (b)   (c)   (d)   (e)

Fig. 4. 2D slice of dendrite data: (a) Sinogram of one slice (b) Sinogram estimated by the method for the same slice (c) Backprojection showing artifacts (d) Initial model obtained by thresholding the backprojection overlaid on the backprojection (e) Final model overlaid on the backprojection

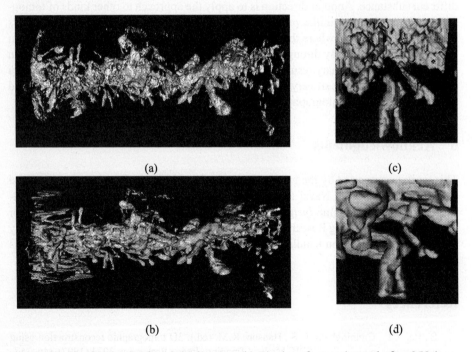

(a)   (c)

(b)   (d)

Fig. 5. 3D results: (a) Surface initialization (b) Final surface estimated after 250 iterations (c) A portion of the initial surface enlarged (d) The corresponding portion in the final surface

3. Caselles, V., Kimmel, R., Sapiro, G.: Geodesic Active Contours. International Conference on Computer Vision, IEEE Computer Society Press (1995) 694–699
4. Chan, T.F., Vese, L.A.: A Level Set Algorithm for Minimizing the Mumford-Shah Functional in Image Processing. UCLA, Department of Mathematics, Technical report, CAM **00-13** (2000)
5. Dorn, O., Miller, E.L., Rappaport, C.: A shape reconstruction method for electromagnetic tomography using adjoint fields and level sets. Inverse Problems: Special issue on Electromagnetic Imaging and Inversion of the Earth's Subsurface **16** (2000) 1119–1156
6. Dorn, O., Miller, E.L., Rappaport, C.: Shape reconstruction in 2D from limited-view multi-frequency electromagnetic data. *to appear* AMS series contemporary mathematics (2001)
7. Frank, J.: Electron Tomography: Three-Dimensional Imaging with the Transmission Electron Microscope. New York Plenum Press (1992)
8. Herman, G.T.: Image Reconstruction from Projections: The Fundamentals of Computerized Tomography. Academic Press, New York (1980)
9. Inouye, T.: Image Reconstruction with Limited Angle Projection Data. IEEE Transactions on Nuclear Science **NS-26** (1979) 2666–2684
10. Malladi, R., Sethian, J.A., Vemuri, B.C.: Shape Modeling with Front Propagation: A Level Set Approach. IEEE PAMI **17(2)** (1995) 158–175
11. Osher, S., Sethian, J.A.: Fronts propagating with curvature-dependent speed: Algorithms based on Hamilton-Jacobi formulations. Journal of Computational Physics (1988) 12–49.
12. Prince, J.L., Willsky, A.S.: Hierarchical Reconstruction Using Geometry and Sinogram Restoration. IEEE Transactions on Image Processing **2(3)** (1993) 401–416
13. Roerdink, J.B.T.M.: Computerized tomography and its applications: a guided tour. Nieuw Archief voor Wiskunde **10(3)** (1992) 277–308
14. Santosa, F: A level set approach for inverse problems involving obstacles. European Series in Applied and Industrial Mathematics: Control Optimization and Calculus of Variations **1** (1996) 17–33
15. Sethian, J.A.: Level Set Methods: Evolving interfaces in Geometry, Fluid Mechanics, Computer Vision, and Material Sciences. Cambridge University Press (1996)
16. Tsai, A., Yezzi, A., Jr., Willsky, A.: A Curve Evolution Approach to Smoothing and Segmentation Using the Mumford-Shah Functional. IEEE Computer Society Conference on Computer Vision and Pattern Recognition (2000) 119–124
17. Whitaker, R.T., Robb, R.A. (ed.): Volumetric Deformable Models: Active Blobs. SPIE Visualization In Biomedical Computing (1994) 122–134
18. Whitaker R.T.: A Level-Set Approach to 3D Reconstruction From Range Data. International Journal of Computer Vision **29(3)** (1998) 203–231
19. Whitaker, R.T., Breen, D.E., Museth, K., Soni, N.: A Framework for Level Set Segmentation of Volume Datasets. *to appear* ACM Volume Graphics Workshop (2001)

An Electro-mechanical Model of the Heart for Cardiac Image Analysis

M. Sermesant[1], Y. Coudière[2], H. Delingette[1], N. Ayache[1], and J.A. Désidéri[2]

[1] EPIDAURE Research Project, INRIA Sophia Antipolis
[2] SINUS Research Project, INRIA Sophia Antipolis

Abstract. A simple electro-mechanical model of the heart is derived to best fit available cardiac images. The model is based on anisotropic linear elasticity and, from the electrical point of view, on the finite-element discretisation of the FitzHugh-Nagumo electric wave-propagation model. Present simulations include static image segmentation. By including biological and physical *a priori* knowledge, more realistic 4D images segmentation of the cardiac motion are expected.

1 Introduction

Cardiovascular pathologies are the first mortality cause in the industrialised countries. Estimating quantitative parameters of the ventricle function from images is a key to reach a better understanding of the cardiac motion but also to detect ischemic zones, to measure the pathology extent and to control the therapy effectiveness. These quantitative parameters, like the ejection fraction, myocardium thickness and local strain and stress constitute the ventricular cardiac function.

Some of these parameters can be efficiently extracted from the deformation of geometric surfaces [12]. But these surfaces do not include any biological and physical *a priori* knowledge to guide their deformations where boundary data is missing [15, 16]. Moreover, only the apparent motion (ie. displacement along the normal direction) can be reconstructed.

In this paper, we propose a framework to extract these parameters of interest from a simplified electro-mechanical model of the heart. Basically, unlike previous approaches, we have constructed an active model of the left and right ventricles; this model is activated by an electrical wave modifying its stiffness and shape and also constrained by the additional geometry originating from medical images. Although this is a work in progress, we believe that the proposed framework will allow a better understanding of the heart's behaviour.

2 Geometric Model

Our geometric model consists of a mesh of the whole myocardium (including both right and left ventricles) and of the myocardium fibre directions. Indeed, the fibres architecture has a great influence on the motion and on the propagation

W. Niessen and M. Viergever (Eds.): MICCAI 2001, LNCS 2208, pp. 224–231, 2001.

of the electrical excitation. It is based on data available from the Bioengineering Research Group of the University of Auckland, New Zealand [9, 13]. This data has been obtained by the dissection of a dog's heart and is composed of a mesh of 256 nodes and 180 hexahedra, and of a fibre direction at each node.

This hexahedral mesh presents the advantage of resulting from the deformation of a 3D regular grid. However, it contains tetrahedra of very different shape and size, and this may cause numerical difficulties. Instead, we are currently using tetrahedral meshes because this allows us to locally refine the mesh in parts of interest and to avoid the use of Gaussian quadrature to build stiffness matrices. In fact, different meshes with varying resolutions are built for the electrical and mechanical aspects of the computation.

To switch from hexahedral to tetrahedral meshes, we first triangulate the surface of the hexahedral mesh, and then refine it to the desired resolution while keeping sufficient quality triangles. Then a tetrahedral mesh is produced based on this triangulated surface and finally, the fibre directions are tri-linearly extrapolated and interpolated.

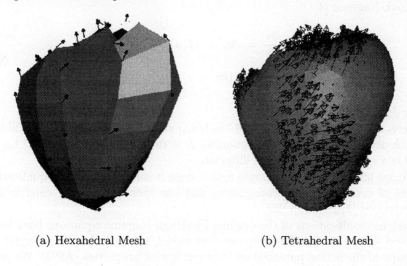

(a) Hexahedral Mesh   (b) Tetrahedral Mesh

Fig. 1. Myocardium meshes of different topologies, with the fibre directions

3   Mechanical Model

The myocardium is a nonlinear viscoelastic anisotropic active material [7, 6]. It is composed of fibre bundles spiralling around the two ventricles. Obviously, the physical model has to be simple enough for computational purposes. Therefore we are limiting ourselves to a linear anisotropic constitutive law. The internal stress-strain relationship in a frame related to the fibre direction is given by:

$$\sigma = \begin{pmatrix} A(\lambda + 2\mu) & \lambda & \lambda & 0 & 0 & 0 \\ \lambda & \lambda + 2\mu & \lambda & 0 & 0 & 0 \\ \lambda & \lambda & \lambda + 2\mu & 0 & 0 & 0 \\ 0 & 0 & 0 & A\mu & 0 & 0 \\ 0 & 0 & 0 & 0 & A\mu & 0 \\ 0 & 0 & 0 & 0 & 0 & \mu \end{pmatrix} \varepsilon,$$

where $\varepsilon = (\mathrm{grad}(U) + \mathrm{grad}(U)^t)/2$ with U the displacement, λ and μ are the Lamé constants and A is a coefficient of anisotropy introduced in Hooke's law.

We have then a linear relationship between the internal body force and the displacement: $F = KU$ where K is the stiffness matrix.

4 Electrical Model

Among the various models for the electric wave-propagation is the system of FitzHugh-Nagumo [4]:

$$\frac{\partial u}{\partial t} = \Delta u + \lambda f(u) - z$$

$$\frac{\partial z}{\partial t} = \epsilon (ku - z) \tag{1}$$

where $f(u) = u(1 - u)(u - a)$.

Here, $x = \bar{x}/L$, $t = \bar{t}/t_{\text{ref}}$, $u = (\bar{u} - u_0)/u_{\text{ref}}$ and z are dimensionless variables. $\bar{u}$ is the actual transmembrane potential, L is the size of the heart and $t_{\text{ref}} = L^2/D$ is a reference time (D the diffusion).

We are interested in this simple model since it correctly captures qualitative aspects of excitation and propagation, and has been successfully used in 3D computations [2, 19, 14, 5, 20].

Various modifications of the original FitzHugh-Nagumo equations have been proposed [8, 18, 11, 1, 10] to improve this model, in particular with respect to the shape of the action potential and the restitution properties (APD). We plan to incorporate one of these in our future work.

The theoretical aspects of (1) have been widely studied [21]: a travelling wave of fixed shape and speed should appear or not, depending on the initial excitation being above or below a threshold.

In a first stage, solutions to (1) have been approximated by using a standard $P1$ Lagrange finite element procedure (with mass lumping and first order numerical integration at vertices), on the given tetrahedral anatomical mesh. The Euler explicit time integration is performed to advance computations:

$$M\frac{u^{n+1} - u^n}{\Delta t} = Ku^n + Mf(u^n) - Mz^n,$$

$$\frac{z^{n+1} - z^n}{\Delta t} = \epsilon(ku^n - z^n),$$

where u^n and z^n are the vector of the nodal values of the approximates u and z at time $t^n = n\Delta t$. K is a stiffness matrix and M is the mass matrix (diagonal here).

In a second stage, anisotropic behaviour will be accounted for by letting the diffusion matrix D depend on the local fibre orientation.

One remaining and crucial problem (of great importance) is that some appropriate boundary conditions must be imposed at the junctions between the special conduction system (Purkinje fibres) and the myocardium, which is not well known so far [5, 17]. We have followed an approach which consists in assuming that the junctions region is located near the apex, below a plane that cuts the main heart axis.

Potential maps are presented at different time steps (Fig. 2), starting after a wave has been initiated at the apex and propagating while taking its complete shape.

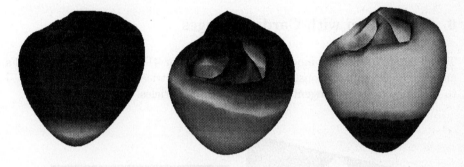

Fig. 2. Surface mapping of the 3D potential at different time steps

5   Activation Model

Each heart-beat cycle, a depolarization wave is initiated and propagates along the myocardium during about 10% of the total cardiac cycle. It induces a contraction of the whole myocardium, which produces a local stress tensor $\sigma_a = \alpha\, f \otimes f$, where f is the fibre direction and α the activation rate, which is directly related to the parameter u of Section 4.

If n is the external normal, by virtue of the Gauss theorem, the equivalent force is:

$$\mathbf{F}_a = \int_V \mathrm{div}(\sigma_a)\,dv = \int_V \mathrm{div}(\alpha f \otimes f)\,dv = \int_S (\alpha f \otimes f)\,\overline{\otimes}\,n\,ds.$$

Therefore, when a fibre is activated, its contraction is modelled as a pressure applied to the surface of the tetrahedron in the fibre direction.

Furthermore, in addition to the extra term σ_f, the electrical activation of the myocardium modifies its elastic properties. To simplify the model, we propose

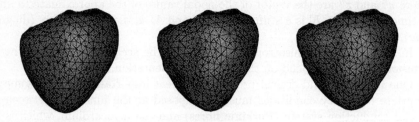

Fig. 3. Effect of the fibres contraction on the model.

to approximate the non-linear behaviour of the myocardium by a series of linear models that are only valid during a small part of the cardiac cycle.

6 Interaction with Cardiac Images

The deformation of our model is guided by 3D or 4D images. The material's anisotropy, through the constitutive law and the electrical activation, is employed to better recover the tangential motion of the ventricles.

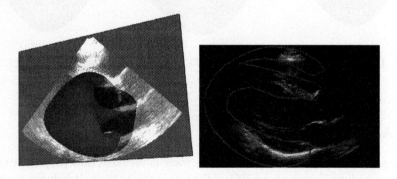

Fig. 4. 3D model in a slice of a 3D ultrasound image.

At time step t, for each node of the mesh surface, we look for the maximum gradient norm along the surface normal direction within a given distance range to find the closest boundary point of the image. We can also use *a priori* knowledge on the image: in ultrasound images, as we know that cardiac structures appear as grey areas on a black background, the gradient direction can help determine if the boundary point found is on the right side of the myocardium. Additionally, we can look for homogeneous areas in a given range of grey values (region approach).

Then, we apply a force $\mathbf{F}_i$ which is proportional to the distance to the closest boundary point of the image from the considered point of the mesh.

We control the effect of those forces with two parameters:

- the proportionality factor to compute those forces from distances;
- the constitutive law of the material (Lamé constants), that controls the stress-strain relationship and the incompressibility;

For the initialisation, we use constants that allow the model to vary importantly, as we adapt the model to the patient heart. Subsequently, during the sequence, we fix the parameters to values found in the literature for the cardiac myocardium, which make it incompressible, for example. As rheological data is complicated to measure in-vivo, this procedure is also a way to adjust the Lamé constants. Furthermore, because of the volumetric nature of our model, it strongly decreases the importance of image's outliers in the motion estimation since it strongly constrains the geometric (for instance the thickness of the myocardium wall) and physical behaviour.

7 Global Heart Model

We use mass-lumping in a Newtonian differential equation with an explicit integration scheme to compute the position $\mathbf{P}$ of each vertex:

$$\left(\frac{1}{\Delta t^2} - \frac{\gamma}{2\Delta t}\right)\mathbf{P}^{t+1} = \mathbf{F}_i + \mathbf{F}_a + \mathbf{F} + \frac{2}{\Delta t^2}\mathbf{P}^t - \left(\frac{1}{\Delta t^2} + \frac{\gamma}{2\Delta t}\right)\mathbf{P}^{t-1},$$

with γ the damping factor and $\mathbf{F}$ the internal forces computed from linear elasticity plus the boundary conditions (in particular the ventricular pressures). The model is activated through the forces $\mathbf{F}_a$ and constrained by the cardiac images through the external forces $\mathbf{F}_i$.

8 Results and Perspectives

This model is really appropriate for the segmentation of ultrasound data, which is sparse and noisy and where *a priori* knowledge is valuable.

The results (Fig. 5) show a rather good match between the mesh and the image data. The radial deformation which is only constrained by the stiffness of the material is however not so accurately adjusted. To improve this, further work on the elastic model and force adjustment is necessary.

In future work, the mechanical model will be improved to better account for normal strength and non linear laws of deformation. Additionally, a realistic simulation of the electric wave-propagation should include, besides the ventricles, the special conduction system (Purkinje Network). Particular efforts will be made in this direction also.

In practice, the model will be forced to fit 4D echocardiographic images sequences synchronised on the electrocardiogram: the electric wave will be deduced from the electrocardiographic measurements, then the activation state will be

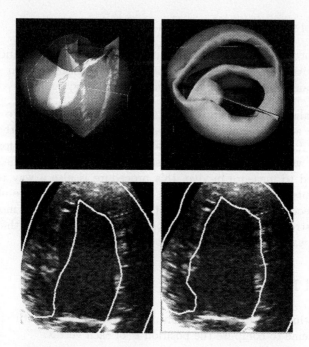

Fig. 5. (Top) 3D model in a slice of a 3D ultrasound image. (Bottom) Intersection of the model and the image, before (left) and after (right) deformation.

known at each time step. Hence, at each time step, the mechanical properties will be evaluated and the model will be deformed to fit the image[1].

Acknowledgements

This work is a part of the multidisciplinary project ICEMA (standing for Images of the Cardiac Electro-Mechanical Activity) a collaborative research action between different INRIA projects which aim is to build a generic dynamic model of the beating heart and a procedure to automatically adjust the parameters to any specific patient [3].

References

[1] R. Aliev and A. Panfilov. A simple two-variable model of cardiac excitation. *Chaos, Solitons and Fractals*, 3(7):293–301, 1996.
[2] A.V. Holden AV and A.V. Panfilov. *Computational biology of the heart*, chapter Modelling propagation in excitable media, pages 65–99. John Wiley & Sons, 1996.
[3] N. Ayache, D. Chapelle, F. Clément, Y. Coudière, H. Delingette, J.A. Désidéri, M. Sermesant, M. Sorine, and J. Urquiza. Towards model-based estimation of the

---

[1] Additional images and videos are available at
http://www-sop.inria.fr/epidaure/personnel/Maxime.Sermesant/heartmodel/

cardiac electro-mechanical activity from ECG signals and ultrasound images. In *Functional Imaging and Modeling of the Heart (FIMH'01)*, 2001 (submitted).

[4] A. L. Bardou, P. M. Auger, P. J. Birkui, and J.-L. Chassé. Modeling of cardiac electrophysiological mechanisms: From action potential genesis to its propagation in myocardium. *Critical Reviews in Biomedical Engineering*, 24:141–221, 1996.

[5] O. Berenfeld and J. Jalife. Purkinje-muscle rentry as a mechanism of polymorphic ventricular arrhytmias in a 3-dimensional model of the ventricles. *Circ. Res.*, 82:1063–1077, 1998.

[6] J. Bestel, F. Clément, and M. Sorine. A biomechanical model of muscle contraction. In *Medical Image Computing and Computer-Assisted intervention (MICCAI'01)*, 2001.

[7] Y. C. Fung. *Biomechanics, Mechanical properties of living tissues*. Springer-Verlag, 1993.

[8] J. Hindmarsh and R. Rose. A model of the nerve impulse using two first-order differential equations. *Nature*, (296):162–164, 1982.

[9] P. J. Hunter and B. H. Smaill. The analysis of cardiac function: a continuum approach. *Biophysical molecular Biology*, 1988.

[10] Z. Knudsen, A.V. Holden, and J. Brindley. Qualitative modelling of mechano electrical feedback in a ventricular cell. *Bulletin of mathematical biology*, 6(59):115–181, 1997.

[11] B. Kogan, W. Karplus, B. Billett, A. Pang, H. Karagueuzian, and S. Khan. The simplified fitzhugh-nagumo model with action potential duration restitution: effects on 2d wave propagation. *Physica D*, (50):327–340, 1991.

[12] J. Montagnat and H. Delingette. Space and time shape constrained deformable surfaces for 4D medical image segmentation. In *Medical Image Computing and Computer-Assisted Intervention (MICCAI'00)*, 2000.

[13] M. Nash. *Mechanics and Material Properties of the Heart using an Anatomically Accurate Mathematical Model*. PhD thesis, University of Auckland, 1998.

[14] A. Panfilov and A. Holden. Computer-simulation of reentry sources in myocardium in 2 and 3 dimensions. *Journal of Theoretical Biology*, 3(161):271–285, 1993.

[15] X. Papademetris, A. J. Sinusas, D. P. Dione, and J. S. Duncan. Estimation of 3D left ventricle deformation from echocardiography. *Medical Image Analysis*, 5, 2001.

[16] Q.C. Pham, F. Vincent, P. Clarysse, P. Croisille, and I. Magnin. A FEM-based deformable model for the 3D segmentation and tracking of the heart in cardiac mri. In *Image and Signal Processing and Analysis (ISPA'01)*, 2001.

[17] A.E. Pollard, N. Hooke, and C.S. Henriquez. Cardiac propagation simulation. *Critical Reviews in biomedical Engineering*, 20(3,4):171–210, 1992.

[18] J. Rinzel. Excitation dynamics: insights from simplified membrane models. *Federation Proceedings*, 15(44):2944–2946, 1985.

[19] J. Rogers, M. Courtemanche, and A. McCulloch. *Computational biology of the heart*, chapter Finite element methods for modelling impulse propagation in the heart, pages 217–233. John Wiley & Sons, 1996.

[20] K. Simelius, J. Nenonen, R. Hren, and B.M. Horacek. Electromagnetic extracardiac fields simulated with a bidomain propagation model. In J. Nenonen, R.J. Ilmoniemi, and T. Katila, editors, *International Conference on Biomagnetism (Biomag'00)*, 2000.

[21] J. Smoller. *Shock Waves and Reaction-Diffusion Equations*. Springer-Verlag (Grundlehren der mathematischen Wissenschaften 258), 1983.

A Mechanical, Three-Dimensional, Ultrasound-Guided Breast Biopsy Apparatus

Kathleen JM Surry[1], Wendy L Smith[1,2], Gregory R Mills[1], Donal B Downey[1,3], Aaron Fenster[1,2,3]

[1]Imaging Research, Robarts Research Institute, London Canada
[2]Medical Biophysics, University of Western Ontario, London Canada
[3]Radiology, London Health Sciences Centre, London Canada
kath@irus.rri.on.ca

Abstract. We have designed a prototype three-dimensional ultrasound (US) guidance apparatus to improve breast biopsy outcomes. Features from stereotactic mammography and free-hand US guided biopsy have been combined with 3D US imaging. This breast biopsy apparatus (BBA) accurately guides a needle into position for firing into target tissue. We have evaluated the BBA in three stages. First, by testing the placement accuracy of a needle in a tissue mimic. Second, with tissue mimic phantoms that had embedded lesions for biopsy. Finally, by comparison to free-hand US-guided biopsy, using chicken breast phantoms. The first two stages of evaluation quantified the mechanical biases in the BBA. Compensating for these, the BBA achieved a 96% success rate in targeting 3.2 mm 'lesions' in chicken breast phantoms. The expert radiologists performing biopsies with free-hand US guidance achieved a 94% success rate. This has proven an equivalence between our apparatus and free-hand biopsy, for 3.2 mm lesions *in vitro*, with a 95% confidence.

1 Introduction

1.1 Breast Biopsy Apparatus (BBA) Development

We have developed a prototype three-dimensional ultrasound (US)-guided breast biopsy apparatus (BBA) to improve patient outcomes (Figure 1). It is based on features from stereotactic mammography and free-hand ultrasound guided biopsy [1-3]. With this apparatus, we avoid the ionizing radiation associated with mammography, but retain the safe needle trajectory, parallel to the chest wall. Also, the real-time imaging associated with US is exploited, with the extra advantage of near real-time 3D US imaging.

A common problem with needle guidance systems for both stereotactic mammography and for the emerging MR breast imaging techniques is the lack of real-time information [4,5]. There are some groups reporting success for needle guidance in interoperative MRI units [6], but these systems are both rare and expensive. A fully robotic breast biopsy system is currently under development for

W. Niessen and M. Viergever (Eds.): MICCAI 2001, LNCS 2208, pp. 232-239, 2001.
© Springer-Verlag Berlin Heidelberg 2001

use within a 1.5T whole body magnet [7], which shows promise, but still requires an expensive and non-portable MRI unit.

The apparatus shown in Figure 1 is a prototype built specifically for testing our biopsy concept with phantoms. The degrees of freedom, apart from the rotational mover for the 3D US scanning, are all manually adjustable. The needle guide (A) and the US probe (B) are kept in the same line by the stage at C (moves in the z-direction). The needle guide may be moved off axis in z (at D) to target a location seen in US at some angle other than zero degrees (straight down). The needle guide is also moved vertically (E, in the y-direction) to target at any depth in the volume. The US probe, in this case a transrectal, side-firing 7 MHz model, is rotated on its axis by the mover at F to collect a 3D volume. It can be moved, on-axis with the needle (the x-direction), by the fourth stage at G. Needle insertion depth, in the same direction, is indicated by a ruler attached to the needle guide.

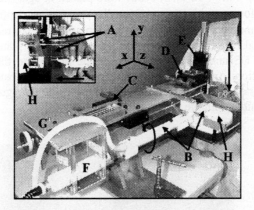

Fig. 1. The prototype three-dimensional ultrasound guided breast biopsy apparatus (BBA), with needle guide shown in inset. **A** Needle guide. **B** US probe. **C, D, E, G** Translational movers. **F** Rotational mover. **H** Compression plate. The system co-ordinates are also indicated as (x, y, z).

2D US images from an Acuson 128 ultrasound machine were digitised and shown as a 3D image within one second by a Power Macintosh 7500 [8]. 3D multi-planar reformatting tools were used to view the 3D volume in any orientation, and to identify a biopsy target point [9-11]. These co-ordinates were used in transformation equations to provide the necessary adjustments to line up the US probe and needle guide with the target. The needle was inserted and positioned under 2D US guidance and the needle gun was fired to acquire a sample of tissue. At any time during the procedure, 3D US images may be acquired to check positioning. A post-biopsy image was often useful, allowing for confirmation that the needle was penetrating the volume.

1.2   BBA Evaluation

We evaluated this apparatus in three stages. First, we determined its accuracy in needle placement at a specified target point in three dimensions. Then, to include the firing of the biopsy gun and the acquisition of a sample, we tested the prototype's biopsy success rates in targeting 'lesions' of known size, between 1.6 mm and 15.9 mm in diameter. Finally, we designed an experiment which compared the biopsy success rates of our 3D US guided BBA with expert radiologists performing free-hand US guided biopsy. In this manner, we have been able to evaluate our prototype BBA so that it may be rebuilt for clinical testing.

2   Methods

2.1   Needle Placement Accuracy

A total of 72 0.79 mm (1/32 inch) beads were placed in agar blocks [12], with a line at each of the four combinations of needle penetration depth (3.5 ± 0.5 mm and 17.5 ± 0.5 mm) and vertical depth (12 ± 0.5 mm and 28 ± 0.5 mm) (Figure 2). These blocks were fixed to the BBA under the top compression plate at H. A target was found using 3D US and the apparatus (both the probe and the needle guide) was moved into position. Another 3D US confirmed the bead's position, and a 14 gauge needle was inserted to these co-ordinates, without 2D US guidance. Another 3D volume was acquired with the needle in place.

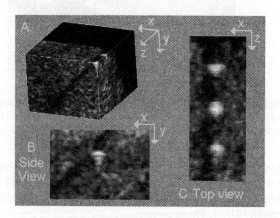

Fig. 2. Small, 0.79 mm beads in an agar phantom, shown here in three-dimensional ultrasound.

Three observers identified the bead's position in the pre-insertion US images, and the needle tip's position in the post-insertion US images. These measurements were made three times by each observer. Needle tip placement relative to bead position was plotted in three dimensions for all combinations of penetration depth and vertical depth. Using 3D principal components analysis (PCA) [13], the maximum variance was found in the needle's placement from the target bead.

2.2   Biopsy Accuracy

To evaluate the biopsy accuracy of the BBA, poly(vinyl alcohol) cryogel (PVA-C) was used as a tissue mimic, due to its robust mechanical properties [14]. Green coloured PVA-C cylinders were embedded as 'lesions' into blocks of white PVA-C (Figure 3). The simulated lesions had equal length and diameter dimensions and were all placed with their centres at the same penetration distance and depth in the US image. The phantoms containing the 1.6 mm, 3.2 mm and 4.8 mm diameter cylinders held 24 samples of each. The phantom with 6.4 mm diameter lesions held 21 samples, the 9.5 mm lesion phantom held 18 and the 15.9 mm lesion phantom held 12. Every lesion was biopsied once only.

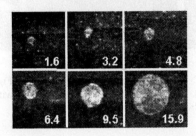

Fig. 3. PVA-C lesions in PVA-C tissue, shown in ultrasound. The lesions' diameters are given in mm.

Similarly to the needle placement study, a 3D US image was acquired and the target identified. The co-ordinates for the centre of the target lesion were used in the transformation equations and the needle inserted. The needle's position was not updated with 2D US guidance. The needle was then fired, using the Bard Magnum biopsy gun (Bard, GA 30014). The biopsy needle acquires a sample by first firing forward a notched central annulus, then a covering sheath which slices off a section of tissue into the notch. This notch is 19 mm long, giving some margin of error in this dimension. A post-biopsy 3D US image was acquired before the needle was removed. The biopsy sample was inspected for green PVA-C and a hit or miss was recorded.

The placement of the needle, relative to the target lesion's centre, was determined using the pre- and post-biopsy 3D images. A 2D PCA analysis was then performed to identify any placement bias in the needle.

2.3   Comparison to Free-Hand US Guided Biopsy

In order to establish whether the BBA is a suitable substitute for free-hand US guided biopsy, we compared the performance of the BBA to that of expert radiologists, in a 'realistic' biopsy task. Chicken breasts were implanted with 3.2 mm diameter PVA-C lesions (Figure 4). Three chicken breasts were sewn together for the radiologists, with 36 lesions in each 3-breast phantom (Figure 5). Each of the two radiologists had to target 55 lesions. Only those lesions which were obvious were targeted (Figure 4). Five smaller phantoms with only a single breast and 15 lesions implanted were made for the BBA testing, as our prototype has a constrained targeting volume (Figure 6).

We also performed 55 biopsies using the BBA. The choice of sample sizes was based on a two group test of equivalence in proportions with large unequal n's [15]. The one-sided test significance level is 10%, and the power was 76%, with a predicted success rate of 90% for both the radiologists and the BBA. This required a sample size of 55 for the test subject (BBA) and 110 samples for the standard for comparison (two radiologists).

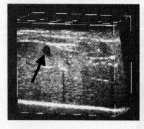
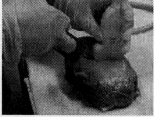
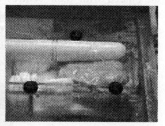

Fig. 4. A 3.2 mm PVA-C lesion in a chicken breast phantom, shown in 3D US.

Fig. 5. Free hand US guided biopsy performed in a chicken phantom.

Fig. 6. BBA biopsy set-up with a chicken phantom.

3   Results

3.1   Needle Placement Accuracy

The largest inter- and intra-observer standard errors of measurement in this study were found for the bead measurement, in the z-direction of our system (see Figure 1), which has the poorest resolution in the reconstructed US image.

The 3D PCA analysis identified that the largest variance (0.73 mm) is found for the deepest beads at the shortest penetration distance. The smallest variance, 0.42 mm, occurs for the shallowest beads, also at short penetration. The axes of maximum variance for each position was not along any of the co-ordinate axes of the machine. Variances along the secondary and tertiary PC axes ranged from 0.31 to 0.13 mm and 0.24 to 0.05 mm, respectively. The largest bias in needle placement was for the deepest beads, at the shortest penetration distance, and was 1.16 mm. The smallest bias was 0.69 mm for the shallowest bead and shortest penetration distance. Also, we can target to within 0.85 mm in the x-y plane, with a 95% confidence.

3.2   Biopsy Accuracy

The post-biopsy 3D US images allowed for identification of the needle's final position. This clearly showed a bias in the placement of the needle's centre line, 0.14 mm too high, and 0.51 mm to the right of centre (Figure 7). No lesions were missed due to misplacement in the needle's axis direction, due to the length of the sampling notch. It was also identified that the needle's sampling notch provided a vertical bias to the tissue sampled. The bevel at the needle's tip directs the tissue at this level down and under the 2 mm diameter shaft and it is this tissue that is sampled by the sampling notch (Figure 8). Since the targeting was done with the central axis of the needle, rather than the bevel tip edge, this contributed to a sampling off-set of 1 mm, and may have affected the results in biopsying the smaller lesions. The biopsy rates are shown in Figure 9. The total variance described by this test was 1.72 mm (standard deviation of 1.31 mm).

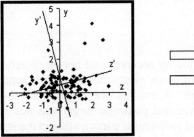

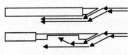

Fig. 7. Scatter plot of needle placement relative to lesion centre (0,0). PCA axes (z', y') are shown at the bias centre.

Fig. 8. Tissue at the needle's tip is directed down under the needle and is sampled by the sampling notch.

Using the minimum and maximum standard deviations along the PC axes, and including the bias caused by the bevel and sampling notch, we developed a model to fit the biopsy values (Figure 9). Using these results, the number of passes needed for a successful biopsy of any lesion size, at a given confidence level can be predicted. The number of passes for 95% confidence in hitting a 3 mm lesion is 5, for example. Six passes are typically used and are well tolerated by patients [2].

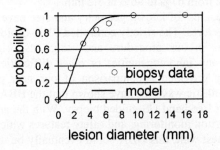

Fig. 9. Biopsy data and the model derived from the PC analysis and the needle notch sampling bias.

3.3   Comparison to Free-Hand US Guided Biopsy

With improvements made based on the first two evaluation experiments, we were able to achieve a 96% success rate with the BBA for 3.2 mm diameter lesions. By a comparison to the expert radiologists, who had a 94% success rate, we have shown our hypothesis, which was that the BBA is equivalent to free-hand biopsy, for this *in vitro* study. The one-sided 95% confidence interval demonstrates that the two biopsy methods are equivalent, within 5%.

The use of chicken phantoms for testing breast biopsy procedures was successful, by providing clearly visible lesions in a tissue-like setting, both when viewed using US and upon biopsy.

4   Discussion

Since our experiments focused on biopsy accuracy and not on detection of 'lesions', our studies avoided any problems of target identification in ultrasound imaging. The targets were always obvious, and, if not, as was sometimes the case in the inhomogeneous chicken breasts, then that particular target was not attempted. This avoided a positive bias for the expert radiologists participating in the study.

We have shown, in three stages, that our breast biopsy apparatus performed well. Through an *in vitro* study, we have shown that this approach is a suitable alternative to free-hand US guided biopsy procedures for 3.2 mm lesions.

By performing the bead targeting study, we were able to establish the targeting accuracy of the BBA's mechanical stages and needle guide under ideal conditions. With the addition of the biopsy part of the procedure, the additional biases were modelled.

It was clear that the 3D US images were important in evaluating the procedure, as they provided information about a placement bias. This was evident in the PVA-C biopsy study, which could have been interpreted without knowledge of the bias, and the low targeting rate attributed solely to a larger scatter in a random normal distribution about the target point. Knowledge of the bias allowed us to improve our targeting success rate from 67% to 96% at 3.2 mm.

Using artificial 'lesions' of known geometry and size have allowed us to compare and rate biopsy procedures. The strictly controlled PVA-C biopsy study allowed us to identify a clear bias in our procedure and assign its origin to the mechanical components, not to any inhomogeneities or other difficulties in the phantom. The chicken breast study provided a comparison of our new procedure to a clinical standard in a more realistic way. We have shown that the BBA provides an equivalent success rate to expert free-hand US guided biopsy. With the additions of 3D imaging, real-time needle insertion monitoring, and safety features which keep the needle away from the patient's chest wall, this BBA could eventually be used in a clinical setting and achieve results equal to an expert using free-hand US guided biopsy.

Improvements must be made to the apparatus before clinical testing. Besides the obvious cosmetic and ergonomic adjustments, we are also automating the movers to increase the speed of the procedure. When a target is identified by the clinician in the 3D US image, the machine will move the US probe and the needle guide into position. We will also be increasing the available target volume, which was suitable for our phantom studies, but not for a clinical setting.

5   References and Acknowledgements

We thank S Odegaard for helping with the US data collection and Dr A Kumar for performing the chicken biopsies. Also, for Dr M Eliasziw's help with the chicken breast statistics. This work was funded by the Canadian Institutes of Health Research (CIHR) and London Health Sciences Centre (LHSC).

1   Roe SM, Mathews JW, Burns RP, Sumida MP, Craft P and Greer MS 1997 Stereotactic and ultrasound core needle breast biopsy performed by surgeons *Am J Surg* **174** 699-704
2   Liberman L, Feng TL, Dershaw DD, Morris EA and Abramson AF 1998 US-guided core breast biopsy: Use and cost-effectiveness *Radiology* **208** 717-723
3   Meyer JE, Smith DN, Lester SC, *et al* 1999 Large-core needle biopsy of nonpalpable breast lesions *JAMA* **281** 1638-1641
4   Dershaw DD 2000 Equipment, technique, quality assurance, and accreditation for imaging-guided breast biopsy procedures *Radiol Clin North Am* **38(4)** 773-789
5   Heywang-Köbrunner SH, Heinig A, Schaumlöffel U, *et al* 1999 MR-guided percutaneous excisional and incisional biopsy of breast lesions *Eur Radiol* **9** 1656-1665
6   Daniel BL, Birdwell RL, Ikeda DM, *et al* 1998 Breast lesion localization: A freehand, interactive MR imaging-guided technique *Radiology* **207** 455-463
7   Kaiser WA, Fischer H, Vagner J, Selig M 2000 Robotic system for biopsy and therapy of breast lesions in a high-field whole-body magnetic resonance tomography unit *Invest Radiol* **35(8)** 513-519
8   Tong S, Downey DB, Cardinal HN and Fenster A 1996 A 3D ultrasound prostate imaging system *Ultrasound Med Biol* **22** 735-746
9   Nelson TR, Downey DB, Pretorius DH and Fenster A 1999 Three-dimensional ultrasound. Lippincott Williams & Wilkins, Philadelphia
10 Fenster A and Downey DB 2000 Three-dimensional ultrasound imaging *In:* Annual Review Biomed Eng 2000: Annual Reviews 457-475
11 Fenster A and Downey DB 1996 3D ultrasound imaging: A review 1996 *IEEE Eng Med Biol* **15** 41-51
12 Rickey DW, Picot PA, Christopher DC and Fenster A 1999 Three-dimensional ultrasound. Lippincott Williams & Wilkins, Philadelphia
13 Drury SA 1993 Image Interpretation in Geology 2nd edition. Chapman and Hall
14 Chu KC and Rutt BK 1997 Polyvinyl alcohol cryogel: An ideal phantom material for MR studies of arterial flow and elasticity *Mag Res Med* **37** 314-319
15 Farrington CP and Manning G 1990 Test statistics and sample size formulae for comparative binomial trials with null hypotheses of non-unity relative risk *Stat Med* **9(12)** 1447-1454

Augmented Reality Guidance for Needle Biopsies:
A Randomized, Controlled Trial in Phantoms

Michael Rosenthal[1], Andrei State[1], Joohi Lee[1], Gentaro Hirota[1],
Jeremy Ackerman[1], Kurtis Keller[1], Etta D. Pisano[2] MD, Michael Jiroutek[3],
Keith Muller[3], and Henry Fuchs[1]

[1]University of North Carolina at Chapel Hill, Department of Computer Science, CB 3175,
Chapel Hill, NC 27599-3175, USA
{rosentha|andrei|lee|hirota|ackerman|keller|fuchs}@cs.unc.edu

[2]University of North Carolina at Chapel Hill, Department of Radiology, CB 7510,
Chapel Hill, NC 27599-7510, USA
etpisano@med.unc.edu

[3]University of North Carolina at Chapel Hill, Department of Biostatistics, CB 7420,
Chapel Hill, NC 27599-7420, USA
mjiroute@bios.unc.edu, keith_muller@unc.edu

Abstract. We report the results of a randomized, controlled trial to compare the accuracy of standard ultrasound-guided needle biopsy to biopsies performed using a 3D Augmented Reality (AR) guidance system. Fifty core biopsies of breast phantoms were conducted by a board-certified radiologist, with each set of five biopsies randomly assigned to one of the methods. The raw ultrasound data from each biopsy was recorded. Another board-certified radiologist, blinded to the actual biopsy guidance mechanism, evaluated the ultrasound recordings and determined the distance of the biopsy from the ideal position. A repeated measures analysis of variance indicated that the head-mounted display method led to a statistically significantly smaller mean deviation from the desired target than did the CRT display method. (2.48mm for control versus 1.62mm for augmented reality, $p < 0.02$). This result suggests that AR systems can offer improved accuracy over traditional biopsy guidance methods.

1 Introduction

Our research group at the University of North Carolina has been working in the area of augmented reality (AR) visualization for ultrasound examinations and ultrasound-guided procedures for nearly a decade [2-5,7,9,10]. The vision for this project is to allow physicians to directly see into a patient, aided by real-time computer graphics and augmented reality technology. The notion of augmenting the view of one's surroundings with computer-generated images has its roots in Ivan Sutherland's seminal paper [12], which described a system with a head-mounted display (HMD) whose synthetic images the user could see optically overlaid on the view of the room around him. Many years of research, both in the general AR field [1] as well as in

W. Niessen and M. Viergever (Eds.): MICCAI 2001, LNCS 2208, pp. 240-248, 2001.
© Springer-Verlag Berlin Heidelberg 2001

specific medical AR applications (for example [6,11]), have resulted in considerable improvement in each of the key technologies.

Using our biopsy guidance system in January 1996, a trained physician (Pisano) was able to guide a needle into a lesion within an artificial breast training phantom and report that the task was "easy" (fig. 1). A subsequent test with a human subject progressed to where the needle was partially inserted towards the target lesion, at which point the physician was forced to abandon the AR guidance and continue the intervention with conventional ultrasound guidance technology. During this and several subsequent experiments it slowly became clear that despite the technological advancements effective patient studies were still not possible. This was mostly due to cumbersome equipment and inadequate tracking technology [3].

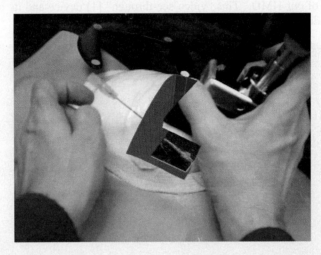

Fig. 1. HMD point of view image from a 1996 AR guidance experiment. The physician has inserted a cyst aspiration needle into a lesion within a breast phantom and holds the ultrasound transducer in her right hand. Correct ultrasound probe calibration and accurate tracking yield lignment between real needle and image of the needle in ultrasound slice. The colored dots in the background are fiducials for head tracking correction (not used in our current system)

We have spent the intervening years developing an enhanced guidance system, which is now being used in live patient studies. In the following sections, we describe the new developments in our guidance system. We also describe the design and report the results of a randomized, controlled study to determine the relative effectiveness of our new AR system versus traditional ultrasound. We conclude with a description of our current and future work.

2 Materials and Methods

Earlier papers have described our system design in detail [3-5,9,10]. In the following sections, we describe the updated components of our system and the design of our recent biopsy accuracy experiment.

2.1 Augmented Reality Guidance System

Our AR guidance system consists of four major components: a head-mounted display (HMD), an instrument tracking system, an ultrasound imaging system, and a graphics and computation platform.

Head-Mounted Display. We have modified a stereoscopic Sony Glasstron LDI-D100 HMD[1] for use as our display system. This HMD provides full color, stereo, SVGA (800x600) resolution displays in a lightweight design. We have added an aluminum superstructure to hold two Toshiba IK-SM43H video cameras for image capture and three infrared LEDs for opto-electronic tracking. Figure 2 shows the latest model of our HMD. This "video see-through" [1] device and its operation are described in detail in [10].

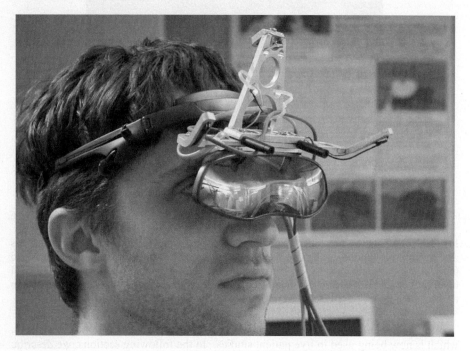

Fig. 2. Video-see-through augmented reality HMD built on the basis of a Sony Glasstron LDI-D100 device. The aluminum superstructure holds two miniature video cameras for image capture and three infrared LEDs for opto-electronic tracking of the HMD

Tracking System. We use an Image-Guided Technologies FlashPoint™ 5000 opto-electronic tracker in our system. The HMD, the ultrasound probe and the biopsy needle are all equipped with infrared LEDs. The FlashPoint delivers sub-millimeter-accurate readings of the positions of these LEDs to the graphics computer. This HMD tracking technology is not quite as accurate as the closed-loop method used in our original 1996 system [8], but it is superior to magnetic technologies and does not

---

[1] Alas, Sony is no longer manufacturing the SVGA stereo version of their Glasstron HMD.

encumber the user's field of view (and the sterile operating field) with fiducials. The ultrasound probe is also tracked opto-electronically. It uses a specially developed 9-LED device that allows rotations up to 80° to any side without losing acquisition, thus freeing the physician to position and orient the probe in the most adequate way for a particular intervention.

Ultrasound Imaging System. We are using a PIE Medical Ultrasound Scanner 350 to acquire ultrasound images during our experiments. This device was donated by PIE Medical.

Graphics and Computation Platform. The system runs on an SGI Onyx2 Reality Monster™ graphics computer equipped with multiple DIVO digital video input/output boards, allowing simultaneous capture of multiple video streams. The software routinely runs at frame rates of 20-30 Hz in stereo on this platform. Fig. 3 shows imagery displayed by our system during an experiment with a breast training phantom in late 2000.

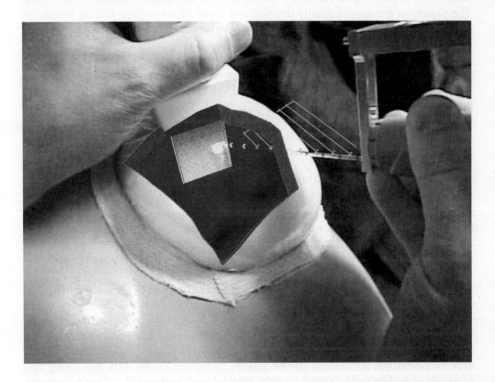

Fig. 3. HMD view during phantom biopsy experiment. Both the ultrasound probe (left hand) and the biopsy needle (right hand) are tracked. The needle aims at the bright lesion visible in the ultrasound slice. The system displays the projection of the needle onto the plane of the ultrasound slice (blue lines) and also displays the projected trajectory of the needle if it were fired at this moment (yellow markers)

2.2 Design of Biopsy Guidance Study

We have performed an experiment to compare our AR guidance system to standard ultrasound guidance for the task of targeting needle biopsies in training phantoms. Our hypothesis was that the two guidance methods would be comparable in terms of needle placement accuracy for this task, indicating that it is safe to evaluate the AR system in humans.

The experimental component of this study was performed using the AR system described above. The control component was performed using only the PIE Medical Ultrasound Scanner 350 component of our system without any computer augmentation.

Biopsy Task. Our task under evaluation was a standard series of core biopsies that would be performed on a solid breast mass. Standard ultrasound training phantoms (Model 52 Biopsy Phantom, Computerized Imaging Reference Systems, Inc., Norfolk, VA) were used as our biopsy subjects. These phantoms each contained six tumor-like targets placed randomly throughout an ultrasound-compatible gel mold. The phantoms are approximately the size and shape of an average human breast. A new phantom was used whenever the radiologist felt that artifacts from previous biopsies were interfering with the current task.

For each selected lesion, biopsies were targeted to the center of the lesion and to the three, six, nine, and twelve o'clock positions around the perimeter of the lesion (as viewed on the plane orthogonal to the axis of the biopsy needle). The biopsies were performed using a 14-gauge Monopty core biopsy needle (C. R. Bard, Inc., Covington, GA). The needle was withdrawn from the phantom after each biopsy attempt. The ultrasound video from each biopsy was reformatted and recorded directly from the ultrasound scanner to DV tape for later evaluation.

Randomization and Control Scheme. This study was designed as a randomized, controlled trial to limit the effects of confounding factors. A single board-certified radiologist (Pisano) performed all of the biopsies in this experiment (fig. 4). Ten targets within the phantoms were sequentially selected; five biopsies were performed on each lesion before selecting the next target. Randomization to the two guidance methods was performed by a coin flip before the selection of each biopsy target.

Evaluation of Accuracy. Another board-certified radiologist (Cherie Kuzmiak, DO) evaluated the ultrasound video to determine the accuracy of each biopsy. The evaluator was blinded to the method of guidance for each biopsy. For each biopsy, she determined the geometric distance (in mm) between the ideal biopsy target point and the actual biopsy positions in the plane orthogonal to the needle. The evaluator also measured the dimensions of the lesions along the needle axis and along two perpendicular directions (approximately vertical and horizontal). These distances were measured on an NTSC display with respect to the reference ruler that was recorded as part of the ultrasound display. The results were later entered into an Excel spreadsheet and associated with the corresponding guidance method.

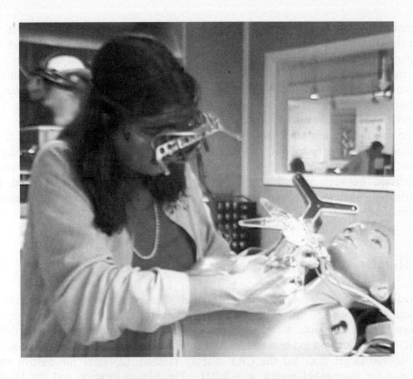

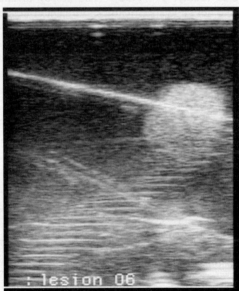

Fig. 4. Lab view (left) and ultrasound image (right) while the physician, wearing the Glasstron-based AR HMD, performs a controlled study with the 2000 AR system. She holds the opto-electronically tracked ultrasound probe and biopsy needle in her left and right hands, respectively. The HMD view was similar to Figure 3

Statistical Analyses. Descriptive statistics (mean ± std) of the error distances were calculated. Separate and combined results were computed for the HMD and CRT display methods for each location, mean error across locations and the mean of the maximum lesion dimension. The primary analysis was a repeated measures analysis of variance (REPM ANOVA) utilized to address the multiple locations targeted within each lesion (a within-'subject' repeated measures dimension). The SAS® procedure GLM was utilized.

To rule out lesion size bias as contributing to the effect attributed to display method in the primary analysis, we performed an exploratory full model in every cell (FMIC) REPM ANOVA analysis to show that the effect due to lesion size was not significant between the display methods. The FMIC was then reduced to a multivariate analysis of covariance (MANCOVA) model and reanalyzed. Maximum lesion dimension (in mm) was the measure we chose to represent lesion size.

3 Results

A total of fifty biopsies were performed: twenty-five in each of the AR guidance and standard guidance groups. The mean error distances for each of these groups are shown in table 1 below. A repeated measures analysis of variance indicated that the HMD display method led to a statistically significantly smaller mean deviation from the desired target than did the CRT display method. (2.48mm for control versus 1.62mm for augmented reality, p < 0.02). The biopsy location and the location-display combination did not yield statistically significant effects upon the accuracy.

Table 1. Results from the phantom biopsy study

(All measures in mm, mean ± std dev)	Standard Guidance	AR Guidance	Combined Results
Error at Center	4.20±1.92	1.50±1.41	2.85±2.14
Error at 3 O'clock	2.00±1.87	1.70±0.67	1.85±1.33
Error at 6 O'clock	1.20±0.84	0.90±1.02	1.05±0.90
Error at 9 O'clock	2.00±1.58	0.80±1.30	1.40±1.51
Error at 12 O'clock	3.00±2.00	3.20±2.05	3.10±1.91
Mean Error across Locations	2.48±0.44	1.62±0.48	2.05±0.63
Mean of Maximum Lesion Dimension	10.50±3.26	12.00±2.09	11.25±2.70

The supportive FMIC ANOVA and MANCOVA analyses of the effects of lesion dimensions upon accuracy indicated that the maximum lesion dimension had no significant effect upon placement error (p > 0.05 for the main effect and all combinations involving maximum lesion dimension).

4 Conclusions

The results of the above study indicate that the AR guidance system yielded statistically improved accuracy as compared to the standard ultrasound guidance method. In fact, we did not expect the AR system to be as good as the conventional guidance technique, especially for the expert user (Pisano). Our goal was to merely demonstrate the system's effectiveness on a procedure that is simple and not dangerous to the patient. The indication that the AR technique may be better even in this comparison, where the advantage should go to the conventional approach, is both surprising and encouraging. Of course, procedures on phantoms may be more advantageous for the new approach than procedures with live patients, since phantoms have simpler tissue characteristics. We may consider user studies with less experienced physicians, which may show an even more dramatic advantage for our new approach.

Additional studies with human subjects are currently underway to confirm that these benefits translate to real improvements in medical care. Beyond that we are considering two possibly parallel paths of research: 1) Exploring the AR approach for relatively simple medical tasks, such as cyst aspiration, for primary care physicians, and 2) Investigating the AR approach for needle placement in more difficult areas of the body (e.g., liver), in which targets are in heavily vascular regions where avoidance of major vessels is a prime consideration.

While results reported here are preliminary and of limited scope, we believe that they suggest the potential of AR visualization to improve patient care. We hope that the next decade of research will continue to explore the potential of augmented reality for both medical and non-medical applications.

5 Acknowledgments

Past and current researchers: Michael Bajura, Andrew Brandt, David T. Chen, D'nardo Colucci, Jessica R. Crawford, William F. Garrett, Jack Goldfeather, Arthur Gregory, Marco C. Jacobs, Mark A. Livingston, Michael J. North, Ryutarou Ohbuchi, Stephen M. Pizer, Paul Rademacher, Chris Tector, Mary C. Whitton.
Past and current medical collaborators: Nancy Chescheir MD, Mark Deutchman MD, Ricardo Hahn MD, Vern Katz MD, Cherie Kuzmiak DO, Matthew Mauro MD, Anthony A. Meyer MD, Melanie Mintzer MD.
Technical assistance: Samuel H. Drake, Caroline K. Green, David G. Harrison, John E. Thomas.
Support: NIH (CA 47982-10), NSF STC for Computer Graphics and Scientific Visualization (NSF Cooperative Agreement ASC-8920219), PIE Medical, and SGI.

References

1. Azuma, Ronald T. A Survey of Augmented Reality. Presence: Teleoperators and Virtual Environments 6, 4 (August 1997), MIT Press, 355-385

2. Bajura, Michael, Henry Fuchs, and Ryutarou Ohbuchi. Merging Virtual Objects with the Real World: Seeing Ultrasound Imagery within the Patient. Proceedings of SIGGRAPH '92 (Chicago, IL, July 26-31, 1992). In Computer Graphics 26, #2 (July 1992), 203-210

3. Fuchs, Henry, Andrei State, Etta D. Pisano, William F. Garrett, Gentaro Hirota, Mark A. Livingston, Mary C. Whitton, and Stephen M. Pizer. (Towards) Performing Ultrasound-Guided Needle Biopsies from within a Head-Mounted Display. Proceedings of Visualization in Biomedical Computing 1996, (Hamburg, Germany, September 22-25, 1996), 591-600

4. Garrett, William F., Henry Fuchs, Mary C. Whitton, and Andrei State. Real-Time Incremental Visualization of Dynamic Ultrasound Volumes Using Parallel BSP Trees. Proceedings of IEEE Visualization 1996 (San Francisco, CA, October 27 - November 1, 1996), 235-240

5. Jacobs, Marco, Mark A. Livingston, and Andrei State. Managing Latency in Complex Augmented Reality Systems. Proceedings of 1997 Symposium on Interactive 3D Graphics (Providence, RI, April 27-30, 1997). Annual Conference Series, 1997, ACM SIGGRAPH, 49-54

6. King, A. P., P. Edwards, C. R. Maurer, Jr., D. A. deCunha, R. P. Gaston, M. Clarkson, D. L. G. Hill, D. J. Hawkes, M. R. Fenlon, A. J. Strong, T. C. S. Cox, M. J. Gleeson. Stereo Augmented Reality in the Surgical Microscope. Presence: Teleoperators and Virtual Environments, 9(4), 360-368, 2000

7. State, Andrei, David T. Chen, Chris Tector, Andrew Brandt, Hong Chen, Ryutarou Ohbuchi, Mike Bajura, and Henry Fuchs. Case Study: Observing a Volume-Rendered Fetus within a Pregnant Patient. Proceedings of IEEE Visualization '94 (Los Alamitos, Calif.: IEEE Computer Society Press, 1994), 364-368

8. State, Andrei, Gentaro Hirota, David T. Chen, William F. Garrett, and Mark A. Livingston. Superior Augmented-Reality Registration by Integrating Landmark Tracking and Magnetic Tracking. Proceedings of SIGGRAPH '96 (New Orleans, LA, August 4-9, 1996). In Computer Graphics Proceedings, Annual Conference Series, 1996, ACM SIGGRAPH, 429-438

9. State, Andrei, Mark A. Livingston, Gentaro Hirota, William F. Garrett, Mary C. Whitton, Henry Fuchs, and Etta D. Pisano (MD). Technologies for Augmented-Reality Systems: realizing Ultrasound-Guided Needle Biopsies. Proceedings of SIGGRAPH '96 (New Orleans, LA, August 4-9, 1996). In Computer Graphics Proceedings, Annual Conference Series, 1996, ACM SIGGRAPH, 439-446

10. State, Andrei, Jeremy Ackerman, Gentaro Hirota, Joohi Lee and Henry Fuchs. Dynamic Virtual Convergence for Video See-through Head-mounted Displays: Maintaining Maximum Stereo Overlap throughout a Close-range Work Space. Submitted for publication

11. Stetten, George, V. Chib. Overlaying Ultrasound Images on Direct Vision. Journal of Ultrasound in Medicine vol. 20, no. 1, 235-240, 2001

12. Sutherland, Ivan E. A Head-Mounted Three-Dimensional Display. AFIPS Conference Proceedings (1968) 33, I, 757-764

Robotic Kidney and Spine Percutaneous Procedures Using a New Laser-Based CT Registration Method

Alexandru Patriciu[1,2], Stephen Solomon MD[1,3], Louis Kavoussi MD[1],
Dan Stoianovici PhD[1,2]

[1]Johns Hopkins Medical Institutions, Brady Urology Institute, URobotics Laboratory
{patriciu, kavoussi, dss} @urology.jhu.edu
[2]Johns Hopkins University, Mechanical Engineering Department
[3]Johns Hopkins Medical Institutions, Department of Radiology

Abstract. We present a simple method for robot registration in computer tomography imaging systems. The method uses the laser markers readily available on any CT scanner and does not require imaging thus eliminating radiation exposure. Its accuracy is inherited from the laser positioning system. This approach does not require additional hardware, laser alignment being performed on the instrument used in the clinical application. Moreover, robotic guidance allows for radiological interventions to be performed on scanners without fluoro-CT capability. Unlike the manual approach, the method allows for performing oblique insertions, for which the skin entry point and the target are located in different slices.

The implementation is realized using the latest version of the PAKY-RCM robot developed in our laboratory. This is an increased precision system based on our new Ball-Worm technology.

The system was successfully used for five CT-guided biopsy and radio-frequency ablation procedures on the kidney and spine and a nephrostomy tube placement. Further investigation will explore its application to other organs and procedures.

1. Introduction

Computer tomography (CT) guided percutaneous procedures are becoming increasingly popular in radiological interventions. CT guided interventions have been facilitated by the development of the CT fluoroscopy (CTF) imaging systems [5]. This new generation of CT-scanners allows for fluoro-imaging of a CT slice. Using the real-time cross-section image the radiologist manually orients and inserts a procedure needle towards the target, provided that the skin entry point and the target are located in the current fluoro slice. Even though the procedure is fast and precise in experienced hands, the major limitation of CTF is the relatively high radiation exposure to patient and physician [6,15]. In order to make the real time adjustments in needle trajectory the physician's hand is in or near the scanning plane. Physician hand exposure has been theoretically and empirically determined to be approximately 2mGy per procedure [11]. Kato et al. [8] have calculated that on the basis of an annual dose limit of 500mSv for the hands, a physician would be limited to performing only *four CTF procedures per year*.

W. Niessen and M. Viergever (Eds.): MICCAI 2001, LNCS 2208, pp. 249-257, 2001.
© Springer-Verlag Berlin Heidelberg 2001

A number of procedural techniques, shields [12], and passive needle holders [1] have been proposed to reduce radiation exposure. Robotic systems have been investigated for eliminating radiation exposure and simultaneously increasing accuracy in radiological interventions [7,19]. A system using CT-fluoroscopy was reported by Loser and Navab [9]. This uses a visual-servoing algorithm to orient the procedure needle based on fluoro-CT images. The approach demonstrated good targeting accuracy by using the procedure needle as a marker, without additional registration hardware. Even though the radiation exposure of the surgeon, which supervises the procedure from the control room, is virtually zero the patient is being exposed to radiation during the robot's image-based servo orientation.

Susil et al. [20] reported a registration method using a localization device (a modified Brown-Roberts-Wells frame [1]) attached to the robot's end-effector, which was further perfected by Masamune [10]. The method presents the advantage of providing the registration data from a single image slice. In addition the method is not restricted to the use of CTF. In our clinical experience implementing their method [13], however, the registration frame was cumbersome in the confined gantry space, and its initial positioning with respect to the CT active field imposed stringent constraints for interventional use.

The proposed method is significantly different from the above two in that it is not an image-based registration method. Similar to the Navab method, it requires no additional hardware and, alike the Susil system, it is not limited to the use of CTF scanners. Its laser-based registration principle insures zero radiation exposure for both the patient and personnel.

2. Methods

The system comprises a CT scanner, a personal computer (PC), and the PAKY-RCM robot [3,14,16,17] attached to the CT table. The PC is equipped with a motion control card for robot control and acquires CT images in DICOM format through a network connection. The laser markers commonly available on the CT scanner are used for robot registration through a needle alignment processes. The radiologist chooses the target in the slice image displayed on the PC monitor, and the robot automatically aligns and delivers the needle. Several software and hardware mechanisms insure the safety of the procedure.

2.1 The Robotic System

The main component of the system is the PAKY – RCM robot. This robot has two components the PAKY (Percutaneous Access of the Kidney) needle driver and the RCM (Remote Center of Motion) robot.

PAKY is a radiolucent needle driver used to guide and actively drive a trocar needle in X-Ray guided percutaneous access procedures. The needle driver is radiolucent thus allowing unobstructed visualization of the anatomical target and radiological guidance of the needle [16]. An electric motor performs automated needle insertion. PAKY has been successfully used in numerous clinical cases [3].

The RCM robot is a compact robot for surgical applications that implements a fulcrum point located distal to the mechanism [17]. The robot presents a compact design: it may be folded into a 171 x 69 x 52 mm box and it weighs only 1.4 Kg. The robot can precisely orient a surgical instrument in space while maintaining the location of one of its points. This kinematic architecture makes it proper for minimally invasive applications as well as trocar/needle orientation in percutaneous procedures. RCM accommodates various end-effectors. The robot was successfully used at the Johns Hopkins Medical Institutions for numerous surgical procedures [1]. The latest version of the RCM robot includes the Ball-Worm Transmission [18] developed in our laboratory and redundant encoding. These significantly enhance the safety, kinematic performance, and rigidity of the mechanism.

In the current setting the PAKY-RCM robot is used to orient a needle while maintaining its initial tip location and perform the insertion of the needle. Two degrees of freedom (DOF) are used for needle alignment and one translational DOF is used for needle insertion. For safety, the orientation and insertion stages may be independently enabled / disabled by hardware means.

The robotic assembly is fixed into a passive arm. This is mounted on a bridge fixture attached over the CT table. The passive arm allows for the support of the mechanism in close proximity of the targeted organ so that the tip of the needle is located at the desired skin entry point. In this setting only two rotations and one translation are required for accessing any nearby target.

2.2 CT-Robot Laser Registration

CT scanners are normally equipped with three laser markers as schematically presented in Figure 1. The Laser Plane 1 (LP1) coincides with the current CT image plane. The Laser Plane 2 (LP2) is parallel with LP1 and positioned at the distance $-z_{12}$

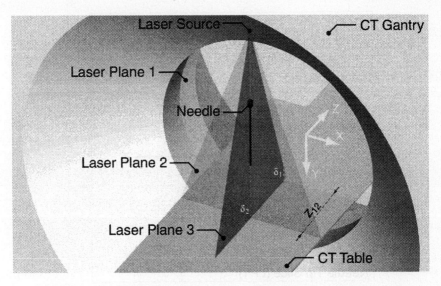

Figure 1: CT Laser Markers and Laser Registration Principle

along the Z-axis of the CT scanner. The Laser Plane 3 (LP3) is perpendicular on LP1 and LP2 and defines the YOZ plane of the CT. The intersection of the LP1 and LP3 defines the vertical direction δ_2 in the CT image space.

The proposed registration method is based on the alignment of the instrument (needle) with the vertical direction δ_2. This is achieved by simultaneously aligning the needle in the LP2 and LP3 laser planes. The central and vertical direction of the current CT image δ_1 is then obtained by a simple z_{12} translation. This alignment with the laser planes provides a 5 DOF registration. The remaining DOF, specifically the Y position of the needle tip is unknown and remains to be determined from the CT image acquired for target specification. Alternatively, a forth laser could be used for providing 6 DOF laser registration by marking a horizontal plane. CT scanners, however, are not normally instrumented with this 4th laser marker. Subsets of this methodology may also be implemented for particular applications and robot kinematic schemes requiring reduced DOF registration.

In our initial implementation we used a combined Laser-Image Registration method. This was required by the limited mobility structure of the PAKY-RCM robot used. The registration procedure involves two main steps, as follows:

Step 1: This defines the current image plane (LP1) in the robot coordinate system by using the laser alignment process. The robot is attached to the mobile CT table through a bridge mount and a passive positioning arm. Using the passive arm, the robot is placed so that the tip of the needle is located at the desired skin entry point. The CT table, together with the robot, is then moved until the tip of the needle is highlighted by the LP1 laser (LP2 and a translation could also be used). Figure 2 presents a schematic of several consecutive needle positions P_1O, P_2O, P_3O, P_4O with the needle point O located in the image and laser plane LP1.

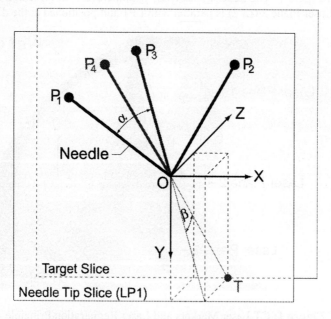

Figure 2: Laser - Image Registration Scheme

The robot is moved under joystick control while observing the laser projection on the needle so that its head is aligned with the laser. During this motion, the RCM robot insures that the needle tip remains in LP1. In the P_1O position of the needle the laser shines its entire barrel. In our approach this was set and inspected by direct observation. For providing automated positioning, a future approach will use a laser detection sensor mounted at the needle head. As such, the needle P_1O is located in the current image and laser plane LP1. The PC acquires this needle orientation by recording the robot joint coordinates.

The process of needle alignment in the laser plane LP1 is then repeated for a dissimilar orientation of the needle P_2O. Joint coordinates are acquired at this position and geometric calculations are employed to define the P_1OP_2 plane in the robot coordinate system. This defines the current image plane in robot space, thus providing the first 2 DOF for the registration process. At this stage the robot may be restricted to move in the LP1 image plane. This could be used to remotely manipulate the needle in the image space, in a similar way that radiologists presently perform CTF manual interventions.

Step 2: The remaining registration data is image-based and uses the image acquired for entry-point / target specification. An image is acquired at the same P_1O orientation of the needle. The combined registration data is then calculated by overlapping the needle P_1O in the image and robot spaces, providing the complete registration data, which will be used for orienting the needle towards the specified target.

2.3 Targeting Methodology

An image slice is acquired through the needle-tip and one through the desired target (Needle Tip Slice and Target Slice in Figure 2). In the particular case that the needle tip and the target are located in the same image plane, only one acquisition is required. The images are acquired in DICOM format and displayed on the PC monitor. The radiologist identifies the target by using the mouse.

The transversal targeting angle (α) is determined by using simple geometric relations in the Target Slice image. The longitudinal targeting angle β is then calculated by using the distance between the two slices retrieved from the DICOM images.

Under the control of the radiologist the robot automatically orients the needle at the position P_4 specified by the angles α and β through the intermediary (in plane) position P_3 (given by α). In the particular case that the target and skin entry point are located in the same slice, all calculations are performed on the same image and $\beta=0$. The needle depth of insertion is calculated by using the image of the target and needle tip in the two slices.

3. Results

Preliminary accuracy testing was performed in-vitro using 1 mm diameter metallic balls. The target was placed in the same image plane with the needle tip and also in different planes. The targeting error achieved over fifty experiments was less than 1 mm in plane and 1.5 mm for out of plane targets. With these satisfactory results, the extensive clinical experience with the PAKY-RCM robot in percutaneous renal access under C-Arm guidance [1,3,17], and the safety of the PAKY-RCM robot rendered by its decoupled needle orientation and insertion capability, we proceeded for the clinical application. For verifying needle-targeting accuracy before needle insertion, in our studies we used a CTF scanner (Siemens - Somatom Plus Four). In addition, in all clinical applications we performed several algorithm-testing steps insuring the functionality of the algorithm in successive phases.

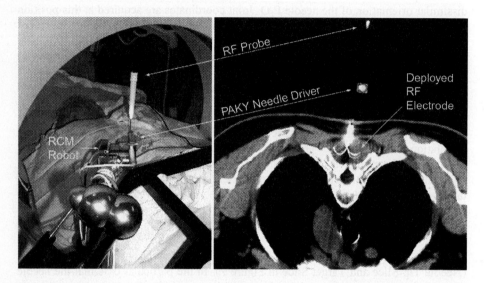

Figure 3: Robotic CT-Guided Spine Radio Frequency Ablation

Five robotic radiological interventions including a nephrostomy tube, kidney and spine biopsy and radio frequency ablation have been successfully performed (Figure 3, Figure 4), as follows:
- The patients were placed in the prone position on the CTF table. A volume scan was initially acquired to localize the lesion and plan the procedure. The patient's back was cleaned with betadine and local lidocaine was administered over the planned entry site. A small nick was made in the skin at the desired entry site.
- The mechanical arm with a sterilized PAKY needle driver holding the needle (Temno 18g/15cm for biopsy and 3.0 Radio Therapeutics for ablation) was placed such that the tip of the needle was located at the skin incision site. The table was then moved, together with the robot, so that the needle tip was located in the laser plane.
- Using the joystick the robot was moved in two different position (P_1 and P_2) located in the laser plane, these directions were acquired by the PC, and used for computing the position of the CT-slice in the robot space. *For testing*, the control was then transferred to the computer and the robot was moved back and forth in the laser plane to insure its correct determination. This was visually acknowledged by observing the laser projection on the barrel of the needle during

the in-plane motion. In all needle orientation phases the tip of the needle was located at the skin site and needle insertion was hardware disabled.

- A scan was that taken with the needle at the first position (P_1). The image was transferred to the PC, the needle tip was identified in the image, and the orientation of the needle in image was determined, finalizing the registration process. *To verify the registration result*, the needle was moved to the vertical in-slice position and a new image slice was acquired for confirmation.

- A second scan was acquired through the targeted lesion. This image was also transferred to the PC and the radiologist indicated the lesion on the PC monitor. The program computed the needle targeting angles (α and β) and the required depth of insertion.

- With needle insertion disabled, under the command of the radiologist the robot oriented the needle towards the target. During this motion the needle was entirely outside the body only its tip being located at the skin level. *Needle orientation accuracy was than verified* by the radiologist under fluoro imaging.

- Finally, the RCM orientation stage was disabled and the PAKY needle driver was enabled on the hardware. At the radiologist's command the needle was inserted under direct fluoro supervision.

- The remaining steps of the procedure were then performed as usual.

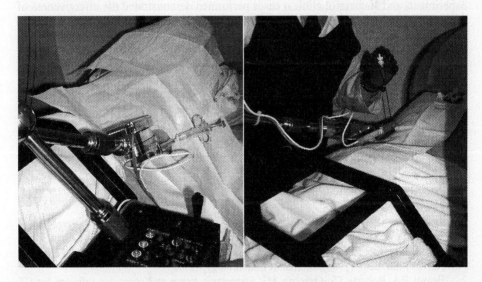

Figure 4: Robotic CT-Guided Kidney Biopsy and Nephrostomy Tube Procedures

The methodology presented above includes numerous verification/confirmation steps that will be eliminated after a complete evaluation of the methodology. This would significantly shorten and speed up the clinical process. The following table summarizes the radiological interventions performed using the above methodology:

Table 1: Robotic CT-Guided Interventions

Case No.	Date	Organ	Procedure
1	February 06, 2001	Kidney	Biopsy
2	February 15, 2001	Kidney	Nephrostomy Tube
3	March 08, 2001	Kidney	Biopsy and RF Ablation
4	March 08, 2001	Spine	RF Ablation
5	March 08, 2001	Spine	RF Ablation

4. Conclusions

We presented a simple CT-robot registration method using the laser markers of the CT scanner and its application to CT-guided interventional procedures. The registration may be used with traditional (non CTF) scanners and it does not involve additional registration devices, using the procedure instrument (needle) as a registration marker. The method allows for performing needle access in an oblique direction, for which the skin entry point and the target are located in different CT slices. This is a significant improvement over the manual method, in which the needle is restricted to the fluoro image of the CTF scanner. The accuracy of the in-vitro experiments and successful clinical cases performed demonstrated the effectiveness of the method. The method's accuracy is inherited from the laser positioning system of the CT scanner. Its clinical implementation on the new PAKY-RCM robot proved safe and reliable in various radiological interventions. It provides null radiation exposure for the radiologist controlling the procedure from the control room and minimizes the exposure of the patient. With the use of the proposed system the radiation exposure does not bound the number of CT interventions a radiologist may safely perform. Moreover, through the use of a specialized algorithm and precise delivery mechanism, the method reduces physician's variability in performing CT-guided percutaneous access. Future applications of this technology to other radiological interventions are in progress.

References

1. Bishoff JT, Stoianovici D, Lee BR, Bauer J, Taylor RH, Whitcomb LL, Cadeddu JA, Chan D, Kavoussi LR: RCM-PAKY: Clinical Application of a New Robotic System for Precise Needle Placement, (1998), Journal of Endourology, 12:82
2. Brown RA, Roberts TS, Osborne AG: Stereotaxic frame and computer software for CT directed Neurosurgical localization. Invest. Radiol. (1980), 15: 308-312
3. Cadeddu JA, Stoianovici D, Chen RN, Moore RG, Kavoussi LR: Stereotactic mechanical percutaneous renal access, (1998), Journal of Endourology, 12:2:121-126.
4. Daly B, Krebs TL, Wong-You-Cheong JJ, Wang SS: Percutaneous abdominal and pelvic interventional procedures using ct fluoroscopy guidance. AJR (1999) 173:637-644
5. Gianfelice D, Lepanto L, Perreault P, Chartrand-Lefebvre C, Milette PC: Value of ct fluoroscopy for percutaneous biopsy procedures. JVIR 2000 (2000) 11:879-884
6. Gianfelice D, Lepanto L, Perreault P, Chartrand-Lefebvre C, Milette PC: Effect of the learning process on procedure times and radiation exposure for ct fluoroscopy-guided percutaneous biopsy procedures. JVIR (2000) 11:1217-1221

7. Glauser D: Neurosurgical robot Minerva, first results and current developments. Proc. Sec. Int. Symp. On Med Rob and Computed Assisted Surgery (1995).
8. Kato R, Katada K, Anno H, Suzuki S, Ida Y, Koga S.: Radiation dosimetry at CT fluoroscopy: physician's hand dose and development of needle holders. Radiology (1996) 201:576-578
9. Loser MH, Navab N: A new robotic system for visually controlled percutaneous interventions under CT fluoroscopy, MICCAI 1999, Lecture Notes in Computer Science, Springer-Verlag (2000) 1935:887-896
10. Masamune K, Patriciu A, Stoianovici D, Susil R, Taylor RH, Fichtinger G, Kavoussi LR, Anderson J, Sakuma I, Dohi T: Development of CT-PAKY frame system - CT image guided Needle puncturing manipulator and a single slice registration for urological surgery, Proc. 8th annual meeting of JSCAS, Kyoto 1999:89-90
11. Nawfel RD, Judy PF, Silverman SG, Hooton S, Tuncali K, Adams DF: Patient and personnel exposure during ct fluoroscopy-guided interventional procedures. Radiology (2000) 216:180-184
12. Nickoloff EL, Khandji A, Dutta A: Radiation doses during ct fluoroscopy. Health Physics (2000) 79:675-681
13. Patriciu A, Mazilu D, Stoianovici D, Stanimir A, Susil R, Masamune K, Fitchinger G, Taylor RH, Anderson J, Kavoussi LR: CT-Guided Robotic Prostate Biopsy, (2000), 18th World Congress on Endourology & SWL, Sept. 2000, Sao Paulo, Brazil.
14. Patriciu A, Stoianovici D, Whitcomb LL, Jarrett T, Mazilu D, Stanimir A, Iordachita I, Anderson J, Taylor R, Kavoussi LR: Motion-Based Robotic Instrument Targeting Under C-Arm Fluoroscopy, (2000), MICCAI, Lecture Notes in Computer Science, Springer-Verlag, 1935:988-998.
15. Silverman SG, Tuncali K, Adams DF, Nawfel RD, Zou KH, Judy PF: CT fluoroscopy-guided abdominal interventions: techniques, results, and radiation exposure. Radiology (1999) 212:673-681
16. Stoianovici D, Cadeddu JA, Demaree RD, Basile HA, Taylor RH, Whitcomb LL, Sharpe W, Kavoussi LR: An Efficient Needle Injection Technique and Radiological Guidance Method for Percutaneous Procedures, (1997), Lecture Notes in Computer Science, Springer-Verlag, 1205:295-298
17. Stoianovici D, Whitcomb LL, Anderson JH, Taylor RH, Kavoussi LR: A Modular Surgical Robotic System for Image Guided Percutaneous Procedures, (1998) Lecture Notes in Computer Science, Springer-Verlag, 1496:404-410
18. Stoianovici D, Kavoussi LR: Ball-Worm Transmission, (1999), Regular U.S. utility and PCT application filled by the Johns Hopkins University (#DM-3512)
19. Stoianovici D: Robotic Surgery, (2000) World Journal of Urology, 18:4:289-295. (http://link.springer.de/link/service/journals/00345/tocs/t0018004.htm)
20. Susil RC, Anderson J, Taylor RH: A Single Image Registration Method for CT Guided Interventions. MICCAI 1999, Lecture Notes in Computer Science, Springer-Verlag (1999) 1679:798-808

Retrospective Evaluation of Inter-subject Brain Registration

P. Hellier[1], C. Barillot[1], I. Corouge[1], B. Gibaud[2], G. Le Goualher[2,3], L. Collins[3], A. Evans[3], G. Malandain[4], and N. Ayache[4]

[1] Projet Vista, IRISA/INRIA-CNRS Rennes, France
[2] Laboratoire SIM, Hôpital de Pontchaillou, Rennes, France
[3] Montreal Neurological Institute, Mc Gill University, Canada
[4] Projet Epidaure, INRIA Sophia-Antipolis, France

Abstract. Although numerous methods to register brains of different individuals have been proposed, few work has been done to evaluate the performances of different registration methods on the same database of subjects. In this paper, we propose an evaluation framework, based on global and local measures of the quality of the registration. Experiments have been conducted for 5 methods, through a database of 18 subjects. We focused more extensively on the registration of cortical landmarks that have a particular relevance in the context of anatomical-functional normalization. For global measures, results show that the quality of the registration is directly related to the transformation's degrees of freedom. However, local measures based on the matching of cortical sulci, did not make it possible to show significant differences between affine and non linear methods.
Key words: Evaluation, non-rigid registration, atlas matching, neuroanatomy, MRI, cortical sulci.

1 Introduction

The comparison of brains of different individuals is an ancient objective in medicine. It has been pursued for a long time and was traditionally treated by paper-based atlases, with generally rather simple transformations. However, during the last few years, the development of electronic brain atlases [4,10,14] has emerged by overcoming some limitations of traditional paper-based atlases. To build such an atlas, it is necessary to compare brains of different individuals, so that each new subject contributes to the evolution and the relevance of the atlas. The comparison of brains requires the development of a registration method, most often with a non-rigid transformation.

An increasing number of authors study this registration problem. As it would be a gargantuan task to quote them all, we refer the reader to [9] for an overall survey on that subject. These methods are generally divided into two groups: intensity-based methods, that rely generally on the matching of voxels having comparable luminance (for mono-modal registration), and feature-based methods that rely on the extraction and matching of sparse landmarks. Feature-based methods dramatically depend on the extraction of features, and are generally valid near these features. In contrast, "photometric" methods use the entire available information, and make it possible to estimate

W. Niessen and M. Viergever (Eds.): MICCAI 2001, LNCS 2208, pp. 258–265, 2001.

transformations with high degrees of freedom. This simple comparison may explain the popularity of intensity-based methods, which has been proved in the particular context of rigid multimodal fusion [16].

Nevertheless, the superiority of "iconic" methods has not been proved in the context of mono-modality inter-individual fusion. As a matter of fact, these methods usually rely on the minimization of an appropriate cost function, that exploits a relationship between voxels' luminance. The different methods mainly differ by the regularization scheme, and by the optimization strategy, which have a crucial consequence on the registration process. Published methods manage to optimize the matching criterion, but we do not really know if the formulation of the problem, combined with the way it is solved, lead to anatomically consistent transformations. Is it relevant to deform one subject toward another? What can we expect from the different registration methods? These questions are the starting point and the motivation of our work.

The evaluation project was conducted for 5 registration methods on a database of 18 subjects. The Vista project (INRIA-CNRS, Rennes) gathered the registration results, i.e. the deformations fields that were used to deform specific anatomical landmarks. The goal of this project is to evaluate how anatomical features are matched by the registration methods.

The paper is organized as follows : section 2 presents briefly the methods that have been evaluated, section 3 presents the data and the evaluation criteria which were used in the evaluation project. Section 4 details the results on a database of 18 subjects with global and local evaluation of the registration methods. Conclusions are drawn in section 5.

2   Participants

This evaluation project is somehow inspired by the Vanderbilt evaluation project [16], since all participants downloaded the data and performed the registration processes in their own laboratory. The results, i.e. the deformation fields, were then sent to our group (Vista Project, IRISA) to be evaluated on the basis of criteria that were not available to the participants of the evaluation project.

So far, 5 methods have been evaluated. We do not describe extensively the different methods, referring the reader to adequate references. We have adopted the following denomination for the methods:

– Method A. The denomination refers to the ANIMAL algorithm developed by L. Collins *et al.* at the MNI [2]. It must be noted that the finest resolution of the method A is 4 mm, for which the deformation field is piecewise constant.
– Method D. The denomination refers to the Demon's algorithm developed by J.P. Thirion in the Epidaure Group at INRIA Sophia-Antipolis [13].
– Method M. This registration is a simple rigid transformation, obtained by maximization of mutual information [8,15]. Although inadequate in that context, this method was implemented as a comparison basis for non-rigid methods.
– Method P. This method is the proportional squaring of Talairach. The method is based on the identification of the points AC-PC, which define a piecewise affine transformation on 12 cubes [12].

– Method R. The method R was developed at INRIA Rennes by P. Hellier *et al.* [7]. It may of course be questionable that the authors of an evaluation project submit their own registration method to the evaluation. Despite this, we hope that the reader would believe that we acted faithfully.

3   Data and Evaluation Criteria

For the evaluation project, we have acquired a database of 18 normal subjects. Each subject underwent a T1-MR (1.5T) SPGR 3D study. We have chosen arbitrarily a particular subject as the reference subject. For all methods, each subject (source image) is registered toward the reference subject (target image), so that all registration results may be compared in the same referential.

From these MR images, we have extracted anatomical features, that will be used to assess the quality of the registration processes. To be objective, the evaluation must rely on features that are independent of the similarity used to drive the registration process.

3.1   Tissue Classification

The most straightforward way to assess the quality of the registration is to evaluate how the tissues are deformed from one subject to the other. We extract grey matter and white matter from the MR volume using the method proposed in [6]. This algorithm consists first in a 3D texture analysis. A clustering technique gives a rough classification that is refined by a bayesian relaxation.

For each subject, we deform the grey and white matter classes toward the reference subject, using the deformation field and trilinear interpolation. The deformed classes are compared to the classes of the reference subject by computing overlapping measures [1]. For sake of concision, we only keep the total performance measure [1], and compute the mean and the variance of that measure over the database of 18 subjects.

3.2   Lvv Volume

We extract differential characteristics from the subjects with the Lvv operator, introduced by Florack *et al.* [5]. The sign of ML_{vv} has a very precise interpretation: it can be demonstrated that when limited to the cortical ROI the crest of a gyrus corresponds to a negative value of the ML_{vv}, while a deep fold like a sulcus corresponds to its positive part. Therefore, the sign of the mean curvature is sufficient to separate sulci from gyri [6].

For each subject, we deform the corresponding Lvv according to the results of a given registration method, using trilinear interpolation. We then compare this deformed Lvv with the Lvv volume of the reference subject, by computing a simple correlation. For each method, we compute the mean and the variance of that measure over the database of 18 subjects.

3.3   Extraction of Cortical Sulci

Cortical sulci are of great interest in the context of that paper, since they are relevant anatomical and functional landmarks. Due to the inter-individual cortical variability, the matching of sulci is crucial to evaluate different registration methods. Several methods have been developped to extract sulcal patterns from MR acquisitions. In this paper, we only describe rapidly the method we have used [6]. After a segmentation of cortical regions and cortical folds via differential operators, a compact and parametric description of a sulcus can be obtained by a medial surface representing the buried part of this sulcus. The method used here consists in modeling this surface by using an "active ribbon" which evolves, in the three-dimensional space, from a 1D curve to a 2D surface. The final position of the ribbon approximates the medial axe of the considered sulcus.

For each subject of the database, we extract 12 major sulci with the method described above. The sulci used for the evaluation project are central sulcus, precentral sulcus, postcentral sulcus, sylvian sulcus, superior frontal sulcus and superior temporal sulcus, for each hemisphere. For each subject, each sulcus is deformed toward the reference subject using the results of a given registration method. As the sulci are modeled by 3D B-splines, we deform each control point of the spline using trilinear interpolation, which naturally defines the deformed sulcus. A "distance" between the deformed sulci of each subject and the corresponding sulcus of the reference subject can be computed.

4   Results

4.1   Global Measures

Average Volume   For each method, we deform each subject toward the reference subject, using the transformation and trilinear interpolation. It is finally possible to compute, for each method, a mean volume by averaging the 17 deformed subjects. A sagittal view of the average volumes are presented on figure 1, and can be compared to the corresponding view of the reference subject. Furthermore, we compute for each method the Mean Square Error (MSE) between the average volume and the reference volume, only for the voxels that belong to the brain of the reference subject (see table 1). The MSE is not a good measure to evaluate the quality of the registration of one subject, but is in that case a more relevant indication as we deal with average volumes.

It must be noted that the registration of the subject 9 has failed for the method A. Therefore, and for all the experiments, the subject 9 has been removed of the results of method A.

Overlapping of Grey and White Matter Tissues   At that stage, the evaluation is not objective, as the MSE is more or less related to the similarity used to drive the registration processes, at least for the methods A, D, M and R. Therefore, we use the segmentation classes (grey matter and white matter) of each subject to evaluate how tissues overlap after registration, as described previously. Table 1 gives the mean and standard deviation of that measure over the database of subjects for each method.

The method M does not give very satisfactory results, whereas he methods D, P and R seem to give better and similar results. The method A seems to be slightly less

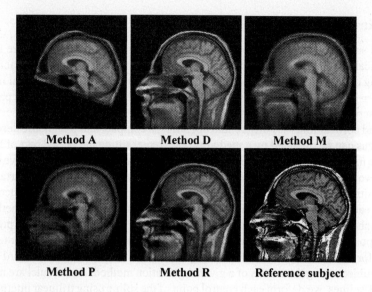

Fig. 1. *For each method, the mean volume is obtained by averaging the 17 deformed subjects, and can be compared to the reference subject.*

efficient, but we must keep in mind that the deformation field is computed at a 4 *mm* grid.

Correlation of Lvv The Lvv operator has been presented in the section 3.2, and provides information related to sulco-gyral patterns. For each method, the mean and standard deviation of the correlation coefficient (between deformed and original Lvv) are presented in table 1.

We first observe that the mean value of the correlation coefficient is quite low for all the registration methods. This might indicate that the matching of cortical features is not very good, but that point will be studied more extensively in section 4.2. The difference between the method M (mean value of 0.01) and other methods is significant. Method D seems to give a slightly better result with a mean correlation of 0.43.

4.2 Local Measures

Visualization of Deformed Sulci We have chosen first to visualize how each left central sulci of the 17 subjects deforms toward the left central sulcus of the reference subject (see figure 2, and associated caption for color code). For a perfect registration, the blue sulci should therefore be superimposed on the yellow sulcus.

It can be observed that the different registration methods seem to give a significant dispersion around the reference sulcus. The postcentral and precentral sulci of the reference subject (in red and green) give the order of magnitude of the dispersion, and indicate that in most cases, the position of the deformed sulci is misleading, with regards to the identification of sulci. If method M seems to give the highest variability, it is quite difficult to distinguish visually the performances of the methods A, D, P and R.

Method	Average volume		Method	Tissue	Mean	St. dev.		Method	Mean	St. dev.
A	987.9		A	grey	91.9	0.08		A	0.17	0.003
				white	89.6	0.07				
D	491.1		D	grey	95.8	0.04		D	0.43	0.005
				white	96.7	0.04				
M	1389.9		M	grey	88.8	0.13		M	0.01	0.001
				white	87.5	0.17				
P	1064.4		P	grey	93.5	0.06		P	0.16	0.003
				white	95.1	0.04				
R	385.6		R	grey	93.9	0.10		R	0.32	0.008
				white	95.0	0.14				

Table 1. Left: *Mean Square Error (MSE) between the average volume and the reference subject. The error is computed only for the voxels that belong to the segmentation mask of the reference subject's brain.* **Middle:** *Overlap between tissues after registration, computed by the total performance measure. For each method, the mean and standard deviation of the measure is computed over the database of subjects.* **Right:** *Mean and standard deviation of the correlation coefficient between reference Lvv and deformed Lvv.*

Numerical Evaluation Beyond visualization, numerical evaluation is needed. In that section, we investigate two measures: one for the global positioning of sulci, and one for shape similarity.

Euclidian distance between registered sulci To assess how sulci are matched, it is possible to compute an euclidian distance between a sulcus, deformed toward the reference subject, and the corresponding sulcus of the reference subject. As explained in section 3.3, sulci are modeled by B-splines, and may therefore be resampled identically. We associate the distance between sulci to the distance between control points.

To present a compact measure, the mean of the distance after registration are computed for all the subjects and all the sulci (we have 12 sulci extracted for each of the 18 subjects). These results are presented in table 2, and the distances are expressed in voxels (the resolution of the voxels is $0.93\ mm$). It can be immediately noticed that the results are not significantly different between rigid and non-rigid methods.

Statistical study of deformed shapes The distance between registered sulci is not a sufficient measure to characterize how sulci deform. We want to evaluate the similarity of deformed sulci in terms of shape, with the use of the Principal Component Analysis (PCA) [3].

For each method, we have a population of shapes that is composed by the corresponding sulci of the different subjects, deformed toward the reference subject by a given registration method. The purpose of the PCA is to analyze the variations of each shape with respect to the reference shape, by decomposition on the eigenvectors of the covariance matrix.

For sake of concision, we have chosen to consider only the trace of the covariance matrix. This measure reflects the entire variation of the population around the reference sulcus, along all the axes of the decomposition. Furthermore, the trace can be compared

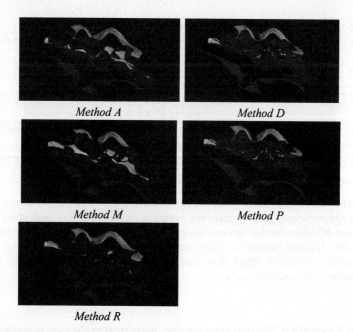

Method A   Method D

Method M   Method P

Method R

Fig. 2. *Left central sulci (in blue) of the database deformed toward the reference subject. The deformed sulci should ideally be superimposed to the left central sulcus of the reference subject (in yellow). The left precentral sulcus (in red) and postcentral sulcus (in green) of the reference subject are also drawn.*

since it is invariant when the axes of the decomposition change. These results are given on table 2. We notice that there is no significant difference between the performances of the different methods.

5   Conclusion

We have proposed in this paper an evaluation framework of methods that aims at registering brains of different subjects. Global and local measures of the registration have been designed to evaluate 5 registration methods on a database of 18 subjects. On the one hand, global measures show the efficiency of non linear methods, and indicate that the quality of the registration increases with the degrees of freedom of the estimated transformation. On the other hand, affine and non-linear methods give surprisingly similar results for local measures, which are based on the matching of major cortical sulci.

To explain these results, we must first keep in mind that the variability of cortical patterns between individuals is very high [11]. We are also tempted to put forward the anatomical "incorrectness" of transformations generated by "computer vision" methods. "Iconic" approaches, which tend to match voxels having the same luminance, fail to apprehend morphological differences between individuals because they use "low level" information. These results also stimulate the introduction of higher anatomical constraints, such as cortical constraints in the registration process.

Method	Average distance		Method	central	superior frontal	sylvian
A	9.9		A	547	736	1172
D	10.3		D	675	767	1046
M	11.5		M	621	622	1373
P	10.7		P	510	859	1233
R	10.8		R	735	741	1064

Table 2. Left: *average distance between registered sulci and corresponding sulci of the reference subject, in voxels. The mean is computed for all the subjects and all the sulci.* **Right:** *for three different population of sulci, the variations of deformed sulci can be analyzed by principal component analysis. The trace of the covariance matrix, normalized by the number of subjects, traduces the entire variation of deformed sulci around the reference sulcus, in the shape space.*

References

1. JH. Van Bemmel, MA. Musen. *Handbook of medical informatics.* Springer, 1997.
2. L. Collins, A. Evans. Animal : validation and applications of nonlinear registration-based segmentation. *IJPRAI*, 8(11):1271–1294, 1997.
3. T. Cootes, C. Taylor, D. Hooper, J. Graham. Active shape models- their training and application. *CVIU*, 61(1):31–59, 1995.
4. A. Evans, L. Collins, B. Milner. A MRI-based stereotaxic atlas from 250 young normal subjects. *Soc. Neuroscience abstract*, 18:408, 1992.
5. L. Florack, B. Romeny, J. Koenderink, M. Viergever. Scale and the differential structure of images. *IVC*, 10:376–388, 1992.
6. G. Le Goualher, C. Barillot, and Y. Bizais. Modeling cortical sulci with active ribbons. *IJPRAI*, 8(11):1295–1315, 1997.
7. P. Hellier, C. Barillot, E. Mémin, and P. Pérez. Hierarchical estimation of a dense deformation field for 3D robust registration. In *IEEE TMI*, 20(5):388-402, 2001.
8. F. Maes, A. Collignon, D. Vandermeulen, G. Marchal, P. Suetens. Multimodality image registration by maximisation of mutual information. *IEEE TMI*, 16(2):187-198, 1997.
9. J. Maintz, MA. Viergever. – A survey of medical image registration. *Medical Image Analysis*, 2(1):1–36, 1998.
10. J. Mazziotta, A. Toga, A. Evans, P. Fox, and J. Lancaster. A probabilistic atlas of the human brain: theory and rationale for its development. *Neuroimage*, 2:89–101, 1995.
11. M. Ono, S. Kubik, C. Abernathey. – *Atlas of the cerebral sulci.* – Verlag, 1990.
12. J. Talairach, P. Tournoux. *Co-planar stereotaxic atlas of the human brain.* Georg Thieme Verlag, Stuttgart, 1988.
13. JP. Thirion. Image matching as a diffusion process: an analogy with Maxwell's demons. *Medical Image Analysis*, 2(3):243-260, 1998.
14. P. Thompson, R. Woods, M. Mega, A. Toga. Mathematical/computational challenges in creating deformable and probabilistic atlases of the human brain. *HBM*, 9:81-92, 2000.
15. P. Viola, W. Wells. Alignment by maximisation of mutual information. *IJCV*, 24(2):137-154, 1997.
16. J. West, J. Fitzpatrick, *et al.* Comparaison and evaluation of retrospective intermodality brain image registration techniques. *JCAT*, 21(4):554-566, 1997.

A Binary Entropy Measure to Assess Nonrigid Registration Algorithms

Simon K. Warfield[1], Jan Rexilius[1], Petra S. Huppi[2], Terrie E. Inder[3],
Erik G Miller[1], William M. Wells III[1], Gary P. Zientara[1], Ferenc A. Jolesz[1],
and Ron Kikinis[1]

[1] Surgical Planning Laboratory, Harvard Medical School and Brigham and Women's
Hospital, 75 Francis St., Boston, MA 02115 USA,
{warfield,rexilius,emiller,sw,zientara,jolesz,kikinis}@bwh.harvard.edu
http://www.spl.harvard.edu
[2] University Hospital of Geneva, Switzerland,
Petra.Huppi@hcuge.ch
[3] Royal Womens and Royal Childrens Hospital, Melbourne, Australia,
indert@cryptic.rch.unimelb.edu.au

Abstract. Assessment of normal and abnormal anatomical variability requires a coordinate system enabling inter-subject comparison. We present a binary minimum entropy criterion to assess affine and nonrigid transformations bringing a group of subject scans into alignment. This measure is a data-driven measure allowing the identification of an intrinsic coordinate system of a particular group of subjects. We assessed two statistical atlases derived from magnetic resonance imaging of newborn infants with gestational age ranging from 24 to 40 weeks. Over this age range major structural changes occur in the human brain and existing atlases are inadequate to capture the resulting anatomical variability. The binary entropy measure we propose allows an objective choice between competing registration algorithms to be made.

1 Introduction

Assessment of normal and abnormal anatomical variability requires a coordinate system enabling inter-subject comparison [1,2,3]. Several nonrigid registration algorithms have been proposed for comparing anatomy or for the construction of statistical atlases [4,5,6,7,8,9,10,11,12,13], and each has advantages that make it attractive for these applications in some circumstances but also disadvantages that potentially may limit the applicability.

We restrict our consideration here to only those nonrigid registration algorithms that attempt to project anatomy from a source to a target with a plausible model of deformation. If we allow arbitrary nonrigid transformations then anatomically implausible deformations can be constructed to generate arbitrarily good alignments. For example, one construction to achieve perfect intensity matching of two volumes is the following: for each voxel of the target, scan across the source until a voxel with matching intensity is found, and then project this

W. Niessen and M. Viergever (Eds.): MICCAI 2001, LNCS 2208, pp. 266–274, 2001.
© Springer-Verlag Berlin Heidelberg 2001

voxel from the source into the target. As long as the source has the same or larger intensity range as the target this will result in a perfect intensity match but will tell us nothing useful about how to project the anatomy of the source to match the target.

We propose below an objective criterion for comparing the quality of a statistical atlas. We define a statistical atlas of anatomy as a group of acquisitions in a common coordinate system. Typical measures available in a statistical atlas are the mean and variance of the underlying acquisition signal intensity at each voxel, and very often, a segmentation of each acquisition is also carried out. In order to assess the quality of the alignment, we require a tissue segmentation of some type be available. The segmentation allows us to compare the spatial distribution of the structures of interest for the particular application or anatomy for which such an atlas is intended.

We define perfect alignment as every voxel of an acquisition being in correspondence with precisely the same anatomy in each scan. Under these circumstances, comparing the segmentations of each scan we would find the same structure identified at each voxel. Variability between the acquisitions can be considered encoded by the transformations that bring them into alignment. For example, a scan of the brain might be brought into alignment with a group of scans, first by an affine transformation correcting for rotation, translation and scale differences, and then a nonrigid transformation correcting for local shape variations. In this case the interesting anatomical variability of the scan is encoded by the nonrigid transformation that brings it into the common coordinate system.

In information theory, the information (or uncertainty) associated with a signal is referred to as the entropy of the signal [14]. Entropy-based methods were first used in medical image registration by [15,16]. Recently Miller et al. [17] proposed using pixelwise entropies across a set of binary images as a measure of their joint alignment. Here, we apply this technique to multi-valued volumes in three-dimensions with the goal of constructing a probabilistic anatomical atlas in an *intrinsic* coordinate system in order to describe anatomical variability. We propose computing the voxelwise entropy of the segmentations of each structure of the scans (as defined below). This measure of entropy is zero for a set of scans in perfect alignment as described above. Under these circumstances, a perfect nonrigid registration algorithm has been able to capture all of the anatomical variability and encode it in the nonrigid transformation, leaving the uncertainty of the atlas (or coordinate system) as zero. For a practical nonrigid registration algorithm, we may expect that the entropy of the atlas does not reach the desirable value of zero, in which case the anatomical variability that the nonrigid registration can capture is encoded in the set of transformations bringing the scans into alignment, and crucially the amount of anatomical variability not captured by the nonrigid registration algorithm is indicated by the entropy of the aligned segmentations.

Therefore, we propose to assess a statistical atlas by measuring the binary entropy of the aligned segmentations voxelwise. We consider the minimum entropy statistical atlas as defining an intrinsic coordinate system for the anatomy under consideration.

2 Method

We consider here the application of constructing a statistical atlas of magnetic resonance images of newborn infants with a gestation age ranging from 24 to 40 weeks. Over this period major developmental changes in the human brain take place [18].

We applied affine (translation, rotation and scale parameters only, no shear parameters were considered) and nonrigid registration to construct a statistical atlas from tissue classifications of the above subjects. We used a minimum entropy criterion as an objective measure of the quality of the statistical atlas generated by affine transformation alone and by affine and nonrigid registration together.

2.1 MRI Acquisition

Spoiled Gradient Recalled Acquisitions in the Steady state (SPGR) with a voxel size of 0.7x0.7x1.5 mm^3 (coronal T1w) and Conventional Spin Echo (axial T2w/PDw) MR acquisitions with a voxel size of 0.7x0.7x3.0 mm^3 of newborn infants are acquired at our institution under a protocol with IRB approval. Twenty two acquisitions of subjects with gestational age (GA) < 34 weeks were analysed. For each subject, T2w and PDw volumes were resampled to align with and have the same voxel size and acquisition order as the T1w volumes.

2.2 Tissue Classification

A sequence of image processing algorithms was used to segment each of the MRI acquisitions into separate tissue classes: cortical graymatter (GM), subcortical GM, unmyelinated white matter (WM), myelinated WM and cerebrospinal fluid (CSF). These algorithms were designed to reduce imaging system noise, and to classify tissue types on the basis of MR intensity and expected anatomy derived from a template. Anisotropic diffusion filtering was used to smooth noise without blurring fine details. Supervised spatially varying template moderated classification was used to identify tissue classes [19]. This analysis is a supervised nonparametric multispectral classification algorithm which identifies tissue classes in the data set by comparison to a set of prototype tissue values selected by an expert operator, knowledgeable in both developmental neuronanatomy and pediatric MR-imaging.

2.3   Minimum Entropy Affine Alignment

Following [17], we define the joint voxelwise entropy of a collection of J binary volumes, $S_j, j \in 1...J$, each brought into alignment by a transform T_j, as

$$E(T_1(S_1), T_2(S_2), ...T_J(S_J)) = \sum_{i=1}^{N} H(v_i)$$

where N is the number of voxels of the volumes, v_i is the binary random variable defined by the values of voxel i across the images and $H(\cdot)$ is the discrete entropy function.

We want an entropy expression for a tissue classification derived from MRI acquisitions of subjects. We treat each tissue class as a separate binary volume, compute the entropy independently for each tissue class as above and sum the entropy for each to obtain the total entropy of a given alignment of a collection of tissue classifications. An alternative entropy expression would be simply the entropy of the multi-valued tissue distributions, i.e. not treating each tissue class independently.

A minimum entropy alignment seeks to identify the set of transforms T_j which minimizes the entropy of the collection i.e.

$$\arg\min_{T_1,...,T_J} E(T_1(S_1), T_2(S_2), ..., T_J(S_J)).$$

A local optimization method has been proposed to solve this optimization simultaneously for each transform [17]. However, here we propose to approximate this by fixing one volume and computing the minimum entropy transform between this and the other tissue classifications using a previously described fast, robust and accurate affine registration method suitable for tissue classifications [20]. We therefore solve the optimization problem :

$$\arg\min_{T_k'} E(I(S_1), T_k'(S_k)), \forall k \in 2...J,$$

where $I(\cdot)$ is the identity transform, and hence we construct the atlas with entropy

$$E(I(S_1), T_2'(S_2), ..., T_J'(S_J)).$$

2.4   Nonrigid Registration

We describe in this section the nonrigid registration algorithm we used for the experiments reported below. However, the primary focus of this work is to describe the method for evaluating any particular nonrigid registration algorithm, and the method we apply here (which is quite successful) is simply one of many that should be evaluated and compared.

Prior to computing a nonrigid registration, the above affine registration is used to remove global rotation, translation and scale differences. The nonrigid registration algorithm we used for our experiments here is a generalization of the method proposed by Ferrant and co-workers [21]. In that work, displacements were estimated from segmentations of two scans by an active surface match, and the nonrigid deformation between surfaces was computed by solving a linear elastic physics-based model. Here we replace the active surface matcher with a brute force normalized cross correlation search from regions of high local structure. Again, displacements away from these regions are computed by solving a linear elastic physics-based model.

Local Structure Detection Sparsely sampled points with regions of high local structure were obtained by smoothing MR acquisitions with an edge-enhancing noise smoothing nonlinear diffusion filter, computing the magnitude of the gradient, and selecting points two standard deviations above the mean magnitude of the gradient.

Correspondence Measurement The normalized cross-correlation function allows comparison of regions of two scans. The function peaks for the displacement that best aligns the two regions. We use a brute force search in a limited search range to identify the best local match for each point of high local structure.

Interpolation with a Linear Elasticity Model The above two procedures identify sparse estimates across the image with known displacements. These are applied as boundary conditions in a linear elastic solver analogously to that previously described [21].

3   Results

Figure 1 and Figure 2 illustrate the construction of statistical atlases using affine only and affine and nonrigid registration. Five tissue class atlases and the corresponding mean SPGR intensity for the recovered transformations are shown. We can observe that the nonrigid registration produces a spatial distribution of tissue classes that is better localized, and indeed, has a lower entropy (measured in bits per voxel) for each of the well-aligned tissue classes (CSF, cortical gray matter, myelinated white matter), and an equivalent entropy for the two tissue classes which remain difficult to spatially localize — unmyelinated white matter and basal ganglia (for which the nonrigid registration produces a better spatial alignment, but due to their small size is not different in the first two decimal places of the entropy measure).

4   Discussion and Conclusion

Two reports have discussed related concepts, described below, for encoding anatomical variability in a statistical atlas. These are the ideas of compact encoding of anatomical variability [13] and a "minimum variance frame" [11]. We observe that the minimum entropy criterion derived from segmentations that we

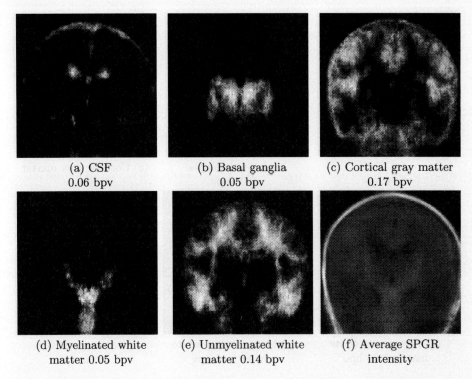

(a) CSF 0.06 bpv	(b) Basal ganglia 0.05 bpv	(c) Cortical gray matter 0.17 bpv
(d) Myelinated white matter 0.05 bpv	(e) Unmyelinated white matter 0.14 bpv	(f) Average SPGR intensity

Fig. 1. Minimum entropy alignment of tissue classifications from subjects with GA < 34 weeks with affine registration. The above figure shows a single slice from class atlases obtained with minimum entropy affine registration for (left to right) CSF, basal ganglia, cortical gray matter, myelinated white matter and unmyelinated white matter. The entropy per voxel for each tissue class atlas independently is noted in units of bits per voxel (bpv).

propose here encapsulates both the concepts of compact encoding of anatomical variability in a formally precise fashion without the requirement of an explicit shape representation, and of maximizing the overlap of corresponding anatomical structures.

Ashburner and Friston [13] proposed a low resolution nonrigid registration algorithm optimizing over a few hundred parameters, justifying this approach as having low computational cost and being sufficiently accurate when correspondence between different individuals (and between structure and function) is not guaranteed. They noted the requirement for a compact encoding of structural variability, suitable for exploitation by a more advanced nonrigid registration algorithm.

Collins [11, pp.28–38] provides an excellent overview of the Talairach atlas and related methods, together with a summary of the primary limitations and restrictions of this form of atlas. These limitations provide motivation to search for an objective criterion with which to identify an intrinsic coordinate system

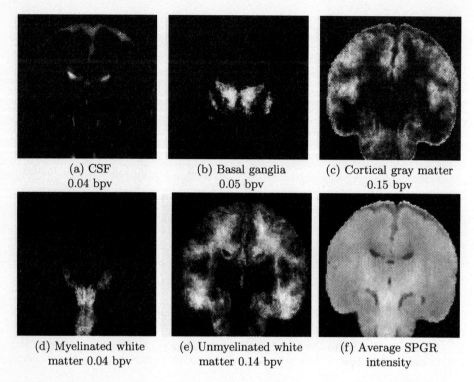

(a) CSF
0.04 bpv

(b) Basal ganglia
0.05 bpv

(c) Cortical gray matter
0.15 bpv

(d) Myelinated white
matter 0.04 bpv

(e) Unmyelinated white
matter 0.14 bpv

(f) Average SPGR
intensity

Fig. 2. This shows the tissue class atlases obtained with nonrigid registration for (left to right) CSF, basal ganglia, cortical gray matter, myelinated white matter and unmyelinated white matter.

in which a probabilistic atlas can be constructed. Collins constructed a mean atlas by aligning and averaging scans of 305 primarily male, primarily young subjects. He found regions of misalignment as compared to the Talairach atlas and attributed these to normal anatomical variability between the subject of the Talairach atlas and those of his cohort. Interestingly, Collins [11, p.36] proposed reconstructing a new atlas in a minimum variance frame as a mechanism for identifying a data-driven "best" coordinate system. This does not yet appear to have been done, possibly due to the difficulty of aligning cortical structures, for which the nonrigid registration algorithm of [11] is explicitly not designed.

Entropy is invariant to the specific label assigned to each tissue. The numeric label assigned to each tissue is irrelevant. It is only the frequency of occurrence of the tissue for a particular voxel that matters. This is not true of the variance measure, which is dependent upon the values assigned to each tissue.

Since entropy is the negative of the average log likelihood, a minimum entropy method can be interpreted as a maximum likelihood method. Minimizing the entropy by transforming a single volume is equivalent to maximizing the mean log likelihood of the voxels in that volume under the distribution implied by the set of scans. So if we view our allowable transformations as being equally likely, then minimum entropy alignment can be interpreted as maximum likelihood alignment under the model implied by the set of volumes [17]. Its maximum value occurs when there is greatest disorder, i.e. an even distribution of labels over a particular voxel (not necessarily true for variance). Its minimum value occurs when there is least disorder, i.e. all labels for a particular voxel are the same. This property is shared by the variance criterion.

A minimum entropy criterion provides a means to obtain a coordinate system intrinsic to the data being studied. Anatomical variability captured by the registration algorithm is encoded in the transformations bringing subject scans into alignment, and the amount of anatomical variability not captured by the registration algorithm is indicated by the binary entropy of segmentations of the aligned data. We propose that this criterion can be applied to assess the alignments obtained by affine and nonrigid registration algorithms. The minimum entropy alignment of segmentations of the subject scans represents the best encoding of the anatomical variability. Hence, this is a principled mechanism for identifying a common coordinate system for a group of subjects under study. The same reasoning applies when other anatomical structures, such as the ventricles or the hippocampal formation are to be studied — again a minimum entropy criterion allows the identification of an intrinsic coordinate system in which to study the structure.

The work described here has not dealt in detail with constraints upon the capacity of the transform aligning the anatomy. It is possible to construct transforms which minimize the entropy of the collection without meaningfully describing anatomical variability. For this reason it is desirable to study the capacity of the transforms allowed. In principle, the transforms should be selected from the group defined by normal anatomical variability, which is unfortunately unknown. An alternative may be to select a class of transforms a priori and seek the minimum entropy atlas constructed with a minimum description length constraint on the allowable transforms.

Applying this approach to scans of newborn infants grouped by age should allow the construction of a spatiotemporal atlas of the developing brain.

Acknowledgements: This investigation was supported by NIH P41 RR13218, NIH P01 CA67165 and NIH R01 RR11747. The authors greatly appreciate the help of Marianna Jakab in enabling this research.

References

1. M. I. Miller, G. E. Christensen, Y. Amit, and U. Grenander, "Mathematical textbook of deformable neuroanatomies," *Proc. Natl. Acad. Sci. USA*, vol. 90, pp. 11944–11948, December 1993.
2. P. M. Thompson, J. N. Giedd, R. P. Woods, D. MacDonald, A. C. Evans, and A. W. Toga, "Growth patterns in the developing brain detected by using continuum mechanical tensor maps," *Nature*, vol. 404, pp. 190–193, 2000.
3. T. Paus, A. Zijdenbos, K. Worsley, D. L. Collins, J. Blumenthal, J. N. Gledd, J. L. Rapoport, and A. C. Evans, "Structural Maturation of Neural Pathways in Children and Adolescents: In Vivo Study," *Science*, vol. 283, pp. 1908–1911, 19 March 1999.

4. P. M. Thompson, D. MacDonald, M. S. Mega, C. J. Holmes, A. C. Evans, and A. W. Toga, "Detection and Mapping of Abnormal Brain Structures with a Probabilistic Atlas of Cortical Surfaces," *Journal of Computer Assisted Tomography*, vol. 21, no. 4, pp. 567–581, 1997.
5. A. W. Toga, ed., *Brain Warping*. Academic Press, San Diego, USA, 1999.
6. R. Bajcsy and S. Kovačič, "Multiresolution Elastic Matching," *Computer Vision, Graphics, and Image Processing*, vol. 46, pp. 1–21, 1989.
7. J. Dengler and M. Schmidt, "The Dynamic Pyramid – A Model for Motion Analysis with Controlled Continuity," *International Journal of Pattern Recognition and Artificial Intelligence*, vol. 2, no. 2, pp. 275–286, 1988.
8. S. K. Warfield, A. Robatino, J. Dengler, F. A. Jolesz, and R. Kikinis, "Nonlinear Registration and Template Driven Segmentation," in *Brain Warping* (A. W. Toga, ed.), ch. 4, pp. 67–84, San Diego, USA: Academic Press, 1999.
9. G. E. Christensen, R. D. Rabbitt, and M. I. Miller, "3D brain mapping using a deformable neuroanatomy," *Phys. Med. Biol.*, vol. 39, pp. 609–618, 1994.
10. J. C. Gee, M. Reivich, and R. Bajcsy, "Elastically Deforming 3D Atlas to Match Anatomical Brain Images," *Journal of Computer Assisted Tomography*, vol. 17, no. 2, pp. 225–236, 1993.
11. D. L. Collins, *3D Model-based segmentation of individual brain structures from magnetic resonance imaging data*. PhD thesis, McGill University, 1994.
12. J. Thirion, "Image matching as a diffusion process: an analogy with maxwell's demons," *Medical Image Analysis*, vol. 2, no. 3, pp. 243–260, 1998.
13. J. Ashburner and K. J. Friston, "Spatial Normalization," in *Brain Warping* (A. W. Toga, ed.), ch. 2, pp. 27–44, San Diego, USA: Academic Press, 1999.
14. T. Cover and J. Thomas, *Elements of Information Theory*. Wiley, 1991.
15. A. Collignon, D. Vandermuelen, P. Suetens, and G. Marchal, "3D multi-modality medical image registration using feature space clustering," in *Computer Vision, Virtual Reality and Robotics in Medicine* (N. Ayache, ed.), pp. 195–204, Springer Verlag, 1995.
16. P. Viola and W. M. Wells, "Alignment by maximization of mutual information," in *Fifth Intl. Conf. Computer Vision (ICCV)*, pp. 16–23, IEEE Press, 1995.
17. E. Miller, N. Matsakis, and P. Viola, "Learning from One Example Through Shared Densities on Transforms," in *Proceedings IEEE Conf. on Computer Vision and Pattern Recognition*, vol. 1, pp. 464–471, 2000.
18. P. Hüppi, S. Warfield, R. Kikinis, P. D. Barnes, G. P. Zientara, F. A. Jolesz, M. K. Tsuji, and J. J. Volpe, "Quantitative Magnetic Resonance Imaging of Brain Development in Premature and Mature Newborns," *Ann. Neurol.*, vol. 43, pp. 224–235, Feb 1998.
19. S. K. Warfield, M. Kaus, F. A. Jolesz, and R. Kikinis, "Adaptive, Template Moderated, Spatially Varying Statistical Classification," *Med Image Anal*, vol. 4, pp. 43–55, Mar 2000.
20. S. K. Warfield, F. Jolesz, and R. Kikinis, "A High Performance Computing Approach to the Registration of Medical Imaging Data," *Parallel Computing*, vol. 24, pp. 1345–1368, Sep 1998.
21. M. Ferrant, S. K. Warfield, A. Nabavi, B. Macq, and R. Kikinis, "Registration of 3D Intraoperative MR Images of the Brain Using a Finite Element Biomechanical Model," in *MICCAI 2000: Third International Conference on Medical Robotics, Imaging And Computer Assisted Surgery; 2000 Oct 11–14; Pittsburgh, USA* (A. M. DiGioia and S. Delp, eds.), (Heidelberg, Germany), pp. 19–28, Springer-Verlag, 2000.

A Methodology to Validate MRI/SPECT Registration Methods Using Realistic Simulated SPECT Data

Christophe Grova[1], Arnaud Biraben[1], Jean-Marie Scarabin[1], Pierre Jannin[1],
Irène Buvat[2], Habib Benali[2], and Bernard Gibaud[1]

[1] Laboratoire IDM, Faculté de Médecine, Université de Rennes 1, France
{christophe.grova,arnaud.biraben,jean-marie.scarabin,
pierre.jannin,bernard.gibaud}@univ-rennes1.fr,
http://idm.univ-rennes1.fr
[2] INSERM U494, CHU Pitié Salpétrière, Paris
{irene.buvat,habib.benali}@imed.jussieu.fr

Abstract. We present a method to validate MRI/SPECT registration methods based on a set of computer-generated SPECT data. The data set was produced through Monte Carlo simulations from an attenuation map and an activity map derived from a manually labeled T1-weighted MRI data set.

Our approach intrinsically provides a gold standard to assess MRI/SPECT registration methods. It was successfully applied to the comparison of four registration methods based on similarity measurements: Mutual Information, Normalised Mutual Information, Correlation Ratio and Woods Criterion.

1   Introduction

Multimodal data fusion has a strong potential to improve diagnosis and treatment preparation in many fields making intensive use of medical images. The accuracy of registration between imaging modalities is central in the technique. That is why the selection of appropriate registration methods should take each clinical context into account (e.g. ictal epileptic state) in order to thoroughly investigate whether the basic assumptions underlying each method (e.g. nature of similarities) are met.

Registration methods have been widely compared and validated for CT, MRI and PET data, particularly in the Retrospective Registration Evaluation Project (RREP) led by Vanderbilt University [1]. However, only few references are specifically geared toward validating SPECT/MRI registration methods [2][3]. In most cases the methods validated for PET/MRI registration are simply applied to register SPECT data [1][4][5].

But in order to validate a method, the precision and accuracy of a registration technique should be assessed by means of a gold standard. The latter provides a reference geometric transformation with which registration methods

W. Niessen and M. Viergever (Eds.): MICCAI 2001, LNCS 2208, pp. 275–282, 2001.
© Springer-Verlag Berlin Heidelberg 2001

can be assessed. Classically, gold standards are provided by fiducial markers [2], stereotactic frames [1][4][5][6] or mean geometric transformation computed from several registration results [3]. But this type of evaluation is limited by the intrinsic accuracy and precision of the registration method used to compute the gold standard. Indeed, the method to be validated cannot yield better performances than the gold standard registration method itself. We suggest that a "perfect" gold standard can be found by using simulated data to validate methods. The main drawback of simulated data is that they are generally too far from clinical reality, possibly causing validation results to be biased by too auspicious test conditions.

We present a validation method based on realistic SPECT simulations to study and compare SPECT/MRI registration methods. We used Monte Carlo simulations to create normal SPECT from an MRI data set. Simulated data were then used to study four MRI/SPECT registration methods based on similarity measurements: Mutual Information (MI)[7][8], Normalised Mutual Information (NMI)[6], Correlation Ratio (CR)[9] and Woods Criterion (WC)[4].

2   Material and Methods

2.1   SPECT Model Construction

Our method is based on the simulation of realistic SPECT data sets from a 3D T1-weighted MRI data set. By constructing simulated SPECT data from an MRI data set, we can be certain that both data sets are perfectly aligned. As a result, our method provides a gold standard for validation. We constructed realistic SPECT data sets by simulating physical processes including both single photon propagation (e.g. Compton scatter, tissue attenuation) and acquisition procedures (e.g. collimator and detector response), using Monte Carlo techniques. Our simulations were performed with the Photon History Generator (PHG) software package created by the Simset team (Simulation System for Emission Tomography[1]) from Washington University [10]. Actually, PHG simulates SPECT data from a theoretical model of brain perfusion. A brain tissue attenuation map and a radioactive tracer activity map are used to build the perfusion model from a high resolution MRI data set.

Spatial Model of Radiotracer Distribution   Our spatial distribution model was based on Zubal's head phantom, which consists of sixty three anatomical entities manually segmented and labeled on a normal T1-weighted MRI data set [11]. These entities were classified into seven different classes (conjunctive tissue, water, brain, bone, muscle, fat and blood), from which the attenuation map was derived.

---

[1] http://depts.washington.edu/~simset/html/simset_main.html

Brain Perfusion Model Using labeled entities of Zubal's phantom, we, along with clinicians, selected eight anatomical structures likely to fix the radioactive tracer (HMPAO-^{99m}Tc) differently: external cortex, occipital lobes, pons, white matter, cerebellum, insula, gray nuclei and caudate nuclei. For each anatomical structure, we extracted eight binary masks from the labeled MRI. Our measurements of normal brain perfusion were performed on the SPECT template provided by the Statistical Parametric Mapping (SPM) software package[2]. This template was generated by Barnden [12] by averaging 22 normal SPECT data sets after spatial normalization. Perfusion measurements were performed on the SPECT template using the eight anatomical entity masks. For this purpose, we spatially normalized Zubal's MRI on the SPM T1 template using SPM [13]. Since the SPM SPECT template is perfectly aligned with the SPM T1 template, the non-linear geometric transformation computed after spatial normalization was applied to our eight binary masks. In order to deal with partial volume effects in SPECT due to different spatial resolutions between SPECT and MRI, we smoothed our binary masks with a Gaussian kernel (full width at half maximum of 15 mm). For each anatomical entity, perfusion measurements consisted in averaging the SPECT template intensities weighted by the smoothed masks. Note that in the white matter, regions of interest were delineated manually before SPECT template measurement, as the smoothed white matter mask included too much gray matter. As a result we generated an activity map mimicking normal brain perfusion.

Normal SPECT Simulation The attenuation and activity maps described above were used by PHG to simulate SPECT data. We chose to simulate photon emission of Technetium ^{99m}Tc. 10^9 photons were simulated. A SPECT acquisition with a parallel hole collimator was simulated (64 projections 128 x 128 over 360°, pixel size = 2.2 mm). Tomographic reconstruction used Filtered BackProjection with a ramp filter and the reconstructed data were postfiltered using a 3D Gaussian filter with full width at half maximum of 8.8 mm. This provided us with a realistic, normal SPECT that was perfectly aligned (on account of its very construction) with a high resolution T1-weighted MRI.

2.2 Application: MRI/SPECT Registration Validation

In this section, we present an application of our simulation environment to validate MRI/SPECT registration methods in the case of non-pathological SPECT and MRI data sets. We decided to study and compare four registration methods based on statistical similarity measurements that are widely used in the context of automatic multimodality registration.

Registration Methods Based on Statistical Similarity Measurements
SPECT/MRI registration is rigid intra-patient registration. The purpose is to

---

[2] http://www.fil.ion.ucl.ac.uk/spm/

assess a rigid geometric T transformation defined by six parameters (three translations and three rotations). Let the reference image R be our SPECT data set and the floating image F our MRI data set. Similarity measurement-based registration relies on the fact that a similarity measurement $S(R, T(F))$ is optimal when the data sets are perfectly registered. We studied four similarity measurements: Mutual Information, Normalised Mutual Information, Correlation Ratio and Woods Criterion.

– *Mutual Information (MI)* [7][8]:

$$S(A, B) = H(A) - H(A|B) = H(A) + H(B) - H(A, B) \qquad (1)$$

where H denotes Shannon entropy.
Mutual Information is a measure of statistical dependence between two random variables, in our case the two images, relying on entropy measurements. Mutual Information makes no assumptions regarding the nature of this dependence.
– *Normalised Mutual Information (NMI)* [6]:

$$S(A, B) = \frac{H(A) + H(B)}{H(A, B)} \qquad (2)$$

Normalised Mutual Information is also an entropy-based measure but invariant to the overlap region of both data sets.
– *Correlation Ratio (CR)* [9]:

$$S(A|B) = \frac{Var[E(A|B)]}{Var(A)} \qquad (3)$$

Correlation Ratio measures the functional dependence between A and B, i.e. it measures how B explains the "energy" of A.
– *Woods Criterion (WC)* [4]:

$$S(A|B) = E_B \left(\frac{\sqrt{Var(A|B)}}{E(A|B)} \right) \qquad (4)$$

Woods Criterion is based on the heuristic that certain structures or organs have a similar uniformity of intensities in both modalities. For each MRI intensity value, this criterion measures the ratio between standard deviation and mean of corresponding SPECT intensity values. As recommended by the author, we segmented brain from the MRI data set before registration.

Given a geometric T transformation, each of these similarity measurements may be computed on the joint histogram of R and $T(F)$. Partial volume interpolation was used to assess joint histograms. To avoid interpolation artifacts that occur when voxel dimensions of both data are multiples [14], we resampled our simulated SPECT data. MRI voxel dimensions being 1.1 mm, we changed SPECT voxel dimensions from 2.2 mm to 4.51 mm, which exactly corresponds to the sampling rate used for our clinical acquisitions. The optimization of these cost functions was then achieved using Powell's multidimensional direction set method and Brent's one-dimensional optimization algorithm for line minimizations [15]. A two-level multiresolution strategy as described by [8] was applied to avoid the pitfall of local optima.

Registration Validation $N = 50$ T^* theoretical transformations were generated by randomly sampling a 6 parameter vector using a Gaussian distribution (Mean = 0, Standard Deviation = 10). T^* was then applied to the MRI data set and a new unregistered MRI was thus created using trilinear interpolation during resampling. We then sequentially launched registration with the simulated SPECT using the four registration methods described above. We called the computed geometric transformation $\hat{T}$.

- *Precision* : For each registration method, precision was assessed by the distribution of $|T^* - \hat{T}|$ values.
- *Accuracy* : For each registration method, accuracy was assessed by computing mean, standard deviation and maximum values of a registration error measured on a set of n P_i points uniformly distributed within the brain and on the skin (identified using labeled MRI) as follows :

$$RMS = \sqrt{\frac{1}{n} \sum_{i=1}^{n} \left\| P_i - \hat{T}^{-1}(T^*(P_i)) \right\|^2} \tag{5}$$

3   Results

Model Construction and SPECT Simulations Fig. 1 presents our normal brain perfusion model or activity map. After simulation, 22 million photons among the 10^9 that were simulated were accepted by the detector. Volume reconstruction of this simulation is represented in Fig. 2.

Results of Registration Validation Distribution of precision measurements ($|T^* - \hat{T}|$) are presented using boxplot representations for MI(Fig. 3), NMI(Fig. 4), CR(Fig. 5) and WC without (Fig. 6) or with (Fig. 7) prior brain segmentation from MRI. Translation errors (Tx, Ty, Tz) were computed in mm whereas rotation errors (Rx, Ry, Rz) were computed in degrees. We used the following reference coordinate system: x axis denotes anterior to posterior axis, y axis denotes top to bottom axis and z axis denotes left to right axis.

Accuracy measurements (mean, standard deviation and maximum values of RMS) are presented in Table 1, for $n = 1600$ points uniformly distributed within the brain and $n = 1400$ points uniformly distributed on the skin. RMS values are given in mm. Distribution of brain and skin RMS values for MI, NMI, CR and WC (with prior brain segmentation) is displayed using boxplot representations (Fig. 8). No registration solution was excluded from these results.

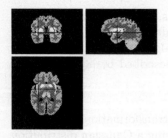

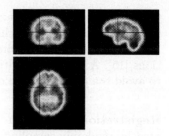

Fig. 1. Normal Brain Perfusion Model

Fig. 2. Monte Carlo Simulations of Normal SPECT

Table 1. Accuracy Measurements

	Brain RMS		Skin RMS	
	Mean ± Std	*Max*	*Mean ± Std*	*Max*
MI	7.75±2.86	21.02	8.67±3.27	22.59
NMI	8.13±2.97	21.43	9.21±3.39	23.17
CR	5.60±2.83	16.63	6.36±3.44	18.05
WC (no segmented brain)	19.87±5.26	36.09	27.29±7.03	50.74
WC (segmented brain)	8.14±2.33	16.57	9.07±2.95	19.23

4 Discussion

Thanks to the method we describe in this paper, we produced a realistic model of SPECT that was perfectly aligned with a T1-weighted MRI data set. The very concept of our approach provides a gold standard to validate MRI/SPECT registration methods. Simulated SPECT data sets were considered realistic because physical processes involved in SPECT acquisition were all closely modeled through PHG. Although our theoretical brain perfusion model does not take detailed physiological knowledge into account, we consider that our simulation results are adequate for registration validation purposes. What we present is a new way to evaluate and compare registration methods using realistic simulated data sets by controlling acquisition procedures (Monte Carlo simulations) and functional information (perfusion model).

Registration precision and accuracy proved very satisfactory for practically every method. Mean registration errors were lower than SPECT data resolution (resolution measurement: 12.4 mm). Some of the less satisfactory results were found when assessing WC with unsegmented brain. This is not surprising since in this case uniformity assumptions made by the Woods Criterion are less valid. No significant differences were found between MI, NMI and WC (with segmented brain). Nevertheless, WC using segmented brain is less automated method, regardless of clinical use. The best results were obtained for CR. We are aware that our simulation approach may implicitly introduce statistical or functional

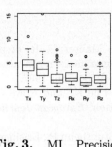

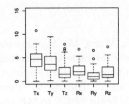

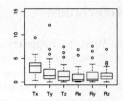

Fig. 3. MI Precision measurements ($|T^* - \hat{T}|$)

Fig. 4. NMI Precision measurements ($|T^* - \hat{T}|$)

Fig. 5. CR Precision measurements ($|T^* - \hat{T}|$)

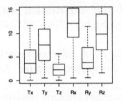

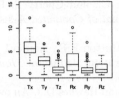

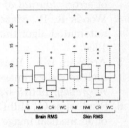

Fig. 6. WC Precision measurements ($|T^* - \hat{T}|$) (no segmented brain)

Fig. 7. WC Precision measurements ($|T^* - \hat{T}|$) (segmented brain)

Fig. 8. Brain and skin accuracy measurements (RMS)

dependence between both data sets. Consequently, results may be better in our study than in real conditions. We plan to study the assumption when creating a pathological perfusion model. Still, our results are qualitatively concordant with literature [2], even though comparing different validation methods is not an easy thing.

We emphasize the generic aspect of our approach. Actually, this study may easily be extended to other registration methods or investigate other aspects such as sensitivity to SPECT reconstruction and correction features (e.g. reconstruction filters, attenuation or scatter correction). Our method may also be applied to study other clinical contexts, in particular by simulating pathological SPECT patterns. Our perfusion model could be improved, however, if it were based on the statistical analysis of a population of subjects (healthy or pathological) rather than on measurements from an averaged SPECT data set. For instance, we plan to study the behavior of the same similarity-based methods in the case of ictal SPECT in epileptic patients because of possibly large dissimilarities between ictal SPECT and MRI data.

5   Acknowledgments

This work was partly supported by a grant from the "Ligue Française Contre l'Epilepsie".

References

1. West J., Fitzpatrick J. M., Wang M. Y., Dawant B. M., Maurer C. R. et al. Comparison and evaluation of retrospective intermodality brain image registration techniques. *Journal of Computer Assisted Tomography*, 21(4):554–566, 1997.
2. Barnden L., Kwiatek R., Lau Y., Hutton B., Thurjfell L., Pile K., and Rowe C. Validation of fully automatic brain SPET to MR co-registration. *European Journal of Nuclear Medecine*, 27(2):147–154, 2000.
3. Pfluger T., Vollmar C., Wismüller A., Dresel S., Berger F., Stuntheim P., Leisinger G., and Hahn K. Quantitative comparison of automatic and interactive methods for MRI-SPECT image registration of the brain based on 3-dimensional calculation of error. *Journal of Nuclear Medecine*, 41:1823–1829, 2000.
4. Woods R. P., Mazziotta J. C., and Cherry S. R. MRI-PET registration with automated algorithm. *Journal of Computed Assisted Tomography*, 17(4):536–546, 1993.
5. Ardekani B.A., Braun M., Hutton B.F., Kanno I., and Iida H. A fully automatic multimodality image registration algorithm. *Journal of Computed Assisted Tomography*, 19:615–623, 1995.
6. Studholme C., Hill D.L.G., and Hawkes D.J. An overlap invariant entropy measure of 3d medical image alignment. *Pattern Recognition*, 32:71–86, 1999.
7. Wells III W.M., Viola P., Atsumi H., Nakajima S., and Kikinis R. Multi-modal volume registration by maximization of mutual information. *Medical Image Analysis*, 1(1):35–51, 1996.
8. Maes F., Collignon A., Vandermeulen D., Marchal G., and Suetens P. Multimodality image registration by maximization of mutual information. *IEEE Transactions on Medical Imaging*, 16(2):187–198, 1997.
9. Roche A., Malandain G., Pennec X., and Ayache N. The correlation ratio as a new similarity measure for multimodal image registration. In *MICCAI 98: Lecture Notes in Computer Science*, 1496:1115–1124, 1998.
10. Harrison R.L., Vannoy S.D., Haynor D.R., Gillispie S.B., Kaplan M.S., and Lewellen T.K. Preliminary experience with the photon history generator module of a public-domain simulation system for emission tomography. In *Conf. Rec. Nucl. Sci. Symp.*, 2:1154– 1158, 1993.
11. Zubal I.G., Harrell C.R., Smith E.O., Rattner Z., Gindi G.R., and Hoffer P.B. Computerized three-dimensional segmented human anatomy. *Medical Physics*, 21(2):299–302, 1994.
12. Kwiatek R., Barnden L., Tedman R., Jarret R., Chew J., Rowe C., and Pile K. Regional cerebral blood flow in fibromyalgia. *Arthritis and Rheumatism*, 43(12):2823–2833, 2000.
13. Friston K.J., Ashburner J., Poline J.B., Frith C.D., Heather J.D., and Frackowiak R.S.J. Spatial registration and normalization of images. *Human Brain Mapping*, 2:165–189, 1995.
14. Pluim J. P. W., Maintz J. B. A., and Viergever M. A. Interpolation artefacts in mutual information-based image registration. In *Computer Vision and Image Understanding: CVIU*, 77(2):211-232, 2000.
15. Press W. H., Teukolsky S. A., Vetterling W. T., and Flannery B. P. *Numerical Recipes in C, 2nd. edition*. Cambridge University Press, 1992.

Correction of Probe Pressure Artifacts in Freehand 3D Ultrasound*

Graham Treece[1], Richard Prager[1], Andrew Gee[1], and Laurence Berman[2]

[1] Department of Engineering, University of Cambridge, Trumpington Street,
Cambridge, UK, CB2 1PZ,
gmt11,rwp,ahg@eng.cam.ac.uk

[2] Department of Radiology, University of Cambridge, Addenbrooke's Hospital,
Cambridge, UK, CB2 2QQ,
lb@radiol.cam.ac.uk

Abstract. We present an algorithm which combines non-rigid image-based registration and conventional position sensing to correct probe-pressure-induced registration errors in freehand three-dimensional (3D) ultrasound volumes. The local accuracy of image-based registration enables the accurate freehand acquisition of high resolution (> 15MHz) 3D ultrasound data, opening the way for 3D musculoskeletal examinations. External position sensor readings guarantee the large-scale positional accuracy of the data. The algorithm is shown to increase both the clarity and accuracy of reslices through *in vivo* volumetric data sets.

1 Introduction

Advances in high resolution ultrasound are increasingly enabling detailed examination of musculoskeletal anatomy [2, 8]. However, typical high resolution ultrasound images (B-scans) have a limited field of view: in order to visualise a larger volume, the B-scans must be combined into a composite data set. The most appropriate technique for this is freehand 3D ultrasound, where the probe is moved by hand, and the resulting sequence of B-scans is registered by either intrinsic (image-based) or extrinsic (position sensing) means.

Current position sensing techniques are not able to correctly register high resolution ultrasound data. Limitations in the accuracy of typical position sensors are not the major problem: movement of the anatomy during scanning is a much greater source of error. Even if the patient is still, variation of the pressure of the probe on the skin causes local deformation of the anatomy on a large scale compared to the pixel size (< 0.1mm) in a high resolution B-scan.

Image-based registration, by contrast, has been used successfully to generate extended-field-of-view images [9]. 3D data sets can be constructed by combining image-based registration with speckle de-correlation [6, 7], the latter providing an estimate of the out-of-plane probe movement. These techniques can achieve

---

* This work was carried out under EPSRC grant GR/N21062. Dynamic Imaging Ltd. provided a modified ultrasound machine to enable digital data acquisition.

W. Niessen and M. Viergever (Eds.): MICCAI 2001, LNCS 2208, pp. 283–290, 2001.

accurate local registration, are fairly robust to noise in the images, and require no user interaction. However, the errors accumulate through a sequence of B-scans.

In this paper, we present a high resolution freehand 3D ultrasound system which uses a combination of non-rigid image-based registration and external position sensing, to provide both local and global accuracy. This robust framework allows us to correct for both pressure-induced and position sensing errors.

To the best of our knowledge, there have been no previous attempts to correct, by non-rigid registration, a sequence of B-scans varying in both time *and* location. Non-rigid registration of two B-scans has been used to track physiological motion [1, 10]. However, such unconstrained registration is only possible if the probe does not move, so all changes can be attributed to tissue movement: even then, substantial regularisation is required. Set in the broader context of image-based registration [3], our work has an important distinguishing feature. While the registration between each pair of images is essentially 2D/2D (the position sensor gives the out-of-plane displacement between consecutive B-scans), we need to make sure that the non-rigid registration corrects only pressure-induced errors, and *not* changes in the image caused by out-of-plane probe movement.

2   Description of the Algorithm

Image-based registration is first performed on a pair of B-scans, the registrations are concatenated over a sequence, then position sensor information is reintroduced to correct any error accumulation.

2.1   Correction of Probe Pressure for a Pair of B-scans

A B-scan is registered to its neighbour by moving it entirely within its own plane, first by a rigid (i.e. x and y) translation, followed by a non-rigid shift in depth (y). Out-of-plane registration is determined solely by the position sensor.

The rigid transformation is calculated from the position of maximum normalised correlation[1] of the pixel intensities within the overlapping region of the B-scans for a range of x and y offsets. Using the whole B-scan, rather than small regions as in block matching [10], de-sensitizes the result to local changes in anatomy. Since the acquisition rate is typically 25Hz, each pair of B-scans is very similar, so the correlation function in x and y approximates the symmetric autocorrelation function, and a simple uphill search for the peak can be used. This symmetry is also useful in interpolating the sub-pixel location of the peak. Given the peak correlation value c_0, and its two neighbours c_{-1} and c_1, the relative offset p from the location of c_0 is given by:

$$p = \begin{cases} \frac{1}{2}\frac{c_1-c_{-1}}{c_0-c_1} & \text{if} \quad c_{-1} > c_1 \\ \frac{1}{2}\frac{c_1-c_{-1}}{c_0-c_{-1}} & \text{if} \quad c_{-1} < c_1 \\ 0 & \text{if} \quad c_{-1} = c_1 \end{cases} \tag{1}$$

which ensures that the angles β are identical.

---

[1] There is no observable effect of using the sum of squared difference (SSD) instead.

This gives the relative x and y translation $\{x_c, y_c\}$ of the centre of the new B-scan. However, we already have an estimate of the relative location of the top left corner of the previous B-scan, from the position sensor. The in-plane component of this, described by a translation $\{x_o, y_o\}$ and a rotation α_o, is found by projecting the location of the previous B-scan along the average normal of the two B-scans. The additional in-plane translation $\{x_r, y_r\}$ which should be applied to the new B-scan is therefore:

$$x_r = x_c - 0.5w\left(\cos(\alpha_o) - 1\right) - 0.5h\sin(\alpha_o) - x_o$$
$$y_r = y_c - 0.5h\left(\cos(\alpha_o) - 1\right) + 0.5w\sin(\alpha_o) - y_o \tag{2}$$

where w and h are the B-scan's width and height respectively.

This rigid registration is applied before calculating the non-rigid registration, and the previous B-scan is resampled so that it can be directly compared to the subsequent B-scan[2]. Several simplifying assumptions are made in order to calculate the non-rigid component of registration:

- Tissue elasticity is assumed to be uniform across the B-scan, such that probe pressure generates deformation in the y (depth) direction only.
- Tissue elasticity is also assumed to vary slowly with out-of-plane movement. Under this assumption, the shift in anatomy between B-scans will be monotonic with depth, i.e. the entire image is either compressed or expanded.
- It is assumed that both speckle and coherent reflections are deformed in the same way by probe pressure, so both can be used for registration.

The pressure estimate for each B-scan is thus a vector, $P_r(y)$, giving the relative shift in depth at each y. This corrects the most significant effects of probe pressure, while imposing suitable constraints on the registration to prevent it simply following changes in the image due to out-of-plane probe motion.

An initial, noisy estimate of $P_r(y)$, $P_n(y)$ (the dots in Fig. 1) is calculated by correlating each line in the B-scan with nearby lines in the previous (resampled) B-scan, and estimating the peak using (1). $P_n(y)$, which is noisy and not monotonic, can be cleaned up by averaging values of $P_n(y)$ in local neighbourhoods, where the size of the neighbourhood depends on the local variance $v(y)$ of $P_n(y)$: a smaller neighbourhood can be used at depths where $P_n(y)$ is tightly clustered (towards the top of Fig. 1). $v(y)$ is estimated for each y using a small number of neighbouring $P_n(y)$ values. Then, starting with the row y with the lowest variance $v(y)$, the cleaned-up pressure estimate is calculated as follows:

$$P_r(y) = \frac{1}{y_{high} - y_{low}} \sum_{i=y_{low}}^{y_{high}} P_n(i) \quad \text{where} \quad \sum_{i=y_{low}}^{y_{high}} \frac{1}{v(i)} > m, \tag{3}$$

where the range $y_{low} \dots y_{high}$ is symmetrically disposed around y, and the constant m determines the acceptable precision in estimating $P_r(y)$. Values of $P_n(y)$

---

[2] Rigid alignment in the y direction is only necessary to limit the search space for non-rigid registration, which itself recalculates the y alignment.

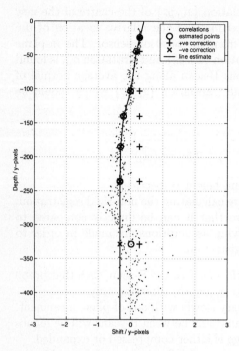

Fig. 1. Estimation of $P_r(y)$.

in the range y_{low} to y_{high} are then discarded, and the process repeated until there are insufficient neighbouring values to satisfy the inequality in (3). The circles in Fig. 1 are seven such estimates of $P_r(y)$: note that there are more in regions where $P_n(y)$ is more tightly clustered.

As these estimates are generated, monotonicity in y is enforced according to the relative depth and value of previous estimates. Both positive and negative adjustments (the crosses in Fig. 1) are investigated: that with the least cost, defined as the sum of the absolute differences between the original and adjusted estimates, is selected. The final $P_r(y)$, shown as a solid line in Fig. 1, is a piecewise linear interpolation of the adjusted pressure estimates. Note that the noisy estimates $P_n(y)$ have been largely ignored at the bottom of the B-scan: this is due to the lack of signal in this region, as apparent in the B-scans in Fig. 2.

2.2   Concatenation of Corrections for a Sequence of B-scans

The final transformation for a B-scan i must take into account all the transformations of the previous B-scans. The location of each B-scan relative to the position sensor reference frame is given by the homogeneous transformation matrix ${}^P\mathbf{T}_{bi}$ [5]. The B-scan can be moved within its plane by *post*-multiplying ${}^P\mathbf{T}_{bi}$ with the matrix $\mathbf{T}_r$, calculated from the translation $\mathbf{t}_r = \{x_r, y_r, 0\}^T$:

$$
{}^r\mathbf{T}_{bi} = {}^P\mathbf{T}_{bi}\mathbf{T}_r, \quad \text{where} \quad \mathbf{T}_r = \left[\begin{array}{c|c} \mathbf{I} & \mathbf{t}_r \\ \hline 0\ 0\ 0 & 1 \end{array}\right] \tag{4}
$$

In order to apply the transformations from previous B-scans without affecting the relative registration, we require the affine *pre*-multiplicative matrix ${}^r\mathbf{T}_{pi}$ which is equivalent in effect to $\mathbf{T}_r$. The final transformation for B-scan i is:

$$
{}^r\mathbf{T}_{bi} = {}^r\mathbf{T}_{pi}{}^P\mathbf{T}_{bi}, \quad \text{where} \quad {}^r\mathbf{T}_{pi} = {}^r\mathbf{T}_{pi-1}{}^P\mathbf{T}_{bi}\mathbf{T}_r{}^P\mathbf{T}_{bi}^{-1} \tag{5}
$$

Unfortunately, the error in ${}^r\mathbf{T}_{bi}$ will accumulate over a sequence of B-scans. This drift can be corrected by examining the in-plane difference in location $\{x_{\varepsilon i}, y_{\varepsilon i}\}$ between the original (${}^P\mathbf{T}_{bi}$) and corrected (${}^r\mathbf{T}_{bi}$) values. In particular, assuming the patient has not moved during the scan, $x_{\varepsilon i}$ should remain within the position sensor tolerance. A simple method of enforcing this constraint is:

- If $x_{\varepsilon i}$ of the last B-scan ($i = N$) is greater than this tolerance (± 1mm in this case), ${}^{r}\mathbf{T}_{bN}$ is reset to ${}^{P}\mathbf{T}_{bN}$, and all previous B-scans are adjusted by $\frac{i}{N}x_{\varepsilon N}$.
- If the maximum remaining $x_{\varepsilon i}$ is still greater than the tolerance, the process is iterated by resetting this B-scan and adjusting all surrounding scans (up to the closest reset scan) in the same way.

Unlike $x_{\varepsilon i}$, $y_{\varepsilon i}$ must be allowed to be greater than the position sensor tolerance in order to correct for pressure. However, if $y_{\varepsilon i}$ measures the change in y location of the deepest data in the B-scans, one similar correction can be made by removing this error from the final B-scan and adjusting the rest by $\frac{i}{N}y_{\varepsilon N}$.

The non-rigid transformation $P_i(y)$ of B-scan i can be calculated simply by adding $P_r(y)$ to the previous non-rigid transformation, allowing for any downward shift y_{offset} in the position of the new B-scan:

$$P_i(y) = P_r(y) + P_{i-1}(y + y_{\text{offset}}) \tag{6}$$

$P_i(y)$ then gives the shift due to pressure relative to the first B-scan. However, $P_i(y)$ may indicate a compression, and we want to *un*-compress the B-scan data. Hence, the B-scan $i = c$ for which $P_i(y)$ caused the most compression is found, and $P_c(y)$ is subtracted from $P_i(y)$ for all i, using (6). This has the effect of re-registering all the B-scans to c.

Instead of overwriting the original data, the application of $P_i(y)$ and ${}^{r}\mathbf{T}_{bi}$ can be toggled in reslice, panoramic, manifold and volume rendering visualisations [4]. This allows a final sanity check on the entire process.

3   Results

B-scans were acquired with a Diasus ultrasound machine[3], using a 10-22MHz linear array probe, on a 4cm depth setting. 8-bit digital log-compressed data was transferred via ethernet at 25Hz to an 800MHz PC running Linux. The probe position was sensed by a Polaris[4] optical tracking system also linked to this PC, and the system calibrated to an accuracy of ± 0.35mm RMS. Calibration, acquisition, processing and display of the data was performed by Stradx [4][5]. Pressure corrections were calculated at between 3 and 4 B-scans per second.

Three *in vivo* tests of varying complexity were performed. Figure 2 shows an examination of the common carotid artery and internal jugular vein. Given only a small sideways movement during the scans, the pressure-corrected version of Fig. 2(b) should be similar to the first B-scan in (a). In Fig. 2(c), the positions of the main features are indeed restored, although the shape of the internal jugular is distorted due to the assumption of uniform tissue elasticity: this vessel is at a much lower internal pressure than the carotid. $P_i(y)$ in Fig. 2(d) also shows a change in gradient at the level of the carotid artery, which correctly reflects the more compressible tissue nearer the surface.

---

[3] Dynamic Imaging Ltd., http://www.dynamicimaging.co.uk/
[4] Northern Digital Inc., http://www.ndigital.com/
[5] http://svr-www.eng.cam.ac.uk/~rwp/stradx/

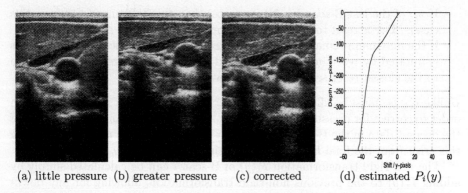

(a) little pressure (b) greater pressure   (c) corrected   (d) estimated $P_i(y)$

Fig. 2. Correction of probe pressure for repeated B-scans at the same location. (a) and (b) are the first and last B-scans from a sequence of 100 acquired with varying pressure. (c) is the same scan as (b) after correction.

Figure 3 shows a panorama [4] of both lobes of the thyroid, constructed by pasting together data from each B-scan of an approximately planar sequence. In Figs. 3(d) to (g), detail of each panorama is compared with one of the original B-scans. Rigid position correction in (b) and (f) removes the 'jitter' in the image, and non-rigid correction in (c) and (g) removes the local deformation, particularly apparent at the skin surface, and in the shape of the carotid. Note that all of the panoramas are slightly compressed in x relative to the original B-scan: this is a consequence of patient movement, for which we do not attempt to correct.

Figure 4 shows four 3D examinations of the arm, acquired in quick succession with the patient remaining still. Variation of probe pressure causing up to 2mm deformation is clear from the top row of Figure 4(a). This variation is nearly eliminated in the corrected data. Reslices parallel to the skin surface are affected by the poor elevational resolution of the ultrasound beam, as apparent in the lower row of Fig. 4(a). However, the corrected reslices in (b) are much clearer: the path of a small (2mm diameter) vein in the arm is particularly well defined.

Figure 5 shows two examples of pressure-correction applied to lower frequency (3MHz) convex array probes. Physically plausible deformations are calculated in both cases. As would be expected, the top of the bladder is deformed whilst the base stays relatively stationary, despite the sparsity of correlatable features in this data. The top right surface of the liver is also straightened out, even in the presence of pulsatile vascular motion lower down. Other changes in the centre of the scan are due to corrections out of the plane of the reslice.

4   Conclusions

We have presented a novel algorithm, combining image-based and position sensing techniques, to correct the most significant effects of probe pressure in free-

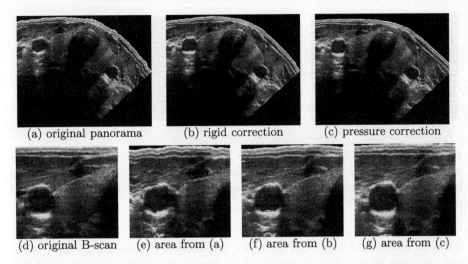

(a) original panorama   (b) rigid correction   (c) pressure correction

(d) original B-scan   (e) area from (a)   (f) area from (b)   (g) area from (c)

Fig. 3. Correction of probe pressure for a panoramic sequence of B-scans. (a) to (c) show a mosaic of the central data from each B-scan. (e) to (g) show an area from each panorama corresponding to one of the original B-scans in (d).

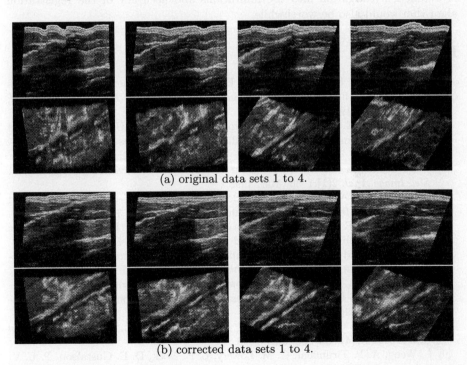

(a) original data sets 1 to 4.

(b) corrected data sets 1 to 4.

Fig. 4. Correction of probe pressure for a freehand 3D volume. (a) shows the same two reslices through four data sets of part of the forearm, the top row perpendicular to the skin surface (and the original B-scans), and the lower row parallel to the skin and about 5mm beneath it. (b) shows the same reslices as in (a) after correction.

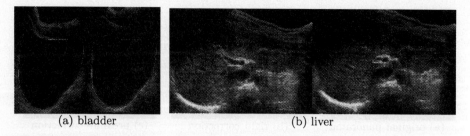

(a) bladder   (b) liver

Fig. 5. Correction of probe pressure for lower resolution data. (a) and (b) show original (left) and corrected (right) reslices through data volumes. Both reslices in (a) show the original outline. (b) was acquired in two sequences, each corrected individually.

hand 3D ultrasound data. This increases the clarity of reslices of such data, without compromising global accuracy. There are many possible extensions of this work, including the correct treatment of probe pressure for convex curvilinear probes, and the use of speckle de-correlation for out-of-plane motion correction. A detailed investigation into the limitations and accuracy of the registration algorithm would also be worthwhile.

References

[1] L. N. Bohs, B. H. Friemel, and G. E. Trahey. Experimental velocity profiles and volumetric flow via two-dimensional speckle tracking. *Ultrasound Med Biol*, 21(7):885–898, 1995.

[2] B. D. Fornage, E. N. Atkinson, L. F. Nock, and P. H. Jones. US with extended field of view: phantom-tested accuracy of distance measurements. *Radiol*, 214(2):579–584, 2000.

[3] J. B. A. Maintz and M. A. Viergever. A survey of medical image registration. *Med Image Anal*, 2(1):1–36, Mar. 1998.

[4] R. W. Prager, A. H. Gee, and L. Berman. Stradx: real-time acquisition and visualisation of freehand 3D ultrasound. *Med Image Anal*, 3(2):129–140, 1999.

[5] R. W. Prager, R. N. Rohling, A. H. Gee, and L. Berman. Rapid calibration for 3-D free-hand ultrasound. *Ultrasound Med Biol*, 24(6):855–869, 1998.

[6] W. L. Smith and A. Fenster. Optimum scan spacing for three-dimensional ultrasound by speckle statistics. *Ultrasound Med Biol*, 26(4):551–562, 2000.

[7] T. A. Tuthill, J. F. Krücker, J. B. Fowlkes, and P. L. Carson. Automated three-dimensional US frame positioning computed from elevational speckle decorrelation. *Radiol*, 209(2):575–582, 1998.

[8] S. Wang, R. K. Chhem, E. Cardinal, and K.-H. Cho. Joint sonography. *Radiol Clin N Am*, 37(4):653–668, July 1999.

[9] L. Weng, A. P. Tirumalai, C. M. Lowery, L. F. Nock, D. E. Gustafson, P. L. V. Behren, and J. H. Kim. US extended-field-of-view imaging technology. *Radiol*, 203(3):877–880, 1997.

[10] F. Yeung, S. F. Levinson, and K. J. Parker. Multilevel and motion model-based ultrasonic speckle tracking algorithms. *Ultrasound Med Biol*, 24(3):427–441, 1998.

In-Vitro Validation of a Novel Model-Based Approach to the Measurement of Arterial Blood Flow Waveforms from Dynamic Digital X-ray Images

Kawal Rhode[1], Gareth Ennew[1], Tryphon Lambrou[1], Alexander Seifalian[2], and David Hawkes[1]

[1]Division of Radiological Sciences and Medical Engineering, Guy's, King's and St. Thomas' Hospitals Medical School, Guy's Hospital, London, U.K., SE1 9RT
[2]University Department of Surgery, Royal Free and University College Medical School, The Royal Free Hospital, Pond Street, London, U.K., NW3 2QG

Abstract. We have developed a blood flow waveform shape model using principal component analysis (PCA) and applied this to our existing concentration-distance curve matching technique for the extraction of flow waveforms from dynamic digital x-ray images. The aim of the study was to validate the system using a moving-vessel flow phantom. Instantaneous recording of flow from an electromagnetic flow meter (EMF) provided the "gold standard" measurement. A model waveform was constructed from 256 previously recorded waveforms from the EMF using PCA. Flow waveforms were extracted from parametric images derived from dynamic x-ray data by finding the parameters of the shape model that minimized the mean value of our cost function. The computed waveforms were compared to the EMF recordings. The model-based approach produced narrower limits of agreement with the EMF data than our previously developed algorithms and, in the presence of increasing noise in the parametric images, it out-performed the other algorithms.

1 Introduction

The algorithms[1] that have been previously reported for the measurement of blood flow in arteries from dynamic digital x-ray images have not fully taken into account the nature of the blood flow in the target artery. At most, investigators have made assumptions about the different velocity profiles that exist radially across an arterial lumen. With the advent of the use of Doppler ultrasound to monitor blood flow in arteries, it became apparent that the shape and content of the Doppler sonogram was characteristic of the artery being investigated and the disease state of this artery. Investigators have attempted to characterize sonograms with a view to distinguish between healthy and diseased states[2-7]. Our method[8] of velocity waveform measurement necessarily over samples the waveform yet is severely noise-limited. The lower bound of the sampling rate is determined by the distance traveled by the blood per sampling interval in relation to the sampled vessel length. Therefore, we hypothesized that the *a priori* knowledge of the nature of the blood flow through a target artery may be used to improve the measurement of blood flow through that

W. Niessen and M. Viergever (Eds.): MICCAI 2001, LNCS 2208, pp. 291-300, 2001.
© Springer-Verlag Berlin Heidelberg 2001

artery using dynamic digital x-ray images. This hypothesis was tested by constructing a blood flow waveform shape model from many waveforms collected by electromagnetic flow meter recordings using a blood flow test circuit under varying conditions of flow. This shape model was then used to constrain the measurement of blood flow in a blood flow circuit using the concentration-distance curve-matching algorithm previously developed[8].

2 Method

2.1 Physiological Blood Flow Circuit

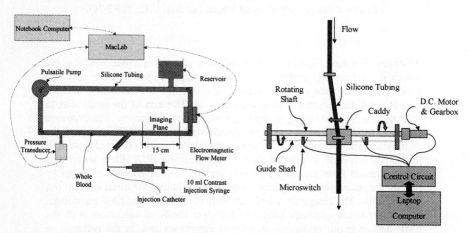

Fig. 1. Physiological blood flow circuit.   **Fig. 2.** Programmable vessel manipulator.

Figure 1 shows a schematic of the physiological blood flow circuit used to simulate pulsatile blood flow in the human circulation. A 15 cm section of silicone tubing was used to simulate a blood vessel. Date-expired whole blood was obtained and used as the circulating fluid. Pulsatile flow was generated using a pulsatile syringe pump (Pulsatile Blood Pump 1405, Harvard Apparatus). This allowed adjustment of mean flow rate by two means: (1) by altering the pumping frequency; (2) by altering the stroke volume. A 6mm calibre electromagnetic flow meter (Electromagnetic Blood Flow Sensor / Electromagnetic Blood Flow and Velocity Meter, Skalar) was placed downstream from the simulated blood vessel. This provided outputs of instantaneous and mean flow rate. These were recorded using an analogue recording system (MacLab 8s, AD Instruments) that was interfaced to a Macintosh notebook. Our x-ray technique was validated by correlating x-ray measurements with those made independently by the EMF. The pressure in the circuit was monitored using a pressure transducer connected to the MacLab. Physiological pressures were maintained by varying the height of the fluid reservoir. A 4-F catheter was inserted just upstream from the blood vessel to allow injection of iodine-based contrast medium using a 10 ml syringe. Figure 2 shows the programmable vessel manipulator that simulated vessel motion such as that seen in the coronary arteries during the cardiac cycle. This consisted of a geared d.c. electric motor driving a caddy on a linear axis. The motor speed was controlled using a pulse-width modulation electronic circuit. The motion of the manipulator could be programmed using a laptop computer that was interfaced to the control circuit. The simulated vessel was mounted with one end on the moving caddy and with the other end fixed. The motion of the manipulator was synchronized to the pulsatile pump.

2.2 Model Waveform Construction

In order to form a model of the blood flow waveforms that are produced by our blood flow circuit, we collected sample waveforms from the EMF under varying conditions of flow. The parameters altered were: (1) the stroke volume of the pump; (2) the pumping frequency; (3) the mean pressure; (4) the output impedance; (5) the vessel size; and (6) the rate of contrast medium injection. For each flow condition approximately 10 seconds of the flow signal was captured that included a 3 second period of contrast medium injection. Figure 3 shows a typical blood flow signal recorded from the EMF. For each recording the individual cycles were isolated. This was performed automatically by software that identified the systolic foot of each cycle in the recording by searching for 5 consecutive positive gradients that exceeded a predefined threshold. The foot was then marked as the first point in this series of gradients. The cycles isolated during the contrast injection phase were used as input to the principal component analysis.

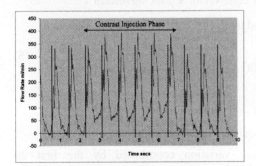

Fig. 3. An example of a recording from the electromagnetic flow meter showing identification of the systolic feet.

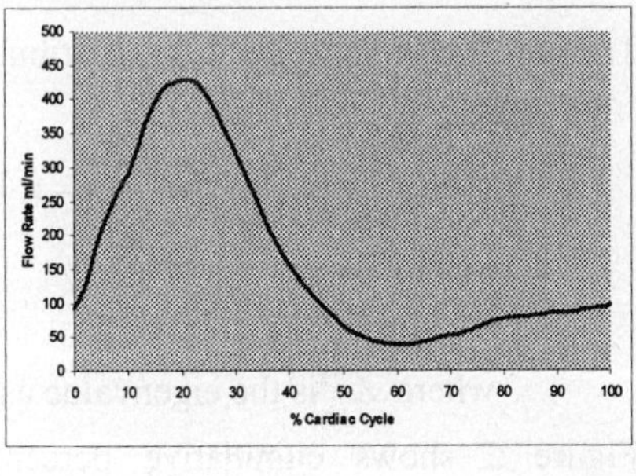

Fig. 4. Mean model waveform shape.

Each cycle was normalized over time by resampling by linear interpolation using $S = 100$ sample points. The mean flow rates ranged from 43 ml/min to 300 ml/min. The instantaneous flow rates ranged from -175 ml/min (reverse flow) to 901 ml/min. In total $N = 256$ input waveforms were used. Each input waveform $\mathbf{P}_i$ consists of S sample points $\{q_{i1}, q_{i2}, q_{i3}, \ldots\ldots, q_{iS}\}$. The input waveforms were averaged to produce a mean waveform shape (figure 4)

$$\overline{\mathbf{P}} = \frac{1}{N} \sum_{i=1}^{i=N} \mathbf{P}_i .$$

(1)

The input waveforms were then transformed by subtracting the mean waveform shape

$$\mathbf{dP}_i = \mathbf{P}_i - \overline{\mathbf{P}} = \{dq_{i1}, dq_{i2}, dq_{i3}, \ldots\ldots, dq_{iS}\} \text{ for } 1 \le i \le N . \tag{2}$$

The $S \times S$ covariance matrix $\mathbf{C}$ was calculated

$$C_{ij} = \frac{1}{N} \sum_{k=1}^{k=N} dq_{ki} \times dq_{kj} \text{ for } 1 \le i, j \le S . \tag{3}$$

Eigen analysis of this real symmetric covariance matrix was performed. This yielded S normalized eigenvectors $\mathbf{e}_j$ with corresponding eigenvalues λ_j $(1 \le j \le S)$. The eigenvectors were sorted in order of decreasing eigenvalue. The eigenvectors form a basis vector set for the transformed input waveforms $\mathbf{dP}_i$. Each eigenvector accounts for one mode of variation of the mean waveform shape $\overline{\mathbf{P}}$ with variance equal to the corresponding eigenvalue. Any of the input waveforms $\mathbf{P}_i$ can now be expressed as the sum of the mean waveform shape and a linear combination of the eigenvectors

$$\mathbf{P}_i = \overline{\mathbf{P}} + \sum_{j=1}^{j=S} w_{ij} \mathbf{e}_j \text{ for } 1 \le i \le N \tag{4}$$

where w_{ij} is the weighting factor for eigenvector $\mathbf{e}_j$ for waveform i .

The percentage variation $v\%_j$ attributed to eigenvector $\mathbf{e}_j$ can be calculated as

$$v\%_j = \frac{\lambda_j}{\sum_{i=1}^{i=S} \lambda_i} \times 100 \text{ for } 1 \le j \le S \tag{5}$$

where λ_j is the eigenvalue associated with eigenvector $\mathbf{e}_j$.

Figure 5 shows cumulative percentage variation contributed by the first 20 eigenvectors. It was found that the first 10 eigenvectors are needed to explain 99.7% of the total variation in the waveform shape. Figures 6 shows the effect of the first eigenvector on the mean shape. It is possible with PCA to see that a particular eigenvector affects a particular aspect of the shape, however, this is not always the case. From the results it can be noted that: (1) the first eigenvector primarily affects the amplitude of the systolic peak; (2) the second eigenvector affects the placement of the systolic peak; and (3) the third eigenvector affects the gradient of the falling edge of the systolic peak. These observations are generalized and each eigenvector has more than just one effect on the waveform shape. The less significant eigenvectors have very little effect on the waveform shape. Therefore, it is possible to reconstruct each of the input waveforms by finding only the weighting factors for the first few eigenvectors. The percentage noise in the input waveform signals was estimated to be 0.5%. Therefore, it was decided to use the first 10 eigenvectors to characterize the waveform shape since this number explained more than 99.5% of the total variation.

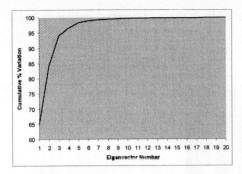

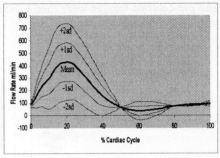

Fig. 5. Percentage cumulative variation accounted for by the first 20 eigenvectors.

Fig. 6. Effect on the mean waveform shape of adding or subtracting 1 and 2 standard deviations of the first eigenvector.

2.3 X-ray Image Acquisition

For the x-ray experiment, a 6 mm internal diameter vessel was used. The vessel manipulator gave a maximum vessel speed of 29 mm/sec and the range of vessel travel was 40 mm. The frequency of motion and of the pump were set to 43 per min. X-ray images were acquired using an Advantx DX (GE Medical Systems) x-ray system. The images were transferred to a PC in real-time by digitisation of the PAL composite video signal normally available for recording of images to a video tape recorder. The x-ray system was set for 5 ms pulsed mode at 25 frames per second. The image acquisition was carried out by a PC workstation using a Pulsar frame capture card (Matrox Imaging). Images were digitised on a 512 x 512 pixel matrix at 8 bits grey depth and image grey level was proportional to the logarithm of the x-ray image brightness. The x-ray tube voltage was 85 kV. The simulated blood vessel was placed in the isocentre of the x-ray system. The stroke volume of the pulsatile pump was adjusted to achieve the required mean flow rate and the system was allowed to reach a steady state. Initially a short sequence of images covering at least 1 cycle was acquired prior to the injection of iodine contrast medium, the pre-contrast sequence. This was followed by the injection of the contrast medium via a catheter just upstream from the segment under investigation. The rate of injection was varied depending on the mean flow rate from 2 ml/sec to 3 ml/sec over 3 seconds. A 3 second acquisition of 75 images was performed during the contrast injection phase. This sequence is known as the post-contrast sequence. Biplanar acquisition was used to determine the three-dimensional course of the blood vessel. For each flow rate, one set of images was acquired with the x-ray c-arm at the L40° position and one at R40°. To calibrate the geometry of the x-ray system, a purpose designed 60 mm Perspex cube with 14 radio-opaque markers at known positions was used. Images of the cube were acquired under the same two projections used for imaging the blood vessel.

To enable quantification of the iodine in the blood vessel, image subtraction was carried out. The technique of phase-match subtraction was used. The images in the pre-contrast sequence were matched in postion of the cardiac cycle to the images in the post-contrast sequence using the extremes of vessel motion for synchronisation.

The pre-contrast images were then subtracted from the post-contrast images to leave just the iodine signal.

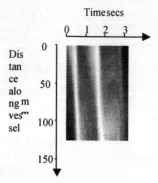

Fig. 7. Example of a parametric image produced from the angiographic data.

The subtracted x-ray images from the biplanar acquisition for each experiment were then analyzed on a computer workstation using a software package developed by our group (SARA – System for Angiographic Reconstruction and Analysis)[9]. This produced a parametric image from the angiographic data in which the image grey level represents contrast material concentration as a function of time and distance along a vessel segment (figure 7). In total 10 experiments were performed for different flow rates. This yielded 19 complete cardiac cycles for comparison with the EMF recordings.

2.4 Extraction of Blood Flow Waveforms from Parametric Images

The concentration of contrast medium along an arterial vessel segment can be expressed as a function of distance along the vessel and of time, $C(x,t)$. The distance x is measured in millimeters and $0 \leq x \leq N$. The segment length is then $(N+1)$ mm. The time t is measured in frames and $0 \leq t \leq T$. This gives rise to a series of concentration-distance curves $C(x,0), C(x,1), C(x,2), \ldots, C(x,T)$ where T is the last frame in the series. If curve $C(x,t)$ is shifted by s mm with respect to curve $C(x,t+1)$, the cost function $\Psi(s,t)$ is calculated as

$$\Psi(s,t) = \frac{1}{N-s+1} \sum_{x=0}^{x=N-s} \left(C(x,t) - C(x+s,t+1)\right)^2 \text{ if } s \geq 0 \tag{6}$$

$$\Psi(s,t) = \frac{1}{N-s+1} \sum_{x=0}^{x=N-s} \left(C(x-s,t) - C(x,t+1)\right)^2 \text{ if } s < 0 .$$

This cost function is the mean sum of squared differences between consecutive concentration-distance curves. The velocity $v(t)$ in millimeters per second for shift s is given by

$$v(t) = s \times FR \text{ where } FR \text{ is the frame rate in frames per second} . \tag{7}$$

The original concentration-curve matching algorithm (ORG algorithm) selects the value of s for which $\Psi(s,t)$ is minimum. This value, s_{opt}, is the value for which there is the best match between consecutive concentration-distance curves. The estimated contrast medium velocity is then given by

$$v(t) = s_{opt} \times FR \ . \tag{8}$$

In order to make this algorithm less susceptible to noise in the angiographic data, polynomials can be fitted to the concentration-distance curves prior to carrying out the curve matching procedure. This is termed the polynomial approximation algorithm (PA algorithm). The order of the polynomial used is dependent on the length of the vessel segment. For this study, fourth order polynomials were found to model the shape of the concentration-distance curves without modeling the noise component.

Instead of choosing the value of the shift that produces the minimum value of the cost function Ψ, the model-based algorithm (MB algorithm) constrains the value of the shift chosen by using the waveform shape information. Let the volumetric flow waveform be $G(t)$ where t is the time measured in percentage cardiac cycle and volumetric flow is measured in millilitres per minute. Using the waveform shape model, $G(t)$ is estimated by

$$\mathbf{G}(t) = \overline{\mathbf{P}} + \sum_{i=1}^{i=S} w_i \mathbf{e}_i \quad \text{where } S \text{ is the total number of eigenvectors .} \tag{9}$$

The model fitting task entails selecting the values of w_i that minimize the mean value of the cost function $\Psi(s,t)$.

Step 1:

The concentration-distance curve function $C(x,t)$ will contain one or more cardiac cycles depending on the cardiac rate and the number of frames acquired. The cycle for which the shape model is to be fitted is identified using the velocity waveform derived from the original concentration-curve matching algorithm. t_s is identified as the starting frame for the cycle and t_e is identified as the end frame of the cycle. The cycle length is then given by

$$T_c = t_e - t_s + 1 \ . \tag{10}$$

The waveform $\mathbf{G}(t)$ is rescaled in the time axis so that $0 \leq t \leq T_c - 1$.

Step 2:

The flow waveform $\mathbf{G}(t)$ is converted into units of mm shift per frame by

$$\mathbf{s}(t) = \frac{\mathbf{G}(t)}{k \times A \times FR} \quad \text{where } A \text{ is the vessel cross-sectional area} \tag{11}$$

and $k = 6$ is the unit conversion factor .

Step 3:
The cost Φ is calculated by

$$\Phi = \frac{1}{T_c} \sum_{t=t_s}^{t=t_e} \Psi(s(t-t_s),t) \ . \tag{12}$$

The values of the weighting factors w_i are found which minimize the cost Φ. This is done by the downhill simplex method. Only 10 eigenvectors were used for the generation of the fitted waveform.

3 Results

Figure 8 shows the model-based x-ray computed flow values and the EMF recording for 1 of the 10 experiments. The waveform produced by the MB algorithm follows the EMF waveform closely and is less noisy than the waveforms produced by the ORG and PA x-ray algorithms.

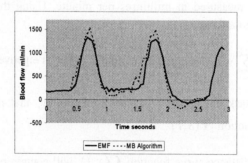

Fig. 8. An example of blood flow waveform produced by the model-based x-ray algorithm and the corresponding waveform from the electromagnetic flow meter.

Figure 9 and figure 10 show scatter plots for instantaneous flow values and average flow rates produced by the MB algorithm. Table 1 summarizes the results obtained using all three algorithms for instantaneous and average flow comparison with the EMF. The correlation between instantaneous and average flow rates between the x-ray measurements and the EMF was highly significant for all three algorithms. Each algorithm produced a mean over-estimation of both instantaneous and average flow but the limits of agreement[10] as expressed by the 95% confidence interval for the difference between x-ray and EMF flow values were narrower for the model-based algorithm.

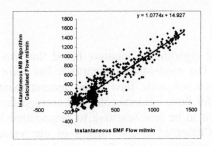
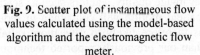
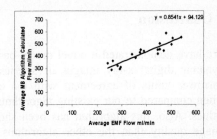

Fig. 9. Scatter plot of instantaneous flow values calculated using the model-based algorithm and the electromagnetic flow meter.

Fig. 10. Scatter plot of average flow values calculated by the model-based algorithm and the electromagnetic flow meter.

	MB Algorithm	ORG Algorithm	PA Algorithm
Instantaneous Flow Correlation	0.934	0.908	0.913
Mean Difference In Instantaneous Flow And 95% CI ml/min (X-Ray – EMF)	44.4 -266.0 to 354.7	17.1 -346.8 to 380.9	29.1 -314.0 to 372.1
Average Flow Correlation	0.906	0.913	0.909
Mean Difference In Average Flow And 95% CI ml/min (X-Ray – EMF)	37.4 -41.5 to 116.3	24.2 -70.2 to 118.7	35.1 -53.8 to 123.9

Table 1. Summary of results of instantaneous and average flow measurement by the x-ray techniques compared to the electromagnetic flow meter measurments. $p < 0.001$ for all correlation coefficients.

In order to study the effect of image quality on the performance of the algorithms, different amounts of Gaussian-distributed noise were added to one of the parametric images obtained. Gaussian noise with standard deviation of 1% to 30% of the maximum pixel grey value in the parametric image was used. Figure 11 illustrates the correlation with the EMF of instantaneous flow values obtained by the three algorithms as function of added percentage noise. It can be seen that there is minimum reduction of correlation for the MB algorithm and maximum for the ORG algorithm, with the PA algorithm performing marginally better than ORG algorithm.

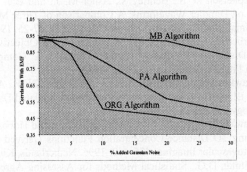

Fig. 11. Variation of correlation between x-ray and electromagnetic flow meter instantaneous values as a function of percentage added Gaussian noise.

4 Conclusion

We have demonstrated a novel model-based algorithm to measure blood flow from dynamic digital x-ray images of arteries. The model-based algorithm has shown narrower limits of agreement with the electromagnetic flow meter measurements when compared to our existing algorithms for both instantaneous and average flow values. Also, this algorithm has been shown to be less sensitive to degradation in image quality than the other algorithms. Compared to the images of our vessel phantom, clinical angiograms will be of poorer image quality. Factors such as scatter, beam hardening, over-lapping vessels, and patient motion will contribute to reduce image quality. The model-based algorithm is therefore likely to give more reliable estimates of blood flow from clinical data than our previously reported techniques. We a view to test this algorithm clinically, we are collecting blood flow waveforms from target arteries in healthy volunteers using Doppler ultrasound. These waveforms will be used to form waveform shape models for these different arteries.

References

1. Shpilfoygel S. D., Close R. A., Valentino D. J., and Duckwiler G. R., X-ray Videodensitometric Methods for Blood Flow and Velocity Measurement: A Critical Review of Literature. Med.Phys. 27[9], 2008-2023. 2000.
2. Evans D.H., Archer L.N.J., and Levene M.I, The Detection of Abnormal Neonatal Cerebral Haemodynamics using Principal Component Analysis of the Doppler Ultrasound Waveform. Ultrasound Med Biol 11, 441-449. 1985.
3. MacPherson D.S., Evans D.H., and Bell P.R.F., Common Femoral Artery Doppler Waveforms: A Comparison of Three Methods of Objective Analysis with Direct Pressure Measurements. Br J Surg 71, 46-49. 1984.
4. Evans D. H., The Interpretation of Continuous Wave Ultrasonic Doppler Blood Velocity Signals Viewed as a Problem in Pattern Recognition. J.Biomed.Eng 6[4], 272-280. 1984.
5. Prytherch D. R., Evans D. H., Smith M. J., and Macpherson D. S., On-line Classification of Arterial Stenosis Severity using Principal Component Analysis Applied to Doppler Ultrasound Signals. Clin.Phys.Physiol Meas. 3[3], 191-200. 1982.
6. Evans D. H., Macpherson D. S., Bentley S., Asher M. J., and Bell P. R., The Effect of Proximal Stenosis on Doppler Waveforms: A Comparison of Three Methods of Waveform Analysis in an Animal Model. Clin.Phys.Physiol Meas. 2[1], 17-25. 1981.
7. Martin T.R.P., Barber D.C., Sherriff S.B, and Prichard D.R., Objective Feature Extraction Applied to the Diagnosis of Carotid Artery Disease: A Comparative Study with Angiography. Clin Phys Physiol Meas 1, 71-81. 1980.
8. Seifalian A.M., Hawkes D.J., Colchester A.C.F., and Hobbs K.E.F., A New Algorithm for Deriving Pulsatile Blood Flow Waveforms Tested using Simulated Dynamic Angiographic Data. Neuroradiology 13, 263-269. 1989.
9. Seifalian A.M., Hawkes D.J., Bladin C., Colchester A.C.F., and Hobbs K.E.F., Blood Flow Measurements Using 3D Distance-Concentration Functions Derived From Digital X-Ray Angiograms. Cardiovascular Imaging, 425-442. 1996. Netherlands, Kluwer Academic.
10. Bland J.M. and Altman D.G., Statistical Methods for Assessing Agreement Between Two Methods of Clinical Measurement. The Lancet 1, 307-310. 1986.

Retrospective Correction of the Heel Effect in Hand Radiographs

G. Behiels, F. Maes*, D. Vandermeulen, and P. Suetens

Katholieke Universiteit Leuven
Faculties of Medicine and Engineering
Medical Image Computing (Radiology - ESAT/PSI)
University Hospital Gasthuisberg, Herestraat 49, B-3000 Leuven, Belgium
Gert.Behiels@uz.kuleuven.ac.be

Abstract. A method for retrospective correction of intensity inhomogeneities induced by the heel effect in digital radiographs is presented.
The method is based on a mathematical model for the heel effect derived
from the acquisition geometry. The model parameters are estimated by
fitting the model to the image intensity data in the background or direct
exposure area only where the heel effect is directly measurable, while
the correction is then applied to the whole image. The method iterates
between background segmentation and heel effect correction until convergence. We illustrate the performance of the method on flat field and
phantom images and demonstrate its robustness on a database of 137
diagnostic hand radiographs.

1 Introduction

Digital radiography offers the possibility for computer aided diagnosis and quantitative analysis using image processing techniques such as segmentation [2,3,4,8].
But intensity-based segmentation of digital radiographs is hindered by intensity
inhomogeneities inherent to the imaging process as illustrated by the hand radiograph shown in Fig. 2a: the background at the left side of the image is clearly
brighter than at the right side. This phenomenon can be largely attributed to
non-uniform X-ray exposure or heel effect. Although the spatially smoothly varying intensity inhomogeneity induced by the heel effect is easily corrected for by
the human visual perception system, its presence complicates the use of automatic processing techniques because the brightness of an object within the image
is position dependent. Intensity rectification based on calibration images is not
feasible in practice because the image acquisition parameters that affect intensity inhomogeneity, such as the positioning of the recording device relative to
the X-ray source, may vary from image to image and can not be recovered from
the acquired image at read out.

In this paper, we present a fully automated retrospective method for intensity
inhomogeneity correction of digital radiographs based on a mathematical model

---

* Frederik Maes is Postdoctoral Fellow of the Fund for Scientific Research - Flanders
(FWO-Vlaanderen, Belgium).

W. Niessen and M. Viergever (Eds.): MICCAI 2001, LNCS 2208, pp. 301–308, 2001.
© Springer-Verlag Berlin Heidelberg 2001

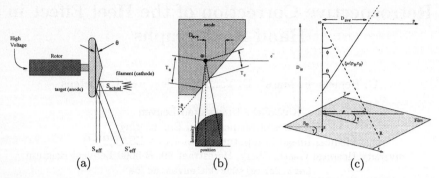

Fig. 1. (a)-(b) Schematic side views of an x-ray tube. The anode angle allows the use of a large focal spot (S_{actual}) for heat-loading considerations and a small projected focal spot (S_{eff}). X-rays are emitted at an average depth D_{ave}; the path length on the anode side $T_a > T_c$ is larger and causes a reduction in intensity. (c) X-ray coordinate system where the X-ray originates at position $(0,0)$ and travels along R to the film at position (p, D_{is}).

for the heel effect derived from the acquisition geometry. Because the heel effect is only directly measurable in the direct exposure area, we first extract the image background and estimate the parameters of the model by fitting it to the image intensity in this region only. Inhomogeneity correction is then applied to the whole image, a new background region is extracted from the corrected data and the model parameters are re-estimated. This is repeated until no significant changes in background and parameter estimation occur. We demonstrate the performance of the method on a database of hand radiographs that were acquired for bone age determination.

2   Modeling the Heel Effect

The heel effect can be understood from the construction of the X-ray tube as schematically depicted in Fig. 1. Electrons originating from the cathode are attracted by the positively charged anode. For better heat dissipation, the anode rotates and is inclined by a small anode angle θ to enlarge the area S_{actual} that is bombarded by electrons while keeping the size of the focal spot S_{eff} fairly small. The X-rays, which can be thought of to originate from a point source ω at a depth D_{ave} below the anode surface S, are therefore attenuated more by the anode material at the anode side than at the cathode side of the beam ($T_a > T_c$). This results in a non-uniform X-ray exposure of the imaging field, which explains the inhomogeneity of the background in the image of Fig. 2a.

A mathematical model for the heel effect can be derived from the simplified one-dimensional model of the anode and beam geometry depicted in Fig. 1c [5]. In the coordinate system (p, z), with p along the anode-cathode axis and z along the vertical direction, the ray R at an angle ϕ from the vertical within the plane

(ω, S) originates at $\omega(0,0)$ and hits the recording device at point (p, D_{is}) with D_{is} the distance between the X-ray source and the recording device and $\tan\phi = p/D_{is}$. The distance r traveled by R through the anode is $r = |\xi - \omega| = \sqrt{p_R^2 + z_R^2}$ with $\xi(p_R, z_R)$ the intersection of R with S. Solving the system of equations

$$\begin{cases} S : p_R = D_{ave} - z_R.\tan\theta \\ R : p_R = z_R.\tan\phi \end{cases}$$

yields:

$$r(p) = D_{ave}\frac{\cos\theta}{\sin(\phi+\theta)} = D_{ave}\frac{\sqrt{1+\left(\frac{p}{D_{ie}}\right)^2}}{\tan\theta + \frac{p}{D_{is}}}$$

The incident radiation along the anode-cathode axis is therefore modeled by

$$M(p, \alpha) = I_0.e^{-\mu.r.(p-p_\omega)} \tag{1}$$

with μ the attenuation coefficient of the anode material, I_0 the radiation originating at ω, p_ω a parameter introduced to account for the fact that the position of the source relative to the recording device is unknown, and α the 5 model parameters $\{I_0, \mu.D_{ave}, \theta, D_{is}, p_\omega\}$. The model predicts that the heel effect behaves exponentially along the anode-cathode axis and assumes that it is constant perpendicular to this axis. This is justified by flat field exposure experiments which show that the difference in intensity perpendicular to the anode-cathode axis is relatively small compared to the intensity differences along this axis (see Fig. 3).

3 Image Partitioning

A typical hand radiograph, as shown in Fig. 2a, consists of three regions: collimation area, direct exposure area and diagnostic regions. Because the heel effect is directly measurable in the direct exposure area only, we first partition the image in order to estimate the parameters of model (1) from this region only. We do this by first extracting the collimation area and then searching the direct exposure area, the remaining areas being diagnostic regions.

We find the boundaries of the collimation area using the Hough transform [6], assuming that these are rectilinear edges as is the case for all hand radiographs in our database. To make this approach more robust, the contributions of each image point to the Hough accumulator are weighted by its gradient magnitude [1] and, for each point, only the lines whose direction is within 10 degrees from the normal to the local gradient direction are considered [7]. The 4 most salient points in Hough space that represent a quadragon with inner angles between 80 and 100 degrees are selected as candidate boundaries of the collimation area. Because not all 4 collimation boundaries are allways present in the image, candidate boundaries along which the image intensity differs from the intensity expected for the collimation region are rejected. A typical result is shown in Fig. 2a.

To extract the direct exposure or background region B, a seed fill algorithm is used that starts from the boundary of the collimation region as determined in

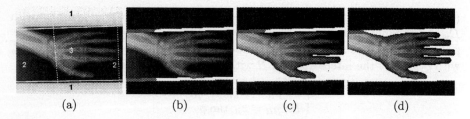

(a)   (b)   (c)   (d)

Fig. 2. (a) Typical hand radiograph with (1) collimation area, (2) direct exposure area, (3) diagnostic areas. The detected collimator edges are displayed as solid white lines and the rejected boundaries as white dotted lines. (b) Seed points for background region growing. (c,d) Intermediate and final stages of background region growing.

the previous step. Appropriate seed points for B are found by considering a small band along each of the collimator edges and retaining all pixels whose intensity is smaller than the mean of the band. This approach avoids choosing pixels that belong to the diagnostic region as candidate seed pixels. B is then grown by considering each 8-connected neighbor n of each pixel b in B and adding n to B if the intensity difference between b and n is smaller than some fixed threshold. A few snapshots of the progress are shown in Fig. 2b-d.

4   Heel Effect Estimation

The orientation γ of the anode-cathode axis and the model parameters α have to be determined such that (1) best fits the image intensity data $N(x,y)$ within the direct exposure area B, with x and y the image coordinates as defined in Fig. 1c. Assuming that γ is known, the average image profile $P_\gamma(p)$ along this direction in the direct exposure region B is given by

$$P_\gamma(p) = \langle N(x,y) \rangle_{(x,y)\in B \,|\, x\cdot\cos\gamma + y\cdot\sin\gamma = p}$$

with $\langle \cdot \rangle$ the averaging operator. We find the optimal model parameters α^* by a least square fit of the expected profile $M(p,\alpha)$ to the measured profile $P_\gamma(p)$:

$$\alpha^*(\gamma) = \arg\min_\alpha \| P_\gamma(p) - M(p,\alpha) \| \tag{2}$$

The fitted one-dimensional model $M(p,\alpha^*(\gamma))$ is then back projected perpendicular to the projection axis γ to obtain a reconstruction $R(x,y,\gamma,\alpha^*(\gamma))$ for the whole image:

$$R(x,y,\gamma,\alpha^*(\gamma)) = M(x\cdot\cos\gamma + y\cdot\sin\gamma, \alpha^*(\gamma))$$

The orientation γ is then determined such that this reconstruction best fits the actual image data within the direct exposure region:

$$\gamma^* = \arg\min_\gamma \| N(x,y) - R(x,y,\gamma,\alpha^*(\gamma)) \|_{(x,y)\in B} \tag{3}$$

or

$$\gamma^* = \arg\min_{\gamma} \left\| \frac{N(x,y)}{R(x,y,\gamma,\alpha^*(\gamma))} - 1 \right\|_{(x,y)\in B}$$

depending on whether we wish to use additive or multiplicative correction. The estimated heel effect is $R(x,y,\gamma^*,\alpha^*(\gamma^*))$ and the corrected image is respectively

$$\hat{N}(x,y) = N(x,y) - R(x,y,\gamma^*,\alpha^*(\gamma^*)) \tag{4}$$

or

$$\hat{N}(x,y) = \frac{N(x,y)}{R(x,y,\gamma^*,\alpha^*(\gamma^*))} . \tag{5}$$

The optimal parameters α^* are found by multidimensional downhill simplex search [9], starting from initial values

$$I_0 = \max_p(P_\gamma(p)), \ \mu.D_{\text{ave}} = 1, \ \theta = 15 \deg, \ D_{\text{is}} = 1\text{m}, \ p_\omega = 0.15\text{m}.$$

In our setup the anode-cathode axis is allways parallel to the image edges or the collimation edges. γ^* is therefore found by exhaustive search over these 8 orientations only, which drastically reduces computation time.

After inhomogeneity correction of the image using (4) or (5), the direct exposure area B is updated by thresholding, using a threshold derived from the histogram of the corrected image intensities $\hat{N}$. Keeping the previously determined anode-cathode orientation γ, new values for the optimal model parameters α^* are determined using (2) taking the newly selected direct exposure region into account. We thus iterate three or four times between background segmentation and heel effect correction until convergence.

5   Results

In all experiments additive correction using (3) and (4) was used. The model (1) was verified using a flat field image and an image of a hand phantom (Fig. 3). The heel effect is clearly visible in the flat field image by inspection of intensity traces along both image axes, showing a smooth degradation along the anode-cathode axis and an almost constant behavior perpendicular to this axis. A similar pattern is visible in the traces of the phantom image. Inspection of the traces of the corrected images shows that most of the background intensity variation is indeed eliminated using model (1). Physical models of X-ray production, recording and read-out predict a Gaussian distribution for the intensity of background pixels. This is not the case for the original flat field and phantom images (see histograms of Fig. 3a,d). However, the distribution of the background pixels of the corrected images is almost perfectly Gaussian (Fig. 3c,f), which is another indication that our model performs very well.

The method was evaluated on 137 digital hand radiographs, recorded with Agfa ADC cassettes and Agfa ADC-MD10 & ADC-MD30 imaging plates and irradiated by X-ray tubes Philips SRM 06 12 - ROT 500 or Siemens Bi 125/40 RL.

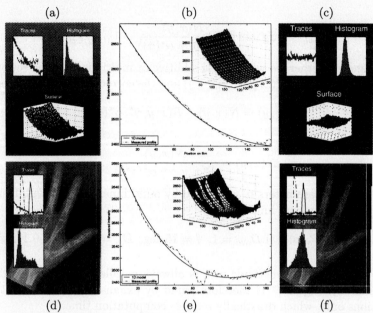

Fig. 3. (a) Flat field image (background) rendered as a surface (bottom) with histogram (top-right) and traces (top-left) along the anode-cathode axis (long solid line) and perpendicular to this axis (shorter dotted line). (b) Average projected data of the flat field (dotted line) and the fitted model (solid line). The sub-image contains back projected data (white grid) on top of the rendered background. (c) Same as (a) for the corrected image. (d) Same as (a) for the phantom image without the background surface and traces taken along the white lines. (e) Same as (b) for the phantom image. (f) Same as (d) for the corrected phantom image.

The images were downsampled by a factor 4 in each direcion to about 512×512 pixels. Visual inspection showed that the image partitioning algorithm was able to give very good estimates of the direct exposure, collimation and diagnostic areas for all images in our database, but erroneously includes some pixels of the soft tissue in the background region. Some results of the intensity correction are shown in Fig. 4. In the first image, the heel effect is clearly visible, while in the second example its presence can be detected from the increased background intensity at the bottom right of the images. For both cases the heel effect smears out the histogram of image background intensities, while after correction the background histogram is Gaussian distributed as it should. Specifying a histogram-derived threshold is sufficient to properly segment the hand after correction (top-right of each image), which is not possible for the original images due to the intensity overlap of diagnostic and background regions. Average computation time on a Pentium III 800MHz processor was 3 seconds, including image partitioning.

The possibly disturbing effect of introducing a hand in the image, thus including some soft tissue pixels coming from the partitioning algorithm and de-

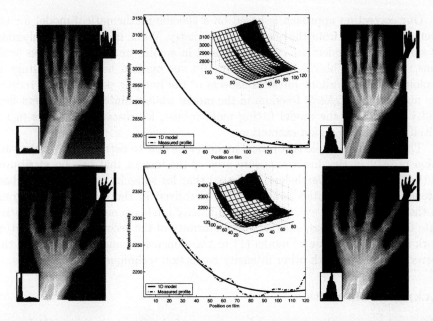

Fig. 4. Left column: original images with corresponding background histogram and histogram based background segmentation. Middle column: one-dimensional projection and back projected model fitted to the image data. Right column: corrected images with corresponding background histogram and histogram based background segmentation.

creasing the robustness of the estimated mean of the heel effect profile of (4), was examined by correcting the flat field image N_{ff} once with parameters computed from the flat field image itself R_{ff} and once with parameters computed from the phantom image R_{ph}. The reconstruction errors $\epsilon_{\mathrm{ff,ph}} = N_{\mathrm{ff}} - R_{\mathrm{ff,ph}}$ are very similar for both cases: $\langle\epsilon\rangle_{\mathrm{ff}} = -3.1$, $\sigma_{\epsilon} = 12.4$, range $(-46.7, 60.8)$ and $\langle\epsilon\rangle_{\mathrm{ph}} = -5.5$, $\sigma_{\epsilon} = 27.1$, range $(-63.9, 49.3)$ respectively, while the dynamic range of N was 800. This indicates that the algorithm can cope well with the presence of diagnostic regions when estimating the background inhomogeneity.

6   Discussion

We presented a fully automated method for heel effect correction of digital radiographs. We demonstrated the reliability of the method on a database of hand radiographs from which we could segment the hand very accurately by simple thresholding after inhomogeneity correction. The method is fast and reliable enough to be used for standardized image display on diagnostic workstations. It can also provide segmentation techniques with properly normalized images whose relative intensity differences are not disturbed by image inhomogeneities. We are currently investigating how this affects the specificity of intensity models constructed for Active Shape Model-based segmentation of the hand bones [2,3].

Our correction approach is based on a specific mathematical model for the heel effect derived from the acquisition geometry. While more general polygonal or spline-based models are commonly used in similar image rectification problems such as MR bias field correction [10], our method has the advantage to exploit knowledge about physical aspects of the imaging process. This reduces the number of degrees of freedom in the model while maintaining sufficient flexibility and makes the model fitting more robust, for instance to errors in the initial background region extraction.

The relatively simple theoretical model (1) is able to correct most of the variation present in the direct exposure area of the images that can be attributed to the heel effect. Nevertheless, we found that for some images in our database intensity inhomogeneities could also be perceived in the direction orthogonal to the anode-cathode axis. Moreover, intensity inhomogeneities may also originate from other sources, such as non-uniformity of the recording device. Future work includes extension of model (1) to two-dimensions and comparison of this correction method with other intensity correction techniques.

Acknowledgments

This work was partly supported by a grant of the Research Fund KU Leuven GOA/99/05 (Variability in Human Shape and Speech).

References

1. D. H. Ballard. Generalizing the hough transform to detect arbitrary shapes. *Pattern Recognition*, 13:111–122, 1981.
2. G. Behiels, D. Vandermeulen, F. Maes, P. Suetens, and P. Dewaele. Active shape model-based segmentation of digital X-ray images. Proc. MICCAI'99, Lecture notes in computer science, vol. 1679, pp. 128–137, 1999, Springer.
3. G. Behiels, D. Vandermeulen, and P. Suetens. Statistical shape model-based segmentation of digital x-ray images. In *IEEE Workshop on Mathematical Methods in Biomedical Image Analysis* (MMBIA'00), pp. 61–68, 2000.
4. S.N.C. Cheng, H.-P. Chan, L.T. Niklason, and R.S. Adler. Automated segmentation of regions of interest on hand radiographs. *Medical Physics*, 21(8):1293–1300, 1994.
5. S.L. Fritz and W.H. Livingston. A comparison of computed and measured heel effect for various target angles. *Medical Physics*, 9(2):216–219, 1982.
6. P. V. C. Hough. Methods and means for recognising complex patterns. U.S. Patent 3 069 654, 1962.
7. C. Kimme, D. Ballard, and J. Sklansky. Finding circles by an array of accumulators. In *Communications of the ACM*, vol. 18, pp. 120–122, 1975.
8. G. Manos, A. Y. Cairns, I. W. Ricketts, and D. Sinclair. Automatic segmentation of hand-wrist radiographs. *Image and Vision Computing*, 11(2):100–111, 1993.
9. J. A. Nelder and R. Mead. A simplex method for function minimization. *The Computer Journal*, 8:308–313, 1965.
10. K. Van Leemput, F. Maes, D. Vandermeulen, and P. Suetens. Automated model-based bias field correction of MR images of the brain. *IEEE Trans. Medical Imaging*, 18(10):885–896, 1999.

SCALPP: A Safe Methodology to Robotize Skin Harvesting

Gilles Duchemin[1], Etienne Dombre[1], François Pierrot[1], Philippe Poignet[1], and Eric Dégoulange[2]

[1] LIRMM UMR 5506 CNRS – UM2, 161 rue Ada, 34392 Montpellier Cedex 5, France
{duchemin, dombre, pierrot, poignet}@lirmm.fr
http://www.lirmm.fr
[2] SINTERS SA, BP 1311, Parc Technologique Basso Cambo, 5 Rue Paul Mesplé, 31106 Toulouse Cedex 1, France
eric.degoulange@tde.alstom.com
http://www.sinters.fr

Abstract. This paper deals with an ongoing research program in robotized reconstructive surgery (especially for skin harvesting) with a mechanical system under force control. The constraints of the process are firstly described in terms of medical and robotic constraints. Then, we present an active mechanical structure which suits to our needs whose interesting features are a simple and closed-form solution to the Inverse Geometric Model (IGM), the ability to handle the tool without collision and a simple mechanical design. In a third part, we present the application and the controller architecture from a working point of view and the force controller chosen. Finally general and particular safety issues for medical robots are discussed and solutions are presented to turn the application intrinsically safe.

1 Introduction

This paper deals with a new robotized medical application for reconstructive surgery with an original active arm, where force control is required.

For severely burnt patients (and for patients suffering from severe orthopedic problems leading to a loss of skin), strips of skin – the thinness ranges from 1/10 to 7/10 mm – are harvested on sound locations with a "shaver-like" device called dermatome (Fig. 1) and are grafted onto burnt locations. A dermatome is a simple mechanical device offering only two adjustable parameters: the blade speed which is modified thanks to a pedal, and the maximum cutting depth which is selected on the dermatome head (Fig. 1). This depth selection does not guarantee at all the actual cutting depth: depending on the user skill, for a given depth selection, the resulting skin strip thinness may range from the selected depth down to zero.

The practitioners used to a daily practice are able to properly perform these grafts. A great discipline in the gestures performed is necessary so as to both get a regular sampling and ascertain a quick healing of the donor area. This speed factor in the epidermis reformation is crucial when the need arises to resample the same area, particularly among the severely burnt population where donor areas are scarce. Many

W. Niessen and M. Viergever (Eds.): MICCAI 2001, LNCS 2208, pp. 309–316, 2001.
© Springer-Verlag Berlin Heidelberg 2001

surgeons having to perform these sampling gestures on an occasional basis –
Orthopedic-Trauma, Surgery, Maxilla-Facial Surgery, ENT Surgery – could be
interested in an automated technique avoiding such intra or postoperative hazards as
skin skipping, occurring when performing a gesture at the origin of unaesthetic scars
in the donor area, or else when performing too deep harvesting which entails difficult
problems of late healing. The robot is designed to help these non-specialized
practitioners, or those who are not performing these gestures on a daily basis.

The goal of this project[1] is then to embed part of a specialized surgeon skill in a
robotic system, called "Système de Coupe Automatisé pour Le Prélèvement de Peau"
(SCALPP), in order to bring this skill to other surgeons who do not practice
harvesting as a routine.

2   Problem Statement

As most human motion or action, a surgeon action consisting in harvesting skin may
be extremely difficult to model accurately [1]. First this is a motion in 3D space,
combined with quite important forces exerted on a non-modeled environment.
Moreover, there is no reason for two different surgeons to cut skin with the same
motion nor the same force (we verified this fact). Finally a surgeon may change his
action depending on his fatigue, and may also adapt his action according to the
patient. The surgeon motion can be divided into four stages (Fig. 1). The surgeon
begins to cut by pressing along z axis with the dermatome blade "not-parallel" to the
skin (the orientation angle of the dermatome blade may change, phase 1); then he
moves along x axis while placing the dermatome blade parallel to a plane tangent to
the skin (phase 2); next, he tries to keep the blade in this plane (phase 3); finally, he
frees the dermatome by a short motion of the hand (phase 4). During the third phase
(cutting phase), the force normal to the skin ranges from 40 N up to 100 N, and is
kept constant; moreover, the torque about x is roughly about zero, meaning that the
surgeon keeps the dermatome blade completely in contact with the skin.

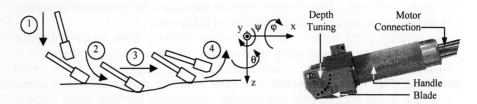

Fig. 1. Different phase of skin harvesting with a dermatome

During surgical operation, the patient is lying on an operating table. For asepsis
considerations, no non-medical equipment must be closer than 400 mm from the
operating table. Moreover, the robot must collide neither with the patient, nor with the
medical staff, nor with the anaesthetic pipes. In our experiment, skin harvesting is

[1] This work has been supported partly by funds from "Ministère de l'Education Nationale et de
la Recherche" and "Région Languedoc-Roussillon".

only considered on the thigh and the head. Indeed, skin harvesting is too much difficult under the armpit and the sole for a scarce result to be worth robotizing. Paths are described as follow: thighs where the path starts from the knee toward the hip or conversely; the length of the sample may vary from few mm to 400 mm (which corresponds to the whole length of a thigh); head, from the neck toward the forehead or conversely, on both sides of the skull. Therefore, due to the thigh zones, it is important to have symmetrical joint limits in order to not favor a thigh compared with the other. Since the surgeon has to manipulate the robot during teaching phase, a good accessibility to the dermatome handle is needed. Finally, note that it is mandatory to keep the robot base fixed for all paths on a given thigh (to avoid time consuming re-arrangement of the system). This motion analysis leads to robotic constraints developed below.

The robot should be able to move along a path, without crossing a singularity position, or without reaching its joints limits. Thus, the t-parcourability of the path (i.e. its continuity) has to be verified prior to start the process. Moreover, during a feasibility pre-study – achieved on pigs with a 7-dof Mitsubishi PA-10 robot, see [1] – we measured that forces involved may reached 100 N, which means that the driving motors should be quite bulky (especially on the wrist). Finally, for the sake of accuracy and safety, a closed-form solution for the IGM is preferred to a numerical algorithm, since its convergence depends on the initial conditions, leading to a non-predictive behavior. That's the reason why redundant robots or 6-dof robots whose IGM has to be solved with polynomial or numerical methods are discarded.

3   Arm Architecture

Under the various constraints mentioned in the previous section, a suitable architecture has been designed, selecting firstly the shoulder, and secondly a convenient wrist. The complete analysis can be found in [2], as well as all the geometric equations of the models.

Two types of shoulders have been considered: anthropomorphic and SCARA (Selective Compliance Assembly Robot Arm), either moving on a track fixed to the ceiling, or fixed to a support mounted on wheels and containing the controller (which provides compactness and stability of the system). A surgery room is usually cluttered with a series of medical equipment and many of them are hung on the ceiling; consequently, the surgeons required that no device would be added on the ceiling: that's the reason why we have discarded hung up shoulders. Anthropomorphic architectures present two main drawbacks for the application at hand: their workspace is spherical while a cylindrical one would be less wasteful; under gravity effects, the robot may collapse patient namely in case of power breakdown, which has to be avoided for safety reasons. To go further, a CAD study shown that it was easier to access all path points with a SCARA robot than with an anthropomorphic robot of equivalent link lengths. For these reasons, a SCARA architecture has been chosen as the shoulder of the robot.

Nevertheless, to avoid the classical singularity of spherical wrists when fully extended, other wrist designs have been investigated. An in-depth study [2] showed us that the non-spherical wrist presented on Fig. 2 fulfilled the four main constraints

312   G. Duchemin et al.

already mentioned in the previous section: absence of singularity in the workspace (the only one appears when q_5 reaches $\pm 90°$), a closed-form solution for the IGM asserted by Pieper's sufficient condition [3] (prismatic and revolute joints with collinear axis), no bulky motor, and sufficient joint position ranges (almost $\pm 90°$ on the fifth joint). Theoretically, four solutions result from the IGM computation, but two of them are out of the mechanical range limits. As a consequence, SCALPP robot features a single singularity in its workspace (the "classical" elbow singularity when q_3 equals $0°$) and a closed-form solution for the IGM (two configurations: "left-elbow" or "right-elbow"). Besides, it provides an easy access to the dermatome handle. Finally, with the Force/Torque (F/T) sensor, the force accuracy of the robot is 0.5 N, its maximum payload is 140 N and tool velocity is about 10 mm.s^{-1}.

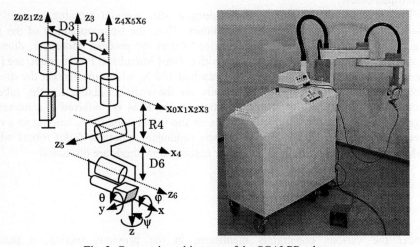

Fig. 2. Geometric architecture of the SCALPP robot

4   The SCALPP Robotic System

As mentioned earlier, SCALPP is a 6-dof SCARA arm with an User Interface (UI), a dedicated controller and a DMS foot pedal. Most of the technical devices come from our experience in specifying and designing robotic equipment [4]. The SCALPP system is fixed to a mobile support mounted on wheels and containing the controller. This last one contains 4 racks: a 550 MHz Pentium industrial PC running QNX^2 for the high level control; a rack including all the resolvers and translators boards for stepper motors control; a power supply unit; a logical unit formatting the I/O signals between user interface, switches, light signals and PC boards.

According to our experience with the Hippocrate system [4], the UI has been developed in close co-operation with physicians, in order to provide user-friendly tools to handle the robotic system. The UI consists of three main control structures. A console desk enables bilateral communications between user and robot. It is made up

---

^{2} A Real Time and Multitasking Operating System (RTMOS).

of three communication sets: control buttons to cancel or validate actions, decrement or increment force applied on skin and to control the arm (respectively esc., enter, - and +, start, free and reconfig.) and lights (powered, active and default). A LCD display indicates the current mode and the faults detected. A Dead Man Switch (DMS) pedal authorizes arm motions in automatic or manual modes (the modes where force control is required).

A detailed analysis of the robot working brought us to choose four functions modes, described bellow: a teaching (or manual) and an automatic modes for process constraints; a reconfiguration mode due to the arm architecture (i.e. its geometric structure); and for safety requirements, a free mode. Teaching mode allows physicians to teach the robot initial and final poses on skin. In this mode, the arm is compliant (the desire force is set to 0 N): the surgeon moves it by holding the dermatome handle and pushing on the DMS foot pedal. Each pose can be recorded or deleted by pressing + or - buttons. When all the points are recorded, the teaching sequence is confirmed or corrected by switching on the enter or esc. buttons. Once the teaching sequence has been recorded, the system switches in the automatic mode: the surgeon first selects a desired force for harvesting (from 0 to 100 N); then, as soon as he pushes on the DMS pedal, the robot begins the harvesting motion. Free mode enables the surgeon to move robot without force control thanks to the reversibility of the mechanism: any movement inside joint limits can be performed since no axes are controlled. This mode, activated by the surgeon by pressing the free button, can be used to place the arm in a "parking" position or to release the arm from the patient. Finally, the reconfiguration mode is selected to pass through arm singularity position: by pressing the reconfig. button, the user can change the arm position from a "left-elbow" to "right-elbow" configuration and conversely.

Since the application requires force control to move the arm in the teaching and automatic modes, the wrist is equipped with a F/T sensor (a laser telemeter is added to control the distance between the wrist and the skin to improve robot behavior when harvesting on the head). Force control schemes have been widely addressed in the past and state of art can be found for instance in [5]. An usual classification consists of dividing force control into two families: passive compliance and active compliance. The first one uses a deformable structure mounted at the arm tip, without force measurement. The second one allows to adapt the robot behavior according to the contact forces; there are three classes of active compliance control laws: without force measurement; with force measurement and without (like explicit force-feedback control); with force measurement and control (active stiffness [6], hybrid [7] and external [8] controls). Due to the task constraints a force control with force measurement is needed. So, we discarded all the controls without F/T sensor. Among the remaining controls, active stiffness and hybrid control have been discarded. Indeed, the first one uses the Jacobian matrix, which could induce numerical problems, and is carried out in joint space whereas our application is a Cartesian task. The second one enables either force control or position control along a direction. The external control (called also nested or cascade structure) is the only suitable force control for our application. Here again, different schemes can be proposed depending on the space where the summation of force and position components is achieved (joint or Cartesian association) and on the position control (joint control by IGM or Jacobian matrix, and Cartesian control). External control with Cartesian summation between force and position components and joint control by IGM have been chosen (Fig. 3). Moreover, the key advantages of external control can be summarized as follow [8]: the joint position servo loop is always activated, providing stability and avoiding switching between the position servo loop and the force control; it works very well with very simple and reliable (thus safe) control laws (like a PID at the joint level and a PI for the external force loop); it is easy to implement on any kind of controller; unless an effort is applied on the dermatome (below the force sensor), the robot will not move; at last, it allows designing the control software in an incremental manner, facilitating the tuning of the parameters and validation (internal joint control, external Cartesian space control with additional force control loop).

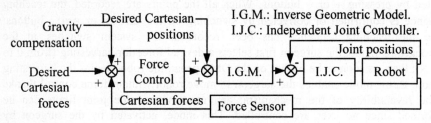

Fig. 3. External force control scheme

5   Safety Issues

A central issue when designing medical robots is safety since the robots cooperate with the surgeons and interact with patient. Consequently, introducing a robot in an operating room must fulfil some elementary rules. Most of these rules have been presented in [9] and [10]. We sum up here the most important ones: the robot should never "run away"; force applied on the patient must be well controlled; the surgeon must supervise the system at any time; the robot working area must be restricted; any automatic motion has to be run under control of a DMS pedal; it mustn't hurt patient, medical staff or instruments; it must be quickly and easily removable from the operating field. In order to satisfy these rules, special cares must be taken when designing mechanical, electrical and software components of the robot.

Thanks to a counterweight on the first axis to compensate gravity, no specific brakes are required. Moreover, the mobile support is counterbalanced to avoid any risk of falling over due to the force exerted during the operation and a locking system under the support prevents him to move once the robot has been placed. As far as actuators are concerned, a stepper technology has been selected; indeed, with conventional DC or AC motors, the rotation speed of the motor shaft depends on the output level of the servo amplifier. If a fault occurs, the motor still continues to rotate: the higher the output at the time of the failure, the faster the output shaft velocity. A stepper motor needs pulses to rotate. If the output of a translator is stuck at a constant value, the motor shaft would receive a holding torque which prevents him rotating. Basically, the output torque decreases as a function of the rotational velocity. Moreover, when the number of pulses per second or the acceleration are too high with respect to the motor type, the output torque is dropped down. Each motor has been chosen to minimize the power transmitted at the joint level and thus increase the safety of the robot. Joints 2 to 5 are equipped with two absolute resolvers, one mounted on the motor output shaft for fine position sensing and the other one mounted on the output reduction gear for coarse sensing of the joint location. While improving robot safety, the combination of the two resolvers suppresses time consuming and potentially hazardous initialisation procedures. The use of reduction gears allows to reduce output axis speed; harmonic drives have been chosen for their low backlash and flexibility and for their high efficiency.

The previous features make SCALPP arm an intrinsically safe mechanical device. We have added several hardware securities, providing very good reliability and safety to the whole system. A description of these securities is presented in the following. On the robot base, an emergency button allows to switch off the arm power in emergency case. The arm is powered on only when the software initialisation procedure is carried out and the emergency button is switched off. A watch-dog board has been developed in order to manage the security from a software point of view. If anything goes wrong in the high level controller, the cyclic signal sent to the watch-dog is stopped, inactivating it and switching off the power. Besides, in order to improve security, two redundant circuits have been wired on the card. Each external module – F/T sensor, laser telemeter and motors – is controlled by a specific board. Each of these boards is separately initialized and can detect a fault on the module: respectively disconnection, saturation, or incoherent data of the F/T sensor; laser measure out of range; tracking error during the arm motion, excessive velocity on a motor, translator or amplifier failure, arm close to the limit of workspace. Moreover, several working LEDs are present on the console desk and on the arm itself and signal to the user any working fault during the motion. Finally, an action on the DMS foot pedal is necessary to authorize a motion of the robot in `automatic` or `teaching` modes; besides, a new motion needs a new action on the pedal.

In addition to the mechanical and electrical securities, the high-level program has been built thanks to a software analysis based on security. The different solutions implemented are presented in this section. We chose the RTMOS QNX dedicated to real-time running on PC. Five processes are running, one for each specific function: security, function modes, force, communication and translators controls. They ran according to a Round-Robin mode and communicate thanks to shared-memory variables in data bases, each one can be read or written only by authorized processes. Of course, all the safety variables are taken into account with higher priority than the other ones. The sampling period of a process is tuned to 1 ms. As we have five processes, if the execution time constraint is respected (i.e. if the five processes are executed in 1 ms or less), the final sampling frequency correspond to 1 KHz. Moreover, every time a fault occurs, all the software and the hardware systems are initialized. Besides, in addition to the above mentioned hardware watch-dog, the dedicated security process checks the activity of the others ones. If anyone of these processes is locked, then the emergency procedure is switched on. In addition, in order to detect jamming of the dermatome blade which can occur during the skin

316   G. Duchemin et al.

harvesting (due for example to a bad lubrication of the mechanism), an algorithm based on a Fast Fourier Transform (FFT) has been implemented. It relies on the analysis of the dermatome noise, namely on the tracking of the resonance frequency of the blade. Finally, in case of a fault or if the DMS pedal is switched off during the automatic mode, different phases of clearing have been planed depending on whether blade is in contact with the skin or not.

6   Conclusion and Perspectives

In this paper, we have described our methodology to design and develop a safe active arm dedicated to skin harvesting. Taking into account several constraints, we designed a SCARA robot with a non-spherical wrist. The robot is force controlled. It is easy to operate thanks to a user-friendly interface. A particular care has been devoted to security at mechanical, electrical and software levels. We are currently at the experimental phase of the project: tests on silicon and on foam rubber (which roughly simulate skin) will be carried out, as well as validation on animals, cadavers before later in vivo graft harvesting.

References

1. Pierrot, F., et al.: Robotized reconstructive surgery: ongoing study and first results. Proc. IEEE Int. Conf. on Robotics and Automation, San Francisco, CA (2000) 1615-1620.
2. Duchemin, G., et al.: SCALPP: a 6-dof robot with a non-spherical wrist for surgical applications. Advances in Robot Kinematics, Piran-Portoroz, Slovenia (2000) 165-174.
3. Pieper, D.L.: The kinematics of manipulators under computer control. Ph. D. Thesis, Stanford University (1968).
4. Pierrot, F., et al.: Hippocrate: a safe robot arm for medical applications with force feedback. Medical Image Analysis (1999) 3(3) 285-300.
5. Yoshikawa, T.: Force Control of Robot Manipulators. Proc. IEEE Int. Conf. on Robotics and Automation, San Francisco, CA (2000) 220-226.
6. Salisbury, K.: Active Stiffness Control of a Manipulator in Cartesian Coordinates. Proc. of the 19th IEEE Conf. on Decision and Control, Albuquerque, New Mexico (1980) 95-100.
7. Pujas, A., et al.: Hybrid position/force control : task description and control scheme determination for a real implementation. IROS'93, Yokohama, Japan (1993) 841-846.
8. Perdereau, V., and Drouin, M.: A New Scheme for Hybrid Force-Position Control. Robotica, 11 (1993) 453-464.
9. Davies, A.: Safety of medical robots. Proc. of 6th ICAR, Tokyo, Japan (1993) 311-317.
10. Dombre, E., et al.: Intrisically safe active robotic systems for medical applications. Proc. of 1st IARP/IEEE-RAS Joint Workshop on Technical Challenge for Dependable Robots in Human Environments, Seoul, Korea (2001).

Surgical Motion Adaptive Robotic Technology (S.M.A.R.T): Taking the Motion out of Physiological Motion

Anshul Thakral, Jeffrey Wallace, Damian Tomlin, Nikesh Seth, and
Nitish V. Thakor

Department of Biomedical Engineering, Engineering Research Center for Computer
Integrated Surgical Systems and Technology
The Johns Hopkins School of Medicine, Baltimore, Maryland 21205 USA
nthakor@bme.jhu.edu

Abstract. In precision computer and robotic assisted minimally invasive surgical procedures, such as retinal microsurgery or cardiac bypass surgery, physiological motion can hamper the surgeon's ability to effectively visualize and approach the target site. Current day stabilizers used for minimally invasive cardiac surgery often stretch or pull at the tissue, causing subsequent tissue damage. In this study, we investigated novel means of modeling Z-axis physiological motion and demonstrate how these models could be used to compensate for this motion in order to provide a more stable surgical field. The Z-axis motion compensation is achieved by using a fiber-optic laser sensor to obtain precise displacement measurements. Using a weighted time series modeling technique, modeling of rodent chest wall motion and heart wall motion was accomplished. Our computational methods for modeling physiological motion open the door for applications using high speed, high precision actuators to filter motion out and provide for a stable surgical field.

1. Introduction

In order to perform accurate surgical procedures, surgeons need a well-exposed and immobilized target site. Creating a well-exposed bloodless surgical field is not as difficult as creating a motionless surgical field. Often moving organs, such as the beating heart, present an added challenge for surgeons to overcome the physiological motion. In cardiac surgery, the heart is traditionally stopped using cardiopulmonary bypass (CPB) to stop this motion. The use of CPB, however, causes many damaging effects to the patient's blood, and often leads to higher costs and recovery times [1]. Even with current day minimally invasive procedures, which are aimed to reduce blood trauma and post-operative complications [2], physiological motion can severely impair the ability of surgeon to effectively operate. During procedures such as minimally invasive direct coronary artery bypass (MIDCAB) surgery, or surgery on a beating heart, sutures placed by a surgeon often rip or tear due to the physiological motion of the heart, which can exceed 1.3 cm of outward expansion [3]. Several methods have been applied to this problem of dealing with motion in the surgical field

W. Niessen and M. Viergever (Eds.): MICCAI 2001, LNCS 2208, pp. 317-325, 2001.

in an attempt to eliminate the hindrances and try to increase the performance of the surgeon.

Current day commercial solutions to the problem of physiological motion involve the use of tissue stabilizers. These stabilizers either use pressure [4] or suction [5] on the tissue to achieve a psuedo-motionless environment. The stabilizers that work by means of pressure only work on grafting to the exterior surfaces of the heart. Suction methods often damage the myocardial tissue, even when used for short periods of time [6]. The use of motion platforms that moves the surgeon's hands in synchrony with either a set of oscillatory motors and pacing the heart [3], or optical and mechanical sensors with feedback [6] have been published. These methodologies have shown that surgeons can perform delicate tasks, such as anastomosis on a moving surface, but include hindrances such as being cumbersome, or invasive.

The ideal solution for motion compensation during surgical procedures would be to provide motion-tracking capabilities using algorithms to filter out the motion, while using high precision robotic systems through minimally invasive ports.

We propose a solution involving the use of novel adaptive motion tracking algorithms to compensate for periodic and quasi-periodic physiological motions. Adaptive filtering, which has been around since the 1950's to study periodic signals [7], allows modeling of the physiological information in an updateable model. By obtaining the tissue surface displacement measurements, we are able to create adaptive models of the both chest wall and heart wall motion from a surgically prepared rodent. In this paper, we compare several different adaptive algorithms and are able to determine the characteristics and uses of the algorithms for the motion compensation problem. Although it is beyond the scope of our experiments, given these adaptive models, a high speed robotic actuator would be able to compensated for the motion by using the models as a motion predictor, and keeping the tissue surface approximately still from the perspective of the tool on the robotic actuator.

2. Methods

A. Rat Chest Wall and Heart Wall Model

In order to simulate physiological motion for our algorithms, rodent chest wall and heart wall motion was exposed during our surgical procedure. To provide controlled breathing patterns, the test subjects (8 Wistar rats, 300 ± 25g) underwent anesthesia and were placed on ventilator systems for intubation. The subjects were anesthetized with 4% halothane and 50:50% nitrous oxide:oxygen, in a small place chamber. Once unconsciousness, the rats was placed in a supine position and two needle electrodes were inserted in the arm and leg of the rat to provide an electrocardiogram (ECG) for reference purposes.

For chest wall motion measurements, the chest of the rat was shaved to provide a smooth and clean surface for measurement. The recording instrumentation was placed next to the rodent, with the extension arm and displacement sensor placed directly 1cm above the chest. Measurements were taken for 2 minutes intervals and repeated 3 times before the sensor was moved to a different portion of the chest. To keep the data synchronized with the ECG data, it was recorded via the same A/D converter and Pentium level computer.

After the chest wall measurements were concluded, the rats were subjected to partial thoracothomy on the left side, about halfway down the ribcage, to provide access to the heart. After this was completed, the heart could be seen and the fiber optic probe attached to the instrumentation could be carefully inserted to within 1cm of the heart wall. Again, measurements were taken for 2 minute intervals and repeated 3 times before recording from a different angle.

B. Instrumentation Setup

For our experiments, we used a M-511 series linear stage micropositioner from Physik Instruments (Waldbronn, Germany), which provides 0.1 micrometer minimum incremental motion and a one micrometer full travel accuracy, as our micropositioner and the basis for our microsurgical robotic arm for recording. This microsurgical robotic arm consists of the micropositioner, a base with an x-z brace that allows for a z-axis setup, an extension arm, and a mount for the displacement sensor (Figure 1). The arm was extended 18 inches out from the faceplate of the M-511, and the fiber optic probe was held in place to record the displacement.

For the recording of biological tissue displacement, we used a D169 fiber optic displacement sensor from Philtec, Inc. (Annapolis, MD USA), which has a linear measurement range of 0.8 to 21.6 mm, with an operating resolution of 3.18μm. The output of the sensor provided a 0 to 5 V analog signal that was directly proportional to the distance being measured. The output was calibrated with a simple $y = m(x) + b$ equation, using several known distances and a simple best fit algorithm.

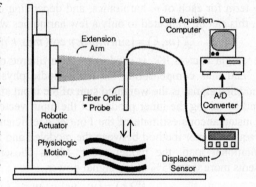

Figure 1: The data acquisition setup for our experiments. The fiber optic probe used to record physiologic motion, was positioned and calibrated with the use of the robotic actuator depicted above.

The analog signal from the fiber optic sensor was converted into a digital signal with the use of a Daytronic 2160 Digital Panel Meter (Daytronic Inc, Dayton, Ohio). The digital signal was then transferred to a computer for recording through a RS232 serial port. The acquisition software was written on a Windows 9X platform using Visual C++ (Microsoft, Redmond, WA.) and the analysis was performed in MATLAB (Mathworks, Natick, MA).

C. Adaptive Algorithms

Adaptive filters and algorithms have been around since the late 1950's as a type of self-learning filter [7]. These filters have a set of predetermined initial conditions, and are able to learn input statistics progressively, and adjust its coefficients in order to minimize error criterion.   In static environment, these filters converge to optimum "Wiener" filters after successive iterations [8].   Windrow and Hoff's least mean square (LMS) algorithm is one of the most widely used adaptive filters [9].

Certain physiological motions, such as heart wall and chest wall motion in our experiments, can be modeled as periodic signals that repeat consistently with a set reference, such as heart beat or respiratory rate.   A discrete Fourier series model (FSM) can be used to represent the periodic components of certain physiological motions [10].   In the FSM equation (Equation 1), w_o is the fundamental frequency, M is the model order required to cover the entire signal bandwidth, and $\{a_m, b_m\}$ are the mth Fourier coefficients of the periodic signal.   The assumption here is that physiological motion can be broken down into discrete sinusoidal components and then can be recomposed by summing weighted versions of the sinusoids.

$$s(k) = \sum_{m=1}^{M} a_m \sin(m\omega_0 k) + b_m \cos(m\omega_0 k) \qquad (1)$$

In the Fourier Linear Combiner (FLC) algorithm, the reference signal is comprised of different harmonics of the defined fundamental frequency (Equation 2).   The reference signal is used to create a model of the input signal. X_k consists of a sine and cosine term for each of m harmonics, and depending on the model order of our input signal, this can be truncated to only a few harmonics without significant distortion.

$$\underline{X}(m,k) = [\sin(m\omega_0 k); \cos(m\omega_0 k)]^T \qquad ; m = 1,..,M \qquad (2)$$

The weight vector, Wk, is used to create a filtered output that models the observed signal, and thus compensating for the periodic physiological motion (Equation 3). The modeled signal is the weighted sum of the input sinusoids, thus the filtered output is found by taking the inner product of the input vector and the weight vector, which is the instantaneous estimate of the Fourier coefficients.   Weights are updated using mean squared error method between the modeled and reference signal.   To reduce the computational load, the model order, M, is chosen so that the truncated series represents more than 95% of the signal power.

$$\underline{W}(k) = [w_1, w_2,...,w_{2M-1}, w_{2M}]^T \qquad (3)$$

The FLC algorithm has been shown to be computationally inexpensive as compared to other adaptive filter [11], have inherently zero phase [12], and has an infinite null [13].   FLC can be viewed as an adaptive notch filter at w_0, with width equal to the adaptive gain parameter, m [13].   The time constant of the filter is a representation of its memory, or the number of sample points it "remembers" in order to compute the estimates.

The FLC, however, operates at a fixed frequency, and cannot compensate for changes in both frequency and amplitude.   The Weighted Frequency Fourier Linear Combiner (WFLC) forms a dynamic truncated Fourier series model of the desired input signal, and adapts to frequency of the model as well as the Fourier coefficients [14].   The fundamental frequency in the FLC algorithm, w_0, is replaced by a set of adaptive frequency weights, w_{0k}.   Thus the modeled signal is no longer represented by inner product of the weights and reference signal, but by Equation 4.   Using the simplified approach underlying the LMS algorithm, an adaptive recursion for w_{0k} can be created in the same amount of time using Equation 5.   An adaptive gain parameter, μ_0, has been added to the frequency weights in order to tune the filter.   Equation 5 is used to update the frequency weights, and the rest of the algorithm proceeds similar to the FLC algorithm. It has been published that for small enough m_0, w_{0k} actually converges to the frequency of the sinusoidal input signal [15]

$$\hat{d}(k) = \sum_{r=1}^{M} [w_{rk} \sin(rw_{0k}k) + w_{r+Mk} \cos(rw_{0k}k)] \qquad (4)$$

$$w_{0_{k+1}} = w_{0_k} - 2\mu\varepsilon_k \frac{\partial \varepsilon_k}{\partial w_{0_k}} \qquad (5)$$

In cases like ours, it is important to have a fast tracking algorithm with minimal misadjustment, to avoid the loss of data. To accomplish this, we added a variable step size LMS algorithm [16] to our adaptive algorithm to create an Adaptive Fourier Linear Combiner (AFLC). The gain parameter, μ in Equation 5, is now represented by a dynamic gain parameter, μ_k as in Equation 6 and is adjusted by square of the prediction error. Since only one more update in needed is each step of the algorithm, the AFLC algorithm is only minimally more complex than the FLC algorithm, but has adaption capabilities.

$$\underline{W}_{k+1} = \underline{W}_k + 2\mu_k e_k \underline{X}_k \qquad (6)$$

For applications, involving complex signals, neither the AFLC Algorithm nor WFLC algorithm alone can compensate for such a signal. To solve this, we employed a technique that uses both the AFLC algorithm and WFLC, in order to model the signal, named the Tiered Fourier Linear Combiner (TFLC) algorithm. In this algorithm, the recorded signal passes through an AFLC routine, which results in a modeled chest wall signal and an error component. This error component is then passed through a WFLC routine to result in a modeled heart wall signal. The two modeled signals are then simply combined to produce the modeled version of the original complex signal.

3. Results and Discussion

A. Characterization of the FLC and WFLC Algorithm for Rat Heart Wall Data

A 30 second segment of the rat heart wall data is run through the FLC algorithm. Trials were run for model order (M) set at 2nd, 3rd, and 4th order. For each value of M, the data was iterated through a series of μ values, which are the adaptive gain factor, and the resulting percent error was recorded. This data is summarized in Figure 2, where we can see that as expected, increasing the μ value helps reduce the error signal. Also we see that at higher μ values, increasing the model order helps lower the percent error; however at lower μ values the difference within model orders is not as significant.

To better understand the advantages of the WFLC over the FLC, the data used in Figure 2 were analyzed using the WFLC algorithm, where the recorded ECG signal is set to the reference signal. The data are summarized in Figure 3, where we can see a drop in percent error with an increase in μ values. With the WFLC algorithm, however, the model order M does not have as much of an effect. The WFLC algorithm's performance is more independent of model order then the AFLC algorithm. Also, we see that with the WFLC algorithm we are able to achieve a lower percent error than with the FLC algorithm, at all model orders.

B. WFLC and TFLC Algorithms Performance Under Varying Signal to Noise Ratios

The efficiency of the AFLC algorithm is dependent on the signal to noise (SNR) ratio of the input signal. In order to determine the performance of the algorithms, we simulated signals with varying SNR. To generate signals with varying SNR, we used recorded pure chest wall (left side of the rat's chest) as the signal, and recorded data of the rat's heart wall to represent the noise on the heart wall. By varying the amplification of the 'noise', several different signals of different SNR were created. Figure 4 shows the performance of the WFLC algorthm compared to the TFLC for different SNR input signals. For the higher SNR signal (Figure 4a), the TFLC had an mean error of 10.3%, while the WFLC resulted in a 12.3% error.

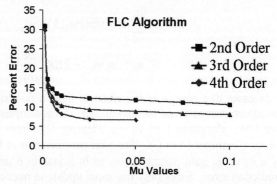

Figure 2: By increasing the value of the adaptation variable μ, the performance of the FLC algorithm was tested for three different M orders (2nd, 3rd, and 4th)

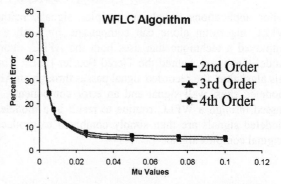

Figure 3: Performance analysis of the WFLC algorithm for different values of μ and different M orders (2nd, 3rd, and 4th). Unlike the FLC algorithm, the WFLC's performance is not as dependent on the order of M.

For the lower SNR case (Figure 4b), the TFLC resulted in a 23.1% error, while the WFLC resulted in a 34.1% error. In both cases, the TFLC outperforms the other showing its resilience within a noisy environment.

C. Modeling of Complex Signal with the TFLC Algorithm

We used chest wall recordings from over the heart as a complex signal to be modeled by the TFLC algorithm. The biological motion recorded by the fiber optic sensor is considered complex because it contains both motion from the respiration and motion from the heart wall underneath the surface of the skin. By taking the FFT of the recorded data from the complex motion, two strong spikes were seen in the spectral plot. The stronger of the two spikes is seen at 0.6 Hz and the second non-harmonic spike was at 5.5 Hz. From this observation, we can see both the chest wall as well as

(A)

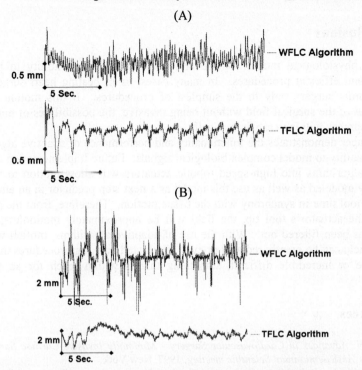

(B)

Figure 4: The comparison of the AFLC and TLC algorithms under different signal to noise ratios (SNR). For the high SNR case (A) where the SNR is –4 dB, the TFLC has a mean error of 10.3% while the WFLC has a mean error of 12.3%. For the low SNR case (B), where the SNR is –9 dB, the TFLC has a mean error of 23.1% and the WFLC has a mean error of 34.1%. In both cases, the TFLC outperforms the WFLC, even in noisy environments (low SNR).

the heart wall motion in the signal. The 0.6 Hz signal corresponds to the chest wall (respiration was set at 45 breaths per minute) and the 5.5 Hz component corresponds to the heart wall motion, (5.5 Hz was the primary frequency in the recorded ECG signal). Modeling the signal using the TFLC algorithm resulted in a signal that had a mean error of only 10%. Figure 5 show the modeled signal plotted with the recorded signal that was used. As demonstrated with this model, even with a complex biological signal, the TFLC can model the signal to a high accuracy.

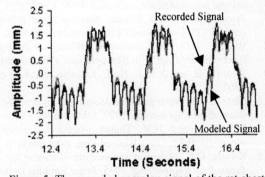

Figure 5: The recorded complex signal of the rat chest wall and heart wall displayed with the resulting modeling signal. The model was generated with the TFLC algorithm.

4. Conclusions

Complex physiological motion can severely limit a surgeon's ability to perform accurate and efficient procedures. In many cases, as in beating heart surgery, the motion limits surgery only to the simplest of procedures. If this motion can be filtered out of the surgical field without being invasive, the possibilities of minimally invasive surgery will increase dramatically.

This paper demonstrates the functionality and performance of adaptive algorithms and their ability to model complex biological signals. Future implementation of these adaptive algorithms into high-speed robotic actuators will allow motion to be both adaptively modeled as well as use this model as a next step predictor in an attempt to move the tool time in synchrony with the tissue motion. Therefore, from the point of view of the actuator's tool tip, the field will be approximately motionless, as the motion has been filtered out. With the use of adaptive algorithms, motion within a surgical field can be greatly reduced or even eliminated, making procedures that were impossible or incredible difficult, something that is within reach for an average surgeon.

References

1. Ko, W. *Advances in Cardiovascular Surgery - Minimally Invasive Cardiac Surgery.* in *1997 CAMS Semiannual Scientific meeting.* 1997. New York.
2. Matsuda, H., *et al., Minimally Invasive Cardiac Surgery: Current Status and Perpective.* Artificial Organs, 1998. 22(9): p. 759-64.
3. Mayer, P.W., *Relative Motion Cancelling,* in *Patent No. 5871017.* 1999: US.
4. Rousou, J.A., *et al., Fenestrated felt facilitates anastomotic stability and safety in & "off-pump" coronary bypass.* Ann Thorac Surg, 1999. 68(1): p. 272-3.
5. Jansen, E.W.L., *et al., Coronary Artery Bypass Grafting Without Cardiopulmonary Bypass Using the Octopus Method: Results in the First One Hundred Patients.* The Journal of Thoracic and Cardiovascular Surgery, 1998. 116(1): p. 60-67.
6. Trejos, A.L., *et al. On the Feasibility of a Moving Support for Surgery on the Beating Heart.* in *Medical Image Computing and Computer-Assisted Intervention - MICCAI'99: Second International Conference.* 1999. Cambridge, UK.
7. Widrow, B. and S.D. Stearns, *Adaptive signal processing.* Prentice-Hall signal processing series. 1985, Englewood Cliffs: Prentice-Hall. xviii, 474.
8. Walter, D.O., *A posteriori Wiener Filtering of average evoked responses.* Electroencephalogr Clin Neurophysiol, 1968. :Suppl(27): p. 61+.
9. Widrow, B. and J. M.E. Hoff. *Adaptive switching circuites.* in *IRE WESCON Conv. Rec.* 1960.
10. Metz, S., *An Intraoperative Monitoring System for the analysis of Evoked Potentials,* in *Biomedical Engineering.* 1999, Johns Hopkins University: Baltimore. p. 159.
11. Vaz, C.A. and N.V. Thakor, *Adaptive Fourier estimation of time-varying evoked potentials.* IEEE Trans Biomed Eng, 1989. 36(4): p. 448-55.
12. Riviere, C.N., *Adaptive suppression of tremor for improved human-machine control.,* in *Biomedical Engineering.* 1995, Johns Hopkins Univesity: Baltimore, Md.
13. Vaz, C., X. Kong, and N.V. Thakor, *An adaptive estimation of periodic signals using a Fourier linear combiner.* IEEE Transactions in Signal Processing, 1994. 42: p. 1-10.
14. Riviere, C.N., R.S. Rader, and N.V. Thakor, *Adaptive canceling of physiological tremor for improved precision in microsurgery.* IEEE Trans Biomed Eng, 1998. 45(7): p. 839-46.

15. Gresty, M. and D. Buckwell, *Spectral analysis of tremor: understanding the results.* J Neurol Neurosurg Psychiatry, 1990. 53(11): p. 976-81.
16. Kwong, R. and E. Johnston, *A Variable Step Size LMS Algorithm.* IEEE Transactions in Signal Processing, 1992. 40(7): p. 1633-1642.

TER: A System for Robotic Tele-echography

Adriana Vilchis Gonzales[1], Philippe Cinquin[1], Jocelyne Troccaz[1], Agnès Guerraz[2],
Bernard Hennion[2], Franck Pellissier[2], Pierre Thorel[2], Fabien Courreges[3,4],
Alain Gourdon[3], Gérard Poisson[3], Pierre Vieyres[3], Pierre Caron[4], Olivier Mérigeaux[4],
Loïc Urbain[4], Cédric Daimo[5], Stéphane Lavallée[5], Philippe Arbeille[6], Marc Althuser[7],
Jean-Marc Ayoubi[7], Bertrand Tondu[8], Serge Ippolito[8]

[1]TIMC/IMAG lab, Faculté de Médecine, Domaine de la Merci, F-38706 La Tronche cedex
[2]France Telecom R&D, 28 chem du vieux Chêne BP 98, F-38243 Meylan cedex
[3]Laboratoire Vision et Robotique, 63 avenue de Lattre de Tassigny, F-18020 Bourges cedex
[4]SINTERS, BP1311, F-31106 Toulouse cedex 01
[5]PRAXIM, Le Grand Sablon, 4 av. de l'Obiou, F-38700 La Tronche
[6]CHU Trousseau, Unité de Médecine et Physiologie Spatiale, F-37044 Tours
[7]CPDPN, CHU de Grenoble, BP 217, F-38043 Grenoble cedex 9
[8]LESIA, Electrical and CS Eng. Dept., INSA, Campus de Rangueil, F-31077 Toulouse
- France -
jocelyne.troccaz@imag.fr

Abstract. The quality of ultrasound based diagnosis highly depends on the operator's skills. Some healthcare centres may not have the required medical experts on hand when needed and therefore may not benefit from highly specialized ultrasound examinations. The aim of this project is to provide a reliable solution in order to perform expert ultrasound examinations in distant geographical areas and for the largest population possible. TER is a tele-robotic system designed and developed by a French consortium composed of universities, hospitals and industrial companies. One originality of TER is the development of a compliant slave robot actuated by muscles. This slave robot is tele-operated by an expert clinician who remotely performs the exam. In this paper, we present the architecture of TER and describe its components.

Introduction

Echography is a difficult examination based on specialized skills. The clinician performing the examination moves the echographic probe on the patient's body to acquire noisy bi-dimensional images. He may perform his diagnosis from static measurements performed on these images and/or from a dynamical behaviour analysis of the organs for instance depending on the pressure exerted by the probe on the body. This is typically the case when diagnosing the presence of thromboses in the lower limbs. Therefore, performing such an examination involves a good eye-hand coordination and the ability to integrate the acquired information over time and space. Some of these highly specialized skills may lack in some healthcare centres or for emergency situations. Tele-consultation is therefore an interesting alternative to conventional care.

W. Niessen and M. Viergever (Eds.): MICCAI 2001, LNCS 2208, pp. 326-334, 2001.

State of the Art

Several projects have been launched worldwide for developing tele-echography. In France, the LOGINAT project [1] based on a multi-centres Visio-conferencing basis has been experimented since 1993 for inter-hospital perinatal care. The project evolved from real-time transmission of the exams to the transmission of static images and related documents. This evolution was due to the limited performance of communication networks at that time. The objective of the TeleinVivo European project [2] was to develop a portable station to allow echographic exams in isolated regions. With a 3D ultrasound probe, a volume of data can be sent to a remote expert who, using a virtual ultrasound sensor, can examine the data in much the same way that he would examine a patient.

Such projects are basically tele-medicine ones. The operator has still to perform the exam on the patient even if he can be guided by the expert; moreover the expert has to perform the diagnosis on a purely visual basis. From our point of view, a tele-echography system has to integrate the ability for the expert to remotely move the echographic probe. The SYRTECH system [3,4] was developed in this spirit. The echographic probe is mounted on a 3 degree of freedom (dof) robot. This system is positioned manually on the patient by an operator. To explore the anatomical region of interest, the 3 rotations are remotely controlled by the expert using a virtual probe which motions are tracked by a magnetic localizer. SYRTECH has been demonstrated by performing from France remote exams on a man participating to a Nepalese expedition. Another system for US tele-intervention and laparoscopic ultrasound tele-manipulation was studied within the MIDSTEP European project [5]. MIDSTEP integrates conventional robotic architectures. Salcudean [6] describes a light robot developed for the assistance of diagnostic ultrasound system; three control schemes have been implemented and tested: motion and force controls and visual servoing. Similarly, [7,8] present HIPPOCRATE, a hybrid force-position controlled robot for assisted echographic diagnosis; such a robot could potentially be integrated in a tele-echography application. Finally, [9] proposes a very original parallel architecture for tele-robotic echography.

Most of these systems are still under development and have been partly validated. For some of them, a specific slave robot has been designed preferring safety and natural compliance to accuracy. This is acceptable because the accuracy requirements are generally lower for tele-robotic echography than for surgical applications; moreover, the operator closes the loop and may compensate for positional errors.

Global Specifications and System Architecture

Figure 1 illustrates the global architecture of TER. A virtual probe is mounted on the master interface device. The real probe is placed on the slave robot end-effector. Position and force information are transmitted bi-directionally. Live visual and audio data are also transmitted in both directions. The system is initialised to match the two environments. Then, mainly based on the echographic images and force information he receives back, the expert operator can move the virtual probe to control the real one. The slave robot executes the orders sent from the master site. A non expert operator is located close to the patient and supervises the procedure that he can interrupt. The patient can at any time communicate with him or with the expert. TER is designed to be used with low-bandwidth widespread networks in order to make it usable on a large scale.

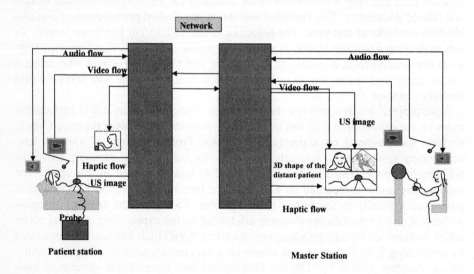

Fig. 1. TER general architecture

TER is under development. The following paragraphs describe the different components and their status of development.

Master System

To accurately reproduce the expert hand movement and the displacement of the ultrasound virtual probe, two solutions of different cost and complexity are being considered and tested. The first one uses a position sensor associated with visual feedback. The other one uses an haptic device that adds force feedback.

Master Position-Based Interface Device

In this version of the master interface device, a magnetic position device is used to track the virtual probe: the Flock of Bird (FOB) localizer from Ascension Technology. This magnetic tracker is a six degree-of-freedom measuring device that can be configured to simultaneously track position and orientation within a ± 130 cm range from the transmitter. A sensor is affixed to the probe.

A second version of this position-based interface system is currently designed in order to integrate a one-direction force feedback rendering to the distant expert the pressure exerted back from the body to the probe.

Master Haptic-Based Interface Device

The haptic-based interface device integrates a SensAble PHANToM haptic system. This device has 6 dof and renders a 3D force information. It can track the position and orientation of the tool within a workspace of 16 cm wide, 13 cm high and 13 cm deep. The maximum exertable force is 6.4 Newton.

The project constraints on the master workstation site are mainly real time information feedback and geometric modelling of the remote patient.

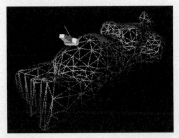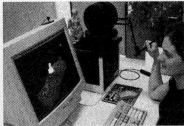

Fig. 2. Master interface device: (left) the local model and (right) the master haptic-based interface device on use

A 3D geometric model of the remote patient is coded with a polygonal mesh. The model is very useful to guarantee a force feedback at a fixed rate compatible with the gesture of the expert. The mesh results from the deformation of standard meshes already recorded and depending on the examination type. For a given patient, the mesh will be re-calculated thanks to registration from measurements on the patient (see [10] for more details). Remarkable points or surface data may be acquired before the exam using the slave robot with a process of tele-calibration[1].

The force feedback is calculated starting from a physical model of the virtual 3D shape. Force feedback computations are refreshed by measurements coming from the slave platform. In the model, the material point is heavy, elastic and viscous. The state of the material point is governed by mechanical equations. The virtual model of the patient is flexible and deformable and its mechanic characteristics - viscosity, stiffness, and mass - can be adjusted. The computation of forces from the contact location may be based (1) on the vertices of the 3D geometric model, or (2) according to the nearest polygon to the contact or (3) integrating its neighbourhood. The third solution is the best one. Experiments and results using this haptic control are encouraging and very realistic on the touch and feel level.

---

[1] Tele-calibration is a process making it possible to gauge an object or a distant 3D form with the help of the haptic flow.

The Slave Robot

Mechanical Architecture

We can roughly decompose the echographic examination in two stages. One stage consists in exploring a large region of the body to localize the structure of interest. During these gross motions, control accuracy is not mandatory. In the second stage, the clinician locally explores the detected structure. These fine motions are mostly composed of rotations relatively to the contact surface of the probe. Therefore, it was reasonable to decouple translation and rotation dof. The TER slave robot is based on two parallel kinematic architectures and on artificial muscle actuation.

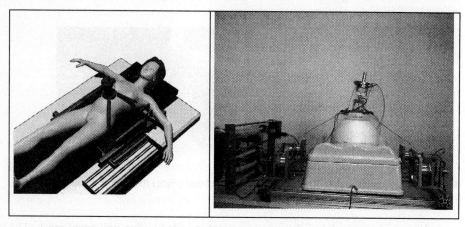

Fig. 3. The slave robot: (left) a sketch of the robot in use - (right) the prototype

As it can be seen on figure 3, a first parallel structure mounted on the consultation bed is composed of four antagonistic muscles enabling translations. They are connected to a ring supporting the probe and the other dof: this second parallel structure is also actuated by four muscles enabling the 3D orientation of the probe and fine translations. Both subsystems can be controlled simultaneously.

Pneumatic Artificial Muscles

The robot is entirely motorized with pneumatic artificial muscles commonly called McKibben artificial muscles. The McKibben muscle was invented in the 1950s to actuate pneumatic arm orthotics [11]; it was redesigned in the 1980s by Bridgestone engineers to obtain more powerful behaviour. The McKibben muscle now appears like one of the most original solution to give a robot a human-like joint softness which is not present in classical industrial robots, and consequently to develop "friendly robots" fully adapted to the new needs of service robotics [12].

The McKibben muscle is made of a thin rubber tube covered with a shell braided according to helical weaving as shown in figure 5. The muscle is closed by two ends, one being the air input and the other the force attachment point. When the inner tube is pressurized to a given pressure P, the flexible pantograph network of the textile shell converts circumferential pressure forces into an axial contraction force which reduces the muscle length while its radius increases.

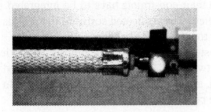 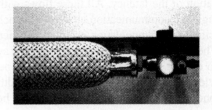

Fig. 4. McKibben muscle: (left) Initial contraction state, (right) maximum contraction state.

McKibben artificial muscles behave like a spring with a variable stiffness directly controlled by pressure P, in analogy with the natural skeletal muscle controlled by the nervous activation as it is expressed in the classical tension-length diagram [13]. This spring character gives to the McKibben muscle its specific softness which can be called "natural compliance". The second aspect of the fundamental analogy between McKibben muscle and natural muscle is that in a given equilibrium position, it is possible to adapt the muscle force and the muscle stiffness by changing the control pressure. This double property of natural compliance and force/stiffness adaptation, combined with a closed-loop control in position or an hybrid position/force control, must lead to an accurate positioning of the probe while controlling the contact force on the body of the patient.

Up to now, the prototype has been designed and realized. It has been modelled and its kinematics has been simulated. Low level control schemes have been implemented for the muscles and tested. [14] reports these experiments.

Communication

The Telecom Flows

As can be seen on figure 1, different flows are necessary in the TER system. Each of these flows requires a specific transmission quality that will be discussed below.

The Visio phonic communication quality has to be as good as possible in order to facilitate the relationship between the patient and local operator and the expert. This includes: high quality bi-directional audio throughput and good transmission of the scene. Specific codec broad are used for this flow. The quality of the medical images that have to be transmitted depends on the phase of the exam: low quality is sufficient for the gross motion phase: high quality may be necessary for fine exploration; high quality is necessary for diagnosis and measurements. Compression algorithms based on wavelet transforms prove to be the best compromise between the image quality, the compression rate and the coding time (cf. [15]). The need for quality may be incompatible with the goal of low bandwidth network and indeed may restrict the application field. Specific codec broad are used for this flow on the remote site. The haptic control flow does not need high bandwidth but low end-to-end latency and very low variation of the latency. All these flows with their constraints have to be integrated in a single telecommunication channel. It is achieved by dedicated software that builds a specific telecommunication protocol in order to allow priority between flows.

The goal of low cost and widely usable system toward French healthcare centre led us to choose, in a first step, native ISDN networking. This telecommunication media provides good guaranty in term of bandwidth, stability of the latency, low latency. In a second step, Next Generation Internet will be considered.

Tele Gesture

We must take into account the physiological constraints of human gesture to make the tele-gesture possible. The haptic loop has to be fed at a frequency of 1kHz because below vibrations would be perceived making the gesture more difficult. We use the local model of the distant patient to calculate the force feedback at this rate. The network will feed the expert master interface device with real measurements at a lower rate. We experimented the transmission of haptic data on the ISDN network. These experiments were performed using two PHANToM systems communicating via the network. Each device sends its position and receives the position of the distant device. We tested the initialisation and shut down of the haptic session, the transmission of the position to the distant device, and the calculation of the efforts at 1khz with a data refresh at the reception with various rates ranging from 10 to 500ms. The first experimental results are reported in table 1.

Table 1. Transmission experiments using the ISDN network

Sample (ms)	10	100	250	500
Flow	100Hz	10Hz	4Hz	2 Hz
Haptic behaviour	Very good	Good	Some vibrations	Some vibrations and oscillations
Command ability	Natural	Restricted in term of the gesture speed	Difficult	Very difficult
Conclusion	Realistic	Realistic for slow gestures	Need to set up finer extrapolators of gesture	Need to set up finer extrapolator and stabilizer of gesture

Conclusion

In this paper, we have presented a system for tele-robotic echography. It combines a master station with or without force feedback with a slave robot which actuation through McKibben artificial muscles makes it naturally compliant. Some elements of the master station are operational. The slave robot has been designed and realized. Low-level control has been implemented. The tele-communication issues related to the transmission of gestures and images have been studied and experimented on an ISDN network. A lot remains to be done concerning system integration and evaluation before assessing that the objective of performing remote echography is reached; nevertheless we think that the development of original robotic architectures and tele-gesture capabilities are already very positive deliverables of such a project.

Acknowledgements

This project is supported by the French Ministry of Research and Technology (action line "ACI Telemédecine"), by France Telecom R&D and by UAEM/CONACyT.

References

[1] on line http://www.irisi-nordpasdecalais.org/acercles/loginat.htm
[2] on line http://www.crcg.edu/projects/teleinvivo.html
[3] A. Gourdon, P. Vieyres, Ph. Poignet, M. Szpieg, Ph. Arbeille, "A tele-scanning robotic system using satellite", in EMBC99 Proceedings, Vienna, November 1999.
[4] A. Gourdon, Ph. Poignet, G. Poisson, P.Vieyres, P.Marché, "A new robotic mechanism for medical application, Proceedings ASME, Atlanta Georgia, September 1999.
[5] D. de Cunha, P. Gravez, C Leroy, E. Maillard, J. Jouan, P Varley, M Jones, M Halliwell, D. Hawkes, P. N. T. Wells, L. Angelini, "The MIDSTEP System for Ultrasound guided Remote Telesurgery", in Proceedings of 20th International Conference of the IEEE Engineering in Medicine and Biology Society. pp 1266 - 1269, 1998
[6] S.E. Salcudean, G. Bell, S. Bachmann, W.H. Zhu, P. Abolmaesumi, P.D. Lawrence, "Robot-assisted diagnostic ultrasound - design and feasibility experiments", in MOCCAI'99, C. Taylor and A. Colchester Eds., LNCS Series, Vol. 1679, pp1063-1071, Springer Verlag, 1999.
[7] Dombre, E., Thérond, X., Dégoulange, E., and Pierrot, E. Robot-Assisted detection of atheromatous plaques in arteries. In Proceedings of the IARP Workshop on Medical Robots, pp 133-140, Vienna, 1996
[8] Boudet, S., Gariepy, J., Mansour S. An Integrated Robotics and Medical Control Device to Quantify Atheromatous Plaques : Experiments on the Arteries of a Patient , in Proceedings of the 10th IROS Conference, Grenoble, 1997
[9] Masuda K., Kimura E., Tateishi N., Ishihara K., Development of remote diagnosis system by using probe movable mechanism and transferring echogram via high speed digital network, in Proceedings of IXth Mediterranean Conference on Medical and Biological Engineering and Computing, MEDICON 2001, Croatia, June 2001

[10] B. Couteau, Y. Payan, S. Lavallée, M.C. Hobatho, "The Mesh-matching algorithm : a new automatic 3D mesh generator for finite element analysis", in MICCAI'99, C. Taylor and A. Colchester Eds., LNCS Series, Vol. 1679, pp1175-1182, Springer Verlag, 1999.

[11] V.L. Nickel, M.D.J. Perry, and A.L. Garret, "Development of Useful Function in the Severely Paralysed Hand", *The Journal of Bone and Joint Surgery*, vol. 45-A, no. 5, pp. 933-952, 1963.

[12] B. Tondu and P. Lopez, "Modeling and Control of McKibben Artificial Muscle Robot Actuators", *IEEE Control Systems Magazine*, vol. 20, no.2, pp. 15-38, 2000.

[13] C. Ghez, "Muscles: Effectors of the Motor System", Chap. 36. in *Principles of Neural Science*, Kandel, E.R., Schwartz., J.H., Jessekk, T.M. (eds), Englewood Cliffs: Prentice-Hall, pp. 548-563, 1991.

[14] A. Vilchis, J. Troccaz, P. Cinquin, F. Courrèges, G. Poisson, B. Tondu, "Robotic tele-ultrasound system (TER): slave robot control", in Proceedings of TA'2001, IFAC Conference on Telematics Application in Automation and Robotics, July 2001

[15] C. Delgorge, P. Vieyres, G. Poisson, C. Rosenberger, P. Arbeille: "Comparative survey of ultrasound images compression methods dedicated to a tele-echography robotic system", in Proceedings of the IEEE EMBS 2001 international conference, 2001

Digital Angioplasty Balloon Inflation Device for Interventional Cardiovascular Procedures

Xin Ma[1], Zhong Fan[2], Chee-Kong Chui*[1], Yiyu Cai[2], James H. Anderson[3], Wieslaw L. Nowinski[1]

1. Biomedical Lab, Kent Ridge Digital Labs, Singapore 119613
2. School of MPE, Nanyang Technological University, Singapore 639798
3. Johns Hopkins University School of Medicine, Maryland 21205, USA
Email: * cheekong@krdl.org.sg

Abstract. Percutaneous transluminal coronary angioplasty (PTCA) is an important interventional procedure performed everyday in major hospitals. In this paper, we describe our new designed angioplasty catheter balloon inflation device. It is a digital system that can be used in the actual PTCA procedure or other balloon angioplasty procedures. It is currently being used to simulate the inflation and deflation of angioplasty balloons in conjunction with an interventional radiology simulator. It also can be used in clinical procedures. The device has several outstanding advantages in addition to it resembling the existing handheld device used in the clinical setting. When used in the clinical procedures, a physician can manipulate the device using one hand with a remote controller as opposed to two-hand operating with the existing device. The manipulation accuracy is high allowing the physician to set the minimum inflation step at the level of 0.1 bar. Being an electromechanical device, it can be integrated better then the existing mechanical device, into the increasing digital clinical environment. New features such as intelligent programming can also be implemented using this new electromechanical device. This new angioplasty catheter balloon inflation device is integrated and validated with our interventional radiology simulator in the clinical setting.

1. Introduction

Since its introduction in the late 70's (1), percutaneous transluminal coronary angioplasty has become an important procedure that is performed daily in major hospitals. This technique consists of a catheter system introduced via a needle puncture in the femoral artery. A pre-shaped guiding catheter maneuvered, under real-time x-ray imaging into the orifice of the coronary artery. An angioplasty balloon catheter is then advanced through this guiding catheter selectively into the stenotic segment of the coronary artery. After traversing the stenotic lesion, the balloon is inflated by a pump-controlled pressure. This pressure compresses the arteriosclerotic material in a direction perpendicular to the wall of the vessel and thereby dilating the vessel lumen. The pressure injector that is used to inflate the balloon is also known as the balloon inflation device. The first balloon inflation device is developed by Dr. Andreas Gruentzig [1]. It is an important component of the PTCA and other related

W. Niessen and M. Viergever (Eds.): MICCAI 2001, LNCS 2208, pp. 335-342, 2001.
© Springer-Verlag Berlin Heidelberg 2001

procedures such as stent placement. Commercially available devices are based on the original mechanical design of the Gruentzig's device.

Physicians have to be careful in performing balloon angioplasty procedures so as to avoid serious injury, such as rupturing or dissecting the wall of the vessel. There are normally two ways to reduce potential injury. One is to provide a better training environment for physicians to acquire the necessary skill levels and experience to avoid injury. Although practicing on live patients can provide excellent training, there exist a limited number of cases and alternative training methods are needed. A realistic vascular catheterization simulation system could provide the type of training the physicians desires [2][3]. The alternative is to improve the performance of medical devices used in the procedures so that they can be used easily by the physician, and are safe to patients.

The balloon injection device currently used in clinical procedures cannot provide the electric signals that are needed for our simulation system. We therefore designed a digital handheld balloon injection device that is an integral component of our vascular catheterization simulator. A challenge is to provide a simulated device that closely resembles the existing device in the clinical setting. It should be able to response by delivering the correct signals corresponding to user's manipulation.

As an additional result, we designed an automatic version of the handheld balloon injection device that can be used not only as a component of our simulation system, but also in real clinical angioplasty procedures. When used in the clinical procedures, physician may use a handheld remote controller to actuate the inflation/deflation procedure allowing for one hand operation. The manipulation accuracy is high allowing physicians to set the minimum inflation steps in the level of 0.1 bar. Finally physicians can operate the device work in an "intelligent" way by setting alarms. For example, physicians can set the rate of balloon inflation alarm and maximum pressure alarm according to their experience and according to manufacture specifications. During the procedure, the micro-controller inside the device can calculate the rate and pressure of inflation. If the value is over the alarm value, a buzzer will alarm the physician. This provides a safety factor to reduce potential balloon overinflation, rupture and serious clinical complications.

In the remaining sections, we will first describe the design and mechanism of our balloon inflation devices (handheld one and automatic one), and then discuss the results from integration with the interventional radiology simulator.

2. Handheld Catheter Balloon Inflation Device

In this section, we will describe the catheter inflation device for simulating balloon inflation and deflation with the interventional radiology simulator. This device is handheld and closely resembles the actual device used in the clinical setting. .

The handheld catheter based balloon inflation device was made for realistic training simulation. It has all the essential components of an existing balloon inflation device, and is different from these currently available handheld syringe pump device by the addition of a digital pressure switch with analog output for PC data interface. Also instead of the standard inflation medium (an X-ray radiopaque contrast based mixture), air is used. In actual clinical setting, air is not injected for fear of balloon rupture and air embolism that could be lethal.

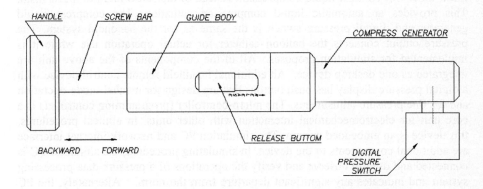

Figure 1. Drawing of handheld digital balloon inflation device

The specifications of the device are listed below:

Specification	Value
Maximum liquid pressure	20 Bar (2 Mpa, 20 ATM)
Compress stroke	Around 2 inches
Pressure switch	Analog output: 1 to 5V

This device can provide up to 20 Bar of compressed liquid by means of a manual screw and nut mechanism. The user can twist the handle (clockwise) and the screw bar forces the piston (inside the compressed liquid generator) forward to compress the liquid which is sealed in the compress generator. The release button can be used to release the compress liquid quickly (balloon deflation).

The digital pressure switch measures the balloon inner pressure directly, and allows one to control the intra-balloon pressure as indicated by the digital LED display more easily. The existed handheld inflation syringe has markers that are used to determine the balloon pressure, but it has more tolerance for actual pressure measurement. Meantime, the digital pressure has analog output and PC can collect this signal to simulate the procedure of inflating/deflating balloon. In addition to the pressure, we are track the rate of inflation and deflation.

3. Automatic Catheter Balloon Inflation Device

The existing handheld balloon inflation device must be held by one hand and twisted by the other hand, during the procedure. One hand operation of the balloon inflation provides the physician cardiologist with an easier means to initiate and monitor balloon inflation. Accordingly, we designed a desktop-based automatic catheter balloon inflation device on the base of our handheld one. It can be used not only with our interventional radiology simulator but also in real clinical procedures.

To convert the manual handheld device to an automatic model, we utilize an AC linear motor for contrast liquid compression instead of the screw and nut mechanism. This provides an automatic liquid compression actuation. The compress liquid generator and digital pressure switch is the same as for the handheld system. The pressure output connects the balloon catheter for actual operation use while it is implemented for simulation proposes. All of the components of the above unit are integrated as one desktop device. An additional handheld remote control device with a digital pressure display has push buttons that are design for manual mode operation and for fine pressure adjustments. The micro-controller (programming controller) is a core unit for electromechanical interaction with other units. In clinical procedures, this device is an embedded system. The simulation PC and network/internet interface are additional components to the device. In simulating procedure, the simulator PC is connected and used to observe and verify the operations of a pressure data processing system and indicates any significant departure from the norm. Alternately, the PC can record data from the practice operation for study and simulation databases. The network/internet interface is intended to connect with other devices, such as respirators and blood pressure monitoring systems utilized in the clinical environment. The system can also be used for remote training and telemedicine. The design of this device is shown in the following schematic block diagram (Figure 2).

The device can work in three modes: manual mode, auto mode and simulation mode. The manual and auto modes allow user to use the device in actual clinical setting. The device has been used in conjunction with our interventional radiology simulator in simulation mode. Nevertheless, it can be used with other simulation systems on PC platform.

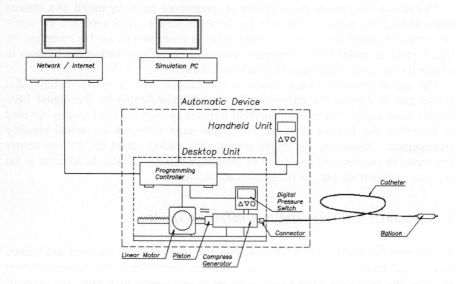

Figure 2. Block diagram of automatic digital balloon inflation device

Manual Mode

In manual mode, the user first selects the maximum pressure to be delivered. This depends on the specific type of catheter balloon device used. The user then starts to increase the pressure by means of a button on the handheld remote control and monitors the pressure display. The monitor PC will check the rate of balloon pressure increase that was pre-selected based on the specific catheter balloon device chosen. If an incorrect action occurs, a buzzer will alarm the user. The system automatically maintains the proper pressure within the balloon during the procedure.

Auto Mode

When in auto mode, the user first selects the type of catheter balloon device to be used. This is done from a library of clinically available catheter balloon device specifications stored in the PC. The user then keys in the maximum pressure as a check. The pre-programming operation will begin after pressing the start button. The user can still monitor the pressure data through the handheld remote control and can stop the programming by means of a stop button located on the remote control. The monitor PC will analyze the data from network I/O to automatically adjust the pressure and increase/decrease speed accordingly.

These two allow the physician to operate the device work more intelligently. Physician can set some alarm values such as balloon inflation rate and maximum inflation pressure alarm according to their clinical experience. If alarm is generated during the clinical procedure, proper steps can be taken by the physician to avoid balloon overexpansion or rupture with subsequentand injury to the patient.

Simulation Mode

In a clinical procedure, the device works as an embedded desktop system. All the information and control signals are processed and generated by the micro-controller inside as shown in Figure 2. For simulation purposes, the device can be connected to a PC. The device can be used as a component of an interventional radiology simulator. The PC also can be used to record data during actual angioplasty procedures. The simulation environmenet is very useful for pretretment planning or training.

The automatic catheter balloon inflation device has three advantages. The first is that physician can complete the whole balloon inflation procedure using one hand. The second relates to the high accuracy of the system in monitoring and displaying inflation pressures. The minimum inflation step is 0.1 bar. The third is that with an intelligent alarm setting, the procedure can prevent balloon overinflation and potential clinical complications.

4. Results

We have integrated the handheld balloon inflation device into our interventional radiology simulator. The pressure switch of the balloon inflation device can apply an analog voltage output in the range of 1-5V. With this analog signal, the device is now used as a component in our TiC (Tactile and Image Control) interfacing system [4]. The analog signal is firstly alternated into digital signal and then inputted into a PC through a serial port. The signal is then used to simulate inflation/deflation of a balloon catheter to treat the stenotic lesion in the virtual blood vessel.

Figure 3 (a) shows the handheld balloon inflation device for simulation purposes. Figure 3(b) illustrates the simulation process using the device. Figures 4 and 5 are snapshots of the graphic display from our interventional radiology simulator [5]. Figure 4, illustrates inflation of the angioplasty in the human cerebral vasculature. Figure 5 shows a stent deployed by balloon inflation at the middle portion of the same cerebral artery. This provides a life-like simulation environment for the user to practice or for pretreatment planning of pertaneous transluminal coronary angioplasty procedures.

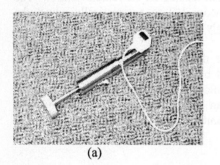
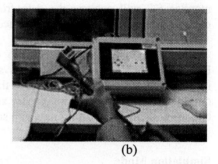

(a)   (b)

Figure 3 (a) Balloon inflation device. (b) Simulating balloon inflation and deflation

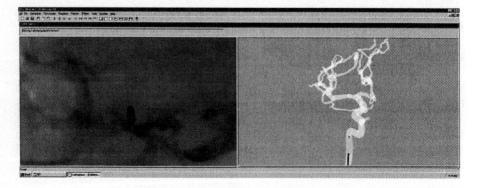

Figure 4. Simulated balloon inflation (Fluoroscopic and 3D views).

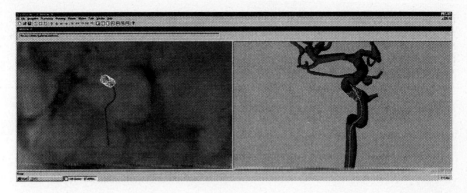

Figure 5. Simulated stent deployment with balloon inflation (Fluoroscopic and 3D views).

5. Conclusion

The catheter balloon inflation device described here, has been successfully used as a component of our interventional radiology simulator. Compared with normally used balloon inflation devices, it provides an electronic output signal that is useful for simulation purposes. We also designed a new desktop-based automatic catheter balloon inflation device that can be used not only in the simulation system, but also in clinical procedures. The manipulation of the device allows the physician to complete the balloon inflation procedure using one hand. The accuracy of the system in recording and displaying inflation pressures is very high. Finally, physicians can control the clinical procedure according to the pressure display on the handheld remote controller and be provided with additional balloon inflation safety alarm features.

Acknowledgement: Support of this research development by National Science and Technology Board of Singapore is gratefully acknowledged. We are grateful to Dr. Anthony C. Venbrux and Dr. Kieran Murphy of Johns Hopkins Hospital, Baltimore, USA for championing the validation effort in the clinical setting.

Reference

[1]. L.A. Geddes and L.E. Geddes, *The Catheter Introducer,* Mobium Press, Chicago, 1997.
[2]. J. Anderson, W. Brody, C. Kriz, Y.P. Wang, C.K. Chui, Y.Y. Cai, R. Viswanathan and R. Raghavan, daVinci- a vascular catheterization and interventional radiology-based training and patient pretreatment planning simulator, *Proc. of Society of Cardiovascular and Interventional Radiology (SCVIR) 21st Annual Meeting,* Seattle, USA, March 1996.
[3]. Y. Wang, C.K. Chui, H.L. Lim et al, *Real-time interactive simulator for percutaneous coronary revascularization procedures.* Computer Aided Surgery, Vol 3, No 5, 211-227, 1998.

342   X. Ma et al.

[4]. C.K. Chui, P. Chen, Y. Wang et al, *Tactile Controlling and Image Manipulation Apparatus for Computer Simulation of Image Guided Surgery*, Recent Advances in Mechatronics, Springe-Verlag, 1999.
[5]. C.K. Chui, J. Anderson, W. Brody, W.L. Nowinski, *Report on Interventional Radiology Simulation Development*, Internal Research Report, KRDL-JHU 2001.

A Computer-Assisted Robotic Ultrasound-Guided Biopsy System for Video-Assisted Surgery

Giuseppe Megali[1], Oliver Tonet[1], Cesare Stefanini[1], Mauro Boccadoro[1], Vassilios Papaspyropoulos[2], Licinio Angelini[2], and Paolo Dario[1]

[1] MiTech Lab – Scuola Superiore Sant'Anna, Pisa, Italy
{g.megali,o.tonet,c.stefanini,m.boccadoro,p.dario}@mail-arts.sssup.it
[2] Dipartimento di Scienze Chirurgiche e Tecnologie Mediche Applicate,
Università "La Sapienza", Roma, Italy
{vassilios.papas, licinio.angelini}@uniroma1.it

Abstract. Current ultrasound-guided biopsy procedures used in video-assisted surgery suffer from limitations due to difficult triangulation and manual positioning of the biopsy needle. We present a prototype computer-assisted robotic system for needle positioning that operates in a synergistic way with the clinician. The performance of the system in terms of positioning accuracy and execution time is assessed. Results suggest suitability for clinical use.

1 Introduction

Intra-operative ultrasonography is used, in surgical practice, for many applications both for diagnostic and therapeutic purposes [1]. Thanks to its specificity and sensitivity, it is of primary importance in disorders of the pancreas [2], biliary tree [3], and liver [4], especially in early stages of the disease.

The diagnostic accuracy of alternative techinques, i.e. pre-operative imaging (angiography, scintigraphy, CT, ultrasonography), bio-humoral surveys, and surgical exploration, does not exceed 60-80% [5]. On the other hand, intra-operative ultrasonography allows early diagnosis and precise localization – and thus accurate and radical surgical treatment – of lesions that are not otherwise detectable.

As intra-operative ultrasonography provides real-time data, it can be applied on demand to assist the surgeon during intervention. A major diagnostic application is providing guidance for percutaneous and endoscopic biopsy.

In current clinical practice, percutaneous ultrasound-guided biopsy is performed either freehand or by means of a *biopsy kit*, consisting of an ultrasound (US) probe equipped with a cylindrical needle guide, hinged at a fixed distance to a beam integral with the probe. This contrivance forces the needle to stay in the imaging plane of the probe, so that the needle tip is always visible in the US image, contrary to what happens in freehand conditions. The hinge on the needle guide allows to vary the needle insertion angle.

W. Niessen and M. Viergever (Eds.): MICCAI 2001, LNCS 2208, pp. 343–350, 2001.

The main drawback of this technique is that, since the needle is anchored to the probe, a difficult compromise is necessary between the probe position that provides the best images and the most convenient insertion point for biopsy.

Small US transducers, mounted in probes of about 1 cm diameter, are of particular interest in minimally invasive surgery. These probes can be introduced directly into the patient's body to obtain better quality images of the internal organs. Anyway, whenever the bioptic procedure cannot be carried out percutaneously, as in the case of video-assisted (laparoscopic or thoracoscopic) interventions, no biopsy kits are available and only freehand approach is possible.

Several systems have been proposed for providing assistance to needle positioning, using ultrasonography [6], or fluoroscopy [7][8].

In this paper we present a prototype *robotic tool* [9] for US-guided biopsy during video-assisted surgery, that operates in a synergistic way with the clinician. The system allows precise 3D localization and visualization of the biopsy target without the need for pre-operative imaging, contrast agents, or intra-operative X-rays. The system is modular and was conceived as feasibility study, for evaluation of the overall performance and suitability for clinical use.

2 System Overview

2.1 A More Accurate Biopsy Procedure

The system, illustrated in Fig. 1, is composed of a robot arm carrying the biopsy syringe, an ultrasonography system, a 3D localizer and a PC-based main processing unit (MPU), which also implements the graphical user interface (GUI).

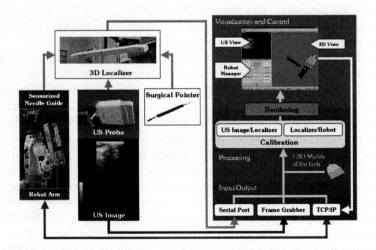

Fig. 1. System architecture and intercommunication between the modules

The biopsy syringe is mounted on the end effector (EE) of the robot arm by means of a needle guide (Fig. 2). When the robot arm is put on place, the guide allows the needle a 1-degree of freedom (DOF) motion along its axis.

The system is designed to provide great accuracy, while keeping the biopsy procedure simple and intuitive: the clinician selects the biopsy target directly on the US image and the insertion point on the patient's body. Subsequently, the robot arm positions the biopsy needle along the defined trajectory. In order to guarantee maximum safety of the procedure, the insertion of the needle and the bioptic sampling is left to the manual execution of the clinician.

From the end user's viewpoint, the procedure consists of the following steps:

target identification: the clinician scans the region of interest with the US probe in order to locate the biopsy target;

target selection: the clinician selects the biopsy target point on the US image shown in the GUI, by clicking on it with the mouse pointer;

insertion point selection: the clinician uses a surgical pointer, connected to the localizer, to select the insertion point for the biopsy needle;

robot positioning: the robot places the EE on the resulting trajectory, so that the needle will reach, at the end of stroke of the guide, the biopsy target;

stop of breath: to avoid the natural movement of the parenchymal structures during respiratory cycle, we considered the anaesthesiological interruption of the patient's breath for the final steps of the procedure;

robot position adjustment: using the US probe and the GUI, the clinician evaluates the accuracy of the needle positioning. If necessary he/she selects the target point again and commands an adjustment of the robot position;

bioptic sampling: the clinician releases the slide which carries the needle, manually slides it down until the end of stroke, and executes the sampling.

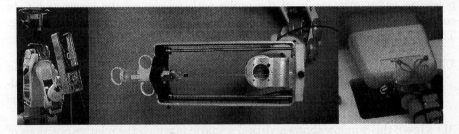

Fig. 2. Hardware components of the system: (a) Dexter arm carrying the (b) sensorized needle guide; (c) sensorized US probe

2.2 Description of the System Components

The robot is an 8-DOF Dexter arm[1]. Whereas it is not designed for surgery applications, its workspace is suitable for this prototype implementation.

---

[1] Dexter arm, S.M. Scienzia Machinale srl, Pisa, Italy.

The ultrasonography system is a portable system[2] equipped with a 7.5 MHz linear probe. In the oncoming clinical trials the system will be replaced by a laparoscopic ultrasonography system with an articulated, sensorized probe.

The localizer is an optical system[3], consisting of three arrays of cameras that detect the pulsed light, emitted by small infrared LEDs, placed on the objects to track: the EE of the robot, the US probe and the surgical pointer.

The position of the objects tracked by the localizer are transmitted to the MPU[4] through a serial port. Bidirectional communication between the MPU and the Dexter arm is established via TCP/IP ethernet. The MPU digitizes and displays the analog video image exported by the ultrasonography system by means of a frame grabber.

The following subsections give some deeper insight on the main custom-made components of the system: the sensorized needle guide and the GUI.

Sensorized Needle Guide This component has to provide a linear motion to the biopsy syringe during insertion. It is positioned at the robot's EE level (see Fig. 2), and is sensorized with four LEDs located in proximity of the guide corners, since large distances allow higher localization accuracy.

The mechanical structure has to fit three requirements: lightness, precision, and smoothness of operation. Lightweight aluminum alloy was used to fabricate the mechanical frame. Linear bearings allow smooth operation. In order to increase the bending stiffness of the system, their shafts are fixed in the seats. The overall weight of the guide is 0.18 kg, widely below the robot payload.

The Graphical User Interface The GUI is displayed on the screen of the MPU and is designed to allow an intuitive visual selection of the biopsy target point, an easier orientation of the probe with respect to the target point, to control the robot movements and evaluate the accuracy of robot positioning. The GUI comprises three windows, as illustrated in Fig. 3:

US view: this window shows the US image captured by the frame grabber. In order to plan the trajectory of needle insertion, a marker, updated in real-time, is displayed on the intersection point between the trajectory of the needle and the US image plane;

3D view: this window shows a virtual scenario in which the relative positions of the CAD models of the sensorized tools are updated in real-time. The target and insertion points, selected by the clinician, are also marked in the scene, simplifying the positioning of the tools relative to them, e.g. for refinding the biopsy target on the US image after having moved the probe;

robot manager: this window contains the "move robot" button and shows all parameters used for robot control. In the final version there will be no

[2] HS-1201 Linear Scanner, Honda Electronics Co., LTD., Toyohashi, Aichi, Japan.
[3] FlashPoint® 5000 3D Localizer, Image Guided Technologies, Inc., Boulder, CO, USA.
[4] TDZ 2000 GX1 workstation, Intergraph Corp., Huntsville, AL, USA.

need for displaying parameters and the clinician will use a pedal to send commands to the robot.

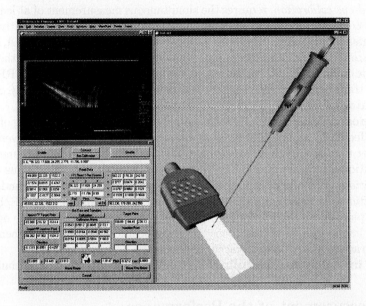

Fig. 3. A screenshot of the graphical user interface, containing the US view (upper left), the 3D view (right) and the robot manager window (lower left)

3   Methods

The biopsy procedure is now illustrated from a methodological point of view:

localization of target point: the user selects the biopsy target point on the US view, with a mouse click. Since the window that displays the image has been calibrated, the pixel coordinates of the chosen point are converted in metric coordinates, referred to the US probe position. The position of the US probe is given in the localizer reference frame (LRF), therefore computation of the 3D position of the biopsy target is straightforward;

localization of insertion point: LRF coordinates of the point on the patient's skin, selected by means of the sensorized surgical pointer, are measured directly by the 3D localizer;

computation of needle guide positioning: the trajectory of needle insertion is the straight line through the target point and the insertion point. The robot EE is positioned so that the needle tip, at end of stroke of the slide, reaches the target point. These requirements lock 5 of the 6 DOF of the EE. The residual 1 DOF, i.e. the rotation of the slide around the needle axis, is chosen so to maximize visibility of the needle guide to the localizer;

hand-eye calibration: selection of insertion and target points is done in LRF
coordinates. To position the robot arm, computation of the corresponding
points in the robot reference frame (RRF) is required. This operation, called
hand-eye calibration, requires the simultaneous measurement of at least three
non-colinear points in the two reference frames. By considering relative movements, the problem can be cast in the form $AX = XB$, where A, B, and
X are 4×4 transformation matrices describing the position of the needle
guide in the LRF, the position of the robot end-effector in the RRF, and
the transformation between the two reference frames, respectively. A least-
squares solution for X can be found in [10];

robot positioning: due to the calibration inaccuracy, the positioning of the EE
is affected by an error, increasing with the magnitude of robot movement. In
order to minimize the amplification of the error due to large movements, the
positioning of the robot involves two phases: first, the robot performs a *coarse
positioning* of the needle guide on the planned trajectory; second, a *fine
positioning* movement corrects the mismatch, measured in the LRF, between
the planned and reached trajectory. This phase, supervised by the operator,
can be iterated to obtain a very accurate positioning, thus implementing an
interactive closed loop for accuracy control;

needle insertion and sampling: performed manually by the clinician.

4   Measurement of the Performance

To evaluate the suitability of the prototype system for clinical use, system performance has been assessed in terms of accuracy and execution time.

Measurements are conducted under ideal conditions (see Fig. 4): the biopsy
target, a fixed and pointed wooden stick, was immersed in water, so to avoid image distortions due to inhomogeneous medium, and needle deformations induced
by contact with solid tissues surrounding the target. To minimize inaccuracy due
to the US image thickness, the biopsy target was placed on the center plane of
the US beam.

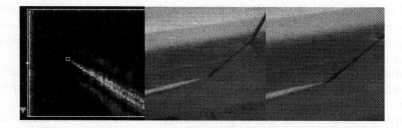

Fig. 4. US View highlighting the biopsy target point and the needle positions
reached after one and two fine positioning cycles

The accuracy of the system has been assessed by measuring, on 30 different target points distributed in the surgical workspace, the deviation of the needle tip from the target point.

The results are presented in the following table, where ε_1, ε_2, and ε_3 are the deviations, measured by the localizer, respectively after one, two, and three cycles of fine robot positioning, while ε_{US} is the deviation, measured on the US image, between the wooden point and the needle tip, after the third cycle:

	ε_1	ε_2	ε_3	ε_{US}
Mean error	1.32 mm	0.85 mm	0.63 mm	2.05 mm
Max error	2.13 mm	1.39 mm	0.88 mm	2.49 mm

The results obtained for the variables $\varepsilon_{1,2,3}$ show that the system achieves sub-millimetric accuracy in the positioning of the needle guide after two fine positioning cycles of the robot. In other words, it is possible to compensate for the inaccuracy of the robot arm (about 2 mm) by means of fine positioning movements; the overall accuracy of the system depends on the accuracy of the localizer [11], on the manufacturing of the frames holding the LEDs, and on calibration and thickness of the US images.

While the error measured by ε_i is relative to the needle guide positioning, ε_{US} is the error measured at the needle tip, when the slide is at end of stroke. The difference between the two is mostly due to the deflection of the needle.

Measurements on time consumption show that the whole procedure, excluding the time spent by the clinician for ultrasonography exploration, requires about 1 min. The breath of the patient has to be stopped only during fine positioning of the robot (i.e. about 15 s for each cycle) and the sampling phase.

5   Conclusions

We presented a prototype robotic US-guided system for video-assisted surgery. The system improves the current US-guided biopsy procedures by offering intuitive selection of the biopsy target point and automated, accurate positioning of the biopsy needle. Featuring needle trajectory locking, the system allows to safely reach the target with a single puncture; this cannot be guaranteed in freehand approach. Experimental results are encouraging and compatible with clinical requirements, in terms of positioning accuracy and execution time.

Accuracy will be further increased by improving the overall stiffness of the robot arm and needle guide. The error due to needle deflection, $\varepsilon_{US} - \varepsilon_3$, will be reduced by adding a second guiding support to the needle, close to the needle insertion point. Oncoming in vitro tests will assess needle deflection and US image distortion due to soft tissue surrounding the biopsy target.

Safety is a very important issue in medical robotics. The current prototype features emergency arrest and leaves to the clinician the execution of needle insertion and sampling. Furthermore, the robot, attaining the target at end of stroke of the needle guide, is kept at maximal distance from the patient.

Future work will also focus on compliant robot control, in order to avoid interference with other devices present in the surgical scene and to prevent potential damage deriving from accidental collision.

Acknowledgements

This work has been carried out with support by the "Progetto Strategico Robotica in Chirurgia", promoted by Consiglio Nazionale delle Ricerche (CNR), Italy. The authors are grateful to Dr. M.C. Carrozza, Dr. B. Magnani, and Dr. S. D'Attanasio for their work in the early stages of the project. The authors would like to thank Dr. C. Laschi, G. Teti, and L. Zollo for providing assistance with the Dexter arm. Thanks to B. Massa and D. Rosti for the CAD drawings.

References

[1] Angelini L. and Caratozzolo M. Intraoperative echography: the state of the art. *Ann Ital Chir*, 70(2):223–30, March-April 1999.

[2] Galiber A.K., Reading C.C., Charboneau J.W., Sheedy P.F., James E.M., Gorman B., Grant C.S., van Heerden J.A., and Telander R.L. Localization of pancreatic insulinoma: comparison of pre- and intraoperative US with CT and angiography. *Radiology*, 166(2):405–8, February 1988.

[3] Orda R., Sayfan J., Strauss S., Barr J., and Oland J. Intra-operative ultrasonography as a routine screening procedure in biliary surgery. *Hepatogastroenterology*, 41(1):61–64, February 1994.

[4] Castaing D., Emond J., Kunstlinger F., and Bismuth H. Utility of operative ultrasound in the surgical management of liver tumors. *Ann Surg*, 204(5):600–5, 1986.

[5] Russo A., La Rosa C., Cajozzo M., Spallitta I., Demma I., Modica G., and Bazan P. Screening for liver metastases of colorectal carcinoma by the routine use of intraoperative echography. *Minerva Chir*, 17(44):1893–900, 1989.

[6] O. Chavanon, C. Barbe, J. Troccaz, and L. Carrat. Computer-ASsisted PERi-cardial punctures: animal feasibility study. *Proc. CVRMed-MRCAS'97, Lecture Notes in Computer Science*, 1205:285–94, March 1997.

[7] Dan Stoianovici, Louis L. Whitcomb, James H. Anderson, Russell H. Taylor, and Louis R. Kavoussi. A modular surgical robotic system for image guided percutaneous procedures. *Proc. MICCAI'98, Lecture Notes in Computer Science*, 1496:404–410, October 1998.

[8] A. Bzostek, S. Schreiner, A. C. Barnes, and J. A. Cadeddu. An automated system for precise percutaneous access of the renal collecting system. *Proc. CVRMed-MRCAS'97, Lecture Notes in Computer Science*, 1205:299–308, March 1997.

[9] P. Dario, M.C. Carrozza, M. Marcacci, S. D'Attanasio, B. Magnani, O. Tonet, and G. Megali. A novel mechatronic tool for computer-assisted arthroscopy. *IEEE Transactions on Information Technology in Biomedicine*, 4(1):15–29, March 2000.

[10] F.C. Park and B.J. Martin. Robot Sensor Calibration - Solving $AX = XB$ on the Euclidean Group. *IEEE Trans. Robotics and Automation*, 10(5):717–721, 1994.

[11] F. Chassat and S. Lavallée. Experimental protocol of accuracy evaluation of 6-d localizers for computer-integrated surgery. application to four optical localizers. *Proc. MICCAI'98, Lecture Notes in Computer Science*, 1496:277–284, October 1998.

Dynamic Brachytherapy of the Prostate Under Active Image Guidance

Gang Cheng[1], Haisong Liu[1], Lydia Liao[2] and Yan Yu[1]

Departments of [1] Radiation Oncology and [2] Radiology, University of Rochester, 601 Elmwood Avenue, Rochester, NY 14642, USA

Abstract. Image-guided brachytherapy is a promising treatment for early stage prostate cancer. Current research emphasizes methods for intraoperative optimized planning and precise implantation of radioactive seeds. Some new technologies for these purposes are described in this paper. A morphological template will overcome pubic arch interference and achieve better-optimized dose coverage under the real-time dynamic dosimetry technique. Auto-segmentation of the prostate anatomy has been implemented for clinical use to reduce operative time. Just-in-time planning and procedure tracking under active image guidance can now be performed in the operating room. Interactive planning and dynamic dosimetry can be achieved based on seed recognition in the live ultrasound images, which permit real-time replanning to eliminate under-dosage. As a result of these advances, prostate brachytherapy of the future will increasingly be practised as a precision procedure rather than an art form.

1 Introduction

In the United States, adenocarcinoma of the prostate is the most common malignancy in man, excluding skin cancer. Prostate cancer is newly diagnosed in over 180,000 men in the US each year. Growing emphasis on prostatic specific antigen (PSA) based early detection and changes in the population demographics suggest that prostate cancer diagnosis, particularly of the early stages, will continue to increase. Standard treatment options at this time for early, localized prostate cancer include prostatectomy, external beam radiation with or without 3D conformal intensity modulation, and interstitial brachytherapy using either permanent implantation of radioactive seeds or temporary placement of high dose rate needle channels. Whereas surgery and external beam radiation therapy offers effective treatment for localized disease, both treatment modalities can cause significant side effects such as urinary incontinence and impotence. In the last few years, there is a rapid growth of interest in interstitial brachytherapy with ^{125}I and ^{103}Pd seeds under the guidance of live ultrasound and needle template. However, it is now widely recognized that interstitial brachytherapy of the prostate is susceptible to great variability due to factors in patient anatomy, dosimetry optimization, and precision of needle placement. Current research emphasis in prostate brachytherapy is therefore to develop methods for intraoperative optimized planning and precise implantation of radioactive seeds for real-time, image-guided prostate brachytherapy.

W. Niessen and M. Viergever (Eds.): MICCAI 2001, LNCS 2208, pp. 351-359, 2001.

In modern prostate brachytherapy, computed tomography (CT), magnetic resonance imaging (MRI) and transrectal ultrasound (TRUS) image guidance have been used to replace free-hand seed implantation. In particular, TRUS permits real time localization of the prostate gland and the needle locations at the same time, which leads to stepwise updating of the actual radiation dosimetry that reflects needle departures from the idealized plan.

2 Treatment Planning Space

The current implantation guidance template is a rectilinear uniform design permitting parallel needle tracks at uniform (5 mm interval) spacing in the left-right and anterior-posterior directions. The square template pattern is an anatomically arbitrary design reflective of the static grid that the early generations of ultrasound machines were capable of displaying on screen. This design artifact led to a long practice of so-called "uniform loading," which for prostate brachytherapy caused excessive dosage to the urethra and the central portions of the prostate gland. Pubic arch interference (PAI) occurs in patients with large prostates where the anterior and/or lateral aspects of the prostate gland are blocked by the pubic bone in the transperineal approach. Although improvisation techniques have been applied to tilt the pelvis in an ad hoc manner, the vast majority of treatment protocols would exclude patients with prostate size greater than 55 to 60 cc, who would undergo hormonal downsizing to reduce the prostate size and therefore the degree of PAI. Though Roy and Wallner developed a methodology permitted semi-automatic optimization of dosimetry and pubic arch avoidance by allowing needle tracks to be positioned with considerable flexibility including angulation, their individual customization of the template does not offer a class solution to the prostate morphology for universal applicability.[1]

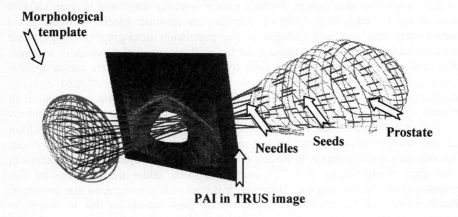

Fig. 1. The morphological template will open up a large solid angle of the implant space for the most effective replanning and optimization in real time.

A morphological template concept (Fig. 1) is being developed as part of the PIPER (Prostate Implant Planning Engine for Radiotherapy) project,[2] which leverages the planning system's active sign guidance capabilities to deliver non-coplanar conformal interstitial brachytherapy. The morphological template will allow patients with pubic arch interference to be treated with brachytherapy or other interstitial ablative therapies of the prostate without first undergoing lengthy hormonal downsizing therapy. In addition, the non-coplanar conformal needle pattern will open up greater degrees of freedom for optimized planning as well as error–feedback/feedforward dynamic brachytherapy. Dynamic re-optimization of the dosimetry plan during brachytherapy seed placement based on real time automatic localization of the prostate boundaries and the implanted seeds on TRUS would benefit from needle adjustments around the periphery of the target volume on the morphologically spaced template where under-dosage usually occurs.

3 Auto-segmentation of Prostate Gland

Prostate volume study using TRUS is an important step for planning optimized dosimetry. In the volume study, transverse cross-sectional images of the prostate are acquired at fixed intervals, e.g., 5 mm increments from the base (superior) of the gland to the apex (inferior). The boundaries of the prostate obtained during the volume study not only result in an accurate determination of the size and shape of the prostate, but also provide important information for adequate dose delivery to the target volume with sparing of dose-sensitive tissues.

Currently, the prostate boundary is manually outlined in each transverse cross-sectional ultrasound image, which is a tedious and time-consuming process, particularly for intraoperative planning. Automatic segmentation is a difficult task due to the inherent noise in the ultrasound image data. However, recent advances in software methodology have made remarkable progress in this area. Arambula has used a genetic algorithm and a constrained prostate model to automatically identify the prostate in ultrasound images.[3] Kwoh used the harmonics method and Radial Bas-Relief (RBR) method to extract a skeletonised boundary from an ultrasound image automatically.[4] Aarnink has investigated multi-scale edge detection algorithm and nonlinear Laplace filtering to improve edge localization in ultrasound images of the prostate.[5][6] We have developed a trainable method for TRUS segmentation and demonstrated its utility in prostate brachytherapy planning and optimization.[7] In this method, the initial ultrasound images are pre-processed to remove noise and increase the contrast. The rectum edge is located from the bottom of the images. Key points on the prostate boundaries are located and connected under the iterative training of a knowledge-based model until the shape of the boundary reaches a stable state. The urethra is segmented near the center of the prostate. In our initial assessment, the automated image segmentation technique will reduce the median operative time for anatomy delineation for intraoperative planning, from 10 min. to 2 min. for complete outline of the prostate, urethra and rectum (Fig. 2).

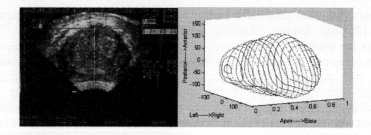

(a) 2D auto-segmentation of prostate gland. (b) 3D reconstruction of prostate surface.

Fig. 2. Auto-segmentation of the prostate gland and 3D reconstruction.

4 Intraoperative Planning Engine

It is now widely recognized that the two-step process of pre-planning (approximately 2-4 weeks prior to implantation) and surgical implantation had several limitations: (a) the pre-planning prostate position often cannot be precisely reproduced in the operating room, especially following relaxation of the pelvic musculature due to anesthesia; (b) time lapse and/or interim hormonal therapy can significantly change the prostate size and shape. These factors limit the efficacy of the pre-plan, often rendering it invalid. Strict adherence to the pre-plan may lead to severe under-dosage and local failure, whereas ad hoc improvisation at the time of implantation can lead to unexpected morbidity.

Compared to pre-planning, the intraoperative planning system refers to the creation of a plan in the operation room just before the implant procedure with immediate execution of the plan, which eliminates separate planning image study with resultant improved efficiency and less patient inconvenience, and reduces the dependence on pubic arch obstruction evaluation study. At the same time, intraoperative planning eliminates the need to reproduce patient and ultrasound probe position as ultrasound images are captured in the OR immediately prior to and during the implant with patient in the treatment position so that it can account for changes in size and shape of the prostate due to hormonal therapy or muscle relaxation. Consequently the best match is obtainable between the planned seed configuration and the actual seed placement locations in the prostate. Thus intraoperative planning reduces the chain of uncertainties to a minimum, thereby minimizing the chance of under-dosage to parts of the cancerous prostate. Real-time dosimetric guidance is a natural extension of intraoperative optimized planning. Based on the use of computer and optimization technologies, dosimetric guidance requires an additional feedback loop following real-time acquisition of seed placement/prostate volume data at selected intervals (e.g. after every 4 needle insertions).

Systematic investigation of treatment planning, seed placement uncertainties and dosimetric consequences of realistic (rather than idealized) implants in the new era of TRUS- and template-guided prostate brachytherapy began in 1993,[8] followed by rigorous efforts to approach dosimetric planning using computerized optimization techniques.[9] This work was later extended to account for the multi-objective nature of treatment planning, including delivering therapeutic dosage to the entire prostate and higher intensity dosage to the tumor foci, sparing the urethra, rectum and neurovascular bundles, and reducing the complexity of needle/seed placement plans.[10] GA optimization and multi-objective decision theory embedded in these early works form the basis of the PIPER (Prostate Implant Planning Engine for Radiotherapy) system for both web-based Internet treatment planning and intraoperative real time dosimetry planning.[2][11] Differential planning to the PTV (planning target volume), GTV (gross tumor volume) and GTF (gross tumor foci) is achievable under the multi-objective optimization framework used by PIPER. In the pilot clinical experience, we demonstrated that intraoperative just-in-time planning using PIPER reduced dosimetric variance that otherwise would occur due to such variabilities as patient pelvic positioning, interim prostate volume change between preplanning and the procedure, and acute edema following the placement of the first three stabilizing needles.[2] Figure 3 shows screen shots of the PIPER system demonstrating the main functionalities designed according to the workflow in actual brachytherapy procedures.

The current PIPER system is designed to connect with the ultrasound machine next to the operating table. When the patient is positioned after anaesthesia induction, ultrasound images of the prostate from base to apex are acquired in registration with the implant template coordinates. The pelvic anatomy is then defined on the images, as shown in Fig. 3a. The anatomy data and the basic radiation dosimetry data are used in the GA planning engine to produce a dose distribution that best complies with the treatment intent, such as prescription dose, dosimetric margin requirements and relative importance of sparing each of the critical structures (Fig. 3b). The needle and seed patterns generated by this treatment planning process are followed during the procedure in an innovative needle tracking design unique to PIPER (Fig. 3c): the live TRUS video signal is imported to the planning system in a real time video window (top right). As each needle insertion occurs, a hyperechoic spot can be identified in this window and is immediately localized. Because the live ultrasound is registered with the planning coordinate system and the template and the planned needle coordinates are accurately known, the needle positioning error in x/y displacements and angular splaying can be quantified immediately. The physician has the option of either accepting the deviations or reinserting the needle. The isodose coverage of the prostate is automatically updated to account for the needle misplacement. It is now a well-known quality problem in prostate brachytherapy that no implant can achieve the planned dose coverage, and that the magnitude of under-dosage to the prostate and/or over-dosage to radio-sensitive critical structures are unknown at the end of the procedure. Implant dosimetry analysis is currently performed using CT post-implant (Fig. 3d); by that time it is already impractical to re-implant sub-optimal treatment or to extract seeds that will cause complications. The needle-tracking feature is the first practical technique to enable online intraoperative dose evaluation and decision-making in ultrasound-guided brachytherapy.

356   G. Cheng et al.

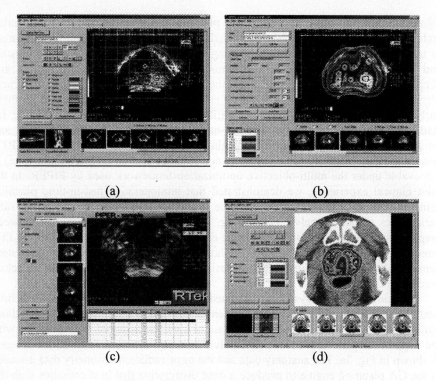

(a)　　　　　　　　　　(b)

(c)　　　　　　　　　　(d)

Fig. 3. PIPER in intraoperative use.

5 Dose Delivery and Dynamic Brachytherapy

5.1 Interactive Planning and Dynamic Dosimetry

Since 1997, a new paradigm of error-feedback/feedforward, dynamic brachytherapy under active, "smart" image guidance was introduced at the University of Rochester. This system continuously acquires volume ultrasound data of the prostate throughout the procedure, perform automatic recognition of the prostate and critical structures, automatically locate each seed as it is implanted into the prostate and perform dosimetry analysis on the fly. During implant progression, an error distribution is computed by comparing the intended seed positions and the detected positions. If the original treatment plan has suffered too much deviation that isolated additional seed placement is not expected to lead to adequate therapy, the GA planning engine can be rerun in the available needle space but taking into account the dosimetric contribution from seeds already implanted in the patient. Dynamic optimization of subsequent seed configurations will take into account the likelihood and extent of misplacement by the convolution of sensitivity analysis and genetic algorithm. Thus the ultimate goal is not only to deliver on-the-fly dosimetric analysis and visualization, but also to recommend subsequent seed placement that anticipates surgical uncertainties rather than chasing after cold spots.

5.2 Active Guidance of Implantation Needles

Targeting of non-coplanar needle placement requires visual guidance on live TRUS, so active guidance sign projected on screen based on the known ultrasound probe locations in space is useful to facilitate pinpoint accuracy in targeted needle placement in any ultrasound view plane at any time.

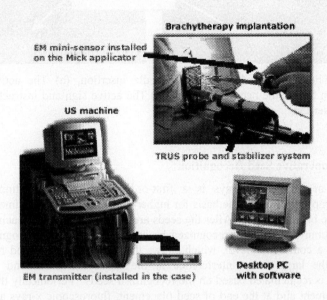

Fig. 4. EM tracking system in the OR.

In PIPER, the electromagnetic (EM) positioning system (Fig. 4) will obtain the 3D physical positions of the needle and the TRUS probe at the same time so that precise registration between the needle and the prostate will be obtained in the physical coordinate system as established by the tracking system. The positions of the needle will be recognized and displayed on the screen with the TRUS image. An active image-subtraction algorithm is developed to analyze whether the needle reaches the pre-planned positions; corresponding instructions will be displayed on the screen at the same time to assist the physician-user in inserting the needle. The active sign and instruction will be shown on the screen to inform the physician-user of the correct steps. Once a needle shadow is found, the TRUS probe will move to the next position unless this needle insertion is completed. If a needle shadow cannot be detected in the viewing window, the needle should be adjusted according to the instructions displayed on the screen based on active seek of the needle path by the tracked ultrasound probe. (Fig. 5)

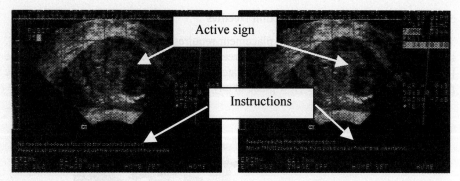

Fig. 5. The active guidance of the needle insertion, (a) The active sign and instruction before the needle insertion; (b) The active sign and instruction after the needle insertion.

5.3. Intraoperative Seed Recognition

Tracking of needle pathways is a first-order dosimetry correction in realistic brachytherapy. It provides the basis for higher-order, seed-based dosimetry necessary in dynamic brachytherapy. After the seeds are implanted in tissue, each seed located in the column of images is recognized by an adaptive-tracking recognition method and given a confidence level, which shows the accuracy of the seed recognition in view of the large noise interference in the transrectal ultrasound images. The dosimetry is recalculated based on the recognized seeds. Periodically throughout the seed placement and at the end of seed placement, fluoroscopic x-rays are taken, and the seed coordinates found in transrectal ultrasound images are matched to the seed coordinates found in fluoroscopic x-ray image. Seed locations with low confidence levels are adjusted based on the x-ray locations, and the dosimetry is recalculated based on these revised seed positions (Fig. 6).

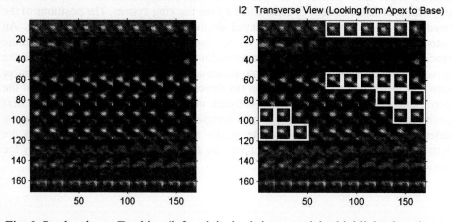

Fig. 6. Seed pathway Tracking (left: original sub-images; right: highlighted seed tracks).

Because angulated needle tracks, used in morphological template, do not necessarily follow any major anatomical planes (e.g., sagittal, coronal), active seek and active guidance of the needle insertion are implemented on live 2D/3D ultrasound, using the needle path recognition algorithm and standard triangulation methodology.

6 Summary and Conclusion

Active image-guidance technologies are now in place to achieve dynamic and quantitative brachytherapy of the prostate in operative conditions with greatly increased surgical implant space and optimized real-time dosimetry planning.

References

1. Roy, J. N., Wallner, K. E., Chiu-Tsao, S. T., Anderson, L. L., and Ling, C. C.: CT-based optimized planning for transperineal prostate planning with customized template. Int. J. Radiat. Oncol. Biol. Phys. 21 (1991) 483-489.
2. Messing, E.M., Zhang, J.B., Rubens, D.J., Brasacchio, R.A., Strang, J.G., Soni, A., Okunieff, P.G. and Yu, Y.: Intraoperative optimized inverse planning for prostate brachytherapy: Early experience. Int. J. Radiat. Oncol. Biol. Phys. 44 (1999) 801-808.
3. Arambula, C. F., Davies, B.L.: Automated prostate recognition: a key process for clinically effective robotic prostatectomy. Med Biol Eng Comput Mar. 37 (1999) 236-243.
4. Kwoh, C. K., Teo, M. Y., Ng, W. S., Tan, S. N., Jones, L. M.: Outlining the prostate boundary using the harmonics method. Med Biol Eng Comput. 36 (1998) 768-771.
5. Aarnink, R. G., Pathak, S. D., de la Rosette, J. J., Debruyne, F. M., Kim, Y., Wijkstra, H.: Edge detection in prostatic ultrasound images using integrated edge maps. Ultrasonics. 36 (1998) 635-642.
6. Aarnink, R. G., Giesen, R. J., Huynen, A. L., de la Rosette, J. J., Debruyne, F. M., Wijkstra, H.: A practical clinical method for contour determination in ultrasonographic prostate images. Ultrasound Med Biol. 20 (1994) 705-717.
7. Cheng, G., Liu, H., Rubens, D.J., Strang, J.G., Liao, L., Yu, Y., Brasacchio, R., Messing, E.: Automatic segmentation of prostate in transrectal ultrasound imaging. Radiology 218 (2001) 612.
8. Yu, Y., Waterman, F.M., Suntharalingam, N., Schulsinger, A.: Limitations of the minimum peripheral dose as a parameter for dose specification in permanent ^{125}I prostate implants. Int. J. Radiation Oncology Biol. Phys. 34 (1996) 717-725.
9. Yu, Y. and Schell, M.C.: A genetic algorithm for the optimization of prostate implants. Med. Phys. 23 (1996) 2085-2091.
10. Yu, Y.: Multiobjective decision theory for computational optimization in radiation therapy. Med. Phys. 24 (1997) 1445-1454.
11. Yu, Y., Zhang, J. B., Brasacchio, R.A., Okunieff, P.G., Rubens, D.J., Strang, J.G., Soni, A., and Messing, E.M.: Automated treatment planning engine for prostate seed implant brachytherapy. Int. J. Radiat. Oncol. Biol. Phys. 43 (1999) 647-652.

Computer-Assisted Soft-Tissue Surgery Training and Monitoring

M.P.S.F. Gomes, A.R.W. Barrett, and B.L. Davies

Mechatronics in Medicine Laboratory, Department of Mechanical Engineering,
Imperial College of Science, Technology and Medicine, Exhibition Road,
London SW7 2BX, UK
{p.gomes, a.r.w.barrett, b.davies}@ic.ac.uk
http://www.me.ic.ac.uk/case/mim/

Abstract. Last year at MICCAI, a computer-assisted surgical training system (CASTS) for Transurethral Resection of the Prostate (TURP), was presented [1]. Unpredictable deformation of the prostate phantom caused unacceptable inaccuracies. Solutions have now been investigated which are described in this paper, namely constraining the phantom, using a different phantom, and tracking the phantom's deformation and movement with ultrasound. Ethics Committee approval was obtained to assess the feasibility of using CASTS as an *in vivo* system for surgical monitoring (CASMS). Pre-operative ultrasound of the patient forms the basis of the computer-generated prostate's model. Per-operative ultrasound is employed to detect and compensate for prostate movement. An optically tracked ultrasound probe is used to relate the images to the optically tracked resectoscope's coordinate system. The CASMS *in vivo* system will help in the assessment of completeness of resection, the provision of information of resection both distal to the verumontanum and near to the capsule. Tests of the CASMS system in the operating room are described.

1 Introduction

In CASTS, the surgeon resects a prostate phantom using real surgical tools (optically tracked), under endoscopic visual guidance (Fig.1). An additional computer display (Fig.2) provides navigational information and shows the progression of the resection.

Whilst evaluating CASTS, it was found that the prostate phantom moved and deformed significantly. This movement has to be taken into account and the graphical model suitably updated. Per-operative ultrasound has been suggested for this and is being evaluated in the laboratory using specially developed gelatine prostate phantoms (Fig.3). Preliminary results are presented in this paper.

The extension of the trainer to the operating room, to be used as an *in vivo* monitoring system (CASMS), is now underway and some results are discussed. This novel two-stage approach aims to bridge the gap between training on a simulator and performing a real surgical procedure.

In CASMS (Fig.4), the surgeon acquires a set of 2D pre-operative transrectal ultrasound scans of the patient's prostate, using an optically tracked ultrasound probe. The scans are then manually segmented by the urologist who delineates the areas to be resected. A 3D model is automatically built and rendered in a computer display.

W. Niessen and M. Viergever (Eds.): MICCAI 2001, LNCS 2208, pp. 360–367, 2001.
© Springer-Verlag Berlin Heidelberg 2001

During the TURP, the display shows the current status of the resection by superimposing a rendering of the resectoscope onto the patient's prostate model. The resected cavity is also rendered. Visual warnings are given if the tip of the resectoscope is outside the resectable volume.

Despite the prostate being anchored to the adjacent anatomical structures, some degree of movement is also to be expected. Per-operative ultrasound can be used to detect and compensate for this movement.

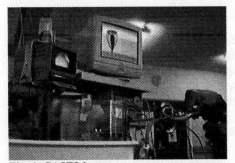

Fig. 1. CASTS in use

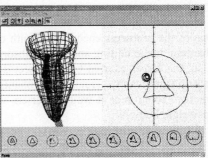

Fig. 2. Graphical User Interface

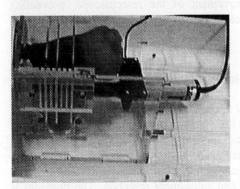

Fig. 3. Perspex profiles and ultrasound

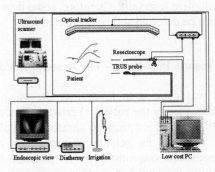

Fig. 4. The *in vivo* monitoring system

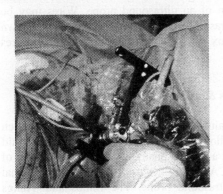

Fig. 5. Mock-up tools in use in the o.r.

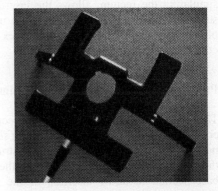

Fig. 6. IRED tool (by Traxtal Technologies)

Mock-ups of instrumentation of the resectoscope have already been tried in the operating room and were found not to interfere with the procedure (Fig.5). Sterilisable tools have been manufactured (Fig.6).

2 Materials and Methods

Constraints to Phantom Movement

One of the problems encountered with the TURP trainer was the deformation of the phantom due to cutting and due to absorption of the irrigating fluid[1] during resection. Also, the forces exerted by the resectoscope on the phantom caused it to move and deform significantly. Tracking the phantom with the optical tracker was not deemed a practical solution as it would interfere with the cutting, and because the phantom is not a rigid body.

A solution that partly solved the problem was the introduction of physical constraints. A set of Perspex profiles was built to limit the severity of the displacements and deformations (Fig.3). Complete constraint of the phantom would be unrealistic and would restrict the movement of the resectoscope, preventing complete resection. Therefore, some degree of motion has to be allowed which must then be detected and compensated for.

Prostate Phantoms – The Resectable Volume

It was decided to investigate the use of ultrasound to track the phantom's (and subsequently the patient's) prostate. Since the phantom being used (Limbs & Things, Bristol, UK) is opaque to ultrasound, an alternative had to be found.

A mould for gelatine phantoms was designed, based on a resection shape from anatomical diagrams [2]. The phantom has a channel, simulating the urethra, that allows the introduction of a resectoscope and subsequent resection. The phantom is inserted into a Perspex box which is filled with gelatine (Figs.7,8). Another channel, simulating the rectum, allows the insertion of an ultrasound probe. Wires may be strung across the phantom so that the ultrasound scans can be acquired in known planes. Replaceable sides on the Perspex box allow the phantom to be cut into slices corresponding to the ultrasound planes.

Prostate Phantoms – The Modified Limbs & Things

The initial design of the phantom contained a straight narrow urethra, which constrained the resectoscope to making shallow cuts, so that the whole volume could not be resected. It was decided to construct a second phantom based on the shape of the Limbs and Things model used in the CASTS trainer system, with an additional base section to allow insertion of the ultrasound probe. The Limbs and Things phantom models the whole of the prostate rather than just the resectable volume and

---

[1] The irrigant for the phantom resections was water.

includes anatomical features such as the verumontanum and bladder neck, thus allowing a laboratory based assessment of the *in vivo* system, more closely mimicking the actual operation.

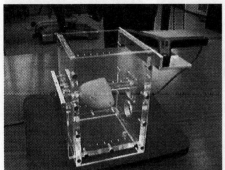

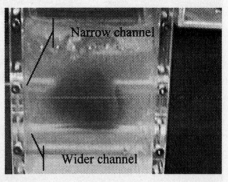

Fig. 7. A wax cast of the prostate phantom inserted into the Perspex box. Two Perspex rods, one through the cast, one below, mark the locations of the simulated urethra and rectum.

Fig. 8. The gelatine prostate in a gelatine bath. The narrow channel through the prostate simulates the urethra. The wider channel below the prostate simulates the rectum.

Formers and moulds for creating the phantom are shown in Figure 9. Three moulds are required for making the phantom. The formers (a,b,c) were provided by Limbs and Things. The first mould (d) models the void of the urethra and bladder neck. This mould is created in two halves by masking off half the former (a) using clay, pouring over silicone rubber which is left to cure, then removing the clay and pouring the second half. A latex skin (Fig.10a) is created by repeated filling of the mould with latex, pouring out the excess and allowing each layer to cure. The second and third moulds (f,g) are made similarly, and model the prostate capsule and surrounding matrix respectively.

The latex skin is filled with water and frozen. The latex skin is then placed in the second mould (e) and gelatine solution is poured into the mould. The solution is 18% gelatine powder (Supercook, Leeds, England) and 9% psyllium husk powder (Regucol, Holland & Barrett Ltd, USA) by weight. The psyllium husk powder scatters the ultrasound beam giving an ultrasound image similar to human tissue [3].

Once set, the gelatine prostate is placed in the third mould which is filled with gelatine solution excluding the psyllium powder. Food colourings are added to the gelatine mixtures to visually distinguish the prostate from its surrounds. Once set, the ice is melted from the latex skin and the skin removed.

The finished phantom is placed inside a latex bladder (Fig.10b) to provide stability and reduce the likelihood of the phantom tearing on deformation. The bladder also provides a reservoir for irrigation fluid to collect, thus ensuring that the urethra is always filled so the ultrasound beam can penetrate the top surface of the phantom. Figure 3 shows the phantom and bladder constrained with Perspex plates and ready for resection.

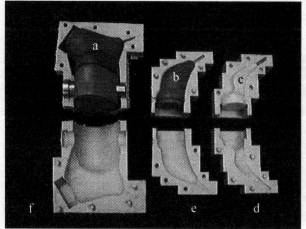

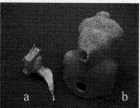

Fig. 10. a) The latex skin for the original cavity. b) The latex bladder which contains the gelatine phantom. Note the large hole at the bottom to allow ultrasound scanning.

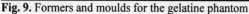

Fig. 9. Formers and moulds for the gelatine phantom

Prostate Modelling from Ultrasound

The procedure for generating a patient-specific prostate model is now described.

The surgeon identifies the limits of resection along the urethra by marking points using the tracked resectoscope. Using a tracked transrectal probe, a series of ultrasound scans with known position and orientation is collected which intersect the resectable region. The surgeon demarcates the region of resection within each scan. Scans may be marked in two ways - with a complete outline if the surgeon can clearly see the resectable region, or a segmented outline if only parts of the region are visible. The complete outline is calculated by spline interpolation through a small number of supplied points.

The outline data consists of a set of points (directly from the segments or interpolated from the complete outlines) lying on the resection volume boundary in a cylindrical coordinate system (linear along the line of the urethra and radial perpendicular to this line). The data is mapped to a 2D data space by assuming that the radius of the points does not vary much over the interpolation range (which is valid for a smoothly varying shape such as the prostate) and unwrapping the cylindrical system onto a flat plane. A 2D Delauney triangulation algorithm is used to construct a triangular mesh with added constraints to ensure that triangles are not created from three points which derive from the same ultrasound slice. The radius of any point on the resection volume surface may be interpolated by finding its containing triangle and interpolating from the vertices.

The algorithms for performing the triangulation and interpolation are extremely fast and the resection volume can be rapidly rendered seconds once outline demarcation is complete. However, the manual outlining process is tedious and time-consuming. Seven algorithms for automatic prostate recognition in ultrasound from the literature are currently being assessed [4-12], however no algorithm has been found which performs faster than manual outlining (many are much slower), and all the algorithms fail on images which do not show the boundary with high clarity. This is particularly problematic since the available ultrasound machine (B&K Medical, Model 1849) is old and produces very poor images when compared to the state-of-the art.

Per-operative Ultrasound

Work is underway to assess the potential of per-operative ultrasound for motion and deformation tracking. In the laboratory, a phantom has been made with a very clear boundary between prostate and non-prostate regions. Figure 11 shows an ultrasound image of the phantom taken in a water bath, and without insertion of a resectoscope. The boundary of the capsule and the urethra cavity are clearly visible. Automated recognition of the phantom boundary, within images captured from the available ultrasound equipment, is feasible. It is expected that image processing and model building time will be short enough to allow rapid update of the computer model as the phantom deforms.

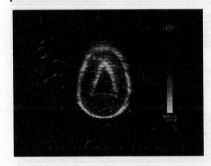

Fig. 11. Ultrasound image of the gelatine phantom taken in a water bath

A motorised holder to traverse the ultrasound probe has been designed so that the phantom may be continually imaged across the region of interest (the resection volume) during the TURP. The holder has one manual linear axis and one manual angular axis so that the probe may be positioned and locked to lie along the direction of the rectum. The motorised axis allows movement of the probe along the rectum using a stepper motor and lead screw under microprocessor control. The ultrasound probe is first clamped to the holder and registered with the optical tracking system by an IRED arrangement on the probe giving initial position and orientation of the probe. The position of the probe during resection can be obtained through the optical tracking system, or by using the initial position and calculating position by counting the steps of the motor. The latter method may be used in the operating theatre where line of sight to the IREDs on the probe will be obstructed.

A preliminary trial of per-operative ultrasound using a stationary probe without positional information has been conducted. Figure 12 shows the prostate outline and slight shadowing caused by the resectoscope within the image. Figure 13 shows the resected cavity with a much brighter edge than the prostate capsule. Figures 14 and 15 show the artefacts introduced when coagulating and cutting respectively.

The shadow caused by the resectoscope does not completely hide the section of prostate boundary behind it. Since the positions of the resectoscope and ultrasound probe within the scan are known, it is possible to anticipate the shadowing and tailor boundary detection methods accordingly. The artefacts caused by current through the resectoscope are far more problematic – indeed they occur at the time when it is crucial to track the prostate's movement. One possibility for overcoming this problem is to momentarily stop the current whilst an image is grabbed, then resume the cutting whilst the ultrasound probe is moved to the next acquisition position.

The cutting and coagulation artefacts do not pose a problem on the gelatine phantom, since resection of the phantom is performed without the current switched on.

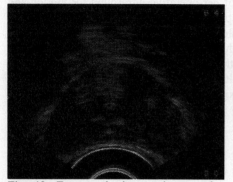

Fig. 12. Transrectal ultrasound scan of a human prostate, showing the shadow cast by the resectoscope

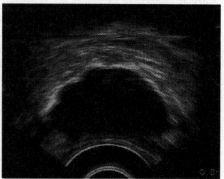

Fig. 13. The cavity formed (darker area roughly in the centre of the image) is easily identifiable

Fig. 14. Artefact whilst coagulating

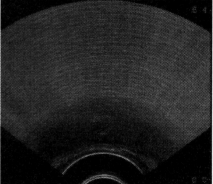

Fig. 15. Artefact whilst cutting

3 Discussion and Conclusions

Prostate phantoms which can be resected with a cutting loop and scanned with ultrasound are described. The procedure for using ultrasound to track prostate movement is presented.

Assessment of tool mock-ups in the operating room has been carried out. This is the first step towards the evaluation of a computer-assisted surgical monitoring system for TURP.

A possible drawback is the difficulty for the surgeon to concentrate on the endoscopic view and also on the computer display simultaneously. The refresh rate needs to be real-time enough for any prostate movement during resection to be detected and compensated for. Line of sight between the optical tracker and the IRED tools needs to be maintained.

The monitoring system can both be used as an assessment and computer-based certification tool and it has scope for surgery planning and as a training tool.

Acknowledgements

The authors would like to thank Mr. Timoney and Mr. Kumar, Southmead Hospital, UK, the Engineering and Physical Sciences Research Council (EPSRC) of the UK, Limbs & Things (UK), and Karl Storz Endoscopy (UK).

References

1. Gomes, M.P.S.F. and Davies, B.L. (2000) Computer-Assisted TURP Training and Monitoring, Medical Image Computing and Computer-Assisted Intervention - MICCAI'00, Pittsburgh, USA, 669-677
2. Blandy, J. (1983) Benign Prostatic Hypertrophy, Springer-Verlag, New York
3. Bude, R.O. and Adler, R.S. (1995) An easily made, low-cost, tissue-like ultrasound phantom material, Journal of Clinical Ultrasound 23, 271-273
4. Aarnick, R., Geisen, R., Huynen, A., Rosette, J., Debruyne, F. and Wijkstra, H. (1994) A practical clinical method for contour determination in ultrasonographic prostate images, Ultrasound Med Biol 20 (8), 705-717
5. Arambula-Cosio, F. and Davies, B. (1999) Automated prostate recognition: a key process for clinically effective robotic prostatectomy, Med Biol Eng Comput 37, 236-243
6. Richard, W. and Keen, C. (1996) Automated texture-based segmentation of ultrasound images of the prostate, Comput Med Imag Graph 20 (3), 131-140
7. Prater, J. and Richard, W. (1992) Segmenting ultrasound images of the prostate using neural networks, Ultrasonic Imaging 14, 159-185
8. Richard, W., Grimmel, C., Bedigian, K. and Frank, K. (1993) A method for three-dimensional prostate imaging using transrectal ultrasound, Comput Med Imag Graph 17(2), 73-79
9. Aarnick, R., Pathak, S., Rosette, J., Debruyne, F., Kim, Y. and Wijkstra, H. (1998) Edge detection in prostatic ultrasound images using integrated edge maps, Ultrasonics 36, 635-642
10. Liu, Y., Ng, W., Teo, M. and Lim, H. (1997) Computerised prostate boundary estimation of ultrasound images using radial bas-relief method, Med Biol Eng Comput 35, 445-454
11. Levienaise-Obadia, B. and Gee, A. (1999) Adaptive segmentation of ultrasound images, Imag Vision Comput 17, 583-588
12. Crivianu-Gaita, D., Miclea, F., Gaspar, A., Margineatu, D. and Holban, S. (1997) 3D reconstruction of prostate from ultrasound images, Int J Medical Informatics 45, 43-51

Towards Dynamic Planning and Guidance of Minimally Invasive Robotic Cardiac Bypass Surgical Procedures

G Lehmann, A Chiu, D Gobbi, Y Starreveld, D Boyd, M Drangova, T Peters

The John P Robarts Resesrch Institute, The University of Western Ontario and the London Health Sciences Centre. London Ontario, Canada

Abstract. Conventional open-heart coronary bypass surgery requires a 30-cm long incision through the breast-bone and stopping the beating heart, which inflict great pain, trauma and lengthy recovery time to patients. Recently, a robot-assisted minimally invasive surgical technique has been introduced to coronary bypass to minimize incisions and avoid cardiac arrest in order to eliminate the medical complications associated with open-heart surgery. Despite its initial success, this innovation has its own limitations and problems. This paper discusses these limitations and proposes a framework that incorporates image-guidance techniques into MIRCAB surgery. We present two aspects of our preliminary work; 1) A Virtual Cardiac Surgical Planning system developed to visualize and manipulate simulated robotic surgical tools within the virtual patient. 2) Our work towards the extension of the static planning system to a dynamic situation that would model the position, orientation and dynamics of the heart, relative to the chest wall, during surgery.

1.1 Background

Traditional coronary artery bypass procedures (CAB) involve the utilization of a blood vessel (bypass graft) from another part of the body and surgically creating an alternate blood supply route, bypassing the blocked part of the artery. Minimally invasive direct coronary artery bypass (MIDCAB) techniques eliminate the need for full sternotomy and cardio-pulmonary bypass (CPB), and are all performed on the beating heart through a small incision in the chest wall. When employed in conjunction with a heart stabilizer, MIDCAB procedures eliminate many of the complications caused by CPB [1;2]. Despite its initial success, MIDCAB has some apparent shortcomings. Due to the small incision, access to the target vessels is limited and the execution of the anastomosis is more challenging. As a result of limited visualization and heart motion, the anastomosis may be less precise [3]. More recently, endoscopic port-access techniques have been incorporated into MIDCAB allowing minimally-invasive procedures to be employed. Nevertheless, a major limitation of these approaches is that the long-handled instruments used in MIDCAB magnify hand tremors, which can make precise suturing difficult and tiring. In addition, the surgeons' natural motion is actually the reverse of the motions of the instruments due to the fact that the instruments pass through a "key hole".

W. Niessen and M. Viergever (Eds.): MICCAI 2001, LNCS 2208, pp. 368-375, 2001.

Robot-assisted telesurgical systems were developed to avoid the restrictions of conventional endoscopic port-access instruments, to remove surgeon tremor, provide a minification factor between the operator's movements and the tools, and permit the surgeon to perform the procedure from a comfortable position.   Currently, two telesurgical robotic systems have been used experimentally and clinically (www.intuitivesurgical.com, www.computermotion.com). Over the past few years, the results of minimally invasive robotic coronary artery bypass (MIRCAB) procedures for closed-chest CPB have been encouraging [4-6].

MIRCAB nevertheless has several technical limitations, including the lack of guidance from conventional 2-D images of patients, possible improper port placement and limited field of view of the operative site from the endoscope. These problems must be overcome to further reduce trauma and risk to patients, which would in turn lead to shorter hospital stays and lower health care expenses.

1.2 A Virtual Environment for Surgical Planning

We believe that a virtual representation of the surgical environment will become an integral part of surgical planning and guidance for minimally invasive robot assisted therapies. Through the use of such simulation, the surgeons can familiarize themselves with new robotic technologies, optimize instrument placement, and plan patient specific procedures. Such virtual planning environments have been proposed by us and others [7,8] that allow the surgeon to simulate and validate incision sites.

Ultimately the goal of this research is to provide the surgeon with a dynamic virtual representation of the patient's thorax in the operating room where the patient's heart motion and positioning are synchronized in the virtual environment. With such a system, the surgeon would always maintain a global view of the operative site, and not be constrained by the small field-of-view of the endoscope.

1.3   Preliminary Work

In this paper we report two aspects of both our preliminary work aimed at providing a virtual cardiac surgical planning environment (VCSP) workstation to plan port placements for MIRCAB, as well as our work to position and animate a virtual heart model within the virtual representation of the patient's thorax. By presenting the VCSP and the virtual heart model together in one paper we hope to give an overview of our preliminary work towards creating a virtual environment for surgical planning of robot assisted coronary by-pass surgery.

2. Cardiac Surgical Planning Platform

The Virtual Cardiac Surgical Planning platform (VCSP) [8] is based on the infrastructure that was developed for the Atamai Surgical Planner (ASP) (www.atamai.com). ASP is written in C++ as well as Python (www.python.org), and relies heavily on the Visualization Tool Kit (VTK) (www.kitware.com) library of C++ classes. A typical computer configuration employed to run the surgical planning platforms is a Pentium III 650 MHz, 256MB RAM, and a 16MB video card with hardware 3-D acceleration. The capabilities of VCSP are as follows:

- Integration of dynamic (ECG-gated) surface and volume-rendered images derived from CT and/or MRI
- Visualization and manipulation of surface models of heart and thorax
- Interactive modeling of the robotic arms and the endoscope
- Interactive distance and angle measurement (3D Ruler)
- Generation of virtual endoscopic images from arbitrary viewpoints
- Interactive zoom of the modeled environment
- Displacement and rotation of individual objects,
- Transparency of overlying structures to expose the target for planning thoracic port placement.

For a bypass operation, the structures that are of most concern to the surgeons are the bypass graft, the coronaries, heart, ribs and the chest wall. The internal thoracic arteries, left coronary artery and the heart are extracted from the MRI images, while the ribs and the chest wall are obtained from the CT images. Segmentation is performed semi-automatically using thresholding and 3-D region-growing [9]. Within this environment, an operator may examine the topology of the patient's thoracic cavity and manipulate simulated surgical tools and endoscope to determine the proper port placement to ensure that they can access the targeted operative site.

2.1 Determination of Port Configuration

It is particularly important to be able to position the inter-costal ports relative to the surgical target(s) such that the surgical tools and endoscopes may interact together without collision. Tabaie *et al.*[10] describe a "magic pyramid" configuration that establishes the optimum configuration of the ports. Using VSCP, an operator can manipulate simulated tools (Fig 1) within the virtual thoracic cavity to determine a workable port configuration. The following steps are used to find the parameters of the pyramid:

1. Examine the topology of the patient through the 3-D thorax model of the patient. Decrease the opacity of the skin to reveal ribs and target.
2. Insert the virtual endoscope. Locate the target via the simulated endoscopic view.
3. Insert left and right thoracic ports. Perform a visual check to ensure the ports do not collide with each other or any of the thoracic structures.
4. Add the simulated trochars to approach the target and make measurements of the "magic pyramid" parameters by using the user interface built into the measurement windows.

At least three fiducial markers must be placed on the surface of the chest for pre-operative image acquisition and kept in place until the operation. The pre-operative 3-D model to the patient is registered to the model during the procedure using a free-hand tracking system. After the patient and model are in registration, the pre-determined incision points can be reproduced on the actual patient. The distances from each incision point to all the markers can be measured by VSCP and the coordinates of the markers can be determined by using the 3-D ruler. The distances between the markers and the incision points can be used to verify the accuracy of the registration.

2.2 Results

Images collected using the muti-modality approach discussed above were displayed in ASP, and were also segmented and reconstructed into 3-D surface models which were displayed in VSCP. The thoracic port placement simulation using the guidelines above was validated using a thoracic phantom. A physical endoscope and thoracic ports were inserted into the phantom to locate the pre-determined targets. A 3-D model of this phantom was imported into VSCP, and the port configurations were simulated and reproduced within the virtual environment. The parameters of the "magic" pyramids of the physical and the simulated port configurations could then be measured and compared.

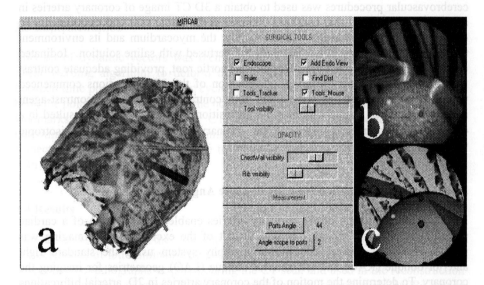

Figure 1. a)VCSP platform incorporating merged thorax and heart images, robotic instruments and endoscope. b) endoscope view of target via real endoscope in physical model, c) virtual endoscope view in VCSP.

The system, as described, can assist the surgeon in the optimal placement of the ports, but relates to a completely static situation, with no movement of the heart between imaging and surgery; no breathing-induced motion and no beating heart. In addition, the patient position on the OR table is generally different from that during imaging. To be effective in the realistic situation, the environment described above must be combined with a means of placing a realistic dynamic model of the heart,

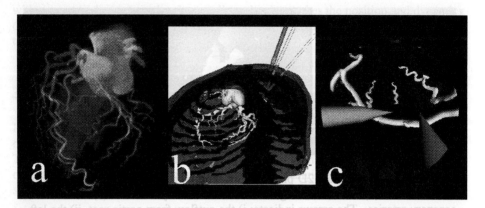

Figure 3. a) an overly of 2 MIPs of the deformed 3D CT images showing the dynamic nature of the model. b) a segmented version of the dynamic 3D CT image integrated into the VCSP platform. c) a virtual endoscopic view of the segmented heart.

The non-linear warping algorithm was then implemented based on the eighteen dynamic landmarks. The fidelity of the deformation algorithm was first evaluated qualitatively by comparing MPRs through the deformed volume images with equivalent MPRs from the original 3D CT image. To demonstrate the dynamics of the coronary-artery model, overlayed MIPs of the 3D images are shown in Figure 3a.

4. Summary

The two themes presented above are both part of a feasibility study aimed at evaluating techniques that could be incorporated into a virtual environment to plan, train and guide robotically-assisted cardiovascular surgery procedures. We have demonstrated that in a static environment, prediction of target positions on the myocardium can be achieved with a precision of 3mm, and that we can animate a static heart model such that the dynamics of the vascular structures can be modeled with approximately the same precision. While here is still much room for improvement, we believe that the combination of the cardiac animation procedure, using gated angiograms acquired in the OR during surgery, can effectively animate a cardiac model within the virtual surgical environment.

The VCSP platform and the virtual heart model will be valuable tools in the development of a dynamic virtual representation of the patient's thorax. While many limitations exist and integrating the virtual heart model into the VCSP will be an important step towards achieving our ultimate goal, our preliminary results are demonstrated in Figure 3. Our ultimate goal is to use the techniques described above to animate a finite-element model of a patients heart which would be integrated with the VCSP environment.

Acknowledgements

We acknowledge support for this project from the Canadian Institute for Health Research (CIHR) and the Heart and Stroke Foundation of Ontario (HSFO). We also acknowledge our college Ravi Gupta for his technical assistance in this project.

Bibliography

1. Subramanian, V. A., McCabe, J. C., and Geller, C. M., "Minimally invasive direct coronary artery bypass grafting: two-year clinical experience," *Ann. Thorac. Surg.*, vol. 64, no. 6, pp. 1648-1653, Dec.1997.
2. Diegeler, A., Falk, V., Matin, M., Battellini, et al., "Minimally invasive coronary artery bypass grafting without cardiopulmonary bypass: early experience and follow-up," *Ann. Thorac. Surg.*, vol. 66, no. 3, pp. 1022-1025, Sept.1998.
3. Pagni, S., Qaqish, N. K., Senior, D. G., and Spence, P. A., "Anastomotic complications in minimally invasive coronary bypass grafting," *Ann. Thorac. Surg.*, vol. 63, no. 6 Suppl, pp. S64-S67, June1997.
4. Loulmet, D., Carpentier, A., d'Attellis, N., et al., "Endoscopic coronary artery bypass grafting with the aid of robotic assisted instruments " *J. Thorac. Cardiovasc. Surg.*, vol. 118, no. 1, pp. 4-10, July1999.
5. Reichenspurner, H., Boehm, D. H., Gulbins, H., et al., "Robotically assisted endoscopic coronary artery bypass procedures without cardiopulmonary bypass," *J. Thorac. Cardiovasc. Surg.*, vol. 118, no. 5, pp. 960-961, Nov.1999.
6. Ducko CT. Robotically – assisted coronary artery bypass surgery: moving toward a completely endoscopic procedure. Edward R.Stephenson, Jr MD1 Sachin Sankholkar MS2 Ralph J. Damiano Jr MD1. Heart Surgery Forum 2[1]. 9-2-1999.
7. Louai, A., Coste-Manière, E., Boissonnat J.D., "Planning and Simulation of Robotically Assisted Minimal Invasive Surgery", MICCAI 2000, 1935, 624-633.
8. Chui, A. M., Dey D., Drangova, M., Boyd, W.D., and Peters, T.M., "3D Image Guidance for Minimally Invasive Robotic Coronary Artery Bypass (MIRCAB)", Heart Surgery Forum, 3(3):224-231, 2000.
9. Slomka, P. J., Hurwitz, G. A., and Stephenson, J. A volume-based image registration toolkit for automated comparison of paired nuclear medicine images. Med Phys 22. 1995.
10. Tabaie,H. A., Reinbolt, J. A., Graper, W. P., et al. "Endoscopic coronary artery bypass graft (ECABG) procedure with robotic assistance." Heart Surgery Forum 2(4): 310-317, 1999.
11. Fahrig, R., Fox, A. J., Lownie, S., and Holdsworth, D. W. Use of a C-arm system to generate true three-dimensional computed rotational angiograms: preliminary in vitro and in vivo results. AJNR Am J Neuroradiol 18 (8), 1507-14. 1997.
12. Bookstein F.L., "Principal warps: Thin-plane splines and the decomposition of deformations," *IEEE Transactions on Pattern Analysis and Machine Intelligence*, vol. PAMI-11, no. 6, pp. 567-585, 1989.

Novel Real-Time Tremor Transduction Technique for Microsurgery

Damian Tomlin[1, 2], Jeffrey Wallace[1, 2], Ralph Etienne-Cummings[1, 3], and Nitish Thakor[1, 2]

[1] Engineer Research Center for Computer Integrated Surgical Systems and Technology, Baltimore, MD, USA
[2] Johns Hopkins University, Department of Biomedical Engineering, Baltimore, MD, USA
nthakor@bme.jhu.edu
[3] Johns Hopkins University, Department of Electrical and Computer Engineering, Baltimore, MD, USA
retienne@jhu.edu

Abstract. Physiological tremor is one of the limiting factors to the scale on which a microsurgeon can operate. The ability to correctly determine the amount of tremor a surgeon has is an invaluable tool both for tremor cancellation and for surgical training. For this reason we have developed a novel tremor transducer using a custom built VLSI motion detection chip connected to the surgical microscope. The chip detects and measures the magnified motion of a microsurgical tool tip under the microscope. This innovative design offers several advantages over conventional methods. It is nonintrusive to the surgeon – not interfering with current microsurgical set-ups; it outputs real-time tremor data, and is small and inexpensive. The system has been implemented in an experimental set-up for analysis of the factors that aggravate tremor. Results presented, include the use of the system as a audio feedback mechanism for tremor reduction – eliciting up to a 16% reduction in tremor.

1. Introduction

Microsurgery involves the performance of surgery on very small blood vessels, nerves and other tissue under microscope magnification. The most dexterous of microsurgeons gain their accolades from their ability to perform very precise procedures on smaller and smaller tissue. As surgeons and clinicians seek to push the limits of microsurgical practice, they encounter several problems – tremor for one. The effect of tremor on microsurgical practice becomes quickly obvious when one looks at the relative scale of microsurgery. With tremor amplitudes on the order of 133 μm [1] working on a 100-μm blood vessel can be quite a formidable task.

Tremor is broadly defined as any involuntary, approximately rhythmic, and roughly sinusoidal movement [3]. More specifically physiologic tremor is defined as a normal involuntary motion accompanying all postures and movements. There are two rhythmic components of physiologic tremor: an 8 to 12-Hz component and a mechanical-reflex component. The frequency of physiologic tremor is classically

W. Niessen and M. Viergever (Eds.): MICCAI 2001, LNCS 2208, pp. 376-383, 2001.

stated to be at 10 Hz but it tends to vary depending on the part of the body from which it is recorded. Although there is no conclusive evidence to support a relationship between the genesis of 8- to 12-Hz tremor and visual feedback, investigations by Isokawa-Akesson and Komisaruk [8] support a correlation between the amplitude and frequency of 8- to 12-Hz tremor and visual feedback.

The methods developed in this paper were used to investigate a correlation between 8- to 12-Hz tremor and audio feedback. This correlation was hypothesized by Harwell and Ferguson [17], who report that with audio feedback of tremor magnitude microsurgical trainees were able to determine which factors aggravate their tremor and make adjustments to minimize it. In effect, the system developed here provides substantial data in the exploration of ways to reduce surgical tremor.

2. System Design and Implementation

2.1 Prior Tremor Sensing Techniques

Prior tremor sensing techniques include *Hall Effect sensors*. The Microsurgery Advanced Design Laboratory Stability, Activation, and Maneuverability tester (MADSAM) is one such system. The MADSAM uses a magnetic field sensor, an analog signal capture board, and customized software routines to correlate magnetic field strength with physical location. The MADSAM can record the position of a small ceramic magnet affixed to a microsurgical instrument, at an accuracy of 1 micron [16]. Norman et al [15] discussed the measurement of tremor using *laser-based transducers*. The measurement principle of a laser transducer is based upon the Doppler effect. Monochromatic laser light, scattered back from a vibrating target, undergoes a frequency shift proportional to the velocity of the target. The frequency of the back-scattered beam is frequency modulated at the so-called Doppler frequency, which is directly proportional to the velocity of the target. *Accelerators* have also been used in tremor-sensing systems. They are highly favored because acceleration is widely considered as a more relevant variable for tremor than is velocity or displacement [15]. Gomez-Blanco et al [14] developed a method for sensing hand tremor in a vitreoretinal microsurgical instrument by attaching three accelerometers to the instrument. Hall Effect sensors and laser-based transducers are not practical for intraoperative use because of their size and mode of operation, and accelerometers intrude on the surgeon by adding some weight to his tool. Our system fills the void created by these different tremor-sensing modalities by offering a completely non-intrusive and easily implemented design.

2.2 Design Criteria

The system is designed to be non-intrusive, to offer the requisite frequency response and artifact rejection, and to be cost-effective. The technique employed does not interfere with the current setup for performing microsurgery. It causes minimal obtrusion to the surgical field. This allows for a test-bed setup that is not cumbersome and that does not introduce undesirable interference to the experiment. The system, as described below, involves only a simply connection to the video output port of the surgical microscope.

Sampling frequency restrictions are also be satisfied. The characteristic frequency of physiologic tremor, on the order of 8-12 Hz, dictates that the sampling frequency of any transducer system must be, at the bare minimum, 24 Hz to comply with the Nyquist sampling theorem and avoid aliasing problems. For our experiment we used a sampling frequency of 250 Hz, which is well above the Nyquist limit.

2.3 Stereomicroscope, DAQ System

Figure 1 shows a schematic of the full system. The shiny tool tip reflects light from the microscope light source. Against a non-reflective background the tool tip is easily identified and differentiated from any other movement within the field of view. This ensures that the chip detects only the tool-tip's motion. Furthermore, during experiments, the tool tip is the only moving object in focus underneath the microscope. The motion of the tool tip is magnified through the microscope and translated onto the surface of the motion detection chip.

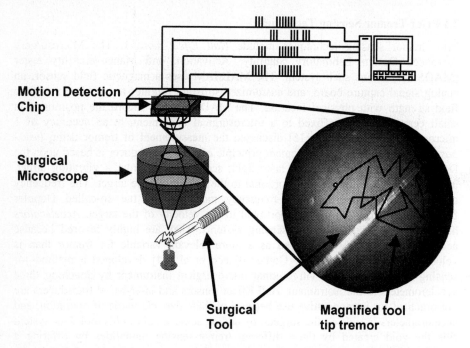

Figure 1: Schematic of the tremor analysis system. The magnified motion of the surgical tool is detected by the motion detection chip. The speed and direction of motion is reported to the data acquisition system. A view of the surgical tool from the chip's perspective is also shown.

The chip has four output lines from the fovea (See Section 2.3). These lines correspond to the Left, Right, Up and Down directions in the plane of the chip. Each line outputs a 5V pulse-train whenever the chip detects an object moving in its direction. In LabVIEW (a visual programming language from National Instruments, Austin, TX), the number of pulses from each output line is averaged over a specific time period. This average (or the density of the pulse-train) is proportional to the speed of the object the chip detects. The average number of Left pulses is subtracted from the average number of Right pulses to yield the X-component of tremor velocity. Similarly, the Y-component is obtained by subtracting the average number of Down pulses from Up pulses. This way a vector representing the velocity of the tremor signal is obtained. The acceleration signal is obtained by a five-point derivative of each component of velocity and, in turn, a vector addition of both resulting acceleration components. The equation below shows the expression used to compute the derivative.

$$df = C_1 f(n) + C_2 f(n-1) - C_2 f(n-2) - C_1 f(n-3)$$

where $C_1 = 1.08144$ and $C_2 = 2.69869$ are coefficients determined from a Gaussian derivative detailed in [19].

The motion detection chip, housed in a 3x2x1 inch box is connected to the video port

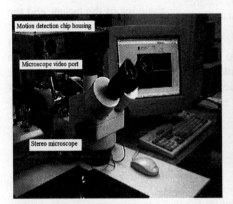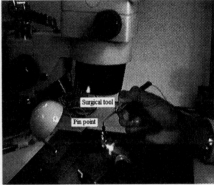

Figure 2. Picture of the setup. The magnified motion of the surgical tool is detected by the motion detection chip connected at the video port of the microscope.

of the microscope through a two-inch C-mount connector (Figure 2). The "focus" knob of the microscope is used to account for the two-inch focal length discrepancy caused by the introduction of the connector. The camera is connected to a PCI-MIO-16E-4 data acquisition card (National Instruments, Austin TX), which is, in turn, accessed from LabVIEW 5.1 software.

2.4 VLSI Motion Detection Chip

Figure 3 shows a picture of the motion detection chip used in the system. The chip is organized into a foveal region and a peripheral region, similar to primate biological systems. It uses compact focal-plane processing to allow for two-dimensional tracking [12]. When a target enters the fovea, an edge detection algorithm determines the edge of the target. The direction of motion of the target is determined by which neighboring pixel the edge reappears after disappearing from one pixel. The motion detection circuit in the fovea produces the pulse train on the Left, Right, Up and Down global motion lines when a target moves away from the center in any of these directions. The chip has two processing stages: phototransduction and edge detection.

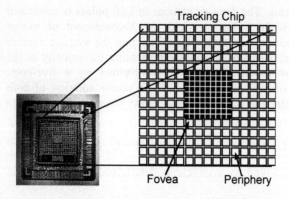

Tracking Chip

Fovea   Periphery

Figure 3: Motion detection chip. The fovea is towards the center of the chip, and the periphery immediately surrounds the fovea.

The *photo-transduction stage* contains the phototransistors and range compression circuits, and the *edge detection* stage computes the edge of the target. A number of issues were considered to ensure that the chip could satisfy the requirements for a tremor transducer. The photoreceptors (photo-transistors) and the edge detection circuitry must be able to correctly determine the edge of the target, and the fovea must be able to report the correct information about the motion of the target. The chip must also possess adequate speed sensitivity. Each of these criterions was tested independently. See [12] for chip performance test results. The chip is operational for ambient intensities ranging over 6 orders of magnitude, targets contrast as low as 10%, and foveal speed ranging from 1.5 to 10K pixels/s.

3. Results and Discussion

Results are presented for the system in operation for two separate experiments: tremor acceleration magnitude versus speed of movement, and tremor acceleration magnitude with and without audio feedback. Figure 4 shows the conversion from

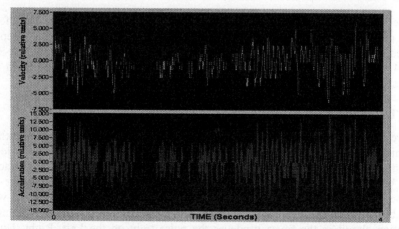

Figure 4. Top graph shows velocity in the X-direction (average Right pulses subtract minus average Left pulses) and bottom graph shows the acceleration in the X-direction (derivative of velocity).

velocity, as determined from the transducer, to acceleration (determined by a Gaussian derivative of the velocity) The top graph in shows the velocity of the tool tip in the X-direction and the bottom graph shows the acceleration in the X-direction. The top graph of Figure 5 shows the magnitude of the acceleration vector and the bottom graph shows a moving average over 50 samples. The magnitude of the acceleration vector is proportional to the amount of tremor present.

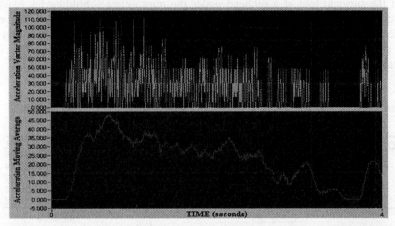

Figure 5. Top graph shows the magnitude of the acceleration vector (vector addition of X and Y components). Bottom graph shows a moving average over 50 samples.

Figure 6 shows results obtained from the system when measuring tremor against a variation in the speed of movement. In this experiment the subject is asked to move a microsurgical tool back and forth in the microscope's field of view at varying frequencies of motion. The speed of oscillation is kept by a metronome. The mean tremor acceleration is recorded for frequencies ranging from 1 to 5 Hz. Figure 6a

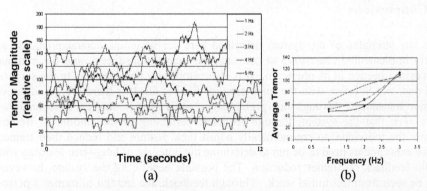

Figure 6. Tremor recorded for voluntary oscillation along a line. The subject is asked to move a microsurgical tool back and forth in the microscope field of view at varying frequency of motion. The frequency (and thus the speed) is kept by a metronome. The mean acceleration recorded increases nearly linearly with increase in the frequency of oscillation.

382   D. Tomlin et al.

shows that at each consecutive increase in frequency, the mean tremor acceleration increases. There is a nearly linear increase in tremor acceleration with frequency (Figure 6b).

Figure 7 shows the results of giving audio feedback of the magnitude of tremor to a subject with no prior surgical training. The results were generated using the Microsoft Excel Analysis of Variance (ANOVA) statistical analysis tool. The subject was asked to point the surgical tool at a pinhead under the microscope – holding his hand as steady as possible – first without audio feedback of tremor magnitude, then with audio feedback. This was repeated five times. Without audio feedback the average tremor acceleration recorded was 35.6 and with feedback it was 30.6. This is a statistically significant decrease in average tremor of 16% (P < .05).

Anova: Single Factor   **NO FEEDBACK**

SUMMARY

Groups	Count	Sum	Average	Variance
Column 1	1301	41994.83	32.27888	310.488
Column 2	1301	57058.87	43.8577	258.6325
Column 3	1301	57167.83	43.94146	262.5986
Column 4	1301	38782.61	29.80984	199.838
Column 5	1301	36724.62	28.22799	159.2528
			35.62318	

Anova: Single Factor   **WITH FEEDBACK**

SUMMARY

Groups	Count	Sum	Average	Variance
Column 1	1301	45577.67	35.0328	483.5768
Column 2	1301	45231.8	34.76695	334.6004
Column 3	1301	15535.66	11.94132	50.27678
Column 4	1301	52235.77	40.15048	124.3033
Column 5	1301	40723.61	31.30178	243.8863
			30.63867	

(a)   (b)

Figure7. Results for audio feedback analysis. The "boxed" figures show the average tremor magnitude for 5 experiments. With feedback there is a 16.5 % decrease in tremor magnitude. (a) the average tremor acceleration is recorded over a 30-second time period for a subject holding the surgical tool steady at one single point. (b) The experiment is repeated while giving audio feedback of acceleration.

4. Conclusions

The key strengths of the system described here are its unique characteristic as an easily implemented alternative to conventional tremor transducers, and the minimal processing needed in its operation. It is also completely non-intrusive to the surgeon and does not interfere with the microsurgical field at all. It is therefore, an effective tremor transducer. Through our preliminary results on non-surgical personnel, we have seen that the system, through feedback pertaining to the amount of tremor, allows the individual to ergonomically adjust their posture and reduce their tremor. More experiments need to be run to determine the outcome of long-term learning with audio feedback on tremor reduction. The possible benefits of the system, however, can be seen from this initial work. Through feedback, the amount of tremor a person has can be minimized for finer, more precise movements during a procedure. This has the ability to improve upon surgical outcomes by decreasing tremor related errors and by decreasing surgery times.

References

1. Riviere CN, Rader RS, Khosla PK. Characteristics of Hand Motion of Eye Surgeons. Prodeedings – 19th International Conference – IEEE/EMBS Oct. 30 – Nov. 2, 1997 Chicago, IL. USA.
2. Silber, SJ. Microsurgery, 1979. The Williams & Wilkins Company, Baltimore, MD
3. Elble R, Koller W. Tremor. Baltimore, MD: Johns Hopkins University Press, 1990
4. Stiles RN. Mechanical and Neural Feedback Factors in Postural Hand Tremor of Normal Subjects. Journal of Neurophysiology 1980; 44:40-59.
5. Wade P, Gresty MA, Findley LJ. A Normative Study of Postural Tremor of the Hand. Archives of Neurology 1982; 39:358-362.
6. Elble RJ. Physiologic and Essential Tremor. Neurology 1986; 36:225-231.
7. Elble RJ, Moody C, Higgins C. Primary Writing Tremor: a form of focal dystonia? Movement Disorders 1990; 5:118-126.
8. Isokawa-Akesson M, Komisaruk BR. Tuning the Power Spectrum of Physiological Finger Tremor Frequency with Flickering light. Journal of Neuroscience Res 1985; 14:373-380.
9. Brumlik J, Yap C-B. Normal Tremor: A Comparative Study. 1970. Springfield, Ill: Charles C Thomas, pp 3-15.
10. Freund H-J. Motor Unit and Muscle Activity in Voluntary Motor Control. Physiological Reviews 1983; 63:387-436.
11. Allum JHJ, Hulliger M. Presumed reflex responses of human first dorsal interosseus muscle to naturally occurring twitch contractions of physiological tremor. Neuroscience Letters 1982; 28:309-314.
12. Etienne-Cummings R, Van der Spiegel J, Mueller P. A Foveated Silicon Retina for Two-Dimensional Tracking. IEEE Trans. Circuits and System II, Vol. 47, No. 6, June 2000.
13. Reichardt W. Autocorrelation: A Principle for the Evaluation of Sensory Information by the Central Nervous System. Sensory Communication, Wiley, New York NY, 1961.
14. Gomez-Blanco M, Riviere CN, Khosla PK. Sensing Hand Tremor in a Vitreoretinal Microsurgical Instrument. CMU-RI-TR-99-39. The Robotics Institute, Carnegie Mellon University, Pittsburgh PA.
15. Norman KE, Edwards R, Beuter A. The measurement of tremor using a velocity transducer: comparison to simultaneous recordings using transducers of displacement, acceleration and muscle activity. Journal of Neuroscience Methods 1999; 92:41-54.
16. Humayun MU, Rader RS, Piermici DJ, Awh CC, de Juan E. Quantitative Measurement of the Effects of Caffeine and Propranolol on Surgeon hand Tremor. Archives of Ophthalmology 1997; 115:371-374.
17. Harwell RC, Ferguson RL. Physiologic Tremor and Microsurgery. Microsurgery 1983; 4:187-192.
18. Taylor R, Jensen P, Whitcomb L, Barnes A, Kumar R et al. A Steady-Hand Robotic System for Microsurgical Augmentation. The International Journal of Robotics Research 1999; Dec.
19. Simoncelli EP. Distributed Representation and Analysis of Visual Motion. PhD Thesis, MIT Dept. of Electrical Engineering and Computer Science, 1993; p95-97.

Computer Assisted Dental Implantology:
A New Method and a Clinical Validation

Julien Dutreuil[1], François Goulette[1] and Claude Laurgeau[1]
Jaime Clavero Zoreda[2] and Stefan Lundgren[2]

[1] Centre de Robotique, Ecole des Mines de Paris, 60 boulevard Saint Michel,
75272 Paris Cedex 06, France
{dutreuil, goulette, laurgeau}@caor.esnmp.fr
[2] Department of Oral and Maxillofacial Surgery, Umeå Universitet, 90187 Umeå, Sweden
jclavero.z@tbc.es, stefan.lundgren@odont.umu.se

Abstract. This paper presents a new method for dental implant surgery. A pre-operative planning software is used to work with CT scanner data. Implant fixtures are placed with the help of a 3D reconstructed model of the patient's jaw. An accurate robot is then used to drill a jaw splint, at the locations determined with the planning software, in order to make a surgical guide. A validation case of this new technique is also presented.

1 Introduction

Dental implants are used in maxillofacial restoration to replace a tooth or a set of teeth. One implant is composed of three parts : a titanium fixture surgically placed into the patient's jaw, a prosthetic crown replacing the missing tooth, and a mechanical part connected between the fixture and the crown, the abutment.

The success of a dental implantation depends directly on the localisation of the fixture in the patient's jaw bone. Firstly, the good adequacy between the axis of the fixture (surgical axis) and the axis of the prosthetic tooth (prosthetic axis) is critical for the good setting of the implant : the angle between both axes must be as small as possible in order to minimise lateral constraints transmitted from the crown to the abutment and then to the fixture [1]. Secondly, the fixture must be precisely implanted in hard cortical bone to assure a good stability. The surgery also requires great accuracy because of particularly sensitive anatomic structures in the neighbourhood of these implants (the mandibular nerve and the maxillary sinus) [1,2].

The new technique we propose improves the accuracy in the fixture placement. It uses a pre-operative planning phase for virtual placement of the fixture, and an accurate robot to drill a jaw splint, exact negative shape of the patient's jaw, in order to create a surgical guide.

Other solutions have already been proposed to improve the accuracy of the fixture placement: using a robot for drilling a splint [1, 3, 4], using stereo-lithography to build the splint from CT scans [5, 6], or using a navigation system during the surgery, coupled with scanner data [7, 8].

W. Niessen and M. Viergever (Eds.): MICCAI 2001, LNCS 2208, pp. 384-391, 2001.

2 Overview of the New Method

This method consists in a 4-stage procedure, presented below and on figure 1.

Stage 1 : a denture impression of the patient's jaw is taken. It is used to make a plaster model of the jaw, and a splint on which the missing teeth are replaced by crowns. Radio-opaque balls are placed at precise locations on the splint, to provide scanner markers [9].

Stage 2 : a CT scan of the patient is taken, with the splint placed in the mouth. The use of CT scans is very classical in dental implantology, because they can provide complete 3D data by tomographic reconstruction, with an excellent sensitivity to bone tissues density [9, 10].

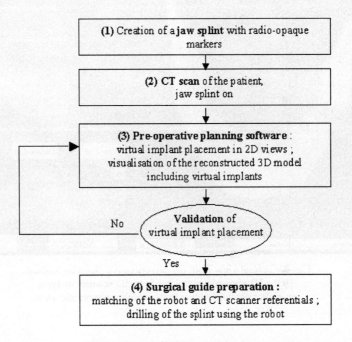

Fig. 1. Sketch of the new method

Stage 3 : the clinician uses the pre-operative planning software and the CT scan data to precisely choose the location of virtual implants. Visual validation of the locations planned is made with the help of 3D reconstructed views of the patient's jaw.

Stage 4 : the splint is placed on the plaster model which is fixed on the robot work plan. Radio-opaque balls located on the splint are visible directly, on the splint and on the CT scanner data : the matching between the robot referential and the CT data referential may be performed. The result of the matching is combined with the information of the desired implant location, expressed in the scanner referential, to compute the implant location in the robot referential. Finally, the splint is drilled by the robot at this precise location to make the surgical guide.

3 Detailed Technical Description of the Method

Some of the stages described above need additional description : the pre-operative planning stage, the method used for 3D visualisation of the scanner data, and the making of the surgical guide including the drilling of the splint.

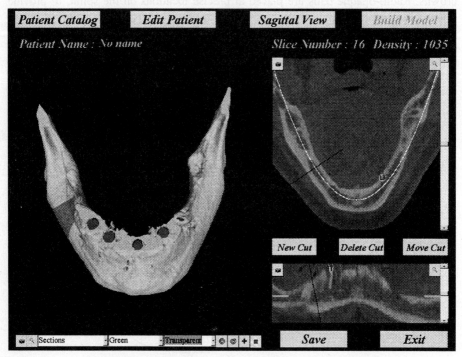

Fig. 2. General view from the pre-operative planning software
(left : 3D view reconstructed from 2D scanner images;
top-right : occlusal view ; bottom-right : panoramic view)

3.1 Pre-operative Planning

To prepare the surgery, a dedicated software that has been especially developed to be adapted to the needs of dental implant surgeons is used (Figure 2). The planning stage consists in identifying the best location to place implants inside the patient's jaw, according to the ideal prosthesis, in order to improve the medical result [11]. The software provides tools and cut views interpolated from the data to optimise this location process.

In a very classical way, dental surgeons work in a local referential fixed on the patient's jaw. This referential defines 3 classical views : the occlusal view, the panoramic view, and the vestibo lingual view.

The occlusal plane is the key reference in the patient's mouth. It is defined by the plane of teeth occlusion. Scanner data are usually acquired in planes parallel to this occlusal plane, so we assimilate occlusal views with these scanner pictures (Figure 2, top-right).

The panoramic view is defined as a view perpendicular to the occlusal plane, curved on a specific way following the jaw shape of each patient. In the software (figure 2, bottom-right), it is defined in the occlusal plane with the help of a 2D curve, which is a 3rd order polynomial. This polynomial is generated by three control points, with a null derivative constraint on the middle point.

The vestibo lingual view is defined locally, as a planar cut view positioned along the panoramic curve, locally perpendicular to this curve. Initially perpendicular to the occlusal plane, it can be inclined from the direction perpendicular to the occlusal plane with a few degrees (+/- 15°), in order to adapt the view to the specific anatomy of the patient and to get more information.

On the planning software, the surgeon visualises the occlusal views, defines the panoramic view by moving the control points, and chooses the vestibo lingual cut views. Implant placements are usually performed initially in the vestibo lingual views. The position, orientation, length and diameter of the implant may be defined interactively, in each view, with a visual feedback in all the graphical windows.

3.2 3D Visualisation of Scanner Data

The 3D model of the patient anatomy gives helpful information on implants location and inclination. In order to build such a 3D model, a pre-processing segmentation stage is performed to identify, for each pixel, the kind of human tissue to which it belongs. For dental surgery, there are soft tissues (mucosa, skin, muscles, fat), bone tissues (soft bone, hard cortical bone, teeth) and metal objects (surgical screws, implants, radio-opaque markers...).

The good sensitivity of CT scans for bone tissues makes it possible to use a simple threshold to segment the raw images, after a simple filtering operation (low pass filter), to eliminate the background noise in the measured data. The comparison of scanner images pixel intensities to standard values gives a good evaluation of the pixel nature. Data obtained by CT scans are expressed in Hounsfield Units (HU), normalised with the air density (-1000 HU) and the water density (0 HU). Therefore, the threshold values are identified universal constants: e.g., bone generally ranged from 200 HU to 1500 HU.

The measure points are regularly distributed on a 3D grid. After the segmentation operation, we generate a skin surface model by extracting a local mesh on each voxel of this 3D grid. Locally, the skin triangulation mesh is obtained using a method based on the "marching-cube" algorithm [12].

For each voxel, the mesh configuration is identified by looking at the tissues recognised on each vertex. For all segments including an intersection with the tissue, the intersection location is estimated by linear interpolation of the threshold between the 2 extremity values. Instead of a reduced number of cases identified by symmetry analysis, we use a complete reference table (256 cases), which speeds up the algorithm and minimises the risk of generating unclosed meshes.

Once the model is built, a post-processing stage is necessary. Generated models are very large. For example, a poor resolution scanner exam (256 x 256 pixels per picture with 30 pictures) can generate more than 250,000 triangles just for bone

388   J. Dutreuil et al.

tissues. For high resolution ones (512 x 512 pixels per picture with 50 pictures), the number of generated triangles can be over 1,500,000. In order to work with such models on a simple PC, a simplification stage is necessary.

Different solutions are possible for mesh simplification, as segment or vertex decimation methods [13] or use of a decimation criterion. In our software, a basic method using vertex decimation, with a threshold criterion on a propagated angular deformation of vertex normals has been implemented. For the next version of the software, a segment decimation method using a parametric representation of the local surface is considered [14].

3.3 Drilling of the Surgical Guide

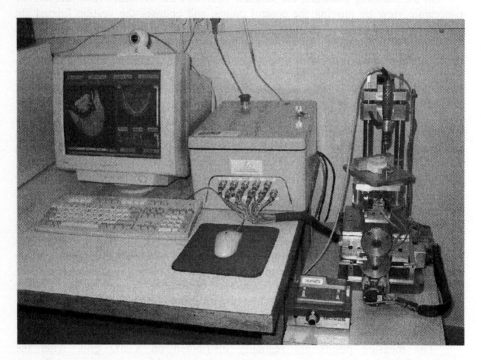

Fig. 3. Complete processing workbench, from pre-operative planning to splint drilling

As presented above, the jaw splint is placed in the mouth of the patient during the scanner acquisition. Radio-opaque balls are placed on this splint, at several specific positions regularly spaced along the jaw arch. These radio-opaque balls are visible in both the scanner images and the jaw splint.

After the virtual implant placement is done, the plaster model is attached to the robot work plan, and the splint is adjusted on the plaster model. The robot is an accurate numerical command machine, with five degrees of freedom (3 translations and 2 rotations). It has a 0.04 mm translation accuracy, and a 0.15° rotation accuracy (Figure 3).

By pointing the radio-opaque balls with the robot, the location of these balls in the robot referential is determined with an accuracy close to 0.3 mm ; by pointing them in the CT scanner images, their location in the scanner referential is also determined, with an accuracy close to 0.25 mm (only limited by the scanner definition).

The radio-opaque balls locations in the two referentials (robot referential and scanner referential) define two sets of control points that have to be matched, by identification of 3 rotation and 3 translation parameters defining the referential frame transformation. This is a non linear problem, which is solved using a least squares minimisation of the sum of distances between each couple of points. The classical Levenberg Marquardt algorithm [15] is used, instead of a simple gradient method to prevent low convergence trouble caused by flat potentials.

We can evaluate that the global accuracy of the complete treatment, from the planning phase to the surgery as presented on figure 3, is lower than 1 mm in location and 1° in orientation.

4 Clinical Validation

A first case has been treated with this new protocol, at the department of oral and maxillo-facial surgery of Umeå University, in Sweden. The patient was an upper jaw edentulous woman. Because of a strong bone resorption, she had a bone graft before the implant surgery.

It is noteworthy that, even if the patient was treated with our new experimental method, there was no additional risk compared to the classical method, as has been pointed out elsewhere for a similar method [1]: a visual expertise was performed by the surgeon on the surgical guide before the surgery.

A 8-implant treatment was planned, using the pre-operative planning software, visible on figure 4-a ; figure 4-b shows the robot drilling the splint ; on figure 4-c, one can see the patient during the surgery, with the surgical guide placed in the mouth, right before drilling the jaw ; figure 4-d displays the position of the fixture implants placed in the jaw after drilling.

This first operation was a success, validating our method : all implants were precisely placed at the right location.

5 Conclusion

A new method for dental implantology has been presented, which is based on the use of a surgical guide, CT scanner imaging, a pre-operative planning software, a robot to drill the splint and a method based on radio-opaque markers to match the implant virtual positions and the actual drilling directions in the splint.

The first clinical case demonstrated the simplicity and the efficiency of the method. Further work is planned with a clinical validation campaign.

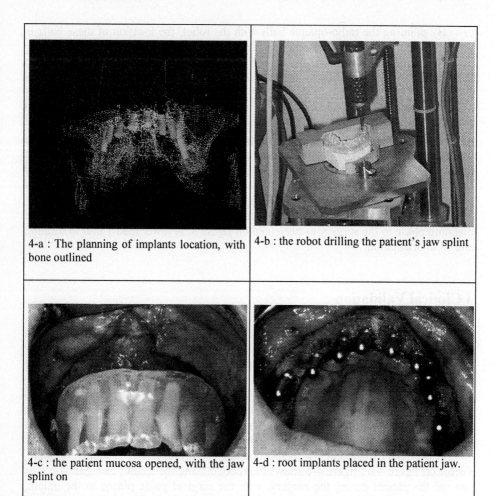

4-a : The planning of implants location, with bone outlined

4-b : the robot drilling the patient's jaw splint

4-c : the patient mucosa opened, with the jaw splint on

4-d : root implants placed in the patient jaw.

Fig. 4. The first validation case.

6 Acknowledgments

This work has been partly supported by the VISIMPLANT Leonardo da Vinci European program (partners: Ecole des Mines de Paris, Umeå University, Techdent, SFO, Imperial College).

References

1. T. Fortin, J.P. Coudert, G. Champleboux et al. : "Computer-assisted dental implant surgery using computed tomography", Journal of image guided surgery, no. 1, p. 53-58, 1995
2. S.L. Bass : "The effects of preoperative resorption and jaw anatomy on implant success: a report of 303 cases". Clin. Oral Impl. Res., no. 2, p. 193-198.
3. G. Champleboux, E. Blanchet, T. Fortin et al. : "A fast, accurate and easy method to position oral implants using computed tomography". In Proc. Computer Assisted Radiology - CAR'98, Elsevier Science, H.U.Lemke Ed., 1998.
4. K. Verstreken, J. van Cleynenbreugel, G. Marchal et al. : "An image guided planning system for oral implant surgery". Proc. of Computer Aided Radiology - CAR '96, p. 888-893, 1996.
5. V. Hietschold, W. Harzer, L. Eckhardt et al. : "Stereolithography of the occlusion plane using MR-tomographic imaging of the set of teeth". In Proc. Computer Assisted Radiology, 1996.
6. J. Lambrecht, C. Besimo, W. Müller et al. : "Precision of presurgical implantological planning with digitised CT and Scanora". In Proc. Computer Assisted Radiology, 1996.
7. P. Solar, S. Rodinger, C. Ulm et al. : "A computer-aided navigation system for oral implants using 3D-CT reconstructions and real time video projection", Int. Conf on Computer Assisted Radiology, 1996.
8. W. Birkfellner, F. Wanschitz, F. Watzinger et al. : "Accuracy of a Navigation System for Computer-Aided Oral Implantology", Proc. MICCAI'00, Lecture Notes in Computer Sciences no. 1935, Springer Verlag, p. 1061-1067, 2000.
9. N. L. Frederiksen : "Diagnostic imaging in dental implantology", Oral surgery, oral medicine, oral pathology, vol. 80, no. 5, p. 540-554, 1995.
10. N. Bellaiche, D. Doyon : "La tomodensimétrie dans le bilan pré-opératoire en implantologie orale", Journal de la Radiologie, tome 73, n°1, 1992.
11. K. Verstreken, J. Van Cleynenbreugel, K. Mertens et al. : "An Image-Guided Planning System for Endosseous Oral Implants", IEEE Transactions on Medical Imaging, 17(5): p. 842-852, 1998
12. W.E. Lorensen, H.E. Cline : "Marching Cube: A High Resolution 3-D Surface Construction Algorithm", Computer Graphics, 21(3): p. 163-169, 1987
13. W.J. Schroeder, J.A. Zarge, W.E. Lorensen : "Decimation of Triangle Meshes", Computer Graphics, 26 (2), p 55-64, 1992.
14. M.J. Diaz, F. Hecht, "Anisotropic Surface Mesh Generation", INRIA, MENUSIN project, research report n° 2672, 1995.
15. D.W. Marquardt, Journal of the society for industrial and applied mathematics, vol. 11, p. 431-441, 1963.

Intra-operative Real-Time 3-D Information Display System Based on Integral Videography

Hongen Liao[1], Susumu Nakajima[2], Makoto Iwahara[3], Etsuko Kobayashi[3], Ichiro Sakuma[3], Naoki Yahagi[3], Takeyoshi Dohi[3]

[1] Department of Precision Machinery Engineering, Graduate School of Engineering
[2] Department of Orthopedic Surgery, Graduate School of Medicine
[3] Institute of Environment Studies, Graduate School of Frontier Sciences
The University of Tokyo, 7-3-1 Hongo, Bunkyo-Ku, Tokyo 113, Japan
{liao, susumu, iwahara, etsuko, sakuma, yahagi, dohi} @miki.pe.u-tokyo.ac.jp

Abstract: A real-time 3-D surgical navigation system that superimposes the real, intuitive 3-D image for medical diagnosis and operation was developed in this paper. This system creates 3-D image based on the principle of integral photography (IP), named "Integral Videography (IV)", which can display geometrically accurate 3-D image and reproduce motion parallax without any need of special devices. 3-D image was superimposed on the surgical fields in the patient via a half-silvered mirror as if they could be seen through the body. In addition, a real-time IV algorithm for calculating the 3-D image of surgical instruments was used for registration between the location of surgical instruments and the organ during the operation. The experimental results of puncturing a point location and avoiding critical area showed the errors of this navigation system were in the range of 2~3mm. By introducing a display device with higher pixel density, accuracy of the system can be improved.

1. Introduction

With the advancements of medical imaging and computer technology, the effective use of diagnostic images and image-guided surgical navigations have been a focus of discussion. They usually show 3-D information in pre-operation images to surgeons, as a set of 2-D sectional images displayed away from the surgical area. Surgeons have to follow some extra procedures to perceive 3-D information of the patient during surgery. Firstly, they need to turn their gaze to the computer display showing the navigation images. Next, they must reconstruct the 3-D information in their minds, with the help of experience and anatomical knowledge. Lastly, they must turn their eyes back to the surgical area and register the 3-D information reconstructed in the minds with the actual patient's body. These procedures interrupt the flow of surgery and the reconstructed 3-D information sometimes differs between individual surgeons. To solve these problems, medical images should be displayed three-dimensionally in the space that coincides with patient's body.

To superimpose images over the observer's direct view of object, a lot of computer display techniques were presented. One of them is image overlay, which is a form of "Augmented Reality" in that it merges computer-generated information with real world images. Blackwell [1] used binoculars stereoscopic vision display system to show 3-D images with this method. This display method reproduces the depth of

W. Niessen and M. Viergever (Eds.): MICCAI 2001, LNCS 2208, pp. 392-400, 2001.
© Springer-Verlag Berlin Heidelberg 2001

projected objects by the fixed binoculars disparity of the images. However, this does not always give the observer a sense of depth and the motion parallax cannot be reproduced without wearing a tracking device. As well as limiting the number of observers, this also causes visual fatigue. Consequently, systems based on binoculars stereoscopic vision are not suitable for surgical display.

In this study, we used 3-D image named Integral Photography (IP), which was first proposed by M.G.Lippmann[2] in 1908. IP records and reproduces 3-D image using a "fly's eye" lens array and photographic film. Masutani et al. recorded an IP of medical 3-D objects on the film and applied it to clinical diagnosis and surgical planning [3]. Igarashi et al. proposed a computer-generated IP method that constructs an image by transforming the 3-D image about the object into 2-D coordinates on the computer display, instead of taking a photograph [4]. However, the computing time for creating IP was so costly that the system could not be practical for rendering medical objects.

To overcome these limitations, we devised a new rendering algorithm for computer- generated IP and developed a practical 3-D display system [5] and applied it to a clinical field of orthopedic surgery [6]. Moreover, in the clinical application, the 3-D image of surgical instrument inserted into the organ also should be shown its real-time location. Consequently, a real-time rendering algorithm for intra- operative image information should be developed, especially for displaying the accuracy location of the intra-operative instrument.

In this paper, we present a real-time 3-D surgical navigation system that superimposes the real, intuitive 3-D image for medical diagnosis and operation. This system creates 3-D image based on the principle of integral photography, named "Integral Videography (IV)", which can be updated following the changes in operator's field of vision. 3-D image was superimposed on the surgical fields in the patient via a half-silvered mirror as if they could be seen through the body. In addition, a real-time Integral Videography algorithm for calculating the 3-D image of surgical instruments was used for registration between the location of surgical instruments and the organ during the operation. The accuracy of the navigation system was evaluated through in vitro experiments with phantoms.

2. Method

2.1 System Configuration

The 3-D real-time surgical navigation system developed in this study consists of the following components:
- Position tracking system POLARIS^{TM} Optical Tracking System, Northern Digital Inc., Ontario, Canada
- 3-D data source collection equipment (such as MRI, CT)
- IP display (consist of LCD with XGA, lens array, half-silvered mirror, supporting stage)
- Personal computer Pentium 800MHz Dual CPU

The source image on the IP display is generated from the 3-D data by the algorithm described later in this paper. Any kind of 3-D data source, such as magnetic resonance (MRI) or Computerized tomography (CT) images can be processed.

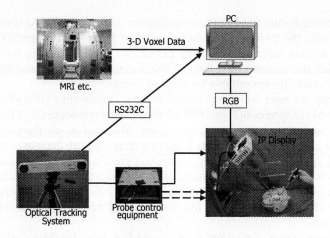

Fig.1 System configuration

We use optical 3-D tracking system to track the position of surgical instrument and organ during the operation. The position and orientation of IP display can be also measured for image registration. With these data, we calculate the relative position of surgical instrument to organ. Both of the patient organ model/target and surgical instrument are represented in the form of IP. The resultant IPs are displayed in real-time on IP display.

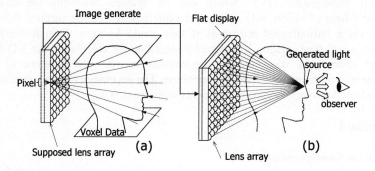

Fig.2 Principle of Integral Videography. The figure shows how to generate and reproduce a 3-D object by IV. Light rays reflected at the first point seen from the observer's side on the 3-D object pass through the centers of all lenses on the array and are redisplayed on the flat display. When the image was lit from behind, light rays intersect at the original point to become a new light point.

In the proposed computer-generated IP, each point showed in a 3-D space is reconstructed by the convergence of rays from pixels on the computer display, through lenses in the array. The observer can see any point in the display from various directions as if it were fixed in 3-D space. Each point appears as a new light source (Fig2.b), and then a 3-D object can thus be constructed as an assembly of such reconstructed light sources. Coordinates of those points in the 3-D object that correspond to each pixel of the flat display (for example: LCD) must be calculated for each pixel on a display. Fig.2a Shows 3-D IP image's rendering method that calculates coordinates of one point for each pixel of the flat display.

The fundamental layouts of this system include the operator, 3-D image on IP display, half-silvered mirror, reflected image, patient in this system, the relations of them are shown in Fig.3.

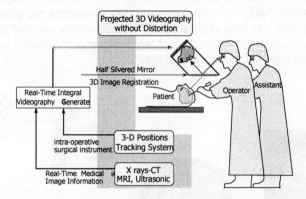

Fig.3 Fundamental layout for surgical registration

2.2 Generate a Real-Time IP for Organ and Surgical Instrument

(1) Method of generating IP for organ and surgical instrument

We can create a clear and detailed stationary IP image by using the fundamental method shown in Fig.2. However, the calculating time of this method for searching the first point seen by observer was too costly to be used as a real-time IP creating. Moreover, the intra-operative situation of the surgical instrument change frequently compared to the organ. It is very difficult to create a real-time intra-operative IP when the surgical instrument is calculated together with the organ. Consequently, we present a new method that creates organ and surgical instrument's IP respectively firstly (Fig.4), and then combine them together. One of integrated IP image of brain and inserted surgical instrument creating with this method is shown in Fig.5.

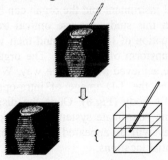

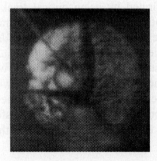

Fig.4 Method for dealing with organ and
surgical instrument for making real-time IP

Fig.5 A cross section and the foci of brain IP

(2) Fast IP rendering algorithm for 3-D object and surgical instrument

Although the fundamental method for IV can achieve all of the image information without any escape, the rendering time for the entire pixel on the flat display is so costly that cannot be used for real-time IP creating. We develop a special rendering method for medical IP, named jump-rendering method (Fig.6). It search the image voxel data every 2^n n=3 or more pixels on the searching line. When the searched position (point on the searching line like A) enter the area of organ, the searching point will return back to the last step, and then re-research the pixel data every one pixel. In addition, we only calculate the IP in the necessary area of lens array (Fig.7). The calculation time with this method will be shorted to below 1 seconds, which is satisfied with the requirements of real-time IP.

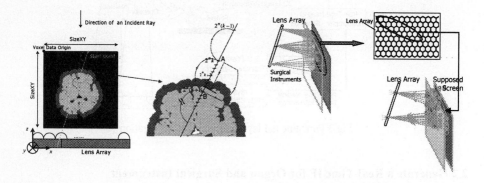

Fig.6 Fast rendering algorithm for IP of organ

Fig.7 Real-time IP rendering algorithm for surgical instrument

2.3 Registration Method

Because the relationship between the location of the projected 3-D image and that of the IP display can be found from calculation, registration between the 3-D image and the patient's body could be performed by registration between the IP display and the patient's body. The relation between the surgical instrument and the organ can be also confirmed by using optical tracking probes. In this study, we use optical tracking probe (Fig.8) to measure the intra-operative situation of IP display, and then we can achieve the display coordinateΣdis form the transform of $\Sigma dis-\Sigma std$. The organ and surgical instrument coordinate Σorg can also be achieved as the same way. With the registration of Σdis and Σorg, we can combine the 3-D image of intra-operative surgical instrument and organ with the patient's body (Fig.8). Once the displayed objects have all been transformed into the same coordinate system via this kind of calibration and registration transformations, they will be appeared to the operator's eyes exactly as if they existed in their virtual spatial locations.

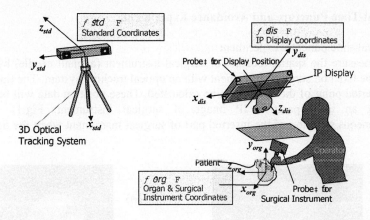

Fig.8 Transformations between coordinate systems

3. Experiments

3.1 Experimental Equipment

Using the registration method shown in 2.3, we can coincides the position of the 3-D image theoretically with that of objects. However, some errors in the recognized positions of the points in the image are inevitable. So we measured the accuracy of the recognized location of the registered image to the real object by using a 80mm cubic phantom objects, which include four MRI markers (a column capsule filled with oil, diameter of about 7mm) on its surface and a ball (diameter 15mm, material in clay, regarded as target in the puncturing experiment), two poles (diameter 2-4mm, regarded as vessel in the avoiding experiment) inside (Fig.9).

The 3-D image generated from MRI was superimposed on the phantom with the registration method mentioned above. The position corresponding to the markers were displayed in the 3-D image and their coordinates were measured three times by the optical tracking system (Fig.10). The mean value of differences between the measured and the true coordinates of four markers M_i (i=1~4) is 1.13mm and the S.D is 0.79mm.

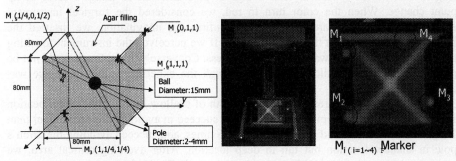

Fig.9 Scheme of the cubic phantom   Fig. 10 Registration result with IP display

398

3.2 Real-Time Puncture and Avoidance Experiment

■ Real-time puncture experiment

We measure the spatial location of surgical instrument (a small needle) by tracking the probe fixed on surgical instrument with an optical tracking system. The tip positions and inserted point of the needle can be calculated. These position data will be used for creating an intra-operative IP image of surgical instrument. Fig.11 show an instantaneous situation of the inserted part of surgical instrument when the tip point of it

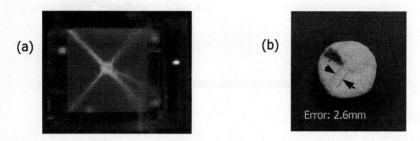

(a)　　　　　　　　　　　(b)

Fig.11 (a): An instantaneous situation of IP image when the tip point of surgical instrument arriving at target. (b): The result of puncture experimentation.

arriving at target in phantom. After finishing puncturing experiment, in order to examine the accuracy, we withdrew the surgical instrument out of phantom and injected colored-ink into the traces of puncture from the entrance point of the needle. The puncture error was 2.6mm by measuring the traces remained in the clay, as shown in Fig.11 (b).

■ Real-time avoidance experiment

In this system, we added feedback information of surgical instrument when it was inserted into the organ. The color of surgical instrument's 3-D image changed automatically from green to red when the tip point of instrument approach critical area as shown in Fig.12 (a). This purpose of experiment was to examine the accuracy of this navigation system by avoiding a set of poles with different diameters. The processes of avoidance experiment are performed as follows. First, we inserted the surgical instrument toward the 3-D image of pole until the IP image's color of tip point change. When the color turn to red, we considered the surgical instrument approached the critical area. In order to confirm our imagination, we inserted the instrument about 2mm at the same direction. If we perceived the instrument touching the pole, the experiment was recognized success. Conversely, if the touch could not be perceived or the color did not change through the experiment, the avoidance was judged as failure.

We conduced procedures four times for both of shallow location and deep location for phantom□and phantom□respectively. We succeed in avoiding the pole bigger than 3 mm both in shallow and deep location for 6 times, and succeed avoiding the 2mm's pole in shallow location but fail in deep location. After avoiding critical area, we continue to insert the surgical instrument, as shown in Fig.12 (b).

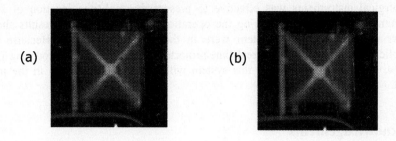

Fig.12 The color on the tip of instrument change to red when the instrument approaching critical area (a). Continue to stick after avoiding critical area (b).

4. Discussion and Conclusions

The navigation system developed in this study is more accurate by using a real-time 3-D guided-image for intra-operative surgical instrument. To minimal invasion surgery, we developed an image-guided surgical system with 2 primary merits by IP.

- It is not necessary for surgeon to look away from the patient to receive guidance. Moreover, it avoid the need of extra devices, such as the wearing of special glasses;
- Geometrical accuracy over the projected objects (esp. depth perspective), visibility of motion parallax over a wide area, simultaneous observation by many people.

Based on the requirements above, we created organ's IP and offer a guidance for surgical instrument by showing the intra-operative location of surgical instrument which cannot be seen by observer when it enter the inside of organ respectively. Because soft tissues may deform during surgery, a method to sense intra-operative organ deformation and to display accurately their shapes and positions will be required. Although the update of organ's IP still costs time and the IP image is not very clear due to the limitation of pixel density of the presently available display device, with the advancement of display technology and computer hardware, it will be possible to register the intra-operative organ's configuration with the surgical instrument in real-time based on the real-time data of organ from Open-MRI or deformation calculation.

The resolution of flat display like LCD in this system is limited to 200 dpi. The spatial resolution of the 3-D image projected is proportional to the ratio of the lens diameter in the lens array to the pixel pitch of display. Thus, both the lens diameter and the pixel pitch need to be made much smaller. One of the possible solutions to realize higher pixel density is the use of multiple projectors to create one image and reduction projection of the resultant image on a small screen with special lens optics. A large computation power is also needed to correspond to multiple-projector system. We are currently developing such a multiple projector system and a parallel-calculation method to accelerate calculation.

In conclusion, our research has shown that the real-time 3-D surgical navigation system can superimpose the real, intuitive 3-D image for medical diagnosis and operation. The newly developed real-time IV algorithm for calculating the 3-D image of surgical instruments was effective to present the real-time location of surgical instruments and the organ during the operation. The experimental results show the errors of this navigation system were in the range of 2~3mm. Because of the simplicity and the accuracy of real-time projected point location by introducing a display device with higher pixel density, this system will be practically usable in the medical field.

Acknowledgements

This studies was partly supported by the research of Future Program JSPS-RFTF 96P00801 by Japan Society for the Promotion of Science.

References

1) M.Blackwell, C.Nikou, A.M.Digioia, T.Kanade, "An Image Overlay System for Medical Data Visualization," Mediacal Image Computing and Computer-Assisted Intervention MICCAI'98, pp.232-240
2) M.G.Lippmann, "Epreuves reversibles donnant la sensation du relief", J. de Phys Vol.7, 4th series, pp821-825, 1908
3) Y.Masutani, M.Iwahara, etc al "Development of integral photography-based enhanced reality visualization system for surgical support. Proc. of ISCAS'95 pp16-17
4) Y.Igarashi, H.Mutrata, M.Ueda, "3-D display system using a computer generated integral photography. Japan J. Appl. Phys. 17 (1978) pp.1683-1684
5) S.Nakajima, K.Masamune, I.Sakuma, T.Dohi, "Three-dimensional display system for medical imaging with compute-generated integral photography", Proc. of SPIE Vol. 3957 (2000) pp.60-67
6) S.Nakajima, S.Orita, K.Masamune, I.Sakuma, T.Dohi, and K.Nakamura "Surgical Navigation System with Intuitive Three-Dimension Display", Mediacal Image Computing and Computer-Assisted Intervention MICCAI 2000, pp.403-411

Towards Motion-Robust Magnetic Resonance Thermometry

M.W. Vogel[1], Suprijanto[3], F.M. Vos[1,3], H.A. Vrooman[1,2], A.M. Vossepoel[3],
P.M.T. Pattynama[1]

[1] Department of Radiology, Erasmus University Rotterdam, The Netherlands
mvogel@rdiag.fgg.eur.nl, p.pattynama@inter.nl.net
[2] Department of Medical Informatics, Erasmus University Rotterdam, The Netherlands
vrooman@mi.fgg.eur.nl
[3] Department of Applied Physics, Delft University of Technology, The Netherlands
{supri, frans, albert}@ph.tn.tudelft.nl

Abstract. Magnetic Resonance Imaging allows for minimally invasive targeting and thermal ablation of tumors while monitoring the temperature distribution. Conventional MR thermometry procedures are hampered by either low accuracy or high sensitivity to motion artifacts due to the use of a reference temperature image. A new, dual-echo technique has been developed to obtain the temperature distribution within a single MR-acquisition. The acquired phase images were post-processed using noise filtering and advanced phase unwrapping, to obtain the two-dimensional temperature distribution. In vitro calibration experiments showed that the accuracy of our newly developed technique is similar to existing thermometry approaches. There was a good linear relationship (r^2=0.99) between the measured phase difference and the recorded temperature up to at least 65°C. The reproducibility of the temperature coefficient ($\Delta\varphi/\Delta T$) was within 5%. Real-time temperature mapping and solving susceptibility inhomogeneity are under investigation.

1 Introduction

On-going improvements in recognition and staging of tumors allow for early management of related morbidity. Tumor size is usually controlled by suppressive chemotherapy. Minimally invasive surgery may be especially beneficial in the early stage of cancer, when lesions are small. Thermal surgery may be an appropriate form of minimally invasive surgery since coagulated tissue allows for regeneration of healthy tissue.

The curative effect of (ablative) hyperthermia on soft tissue tumors has been known for over half a century. The resulting heat distribution, however, is difficult to predict. Due to the *a priori* unknown differences in thermal conductivity, diffusion and physiological cooling effects, the efficiency of hyperthermic applications is greatly reduced. Models for predicting the temperature distribution, especially in the higher temperature range used for ablative therapy, are not yet fully established [1]. With the availability of advanced imaging equipment, temperature changes during treatment can be visualized using ultrasound [2] or Magnetic Resonance Imaging

W. Niessen and M. Viergever (Eds.): MICCAI 2001, LNCS 2208, pp. 401–408, 2001.

(MRI) [3,4]. Use of temperature information allows for monitoring and controlling temperature related events [5,6]. Registering changes in temperature for specific pixels allows for precise thermal dose calculation [7].

MRI has been favored for monitoring local hyperthermia therapy, since it offers both target visualization and temperature sensitivity. Temperature sensitivity by MRI has been demonstrated for the apparent diffusion constant, the spin-lattice relaxation time (T_1), and the water proton resonance frequency shift. The frequency shift approach is accurate, but very sensitive to motion artifacts that may lead to corrupted temperature information.

The objective of this paper is to show that sufficiently accurate temperature information can be collected in a single MR-acquisition using a newly developed procedure, which may apply for thermometry purposes in vivo.

2 Materials & Methods

There is a direct relationship between tissue temperature and proton (spin) mobility [8-10]. For diamagnetic materials, such as soft tissues in the human body, the moving electrons around the proton spin result in a small local magnetic field, opposing the applied field (B_0). This shielding is temperature dependent. For water, the screening constant α shows a linear increase with increasing temperature over a broad range ($T\epsilon[0,83°C]$) [9,11].

2.1 Conventional Phase Shift Thermometry

The change in the local magnetic field causes a change in the Larmor frequency, resulting in phase differences in the acquired MR phase image. The measured phase $\Delta\phi$ can be used for calculating differences in temperature ΔT, according to [12]:

$$\Delta\varphi = \gamma \cdot \alpha \cdot B_0 \cdot \Delta T \cdot te \tag{1}$$

where γ is the gyromagnetic ratio, α the temperature coefficient, te the echo time, and B_0 the main magnetic field.

Measured phase is relative to the phase at initial temperature and therefore easily invalidated when voxels are displaced by patient breathing or patient movement. Recent studies have shown the feasibility of MR-controlled hyperthermia using the phase shift method, albeit in the absence of tissue motion [13]. In order to be able to employ the phase shift, the method should be robust for phase changes that result from motion.

2.2 Dual-Echo Phase Shift Thermometry

Because currently not all movement artifacts can be corrected for, we investigated the use of the phase that develops between two subsequent echoes for the measurement of temperature, instead of referencing to the static phase reference from a fixed geometry that was acquired prior to heating. The difference between two sampled phases for the same region yields, with a given period, a specific frequency for that region, which translates into local temperature differences.

We modified the standard spoiled gradient echo sequence to incorporate a second readout period. If two echoes are acquired successively using one excitation only, this yields:

$$\varphi_1 - \varphi_0 = \gamma \cdot \alpha \cdot B_0 \cdot (T_1 - T_0) \cdot te_1,$$

$$\varphi_2 - \varphi_0 = \gamma \cdot \alpha \cdot B_0 \cdot (T_2 - T_0) \cdot te_2 .$$

(2)

Now if we assume that

$$T_1 \approx T_2 \Rightarrow \Delta\varphi_{2-1} = k \cdot \Delta T \cdot (te_2 - te_1),$$

(3)

where k incorporates the constant terms, temperature relates directly to the phase evolution. When we take into account the surroundings of the object, for which we assume identical shielding and main magnetic field, we can normalize the evolution of phase to the pixels in the vicinity, rather than using base images.

Analysis of the local magnetic field in a chemically homogeneous sphere, shows that the macroscopic susceptibility is approximated by $H*(1-2*(\mathcal{X}_e - \mathcal{X}_o)/3)$ [14]. At the microscopic level, we arrive at an expression for the local magnetic field that is only a function of the temperature dependent screening constant.

2.3 Experiments

To demonstrate the reproducibility of the conventional thermometric procedure and to compare the measured α with values in the literature, an experiment was carried out in which phase images from a phantom (n=10) were acquired (Experiment 1). The used phantom was a gel (5% agar, Sigma; 95% distilled water) that was heated in a water bath up to 70°C and was put in a Styrofoam box. This setup was placed in the MR-scanner, where it was allowed to cool down to 30°C during continuous acquisition of MR images. In total, more than 100 time samples were acquired. MR hardware consisted of a GE CV/i 1.5T scanner (slew rate 150 $Tm^{-1}s^{-1}$, gradient strength $40*10^{-3}$ Tm^{-1}, rise time $268*10^{-6}$ s). Scanning was done using a conventional gradient echo scanning technique (Table 1). Gel temperature was simultaneously recorded using a fiber optic measurement device (Luxtron 790, Luxtron, Santa Clara, USA). The fibers were positioned in both the phantom and a reference gel.

To be able to make comparisons between the temperature sensitivity of the conventional and the newly developed dual-echo method, two experiments (Experiment 2 and 3) were carried out, with identical experimental setup and comparable imaging settings. In Experiment 2 (n=10), a spoiled gradient recalled echo sequence was employed to assess the conventional phase difference versus temperature. The procedure was repeated for Experiment 3 (n=10) employing the newly developed dual-echo pulse sequence.

Table 1. Imaging parameters for the different experiments. All sequences were steady state incoherent.

Parameter	Experiment 1	Experiment 2	Experiment 3
Sequence	Conv. GRE	Conv.GRE	Dual-echo GRE
TR (msec)	40	40	40
te_1 / te_2 (msec)	6.8 / NA	20 / NA	20.0 / 30.0
Temporal resolution (sec)	10	10	10
Flip angle (°)	20	20	60
Number of excitations	1	1	1
Slice thickness (mm)	10	10	5
Field of view (mm^2)	480 x 480	240 x 240	240 x 240
Bandwidth (kHz)	16	16	16
Matrix	256 x 256	256 x 256	256 x 256

To assess the generalizability of referencing the temperature using the phase difference between the current pixel and neighboring pixels, a final experiment was carried out, using a homogeneous spherical phantom, positioned at the iso-center of the MR-bore. According to the theory, there should be a uniform phase over a homogeneous sphere. Two phase images were acquired, using the same pulse sequence as was used in the Experiment 3, with identical processing.

2.4 Image Post-processing

Images were transferred off-line from an SGI Octane (SGI, Mountain View, CA, USA) to a PC using the DICOM transfer protocol. Further processing was carried out using IDL 5.3 for Windows (Research Systems Inc, Boulder, CO, USA). Phase values are normally computed by taking the arctangent of the real and imaginary part of the MR image, yielding phase values modulo 2π. Further post-processing of the data is hampered by the resulting phase jumps (transitions from π to -π). An example of a phase image is shown in Fig. 1. The central object is the heated agar gel. The surrounding objects are reliability markers to correct for main field drift.

To correctly restore the original linear phase in a pixel, its direct surrounding can be used. The solution to this problem, however, is not trivial. We unwrapped the phase images using Flynn's Minimum Discontinuity Method [15]. In addition to Flynn's algorithm, quality maps and noise filtering (of the real and imaginary part of the signal) were used to optimize the unwrapping process. Afterwards, phase maps were calculated by subtracting the reference image from consecutive phase images. From these phase maps a pixel was selected within the heated gel nearby the inserted Luxtron fiber. The local phase evolution was compared with the measurements of the Luxtron device for the times at which the echoes were acquired. For the dual-echo technique a similar procedure was followed, except that the difference was computed from the phase images that were acquired in one single acquisition.

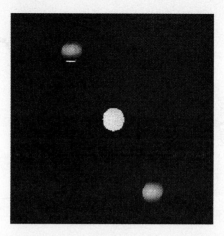

Fig. 1. A typical resulting phase image with three gels in the field of view. The outer two function as magnetic field markers. The temperature over the central gel changed during the course of the experiment. Phase of the background is masked out in this image, to improve visibility. Note the small phase jump in the upper marker.

In both experiments the mean heat coefficient was determined by linear regression. The temperature uncertainty was defined as ± SD of the temperature difference between MR and the fiber optic measurements. Phase noise was estimated from the ± SD of the phase signal in the non-heated reliability markers.

3 Results

To validate the newly developed procedure for MR thermometry, the reproducibility and accuracy of the measured temperature coefficient α was determined from the experiments mentioned above.

3.1 Reproducibility of the Temperature-Dependent Screening Constant

The temperature-dependent screening constant α (Table 2) was within the range of values from the literature [16], and showed low standard error for the conventional as well as the dual-echo technique. The variation of the screening constant using the conventional method was about 5%, which may be caused by a variety of sources and is generally acceptable.

3.2 Temperature Sensitivity

The linearity and sensitivity for the dual-echo technique are depicted in Fig. 2. There was good linearity ($r^2=0.99$) with temperature that holds up to at least 65°C.

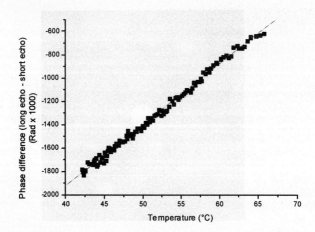

Fig. 2. The evolution of phase difference from the dual-echo technique is plotted against temperature.

The sensitivity of the dual-echo technique was slightly less than that of the conventional technique (see Table 2), as it was the result of two measurements with unrelated errors. The dual-echo sequence suffered from lower SNR due to a smaller voxel size and a relatively high flip angle.

Table 2. Temperature uncertainties, noise, and coefficients for both the conventional and the dual-echo method.

Parameter	Experiment 2	Experiment 3
Sequence	Conventional GRE	Dual-echo GRE
MR versus Luxtron	± 0.57 °C	± 1.20 °C
MR noise	± 1.10 °C	± 0.89 °C
Temperature coefficient	0.0106 ± 0.0001 ppm / °C	0.0098 ± 0.0001 ppm / °C

3.3 Spatial Stability of the Dual-Echo Phase Difference

As seen in Fig. 3, the spatial stability of the phase was low. The dual-echo sequence used did not compensate for sampling errors during the two different readout periods. The conventional method is compensated for this type of errors, since it acquires images, which will be compared against each other, using the same gradient waveforms. Controlling and compensating for the sampling error due to the gradient waveforms of the dual-echo sequence is the topic of current research.

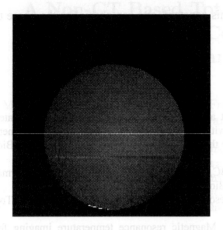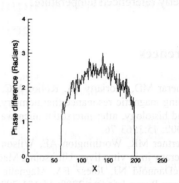

Fig. 3. Clearly visible is the change of phase value over the spherical phantom (left). In the right graph, the intensity (phase difference) profile along the horizontal line is shown. Again the background phase is masked for improved visualization. Sampling errors lead to such a pattern, and can be compensated for.

4 Discussion

In this paper, we have shown that the dual-echo sequence may allow for temperature encoding using the information from one MR acquisition only. Phase difference between the two generated images, varies linearly with temperature. The accuracy is slightly less when compared with the conventional thermometry method. The reproducibility of the temperature coefficient, however, was good. The inconsistency between the screening constants from the conventional method versus the dual-echo method may be explained by a slightly different makeup of the fabricated gel. Minuscule bubbles of air, may affect the evolution of phase approaching the order of the heating constant. However, *in vivo* micro-bubbles are not an issue. The expectation is that temperature changes can be calculated using the established screening constant of -0.0101 ppm°C^{-1} [16].

The found temperature resolution is sufficiently close to 1 °C, and therefore within the acceptable range for hyperthermia applications. Several reports [17,18] have shown a decreased sensitivity in actual *in vivo* settings. Consecutive experiments will include *in vivo* measurements to determine whether the sensitivity of the proposed dual-echo technique suffices for *in vivo* application.

Due to sampling error, variations in the spatially localized signal occur. These imperfections cannot be estimated from the acquired images. Theoretically they can be assessed when using a slightly adapted version of the dual-echo sequence, incorporating refocusing pulses. Removing these imperfections is the strategy to overcome the spatial limitation of the dual-echo technique. In order to allow quantification of temperature from pixels relative to others in the same image, the

2   Methods

An optical tracking device is placed in the operating theater to track relative motions between femur, tibia, and instruments. For this purpose dynamic reference bases are attached to each of these objects.

The first step during the intraoperative usage of the system is the registration of the patient's anatomy using the technique of "surgeon defined anatomy", as it was introduced in the area of computer assisted total knee arthroplasty by Leitner et.al in 1997 ([4], [5], [7]). Additionally ligament behavior is taken into account. This allows to navigate soft-tissue balancing and to include an intra-operative planning step, which contains both, a manual and an automatic planning option. Finally the planned resection planes are executed by means of adapted cutting jigs.

3   Registration of the Patient's Anatomy

For successful navigation during total knee replacement, the axes of femur and tibia (defined by the centers of hip, femoral knee, tibia knee, and ankle) as well as certain geometric features of the knee have to be determined. For the hip center registration a pivoting method is used, similar to the one presented by Piccard et.al ([6]). However, we implemented an alternative to track possible pelvis motion by using a pointer placed onto the spina iliaca rather than an invasivly fixated reference base. During the rotation of the femur the system records the orientation of the femur and the position of the pointer tip and calculates the pivoting center according to these values. The registrations of the knee centers and the ankle center are based on anatomical structures, which are intraoperativly digitized by the surgeon using specially designed instruments. On the femoral knee side the surgeon palpates the attachment areas of the collateral ligaments. The system determines the most prominent points within these areas and calculates the epicondylar femoral axis based on its finding. The center of this axis marks a reference point for the latero-medial location of the femoral knee center. Depending on the prosthesis design this center can be corrected anterior-posteriorly towards the center of the femoral shaft, which is calculated by palpated points on the ventral and dorsal cortexes. The tuberosity and eminentia are the reference landmarks taken for the tibial knee center. One of the measurements for the ankle center calculation is the transmalleolar axis. The surgeon defines it by digitalization of both malleoli. For the location of the ankle center on the transmalleolar axis the surgeon identifies an additional reference like the ligament tibiales anterior or then second toe.

Additionally digitized landmarks are used for the calculation of the anatomically best fitting component size, the defect-management, the restoring of the natural joint line, and the synchronization of the natural tibial rotation and the postoperative rotation of the tibial component.

4 Intraoperative Planning and Soft-Tissue Balancing

The registration of the patient's anatomy allows alignment of the component according to the mechanical axes, but obtaining an ideal knee kinematics requires an intraoperative planning step. The major aims of this planning step are

1. Creation of a uniform extension gap
2. Creation of a uniform flexion gap
3. Balancing the distances of both gaps

To create a uniform extension gap the soft tissue behavior has to be taken into account by loading both collateral ligaments, which can be performed in two different ways, either by manually stressing the knee in varus/valgus directions or by using distractors that hold both collateral ligaments under the same tension. Based on this recorded ligament behavior the system displays the varus/valgus angle between the femoral and tibial mechanical axes. The surgeon can use this information to perform a soft tissue balancing. In case that it is not possible to completely align the extension gap by manipulating the soft tissues, the system offers to modify the varus or valgus angle of the planed femoral distal and/or tibial resection plane. This allows the creation of a stable knee in extension even in difficult preoperative knee situations.

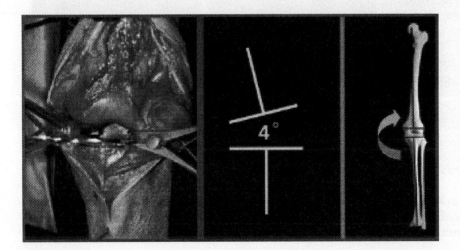

Fig. 1. Soft tissue balancing in extension. Left side: Use of distrators to bring collateral ligaments in tension. Right side: The system displays varus or valgus angle to help the surgeon performing soft tissue balancing.

For the following planning step the final ligament behavior in both extension and flexion will be taken into account by the same procedure, which was described before. The recorded information about the ligament behavior in flexion is used in the intraoperative planning step to define the outside rotation of the femoral component. The result of the patient-depend determination of the outside rotation is a postoperatively stable flexion gap. The planned situation now features uniform extension and flexion gaps. However, both gaps have to be balanced for a successful arthroplasty. For this purpose additional manual planning features are implemented. To facilitate the complex adjustment of the considerable number of parameters, we introduced an automatic planning step, which proposes an initial planning situation in the following manner: The flex-

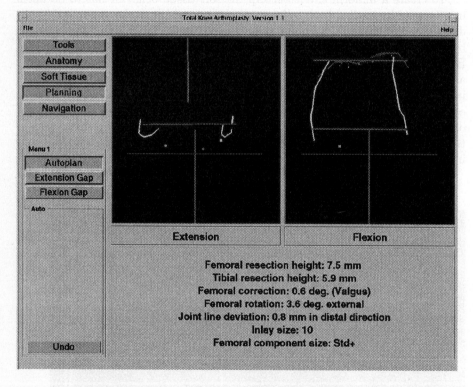

Fig. 2. Auto-Planner after calculation. The system suggests optimal positioning of the prosthesis components and simulates numerically and graphically the resulting postoperative situation in extension and flexion.

ion gap is defined based on the recorded ligament behavior, the planned femoral component size, and a predefined minimal tibial resection height. According to the recorded ligament situation in extension the transfer of this flexion gap into extension results the femoral distal resection height. Next the system gives information about the deviation of the planned joint line from the natural joint line and navigates the surgeon to up- or downsize the femoral component. As a consequence this modification of the flexion gap changes also the planned femoral resection height for a better restoring of the natural joint line. Figure 2 shows the in interface for such a autoplanning step.

The outcome of the automatic planning can be used by the surgeon as an initial situation for the manually planning. This allows both, a fast intraoperative planning without loosing of surgery time and the including of the surgeon's experience into the plan. After the surgeon has performed the planning step the system helps with a graphical interface to accurately perform the planned resection planes. For this purpose the conventional cutting jigs are equipped with LED's. The system presents the deviation between the target plane and the real resection plane in different views.

5 Results

We collected early experiences with the system in a number of in-vivo and in-vitro tests. Table 1 summarizes the results of a study, which was performed on three fresh frozen cadaver specimens. This kind of specimen-preperation also allowed us to test the soft-tissue balancing in a realistic situation. During this process we performed the qualitative evaluation with trial prostheses and measured also the postoperative instability in extension.

Table 1. First results of in-vitro tests

| Nr. | Passive Extension | | | | Varus/Valgus Stress |
| | Coronal | | Sagittal | | |
	Pre	Post	Pre	Post	Post. Instability
1	0°	−1.5°	0.1° Varus	0.5° Valgus	1.5° Varus
2	−14.0°	−1.5°	1.5° Varus	1.1° Valgus	1.7° Varus
3	−10.0°	+0.6°	8.3° Varus	0.5° Valgus	0.7° Varus

Table 2 lists the postoperative data of 10 patients, who recieved a total knee arthroplasty with the help of our system. The values were measured directly after the surgery, whithout loading. For measuring Varus/Valgus angle in passive extension postoperative radiographs were used. The varus valgus stress was determined with help of the system.

The presented values are the result of a first clinical trial phase of the system. We are now going to evaluate the system by performing full clinical studies.

Table 2. First results of in-vivo tests

Passive Extension		Varus/Valgus Stress
Coronal	Sagittal	Post. Instability
$0.8° - 4.2°$ (av. $1.9°$)	$0.2° - 3.9°$ (av. $1.8°$)	Av. $7.2°$

6 Conclusions

The presented system is based on the registration of the mechanical limb axes, which does not require a CT scan, equivalent to the systems presented by Piccard et al., Krakow et al ([3], [4], [5], [7]), and Ritschl et al. ([2]). In order to realize accurate results the calculation of the mechanical axes must not depend on anatomical landmarks, which are influenced by the pathological situation of the knee. In addition to respecting the bony anatomy we introduced the soft tissue consideration into the intraoperative planning step, which allows producing a postoperative result, that is optimized regarding anatomy and kinematics. For this purpose also the anterior and posterior femoral resection planes are navigated by the system.

References

1. Andriacchi, T.P.: Dynamics of Knee Malalignment. Orthopaedic Clinics of North America **25(3)** (1994) 395–403
2. Ritschl, P., Fuiko, R., Broers, H., Wurzinger, A., Berner, W.: Computerassisted navigation and robot-cutting system for total knee replacement. In Proceedings of the 1st Annual Meeting of the International Society for Computer Assisted Orthopaedics Surgery, Davos (2001) 94
3. Krackow, K., Bayers-Thering, M., Phillips, M., Mihalko, W.: A new technique for determining proper mechanical axis alignment during total knee arthroplasty: progress toward computer-assisted TKA. Orthopedics **22(7)** (1999) 698–702
4. Leitner, F., Picard, F., Minfelde, R., Schulz, H.-J., Cinquin, P., Saragaglia, D.: Computer-Assited Knee Surgical Total Replacement. In CVDMed-MRCAS '97. J. Troccaz, E. Grimson, and R. Moesger, editors. Springer Verlag, Berlin Heidelberg New York (1997) 629–637
5. Miehlke, R.K., Clemens, U., Kershally, S.: Computer Integrated Instrumentation in Knee Arthroplasty - A comparative study of conventional and computerized Technique. In CAOS USA 2000 - Conference Proceeding, June 15-17, 2000, Pittsburgh, Pennsylvania, USA. A.M. DiGioia and L.P. Nolte, editors. Centers for Medical Robotics and Computer Assisted Surgery, Western Pennsylvania Institute for Computer Assisted Surgery, Pittsburgh (2000) 93–96
6. Moreland, J.R.: Mechanisms of Failure in Total Knee Arthroplasty. Clinical Orthopaedics and Related Research **226** (1987) 49–63
7. Picard, F., Leitner, F., Saragaglia, D., Raoult, O., Chaussard, C., Montbarbon, E.: Intraoperative Navigation for TKA: Location of a rotational center of the knee

A Non-CT Based Total Knee Arthroplasty System   415

and hip. In CAOS USA 2000 - Conference Proceeding, June 15-17, 2000, Pittsburgh, Pennsylvania, USA. A.M. DiGioia and L.P. Nolte, editors. Centers for Medical Robotics and Computer Assisted Surgery, Western Pennsylvania Institute for Computer Assisted Surgery, Pittsburgh (2000) 91–92.
8. Sathasivam, S. Walker, P.S.: The conflicting requirements of laxity and conformity in total knee replacement. Journal of Biomechanics **32** (1999) 239–247

A Statistical Atlas of Prostate Cancer for Optimal Biopsy

Dinggang Shen[1], Zhiqiang Lao[1], Jianchao Zeng[2], Edward H. Herskovits[1],
Gabor Fichtinger[3], Christos Davatzikos[1,3]

[1] Department of Radiology, Johns Hopkins University
[2] ISIS Center, Radiology Department, Georgetown University Medical Center
[3] Center for Computer-Integrated Surgical Systems and Technology, Johns Hopkins University
Email: dgshen@cbmv.jhu.edu, hristos@rad.jhu.edu

Abstract. This paper presents a methodology of creating a statistical atlas of spatial distribution of prostate cancer from a large patient cohort, and uses it for designing optimal needle biopsy strategies. In order to remove inter-individual morphological variability and determine the true variability in cancer position, an adaptive-focus deformable model (AFDM) is used to register and normalize prostate samples. Moreover, a probabilistic method is developed for designing optimal biopsy strategies that determine the locations and the number of needles by optimizing cancer detection probability. Various experiments demonstrate the performance of AFDM in registering prostate samples for construction of the statistical atlas, and also validate the predictive power of our atlas-based optimal biopsy strategies in detecting prostate cancer.

1 Introduction

Prostate cancer is the second leading cause of death for American men. Transrectal Ultrasonography-guided symmetric needle biopsy has been widely used as a gold standard for the diagnosis and staging of prostate cancer. However, biopsy is currently performed in a rather empirical way, since cancer is mostly undetectable in the routinely used ultrasound images. This results in a significant number of prostate cancer cases being undetected at their initial biopsy. For example, the systematic sextant biopsy protocol [1] is the most common biopsy protocol. However, some studies have shown that this protocol results in a positive predictive value of only around 30% [2]. Other clinical studies have suggested that the sextant technique may not be optimal and have investigated new biopsy protocols that might yield significantly better results [3,4]. Obviously, if the biopsy protocol can be optimized to increase the chances of detecting prostate cancer, according to some objective and quantitative criteria, then significant improvement in diagnostic accuracy should be expected.

Some researchers have investigated the possibility of using a large number of patient histopathological images to determine prostate regions that are most likely to develop cancer, and therefore should be sampled during biopsy [5]. Those techniques, however, are limited by inter-individual morphological variability, which reduces both the statistical power in detecting associations and the spatial specificity of these methods, which is often limited to relatively coarse subdivisions of the prostate. In this paper, we propose a methodology that overcomes both of these limitations. In order to reduce inter-individual variability, we use AFDM [6,7], which spatially normalize the prostate images to a canonical coordinate system with high accuracy. With accurate

W. Niessen and M. Viergever (Eds.): MICCAI 2001, LNCS 2208, pp. 416-424, 2001.

registration of the prostate images of a large number of patients, a statistical atlas of cancer distribution can be created and further applied in suggesting optimal biopsy strategies. As to the statistical analysis, we not only look at the probability of developing cancer at individual locations, but also develop a full statistical predictive model that takes into account the spatial correlation of cancer incidence between different prostate regions. Our rationale is that regions between which cancer incidence is very highly correlated need not be sampled simultaneously, as opposed to regions between which cancer occurrence is relatively independent. These models are used in an optimization framework for estimation of optimal needle biopsy strategies.

This paper is organized as follows. In Section 2, we build a methodology for deformable registration and normalization of prostate samples. In Section 3, we create a statistical atlas of the spatial distribution of prostate cancer and develop a probabilistic method for designing optimal biopsy strategies that best predict the presence of prostate cancer in a particular patient. In Section 4, we demonstrate the performance of AFDM in registering prostate samples, and validate the predictive power of our atlas-based optimal biopsy strategies in detecting clinically significant cancer in our existing prostate database.

2 Spatial Registration and Normalization of Prostate Samples

The major problem in developing a spatial normalization method is determining correspondences. We have developed a deformable shape modeling framework, for segmentation and reconstruction of anatomical shapes, and for determining morphology-based correspondence across individuals, from tomographic images [6,7]. This framework is based on our AFDM. In AFDM, for a given set of structures, a shape model is first constructed to represent a typical shape of these structures. This shape model includes two kinds of information: information about the geometry of the structures and information about the statistical variation of these structures within a given population. In the application stage, the deformable shape model is placed in an image with the structures of interest, and is subsequently let free to deform according to features extracted from the images, seeking objects that have similar geometry, but also objects that fall within the expected range of shape variation.

In this section, we use AFDM as a registration method to spatially normalize the external and internal structures of the prostate samples, such as the capsule and the urethra. In particular, we select one typical prostate as the template (Fig. 1a), and other subjects are warped into the space of this template. The warping is performed in two stages. First, AFDM is used to reconstruct the shape of each structure and to determine point correspondences between the subjects and the template. Second, these point correspondences are interpolated elsewhere in the space of the prostate by using an elastic warping technique [8]. Since AFDM is the cornerstone of our deformable registration method, it is particularly redesigned for prostate application next.

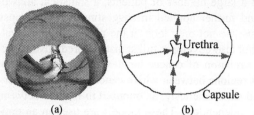   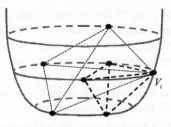

Fig. 1. A prostate surface model. (a) 3D display, and (b) a cross-section.

Fig. 2. Attributes defined as volumes of tetrahedra in 3D.

2.1 Spatial Connections between Distant Structures of the Prostate Surface Model

AFDM comprises several inter-connected surfaces, each representing the anatomy of a structure of interest. Fig. 1a shows a 3D prostate model with two surfaces that represent the capsule and the urethral boundaries. In order to allow a deformation imposed on a segment of one surface (such as the capsule) to rapidly propagate to the segments of the other surface (such as the urethra) in a hierarchical fashion, connections between these two surfaces are added (gray arrows in Fig. 1b), effectively rendering distant surface patches as neighbors. Therefore, at a coarse scale, large segments are connected together, and thus deformations have a strong effect on the distant segments. At a finer scale, the deformations have a more local character.

2.2 Affine-Invariant Attribute Vector on Each Model Point

In order to capture the geometry of anatomical structures in a hierarchical fashion, we introduced the concept of an attribute vector that is attached to each point of the prostate surface model and reflects the geometric structure of the model from a global scale to a local scale. The attribute vectors are an important aspect of AFDM, since they provide a means for finding correspondences across individuals by examining the similarity of the underlying attribute vectors. In 3D case, each attribute is defined as the volume of a tetrahedron (see Fig. 2), formed by a model point V_i and any three points in its certain neighborhood layer. For each model point V_i, the volumes that are calculated from different neighborhood layers of its surface segment can be stacked into an attribute vector $F(V_i)$, which can be made affine-invariant as $\hat{F}(V_i)$ by normalizing it over the whole model [6,7].

2.3 Energy Definition of Prostate Surface Model

Our deformable model is very robust to local minima, since the local energy term E_i [7], that is composed of two terms E_i^{model} and E_i^{data}, is defined on the surface segment of the model point V_i, rather than a single model point V_i. The model energy term E_i^{model} is defined to allow AFDM determine correspondences, in addition to segmenting structures of interest. In particular, the model energy term E_i^{model} is defined as the difference between the attribute vectors of the model and its deformed configuration, and it is given by $E_i^{model} = \left\| \hat{F}^{Def}(V_i) - \hat{F}^{Mdl}(V_i) \right\|^2$, where $\hat{F}^{Def}(V_i)$ and $\hat{F}^{Mdl}(V_i)$ are respectively the normalized attribute vectors of the deformed model configuration and the model at the point V_i. As to the data energy term, E_i^{data}, it is designed to move the deformable model towards an object boundary. Since our deformation mechanism deforms a surface segment around each model point V_i at a time, we design a data energy term E_i^{data} that reflects the fit of the whole surface segment, rather than a single model point, with image edges.

2.4 Adaptive-Focus Deformation Strategy

In our previous work we have determined that model adaptivity is very important for robust segmentation and correspondence estimation. Adaptivity was embedded in AFDM by employing an external force mechanism in a hierarchical way, starting with relatively easier to find structures and gradually shifting focus to other structures, as the model deforms into a configuration closer to the shape of an individual structure. We explore the utility of adaptive modeling further in the registration of prostate samples (see Fig. 3). Two types of prior knowledge about the prostate shapes are available. First, the attribute vectors of the model points along the two open surface boundaries of the prostate shape model are very distinct, compared to other attribute vectors of other model points, such as in the middle cross-section of the prostate model. With this prior knowledge, we will focus on the two open surface boundaries in the initial deformation stages, which will lead to a rough match between the prostate model and the subject. Second, the prostate capsule is more accurately and reliably outlined in the histopathological samples, compared to the urethra that does not include soft tissue and therefore is very deformed in the specimens. This prior knowledge suggests us to focus on the prostate capsule first, and then shift focus to the urethra, as more information about the urethral shape is gathered from the subject.

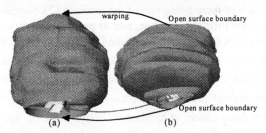

Fig. 3. The procedure of warping a prostate subject to the template. (a) Side view of the template given in Fig. 1, (b) Side view of the subject that is the same as the one in Fig. 4(b1).

3 Optimal Needle Biopsy Strategy

After warping all prostate subjects into the space of the template by AFDM, we construct the 3D statistical atlas of spatial distribution of prostate cancer, and we further design optimal needle biopsy strategies for diagnosing prostate cancer in a patient. In the next, we describe an algorithm to design optimal K-biopsy (biopsy with a number K of needles) strategy by minimizing the probability of missing the cancer.

3.1 Optimization

A K-biopsy strategy can be optimized by minimizing the probability that none of the K needles detects cancer. This probability is defined by

$$P(B(x_i) = \text{NC}, i = 1,..,K), \qquad (1)$$

where $B(x_i)$ is the biopsy outcome at location x_i, and NC denotes a negative cancer detection result. Location x_i can be anywhere inside of a 3D prostate template. We can find the configuration that minimizes this probability by using standard optimization methods. Since the probability in (1) is likely to have many local minima, we use the simulated annealing technique to find globally optimal values for $x_1 \ldots x_K$. We start with an initial guess for the coordinates of the K needles, and then we iteratively change these values toward a direction that decreases the probability function in (1). Initially, changes in the direction that increases the probability in (1) are allowed, but these steps are progressively discouraged more and more as the algorithm proceeds, as customary in random optimization methods.

3.2 A Fast Heuristic Method

The search space in our optimization problem is very large, since each of the K needle coordinates can be any voxel within the prostate template. Therefore, in order to make the simulated annealing technique practical, we need to find a good initial guess to be used as a starting point for this algorithm. In the following, we describe a very fast heuristic method.

The probability of missing the cancer can be expressed as a product of conditional probabilities,

$$P(B(x_i)=\text{NC}, \ i=1,..,K) = P(B(x_1)=\text{NC}) \bullet P(B(x_2)=\text{NC} \mid B(x_1)=\text{NC}) \bullet$$
$$\cdots \bullet P(B(x_K)=\text{NC} \mid B(x_i)=\text{NC}, \ i=1,...,K\text{-}1). \qquad (2)$$

Our heuristic method sequentially minimizes a series of the conditional probabilities of missing cancer, each of them being one of the terms in (2). Suppose that there are N different locations in the prostate template, and M prostate samples in the training set. To minimize (2), one of K biopsies, let's say the first biopsy $B(x_1)$, will be taken from the location x_1 where the likelihood of cancer is the highest, that is, the first term in (2), $P(B(x_1) = \text{NC})$, is the lowest. Knowing the location of the first biopsy x_1, in order to calculate the conditional probability $P(B(x_2)=\text{NC} \mid B(x_1)=\text{NC})$, we remove those prostate samples that have cancer at location x_1, since those do not satisfy the condition $B(x_1)=\text{NC}$, and recalculate the probability at each location. It is important to note that if the incidence of cancer at a location other than x_1 is strongly related with the incidence of cancer at location x_1, then the cancer occurrence probability of this location will become very low in the conditional probability $P(B(x_2)=\text{NC} \mid B(x_1)=\text{NC})$. This is because all subjects with cancer at x_1 have been excluded in calculating the conditional probability $P(B(x_2)=\text{NC} \mid B(x_1)=\text{NC})$. This implies that the second biopsy will most likely not be placed at the cancer locations strongly related with the location x_1. With this new conditional probability, the biopsy location x_2 can be determined by selecting the location where the likelihood of cancer is highest, i.e. the conditional probability $P(B(x_2)=\text{NC} \mid B(x_1)=\text{NC})$ is lowest. Using the same procedure, the locations of other biopsy sites can be similarly determined. Effectively, this procedure minimizes each of the terms in (2) sequentially, rather than operating at the full joint distribution, and is therefore extremely fast.

3.3 Increasing Robustness of Our Biopsy Strategy

In order to make our biopsy strategy robust to the errors from needle placement, each cancer probability (or conditional cancer probability) function is spatially smoothed prior to finding optimal needle locations. This is specifically designed to avoid the cases that optimal needle locations are determined to be on isolated, high-probability regions, since those regions might be difficult to accurately sample in practice due to unavoidable errors in placing needles. With this formulation, our biopsy strategy is robust, since we guarantee that the optimal needle locations be on the regions with both high cancer probability and relatively wider spatial extent. Therefore, even a needle is wrongly placed in the neighborhood around the expected location, we still have very higher probability in detecting cancer.

4 Experiments

Two groups of experiments are performed in this section, in order to 1) test the performance of our deformable registration, 2) validate the predictive power of our atlas-based optimal biopsy strategies in detecting prostate cancer. These two experiments were performed on 64 of the 281 prostate subjects in our database.

4.1 Performance on AFDM-Based Deformable Registration

Fig. 4 demonstrates a procedure of registering and warping a representative prostate subject (Fig. 4(b1)) to the space of the prostate template (Fig. 4(a1)). In both of Figs. 4(a1) and 4(b1), the orange surfaces denote the prostate capsule, and the yellow surfaces denote the urethra. The red region in the subject denotes the positions of cancer. The side views of the template and the subject are shown in Fig. 3. The spatially normalized version of the subject is shown in Fig. 4(c1), where the white mesh corresponds to the capsule of the template and the red mesh corresponds to the capsule of the subject. Fig. 4(a2) shows a typical cross-sectional image of the template prostate. The corresponding cross-sectional image of the subject's prostate is shown in Fig. 4(b2). Notable are the shape differences between these two cross-sections. After using the warping algorithm, we obtain the warped image of Fig. 4(c2), whose shape is very similar to that of the template prostate in Fig. 4(a2).

We also measured the registration accuracy of AFDM. We did this by measuring the percent overlap and average distance between the prostate structures in the 64 images and their counterparts in the prostate template, after all prostate subjects had spatially normalized to the template. Note that these images are all labeled, and therefore overlap of the various prostate structures across subjects can be readily computed. For 64 prostate samples, their percent overlap measures ranged from 96.4% to 98.4%, with the mean overlap 97.7%. Their average boundary distances ranged from

1.7 to 3.0 pixels, which is very small compared to the prostate image with the size of 256x256x124 pixels.

4.2 Testing Predictability of the Statistical Atlas

Using the registration and warping algorithm, we can eliminate the overall shape differences across individuals. In this way, we can find the spatial distribution of cancer within the space of the prostate template, which can be used to determine the needle biopsy strategy. We tested the heuristic sequential optimization procedure on 64 subjects (M=64). All N=256x256x124 voxels were considered to be candidate biopsy locations. In Fig. 5(a), the optimal biopsy sites are shown as small red/yellow spheres and the underlying spatial statistical distribution of cancer is shown as green. Brighter green indicates higher likelihood for finding cancer in that location. The viewing angle of the statistical distribution is similar in both of Figs. 5(a) and 5(b), to facilitate comparison. In Fig. 5(b), the prostate capsule is shown as red. A typical cross-section of the 3D cancer distribution is also shown in Fig. 5(d). Six needles were adequate to detect the tumor 100%, in those 64 subjects. The locations of 6 needles with depth information are shown in Fig. 5(c). Of course, this will likely not be the case as we increase the number of subjects. But, an important implication is that optimized needle placement is not necessarily on regions that have high likelihood of cancer. As we can see from Fig. 5(a), only first three yellow needles were placed in brighter green (high likelihood) regions. The rest three were placed in regions that were almost statistically independent from the first three.

We validated the predictive power of our statistical atlas using the leave-one-out method. For each time, we selected one subject from our 64 prostate samples, and we regenerated the statistical atlas by leaving this subject out. We then determined again the optimal biopsy sites, and we applied them to this left-out subject. This way, we measured the probability of missing the cancer. For 6-biopsy strategy, the leave-one-out method showed that the rate of success was 96.9%.

In Fig. 6, we also provide the rates of success, as a function of the number of the needles (K) and the volume of tissue that the needle actually extracts from the patient. Suppose that the volume extracted by a needle is V. In the reality there are errors in placing a needle, or in determining angle. Accordingly, we assume that the needle will actually extract only a part of the tissue thought to be extracted under ideal conditions in the optimized K-biopsy. If each needle actually extracts 60%~100% of V around its optimized location, then identical curves of success rates are obtained, as shown as the curve with 'o'. 6 needles are adequate to detect the tumor 100%, while five needles can detect the tumor in 63 out of 64 cases. For other percentages of actual vs. theoretical volume extraction, i.e. 50%, 30%, 10%, the rates of success with the number of the needles are shown as curves with '♦', '△', '■'. For all these cases, 7 or 8 needles are adequate to detect the tumor 100%. This numerical figure of success rate is very valuable for clinicians using our method, since they will be able to quantitatively evaluate the trade-off between success rate and patient discomfort.

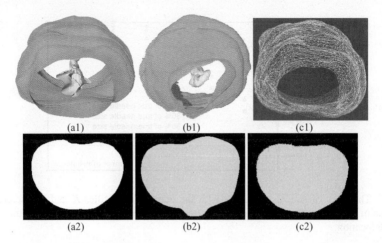

Fig. 4. Results of the deformable registration technique in registering prostates. (a1) A prostate template to which all subjects are warped, (b1) a selected subject, (c1) overlay of the prostate boundary of the subject of b1 (red) after deformable registration with the template prostate (white). Figs. (a2-c2) are representative cross-sectional images corresponding to (a1-c1).

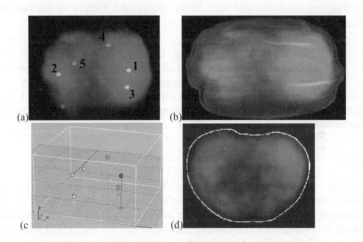

Fig. 5. Optimal biopsy strategy using statistical atlas of cancer distribution. The 6 biopsy positions are shown as small color spheres in (a,c), with the statistical atlas of cancer shown as green in (a,b,d). Prostate capsule is shown as red in (b) for comparison. The cross-sectional image of the statistical atlas of cancer is shown in (d), where prostate capsule is shown as white.

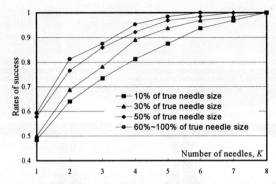

Fig. 6. The rates of success changing with the number of needles K and the percentages of volume of tissue that the needle actually extracts from the expected neighbor of the optimized needle location.

5 Summary and Conclusion

We have presented a methodology to create a statistical atlas for designing optimal needle biopsy strategies. We have applied this method on 64 subjects. We will finally test this method on the whole database of 281 prostate subjects. We will also study the method of warping the statistical atlas to the ultrasound images of the patients' prostate, for image-guided biopsy and therapy.

Acknowledgments: We thankfully acknowledge the collaborations of John Bauer (Walter Reed Army Medical Center), Wei Zhang and Isabell Sesterhenn (Armed Forces Institute of Pathology), Judd Moul (Center for Prostate Disease Research), and Seong K. Mun (Georgetown University Medical Center). This work was supported in part by a grant from the National Science Foundation to the Center for Computer Integrated Surgical Systems and Technology. J. Zeng was supported by the Whitaker Foundation.

References

1. K.K. Hodge , J.E Mcneal, M.K. Terris, T.A. Stamey. Random systematic versus directed ultrasound guided transrectal core biopsies of the prostate. *J. Urol.*, 142: 71-74, 1989.

2. R.C. Flanigan, W.J. Catalona, J.P. Richie, *et al*. Accuracy of digital rectal examination and transrectal ultrasonography in localizing prostate cancer. *J. Urol.*, 152: 1506-1509, 1994.

3. A.L. Eskew, R.L. Bare, D.L. McCullough. Systematic 5-region prostate biopsy is superior to sextant method for diagnosing carcinoma of the prostate. *J. Urol.*, 157: 199-202, 1997.

4. M.E. Chen, P. Troncoso, D.A. Johnston, K. Tang, R.J. Babaian. Optimization of prostate biopsy strategy using computer based analysis. *J. Urol.*, 158(6): 2168-2175, Dec 1997.

5. J. Zeng, J.J. Bauer, A. Sofer, *et al*. Distribution of prostate cancer for optimized biopsy protocols. *MICCAI*, Pittsburgh, Oct. 2000.

6. D. Shen, C. Davatzikos. An adaptive-focus deformable model using statistical and geometric information. *IEEE Trans. on PAMI*, 22(8):906-913, August 2000.

7. D. Shen, E. Herskovits, and C. Davatzikos. An adaptive-focus statistical shape model for segmentation and shape modeling of 3D brain structures. *IEEE Trans. on Medical Imaging*, 20(4):257-270, April 2001.

8. C. Davatzikos. Spatial transformation and registration of brain images using elastically deformable models. *Comp. Vis. and Image Understanding*, 66(2):207-222, May 1997.

A New Approach to Cutting into Finite Element Models

D. Serby, M. Harders, and G. Székely

Swiss Federal Institute of Technology
Communication Technology Laboratory
ETH Zentrum, CH-8092 Zürich, Switzerland
{dserby, mharders, szekely}@vision.ee.ethz.ch

Abstract. Virtual reality based surgical simulators offer a very elegant approach to enhancing traditional training in endoscopic surgery. In this context a realistic soft tissue model is of central importance. The most accurate procedures for modeling elastic deformations of tissue use the Finite Element Method to solve the governing mechanical equations. Therapeutic interventions (e.g. cutting) require topological changes of the Finite Element mesh, thus making a non-trivial remeshing step necessary. This paper describes a new approach to cutting in Finite Element models. The central idea is not to introduce new nodes/elements but to displace the existing ones to account for the topological changes introduced by a cut. After the displacement of the nodes/elements the mesh is homogenized to avoid tiny elements which destabilize the explicit time integration necessary for solving the equations of motion.

1 Introduction

Endoscopic operations have become a very popular technique for the diagnosis and treatment of many kinds of human diseases and injuries. The basic aim of endoscopic surgery is to minimize the damage of the surrounding healthy tissue that is caused by conventional surgery. By employing minimally invasive surgical techniques, the surgeon loses direct contact with the operation site. Performing operations under these conditions demands very specific skills that can be gained only with extensive training. Virtual reality (VR) surgery simulators provide an elegant training possibility.

Within the framework of an earlier project at our institute a realistic, VR-based, endoscopic surgery simulator has been developed [10]. The soft tissue deformations are determined using a complex, non-linear, explicit Finite Element (FE) model. A reduced volume integration scheme (total hourglass control) [5] was applied in order to reduce the computational burden. Furthermore, a parallel computer was built to maintain real-time performance. At present, the simulation is limited to diagnostic interactions. It is, however, desirable to allow also for interactive modifications of the model, especially cutting procedures.

The aim of this paper is to investigate some of the problems that arise while cutting through a FE mesh in a real-time application. We will focus on the

W. Niessen and M. Viergever (Eds.): MICCAI 2001, LNCS 2208, pp. 425–433, 2001.
© Springer-Verlag Berlin Heidelberg 2001

necessary remeshing caused by the topological changes and present a new cutting algorithm.

1.1   Previous Work

Realistic simulation of tissue behaviour during interventions is one of the most challenging tasks in surgical simulations. Several different methods for elastic tissue modeling have been proposed. [11] for instance solves the linear elasticity equations of elastic surface models to calculate deformations.

The two most popular approaches to model soft tissue are physically based mass-spring models and FE models, which are based on continuum mechanics. Whereas the former suffer from poor precision and configuration problems the latter are computationally expensive. There is rich literature on both methods available.

[2] dealt with the interactive simulation of surgical cuts through 3D soft tissue modeled by mass-spring systems. They performed free-form cuts through tetrahedral meshes by applying dynamically adaptive subdivision schemes during the simulation. Any element that is intersected is split into 17 smaller elements once the cutting tool leaves the element, thus dramatically increasing the number of tetrahedra by an average factor of six. [6] has implemented ordinary mass-spring models. In principle using surface models, he adds some additional interior nodes in order to model the volumetric behaviour of the objects. Cutting can only be done along the springs. [4] adopted multi-resolution techniques to optimize the time performance by representing at high resolution only the object parts considered more important. Their approach also allows for topological modifications of tetrahedral mass-spring meshes.

[8] dealt with the simulation of deformable objects using 3D linear FE models. They used various precomputation techniques to achieve real-time performance. Cutting is implemented by removing tetrahedral elements that collide with a virtual scalpel. However, the removal violates the principle of mass conservation. [3] decomposed the anatomical structure into two sections: one onto which they plan to perform cuts and one that will not be affected. Therefore, they propose to apply different elastic models to each section of the anatomy: the more expensive dynamic model is applied only to the section that the user will probably cut. [7] presented a method to cut through soft tissue modeled by a tetrahedral mesh. The tissue deformations are calculated using a linear FE model. The latter can become unstable when the cut is resulting in small elements, which is usually the case. Their examples were not real-time, because they had to run the simulation with a very small integration time step to ensure the stability of the soft tissue model.

After an illustration of the applied FE method in section 2, we will present in section 3 a new cutting algorithm to circumvent some of the problems encountered above. Section 4 describes our results. Finally, we will discuss the improvements and limitations of the new cutting algorithm and future work will be addressed.

2   FE Method

2.1   Physical Model

In this section we will describe the model which we use to simulate elastic deformation of an object. Within FE methods, a body is subdivided into a number of finite elements (such as tetrahedra in 3D or triangles in 2D). Displacements and positions in an element are interpolated from discrete nodal values. For every element, the partial differential equations governing the motion of material points of a continuum can be formulated, resulting in the following discrete system of differential equations [1]:

$$M\ddot{U} + C\dot{U} + KU = R \tag{1}$$

where U is the vector of nodal displacements, M is the mass matrix, C is the damping matrix, K is the stiffness matrix and R is the vector of external node forces. Given an isotropic solid no time-consuming, numerical integration is necessary to determine the stiffness matrix.

The time integration of the above system of equations can be performed using implicit or explicit integration schemes. For the implicit method, the solution has to be calculated iteratively at every discrete time step. In contrast to this, the explicit time integration can be performed without iteration and without solving a system of linear algebraic equations. This integration scheme is only conditionally stable. The critical integration step Δt_{cr} is given by the Courant-Friedrichs-Lewy condition. It is approximately proportional to the characteristical element length ΔL_{min} of the model:

$$\Delta t_{cr} \approx \frac{\Delta L_{min}}{c} \tag{2}$$

where c is the speed of sound in the medium.

In order to calculate a solution for (1) the time-dependent variables must be discretized. We use the explicit Euler central difference terms as estimates of the continuous variables and formulate the equation of motion at the time t:

$$\left(\frac{1}{\Delta t^2}M + \frac{1}{2\Delta t}C\right)^{t+\Delta t}U =$$

$$^tR - \left(K - \frac{2}{\Delta t^2}M\right){}^tU - \left(\frac{1}{\Delta t^2}M - \frac{1}{2\Delta t}C\right)^{t-\Delta t}U \tag{3}$$

Assuming lumped masses at the nodes, we can use diagonal damping and mass matrices. In this case, (3) can be easily solved for the unknown nodal displacements at the time $t + \Delta t$.

2.2   Problems when Cutting in FE Meshes

Purely diagnostic interactions require only one generation of the FE mesh at the beginning of the simulation. In contrast to this, cutting into a FE mesh results in topological changes which demand a remeshing process after each cut. In order to conserve the stability of the integration scheme it is crucial to prevent the element size ΔL_{min} from decreasing rapidly during the cutting process as this requires the adequate adjustment of the critical integration step Δt_{cr}. To this end, an appropriate remeshing has to be performed after each cut.

Another issue, when cutting into a FE mesh, is the dimension of the system matrices. If during the cutting process the number of elements is increasing, the calculation effort to set up the system matrices as well as to solve the corresponding equations of motion increases, too. Again, an appropriate remeshing should prevent this.

In the next section a new cutting algorithm will be introduced. In order to understand the performance as well as the limitations of our concept we performed an initial study in the 2D case. Nevertheless, we always ensured the extensibility of our approach to the third dimension.

3   Cutting Algorithm

3.1   Overview

In order to avoid a rapid growth of the number of nodes/elements, no new nodes, except for the necessary duplicates on the cut line, are introduced after performing a cut. Instead, the nearest existing nodes will be displaced into the cut points to account for the topological changes caused by a cut. The displacements result in a more or less distorted mesh. Several edges can become quite small, bringing about instabilities when integrating the equations of motion. Therefore, it is necessary to homogenize the mesh in a subsequent step. To this end, a combination of a linear mass-spring and a particle system is applied.

The particle system provokes a relatively homogeneous arrangement of the nodes. However, it does not ensure the preservation of the mesh topology. The mass-spring system is well suited for this task but it fails to completely rectify the mesh. For these reasons, a suitable combination of both systems will be utilized. After this brief presentation of our concept, we will give an in-depth explanation of the necessary steps performed by the cutting algorithm.

3.2   Detailed Description

We start from a triangular mesh through which a straight cut is laid (see Fig. 1(a)). First of all, the cut is divided into a number of segments of equal length. In a next step the number of cut points, which was deliberately chosen too high, has to be adapted to the present mesh. To this end, the distance between each cut point and its nearest neighbour is determined. If any two cut points have the same nearest neighbour, the number of cut points is reduced by one and the new cut points are determined. This process is repeated until no two cut points have the same nearest neighbour (see Fig. 1(b)). Thereupon, the nearest neighbours are displaced to the cut point positions (see Fig. 2(a)).

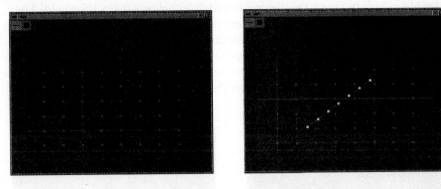

(a) Cut through initial mesh   (b) Adaption of number of cut points to current mesh

Fig. 1. First steps of the cutting algorithm

The adaption process prevents the occurrence of all but two mesh errors. First, a cut line segment can sometimes be intersected by another element edge. The second error occurs when all three nodes of an element are displaced into cut points, causing it to degenerate into a line. Both kinds of errors are traced and corrected. In the next step, the combined mass-spring/particle system is applied. Since the mesh distortion occurs mainly in a neighbourhood of the cut, we have limited the homogenization process to the vicinity of the cut to reduce the computational cost. Nodes are considered as mass points resp. particles and element edges as springs. There are two kinds of internal forces that affect the nodes: On the one hand the spring forces g_{ij}, on the other hand the forces f_i^{int} resulting from the potential energy function ϕ of the particle system:

$$g_{ij} = k_{ij}(\|x_j - x_i\| - l_{ij})\frac{(x_j - x_i)}{\|x_j - x_i\|} , \qquad f_i^{int} = -\nabla_{x_i}\phi \qquad (4)$$

We used the Lennard-Jones potential ϕ_{LJ} [9] because it creates long-range attractive forces and short range repulsive forces which encourage particles to maintain equal spacing. The Lennard-Jones energy function ϕ_{LJ} is defined as a function of separation distance r between a pair of particles:

$$\phi_{LJ}(r) = \frac{B}{r^n} - \frac{A}{r^m} \qquad (5)$$

A single node i of the combined mass-spring/particle system is governed by the following equation of motion:

$$m_i\ddot{x}_i + c_i\dot{x}_i + \left(s_{spring}\sum_j g_{ij} + s_{particle}f_i^{int} \right) = f_i \qquad (6)$$

where s_{spring} and $s_{particle}$ are scaling factors. In order to solve the above dynamic problem the explicit Euler scheme is applied. The new positions of the movable nodes are calculated until the displacements drop below a given threshold. Then, additional postprocessing-steps are performed, which optimize the area of the elements. The result of the whole remeshing process is shown in Figure 2(b). Finally, in order to allow the mesh to open a partner node is generated for each cut point. The original node belongs to elements on one side of the cut and the duplicated node belongs to elements on the other side of the cut.

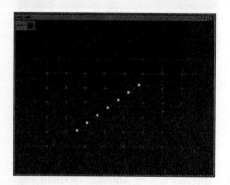

(a) Neighbours dislocated into cut points

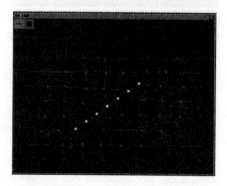

(b) Mesh after homogenization process

Fig. 2. Dislocation and homogenization process

4   Results and Discussion

Several different configurations regarding the kind of mesh and the run of the cut were examined. In order to analyze the quality of the remeshing process a number of statistical values were determined: the number of nodes $\#N$, the number of elements $\#E$, the minimum element area A_{min} and edge length E_{min}, the maximum element area A_{max} and edge length E_{max}, the median element area A_{med} and edge length E_{med}, the standard deviation of the element area A_σ and of the edge length E_σ and the computing time t. All the statistical values were determined before (I) and after (NR) the cut was performed. In the case of the regularly meshed rectangle, these values were also determined for another kind of remeshing (OR) for comparison purposes. Within the OR, at every intersection of the cut line with the mesh a new node is introduced together with the necessary corresponding elements.

All experiments were carried out on a one-processor SGI Octane (195 MHz; 128 MB RAM). An excerpt of the examples is listed in table 1. Figure 3(a) shows as an example a homogeneous mesh through which a cut was laid. In order to do a FE calculation boundary and initial conditions were applied and material and geometric parameters were allocated. Subsequently, the equations of motion were solved by means of a commercial FE software. A snapshot of the solution at a certain point in time is shown in Figure 3(b).

Table 1. Statistical values of the example configurations

Config.	Mesh	#N [−]	#E [−]	A_{min} [mm^2]	A_{max} [mm^2]	A_{med} [mm^2]	A_σ [mm^2]	E_{min} [mm]	E_{max} [mm]	E_{med} [mm]	E_σ [mm]	t [s]
1	I	80	126	22.22	22.22	22.22	0.00	5.7	9.7	7.7	1.4	
	OR	106	152	2.24	22.22	18.42	7.10	2.2	9.7	6.9	2.2	
	NR	85	126	14.46	33.01	22.22	3.10	4.8	10.6	7.7	1.5	3.09
2	I	320	570	4.91	4.91	4.91	0.00	2.7	4.6	3.6	0.7	
	OR	376	626	0.00	4.91	4.47	1.29	0.1	4.6	3.4	1.0	
	NR	326	570	3.56	7.62	4.91	0.24	2.3	4.9	3.6	0.7	23.30
3	I	76	119	26.20	26.20	26.2	0.00	7.8	7.8	7.8	0.0	
	NR	83	312	13.88	39.88	26.20	4.43	4.8	11.2	7.8	0.9	2.75
4	I	312	555	5.88	5.88	5.88	0.00	3.7	3.7	3.7	0.0	
	NR	327	555	2.45	8.26	5.88	0.61	2.2	4.9	3.7	0.3	35.96
5	I	45	69	3.37	53.54	24.59	12.33	2.8	13.6	7.6	2.3	
	NR	48	69	3.37	53.54	24.59	12.48	2.8	13.6	7.7	2.3	0.77
6	I	120	200	0.83	20.87	8.82	4.78	1.2	9.9	4.6	1.6	
	NR	124	200	0.83	23.84	8.82	5.00	1.2	9.2	4.6	1.6	3.05

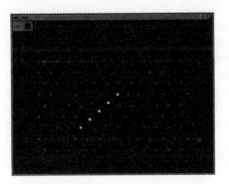

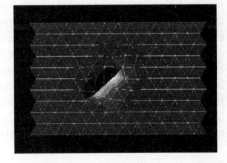

(a) Result of the remeshing with the cutting algorithm

(b) Output of the FE calculation at a certain point in time

Fig. 3. Example showing the result of the remeshing and the FE calculation

The following remarks refer to specific configurations but they are valid in general. Configuration 1 in the table 1 shows that there were 80 nodes and 126 elements before cutting, and 85 nodes and the 126 elements afterwards when using the NR. This compares very favorably to the same cut performed by the OR. While the minimum element area and the minimum edge length are heavily decreasing with the OR, there is only a slight decline with the NR. Configuration 2 points out that the median values and the standard deviations remain approximately the same before and after cutting with the NR. In contrast to this, the

OR results in considerably different median values and standard deviations. Regarding the computing time, it has to be noted, that there is a disproportionate increase from smaller to larger meshes. This is due to the currently inefficient implementation of the post-processing step, which unnecessarily investigates the whole mesh. Due to the local nature of the homogenization process, it is sufficient to also limit the subsequent optimization to the vicinity of the cut, thus making the running time of this step directly proportional to the number of cut points and not to the mesh size.

5   Conclusion and Perspectives

We have presented a new algorithm for cutting into a FE mesh. The technique of dislocating the nodes prevents the number of elements from increasing. The additional nodes that are generated, are the unavoidable partner nodes at the cut points. Therefore, the size of the system matrices stays at a reasonable level, while cutting the mesh. The homogenization procedure restores a more or less homogeneous mesh after the node dislocations. Thus, the problem of decreasing element size is minimized and consequently the stability of the solution of the equations of motion is increased. The computing time necessary for the remeshing takes up only a small fraction of the overall time our surgery simulator needs for the FE calculations and the collision detection, respectively. Due to the fact, that the computing time of our approach is only dependent on the number of cut points, its real-time capability is guaranteed even for larger models.

Future work will focus on analyzing the inter-dependence of the parameters of the combined system (e.g. spring constants) in order to adjust them optimally for a specific mesh, thereby improving the homogenization process. Also the possibility of combining progressive cutting with the current algorithm will be investigated. Finally, we will research further into the problems arising in the 3D case, where whole tetrahedral faces have to be dislocated into the cutting plane.

References

1. Klaus-Jürgen Bathe. "Finite-Elemente-Methoden". *Springer Verlag, Berlin Heidelberg*, 1990.
2. Daniel Bielser, Volker. A. Maiwald, and Markus H. Gross. "Interactive Simulation of Surgical Cuts". *Proceedings of Pacific Graphics 2000, IEEE Computer Society Press*, 2000.
3. Stéphane Cotin, Hervé Delingette, and Nicholas Ayache. "Efficient Linear Elastic Models of Soft Tissues for real-time surgery simulation". *Research Report No. 3510, INRIA Sophia Antipolis*, 1998.
4. Fabio Ganovelli, Paolo Cignoni, Claudio Montani, and Roberto Scopigno. "A Multiresolution Modell for Soft Objects supporting interactive cuts and lacerations". *EUROGRAPHICS 2000*, 2000.
5. Roland Hutter, and Peter F. Niederer. "Fast Accurate Finite Element Algorithm for the Calculation of Organ Deformations". *ASME Summer Bioengineering Conference, Big Sky, Montana*, 1999.

6. Christian Kuhn. "Modellbildung und Echzeitsimulation deformierbarer Objekte zur Entwicklung einer interaktiven Trainingsumgebung für die Minimal-Invasive Chirurgie". *Dissertation, Fakultät für Informatik, Universität Karlsruhe*, 1997.
7. Andrew B. Mor and Takeo Kanade. "Progressive Cutting with Minimal New Element Creation". *In Proceedings MICCAI 2000, Third International Conference, Pittsburgh, PA*, 2000.
8. Morten-Bro Nielsen. "Finite Element Modelling in Surgery Simulation". *In Proceedings MMVR 1997, San Diego, CA*, 1997.
9. David Love Tonnesen. "Dynamically Coupled Particle Systems for Geometric Modeling, Reconstruction, and Animation". *Thesis, Graduate Department of Computer Science, University of Toronto*, 1998.
10. G. Székely et al. "Virtual Reality-Based Simulation of Endoscopic Surgery". *Presence, Vol. 9, June 2000, 310-333, Massachusetts Insitute of Technology*, 2000.
11. Demetri Terzopoulos, John Platt, Alan Barr, and Kurt Fleischer. "Elastically Deformable Models". *Computer Graphics, Volume 21, Number 4, July 1987*, 1987.

Methodology of Precise Skull Model Creation

James Xia[1], Jaime Gateno[1], John Teichgraeber[2], Andrew Rosen[3]

1. Department of Oral and Maxillofacial Surgery
2. Department of Pediatric Surgery
3. Department of Orthodontics
University of Texas Health Science Center at Houston
Houston, Texas, U.S.A.
{James.J.Xia, Jaime.Gateno, John.F.Teichgraeber}@uth.tmc.edu

Abstract: While CT imaging is excellent for demonstrating bone structures, it is unable to display an accurate rendition of the teeth. To address this problem, a method of incorporating accurate teeth into the CT scan was developed. This method combined a 3D CT bone model with digital dental models creating a "precise skull model". An experiment was completed to test the accuracy with which the digital dental models were incorporated into the CT bone models.

1 Introduction

Computed Tomography (CT) imaging is excellent for generating bone models. However, a significant disadvantage of CT is that it is not capable of accurately representing the teeth. The current maxillofacial surgical planning systems still need to employ conventional dental model surgery to establish the occlusion and fabricate surgical splints. Plaster dental models, mounted on articulators, are the most accurate replicas of the patient's teeth. However, the models themselves lack bony support. The limitation of conventional dental model surgery is that the planner cannot visualize the surrounding bony structures, which is critical in the treatment of complex cranio-maxillofacial deformities.

The purpose of this study was to create a "precise skull model", which accurately represents both bony structures and teeth. The authors developed a technique to create a computer bone model with accurate teeth by incorporating digital dental models into a CT bone model, called "precise skull model". This was done to avoid the need for dental model surgery, or the need for incorporating plaster dental model into a stereolithographic model. The digital dental models were obtained by laser surface scanning dental impressions, and they were incorporated into the CT bone models by using fiducial markers.

2 Materials and Methods

The study was completed in three steps. The first step was to create digital dental models. The second step was to incorporate the digital dental models into 3D CT skull

W. Niessen and M. Viergever (Eds.): MICCAI 2001, LNCS 2208, pp. 434-440, 2001.

model, creating a "precise skull model". The final step was to assess the accuracy of this "precise skull model".

2.1 Creation of Digital Dental Models

Prior to obtaining dental impressions, fiducial markers were inserted into a radiolucent full-arch dental impression tray (triple-tray, *ESPE America*, Norristown, PA) (Fig.1). This triple-tray was used to take simultaneous impressions of the maxillary and mandibular arches. Four fiducial markers were mounted on the tray. One pair was at right and left canine region, another pair was at right and left molar region (Fig.2). Dental impressions were then taken in the conventional manner.

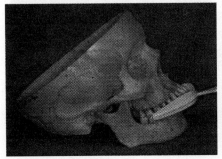
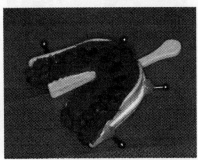

Fig.1 Triple tray   **Fig.2** Fiducial markers

The dental impressions with the four fiducial markers were scanned using a 3D laser surface scanner. Using a custom program, the scanned impression was turned inside out to generate from the negative model of the impression a positive model of the teeth. A digital dental model with four fiducial markers was created.

2.2 Incorporation of Digital Dental Models into a 3D CT Bone Model

With the same dental impressions and fiducial markers in place, a CT scan was taken at a thickness of 1.0 mm. The digital CT data was directly transferred from the CT scanner to a personal computer using a 5.25" MO disk drive.

A 3D CT skull model with four fiducial markers was reconstructed via *Marching Cubes* algorithm and the total numbers of triangles were reduced to 210,000 via *Decimation* algorithm. These fiducial markers were located in the exactly same position as they were on the digital dental models.

Using another custom computer program, interactive alignment of these corresponding fiducial markers was made between the bone model and the digital dental models. After the fiducial markers were aligned, the less than accurate dentition in the 3D skull model was replaced by the accurate dentition of the digital dental models. The fiducial markers were then removed and a "precise skull model" was created (Fig.3).

2.3 Assessment of Accuracy of "Precise Skull Model"

A dry skull with intact dentition was employed. Digital dental models were first created. The dry skull was then CT scanned in order to generate 3D bone model. The digital dental models were incorporated into the CT bone models to create a "precise skull model".

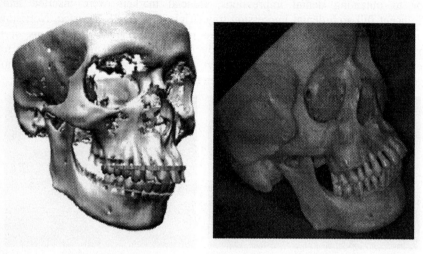

Fig.3 Comparison between "Precise skull model" and dry skull

Measurements were made on the "precise skull model". The measurements were grouped into three categories: bone-to-bone, tooth-to-tooth and bone-to-tooth measurements (Table 1). The bone-to-bone measurements were made between two bony landmarks and were used to assess the accuracy of the 3D bone model. The tooth-to-tooth measurements were made between two dental landmarks and were used to assess the accuracy of the digital dental models. The bone-to-tooth measurements were made from a bony landmark to a dental landmark and were used to assess the accuracy of the alignment of the digital dental models to the 3D CT bone model. The same measurements were made directly on the dry skull utilizing a Boley gauge. All measurements were performed by the same investigator (A.R.) and each measurement was repeated three times on different days.

The means, standard deviations and variances of the measurements of the 3D model and the dry skull were computed respectively. *Person's* correlation coefficient of variance was performed to identify any possible differences between the 3D model and the dry skull.

3 Results

A "precise skull model" was created. This computer model not only represented bony structures from CT data, but also represented dentition from digital dental models.

The intra-observer variances ranged from 0.00 to 0.42 on "composite skull model" and from 0.00 to 0.09 on dry skull. There were no significant differences among the three measurements made by the investigator. Therefore, the three measurements were averaged for each item.

The mean differences between the computerized "precise skull model" and the dry skull were also calculated. Their means and standard deviations were then computed. For the bone-to-bone measurements, the average difference was 0.50mm ± 0.62mm. For the tooth-to-tooth measurements, the average difference was -0.06mm ± 0.19mm. For the bone-to-tooth measurements, the average difference was 0.23mm ± 0.30mm. The average difference for all measurements was 0.24mm ± 0.48mm (Table 2).

The Pearson's correlation coefficient of variance was calculated for each group of measurements. It was 0.9997 for the bone-to-bone measurements, 0.9999 for the bone-to-tooth measurements, and 0.9999 for the teeth-to-teeth measurements. There is no statistical significant difference between the 3D skull model and the dry skull.

4 Discussion

Three-dimensional CT modeling for diagnosis and treatment planning in orthognathic surgery has demonstrated significant potential.[1] It has the ability to simplify surgical procedures, decrease anesthesia time, and increase the accuracy of the intended surgical outcomes.

Three-dimensional CT bone model is excellent at representing bony structures, but it is only an approximation of the patient's actual structures. The precision of a 3D CT model is limited by the layer thickness during CT scanning. CT scanners are only able to capture images layer by layer, data between the image layers is reconstructed by mathematic algorithms, i.e. *Marching Cubes*. Interocclusal relationship of maxillary and mandibular arches plays a major role as reference and is the key to an excellent surgical outcome. However, the 3D CT model is not accurate enough to reproduce interocclusal relationships because of the complexities of dental anatomy. Furthermore, it is not possible to remove scattering, which was caused by metal orthodontic brackets, dental filling or prosthesis during CT scanning. The current surgical planning systems still need to employ conventional dental model surgery to establish the occlusion and fabricate surgical splints.

Plaster dental models, mounted on articulators, are the most accurate replicas of the patients' teeth. However, the models themselves lack bony support. The surgical plan for a plaster dental model is only based on the physical examination, radiography and photography. The limitation of this approach is that the planner cannot visualize the surrounding bony structures, which are critical in the treatment of complex maxillofacial deformities. Stand-alone digital dental models, generated by a laser scanner, have the same shortcoming as plaster dental models.

Several investigators have attempted to incorporate dental models into a CT bone model.[6,7] In order to accomplish this, they developed different methods for replacing the teeth in 3D stereolithographic models with plaster dental models. The existing dentition in the stereolithographic model was removed and plaster dental models were physically inserted. A specially designed face-bow was used to align the plaster dental models to the stereolithographic model. However, these methods were based on physical models, which were not suitable for virtual osteotomies.

The authors have created a three-dimensional "precise skull model" for orthognathic surgical planning. This computerized model precisely represents both bony structures and dentition. By using the authors' method, digital dental models with accurate occlusal relationships can be directly incorporate into a 3D CT bone model, traditional plaster dental model surgery will be unnecessary and totally replaced by computerized virtual osteotomies. The accuracy of the "precise skull model" was demonstrated by *Pearson's* correlation coefficient. The tooth-to-tooth and the bone-to-tooth measurements demonstrated a high degree of accuracy in the digital dental models and their incorporation into 3D CT bone model. There was only a small degree of variance in bone-to-bone measurements (0.5mm ± 0.6mm) between the computerized "composite skull model" and the dry skull, which was due to the limitation of current CT technology. The accuracy of this precise skull model is also superior to other methods.[2-7] *Terai* et al published an error of 4.2 mm while incorporating plaster dental models into a 3D stereolithographic model.[7]

This "precise skull model" can be used for accurate computer diagnosis and treatment planning. It also can be used to generate a stereolithographic model of the patient's craniofacial skeleton and dentition. The next logical step is to determine whether surgical splints can be fabricated from this "precise skull model".

5 References

1. Bill J Reuther JF, Betz T, Dittmann W and Wittenberg G. Rapid prototyping in head and neck surgery planning. *J Cranio Maxillofac Surg.* 24:20-1, 1996

2. Karcher H. Three-dimensional craniofacial surgery: transfer from a three-dimensional (Endoplan) to clinical surgery: a new technique (Graz). *J Cranio Maxillofac Surg.* 20:125-31, 1992

3. Lambrecht JT. 3D modeling technology in oral and maxillofacial surgery. *Quintessence: Chicago, IL.* Pp61-4, 1995

4. Okumura H, Chen LH, Yokoe Y, Tsutsumi S, Oka M. CAD/CAM fabrication of occlusal splints for orthognathic surgery. *J Clin Orthodont.* 23:231-5, 1999

5. Rose EH, Norris MS, Rosen JM. Application of high-tech three-dimensional imaging and computer-generated models in complex facial reconstructions with vascularized bone grafts. *Plast Reconstr Surg.* 91:252-64, 1993

6. Santler G. The Graz hemisphere splint: a new precise, non-invasive method of replacing the dental arch of 3D-models by plaster models. *J Cranio Maxillofac Surg.* 27:169-73, 1999

7. Terai H, Shimahara M, Sakinaka Y, Tajima S. Accuracy of integration of dental cases in three-dimensional models. *J Oral Maxillofac Surg.* 57:662-5, 1999

GROUP	LANDMARKS	DEFINITIONS
BONE TO BONE	R Po-Me	Right porion to menton
	L Po-Me	Left porion to menton
	L Go-Me	Left gonion to menton
	R Go-Me	Right gonion to menton
	Go-Go	Right gonion to left gonion
	Zy-Zy	Right zygomatic arch to left zygomatic arch, smallest distance
	L Po-L Or	Left porion to left orbitale
	R Po-R Or	Right porion to right orbitale
	Max width	Smallest width of maxilla at Lefort 1 level
	Man width	Smallest width of mandible, ramus to ramus
TOOTH TO TOOTH	U3-U3	Upper right cuspid to upper left cuspid, buccal surfaces
	L3-L3	Lower right cuspid to lower left cuspid, buccal surfaces
	U6-U6	Right upper first molar to left upper first molar, buccal surfaces
	LL6-LR3	Lower left first molar to lower right cuspid, buccal surfaces
	LR6-LL3	Lower right first molar to lower left cuspid, buccal surfaces .
	UR6-UL3	Upper right first molar to upper left cuspid, buccal surfaces
	UL6-UR3	Upper left first molar to upper right cuspid, buccal surfaces
	U2-U2	Upper right lateral to upper left lateral, distal surfaces
BONE TO TOOTH	RL3-Me	Right lower cuspid tip to menton
	LL3-Me	Left lower cuspid tip to menton
	LU3-L Or	Upper left cuspid tip to left orbitale
	RU3-R Or	Upper right cuspid tip to right orbitale
	Na-RU3	Nasion to upper right cuspid
	Na-LU3	Nasion to upper left cuspid
	Na-RU6	Nasion to upper right first molar
	Na-LU6	Nasion to upper left first molar

Table 1 Definitions of measurement landmarks by group

GROUP	LANDMARK	3D MODEL Average	SKULL Average	Difference
BONE TO BONE	R Po-Me	129.30	129.62	0.32
	L Po-Me	127.81	129.15	1.34
	L Go-Me	80.04	81.54	1.50
	R Go-Me	79.54	78.87	-0.67
	Go-Go	95.03	95.79	0.76
	Zy-Zy	120.86	121.51	0.65
	R Po-R Or	80.21	80.54	0.33
	L Po-L Or	80.39	80.58	0.19
	Max width	66.38	66.66	0.28
	Man width	95.49	95.75	0.26
Average difference				0.50
SD				0.62
TOOTH TO TOOTH	U3-U3	43.71	43.78	0.07
	U6-U6	60.81	60.90	0.09
	L3-L3	32.13	32.04	-0.09
	LL6-LR3	49.91	49.49	-0.42
	LR6-LL3	50.53	50.66	0.13
	UR6-UL3	57.73	57.59	-0.14
	UL6-UR3	58.75	58.52	-0.23
	U2-U2	34.54	34.63	0.09
Average difference				-0.06
SD				0.19
BONE TO TOOTH	RU3-R Or	53.92	54.59	0.67
	LU3-L Or	55.10	55.10	0.00
	RL3-Me	46.83	47.04	0.21
	LL3-Me	46.72	47.42	0.70
	Na-RU3	85.69	85.70	0.01
	Na-LU3	85.93	86.02	0.09
	Na-RU6	86.30	86.25	-0.05
	Na-LU6	87.03	87.28	0.25
Average difference				0.23
SD				0.30
Average difference for all groups				0.24
SD for all groups				0.48

Table 2 Comparison of "precise skull model" and dry skull

Medial Axis Seeding of a Guided Evolutionary Simulated Annealing (GESA) Algorithm for Automated Gamma Knife Radiosurgery Treatment Planning

David Dean[1], Pengpeng Zhang[2], Andrew K. Metzger[1], Claudio Sibata[3], and Robert J. Maciunas[1]

[1] Department of Neurological Surgery, and The Research Institute, University Hospitals of Cleveland, and Department of Neurological Surgery, Case Western Reserve University
10900 Euclid Avenue, Cleveland, OH 44106-5042 USA
{dxd35, rjm31, akm8}@po.cwru.edu
[2] Department of Biomedical Engineering, Case Western Reserve University
10900 Euclid Avenue, Cleveland, OH 44106-7207 USA
pxz11@po.cwru.edu
[3] Department of Radiation Oncology, and The Research Institute, University Hospitals of Cleveland, and Department of Radiation Oncology, Case Western Reserve University
10900 Euclid Avenue, Cleveland, OH 44106-6068 USA
cxs81@po.cwru.edu

Abstract. We present a method to optimize Gamma Knife™ (Elekta, Stockholm, Sweden) radiosurgery treatment planning. A Guided Evolutionary Simulated Annealing optimization algorithm is used to maximize the therapeutic benefit through a probability model that dissects a patient volume image into three components: normal, critical normal, and tumor tissue. This evolutionary optimization algorithm may be seeded randomly or via an automatically detected medial axis. We use indices of dose conformality, level, and homogeneity to evaluate the degree to which a treatment plan has been optimized. Two clinical examples compare the GESA algorithm with current manual methods. GESA optimization shows therapeutic advantage over the treatment team's manual effort. We find that computation of treatment plans with more than 8 shots require initial medial axis seeding (i.e., shot: number, size, and position) to complete within 8 hours on our workstation.

1 Introduction

The Leksell Gamma Knife™ (LGK) is a tool for providing highly accurate stereotactic radiosurgical treatment of brain tumors. It conforms radiation beams to a lesion from 201 ^{60}Co sources through four different size collimators. Typically, a neurosurgeon, a radiation oncologist, and a medical physicist collaborate to form a unique treatment plan for each patient. Each application of radiation, a "shot," has an ellipsoid shape dose distribution that varies with the location of the isocenter. Typically, more than one shot is usually required to irradiate the tumor. The clinicians provide each shot in the plan to the stationary patient as a separate procedure.

W. Niessen and M. Viergever (Eds.): MICCAI 2001, LNCS 2208, pp. 441–448, 2001.

The tumor portion, and perhaps nearby critical structures, are most often segmented (labeled) in a series of 2D MRI images. The planning team prescribes a radiation dose (D_{pd}, usually 50% of D_{pmax}) based in large part on tumor type and volume. Now the number of shots, shot size (only four radiation collimators are available, with diameters of 4mm, 8mm, 14mm, or 18mm respectively), shot weight (irradiation level), and shot position are determined.

Treatment parameters which a computer is better suited to optimize than the treatment team are best handled through inverse-planning. These tasks include determining the location of shots which best conform to, and provide homogeneous irradiation to, the lesion at a prescribed level. Highly conformal plans also contribute to minimization of normal tissue damage. The shot positioning problem can be viewed as a combinatorial packing problem; a search for a group of roughly 3D Gaussian functions (shots) that conform to the 3D tumor shape under the constraint of minimized spread out to the adjacent volume. However, the limited number of LGK shot sizes and weights (dose level) require complex compromise between the goal of irradiating tumor and sparing normal tissue. The physician specifies where critical structures next to the tumor demand a rapid dose drop-off (steep gradient).

When multiple shots are applied in the treatment plan, the dose is normalized to the maximum dose in the Volume of Interest (VOI). For a treatment plan that includes N_s shots, each with weight w_s, size r, isocenter (i,j,k), the dose delivered to the voxel A in the VOI, can be written as:

$$D_A = \frac{\sum_{s=1}^{N_s} D_{sA}(w,i,j,k,r)}{\max\left\{\sum_{s=1}^{N_s} D_{sB}(w,i,j,k,r), \quad \forall B \in VOI\right\}} \times D_{p\max} \quad (1)$$

where D_{pmax} is the prescribed maximum dose by the treatment planning team, and $D_{sA}(w,i,j,k,r)$ is dose contributed to point A via shot s. The goal is to maximize tumor are covered with greater than 50% of D_{pmax}, and minimize the normal tissue damage by delivering less than 50% of D_{pmax} there, much less to adjacent critical structures.

Elekta's LGK treatment planning software, GammaPlan[TM], asks the treatment planning team to manually choose shot size, weight, and position based on the patient's 2D MR-scan series. The team re-computes the cumulative dose and dose distribution as each new shot is added to the treatment plan, until a sufficient dose acceptably conforms to the lesion. In our experience this iterative procedure ranges from 45 minutes to over 5 hours.

1.1 Automated Radiosurgery Planning

Several other groups have presented inverse planning of LGK treatment variables. Shu et. al.[1] present a solution the shot packing problem that uses multiplier penalty methods. Gibon et al.[2] solve the same LGK shot positioning problem with a conjugate gradient and simulated annealing approach. Wu et al.[3] and Wagner et al.[4] treat LINAC radiosurgery planning as a "shot packing" problem using a depth map similar to our medial axis seeding algorithm. Leichtman et al.[5] use an adaptive simulated annealing method to refine an initial plan generated automatically by computer or manually by the physician. Our Guided Evolutionary Simulated Annealing (GESA) algorithm[6] hybridizes the evolutionary nature of genetic algorithms with parallel computing (i.e., parallel processing of competing treatment plans), and objective function optimization procedures. The optimized objective function represents a biological model of all treatment criteria. This algorithm discovers a near-optimal solution after examining a small fraction of the possible solutions.[7]

2 Treatment Criteria Model

Our mathematical model simulates all treatment criteria. For each ijk^{th} voxel in a VOI identified by the surgeon. The therapeutic benefit is modeled by probability P^+_{ijk}:

$$P^+_{ijk} = \frac{e^{K_{ijk} \times \Delta d_{ijk}}}{e^{K_{ijk} \times \Delta d_{ijk}} + e^{-K_{ijk} \times \Delta d_{ijk}}} \qquad (2)$$

where $\Delta d_{ijk} = (D_{ijk} - D_{PD})/D_{PD}$, D_{ijk} is the dose delivered to the ijk^{th} voxel; D_{pd} is assigned as 50% of D_{pmax}; and K_{ijk} is a scale factor (imposing the importance of fitting the desired dose to the voxel). Our goal is to maximize therapeutic benefit (i.e., tumor destruction and normal tissue sparing). For a voxel classified as tumor, the associated K_{ijk} is positive. Dose that is between the prescribed and maximum levels results in a large P^+_{ijk}. For a voxel classified as normal tissue, the associated K_{ijk} is negative. Normal tissue dose below the prescribed minimum tumor level results in a beneficial (large) P^+_{ijk}. For a voxel classified as critical structure, the associated K_{ijk} is yet more negative than other normal tissue; the corresponding D_{pd} would be assigned an even lower value (i.e., 30% of D_{pmax}) relative to the prescribed tumor dose. Therefore, a large dose (compared to its own D_{pd}) delivered to critical structure voxels will result in a very small P^+_{ijk} value, counter to our goal of maximizing P^+_{ijk}. The choice of each K_{ijk}, especially the ratio different tissue type K_{ijk}'s, determines the compromise between irradiating the entire tumor and sparing adjacent normal tissue.

3 Objective Function

An objective function is used to achieve the goal of optimizing the initial plan to match the clinician-specified treatment criteria. As noted, the goal of our objective function is to maximize the plan's therapeutic benefit, modeled as a probability, P^+_{ijk}, at each voxel. The objective function to be minimized (i.e., annealed) is written as:

$$E = -\frac{1}{N} \sum_{ijk} (P^+_{ijk})^2 \qquad (3)$$

where N is the number of voxels in the VOI. Maximizing P^+_{ijk} also works towards another planning goal, homogeneous dose distribution (i.e., no hot or cold spots).

444   D. Dean et al.

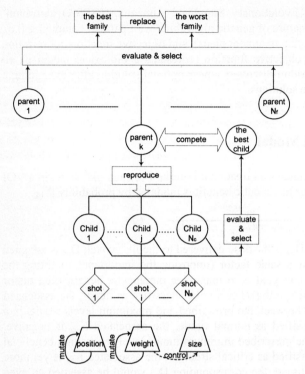

Fig. 1. GESA Evolutionary Procedure. See text for explanation.

3.1 GESA Optimizes Objective Function

The GESA algorithm (Figure 1) begins by first choosing N_p parents from the search space. Each parent generates N_c children. There is a small random mutation between the parent and its children. The child is accepted only if it satisfies:

$$e^{-|x_c-x_p|/T_3} > p \quad (4)$$

where x_c is the child, x_p is the parent, T_3 is a temperature parameter, and p is random between 0 and 1.

There are two levels of competition in our GESA algorithm. First, within a family, children compete with their parents for a position as a parent in the next generation. The objective function value of the best child in the family is y_{bc}, y_p is the objective function value of the parent, T_1 is a temperature parameter, and p is a random number. The best child in the family is qualified to replace its parent if it satisfies:

$$y_{bc} < y_p \quad or \quad e^{(y_{bc}-y_p)/T_1} > p \quad (5)$$

Second, there is also competition among families. We evaluate the quality of each family. There are different criteria for inter-family competition.

There are three temperature parameters for the optimization procedure, T_1, T_2, and T_3. Between successive generations, the temperature decreases linearly:

$$T(n) = T(0) - n(T(N) - T(0))/N \quad (6)$$

where $T(0)$ is the initial temperature, N is the designed maximum generations, and $T(N)$ is the final temperature.

4 Seeding the GESA Radiosurgery Treatment Planning Algorithm

Since the discrete shot number and size are not fixed during the optimization process, there is evolutionary mutation of these parameters in the GESA procedure. Evolution requires variation, therefore we seed GESA with multiple species (i.e., initial treatment plans with different shot number and size) and let them compete for survival. For different levels of tumor complexity (i.e., size and geometry), the optimization task utilizes different GESA strategies. For a small tumor with regular shape (i.e., requiring less than 8 shots to cover the tumor), the GESA algorithm begins with a randomly determined initial plan with a maximum number of shots of uniform size by the treatment planning team. From this starting point the treatment plan adapts an evolutionary strategy that is able to mutate the shot number and size. For a big tumor with irregular shape, multiple initial treatment plans with different number of shot and shot size are generated via our medial axis guided algorithm.[8] These plans evolve and compete as potentially optimal plans within the GESA analysis.

4.1 Medial Axis GESA Seeding

Medial axis detection is an image processing technique that is used to model the geometrical shape of an object of interest. The medial axis is a line representation of an object where all points are equidistant from at least two points along the object's border. One means of detecting the depth of voxels from the surface of the segmented tumor is the Grassfire Based Euclidean Distance Transform. A Euclid Distance Transform (EDT) of a binary image can be simulated as the propagation of the grass fire wave front. The fire is ignited all about the object's periphery and is extinguished at the innermost area where convergent fires create the highest local heat value. A sequential algorithm, based on Danielsson's work[3,8] efficiently produces the EDT. First, distance values are assigned to the boundary points (i.e., at least one of the 8-connected neighbors is a member of non-object), the fire source of the binary image object. These values are assigned by:

$$EDM(p) = \min[L(p, p') + EDM(p')] \quad \forall p' \in N \cap S' \quad (2)$$

where O is the object, O' is the non-object, $p \in O$, $p \in O'$, N is the point set of 8-connected neighbors of p, L is the real distance between p and p'. Next, the binary object is peeled away, one layer at a time. Old boundary points become members of a non-object, and new boundary points are exposed. For each set of new boundary points p, the distance values are also calculated by Eq. 2. This calculation continues until it reaches the final layer of the object. The accuracy of grass fire-based EDT is improved by using a floating value instead of an integer value. The result better approximates a binary segmented object in digitized space.

Medial axis points may be detected as ridge points on an EDM surface via our Gradient Phase Operator.[8] We define the phase gradient of a point on a 3D EDM surface:

$$G(S, r, \varphi) = (EDM(S) - EDM(P)) / \Delta L \quad (3)$$

where S is a point of the object, P is a point on a circle centered at S with radius of r, φ is the angle between line SP and the vertical direction, and ΔL is the real distance between S and P. The medial axis is an optimal location for LGK shot centroids.

4.2 GESA Optimization

Whether randomly or medial axis-generated, once seeded with 20 initial treatment plan families, the evolution process toward an optimal plan occurs automatically.

Given the shape and volume of the tumor, the treatment planning team determines maximum shot number, initially uniform shot size. Then shot weight (w) and position (pos[i,j,k]) are chosen randomly in the 20 initial plan domains, where $w \in [0.2, 1.5]$, and $pos \in \{tumor\ voxel\}$. For each family, twenty children are reproduced, each slightly mutated from its parent (Equation 4). Note that the reproduction the size of each shot can also mutate. If the weight of the shot falls under 0.2, the shot size will change to the next smaller available size. Shot weight is assigned:

$$w_{mutated} = w_{current} \times \frac{size_{current}}{size_{mutated}} \quad (7)$$

A 4mm shot with weight below 0.2 would be removed from the treatment plan to reduce redundancy, thus change the total number of shots in the treatment plan. The initialized families are sent to GESA. After evaluating the fitness of each child (Equation 3) in each family, the best child competes with its parent for the parent position of the next generation based on Equation 5. Competition at the inter-family level results in replacement of parents of the worst performing family by that with the best treatment plan. This ensures that a family with the highest quality gets more chances to reproduce. This evolutionary procedure continues until the parents of each family change little (i.e., an objective function reaches an acceptable value).

Plan Origin	Tumor Tiss. Vol.	Normal Tiss. Vol. (Critical Structure)	Shot #	Tumor Dose Avg	Tumor Dose Std. Dev	Planning Time
CASE 1: Acoustic Tumor						
Manual	6.69 cm³	2.01	8	0.62D$_{pmax}$	0.09	45 min
GESA	6.77 cm³	1.32	7	0.65D$_{pmax}$	0.08	1 hour
CASE 2: Meningioma Tumor						
Manual	5.40 cm³	4.77 (0.03)	19	0.60D$_{pmax}$	0.10	5.5 hrs
GESA	5.47 cm³	3.16 (0.02)	15	0.62D$_{pmax}$	0.11	7.5 hrs

Table 1. Manual Plan and Optimized Plans for Cases 1 and 2.

5   Brain Tumor Treatment Planning Experiment

Our goal is to obtain an optimal treatment plan via GESA in less than one work day's (8 hours) computation time. We present two of the cases that test the effectiveness of our GESA treatment planning algorithm, especially where initial seeding is helpful.

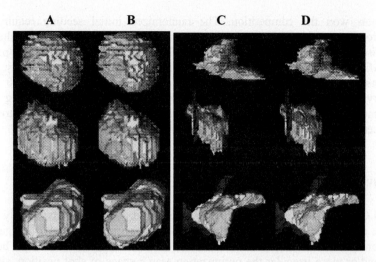

Figure 2. Comparison of Acoustic Tumor treatment plan (Columns A and B) and Meningioma Tumor treatment plan (Columns C and D) generated by GESA algorithm (Columns A and C) and that manually generated by a treatment planning team (Columns B and D). Views: Sagittal (Row 1), Coronal (Row 2), Axial (Row 3). The original tumor surface is opaque yellow. The surface of the volume receiving than 50% of D_{pmax} is assigned transparent blue.

5.1 Case 1: A Small Acoustic Tumor with Simple Shape

After determining the tumor volume, the attending treatment planning team set the initial shot number at 8 utilizing uniform shot size of 14 mm, and uniform shot weight of 0.8. The GESA began its search for a treatment plan with random shot location (i.e., no seeding). After 38 generations, a 7-shot treatment plan was generated (Table 1). The GESA treatment plan improved conformality (Figure 2) as evidenced by 0.08cm^3 more tumor irradiation, and 0.69cm^3 more normal tissue spared. The GESA optimized plan required 1 less shot and resulted in a higher tumor dose average which was closer to the desired dose (0.8), and a lower tumor dose standard deviation between voxels (i.e.,. homogeneity). over the manual shot packing plan (Figure 1). It took 1 hour to process the 38 GESA generations involved on a Silicon Graphics Inc. (Mountain View, CA) ORIGIN 200^{TM} SGI workstation with an R10000, 250MHz CPU. This unsupervised computation may be compared to the treatment planning team's 45 minutes spent manually generating the plan that the patient received.

5.2 Case 2: A Large Meningioma Tumor with Complex Shape

To initiate the GESA algorithm, the tumor's medial axis was located for a segmented meningioma tumor. Seven treatment plans with various shot number and shot size were based on the medial axis and provided as seeds to the GESA algorithm. Each of these seeds resulted in six families, each with twenty children. After 58 generations, the species with 15 shots that includes three 14mm-shots, nine 8mm-shots and three

4mm-shots won the competition. The randomized initial seeding required 214 generations (days) for GESA to reach an acceptable treatment plan. Table 1 shows the comparison between the plan generated by GESA and that generated by the planning team. GESA algorithm achieved better conformality and similar homogeneity. It took 7.5 hours to process the 58 GESA generations on the same SGI ORIGIN 200^{TM}. This unsupervised computation should be compared to the treatment planning team's requirement of 5.5 hours to manually generate their plan. Movies of the treatment plans seen in Figure 2 may be found at http://neurosurgery.cwru.edu/imaging.

6   Discussion and Conclusion

The 3D GESA algorithm searches the shot parameter space more thoroughly than is possible during manual shot packing. We note that, where beneficial to the patient, a reduction of shot number reduces treatment time. Also, as tumor shape becomes larger and/or more irregular the optimization search space of shot position, size, and weight expands exponentially. Medial axis seeding reduces that space by providing several good initial shot packing plans.

References

1. Shu, H., Yan, Y., Luo, L., Bao, X.: Three-dimensional optimization of treatment planning for gamma unit treatment system. Med. Phys., 25 (1998) 2352-2357.
2. Gibon, D., Rousseau, J., Castelain, B., Blond, S., Vasseur, C., Marchandise, X.: Treatment Planning Optimization by Conjugate Gradients and Simulated Annealing Methods in Stereotactic Radiosurgery. Int. J. Radiation Oncology Biol. Phys. 33 (1995) 201-210.
3. Wu, Q.J., and J. D Bourland "Morphology-guided radiosurgery treatment planning and optimization for multiple isocenters", Med. Phys. 26, October, pp. 2151-2160, 1999.
4. Wagner, T.H., Taeil, M.E., Ma, S.F., Meeks, S.L., Bova, F.J., Brechner, B.L., Chen, Y., Buatti, J.M., Friedman, W.A., Foote, K.D., Bouchet, L.G., A Geometrically Based Method for Automated Radiosurgery Planning. Int. J. Radiation Oncology Biol. Phys., 48 (2000) 1599-1611.
5. Leichtman, G.S., Aita, A.L., Goldman, H.W.: Automated Gamma Knife dose planning using polygon clipping and adaptive simulated annealing. Med. Phys., 27 (2000) 154-162.
6. Yip, P.P.C., Pao, Y.: Combinatorial Optimization with Use of Guided Evolutionary Simulated Annealing", IEEE Trans. Neural Networks, 6 (1995) 290-295.
7. Zhang, P., D. Dean, A. Metzger, and C. Sibata, "Optimization of Gamma Knife Treatment Planning via Guided Evolutionary Simulated Annealing", Med. Phys., 28 (2001), in press.
8. Dean D, Metzger A, Duerk J, Kapur V, Zhang P, Chou H, Sibata D, and Wu J: Accuracy and Precision of Gamma Knife Procedure Planning and Outcomes Assessment. Computer Aided Surgery. 5 (1999) 63.

A Software Framework for Creating Patient Specific Geometric Models from Medical Imaging Data for Simulation Based Medical Planning of Vascular Surgery

Nathan Wilson[1], Kenneth Wang[2], Robert W. Dutton[3], Charles Taylor[4]

[1] CISX 305, Stanford University, Stanford, CA, 94305-4075
nwilson@stanford.edu
[2] CISX 332, Stanford University, Stanford, CA, 94305-4075
wang@gloworm.stanford.edu
[3] CISX 333, Stanford University, Stanford, CA, 94305-4075
dutton@gloworm.stanford.edu
[4] Division of Biomechanical Engineering, Durand 213,
Stanford University, Stanford, CA 94305-3030
taylorca@stanford.edu

Abstract. The primary purpose of vascular surgery is to restore blood flow to organs and tissues. Current methods of vascular treatment planning rely solely on diagnostic and empirical data to guide the decision-making process. This paper details a simulation-based medical planning system for cardiovascular disease that use computational methods to evaluate alternative surgical options prior to treatment using patient-specific models of the vascular system. A software framework, called Geodesic, is introduced that reduces the time required to build patient-specific models from medical imaging data from several weeks to less than one day.

1 Introduction

The current paradigm for surgery planning for the treatment of cardiovascular disease relies exclusively on diagnostic imaging data to define the present state of the patient, empirical data to evaluate the efficacy of prior treatments for similar patients, and the judgment of the surgeon to decide on a preferred treatment. This paper details a simulation-based medical planning system for cardiovascular disease that uses computational methods to evaluate alternative surgical options prior to treatment using patient-specific models of the vascular system. The blood flow (hemodynamic) simulations enable a surgeon to see the flow features resulting from a proposed operation and to determine if they pose potential adverse effects such as increased risk of atherosclerosis and thrombosis formation. A significant bottleneck for simulation-based medical planning, however, is the lengthy time required to build patient specific geometric models and associated difficulties in discretization and numerical simulation. This paper details a software framework, called Geodesic, that reduces the time required to build patient-specific geometric models from medical imaging data from several weeks to less than one day. Geodesic includes an integrated level set kernel

W. Niessen and M. Viergever (Eds.): MICCAI 2001, LNCS 2208, pp. 449-456, 2001.

for image segmentation of blood vessel (lumen) boundaries and prepares the appropriate input files for hemodynamic simulation.

Cardiovascular surgeons currently rely on medical imaging data and past experience to form an operative plan. Taylor et. al. [1] proposed a new paradigm in vascular surgery, namely that computer simulation could be used to provide a surgeon with quantitative and qualitative comparisons of different operative plans prior to surgery to augment the information already available. This requires a software system that can be used by medical technicians in conjunction with vascular surgeons to perform numerical simulations predicting the blood flow for several different operative procedures.

2 Simulation Based Medical Planning

The first system developed for simulation based medical planning (SBMP) of vascular surgery was the "Stanford Virtual Vascular Laboratory" [2]. This system predominantly relied on idealized models of the vascular system. Specifically, circular cross-sections were used to describe the surface of each artery branch to be included in the model and these individual artery models were joined (boolean union) together to create a solid model representing the vascular system. This solid model could then be automatically meshed with unstructured tetrahedral elements using an automatic mesh generator. Finally, input files were automatically created for a finite element fluid mechanics solver to perform hemodynamic simulation of the given vascular system.

A major advantage of using idealized models was the ability to use parametric models, which enabled studies of a wide variety of vascular anatomy to be performed in a short period of time. The major shortcoming of the SVVL was its inability to build patient specific preoperative geometric models from medical imaging data. A second generation system for vascular surgery planning (named ASPIRE) is detailed in [2]. This system had an internet-based user interface specifically designed for a vascular surgeon. However, like the SVVL this system also lacked the ability to build 3-D patient-specific geometric models from medical imaging data.

This paper will detail recent advances in the development of a software system, named Geodesic, which is a modular framework that greatly simplifies the process of building preoperative vascular models from medical imaging data and performing subsequent postoperative planning. The Geodesic framework consists of several key modules including: a level set module for segmentation of imaging data, a solid modeling module for geometric computation, a meshing layer for querying meshes for information required to specify boundary conditions and creating input files for hemodynamic solvers, and an interactive graphical user interface (GUI) for easily creating alternative post operative plans.

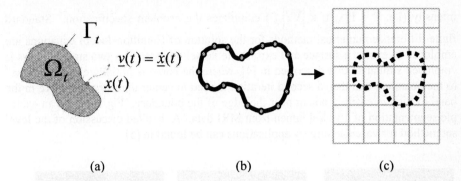

Fig.1: The level set function. Figure (a) shows the abstract mathematical representation, while (b) shows 1-D boundary edges being embedded in a 2-D uniformly spaced grid (c).

3 Image Segmentation Using Level Set Methods

Numerous methods exist for segmentation of boundaries from medical imaging data. For example, thresholding is a technique that defines boundary edges as a given value of image intensity. A contouring algorithm, such as marching cubes, is then used to extract the iso-surface yielding the boundary. A more powerful and increasingly popular approach, introduced by Osher and Sethian [3], is known as the level set method. Briefly, the level set method imbeds a boundary of interest in a higher dimension space, and solves a partial differential equation governing the evolution of the interface (see Fig. 1). That is, we define a scalar function ϕ such that:

$$\phi(\underline{x}(t),t) = 0 \qquad \underline{x} \in \Gamma \tag{1}$$

Using the chain rule and taking the time derivation of (1), the definition of the normal from differential geometry, and projecting the velocity function along the normal to the boundary, transforms the expression of (1) into the standard partial differential equation of the level set method:

$$\phi_t + \underline{v}(t) \cdot \nabla\phi = 0 \quad \Rightarrow \quad \phi_t + F|\nabla\phi| = 0$$

$$where \quad \underline{n} = \frac{\nabla\phi}{|\nabla\phi|} \quad and \quad \underline{v} = F\underline{n} \tag{2}$$

Choosing ϕ as the signed distance function (i.e. $|\nabla\phi| = 1$) and making the velocity normal to the curve depend on boundary curvature and the gradient of the image data intensity (i.e. $F = F(\underline{x}, t, \kappa, |\nabla I|)$)) completes the problem specification. Standard finite-difference numerical methods for the solution of Hamilton-Jacobi equations are employed to evolve a surface and extract the vessel boundary. A two stage process is employed similar to that described in [4], where the curve is initially evolved "close" to the boundary and then a second iteration is used to center the extracted curve in the band of high intensity gradient near the edge of the boundary. Fig. 2 shows an example segmentation of a vessel lumen from MRI data. A detailed discussion of the level set method for vascular surgery applications can be found in [5].

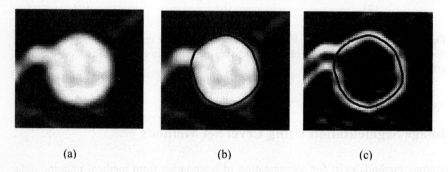

(a)   (b)   (c)

Fig. 2: Level set segmentation of a vessel boundary. (a) shows the original MR image slice, (b) shows the final boundary on the image data, and (c) shows the final boundary on a plot of the magnitude of the gradient of the image intensity (where white represents a larger absolute value of the gradient). This example shows the need for curvature feedback when evolving the surface, that is the curvature dependence prevents the boundary from "leaking" into the smaller adjacent branch vessel.

4 Preoperative Patient-Specific Model Construction

The level set method discussed previously can be used in any number of spatial dimensions, and Geodesic has an integrated multi-dimensional level set kernel. While using the 3-D level set method theoretically has many advantages such as the ability to directly extract volumetric geometry from image data, it has several significant practical disadvantages. First, the method imbeds the evolving boundary in a higher dimension space (i.e. a surface defining a volume represented using triangular facets requires a 3-dimensional grid). Thus memory and computational cost scale roughly by $O(n^3)$. Additionally, the variability in the image data can make the constants found in the boundary velocity functions used to do the segmentation a function of position. Finally, the human body contains a vast network of arteries, but it may be desired to simulate only a subset of them. It is difficult to extract an accurate geometric representation using the level set method in 3-D while preventing the front from advancing into undesired branches.

For these reasons, the technique used in the current work is to extract 2-D cross sections of the lumen boundary along the path of a given arterial branch, and then use solid modeling operations to "loft" an analytic (NURBS) surface skinning the surface of the contours. This process can be seen in Fig. 3. The process is repeated for each desired branch in the image data. In more detail, the first step is for the user to define a path for a given branch. This can be done in two ways, with the user selecting multiple points defining the path or automatically using a custom program to extract the path given an initial and final point. Once the path is obtained, level set simulations are performed on selected cross sections along the path. Typically, a subset of these cross-sections are chosen by the user to create a lofted solid model of the given branch.

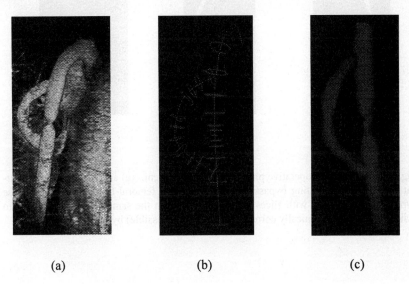

(a)   (b)   (c)

Fig. 3: Solid model construction of a bypass model for a pig with an artificially created stenonsis. (a) shows the image data, (b) shows the paths along which selected level set curves have been extracted, and (c) shows the resulting solid model after the joining of the bypass and aorta branches.

When desired branches have been created, they are joined (i.e. boolean union) together in the solid modeler to create a single solid representing the vascular system. This solid model is then meshed using automatic mesh generation methods [6], and hemodynamic solver input files are automatically created (see Fig. 5). Note that an additional advantage of building the system from a set of branches is the information needed to assign boundary conditions for simulation is implicitly specified during the creation of the resulting solid. That is, the "cap" of each branch is a planar cross section tagged with an integer id and the branch name (the tagged parameters are called "attributes"). The solid modeler being used propagates the attributes during boolean operations, so when the final solid is being created all of the outflow boundaries are automatically marked. This is because for all branches, except possibly the aorta, one of the two caps will be absorbed (i.e. eliminated) in the final solid. The remaining named surface is then assumed to be the outflow boundary. This eliminates the user from needing to interact with the mesh to select element faces or nodes for boundary conditions, which is key to going automatically from patient geometric models to simulation results.

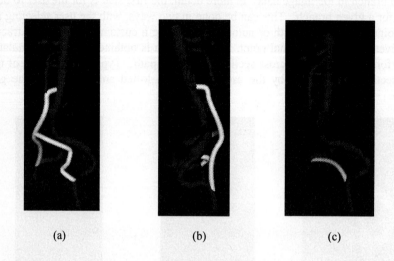

(a)   (b)   (c)

Fig. 4: Two different operative plans for a human patient. (a) and (b) show two different views of a bifurcating bypass, while (c) shows a femoral-femoral bypass. These bypasses were created with slices of the image data in the same rendering window to assist in making anatomically correct (i.e. physically possible) bypasses.

5 Creating Alternative Operative Plan Models

The ability to evaluate different treatment options and predict the impact of different procedures on a given patient is of critical importance in patient specific vascular surgery planning.   Additionally, these procedures should be planned in the presence of the imaging data so that the validity of the proposed procedure is insured. Fig. 4 shows several different images of potential treatment options for an individual patient. The operative planning GUI inside of Geodesic is simple, yet powerful. Slide bars control the location of three image slices (x, y, z) oriented in the image volume. In addition, a cursor is controlled by slide bars and positioned in 3-space. The user selects desired points by moving the cursor, and the path is highlighted in the rendering window as the user selects points.   This allows the user to verify that the proposed operation is physically possible given the patient anatomy. Currently this operation requires significantly less time than the preoperative model construction, as three or four clinically relevant operation alternatives can be created in less than one hour.

6 Mesh Generation and Simulation

As a first approximation, it can be assumed that the vessel walls do not deform (i.e. are rigid) and that blood can be approximated as a Newtonian fluid with constant material parameters. In addition, it is assumed that the outlet pressure of each of the branches is known and can be set to a constant pressure (i.e. p=0). With these assumptions, the hemodynamic simulation reduces to solving the Navier-Stokes equations of fluid mechanics with periodic inflow boundary conditions. Two types of boundary conditions have been explored. First, as an approximation the analytic inflow profile (which assumes fully developed, axisymmetric flow) proposed by Womersley [7] can be prescribed on the inflow boundary. The only required input for the analytic profile is the volumetric flow rate as a function of time. Second, the inlet velocity can be directly determined from physiologic data using phase-contrast MRI.

Fig. 5 shows a mesh of a pig that underwent an aortic bypass, as well as a simulation of blood flow in the system. This model was created completely inside of Geodesic and is currently being compared with *in vivo* experimental results.

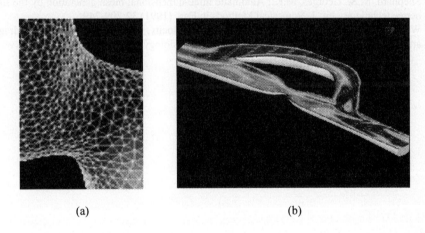

(a)   (b)

Fig.5: Mesh and simulation results of a pig aortic-bypass. (a) shows a close up of the surface mesh near the stenonosis, while (b) shows the magnitude of the flow velocity (blue low, red high) in the aorta and bypass.

7 Conclusions and Future Work

A software framework, called Geodesic, was introduced that reduces the time required to build patient-specific models from medical imaging data from several weeks to less than one day. Further improvements in the model construction, mesh generation and flow solution processes are essential for these simulation-based medical planning methods to be clinically feasible. In addition, work still remains in automating the

456   N. Wilson et al.

specification of physiologic inflow boundary condition data from PC-MRI. *In vivo* studies comparing animal (pig) experiments and the simulation results to validate the assumptions being used are currently underway.

References

1. Taylor, C. A.: A Computational Framework for Investigating Hemodynamic Factors in Vascular Adaptation and Disease. Phd thesis, Stanford University (1996)
2. Taylor, C.A., Draney, M.T., Ku, J.P., Parker, D., Steele, B.N., Wang, K., Zarins, C.K.: Predictive Medicine: Computational Techniques in Therapeutic Decision-Making. Computer Aided Surgery (1999) 4:231-247
3. Osher, S., Sethian, J.A.: Fronts propagating with curvature-dependent speed: Algorithms based on Hamilton-Jacobi formulations. J. Computational Physics (1988) 79:12-49
4. Malladi, R., Sethian, J.A.: A Real-Time Algorithm for Medical Shape Recovery. Proc. Intl. Conf. Computer Vision (1998) 304-310
5. Wang, K.: Level Set Methods for Computational Prototyping with Application to Hemodynamic Modeling. Phd thesis, Stanford University (expected 2001)
6. Shephard, M.S., Georges, M.K.: Automatic three-dimensional mesh generation by the finite octree technique. Int. J. Numerical Methods in Eng. (1991) 32:709-749
7. Womersley, J.R.: Method for the calculation of velocity, rate of flow and viscous drag in arteries when the pressure gradient is known. J. Physiology (1955) 53:502-514

Interactive Catheter Shape Modeling in Interventional Radiology Simulation

Zirui Li[1], Chee-Kong Chui*[1], Yiyu Cai[2], James H. Anderson[3],
Wieslaw L. Nowinski[1]

1 Biomedical Lab, Kent Ridge Digital Labs, Singapore 119613
2 School of MPE, Nanyang Technological University, Singapore 639798
3 Johns Hopkins University School of Medicine, Baltimore, Maryland 21205, USA
*cheekong@krdl.org.sg

Abstract. Vascular catheterization provides a less invasive, non-surgical approach for treatment of vascular diseases. Although preformed catheters with diverse shapes and specific features are commonly available, clinicians still often use devices such as mandrels to modify the shape of catheters at the time of the clinical procedure. In this paper, we describe catheter shape modeling techniques. The purpose of catheter shape modeling is to provide clinicians with a means to modify catheter shape using a computer, and to practice catheterization procedures with this modified catheter on a computer based interventional radiology simulation system. We have proposed a 2-level design approach with the support of shapes and properties databases. In the first level, the shape of catheter is defined as a series of smoothly joined element segments. In the second level, we introduce catheter shaping algebraic operations recursively on the segments including merging, splitting, inserting and removing. We present our results by demonstrating the creation of right coronary artery catheters for different size and shape of aortic roots. The correctness of these catheters is validated with our catheter navigation simulator.

1. Introduction

Catheterization, the least invasive, non-surgical approach for treating vascular and other diseases, provides effective and quality patient care by significantly reducing patient discomfort, hospital stay and medical cost. It often requires the ability to enter the vascular system through needle puncture sites and to maneuver therapeutic or diagnostic devices through the vascular system, using x-ray imaging, to the target lesion in the body. With the smallest possible circular cross-sections, catheters are the most widely used devices in cardiovascular interventional procedures. The Catheters used in the interventional procedures are extremely diverse in shapes and specific features [1].

Specific catheter tip shaping is often required because of the wide variety of sizes and anatomical configurations of blood vessels and because the vascular characteristics of lesion vary significantly between different people. For example, in the field of interventional cardiology, there are at least three types of aortic configurations to be considered: normal, unfolded, and post-stenotic. The catheter

W. Niessen and M. Viergever (Eds.): MICCAI 2001, LNCS 2208, pp. 457-464, 2001.

shapes and dimensions have to be modified appropriately to accommodate different configurations. In the 1960s, before the availability of preformed angiographic catheters, Dr. Melvin P. Judkins shaped catheters at the time of each examination [2]. He placed a polyurethane tubing over a stiff wire bent to conform to the shape of the vessel, and then immersed the catheter in boiling water to soften it. When the assembly cooled, he withdrew the wire, and the catheter retained its shape. Although there are now many commercially available preformed catheters, clinicians still use devices like "Steam Shaping Mandrel" to modify the shape on the tip of the catheter.

In conjunction with development of our interventional radiology simulators[3-5], we developed a software system to design the shape of the catheter. The process is similar to the steam shaping and mandrel process, but instead of working with a physical device, the users create and test new catheter designs through software simulation. In such a system, the user can choose a catheter from the database with preformed shape and predefined material composition, and then modify its shape and size through a series of mouse clicks. In the next step, the clinician can use the interventional radiology simulator for pretreatment planning purpose[6] to determine the optimal shape of a catheter for a specific patient application and make the desired modifications in catheter shape using the method described in this paper.

We call our software system for shaping catheters "Digital Catheter Shaping Mandrel" or DCSM. Unlike our previous work [7], it is designed as a simple and user friendly system for training and planning through simulation. In this system, operations related to the manipulation of the piecewise curves are defined and implemented. Handy tools to carry out these operations are provided. Database of catheter shapes and materials are built. The output of the system is a finite element model (FEM) comprising a series of nodes in a format compatible with our simulator. Initial results of its application to interventional cardiology are described.

2. Methods

In DCSM, the catheter is defined as smoothly linked segments. For the convenience of manipulation, the catheter shape is represented by a tree structure as explained in the following subsection. In such a shape tree, a node corresponds to a subset of consequent segments and the leaf represents the element shape. The element shape is defined by parameters such as length, cross sectional radius, curve radius, *etc*. The modification of the catheter's shape is carried out through changing of the shape tree structure and/or changing of the element shape parameters. We have implemented handy tools to carry out these tasks. For example, the manipulation of the element shape such as elongation, bending and twisting are performed through mouse dragging. The manipulation on the element segment defined the first level of our 2-level design approach. In the second level, there are arithmetic operations including merging, splitting, inserting and removing segments that have been defined mathematically. Interactive tools to carry out these operations are provided.

Figure 1 illustrates the process of catheter shape modification. The user starts the process by selecting an existing catheter from databases of catheter shapes and materials. He/she then modifies the shape through adjusting the element shape parameters or a combination of arithmetic operations such as merging and splitting.

User friendly graphical display and intuitive interactions are provided to facilitate the execution of such operations.

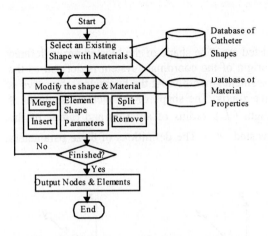

Figure 1. Flow chart of catheter shape modification

Material properties are critical to the behavior of the catheter. Physical parameters of the materials are stored in a database. These parameters are defined for each catheter element and are used in the finite element analysis of catheter navigation process. The purpose of finite element analysis is to determine the interactions between the catheter and guidewire, and between the catheter and the blood vessel wall with or without consideration of blood flow.

2.1 Catheter Shape Representation

A catheter is defined as a series of curved arc segments joined smoothly one after another. We use the operation " $|$ " as the joining of two segments. For example, $S = S_1 | S_2$ means we join smoothly the head of S_2 to the tail of S_1. The shape of the catheter can be defined as

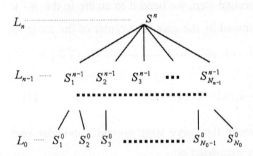

Figure 2. Tree representation of catheter shape

$S = S_1 | S_2 | \cdots | S_N$, where N is the number of segments used to define the shape of the catheter. In addition, each segment in this expression can be formed by joining several component segments. Therefore the catheter shape could be represented as a tree shown in Figure 2. In such a tree, a node represents a shape segment. Siblings from left to right join subsequently to form the shape

of their parent in the upper level. For example, $S_i^k = S_{i_1}^{k-1} | S_{i_2}^{k-1} | \cdots | S_{i_{ni}}^{k-1}$ means that the ith segment in level k consists of $i_{ni} - i_1 + 1$ segments in the level k-1. The sequence numbers of these segments are $i_1, i_2, \cdots, i_{ni}$, respectively. If a node in the middle level of the tree contains only one segment, the same segment is are defined as the descendant of this node at each lower level. In such structure, every level of the nodes could be joined together to represent the final shape.   We represent such a structure as $S = S_1^k \mid S_2^k \mid \cdots \mid S_{N_K}^k$, $k = 0,1,2,\cdots,n$, where N_k is the number of sub-shapes defined in the kth level.

2.2 Element Definition

An element shape is defined as a twisted arc. The shape of the twisted arc is defined in its own coordinate system. The origin of the coordinate system is defined as the point where the curve joins to other segment smoothly. At the beginning, the curve is straight and located along the positive x-axis. The shape of the element segment is defined by three parameters, the length (L), radius of arc (r) and radius of the cylinder around which the curve is twisted (r_c). The definitions of these parameters are shown in Figure 3.

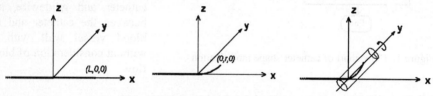

Figure 3. Definition of element shape

If L is the total length of the catheter curve element, each point on the curve can be assigned parameterized coordinates $C(s) = (x(s), y(s), z(s))$. The determination of these coordinates is carried out in three steps. In the first step, we determine the length of a straight line segment (L). In the second step, we bend it to an arc in the x-y plane. The radius of the arc r is determined by the user. The center of the arc is (0, r,0). By such definition, for $0 \le s \le L$, the parameterized coordinate of the arc can be expressed as,

$$(u(s), v(s), w(s)) = (r\sin(\frac{s}{r}), r(1-\cos(\frac{s}{r})), 0) \qquad (1)$$

In the third step, we twist the arc to make the curve wrap around a cylinder with radius r_c, the points on the curve can be expressed as:

$$(x(s), y(s), z(s)) = (r_c \sin(\frac{u(s)}{r_c}), v(s), r_c (1-\cos(\frac{u(s)}{r_c}))) \qquad (2)$$

2.3 Catheter Shaping Algebra

Typically, a catheter consists of several curves. For example, the left and right coronary catheters developed by Dr. Melvin P. Judkins[2] comprise primary, secondary and tertiary curves. In our model, each of these curves corresponds to an element segment or a segment formed by several elements. Catheter Shaping Algebra comprises of arithmetic operations that are developed to carry out operations such as merging, splitting, removing and inserting segments. For convenient of illustration, we use sub-shape to describe the segments that form a new catheter curve.

Merging

There are two sub-shapes S_i and S_j with lengths of L_i and L_j. Their shapes are defined in their own coordinate systems are $(x^i(s), y^i(s), z^i(s))$ and $(x^j(s), y^j(s), z^j(s))$ respectively. The merging operation $S = S_i | S_j$ will join the head the S_j to the tail of S_i smoothly. The length of the new curve is $L = L_i + L_j$. For sub-shape S_i, the coordinates of the curve remain unchanged, that is, for $s \le L_i$, $(x(s), y(s), z(s))) = ((x^i(s), y^i(s), z^i(s)))$.

The sub-shape S_j should be transformed to the new coordinate system through the following matrix. For $L_i < s \le L_i + L_j$,

$$\begin{Bmatrix} x(s) \\ y(s) \\ z(s) \\ 1 \end{Bmatrix} = \begin{bmatrix} r_{11} & r_{12} & r_{13} & U_i \\ r_{21} & r_{22} & r_{23} & V_i \\ r_{31} & r_{32} & r_{33} & W_i \\ 0 & 0 & 0 & 1 \end{bmatrix} \begin{Bmatrix} x^j(s) \\ y^j(s) \\ z^j(s) \\ 1 \end{Bmatrix} \tag{3}$$

The transform matrix must satisfies:

$$(U_i, V_i, W_i) = (x^i(L_i), y^i(L_i), z^i(L_i)) \tag{4}$$

$$\left(\frac{\partial x(s)}{\partial s}, \frac{\partial y(s)}{\partial s}, \frac{\partial z(s)}{\partial s} \right)s = L_i^- = \left(\frac{\partial x(s)}{\partial s}, \frac{\partial y(s)}{\partial s}, \frac{\partial z(s)}{\partial s} \right)s = L_i^+ \tag{5}$$

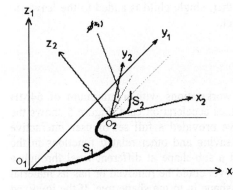

Figure 4. Merging of segments

It should be noted that Equation (5) determines only the vector of x-axis of local coordinate system of ith segment. The rotation angle $\phi_i^{(x)}$ is to be defined by the user to determine the direction of local y-axis. In Figure 4, origin of the segment S_2 is on the end point the segment S_1. The local x-axis of the segment S_2 is the tangential direction of S_1 at the tail. $\phi^{(x)}$ is defined as the angle between y_2 axis and its projection on the x_1-y_1 plane. The vector for the direction of S_2 's local z-axis and the rotation matrix can be determined accordingly.

The merging of more than two segments is carried out from left to right, and the final curve is defined in the same coordinate system as that of segment 1.

Splitting

The splitting of a segment works with the sub-shapes that are formed through merging. Users can not split an element shape. For a curve shape $S = S_1^k \mid S_2^k \mid \cdots \mid S_i^k \mid \cdots \mid S_{N_K}^k$ and $S_i^k = S_{i_1}^{k-1} \mid S_{i_2}^{k-1} \mid \cdots \mid S_{i_{ni}}^{k-1}$, the splitting can be expressed as $S = S_1^k \mid S_2^k \mid \cdots \mid S_{i_1}^{k-1} \mid S_{i_2}^{k-1} \mid \cdots \mid S_{i_{ni}}^{k-1} \mid \cdots \mid S_{N_K}^k$. The resulted shape contains $N'_k = N_k + i_{ni} - i_1$ segments.

Removing Segment

Removing a segment can be applied to the element shape or a sub-shape in any level of the shape tree. For a curve shape $S = S_1^k \mid S_2^k \mid \cdots \mid S_i^k \mid \cdots \mid S_{N_K}^k$, the result of removing S_i^k can be expressed as $S = S_1^k \mid S_2^k \mid \cdots \mid S_{i-1}^k \mid S_{i+1}^k \mid \cdots \mid S_{N_k}^k$. In the tree structure shown in Figure 2, all children of S_i^k are removed accordingly. The catheter shape could be updated accordingly at any level of the shape tree.

Inserting Segment

Inserting a sub-shape can happen in any level of the shape tree. For a curve shape $S = S_1^k \mid S_2^k \mid \cdots \mid S_i^k \mid \cdots \mid S_{N_K}^k$, the results of inserting a shape $\overline{S}$ at position i could be expressed as $S = S_1^k \mid S_2^k \mid \cdots \mid \overline{S} \mid S_i^k \mid \cdots \mid S_{N_K}^k$. If an element shape is inserted in an upper level, we define it as its children until the lowest level of the shape tree currently under design. On the other hand, if the inserted shape is a sub-tree, its branches are inserted to the corresponding level of the current shape tree. If the depth of any sub-tree is less then the other, single child is added to the leaves to make the two sub-trees having the same level.

3. Results

The DCSM works on consumer PCs or workstations with a minimum of 64MB memory, preferably with an OpenGL graphics acceleration card. Figure 5 shows the graphics user interface of DCMS. We have provided a full set of user interactive functions to facilitate loading, modifying, saving and other related functions in the design of the catheter. The user can select a sub-shape at different level through a several mouse clicks. A sub-shape at any level could be removed or has its material property changed. Users can insert another shape in to the shape tree. If the involved shape is a sub-shape, it can be split at different level. However, if it is an element shape at the lowest level, its shape parameters can be adjusted freely. Editing functions includes changing of the following parameters: length, radius of arc, radius of twist cylinder. These functions include elongation/shortening, bending/straighten, and twisting/flatten. Rulers/grids can be displayed when users are modifying the shape of the element shape.

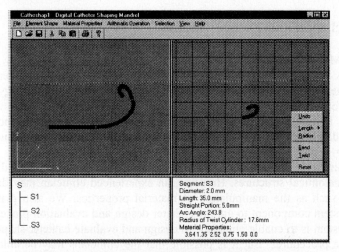

Figure 5. Graphical user interface for catheter shape design

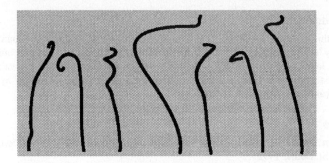

Figure 6. Examples of catheter shapes designed using DCSM

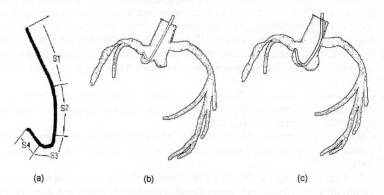

Figure 7. Right coronary catheter shape model and its navigation in heart model

Figure 6 shows some of the resultant catheter shapes we have modified from a straight catheter. Figure 7(a) illustrates the contributing components of our catheter shape model. Figure 7(b) and (c) show navigation of these right coronary catheters in a heart model having different size and shape of aortic roots.

4. Conclusion and Future Works

The DCMS is developed as a low-cost, user friendly and powerful tool for the clinicians to design and modify the catheter shapes in a computer simulation environment. It has been integrated into our interventional radiology simulation system for pretreatment planning. This software system has been validated by clinicians in the clinical context. This validation proves the usefulness and correctness of the underlying catheter shaping technique that has been defined mathematically in this paper.

The clinicians can use DCMS to modify catheter shape to allow for differences in human anatomical structures. However, an experienced clinician may demand more features, such as the manipulation of material properties. We also plan to add an expert system component to aid the catheter design and evaluation process. The goal of this system is to enable clinicians to design and evaluate catheter shape prior to its use in the procedures. But it is possible that the clinicians may be able to use this system to invent new catheters and/or a new procedure.

Acknowledgements

Support of this research development by National Science and Technology Board of Singapore is gratefully acknowledged. We are grateful to Dr. Anthony C. Venbrux and Dr. Kieran Murphy of Johns Hopkins Hospital, Baltimore, USA for championing the validation of our software systems in the clinical context. The project is partially sponsored by the Nanyang Technological University (SDS 15/2000).

References

[1]. D. Kim and D.E. Orron, *Peripheral Vascular Imaging and Intervention*, Mosby-Year Book, St. Louis, 1992.

[2]. L.A. Geddes and L.E. Geddes, *The Catheter Introducers*, Mobium Press, Chicago, 1997.

[3]. J. Anderson, W. Brody, C. Kriz, Y.P. Wang, C.K. Chui, Y.Y. Cai, R. Viswanathan and R. Raghavan, daVinci- a vascular catheterization and interventional radiology-based training and patient pretreatment planning simulator, *Proc. of Society of Cardiovascular and Interventional Radiology (SCVIR) 21st Annual Meeting*, Seattle, USA, March 1996.

[4]. Y. Wang, C.K. Chui, H.L. Lim et al, *Real-time interactive simulator for percutaneous coronary revascularization procedures*. Computer Aided Surgery, Vol 3, No 5, 211-227, 1998.

[5]. C.K. Chui, P. Chen, Y. Wang et al, *Tactile Controlling and Image Manipulation Apparatus for Computer Simulation of Image Guided Surgery*, Recent Advances in Mechatronics, Springe-Verlag, 1999.

[6]. C.K. Chui, J. Anderson, W. Brody, W.L. Nowinski, *Report on Interventional Radiology Simulation Development*, Internal Research Report, KRDL- Johns Hopkins University, 2001.

[7]. Y.Y. Cai, Y. Wang, X. Ye, X., C.K. Chui et al, *Catheter designing, presenting and validating using CathWorks*, International Journal of Robotics and Automation, February 2000.

Parametric Eyeball Model for Interactive Simulation of Ophthalmologic Surgery

Yiyu Cai*[1], Chee-Kong Chui[2], Yaoping Wang[2], Zhenlan Wang[2],
James H. Anderson[3]

[1]School of MPE, Nanyang Technological University, Singapore 639798
[2]Biomedical Lab, Kent Ridge Digital Labs, Singapore 119613
[3]Johns Hopkins University School of Medicine, Maryland 21205, USA
Email: myycai@ntu.edu.sg

Abstract. In this paper, we describe a parametric eyeball modeling system for real-time simulation of eye surgery. A knowledge-based approach is used to parametrically model the ophthalmologic structures. Together with the parametric eye modeling and the integration of patient-specific disease images, the ophthalmologic knowledge databases of eye diseases, eye material properties, and eye surgical instruments and procedures can help to provide better maneuverability and more realistic scenarios for eye surgical simulation. A customized Finite Element Method (FEM) is developed to analyze the deformation of the eyeball and the interactions between the bio-structures and the instruments in the surgery simulation. A phantom haptic and force feedback virtual environment is used for real-time interactive ophthalmologic surgical simulation.

1. Introduction

Eye diseases are among the most common and rapidly growing public health concerns. Eye surgery involves very dedicated procedures, and new techniques and device are being constantly introduced to the ophthalmology community [1-2]. The complications of ophthalmologic diseases, however, often pose difficulties for surgeons to make both timely and accurate critical decisions. Subsequently, very intensive training is required for ophthalmologic professionals in order to provide high quality standard surgical services.

Computer eye surgical simulation has been developed to provide better training for the ophthalmologic students or junior eye surgeons. Hanna et al reported their simulation work of arcuate keratomomy for astigmatism [3-4]. Sagar et al built an eye surgical simulator within a virtual reality environment [5-6]. Bio-mechanical studies for eye anatomy and pathology play a vital role in eye surgical simulation [7-10].

In this work, we aim to develop a more realistic eye surgical simulator. Patient-specific eye diseases will be considered with the simulation. This information is further enhanced by the knowledge database providing typical information and scenario in eye diseases, diseased eye material properties and eye surgery instruments and procedures. The work focuses on the Asian populations. A parametric eyeball

W. Niessen and M. Viergever (Eds.): MICCAI 2001, LNCS 2208, pp. 465-472, 2001.

model including the cornea, lens, sclera, retina, and choroid, etc, are developed with the capability of 3D variational change of the ophthalmology. A customized computational engine using FEM method is provides real-time analysis for deformation and interaction in eye surgery. The graphical simulation is seamlessly integrated with the FEM based physical modeling on the advanced OpenGL architecture and virtual haptic environment.

2. Parametric Eyeball Modeling Using Ophthalmologic Knowledge Guidance

2.1 Ophthalmologic Knowledge Base

Our online survey on eye disease was conducted in Singapore recently that shows about 80% of the 168 voting people have myopia (Figure 1). There is also a trend in the average age of the onset of pupils diagnosed with eye diseases. Eye surgery is becoming more common and popular. Traditionally, eye surgery trainees practice using animal eyeballs. There approach presnts problems. First, animals don't suffer from the same disease as humans. Next, animal eyeballs are not reusable and if a mistake is made, the eyeball must be discarded and a new one used. Also, there are differences in terms of ophthalmologic anatomy and pathology between different races, sex, age, etc.

We are building an ophthalmologic knowledge database for Asian races. The data is obtained from published literature, public domain eye disease data, and interviews including online survey. Typical data include (1) Asian eye diseases; (2) Asian eye biomechanical material property; and (3) Eye surgical instrument and procedures. The knowledge database will capture various eye diseases for the Asian population (Figure 2). The eye disease database captures information of geometry and pathology. The eye material property database keeps biomechanical values such as Young's and Shear's modules for various parts of the bio-structure. The eye instrument and procedure database include typical surgical devices and procedures used for a particular operation. With such an ophthalmologic knowledge database, simulation of different eye disease scenario becomes feasible.

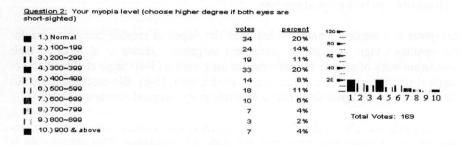

Figure 1. Online survey on eye disease in Singapore

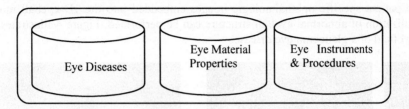

Figure 2. Ophthalmologic Knowledge Database

2.2 Parametric Eyeball Modeling

We model the eyeball parametrically. This allows variational change of eyeball geometry and anatomy. The cornea is transparent, and resembles a little watch-glass [7-8]. In the anterior aspect, the cornea is transversely ellipsoid, whereas its posterior aspect is circular. Looked from in front, the cornea is elliptical. From the behind, the cornea appears circular. This difference is due to the fact that the sclera and conjunctiva overlap the cornea anteriorly more above and below than laterally. Ideally, the cornea forms part of the surface of a sphere. In diseased condition such as astigmatism, it is more curved in the vertical than in the horizontal meridian. The sclera forms the posterior opaque approximately five-sixths of the fibrous tunic of the eye. Its anterior portion is visible, and constitutes the "white" of the eye. The sclera is thickest behind and gradually becomes thinner when traced forwards. The choroid is firmly attached to the margin of the optic nerve, and slightly placed at the points where vessels and nerves enter it. The lens of the eye is a transparent bi-convex body of crystalline appearance placed between the iris and the vitreous. Its axial diameter varies markedly with accommodation. Like all lenses, that of the eye presents two surfaces: anterior and posterior, and a border where these surfaces meet, known as the equator. The anterior surface is the segment of a sphere.

Figure 3 illustrates the eyeball model represented in a polygonal mode. Individual parts of the eyeball are parametrically represented and variation of the geometry is possible. With the ophthalmologic knowledge database, the parametric modeled eyeballs can provide high fidelity platforms for eye surgical simulation.

2.3 Patient-Specific Image Registration

To improve the realism of eye surgery simulation, it is high important to integrate patient-specific eye disease information into the simulator. Ophthalmologic images are embedded inside the 3D parametric model using the atlas-based image alignment algorithm [11-12]. A uniform polar coordinate system of the eyeball is used in the process. A texture mapping technique is applied to match the ophthalmologic images and the eyeball structure. Alignment of the ophthalmologic image with the eyeball under the guidance of eye atlas is thus turned into an optimization task.

With patient specific ophthalmologic images embedded into the 3D eyeball model, visualization of abnormal eyeball structure can be performed. Figure 4 illustrates the visual field of a glaucoma eye disease.

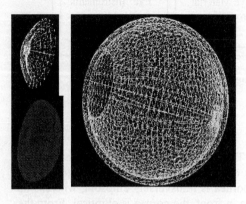
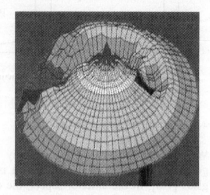

Figure 3. Parametric representation of   Figure 4. Visualization of eye abnormal
        eyeball model

3. FEM-Based Physical Modeling for Eye Surgery

We are developing a computer-based simulator for eye surgery to help medical students and junior ophthalmologists impeove their surgical skills. We have built a physical based model with finite element method to simulate the real movement of bio-structures in response to the manipulation of the instruments during the surgical procedure. The visco-elasticity biomechanics is adopted to describe the deformation of the bio-structures [13-15]. In the 3D ocular model, we have considered the following structures: (1) Cornea, (2) Lens, (3) Sclera, (4) Choroids, and Iris, (5) Retina, (6) Muscles.

All the structures are parametrically modeled with reference to the ophthalmologic knowledge base. Emphasis, however, will be placed upon the cornea, lens, and choroids since these are the primary structures involved in common practices. In the following sections, we describe the bio-mechanical modeling of instruments and eye bio-structures.

3.1 Movement of Instrument

It is noted that the elasticity of all the instruments in practices are much harder then all the bio-structures involved in the operation. It is assumed that a rigid structure with six-degree of freedom is used to represent the instruments. The movements of the instruments are then the sum of rigid body displacements as

$$\Re = \Re(R_x, R_y, R_z, R_\theta, R_\rho, R_\omega) \tag{1}$$

where R_x, R_y and R_z are the coordinates of the end of the instruments at the global space. R_θ, R_ρ and R_ω represent the two rotations of the tip of the instruments with respect to the axis of the global system and a rotation with regard to its logistical axis.

3.2 Governing Equation of Deformation of Biostructures

From studies, 90% of corneal thickness is formed by the stroma. We assumed that this controls the majority of the biomechanical behavior of the cornea and mainly consists of water (78%) and layered protein fibres (16%), which provides strength, elasticity and form. Ideally, it is assumed as the visco-elasticity material in the deformation analysis.

A visco-elastic material is one which exhibits properties of both viscous fluids and elastic solids. Many materials exhibit properties of elastic and viscous behavior dependent on stress. Examples include metals and Bingham plastics. However, visco-elasticity describes a material which exhibits a combination of viscous and elastic behavior simultaneously. Visco-elastic materials can appear to be either solid or liquid, depending on whether the dominant property is elastic or viscous. Visco-elasticity is common among macromolecular materials and is often the result of molecular entaglement between macromolecules. Visco-elastic materials are characterized by two particular behaviors: Creep and Stress Relaxation.

When a sudden load is applied, there is an initial rapid extension but instead of having a fixed extension as with an elastic solid, it continues to extend with time. When the load is removed, there is an initial rapid contraction that quickly slows down. Conversely, the stress required to maintain constant strain decreases with time. This is known as stress relaxation. And the deformation problem we encountered here is a multi-structures stress relaxation problem.

3.3 FEM Formulation

We consider the FEM analysis of this multi-structures stress relaxation problem. The materials here is a time-dependent "flow" occurrence due to the intervention of the instruments. The given equation can be given as, using Hamilton's principle,

$$F(x_i, t) = \int_{t_0}^{t_1} L\,dt = \int_{t_0}^{t_1} (\Pi - \Lambda)\,dt \tag{2}$$

Where the Lagrangian function L is defined in terms of the potential energy (Π) and the Kinetic energy (Λ).

The calculation of Π can be made:

$$\Pi = \frac{1}{2} d^T \int_0^v B^T DB\,dv\,d \tag{3}$$

where

$$d = [d_{1x} d_{1y} d_{1z}, d_{1x} d_{1y} d_{1z}, \cdots, d_{Nx} d_{Ny} d_{Nz}]^T \tag{4}$$

d_{ix}, d_{iy}, d_{iz} are the displacements at x,y,z directions at i^{th} FEM node. B is the standard strain matrix and D is the material matrix. Π can be further written as

$$\Pi = \frac{1}{2}d^T K\, d \tag{5}$$

where

$$K = \int_0^v B^T DB\, dv \tag{6}$$

K is the stiffness matrix of the bio-structures.

The kinetic energy Λ can be given as

$$\Lambda = \frac{1}{2}\int_0^v \rho(\frac{\partial d}{\partial t})^2 dv \tag{7}$$

ρ is the mass density of the individual material.

Our problem here is a First-order problem as

$$K\dot{d} + K\, d = Q \tag{8}$$

where

$$\dot{d} = \frac{\partial d}{\partial t} \tag{9}$$

and these derivatives can be replaced by finite difference approximations. In the Crank-Nicokon scheme, a time-stepping technique,

$$d = \frac{d_{n+1} + d_n}{2} \tag{10}$$

$$\dot{d} = \frac{d_{n+1} - d_n}{\delta} \tag{11}$$

where δ is the finite step length.

Hence the recurrence relation is obtained as

$$(K + \frac{2}{\delta}K_d)d_{n+1} = Q_{n+\frac{1}{2}} + (\frac{2}{\delta}K_d - K)d_n \tag{12}$$

It is implemented, for consistency, equation (10) should be used for Q. And using backward difference for (11) giving

$$(K + \frac{1}{\delta}K_d)d_{n+1} = Q_{n+1} + \frac{1}{\delta}K_d d_n \tag{13}$$

In this case, the displacement increments d are calculated using the equilibrium iteration.

4. Virtual Reality Supported Eye Surgical Simulation

We developed a computer-based simulator for eye surgery with the parametric eyeball model to help medical students and ophthalmologists improving their surgical skills.

Figure 5(a) is an image of the rendered eyeball model. Figures 5(b) is a snapshot of the graphical user interface. It shows the interaction between the device and the cornea surface of the eyeball modeled. User can feel the force feedback on the device via the force feedback device (PHANToM) in our simulation environment shown in Figure 6.

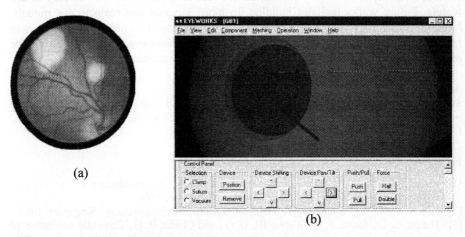

(a)

(b)

Figure 5. (a) Eyeball model (b) Snapshot of graphical user interface of simulator

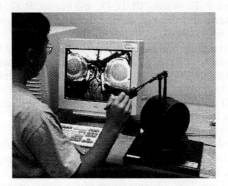

Figure 6. Eye surgical simulation environment

The simulation system provides direct interaction with patient-specific model and volumetric data set while delivering haptic feedback to the user. A real-time volume rendering technique based on ray casting, trilinear interpolation, and per-sample gradient estimation algorithms was employed to visualize the patient-specific volume data. Our physical-based eyeball model and the associated FEM analysis provide the realistic haptic rendering. User feels the force through the PHANToM. With the guidance of see-able and magnified internal eyeball 3D representations of the patient-specific data, a trainee can easily interact with the abnormal eye structures such as slightly cutting some cornea with a virtual scalpel. In Figure 6, a user is manipulating the PHANToM to interact with a patient's eyeball volume MRI data sets under the assistance of a variety of virtual tools.

5. Conclusion

To meet the needs of training for ophthalmological professionals, a prototype for eye surgery simulation is described using the physical-based parametric eyeball model. It enables simplified eye surgery simulation in a real-time mode and with an easy-to-use feature. Future works includes building up more accurate and realistic eye models. More devices and eye surgical operations will be developed. In order to allow users to realistically operate the simulated tools, appropriate hand-eye co-ordination will be enhanced through continue application of virtual reality technologies.

Acknowledgements

Support of this research development by National Science and Technology Board of Singapore is gratefully acknowledged. The project is partially sponsored by the Nanyang Technological University (SDS 15/2000).

Reference

[1] Mann, I. C., "Culture, Race, Climate and Eye Disease : An Introduction to The Study of Geographical Ophthalmology", Springfield, Ill. : Thomas, 1966.
[2] Lim A. S. M., "Ophthalmology", Singapore Society of Ophthalmology , Singapore, 1982.
[3] Hanna, K. D., Jouve, F. E., Waring III, G. O., and Ciarlet, P. G., Computer simulation of arcuate and radial incisions involving the corneoscleral limbus, Eye, 1989, No. 3, pp. 227-239.
[4] Hanna, K. D., Jouve, F. E., Waring III, G. O., and Ciarlet, P. G., Computer simulation of arcuate and keratotomy for astigmatism, Refractive & Corneal Surgery, Vol. 8, March/April 1989, pp. 152-163.
[5] Sagar, M. A., Bullivant, D., Mallinson, G. D., Hunter, P. J., and Hunter, I. W., A virtual environment and model of the eye for surgical simulation, Proceedings of SIGGRAPH Annual Computer Graphics Conference 1994, Orlando, Florida, July 24-29, pp. 205-211.
[6] Hunter, I. W., Doukogiou, D., Lafontaine, S. R., Charette, P. G., Jones, L. A., Sagar, M. A., Mallinson, G. D., and Hunter, P. J., A teleoperated microsurgical robot and associated virtual environment for eye surgery, Presence, Vol. 2, No. 4, MIT, Fall 1993, pp. 265-280.
[7] Davson, H., "The Eye", Academic Press, Cincinnati, New York, USA, 1984.
[8] Spencer W. H., "Ophthalmic Pathology", W.B. Saunders Co., Philadelphia, 1996.
[9] Duane, T. D. and Jaeger E. A., "Biomedical Foundations of Ophthalmology", Harper & Row , Philadelphia, PA, 1986.
[10] Freberg, T. R. and Lace, J. W., A comparison of the elastic properties of human choroids and sclera, Experiment Eye Research, Vol. 47, 1988, pp. 429-436.
[11] Richard, K. and Parrish II, Bascom Palmer Eye Institute's Atlas of Ophthalmology, Philadelphia, PA, Current Medicine, 1999.
[12] Perkins, E. S., An Atlas of Diseases of the Eye, Churchill Livingstone, Edinburgh, 1987.
[13] van Alphen, G. W. H. M., and Graebel, W. P., Elasticity of tissues involved in accommodation, Vision Research, Vol. 31, No. 7/8, 1991, pp. 1417-1438.
[14] Gallagher R. H., et al, "Finite Elements In Biomechanics", Wiley, New York, USA, 1982.
[15] Pinsky, P. M., and Datye, D. V., A microstructureally-based finite element model of the incised human cornea, Bio-mechanics, Vol. 24, No. 10, 1991, pp. 907-922.

Improved 3D Osteotomy Planning
in Cranio-maxillofacial Surgery

Stefan Zachow[1], Evgeny Gladilin[1], Hans-Florian Zeilhofer[2], and Robert Sader[2]

[1] Konrad-Zuse-Zentrum für Informationstechnik Berlin (ZIB)
http://www.zib.de/visual/projects/cas
[2] Department of Oral & Maxillofacial Surgery, University of Technology Munich

Abstract In this paper we present two clinical cases in maxillofacial surgery, where complex surgical interventions have been pre-operatively planned on 3D models of the patients' heads. Our goal was to provide surgeons with an additional planning criterion, i.e. the prediction of the post-operative facial appearance. In our first study a two step mandibular distraction has been planned, and in the second one a bimaxillary operation with a high Le Fort I osteotomy of the maxilla according to Bell, as well as a sagittal split osteotomy on both sides of the mandible, according to Obwegeser–Dal Pont. Within our study we did focus on the three dimensional soft tissue simulation using finite element methods. For the provision of such a planning aid, concepts for an integrated 3D surgery planning system are proposed that are partially implemented and demonstrated.

Keywords: Computer-Assisted Cranio-Maxillofacial Surgery, Osteotomy, Osteodistraction, Soft Tissue Prediction, Finite-Element Methods

1   Introduction

The planning of *complex* osteotomies and multidirectional osteodistraction in cranio-maxillofacial surgery requires a high degree of experience and expertise for retrieving an optimal rehabilitation. Live size skull facsimiles are very helpful, and currently an established and very valuable 3D planning aid. Soft tissue in its entirety, however, cannot be taken into account for pre-operative planning in clinical practice right now. Techniques for two dimensional profile analysis from lateral cephalograms including video overlays are giving a rough estimation on how the patient might look after an operation, but a full spatial prognosis of the patients' post-operative appearance is the most desired feature of an enhanced 3D planning system for computer assisted cranio-maxillofacial surgery.

First concepts of 3D planning in cranio-maxillofacial surgery including soft tissue prediction can be found in [1]. Active research started approximately 10 years ago [2, 3, 4]. Other research groups have continued working on the simulation of soft tissue deformation for maxillofacial surgery [5, 6]. To our knowledge, a surgical planning system, integrating all *essential* requirements for a sound clinical use does not yet exist. However, the combination of the latest results in this field of work is getting close to the envisioned goal [7, 8, 9, 10, 11].

W. Niessen and M. Viergever (Eds.): MICCAI 2001, LNCS 2208, pp. 473–481, 2001.
© Springer-Verlag Berlin Heidelberg 2001

2   Material and Methods

At our institute (ZIB) a prototype system has been developed that allows the planning of osteotomies including bone rearrangement on 3D patient models, derived from tomographic data. At the moment, our focus is on the prediction of the post-operative appearance by means of 3D soft tissue simulation [11]. The development platform is our 3D modeling and visualization system Amira [12]. A finite element approach on a tetrahedral grid of the *entire* facial soft tissue allows the prediction of the post-operative facial appearance, induced by the relocation of underlying bony structures [13, 14]. To improve our planning environment, a task level analysis lead to the following requirements for computer assisted 3D planning in maxillofacial surgery:

- New concepts for 3D cephalometry under provision of appropriate measuring tools and normative data are required [1, 10, 15].
- Tools for an intuitive definition of osteotomy lines on a 3D model of the skull are necessary (electronic pen, virtual saw).
- Drill, saw and plane operations must be incorporated into the planning. Material reduction has to be taken into account.
- Bony structures of the model have to be split or cut in consideration of vulnerable structures, like nerves and vessels. Individual parts have to be transformed quantifiably.
- 3D implant models (miniplates, screws and distraction devices) must be selectable from a toolbox. These items have to be positioned and fixed on the skull model in consideration of bone thickness and geometry. Planning aids for the assessment of optimal access paths or mount points are required [16].
- The prognosis of the patients' post-operative facial appearance induced by the planned rearrangement of bony structures has to become an additional aspect for pre-operative assessment of the surgical plan.

An improved 3D surgery planning system thus requires: a) techniques for the generation of adequate patient models, b) methods for intuitive and exact measurements and surgical manipulations on basis of such models, and c) the incorporation of fast and reliable soft tissue simulation into the planning.

2.1   Modeling

Prerequisite for the generation of anatomical correct volumetric patient models are tomographic data. An exact reconstruction of diverse tissue regions still requires semi-automatic techniques to avoid misclassification of fine structures or non-distinguishable tissue types. Appropriate tools for an efficient and accurate segmentation are provided with our planning environment as shown in figure 1.

After classification of all relevant structures an automatic reconstruction of a topological correct, *non-manifold* surface model with subvoxel accuracy is generated [17, 18]. This model can be automatically simplified with arbitrary, adaptively chosen resolution to preserve relevant details but allow interactive manipulation on conventional computer

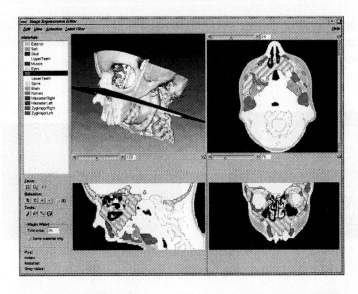

Fig. 1. Segmentation in three projections including 3D model view

systems. From the surface model, describing *all classified* tissue regions, a tetrahedral grid is generated automatically using a 3D advancing front algorithm [19]. In view of a finite-element simulation of soft tissue deformation, the mesh quality has to be optimized in a final step [11]. Surface and grid model are the basis of all subsequent planning (Fig. 2).

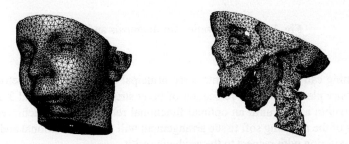

Fig. 2. 3D patient model with local adaptive resolution

2.2 Diagnosis and Planning

Two- and three-dimensional visualization techniques allow a multifarious interpretation of tomographic image data for diagnostic purposes. Currently the following techniques are used with our planning environment, either separately or in combination: a) 2D views of orthogonal or oblique slices, b) lateral, frontal and transversal radiographic views using intensity projections, c) volume rendering and d) surface rendering including texture mapping (Fig. 3).

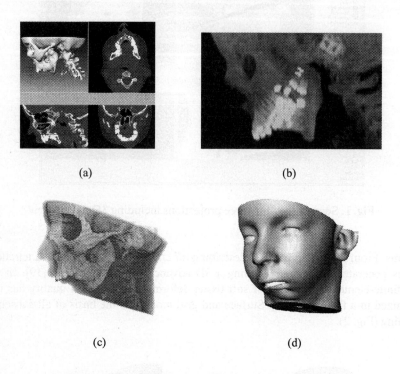

(a)   (b)

(c)   (d)

Fig. 3. 3D visualization for diagnosis and planning

The planning can be subdivided into three principal tasks: 1) cephalometric analysis, 2) osteotomy planning and 3) relocation of bony structures. Step 1 and 3 are usually repeated within a loop until an optimal functional rehabilitation is achieved. The 3D prognosis of the resulting soft tissue arrangement will give an additional and important planning criterion with respect to the aesthetic result.

3D Cephalometry

For the quantitative assessment of maxillofacial dysmorphisms on a 3D model of the skull, orthodontic and orthognatic specifications have to be taken into account. The most important criteria are facial symmetry and dental occlusion. The combination of 2D profile analysis with 3D visualization techniques, under provision of 3D measuring tools for angles and distances [10], as well as methods for the comparison of pathologic and normative data [1, 15] will enhance the planning process tremendously. Therefore, methods of conventional 2D cephalometry have to be adopted to 3D and normative data as well as new paradigms for a 3D cephalometry have to be found.

Currently, 3D measurements of distances and angles are implemented with our proto-type system, as well as the visualization of 3D models in combination with planning planes, like profile projection, occlusional plane, medial plane or the eye-ear plane. Distances can be generally measured either in a projective, euclidean or geodaesic way.

Osteotomy Planning

Osteotomy planning depends on the patient specific situation as well as on standard procedures in maxillofacial surgery. For a 3D planning, arbitrarily shaped cut paths have to be defined, whereas vulnerable structures have to be preserved. Two different approaches are conceivable: 1) Osteotomy lines can be directly drawn onto the surface model of the skull using a 'virtual pen' or 2) a 3D cut path can be defined using a 'vir-tual saw'. Both methods require 3D input devices, two-handed interaction techniques, collision detection and force feedback for an intuitive use. In both cases the result will be either a 3D *cut plane* or a *cut volume* (according to the thickness of the saw blade) that separates parts and eventually removes material from the model. Performing cuts on the raw image data is a simple operation, but always requires the generation of a new 3D model for further planning. Cutting the surface model or the tetrahedral grid is much more difficult to implement, but speeds up the planning process, so that different strategies can be taken into account. Having such a *cut plane* or *cut volume*, we are also able to consider vulnerable structures, that are not already segmented within the modeling stage, by placing it into the 3D image data or mapping these data onto the respective surface.

Bone Rearrangement

The relocation of bony structures can either occur interactively under visual control (pick and transform), or via specification of numeric values (distances and angles) de-rived from the cephalometric analysis. Both methods are implemented with our plan-ning system. An automatic correction of malformations, e.g. via statistical analysis, requires 3D craniofacial reference data that are currently not available. As result of the bone rearrangement we obtain displacement vectors for all nodes of our 3D model. These displacements serve as boundary conditions for our finite-element analysis, where the resulting 3D soft tissue deformation will be approximated.

2.3   Soft Tissue Prediction

The prediction of the *entire* spatial arrangement of the facial soft tissue will give the planning physician an additional, very important criterion for the assessment of the aesthetic impact of bone relocation. One can differentiate between two modes of simu-lation: 1) Deformation at interactive speeds with simple geometric or spring-mass mod-els, and 2) consequent physics based deformation, using an elastomechanical model of biological tissues, a volumetric discretization of soft tissue and a finite-element ap-proximation. The latter has been successfully integrated into our planning system, and has been discussed in detail within [11, 13, 14]. For a residual error norm, i.e. the ap-proximation accuracy, of 10^{-6}, simulation speed is between 30 and 180 s for 100.000 – 500.000 tetrahedra, even on a conventional 500 MHz Pentium PC with more than 256 MB RAM to avoid memory swap.

3   Results

With our planning environment it is possible to generate adequate 3D patient models for surgery planning and soft tissue simulation. Graphical planning aids are integrated for simple cephalometric analysis. Osteotomy lines can be specified, and separated bone parts can be relocated according to the surgeon's guidelines. The bone rearrangement is the basis for the prediction of the patient's post-operative appearance as described above. For two clinical cases a complete planning including soft tissue simulation has been performed at our institute in a tele-collaboration with surgeons in Munich.

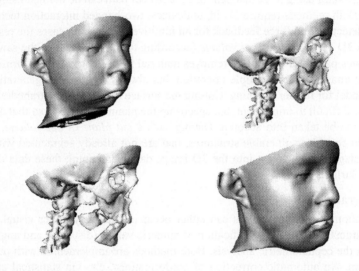

Fig. 4. 3D Planning of a bidirectional osteodistraction of the mandible: (top) pre-operative situation, (bottom left) end position of the distractors, (bottom right) predicted facial appearance.

In the first case (Fig. 4) a bidirectional osteodistraction has been planned for a patient with a severe congenital mandibular hypoplasia. The *rami mandibulae* were separated horizontally and the *corpus mandibulae* has been separated on both sides with vertical cuts. The position of the simulated cuts do not exactly correspond to the surgical rules, and the mandibular nerve has not been addressed because in this case we were only interested in the post-operative appearance of the patient's face after reaching the end position of the distraction devices.

The initial surgical guidelines for the distraction vectors were: 30 mm in vertical direction (because of the limitation of available distraction devices), and 22 mm in horizontal direction. These displacements have been applied to the separated parts of the mandible, visually assessed and modified with respect to the soft tissue implication. The maximum displacements (vector norm) for a visually pleasing result have been 34 mm in vertical and 24 mm in horizontal direction (Table 1). The reference coordinate system is centered in the patient's head and the axes are: x) left-right, y) posterior-anterior and z) cranial-caudal.

Table 1. Distraction vectors and angles of all relocated bone parts

bone part		translation in mm (LR/PA/CC)			rotational axis (LR/PA/CC)			angle in °
ramus	right	1,50	-3,13	4,88	-0,93	0,02	0,34	2,24
	left	0,02	-0,52	1,34	-1,00	-0,07	0,00	0,48
corpus	right	2,48	-8,19	16,99	-1,00	0,02	0,07	14,47
	left	3,77	-2,65	23,92	-1,00	-0,08	-0,01	21,04
	front	-6,22	1,97	33,84	-1,00	0,06	-0,14	29,99

In the second case (Fig. 5) for a patient with maxillary retrognathism and mandibular prognathism a bimaxillary operation has been planned, i.e. a high Le Fort I osteotomy of the maxilla, according to Bell and a sagittal split osteotomy on both sides of the mandible, according to Obwegeser-Dal Pont. The surgical guidelines were obeyed and the mandibular as well as the infraorbital nerve have been taken into account. The surgical guidelines for the bone transposition were: Advancement of the maxilla by 10 mm and back relocation of the mandible by 12 mm. The visual assessment lead to a correction of the advancement to only 7 mm, due to an over accentuated cheek and nose. However, the simulated results had no influence on the operation itself, but will be used for retrospective validation.

4   Conclusion

The quantification of the exact bone displacements as well as the validation of the simulated soft tissue deformation is still open. For the first case a second operation is scheduled in summer, where the horizontal distraction will be prepared. The availability of post-operative CT data will enable us to retrospectively simulate the same patient again, using the initial model but applying the real distraction values. Thus we are able to compare our simulation with the post-operative results qualitatively *and* quantitatively. A quantification of the difference between simulated and real soft tissue arrangement allows an inverse determination of the elasticity parameters, lying in a wide range for different tissue types (Poisson's Ratio $\nu \in [0.3, 0.49]$ and Young's modulus $E \in [2, 150]$ kPa) [20].

We believe that 3D soft tissue prediction on basis of a volumetric discretization of a patient's head and FE methods has the potential for being an important criterion in surgery planning. A simulation time of a few minutes is neglectable in relation to the time needed for pre-operative planning. The most time consuming task is the segmentation, currently taking several hours. However, the segmentation result can be directly exported in STL format for the production of a stereolithographic model, thus conven-

480   S. Zachow et al.

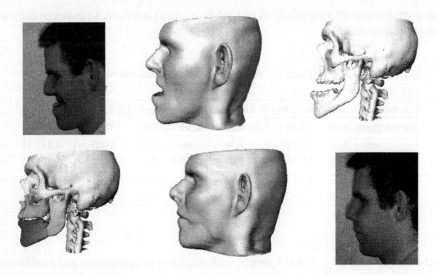

Fig. 5. 3D Planning of a bimaxillary osteotomy: (top) pre-operative situation, (bottom left) relocation of maxilla and mandible, (center) predicted facial appearance, (right) postoperative result

tional planning is still supported to assess different strategies in a non-destructive way, before applying the optimal one to a life size replica of the patient's skull.

References

[1] Cutting, C. ; Bookstein, F.L. ; Grayson, B. et'al.: *Three-Dimensional Computer-Assisted Design of Craniofacial Surgical Procedures: Optimization and Interaction with Cephalometric and CT-Based Models.* J. Plast. Reconstr. Surg. 77(6), pp. 877–885 (1986)

[2] Yasuda, T. ; Hashimoto, Y. ; Yokoi, S. and Toriwaki, J.-J.: *Computer System for Craniofacial Surgical Planning Based on CT Images.* IEEE Trans. Med. Imag. 9(3), pp. 270–280 (1990)

[3] Pieper, S.: CAPS: *Computer Aided Plastic Surgery.* Ph.D. thesis, MIT (1991)

[4] Altobelli, D.E. ; Kikinis, R. ; Mulliken, J.B. et al.: *Computer-assisted three-dimensional planning in craniofacial surgery.* J. Plast. Reconstr. Surg., Sep 92(4), pp. 576–587 (1993)

[5] Girod, S. ; Keeve, E. ; Girod, B.: *Advances in interactive craniofacial surgery planning by 3D simulation and visualization.* Int. J. Oral Maxillof. Surg. 24(1), pp 120–125 (1995)

[6] Koch, R.M. ; Gross, M.H. ; Carls, F.R. et al.: *Simulating Facial Surgery Using Finite Element Models.* Computer Graphics, Proc. ACM Siggraph, pp. 421–428 (1996)

[7] Teschner, M.: *Direct Computation of Soft-Tissue Deformation in Craniofacial Surgery Simulation.* Ph.D. thesis, Friedrich-Alexander-Universität Erlangen-Nürnberg (2000)

[8] Schutyser, F. ; Van Cleynenbreugel, J. ; Ferrant, M. et al.: *Image-Based 3D Planning of Maxillofacial Distraction Procedures Including Soft Tissue Implications.* In: Delp, S.L. et al. (eds.) Medical Image Computing and Computer-Assisted Intervention (MICCAI), pp. 999–1007 (2000)

[9] Everett, P.C. ; Seldin, E.B. ; Troulis, M. et al.: *A 3-D System for Planning and Simulating Minimally-Invasive Distraction Osteogenesis of the Facial Skeleton*. In: Delp, S.L. et al. (eds.) Medical Image Computing and Computer-Assisted Intervention (MICCAI), pp. 1029–1039 (2000)

[10] Bettega, G. ; Payan, Y. ; Mollard, B. et al.: *A simulator for maxillofacial surgery integrating 3D cephalometry and orthodontia*. J. Comp. Aid. Surg. 5(3), pp. 156–165 (2000)

[11] Zachow, S. ; Gladilin, E. ; Hege, H.-C. and Deuflhard, P.: *Finite-Element Simulation of Soft Tissue Deformation*. In: Lemke, H.U. et al. (eds.): Computer Assisted Radiology and Surgery, pp. 23–28 (2000)

[12] Stalling, D. ; Hege, H.C. ; Zöckler, M. et. al.: *Amira - An Advanced 3D Visualization and Modeling System*, URL: http://amira.zib.de

[13] Gladilin, E. ; Zachow, S. ; Deuflhard, P. and Hege, H.-C.: *Validation of a Linear Elastic Model for Soft Tissue Prediction in Craniofacial Surgery*. SPIE Medical Imaging, San Diego, (2001)

[14] Gladilin, E. ; Zachow, S. ; Deuflhard, P. and Hege, H.-C.: *A Biomechanical Model for Soft Tissue Simulation in Craniofacial Surgery*. Medical Imaging and Augmented Reality, Hong Kong, China (2001)

[15] Brief, J. ; Hassfeld, S. ; Däuber, S. et al.: *3D Norm Data: The first step towards Semiautomatic Virtual Craniofacial Surgery*. J. Comp. Aid. Surg. 5(3), pp. 353–358 (2000)

[16] Zachow, S. ; Lueth, T.C. ; Stalling, D. et al.: *Optimized Arrangement of Osseointegrated Implants: A Surgical Planning System for the Fixation of Facial Prostheses*. In: Lemke, H.U. et al. (eds.): Computer Assisted Radiology and Surgery (CARS), pp. 942–946 (1999)

[17] Hege, H.C. ; Seebaß, M. ; Stalling, D. ; Zöckler, M.: *A Generalized Marching Cubes Algorithm Based On Non-Binary Classifications*. ZIB Preprint SC-97-05 (1997)

[18] Stalling, D. ; Zöckler, M. ; Hege, H.-C.: *Interactive Segmentation of 3D Medical Images with Subvoxel Accuracy*. In: Lemke, H.U. et al. (eds.), Computer Assisted Radiology and Surgery, pp. 137–142 (1989)

[19] Jin, H. and Tanner, R.I.: *Generation of Unstructured Tetrahedral Meshes by Advancing Front Technique*. Int. J. Numer. Methods Eng. 36, pp. 1805–1823 (1993)

[20] Duck, F.A.: *Physical Properties of Tissue – A Comprehensive Reference Book*. Academic Press, Chap. 5, pp. 151 ff. (1990)

Combining Edge, Region, and Shape Information to Segment the Left Ventricle in Cardiac MR Images

Marie-Pierre Jolly

Imaging and Visualization Department
Siemens Corporate Research
Princeton, NJ
jolly@scr.siemens.com

Abstract. This paper describes a segmentation technique to automatically extract the myocardium in 4D cardiac MR images for quantitative cardiac analysis and the diagnosis of patients. An approximate outline of the left ventricle is obtained either from automatic localization based on the maximum discrimination method or from copying a template shape during propagation. The histogram of the image is analyzed and divided into peaks using the EM algorithm to produce a region-based segmentation. This result and the image gradient are combined to obtain candidate boundaries for the left ventricle by deforming the contour using a graph search active contour approach. The final boundary is chosen using a minimum cut graph algorithm, spline fitting, or point pattern matching to maintain the shape of the template. We have experimented with the proposed method on a large number of patients and present some quantitative and qualitative results.

1. Introduction

Cardiovascular disease is the leading cause of death in the United States. Mortality has been declining over the years as lifestyle has changed, but the decline is also due to the development of new technologies to diagnose disease. One of these techniques is magnetic resonance imaging (MRI) which provides time-varying three-dimensional imagery of the heart. To help in the diagnosis of disease, the physicians are interested in identifying the heart chambers, the endocardium and epicardium, and measuring the change in ventricular blood volume (ejection fraction) and wall thickening properties over the cardiac cycle. The left ventricle is of particular interest since it pumps oxygenated blood out to distant tissue in the entire body.

There has been a large amount of research on the analysis of medical images [1] and the segmentation problem has been particularly challenging. In the early nineties, researchers have realized that tracking the cardiac wall motion in MR images was important to characterize meaningful functional changes. The system proposed by Fleagle *et al.* [2] was able to delineate the borders of the myocardium using a minimum cost path graph search algorithm after the user indicated the center of the left ventricular cavity and the area of interest with a few mouse clicks. Geiger *et al.* [3] used a dynamic programming approach to refine the contours specified by the user. Goshtasby and Turner [4] proposed a two step algorithm combining intensity

W. Niessen and M. Viergever (Eds.): MICCAI 2001, LNCS 2208, pp. 482–490, 2001.

thresholding to recover the bright blood and local gradient to outline the strong edges using elastic curves. Weng *et al.* [5] thresholded the image based on parameters estimated during a learning phase to get a good approximate of the segmentation. Although we have not directly used any of these techniques, all of these papers have greatly influenced our work.

Argus is a cardiac analysis package developed by Siemens which offers a complete system of drawing tools and automatic segmentation algorithms to allow the physician to outline the myocardium in each image in the patient data set, compute volumes, ejection fraction, and perform a thickening analysis. In this paper, we present the segmentation module which combines edge, region, and shape information in a deformable template approach.

2. Approximate Localization of the Left Ventricle

As for any deformable template based algorithm, our method requires an approximate delineation of the object of interest to be provided. We have developed an algorithm to automatically hypothesize two concentric circles at the location of the left ventricle in a new image. We use a method similar to the maximum discrimination method proposed by Colmenarez and Huang [6]. However, due to the relative symmetry of the left ventricle and computational constraints, we have only used the gray values of the pixels along the main four cross sections through the ventricle instead of the entire region to derive the feature set. More details are given in [7] and [8].

The system models patterns as a Markov process. In the learning phase, positive and negative examples are presented and the system finds the ordering of the Markov process that maximizes the separation (minimizes the Kullbach distance) between the two classes in the training set. In the detection stage, the test image is scanned and each location is assigned to the closest class based on the log-likelihood ratio.

Neighboring positions classified as left ventricle are partitioned into clusters. We define 8 salient points in the gray level profiles as the intersection of the 4 cross sections with the ventricle's medial axis. Average profiles were built from training example profiles which were aligned using the curve registration technique proposed by Ramsay and Li [9]. The cross sections of each of the cluster candidates are warped onto their corresponding average profiles. The location of the salient points in the image are then accumulated using a Hough transform array to vote for the most likely center position and radius for the myocardium centerline.

Typically, the user segments one image, usually the slice closest to the valves at end-diastole (ED base) and propagates the segmented contours to all the slices in the ED phase (ED propagation). Then, all the ED contours are propagated to the end-systole (ES) phase (ES propagation) to compute the ejection fraction. For a more detailed analysis, the user can also propagate all the ED contours to all the images in all the phases using temporal propagation.

For ED propagation, we use the automatic localization algorithm just described, but since the ventricle size is approximately known from the template image, we limit the scale search to 0.85 to 1.15 times the size of the template. We also limit the search space for the location of the ventricle to 30 pixels around the location of the template, instead of the entire image. For ES propagation, we know that the location of the left ventricle has not changed, so we simply scale the template contours. The endocardium is scaled by 0.6 and the epicardium by 0.9. In the case of temporal propagation, both the location and scale of the contours barely change. So, we simply copy the contours from one image to the next.

These contours, obtained either through automatic localization or propagation (see Fig. 1) are the starting point to our local deformation process.

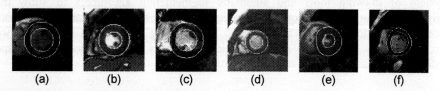

(a)   (b)   (c)   (d)   (e)   (f)

Fig. 1. Examples of approximate contours: (a)-(c) From automatic localization; (d) From ED propagation; (e) From ES propagation; (f) From temporal propagation.

3. Local Deformations

3.1 Region Segmentation

In MR imaging, the intensity of a pixel depends on the properties of the tissue being imaged. In our MR sequences of the left ventricle, the blood is very bright, the muscles are somewhat dark, but not as dark as the air-filled lungs. This fact can be verified by looking at the histogram of a region around the myocardium (see Fig. 2). We use the Expectation-Maximization (EM) algorithm [10] to fit a mixture of 3 Gaussians to the histogram. We then create a myocardium response image, showing the probability that a pixel belongs to the middle Gaussian which corresponds to the myocardium. It can be seen from Fig. 2(c) that the left ventricle myocardium is nicely highlighted, but neighboring organs are highlighted too.

3.2 Active Contours

To complement the results of region segmentation, we use an active contour formulation similar to Geiger *et al.*'s [3] dynamic programming approach or Mortensen and Barrett's [11] Dijkstra's approach. The advantage of these graph theoretic methods over the traditional gradient descent approach proposed by Kass *et al.* [12] is that they are able to recover the global optimum of the energy function and are therefore insensitive to the initial contour position.

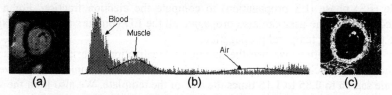

(a)   (b)   (c)

Fig. 2. Region segmentation and myocardium response image.

Geiger *et al.* [3] define the energy of a contour $(p_1,...p_n)$ as:

$$E(p_1,...,p_n) = \sum_{i=1}^{n} \frac{1}{\|\nabla I(p_i)\| + \varepsilon} + \alpha \sum_{i=2}^{n} |\vec{\nabla} I(p_i) - \vec{\nabla} I(p_{i-1})| \tag{1}$$

where $\|\nabla I(p)\|$ is the magnitude and $\vec{\nabla} I(p)$ the direction of the image gradient at pixel p. This is equivalent to finding the shortest path in a graph where nodes correspond to pixels and the cost of a link between two neighboring pixels is defined as:

$$e(p_1, p_2) = \frac{1}{\|\nabla I(p_2)\| + \varepsilon} + \alpha |\vec{\nabla} I(p_2) - \vec{\nabla} I(p_1)| \tag{2}$$

Given an approximate contour in an image as in Fig. 3(a), we place a symmetrical search space around it and define a line of source nodes (all connected to a "pseudo" source node) and sink nodes as in Fig. 3(b). Dijkstra's algorithm then finds the shortest path between the pseudo source node and one of the sink nodes as seen in Fig. 3(c). Unfortunately, there is no guarantee that this contour will be closed. So we define a new single source point in the middle of the recovered contour as in Fig. 3(d) and do a second pass of Dijkstra's algorithm to produce the final closed contour as in Fig. 3(e).

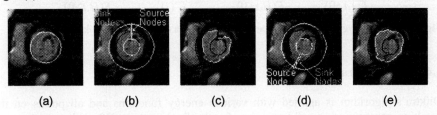

(a)   (b)   (c)   (d)   (e)

Fig. 3. Two passes of Dijkstra's algorithm are used to recover a closed contour.

3.3 Energy Function

To combine the information provided by both the image and the myocardium response image, we have chosen to run Dijkstra's algorithm with two different energy functions. Each run gives different candidate points for the contours, along with a confidence value based on the contribution of that point to the total energy function. One energy function combines gradient magnitude and direction using the cross product of the gradient direction and the contour direction. In our case, the contour is built clockwise by the Dijkstra process and the image gradient points from bright to dark. To separate a bright region inside from a dark region outside (resp. a dark region inside from a bright region outside), the z component of the cross product between the image gradient and the contour direction should be positive (resp. negative). Thus, we set the energy to a large number otherwise. The cost of a link between two pixels is:

$$e(I, z > 0, p_1, p_2) = \begin{cases} \dfrac{1}{\|\nabla I(p_2)\|^2 + \varepsilon} & \text{if } z = \begin{aligned} &(x_2 - x_1)\sin(\vec{\nabla} I(p_2)) - \\ &(y_2 - y_1)\cos(\vec{\nabla} I(p_2)) > 0 \end{aligned} \\ 1/\varepsilon & \text{otherwise} \end{cases} \tag{3}$$

486   M.-P. Jolly

where ε is a small constant (0.001) to bound the energy function. We use $E(I,z>0)$ and $E(H,z<0)$ for the endocardium, where I is the input image and H is the myocardium response image. For the epicardium, we use $E(H,z>0)$. Since the gradient direction in I outside the myocardium flips between the bright right ventricle and the dark lungs, we also use the energy function based on gradient magnitude only $E'(I)$ defined by the cost between two pixels:

$$e'(I, p_1, p_2) = \frac{1}{\left\|\nabla I(p_2)\right\|^2 + \varepsilon} \tag{4}$$

In Fig. 4 it can be seen that different energy functions highlight different features of the myocardium. In particular, $E(I,z>0)$ for the endocardium outlines the papillary muscles while $E(H,z<0)$ does not. Also, $E'(I)$ for the epicardium outlines the fat while $E(H,z>0)$ outlines the true border of the myocardium.

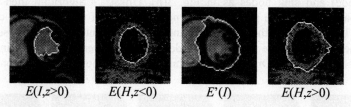

$E(I,z>0)$ $E(H,z<0)$ $E'(I)$ $E(H,z>0)$

Fig. 4. Various energy functions can be used to recover a contour using Dijkstra's algorithm.

3.4 Shape Constraint

Dijktra's algorithm is applied with various energy functions and all points on the resulting contours are candidate points for the final contour. When the contours are propagated from one image to the next, either spatially or temporally, the shape of the contours does not change drastically. Based on this assumption, we can decide which parts of which contours are correct.

We use the shape alignment method proposed by Duta et al. [13] to establish the correspondence between a subset A' of the template points $A=\{A_j\}_{j=1,...,a}$ and a subset B' of the candidate test points $B=\{B_k\}_{k=1,...,b}$. Best results are obtained when endocardium and epicardium are considered together as one shape. Given a pair of "corresponding" points in A and B, we hypothesize a rigid similarity transform to align them. We then determine a one-to-one match matrix M by assigning every point in B to its closest neighbor in A (if the distance is less than a threshold). This allows us to compute the distance:

$$f(M) = \frac{1}{n^2} \sum_{j=1}^{n} w_j \left[(x_{A_j} - ax_{B_j} + cy_{B_j} - b)^2 + (y_{A_j} - ay_{B_j} - cx_{B_j} - d)^2 \right] + \frac{2}{n} \tag{5}$$

where n is the number of correspondences. We set the weight w_j to be the confidence value of test point B_j which is the inverse of the contribution of this point to the entire contour energy. The goal is to find the coefficients (a,b,c,d) of the similarity transform which minimize $f(M)$. Of course, it is not possible to evaluate all possible quadruplets of points, so we choose the 10% of the points with largest confidence in the test set and pair them with points from the same contour in the template set.

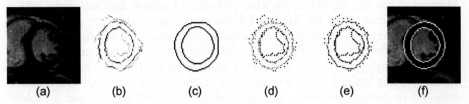

(a)   (b)   (c)   (d)   (e)   (f)

Fig. 5. Applying shape constraints to recover the myocardium contours.

Fig. 5(a) shows the input image and Fig. 5(b) the 4 recovered contours where darker points show higher confidence. Fig. 5(c) shows the template shape being propagated. Fig. 5(d) shows the established correspondences for the best similarity transform. The shape constraints allow the system to choose the outside candidate points for the endocardium (rather than the inside points that outline the papillary muscles) and the inside candidate points for the epicardium (rather than the outside points that outline the fat). Once the correspondences are established, the template shape is warped by moving the template points to their corresponding test points as in Fig. 5(e). Finally, the contours are smoothed using the method proposed by Xu *et al.* [14] that minimizes shrinkage. The final segmentation result is shown in Fig. 5(f).

3.5 No Shape Constraint

When an image needs to be segmented on its own (not in the context of propagation), there is no shape information available to the system. In this case, we use the techniques that were used in the previous version of our segmentation algorithm presented in [8]. The confidence values of every point on candidate contours are modified by:

$$C_{endo}(p) = C(p) \left(\frac{d(p, \Omega)}{\max_p d(p, \Omega)} \right)^3 \qquad C_{epi}(p) = C(p) \left(\frac{d(p, endo)}{\max_p d(p, endo)} \right)^3 \qquad (6)$$

so that endocardium points far away from the centroid Ω are emphasized and epicardium points closer to endocardium points are also emphasized.

Then, for the endocardium, we want to find the cycle with maximum confidence. We define a graph where each node corresponds to connected component regions between confidence pixels. The weight of an edge between two nodes is inversely proportional to the confidence of pixels on the common boundary. Then, we seek the minimum cut between the center node and the outside node. For the epicardium, we mostly want the contour to be smooth since there is no clear edge between the myocardium and the liver and the right ventricle myocardium appears to merge into the left ventricle myocardium. So, we simply fit a spline through the points of the 2 candidate contours. More details on these techniques are given in [8].

4. Results

In order to test our algorithm, we have collected 29 patient data sets along with a manual segmentation of the ED and ES phases by radiologists, for a total of 458 segmented images. The images were acquired on Siemens MAGNETOM systems using two different pulse sequences. FLASH pulse sequences were traditionally used for MR cineangiography. Siemens recently pionneered the TrueFISP pulse sequences for cardiac cine imaging which present higher contrast-to-noise ratio without affecting temporal or spatial resolution. We collected 22 TrueFISP patients and 7 FLASH patients. Our database presents a great variety of heart shapes, image contrast, and edge crispness. The difficulty with FLASH images (Fig. 9(a) or (c)) is that the edges are very blurred. The challenge with TrueFISP images is that the papillary muscles are so well defined that it can be difficult to avoid outlining them. Most of the time, the user does not want to outline them and we will see that the shape constraint greatly helps in this task.

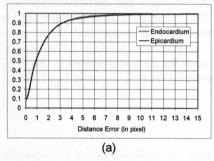 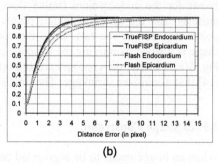

(a)   (b)

Fig. 6. Cumulative distribution of error distances between the true contours and the segmented contours, over all points, over all images, and over all patients.

We ran our algorithm to automatically segment the ED and ES phases of all the datasets. To compare the automatic contours A with the true contours B, we compute the distances $d(a,B)=\min_{b \in B} \|a-b\|$ for all points a in the automatic contour. Similarly, we compute $d(b,A)$ for all points b in the true contour. Fig. 6(a) shows the cumulative distribution of these error distances over all ED and ES images of all 29 datasets. It can be seen that, on the average, the error is less than 1 pixel and an error of 5 pixels or more is made less than 5% of the time. Fig. 6(b) shows the same curves separately for TrueFISP and FLASH data. It can be seen that the system performs better for TrueFISP data which is the standard acquisition mode on the new Siemens systems. The accurate localization of the epicardium on FLASH images is particularly difficult due to the weak edges. Nevertheless, in 90% of the cases, the error was less than 5 pixels.

Fig. 7 shows the segmentation of the whole heart, for all the slices in the ED phase. In a similar manner, Fig. 8 shows a temporal propagation for all the phases of a particular slice. Fig. 9(a) shows an example of ES propagation. It can be seen that the papillary muscles are kept inside the blood pool in the ES phase so that the shape of the endocardium is close to the shape defined in the ED phase. Fig. 9(b) shows another segmentation example. Fig. 9(c) shows a diseased heart where the cross section of the left ventricle appears elongated. Fig. 9(d) shows an example at the valve plane where the endocardium and the epicardium coincide. Fig. 9(e) shows an example where the myocardium is very thick and the papillary muscles very large. All these examples demonstrate the strength of our algorithm in handling different cases.

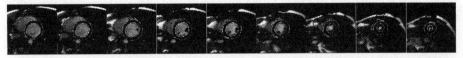

Fig. 7. Automatic localization followed by ED propagation for all the slices of the ED phase.

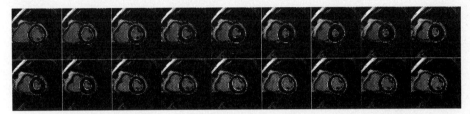

Fig. 8. Temporal propagation for all the phases of a particular slice.

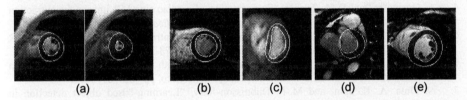

(a)   (b)   (c)   (d)   (e)

Fig. 9. ES propagation and other segmentation examples.

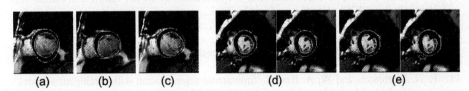

(a)   (b)   (c)   (d)   (e)

Fig. 10. Shape information is propagated to achieve the desired segmentation (see text).

Figure 10 illustrates the importance of the shape constraints. In Fig. 10(a) the left ventricle was automatically localized and local deformations were applied. Unfortunately, this patient has suffered an infarct in the past and the lower right side of the myocardium is very thin. In addition, there is no clear edge in the image between the myocardium and the liver. Thus, the resulting segmentation is wrong. Fig. 10(b) shows the previous slice in the volume where we have defined the desired contour manually. When the contour is propagated to the next slice, the shape constraint is enforced and the segmentation result is correct (as seen in Fig. 10(c)). Fig. 10(d) and (e) show temporal propagation. In Fig. 10(d) we chose to not outline the papillary muscle, whereas in Fig. 10(e), we decided to include the papillary muscle with the myocardium. In both cases, the contour propagated to the next image kept the shape outlined by the user.

5. Conclusions

We have presented an algorithm to segment the left ventricle in cardiac MR images. The algorithm combines edge information, region information obtained from an EM fitting of a mixture of Gaussians to the histogram, and shape information through a point pattern matching strategy. We have obtained excellent results with this technique and integrated this algorithm with the next version of the cardiac analysis package Argus commercialized by Siemens.

References

1. J. S. Duncan and N. Ayache, "Medical image analysis: Progress over two decades and the challenges ahead", *IEEE Trans. PAMI*, 22(1):85-106, 2000.
2. S. R. Fleagle, D. R. Thedens, J. C. Ehrhardt, T. D. Scholz, and D. J. Skorton, "Automated identification of left ventricular borders from spin-echo resonance images", *Investigative Radiology*, 26:295-303, 1991.
3. D. Geiger, A. Gupta, L. A. Costa, and J. Vlontzos, "Dynamic programming for detecting, tracking, and matching deformable contours", *IEEE Trans. PAMI*, 17(3):294-302, 1995.
4. A. Goshtasby and D. A. Turner, "Segmentation of cardiac cine MR images for extraction of right and left ventricular chambers", *IEEE Trans. Medical Imaging*, 14(1):56-64, 1995.
5. J. Weng, A. Singh, and M. Y. Chiu, "Learning-based ventricle detection from cardiac MR and CT images", *IEEE Trans. Medical Imaging*, 16(4):378-391, 1997.
6. A. Colmenarez and T. Huang, "Face detection with information-based maximum discrimination", *Proc. IEEE CVPR*, San Juan, Puerto Rico, pp 782-787, 1997.
7. N. Duta, A. K. Jain, and M.-P. Dubuisson-Jolly, "Learning-based object detection in cardiac MR images", *Proc. ICCV*, Corfu, Greece, pp 1210-1216, 1999.
8. M.-P. Jolly, N. Duta, and G. Funka-Lea, "Segmentation of the left ventricle in cardiac MR images", *Proc. ICCV*, Vancouver, Canada, 2001.
9. J. O. Ramsay and X. Li, "Curve registration", *Journal of the Royal Statistical Society Series B*, 60:351-363, 1998.
10. R. A. Redner and H. F. Walker, "Mixture densities, maximum likelihood and the EM algorithm", *SIAM Review*, 26:195-239, 1984.
11. E. N. Mortensen and W. A. Barrett, "Interactive segmentation with intelligent scissors", *Graphical Models and Image Processing*, 60:349-384, 1998.
12. M. Kass, A. Witkin, and D. Terzopoulos, "Snakes: Active contour models", *International Journal of Computer Vision*, 2:321-331, 1988.
13. N. Duta, A. K. Jain, M.-P. Dubuisson-Jolly, "Learning 2D shape models", *Proc. IEEE CVPR*, Fort Collins, CO, vol. II, pp. 8-14, 1999.
14. C. Xu, A. Yezzi Jr., J. L. Prince, "On the relationship between parametric and geometric active contours", *Asilomar Conf. Signals, Systems, and Computers*, pp. 483-489, 2000.

Vessel Segmentation for Visualization of MRA with Blood Pool Contrast Agent

S. Young, V. Pekar, and J. Weese

[1] Philips Research Laboratories, Technical Systems Hamburg
Röntgenstrasse 24–26, D-22335 Hamburg, Germany
[2] Medical University of Lübeck, Institute for Signal Processing,
Seelandstrasse 1a, D-23569, Germany
{stewart.young, vladimir.pekar, juergen.weese}@philips.com

Abstract. We present a method for the segmentation of vessel structures in 3D magnetic resonance angiography (MRA) images with blood-
pool contrast agent, allowing artery–vein separation for occluding vessel
removal from MIP visualization. The method first uses a front propagation algorithm to select a path along the vessel of interest. Two controlling speed functions are considered, a multi–scale vessel filter, and an
approach based on a cylinder shape model. The cylinder based method
uses orientation information which is propagated with the front and iteratively updated as the surface expands. Once a vessel of interest is
selected, orientation and radius parameters are used to construct a deformable model of the vessel, which is then adapted to the image borders
to refine the segmentation of the selected vessel. The results of a comparison with manual segmentations are presented. The extracted centre
lines are compared with those from the manual segmentations, showing a mean deviation of 2.55mm for the multi–scale filter, and 1.06mm
for the cylinder model, compared to voxel dimensions of 0.93mm. The
mean deviation of the final segmentation from the surface of the manual
segmentation was 0.59mm.

1 Introduction

MRA images provide important information for the diagnosis of vascular diseases
such as arterial stenosis and aneurysm. The visualization of the vessel pathways
is crucial to allow quick and reliable assessment of any potential problems. The
most common visualization method is to construct a maximum intensity projection (MIP). The recent development of MR blood-pool contrast agents which
have extended intravascular halflife allows the acquisition of high resolution,
high contrast 3D images of the vascular system. The longer scan times necessary
to achieve higher resolution require imaging during the steady state of contrast
agent diffusion. Therefore both arteries and veins are enhanced, and diagnostically important information (typically the arteries, where stenosis occurs) may
be fully or partially occluded in the MIP.

Our work is aimed at semi-automated artery-vein separation. User selected
seed and end points identify a vessel of interest, which is then automatically

W. Niessen and M. Viergever (Eds.): MICCAI 2001, LNCS 2208, pp. 491–498, 2001.
© Springer-Verlag Berlin Heidelberg 2001

segmented. After segmentation, the vessel may be suppressed during generation of the MIP, revealing any previously occluded structure [10]. There are two important issues to be considered when selecting a suitable approach. Firstly, the vessel boundary should be accurately identified, since even small segmentation errors can cause residual artifacts in the MIP. Secondly, venous and arterial pathways are often close together, so methods should be able to discriminate between very closely separated structures, in order that only anatomically connected pathways are selected. A further consideration is that the segmentation method should be able to detect vessels across a range of scales, since the width of vessels can vary significantly.

Several vessel detection criteria have been proposed in the literature. A straightforward approach is to rely on image contrast, applying an intensity threshold followed by morphology analysis [8]. However, non-uniform distribution of contrast agent can lead to significant intensity variations along vessels, defeating such methods. A widespread approach for vessel enhancement is to use multi-scale orientation selective filters, based on eigen–analysis of the Hessian matrix [3,6]. Though it is asserted that these filters give their maximum response on the vessel axis, results presented here indicate this is not always observed. Krissian *et al.* [4] detect vessels with a boundary model based on scale and direction parameters from such a filter. An alternative boundary detection method was proposed in [12], using planar reconstructions based on orientation estimates obtained from a centre line tracking module.

As in [1], our method extracts the vessel path using a front propagation approach. However, we propose a shape–model based response as a speed function, as opposed to a purely intensity–based response which is not necessarily maximal on the vessel axis. After centre line extraction the path is combined with radius information, assuming a circular cross–section, to build a deformable model, which is then adapted to refine the segmentation. In contrast to Bulpitt and Berry [2], where the mesh structure adapts from an initial ellipsoid, our model is initialized relatively close to the object of interest, and has a fixed structure.

The next section describes the two alternative vesselness responses considered. Section 3 describes the front propagation, and the refinement method is discussed in section 4. Validation results are presented in section 5, and conclusions are drawn in section 6.

2   Vessel Response

Vessels are characterized by their axial symmetry - they are extended in one direction, along their axis, but not in the directions orthogonal to this. This morphological property may be exploited to distinguish vessel voxels from other image structures.

2.1   Multi–scale Vessel Filter

This approach is based on analysis of local grey–value curvature, where a vessel is characterized by low derivatives along its axis, and high derivatives in orthogonal directions. The Hessian matrix captures information on local second–order derivatives, and its eigenvalues reflect the degree of curvature. The eigenvector associated with the smallest eigenvalue indicates the direction of minimum curvature at a point. Therefore, assuming that the eigenvalues are ordered such that $|\lambda_1| \leq |\lambda_2| \leq |\lambda_3|$, and that objects of interest are brighter than the background, the response of a vesselness filter may be defined as [3]:

$$F(\mathbf{p}) = \begin{cases} 0, & \text{if } \lambda_2(\mathbf{p}) > 0 \text{ or } \lambda_3(\mathbf{p}) > 0; \\ (1 - \exp\{\frac{-|\lambda_2|^2}{2|\lambda_3|^2\alpha^2}\}) \exp\{\frac{-|\lambda_1|^2}{2|\lambda_2\lambda_3|\beta^2}\}(1 - \exp\{-\frac{\sum_{j=1}^3 \lambda_j^2}{2c^2}\}), & \text{else} \end{cases} \quad (1)$$

where α, β and c control the sensitivity of the filter to their respective terms. The multi-scale response is defined as the maximum response over an appropriate scale range, using a scale-space representation of the image, $I(\mathbf{p}, \sigma)$, and its γ-*normalized* derivatives, defined as [5],

$$\begin{aligned} \mathcal{I}(\mathbf{p}, \sigma) &= I(\mathbf{p}) * G(\mathbf{p}, \sigma), \\ \frac{\partial^i}{\partial p_j}\mathcal{I}(\mathbf{p}, \sigma) &= \sigma^{i\gamma/2} I(\mathbf{p}) * \frac{\partial^i}{\partial p_j}G(\mathbf{p}, \sigma) \end{aligned} \quad (2)$$

where $G(\mathbf{p}, \sigma)$ is a Gaussian kernel of width σ, and γ is a normalization parameter. An appealing feature of this filter is that it requires no prior orientation estimate. However, the accuracy of the resulting radius estimate is typically low, since considerations of complexity, and memory requirements, restrict the number of scales which it is feasible to search. Furthermore, discrimination between nearby structures is reduced at coarser scales.

2.2   An Adaptable Cylinder Model

A short section of vessel may be modeled using a simple geometric cylinder representation. The cylinder is parameterized by its length, L, radius, r, and axis orientation, $\boldsymbol{a}$. Its surface, at an image position $\boldsymbol{p}$, is then specified according to

$$\mathbf{s}(l, \theta) = \boldsymbol{p} + l\,\boldsymbol{a} + r(\cos\theta\,\boldsymbol{b} + \sin\theta\,\boldsymbol{c}) \qquad \text{for } \begin{array}{c} -\frac{L}{2} \leq l \leq \frac{L}{2}, \\ 0 \leq \theta \leq 2\pi \end{array} \quad (3)$$

where $\boldsymbol{b}$ and $\boldsymbol{c}$ are orthonormal vectors in the plane perpendicular to the axis, such that $\boldsymbol{a} \cdot \boldsymbol{b} = \boldsymbol{a} \cdot \boldsymbol{c} = \boldsymbol{b} \cdot \boldsymbol{c} = 0$. In practice a discrete sampling of this surface, $\mathbf{s}(l_i, \theta_j) = \mathbf{s}_{i,j}$ (where $i = 1, \dots N_l, j = 1, \dots N_\theta$) is used. Agreement between the model and the image at $\boldsymbol{p}$ can be measured by integrating the image gradient across the surface (disregarding the ends of the cylinder). Ideally, the response at $\boldsymbol{p}$ is obtained by maximizing this measure with respect to the model parameters. However, considerations of computational complexity rule out such a direct approach.

An alternative response is defined based on model adaptation, inspired by a method for deformable mesh model adaptation [11]. Assuming that an approximate direction estimate is available, a set of feature points, $\tilde{\mathbf{x}}_{i,j}$, are identified via a search along the surface normals, $\boldsymbol{n}_j (= \cos\theta_j\,\boldsymbol{b} + \sin\theta_j\,\boldsymbol{c})$, according to

$$\tilde{\mathbf{x}}_{i,j} = \mathbf{p} + l_i\,\boldsymbol{a} + \delta\,\boldsymbol{n}_j \operatorname*{arg\,min}_{k=1\dots r_{\max}} \{Dk^2\delta^2 - f(\mathbf{p} + l_i\,\boldsymbol{a} + k\,\delta\,\boldsymbol{n}_j)\} \quad (4)$$

where δ is the spacing between points on the searched profile, D is a weighting factor, r_{max} is the maximum search radius, and $f(\mathbf{x})$ is the feature value (we use the gradient in the direction of the cylinder normal). After feature point detection, cylinder parameters are updated as follows. A new axis orientation is determined as the mean orientation over all vectors between feature points at opposite ends of the cylinder for the same orientation, $d_j = \tilde{\mathbf{x}}(l_1, \theta_j) - \tilde{\mathbf{x}}(l_{N_l}, \theta_j)$. The updated radius is then calculated as the mean perpendicular distance of the feature points to the updated axis.

The vesselness response should be largest on the vessel axis. Therefore, we use the RMS value of the residual distances between the feature points and the adapted cylinder surface, $\tilde{\mathbf{s}}$,

$$R = \sqrt{\frac{1}{N_l N_\theta} \sum_{i,j} \|\tilde{\mathbf{x}}_{i,j} - \tilde{\mathbf{s}}_{i,j}\|^2 / \|\tilde{\mathbf{s}}_{i,j}\|^2} \tag{5}$$

where $\tilde{\mathbf{s}}_{i,j}$ are points at which the search profiles intersect the adapted model's surface. This is combined with the feature strengths, to define the speed function

$$F(\mathbf{p}) = \exp\{-R^2/\mu^2\}(1 - \exp\{-\frac{1}{N_l N_\theta}(\sum_{i,j} f(\tilde{\mathbf{x}}_{i,j}))/\nu\}) \tag{6}$$

where the constants μ and ν serve to normalise the exponential terms around expected values for the RMS fractional deviation and mean feature value respectively, and to control the sensitivity of surface evolution to the respective terms. In our experiments, these values were set to $\mu=0.17$ and $\nu=30.0$.

3   Centre Line Extraction via Front Propagation

A front propagation approach is well suited to selecting vessel structures, where a simple local structure is repeated to form a complex pattern at larger scales. The method [7] is initialized by selecting a seed point inside the object of interest. The initial state of a time field, $T(\mathbf{x})$, is defined as zero at the ('selected') seed point, and infinity at all other ('un–selected') locations. Subsequently, the propagation of the front proceeds by iterating the following operations:

1. Voxels in the un–selected region which border the selected region are labeled as border, and their time values are updated according to the governing equation:

$$|\nabla T| F = 1 \tag{7}$$

2. The voxel in the border with the lowest time value is moved to the selected region.

The use of the multi–scale Hessian filter as the speed function is straightforward. In the case of the cylinder model based response, initial orientation parameters are estimated at the seed point via an exhaustive search, then propagated as voxels are moved into the *border* set, and updated whenever the time is computed.

If an end-point is selected before propagation, the process is terminated when this point is reached. Otherwise, a fixed number of iterations are used, and an end point is then interactively obtained from the selected region. A path may be constructed between the seed and end points, by following the minimum time connections in the time field.

4   Deformable Model Refinement

The centre line extracted via front propagation is used to reconstruct the vessel volume. If the cylinder–based speed function is used, orientation and radius estimates are available directly, otherwise cylinder models may be oriented along the path and adapted to retrieve these estimates. However, a vessel's cross sectional profile often deviates from circular. Visualization applications require accurate detection of the vessel wall, in order to avoid residual regions appearing in the MIP. Therefore, we construct a deformable model [9] using the centre line and radius estimates, which can be adapted to refine the segmentation.

The vessel is represented using a triangulated mesh, which is adapted according to image features while also imposing shape based constraints on the deformation. The chosen method [11] maintains the underlying triangle structure, and uses the initialising configuration as a guiding shape model to avoid excessive deformation. Adaptation is an iterative procedure consisting of a surface detection step, similar to the feature detection described in equation (4), followed by minimization of an energy function. The energy is composed of an external, image-related energy, and an internal, shape-related term:

$$E(\mathbf{x}) := \alpha E_{int}(\mathbf{x}) + E_{ext}(\mathbf{x}) \qquad (8)$$

where α weights the relative influence of each term. The external energy attracts the mesh towards the surface points. The internal energy is defined with respect to changes of the difference vectors between neighbouring mesh vertices, penalizing large deviations from the initial shape. Energy minimization uses the conjugate gradients method.

5   Results

The approach was tested with blood–pool MR images, and a validation performed via comparison with manual segmentations. Reference segmentations of the major venous and arterial pathways were available for two images. The images were re-sampled to obtain isotropic data from original image dimensions of 512x512x60 voxels of size 0.9x0.9x1.8 mm.

Centre lines estimates extracted for both speed functions were compared to vessel axes obtained from the manual segmentations. Two scales were used for

496   S. Young, V. Pekar, and J. Weese

Data set	Mean deviation (mm)		Max. deviation (mm)		Path length (mm)	
	CYL	MULTI	CYL	MULTI	CYL	MULTI
1 - right vein	1.110	2.836	3.085	10.230	486.4	479.0
left vein	0.910	2.458	2.941	7.143	501.3	475.2
2 - right vein	0.900	2.582	3.222	6.307	535.7	537.5
left vein	1.330	2.342	8.823	9.206	458.5	439.9

Table 1. Comparison of mean and maximum deviations of steepest descent path with respect to centre-line of manually segmented data

the multi-scale filter response, the original image resolution and $\sigma=2$, and the parameters were set to $\alpha=\beta=0.5$, $c=5$, while for the cylinder model approach, the parameters used were $L=4$, $D=0.1$. Reference paths were extracted using front propagation, with a speed function defined using the distance map of the manual segmentation, such that propagation was fastest at voxels furthest from the background. Then the minimal time path between the seed and end point was computed to define the reference centre line. For each point of the automatically determined centre line, the minimum distance to the reference centre line was computed. Comparison results for the two speed functions are given in table 1. The mean error for the cylinder fitting method is 1.06mm, compared to 2.55mm for the multi–scale vessel filter.

The paths extracted using the cylinder–based speed function were used to construct deformable models. The final segmentations after model adaptation were compared to the manual segmentations in two ways: using the overlap between the volumes, and the mean Euclidean distance between the surfaces of the two volumes. Since each manual segmentation also included several other vessel sections connected to the vein of interest at bifurcations, the regions near bifurcations were masked from the following results, in order to avoid ambiguity in defining voxels belonging to the vessel of interest. Comparison results are shown in table 2. Rather than considering the total proportion of falsely selected background voxels, we compute the fraction of artery falsely included since this is the important information regarding the appearance of the MIP. There are two important considerations when assessing these results. Firstly, there is a degree

Data set	Vein volume (voxels)	Vein segmented (% of total)	Artery included (% wrt vein volume)	Mean Deviation (mm)
1 - right vein	40783	87.86	1.10	0.586
left vein	42510	88.94	0.68	0.516
2 - right vein	52593	85.49	0.47	0.632
left vein	40845	87.24	0.59	0.622

Table 2. Comparison of the overlap, and Euclidean distances, between the final and the manual segmentations.

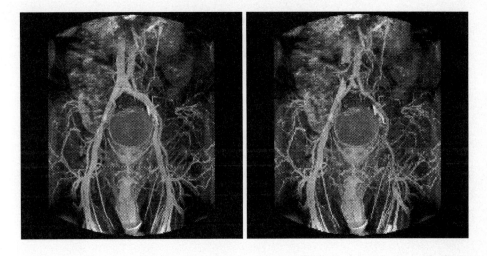

Fig. 1. MIPs before (left) and after (right) suppression of the right hand vein selected using our method, with the cylinder–model based speed function.

of subjectivity during hand segmentation, regarding the placement of the vessel border. Secondly, vessel structures have a large surface area to volume ratio, and so small errors in the radius estimate can lead to a significant error in the segmented volume. For example, the veins considered here have an average radius of approximately 5mm, and an error of 0.5 mm in the average radius estimate would result in a 20% error in the selected volume. The mean distance between the automatic and reference surface, which is less than the voxel dimensions, shows that the final segmentation accurately identifies the vessel boundaries. Figure 1 shows two MIPs, before and after suppression of right hand vein, where the cylinder model based speed function was used. Apart from a small region of unselected vein seen just below the artery bifurcation, where the deformable model failed to identify the vein border, the artery pathway is clearly seen after suppression.

6   Conclusions

A method for vessel selection has been described which allows individual vessels to be suppressed from MIP visualizations. First, a centre line is determined using a front propagation method guided by a cylinder model based response, where model parameters are propagated with the front, and then updated. The resulting centre line is combined with radius and orientation information to construct a deformable model which is adapted to refine the segmentation. The cylinder–based vessel detection criterion improves discrimination between the vessel of interest and other nearby structures, compared to a multi-scale filtering criterion. A validation of the method shows that the centre line extracted has a mean deviation of 1.06mm, and that the final segmentation has a mean error of 0.59mm. While further improvements are necessary, for example for accurate border selection in regions near bifurcations, we have demonstrated the feasibility of artery–vein separation.

Acknowledgments

The authors thank Dr. Toombs and Dr. Flamm from St. Luke's Episcopal Hospital, Houston, USA for providing MRI blood pool contrast images. We would also like to thank Arianne van Muiswinkel and Jan de Becker from Philips Medical Systems, Best, Netherlands for their support.

References

1. B. B. Avants and J. P. Williams. An adaptive minimal path generation technique for vessel tracking in CTA/CE-MRA volume images. In *MICCAI'00*, pages 707-716, Pittsburgh, PA, 2000.
2. A. Bulpitt and E. Berry. An automatic 3D deformable model for segmentation of branching structures compared with interactive region growing. In *Med. Image Understanding and Analysis*, pages 25-28, Leeds ,UK, 1998.
3. A. Frangi, W. Niessen, K. Vincken, and M. Viergever. Multiscale vessel enhancement filtering. In *MICCAI'98*, pages 130-137, Cambridge, MA, 1998.
4. K. Krissian, G. Malandain, N. Ayache, R. Vaillant, and Y. Trousset. Model based detection of tubular structures in 3D images. Technical Report TR-3736, INRIA, July 1999.
5. T. Lindeberg. Edge detection and ridge detection with automatic scale selection. *International Journal of Computer Vision*, 30(2), 1998.
6. C. Lorenz, I.-C. Carlsen, T. Buzug, C. Fassnacht, and J. Weese. Multi-scale line segmentation with automatic estimation of width, contrast and tangential direction in 2D and 3D medical images. In *Proc. of CVRMed-MRCAS '97*, pages 233-242, Grenoble, France, 1997.
7. R. Malladi and J. A. Sethian. A real-time algorithm for medical shape recovery. In *Proc. 8th Int. Conf. on Computer Vision*, pages 304-310, Bombay, India, 1998.
8. Y. Masutani, T. Schiemann, and K.-H. Höhne. Vascular shape segmentation and structure extraction using a shape-based region-growing model. In *MICCAI'98*, pages 1242-1249, Cambridge, MA, 1998.
9. T. McInerney and D. Terzopoulos. Deformable models in medical image analysis: A survey. *Medical Image Analysis*, 1(2):91-108, 1996.
10. W. Niessen, A. Montauban van Swijndregt, B. Elsman, O. Wink, M. Viergever, and W. Mali. Improved arterial visualization in blood pool agent MRA of the peripheral vasculature. In *CARS'99*, pages 119-123, 1999.
11. J. Weese, M. R. Kaus, C. Lorenz, S. Lobregt, R. Truyen, and V. Pekar. Shape constrained deformable models for 3-D medical image segmentation. Accepted for IPMI 2001, June 2001.
12. O. Wink, W. J. Niessen, and M. A. Viergever. Fast delineation and visualization of vessels in 3D angiographic images. *IEEE Trans. Medical Imaging*, 19(4):337-346, 2000.

Segmenting Articulated Structures by Hierarchical Statistical Modeling of Shape, Appearance, and Topology

Rok Bernard, Boštjan Likar, Franjo Pernuš

University of Ljubljana, Faculty of Electrical Engineering, Tržaška 25, Ljubljana, Slovenia
{rok.bernard, bostjan.likar, franjo.pernus}@fe.uni-lj.si

Abstract. This paper describes a general method for segmenting articulated structures. The method is based on statistical parametrical models, obtained by principal component analysis (PCA). The models, which describe shape, appearance, and topology of anatomic structures, are incorporated in a two-level hierarchical scheme. Shape and appearance models, describing plausible variations of shapes and appearances of individual structures, form the lower level, while the topological model, describing plausible topological variations of the articulated structure, forms the upper level. This novel scheme is actually a hierarchical PCA as the topological model is generated by the PCA of the parameters obtained at the lower level. In the segmentation process, we seek the configuration of the model instances that best matches the given image. For this purpose we introduce coarse and fine matching strategies for minimizing an energy function, which is a sum of a match measure and deformation energies of topology, shape, and appearance. The proposed method was evaluated on 36 X-ray images of cervical vertebrae by a leave-one-out test. The results show that the method well describes the anatomical variations of the cervical vertebrae, which confirms the feasibility of the proposed modeling and segmentation strategies.

1   Introduction

Ascertaining the detailed shape and organization of anatomic structures is important not only within diagnostic settings but also for tracking the process of disease, surgical planning, simulation, and intraoperative navigation. Accurate and efficient automated segmentation of articulated structures is difficult because of their complexity and inter-patient variability. Furthermore, the position of the patient during image acquisition, the imaging device itself, and the imaging protocol induce additional variations in shape and appearance. To deal with the variations, a segmentation method should use as much available prior information on shape, location, and appearance of the analyzed structures as possible. When segmenting articulated structures, like the spine, knee, or hand, prior knowledge on topology, i.e. organization of anatomical structures, should also be considered.

In recent years, a great variety of shape and appearance models have been proposed as a source of prior knowledge and applied to various tasks in medical image analysis [1]. Efficient models should be general to deal with inter-patient variability and yet specific to maintain certain anatomical properties [1, 2]. Models,

W. Niessen and M. Viergever (Eds.): MICCAI 2001, LNCS 2208, pp. 499-506, 2001.
© Springer-Verlag Berlin Heidelberg 2001

which are trained on a set of labeled training images meet these requirements and have therefore received much attention. For example, point distribution models, active shape models, and active appearance models, all proposed by Cootes *et al.* [3, 4], were successfully applied to bony structures, e.g., vertebrae [5], spine [6], knee joint [4], hand [7], rib cage [8] or hip and pelvis [9], most often for segmentation purposes.

Articulated structures exhibit two kinds of shape variations, i.e. variations in shapes of individual parts and variations in spatial relationships between the parts. Such combined variations cannot be optimally described by a single linear model unless variations of spatial relationships are sufficiently small and a sufficiently large training set is used [6]. Therefore, alternative approaches are required to describe the non-linear shape variations. This can be assessed by a piecewise linear models [10] or by separately modeling the variations of spatial relationships and variations of shapes of individual parts [7]. The problem with piecewise linearization is that it can only approximate the non-linear shape variations without using prior knowledge on organization of articulated structures, while in [7] the prior knowledge is used only for model initialization and not throughout the matching process.

In this paper we propose a general statistical hierarchical modeling of shape, appearance, and topology of articulated structures, which efficiently deals with non-linear shape variations and incorporates prior knowledge on organization of articulated structures. The hierarchical scheme is comprised of two levels. Shape and appearance models, which describe individual structures form the lower level, while the topological model, which describes the organization of anatomical structures, forms the upper level and supervises spatial relations between individual models at the lower level. The proposed method is applied to the segmentation of cervical spine vertebrae.

2   Hierarchical Scheme

To build up a general scheme that can describe the shape and appearance variations of anatomical structures, such as vertebrae, and the topological variations of the articulated structures, e.g. the cervical spine, we use the principal component analysis (PCA), which is a well-known statistical tool [11]. By PCA the principal variations of average shape, appearance, and topology can be derived from a set of representative training images.

2.1   Principal Component Analysis

Principal component analysis (PCA) is based on the statistical representation of a random variable [11]. Suppose we have a random vector population $\mathbf{x}$ and the mean of that population is denoted by $\bar{\mathbf{x}}$; $\bar{\mathbf{x}} = E(\mathbf{x})$. The covariance matrix of the same data set is $\mathbf{C}$:

$$\mathbf{C} = E\left((\mathbf{x} - \bar{\mathbf{x}})(\mathbf{x} - \bar{\mathbf{x}})^T\right) . \tag{1}$$

From a symmetric matrix such as $\mathbf{C}$ we can define an orthogonal basis by finding its eigenvalues and eigenvectors. By ordering the eigenvectors $\varnothing_i$ in the order of descending eigenvalues $\lambda_i \geq \lambda_{i+1}$, one can create an ordered orthogonal basis with the first eigenvector having the direction of largest variance of the data. Data may be reconstructed by a linear combination of orthogonal basis vectors. Instead of using all the eigenvectors of the covariance matrix, we may represent the data in terms of only a few basis vectors of the orthogonal basis. Let t largest eigenvalues and corresponding eigenvectors be retained to form the matrix $\mathbf{\Phi}$; $\mathbf{\Phi} = (\varphi_1 | \varphi_2 | \ldots | \varphi_t)$. Knowing $\overline{\mathbf{x}}$ and matrix $\mathbf{\Phi}$, we can reconstruct the input data vector $\mathbf{x}$:

$$\mathbf{x} \approx \overline{\mathbf{x}} + \mathbf{\Phi}\mathbf{y} , \tag{2}$$

from the parameters $\mathbf{y}$ of the statistical model. If the data is concentrated in a linear subspace, this provides a way to compress data without losing much information and simplifies the representation. Alternatively, the input data vector $\mathbf{x}$ can be transformed into vector $\mathbf{y}$:

$$\mathbf{y} = \mathbf{\Phi}^T (\mathbf{x} - \overline{\mathbf{x}}) . \tag{3}$$

By the above statistical model we can describe shape, appearance, and topology of an articulated structure as shown below.

2.2   Shape

Each structure is described by a statistical shape model as proposed by Cootes *et al.* [3]. The model is derived from a set of training shapes. Each training shape is composed of anatomical points defined in training images. Prior to defining the mean shape of a structure, the training shapes are rigidly aligned [3]. Shape variations are found by the PCA of training sets of anatomical points and represented by the most significant eigenshapes.

2.3   Appearance

The appearance, i.e., the texture of each structure is modeled on shape-free training images, obtained by elastic registration of training shapes and mean shape. Thin-plate splines interpolation between corresponding anatomical points is used for this purpose [12]. By applying PCA to the set of shape-free training images, defined on a region of interest covering a structure, the mean image and the most significant eigenimages are extracted.

2.4   Topology

To describe topological variations of an articulated structure we need to correlate variations in pose and shape of all structures. We propose to apply the PCA on pose and shape parameters of all structures, which were obtained in the shape model generation step. In this way, the most significant eigentopologies describe the anatomically plausible topological variations. This novel strategy can be viewed upon as a hierarchical PCA. The topological PCA (upper level of hierarchy), describing plausible topological variations of an articulated structure, is constructed from sets of parameters generated by shape PCAs and corresponding pose parameters (lower level of hierarchy) that describe plausible variations of shapes and poses of individual structures. In this way, the topological PCA enables the supervision of the spatial relations between shapes of structures, which form the articulated structure.

3   Segmentation

The above hierarchical scheme consists of parametrical models that describe shape, appearance, and topology of an articulated structure. Once extensively trained, it incorporates a valuable prior knowledge that can be used efficiently for describing the image of the articulated structure. We consider model-based image segmentation by searching the configuration $\mathbf{L}$ of the model instances that best match the given image I. The best configuration $\mathbf{L}^*$ may be found by the maximum a posteriori (MAP) estimation:

$$\mathbf{L}^* = \arg\max_{\mathbf{L}} P(\mathbf{L} \mid I) \ . \tag{4}$$

Bayes rule then implies:

$$\mathbf{L}^* = \arg\max_{\mathbf{L}} P(\mathbf{L})P(I \mid \mathbf{L}) \ . \tag{5}$$

The prior $P(\mathbf{L})$ is given by the probability distributions of shapes, appearances, and topology. The likelihood function $P(I|\mathbf{L})$, measures the probability of observing image I given a particular configuration $\mathbf{L}$. The standard approach to finding the MAP estimation is to minimize the energy function $F(I,\mathbf{L})$ obtained by taking the negative logarithm of a posteriori probability:

$$\mathbf{L}^* = \arg\min_{\mathbf{L}} F(I,\mathbf{L}) \ . \tag{6}$$

The required matching strategy and the energy function are given in the following sub-sections.

3.1   Matching Strategy

Consider the configuration $\mathbf{L}$ describing an articulated structure composed of N structures where each structure is described by t_s shape, t_a appearance, and t_p pose parameters. The number of all parameters is $N^*(t_s + t_a + t_p)$, possibly causing a demanding optimization problem. To overcome this problem, we can elegantly omit the appearance parameters as they may be estimated from the image patch defined by the shape model. This reduces the number of parameters to $N^*(t_s + t_p)$. We name this optimization strategy a fine matching strategy. We consider also a coarse matching strategy by which the number of parameters can be further significantly reduced to $t_P + t_T$ by tuning only t_P global pose and t_T topological parameters of the articulated structure at the upper level in the hierarchy. Global pose and topological parameters then drive pose and shape parameters of individual structures at the lower level of hierarchy. The coarse and fine matching strategies are considered in the following.

3.1.1   Coarse Matching

In the coarse matching step, illustrated in Fig. 1a, we tune only global pose and topological parameters that in turn drive pose and shape parameters of the structures. According to these parameters, each shape model, describing a corresponding structure, generates a shape that defines a patch on the underlying image. The patch is then elastically transformed to the shape-free form, which is fed into the appearance model that yields appearance parameters and approximates the given shape-free image patch. Finally, the match measure between the shape-free image patch and its approximation is calculated. The obtained match measure is part of the energy function that is used for selecting the global pose and topological parameters for the next iteration in the optimization process. The energy function, which considers also topology, shape, and appearance deformation energies, is described latter.

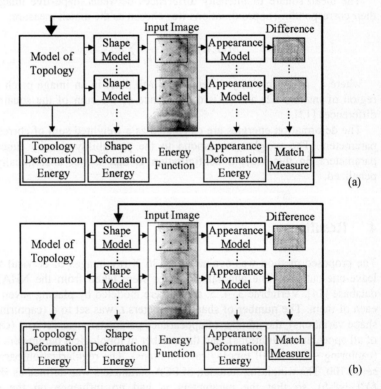

Fig. 1. Coarse matching strategy (a): global pose and topological parameters are optimized and fine matching strategy (b): pose and shape parameters of all structures are optimized simultaneously

3.1.2   Fine Matching

In a fine matching strategy, illustrated in Fig. 1b, the pose and shape parameters of all structures are optimized simultaneously, whereas the model of topology only supervises the spatial relations between shapes of structures via the topology deformation energy in the energy function.

3.2   Energy Function

To suppress anatomically implausible configurations we define the energy function $F(I,\mathbf{L})$ as a weighted sum of match measure $M(I,\mathbf{L})$ and topology $F_T(\mathbf{L})$, shape $F_S(\mathbf{L})$, and appearance $F_A(\mathbf{L})$ deformation energies:

$$F(I,\mathbf{L}) = \alpha \cdot M(I,\mathbf{L}) + F_T(\mathbf{L}) + F_S(\mathbf{L}) + F_A(\mathbf{L}) \ , \tag{7}$$

where α is a regularization parameter weighting the match measure against deformation energies.

The mean square of intensity differences between shape-free image patches and their corresponding approximations was chosen as the match measure:

$$M(I,\mathbf{L}) = \sum_{i=1}^{N} \frac{1}{\Omega_i} \frac{1}{V_i} \sum_{j \in \Omega_i} r_{i,j}^2 \ , \tag{8}$$

where $r_{i,j}$ is the intensity difference of j-th pixel in an image patch i defined on a region of interest Ω_i and V_i is the variance of the sum of the squares of intensity differences [13].

The deformation energies are calculated as a weighted sum of corresponding PCA parameters. The weights correspond to the probability density functions of PCA parameters. In this way, a configuration $\mathbf{L}$ that is not anatomically plausible is penalized.

4   Results

The proposed method was evaluated on 36 X-ray images of cervical vertebrae by a leave-one-out test. The annotated images were taken from the NHANES II X-ray database [14]. Vertebrae 3, 4, 5, and 6 were modeled by placing seven landmarks on each of them. The number of shape parameters t_s was set to 4 (capturing ~72% of all shape variations), the number of appearance parameters was set to 3 (capturing ~85% of all appearance variations), and the number of topological parameters t_T was set to 2 (capturing ~40% of all topological variations). The regularization parameter α was set to 100. The weighting function of PCA parameters was defined as $W(y_k)=sign(|y_k|-b)*(\ |y_k|-b)$, so that the parameters y_k had no influence on the corresponding deformation energy if lying inside the interval $[-b, b]$. The values of b were 1, 0, and 1 for shape, appearance and topological parameters, respectively. The simulated annealing global optimization method was used for energy minimization [14].

In the leave-one-out test the method was trained on 35 images and then tested on the remaining image. The initialization of the method, which provided global pose parameters of the cervical spine model, was performed by selecting two points, one on vertebra 3 and one on vertebra 6. Points were selected in centers of the vertebrae and then perturbed by a constant distance, which was quarter of the vertebra size, in 10 different directions. After applying the method, the resulting landmark positions were compared to the manually defined gold-standard positions by calculating root mean square (RMS) error separately for each of the vertebrae. The RMS errors were calculated for the initial landmark positions and after the coarse and fine matching steps. In 80% of the cases the initial RMS error was reduced. Fig. 2 shows two cervical spine X-ray images. In Fig. 2a the landmarks were accurately placed by the proposed method, while in Fig. 2b the method failed because of the poor contrast on vertebrae 3 and 4, large osteophyte on vertebra 5, and partial overlapping of vertebra 6 and shoulder. Also a well-trained human operator hardly identifies vertebrae landmarks on such images.

The initial RMS errors and RMS errors after coarse and fine matching steps are shown in Fig. 3. The resulting RMS errors were on the average 2.2 pixels, while the initial RMS error ranged on the average from 5.5-7.5 pixels. The coarse matching step succeeded to locate the landmarks to pixel accuracy, while the fine matching step only slightly improved the localisation.

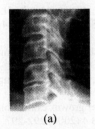 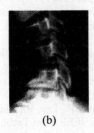

| (a) | (b) |

Fig. 2. Cervical spine X-ray images on which the method was successful (a) and on which the method failed (b)

Fig. 3. Mean RMS errors and corresponding standard deviations (in pixels) for initial landmark positions (dark gray) and after coarse (light gray) and fine (white) matching steps

5   Conclusion

In this paper we presented a general method for segmenting articulated structures exhibiting variations in shape, appearance and topology. The method is based on statistical parametrical models that are incorporated in a two-level hierarchical scheme. The lower level describes the shape and appearance of individual structures, while the upper level controls the topology of the articulated structure. When segmenting a given image, the anatomically plausible configuration of the models is searched for in coarse and fine matching steps. The segmentation results on 36 X-ray images confirmed the applicability of the proposed modeling and segmentation strategies. We will focus our future efforts on extensive evaluation of the method on a larger number of spine X-ray images. The proposed hierarchical statistical modeling of shape, appearance, and topology is an important breakthrough for describing non-linear shape variations of articulated structures. Further development and refinement of this methodology should remain an important area of research in the near future.

Acknowledgements

This work was supported by the Ministry of Science and Technology of the Republic of Slovenia under grant J2-0659-1538 and by the IST-1999-12338 project, funded by the European Commission.

References

1. McInerney, T., Terzopoulos, D.: Deformable models in medical image analysis: A survey. Medical Image Analysis 1 (1996) 91-108.
2. Jain, A.K., Zhong, Y., Dubuisson-Jolly, M.P.: Deformable template models: A review. Signal process 71 (1998) 109-129
3. Cootes, T.F., Hill, A., Taylor, C.J., Haslam, J.: Use of active shape models for locating structures in medical images. Image Vision Comput 12 (1994) 355-365
4. Cootes, T.F., Edwards, G.J., Taylor, C.J.: Active appearance models. In: Burkhardt, H., Neumann, B. (eds.): European conference on computer vision, Vol. 2. Springer (1998) 484-498
5. Hill, A., Cootes, T.F., Taylor, C.J.: Active shape models and the shape approximation problem. Image Vision Comput 14 (1996) 601-607
6. Smyth, P.P., Taylor, C.J., Adams, J.E.: Automatic measurement of vertebral shape using active shape models. Image Vision Comput 15 (1997) pp. 575-581
7. Mahmoodi, S., Sharif, B.S., Chester, E.G., Owen, J.P., Lee, R.: Skeletal growth estimation using radiographic image processing and analysis. IEEE T Inf Technol B 4 (2000) 292-297
8. van Ginneken, B., Haar Romeny, B.M.: Automatic delineation of ribs in frontal chest radiographs. In: Hanson, K.M. (ed.): Image processing. Medical Imaging Vol. 3979. SPIE San Diego (2000) 825-836
9. Bernard, R., Pernuš, F.: Statistical approach to anatomical landmark extraction in AP radiographs. In: Sonka, M., Hanson, K.M. (eds.): Image processing. Medical Imaging Vol. 4322. SPIE San Diego (2001) in press
10. Heap, T., Hogg, D.: Improving specifity in PDMs using hierarchical approach. In: Clark, A.F. (ed): British Machine Vision Conference. Essex, UK (1997) 80-89
11. Gonzalez, R.C., Woods, R.E.: Digital image processing. Addison Wessley (1992)
12. Bookstein, F.L.: Principal warps: thin-plate splines and the decomposition of deformations. IEEE T Pattern Anal 11 (1989) 567-585
13. Cootes, T.F., Page, G.J., Jackson, C.B., Taylor, C.J.: Statistical grey-level models for object location and identification. Image Vision Comput 14 (1996) 533-540
14. Long, L.R., Pillemer, S.R., Lawrence, R.C., Goh, G-H., Neve, L., Thoma, G.R.: World Wide Web platform-independent access to biomedical text/image databases. In: Horii, S.C., Blaine, G. (eds.): PACS design and evaluation: Engineering and clinical issues. Medical Imaging Vol. 3339. SPIE San Diego (1998) 52-63
15. Press, W.H., Teukolsky, S.A., Vetterling, W.T., Flannery, B. P.: Numerical recipes in C, The art of scientific computing. University Press, Cambridge (1992)

Validation of Nonlinear Spatial Filtering to Improve Tissue Segmentation of MR Brain Images

Siddharth Srivastava, Koen Van Leemput, Frederik Maes, Dirk Vandermeulen, and Paul Suetens

Medical Image Computing (Radiology + ESAT/PSI)
Katholieke Universiteit Leuven, Faculties of Medicine and Engineering
University Hospital Gasthuisberg, Herestraat 49, B-3000, Leuven, Belgium

Abstract. Intensity-based tissue segmentation of MR brain images is facilitated if the image noise can be effectively reduced without removing significant image detail. Signal to noise ratio can be increased by averaging multiple acquisitions of the same subject after proper geometric alignment, but this penalizes acquisition time. In this paper we evaluate the effect of nonlinear spatial filtering of single scans prior to tissue classification. Spatial filtering is performed iteratively by nonlinear intensity diffusion to suppress noise in homogeneous tissue regions without smoothing across tissue boundaries. We validate the impact on segmentation accuracy using simulated MR data with known ground-truth, demonstrating that the performance obtained with spatial filtering of single scans is comparable to that of averaging multiple coregistered scans. The performance can be further improved by tuning the filter parameters towards optimal segmentation accuracy.

1 Introduction

Accurate brain segmentation and brain tissue quantification from high resolution three-dimensional (3-D) magnetic resonance (MR) images is of paramount importance for the reliable detection of morphological abnormalities by automated image analysis procedures in the study of a variety of neurological diseases. State-of-the-art computational strategies for brain tissue segmentation apply intensity-based pixel classification to assign to each voxel a probability value of belonging to either white matter, grey matter, CSF or 'other', modeling the intensity of each brain tissue class by a Gaussian distribution whose parameters are estimated from the image data [7]. Because this estimation is highly sensitive to noise, especially when only single channel data are considered, and because small changes in the parameter estimates may result in significant changes in the classification and in the tissue volumes computed from it, the reliability of the results is obviously improved when the images under study have less noise, more contrast and higher signal to noise ratio (SNR).

MR image contrast and SNR can be optimized at acquisition, but this generally results in an increase in measurement time which may not be clinically

W. Niessen and M. Viergever (Eds.): MICCAI 2001, LNCS 2208, pp. 507–515, 2001.
© Springer-Verlag Berlin Heidelberg 2001

acceptable and which also increases the possibility of the presence of imaging artifacts, due to subject motion for instance, that may affect overall image quality. Alternatively, image noise can be reduced by temporal averaging of multiple similar scans obtained by repeated acquisitions, provided that all scans were properly aligned. Another approach, which is investigated here, that does not penalize acquisition time and that is not affected by misregistration, is spatial filtering of the image intensities prior to tissue segmentation using filters based on nonlinear anisotropic intensity diffusion, aiming at reducing noise in homogeneous regions while at the same time preserving or even sharpening the image edges that are indicative for the true object boundaries.

In this paper we evaluate the effect of noise suppression by nonlinear diffusion prior to tissue classification on the accuracy of the segmentation result for simulated MR data with known ground truth. We compare the segmentation of the filtered images with that obtained for the original data and for temporally averaged images, showing that spatial filtering of the data yields the best performance without the need for multiple acquisitions. We also illustrate the performance of the method on actual patient data of a study aiming at detecting cortical malformations in epilepsy patients.

2   Spatial Filtering by Nonlinear Anisotropic Diffusion

2.1   The Perona-Malik Nonlinear Diffusion Filter

Analogous to the physical notion of diffusion as a process that equilibrates concentration differences by transporting mass without creating or destroying it, diffusion of image intensities over the image domain is described by the diffusion equation:

$$\partial_t u(\bar{r}, t) = div(G(\bar{r}, t).\nabla u(\bar{r}, t)) \tag{1}$$

with $u(\bar{r}, t)$ the image intensity at position $\bar{r}$ and time t, ∇u its spatial gradient, $\partial_t u$ its temporal derivative and $G(\bar{r}, t)$ the conductance parameter. Setting $G = 1$ results in linear diffusion, which has been shown to be equivalent to smoothing the image data with a family of Gaussian filter kernels whose scale evolves in relation to t [3]. Perona and Malik [6] proposed letting G vary over the image domain and to make it depend on the local intensity gradient ∇u, such that the diffusion process achieves piecewise smoothing while preserving the relevant image edges. The conductivity model suggested in [6] that we used in our experiments is:

$$G(\bar{r}, t) = \exp\left[-\left(\frac{\|\nabla u(\bar{r})\|}{\kappa} \right)^2 \right] \tag{2}$$

The parameter κ determines the local behavior of the filter: smoothing if $\|\nabla u\| \leq \kappa$ and edge sharpening if $\|\nabla u\| > \kappa$.

2.2 Discrete Implementation

Discretization of the diffusion equation is required in order to apply it to digital images, estimating the spatial gradients as differences between neighboring data elements. Following the approach of Gerig *et al.* [2], the discrete version of equation (1) in 1-D is given by:

$$\partial_t u(x,t) = \frac{1}{\Delta x^2}\left[G\left(x+\frac{\Delta x}{2},t\right).(u(x+\Delta x,t)-u(x,t))\right.$$
$$\left. -G\left(x-\frac{\Delta x}{2},t\right).(u(x,t)-u(x-\Delta x,t))\right] \tag{3}$$

Defining the flow $\Phi = G.\nabla u$ [2] and setting $\Delta x = 1$, this can be written as $\partial_t u = \Phi_{x_+} - \Phi_{x_-}$ with Φ_{x_+} the signal flow from the right neighbor and Φ_{x_-} the signal flow to the left neighbor. The evolution of the image intensity over time is computed as:

$$u(x,t+\Delta t) \approx u(x,t) + \Delta t.\partial_t u(x,t) = u(x,t) + \Delta t.(\Phi_{x_+} - \Phi_{x_-}) \tag{4}$$

with Δt the time step parameter which should be small enough to assure stability of the process. Following [2], we select $\Delta t \le 1/(n+1)$ with n the number of neighbors used to calculate the flow.

As we are dealing with 3-D isotropic volume data, we extend equation (4) to 3-D by considering flow contributions from the six nearest neighbors:

$$u(x,t+\Delta t) = u(x,t) + \Delta t.\left((\Phi_{x_+} - \Phi_{x_-}) + (\Phi_{y_+} - \Phi_{y_-}) + (\Phi_{z_+} - \Phi_{z_-})\right) \tag{5}$$

This iterative scheme eventually converges to a constant in the limit of infinite time, such that the process has to be terminated at some intermediate stage to obtain the desired filtering effect. Rather than prescribing a specified number of iterations, we adopt the "biased anisotropic diffusion" approach proposed by Nordström [5] and alter equation (5) into:

$$u(x,t+\Delta t) = u(x,t) + \Delta t.\left[\Phi_{xyz} + \lambda.(u(x,0) - u(x,t))\right] \tag{6}$$

with Φ_{xyz} the sum of the flow contributions in the three directions and λ a weight factor which was set to $\lambda = 1$ in all our experiments. We stop iterating equation (6) when the root mean square norm $\|\partial_t u\| = \|\Phi_{xyz} + \lambda.(u(x,0) - u(x,t)\|$ over the whole image domain has sufficiently converged to zero.

2.3 Selecting the Conductance Parameter

The choice of the conductance parameter κ in (2) is critical for good performance of the filter. Proper selection of κ requires a reliable estimate for the image noise. We obtain such an estimate using the approach proposed in [2] by computing the mean and standard deviation (SD) of the image intensity within subvolumes centered at each voxel. The image intensity is quantized into a set of intervals and for each interval the minimal SD is determined over all subvolumes whose mean intensity falls within the range spanned by this interval. We take the resulting SD value for the lowest intensity interval as estimate for the background noise σ_b and the minimal SD value over all other intervals as estimate for the tissue noise σ_t. Gerig *et al.* [2] determined σ_t in a similar way and found that a good choice for κ was $\kappa = \alpha \times \sigma_t$ with $1.5 \leq \alpha \leq 2.0$.

3   Validation

We validated the effect of spatial filtering on segmentation accuracy using simulated 1 mm isotropic T1-weighted $181 \times 217 \times 181$ MR images generated by the BrainWeb simulator of Cocosco *et al.* [1]. Five similar images with noise levels of 0, 3, 5, 7 and 9% were obtained, which we denote by n_0, n_1, n_2, n_3 and n_4 respectively. Nonlinear spatial filtering was applied to the noisy images with $\kappa = \alpha \times \sigma_t$ for various choices of α and with the tissue noise σ_t determined as described in section 2.3.

White and grey matter maps are segmented from the images using the fully automated intensity-based pixel classification method of Van Leemput *et al.* [7]. This method assumes that the intensities of each tissue class obey a Gaussian distribution, the parameters of which are estimated during classification. The method corrects for global MR intensity inhomogeneities by including a model for the MR bias field whose parameters are iteratively updated during classification. Prior knowledge about the expected distribution of the various tissue classes in the image is derived from a digital brain atlas that is co-registered with the image under study. The method also allows incorporation of contextual information in the classification procedure by modeling spatial interactions between neighboring pixels as a Markov Random Field (MRF), providing local spatial regularization of the tissue maps which makes the segmentation less sensitive to noise.

The resulting fuzzy tissue maps indicate the probability of each voxel belonging to a certain tissue type. A binary classification was obtained by assigning each voxel to its most likely class. Volumes were then computed as voxel counts. The segmentation of the noise-free image n_0 yields the ground-truth tissue maps and ground-truth volumes V_g for each tissue class. The performance of the spatial filtering and its effect on segmentation accuracy is assessed by comparing the estimated volumes V_e obtained for the noisy and the filtered images to the ground-truth volumes V_g using three different similarity measures: the relative volume error $\delta V = (V_e - V_g)/V_g$, the similarity index $2.V_o/(V_g + V_e)$ and the overlap index $V_o/(V_g + V_e - V_o)$, with V_o the volume of overlap of the maps that are being compared [8].

4   Results

4.1   Influence of Spatial Filtering on Segmentation Accuracy

The tissue and background noise levels in the original and filtered simulated images are tabulated in table 1 for three values of α: $\alpha = 1.75$ midway the range suggested in [2], $\alpha = 2$ at the high end of the range and $\alpha = 3$ beyond this range. Figure 1 illustrates the effect of nonlinear spatial filtering on the most noisy image n_4. The filtered images show an increase in contrast, as well as sharper boundaries between gray and white matter. Figure 2 shows the tissue maps obtained for image n_3 before and after filtering, as well as the ground-truth maps extracted from the noise-free image n_0.

Grey matter volume was underestimated in the original images as well as in the filtered images by a volume error δV of about 5% for all noise levels and both values of α. White matter volume was overestimated by 10% for n_1 up to 15% for n_4 for the original images, which improved to about 5% after filtering with $\alpha = 2$. The overlap and similarity indices for all experiments are summarized in table 2.

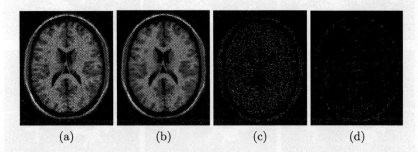

(a)   (b)   (c)   (d)

Fig. 1. Effect of nonlinear spatial filtering using (6): (a) original axial slice of image n_4; (b) image after filtering with $\alpha = 2$; (c) absolute difference between (a) and n_0; (d) absolute difference between (b) and n_0.

	σ_t				σ_b			
α	0	1.75	2	3	0	1.75	2	3
n_1	3.63	0.83	0.74	0.67	2.28	0.42	0.41	0.41
n_2	5.82	1.32	1.15	1.07	3.71	0.68	0.66	0.65
n_3	7.90	1.76	1.51	1.47	5.07	0.91	0.92	0.90
n_4	9.66	2.10	1.92	1.81	6.13	1.13	1.05	1.00

Table 1. Tissue and background noise levels σ_t and σ_b in the original noisy images n_1 to n_4 ($\alpha = 0$) and after filtering with $\kappa = \alpha \times \sigma_t$.

4.2   Spatial Filtering versus Temporal Averaging

To investigate how noise suppression by spatial filtering of a single MR scan compares to SNR improvement by temporal averaging of multiple repeated scans, a set of such scans was artificially generated by applying small translational and rotational offsets to one image to simulate inter-scan subject motion. Motion parameters were derived from a set of four repeated real patient 3-D volume

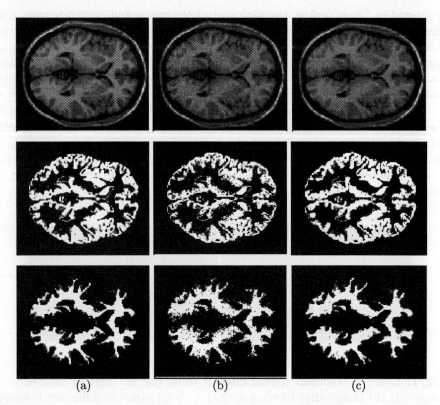

(a)   (b)   (c)

Fig. 2. Tissue maps obtained by automated pixel classification for simulated MR images, followed by hard classification: (a) noise-free ground-truth image n_0; (b) original image n_3; (c) filtered image n_3 ($\alpha = 2$). Top: MR data; middle: grey matter map; bottom: white matter map.

Overlap index

	Grey matter						White matter					
	with MRF			without MRF			with MRF			without MRF		
α	0	1.75	2	0	1.75	2	0	1.75	2	0	1.75	2
n_1	0.896	0.914	0.917	0.824	0.897	0.902	0.881	0.908	0.913	0.711	0.901	0.909
n_2	0.847	0.878	0.879	0.793	0.871	0.874	0.824	0.863	0.874	0.675	0.862	0.872
n_3	0.808	0.851	0.864	0.761	0.848	0.860	0.775	0.835	0.857	0.642	0.833	0.855
n_4	0.769	0.836	0.855	0.732	0.829	0.849	0.729	0.824	0.851	0.611	0.816	0.847

Similarity index

	Grey matter						White matter					
	with MRF			without MRF			with MRF			without MRF		
α	0	1.75	2	0	1.75	2	0	1.75	2	0	1.75	2
n_1	0.945	0.955	0.956	0.903	0.946	0.948	0.937	0.952	0.955	0.831	0.948	0.953
n_2	0.917	0.935	0.936	0.884	0.931	0.933	0.903	0.927	0.933	0.806	0.926	0.932
n_3	0.894	0.920	0.927	0.865	0.917	0.921	0.873	0.910	0.923	0.782	0.910	0.922
n_4	0.870	0.910	0.921	0.845	0.907	0.918	0.843	0.900	0.917	0.759	0.876	0.917

Table 2. Similarity measures for the tissue maps of the original ($\alpha = 0$) and filtered noisy images n_1 to n_4 compared to the ground-truth maps of the noise-free image n_0 obtained with and without including spatial context during classification.

scans that were carefully aligned using an automated procedure [4]. Identical displacements were then applied to the simulated MR images such that each time a set of four similar volumes was obtained with identical noise characteristics and with the same misregistration as the patient images. Temporal averaging of each such quadruple of simulated images was then performed either without or with prior geometric alignment of the images. The averaged images were then segmented with the MRF enabled and the resulting tissue maps compared to the ground truth obtained for the noise-free images as in section 4.1.

The results are summarized in table 3. Spatial filtering performs obviously better than temporal averaging without correcting for misregistration and not worse than temporal averaging after misregistration correction.

Overlap index						Similarity index					
Grey matter			White matter			Grey matter			White matter		
(1)	(2)	(3)	(1)	(2)	(3)	(1)	(2)	(3)	(1)	(2)	(3)
n_0 0.821			0.873			n_0 0.902			0.932		
n_2 0.788	0.844	0.886	0.825	0.858	0.881	n_2 0.882	0.916	0.940	0.904	0.924	0.937
n_4 0.766	0.807	0.853	0.709	0.810	0.858	n_4 0.867	0.893	0.921	0.829	0.895	0.923

Table 3. Similarity measures comparing the influence of temporal averaging of multiple scans and of spatial filtering of a single scan on the segmentation accuracy for simulated MR data: (1) temporal averaging without correcting for misregistration; (2) temporal averaging after misregistration correction; (3) nonlinear spatial filtering using $\kappa = 2 \times \sigma_t$. The MRF was enabled during voxel classification in all experiments.

4.3   Patient Data

A set of four identically repeated 3-D volume scans was acquired for a real subject as part of a study aiming at detecting cortical malformations in the brain of epilepsy patients. All 4 images were segmented before and after nonlinear spatial filtering using $\alpha = 1.75$ and $\alpha = 2$ as before. Although no ground truth is available for these data, the effect of spatial filtering can be evaluated from its impact on the variability of the tissue volumes obtained from repeated scans. The coefficient of variation (i.e. standard deviation divided by the mean) was 0.8% for gray matter, 1.15% for white matter and 0.48% for gray and white matter combined when no filtering was applied. After filtering with $\alpha = 2$, these values were 0.87%, 3.15% and 0.68% respectively.

5   Discussion

The effect of nonlinear spatial filtering on segmentation accuracy was evaluated by comparing tissue maps obtained for noisy simulated MR brain images and their filtered versions with ground-truth maps obtained for the corresponding noise-free image. The results of table 2 indicate that spatial filtering indeed improves segmentation accuracy, and its impact is larger than explicitly including spatial contextual constraints, modeled as an MRF, in the classification algorithm itself.

We compared the impact on segmentation accuracy of spatial filtering of single scans with that of averaging of multiple scans. Our results on simulated data (table 3) show that spatial filtering performs equally well as temporal averaging with misregistration correction, but without penalizing acquisition time. But on actual patient data, contrary to what was expected, spatial filtering increased the variability of volume measurements in repeated scans. We found that the tissue specific intensity histograms are less well modeled by a Gaussian distribution after filtering. Further investigations are needed to explain why the filtering seems to have different effect on each scan.

6   Conclusion

In this paper we demonstrated using simulated data with known ground-truth that nonlinear spatial intensity filtering improves the accuracy of tissue segmentation in MR brain images. A more robust validation of the approach on clinical data is necessary for its deployment as an alternative preprocessing methodology. Our future reports will focus on this aspect of the work.

7   Acknowledgements

This work was funded by grant KU Leuven IDO/A5018. The authors thank Wim Van Paesschen, Patrick Dupont and Kristof Baete for stimulating discussions on the clinical and engineering aspects of the work. Thanks are due also to the anonymous reviewers for their comments and suggestions.

References

[1] C.A. Cocosco, V. Kollokian, R.K.-S. Kwan, and A.C. Evans. BrainWeb: Online Interface to a 3D MRI Simulated Brain Database. *NeuroImage*, 5(4): part 2/4, S425, 1997.
[2] G. Gerig, O. Kübler, R. Kikinis, and F.A. Jolesz. Nonlinear anisotropic filtering of MRI data. *IEEE Transactions on Medical Imaging*, 11(2):221–232, 1992.
[3] J. J. Koenderink. The structure of images. *Biological Cybernetics*, 50:363–370, 1984.
[4] F. Maes, A. Collignon, D. Vandermeulen, G. Marchal, and P. Suetens. Multi-modality image registration by maximization of mutual information. *IEEE Transactions on Medical Imaging*, 16(2):187–198, 1997.
[5] K.N. Nordström. Biased anisotropic diffusion: a unified regularization and diffusion approach to edge detection. *Image and Vision Computing*, 8(4):318–327, 1990.

[6] P. Perona and J. Malik. Scale-space and edge detection using anisotropic diffusion. *IEEE Transactions on Pattern Analysis and Machine Intelligence*, 12:629–639, 1990.

[7] K. Van Leemput, F. Maes, D. Vandermeulen, and P. Suetens. Automated model-based tissue classification of MR images of the brain. *IEEE Transactions on Medical Imaging*, 18(10):897–908, 1999.

[8] A.P. Zijdenbos, B.M. Dawant, R. Margolin, and A.C. Palmer. Morphometric analysis of white matter lesions in MR images: method and validation. *IEEE Transactions on Medical Imaging*, 13(4):716–724, 1994.

Valmet: A New Validation Tool for Assessing and Improving 3D Object Segmentation

[1,2]Guido Gerig, [1]Matthieu Jomier, [2]Miranda Chakos

[1]Department of Computer Science, UNC, Chapel Hill, NC 27599, USA
[2]Department of Psychiatry, UNC, Chapel Hill, NC 27599, USA
Software: http://www.ia.unc.edu/public/valmet
email: gerig@cs.unc.edu

Abstract. Extracting 3D structures from volumetric images like MRI or CT is becoming a routine process for diagnosis based on quantitation, for radiotherapy planning, for surgical planning and image-guided intervention, for studying neurodevelopmental and neurodegenerative aspects of brain diseases, and for clinical drug trials. Key issues for segmenting anatomical objects from 3D medical images are validity and reliability. We have developed VALMET, a new tool for validation and comparison of object segmentation. New features not available in commercial and public-domain image processing packages are the choice between different metrics to describe differences between segmentations and the use of graphical overlay and 3D display for visual assessment of the locality and magnitude of segmentation variability. Input to the tool are an original 3D image (MRI, CT, ultrasound), and a series of segmentations either generated by several human raters and/or by automatic methods (machine). Quantitative evaluation includes intra-class correlation of resulting volumes and four different shape distance metrics, a) percentage overlap of segmented structures (R intersect S)/(R union S), b) probabilistic overlap measure for non-binary segmentations, c) mean/median absolute distances between object surfaces, and maximum (Hausdorff) distance. All these measures are calculated for arbitrarily selected 2D cross-sections and full 3D segmentations. Segmentation results are overlaid onto the original image data for visual comparison. A 3D graphical display of the segmented organ is color-coded depending on the selected metric for measuring segmentation difference. The new tool is in routine use for intra- and inter-rater reliability studies and for testing novel automatic machine-segmentation versus a gold standard established by human experts. Preliminary studies showed that the new tool could significantly improve intra- and inter-rater reliability of hippocampus segmentation to achieve intra-class correlation coefficients significantly higher than published elsewhere.

1. Scoring Measurement Methods

The computer vision community started several efforts with a number of workshops, conferences, and special issues of journals on the topic of empirical evaluation technique, see for example [Bowyer 1998], [Niessen 2000], [Vincken 2000], [Chalana 1997], and [Remiejer 1999]. Measuring performance of algorithms or human raters in image segmentation requires an appropriate metric, a "goodness" index that gives us a

W. Niessen and M. Viergever (Eds.): MICCAI 2001, LNCS 2208, pp. 516-523, 2001.
© Springer-Verlag Berlin Heidelberg 2001

valid measure of the quality of a segmentation result. A good source and discussion of techniques is found in the most recent book, *Performance Characterization in Computer Vision* [Klette 2000]. Typical procedures for validation of computer-assisted segmentation are listed in [Kapur 1996]: Segmentation results are validated by a) visual inspection, b) comparison with manual segmentation, c) tests with synthetic data, d) use of fiducials on patients, and e) use of fiducials and/or cadavers. The problem is not that there is no ground truth for medical data, but that the ground truth is not typically available to the segmentation validation system in any form that can be readily used. For some structures or parts of structures the boundary can only be known with non-negligible tolerance. For other structures, the ground truth/gold standard is in reality barely fuzzy.

The following list covers metrics to measure the differences of segmentation results for measuring and comparing the reliability of intra-rater, inter-rater and machine-to-rater segmentations. We have developed a new tool called VALMET [freely avaible at http://www.ia.unc.edu/public/valmet] that reads an original 3D image to be segmented and a series of 3D segmentation results. Valmet calculates different metrics to assess pairwise segmentation differences and differences between groups. It further displays volumetric images with overlaid segmentations as 3 orthogonal sections with coupled cursors and as 3D renderings (see Fig. 2).

1.1 Volumes

A feature most easily accessible is the total volume of a structure. This is the simplest morphologic measure and often used in reliability studies in neuroimaging applications. For binary segmentations, we calculate the number of voxels adjusted by the voxel volume. More precise volumetric measurements can be obtained by fitting a surface (marching cubes, e.g.) with sub-voxel accuracy and calculating the volume by integration. Comparing volumes of segmented structures does not take into account any regional differences and does not give an answer to the question where differences occur. Further, over- and underestimation along boundaries or surfaces cancel and can give excellent agreement even if the boundary segmentation is poor [Niessen 2000].

1.2 Volumetric Overlap (True and False Positives, True and False Negatives)

One approach for taking in to account the spatial properties of structures is a pair-wise comparison of two binary segmentations by relative overlap. Assuming spatial registration, images are analyzed voxel by voxel to calculate false positives, false negative, true positive and true negative voxels. Well accepted measures are the intersection of subject and reference divided by the union, $(S \cap R)/(S \cup R)$, or intersection divided by reference $(S \cap R)/R$. Both measures give a score of 1 for perfect agreement and 0 for complete disagreement. The first is more sensitive to differences since both denominator and numerator change with increasing or decreasing overlap. The measure gives comparable results if applied at different institutions if structures and resolution of image data are standardized. However, the overlap measure depends on the size and the shape complexity of the object and is related to the image sampling. Assuming that most of the error occurs at the boundary of objects, small objects are penalized and get a much lower score than large objects.

1.3 Probabilistic Distances between Segmentations

In a lot of medical image segmentation tasks there are no clear boundaries between anatomical structures. Absolute ground truth by manual segmentation does not exist and only a 'fuzzy' probabilistic segmentation is possible. Manual probabilistic segmentations can be generated by aggregating repeated multiple segmentations of the same structure done either by a trained individual rater or by multiple raters. We have developed a probabilistic overlap measure between two fuzzy segmentations derived from the normalized L^1 distance between two probability distributions. The probabilistic overlap is defined as

$$POV(A, B) = 1 - \frac{\int |P_A - P_B|}{2 \int P_{AB}},$$

where P_A and P_B are the probability distributions representing the two fuzzy segmentations and P_{AB} is the pooled joint probability distribution.

1.4 Maximum Surface Distance (Hausdorff Distance)

The Hausdorff-Chebyshev metric defines the largest difference between two contours. Given two contours C and D, we first calculate for each point c on C the minimal distance to all the points on contour D, $d_c(c, D)$, $d_C(c, D) = \min\{d_{ps}(c, s), s \subset D\}$. We calculate this minimal distance for each boundary point and take the maximum minimal distance as the "worst case distance", $h_C(C, D) = \max\{d_C(c, D), c \in C\}$. The Hausdorff metric is not symmetric and $h_c(C, D)$ is not equal to $h_c(D, C)$ (see drawn figure), which is accounted for by finally calculating $H_C(C, D) = \max\{h_C(C, D), h_C(D, C)\}$. The Hausdorff metric calculation is computationally very expensive, as we need to compare each contour point to all the other ones. A comparison of complex 3D surfaces would require huge number of calculations. The VALMET implementation uses 3D Euclidean distance transform calculation on one object and overlay of the second object to efficiently calculate the measure. The measure is extremely sensitive to outliers and does not reflect properties integrated along the whole boundary or surface. In certain cases, however, where a procedure does have to stay within certain limits, this measure would be the metrics of choice.

1.5 Mean Absolute Surface Distance

The mean absolute surface distance tells us how much on average the two surfaces differ. This measure integrates over both over- and under-estimation of a contour, and results in an L^1 norm with intuitive explanation [Chalana 1997]. The calculation is not straightforward if point to point correspondence on two surfaces is not available. We use a similar strategy as for the Hausdorff metric calculation, namely signed Euclidean distance transforms on one object and overlay of the second object surface. We then trace the surface and integrate the distance values. This calculation is not symmetric, since distances from A to B are not the same as B to A (see discussion Hausdorff distance above). We therefore derive a common average by combining the two averages. The mean absolute distance, as opposed to binary overlap, does not depend on the object size. As a prerequisite, however, it requires existing surfaces and is therefore only suitable for single object comparison.

1.6 Interclass Correlation Coefficient for Assessing Intra-, Inter-rater and Rater-Machine Reliability

A common measure of reliability of segmentation tasks is the intraclass correlation coefficient. The measure calculates the ratio between the variance of a normally population and the "population of measurements", i.e. the variance of the population $\sigma_b^{\,2}$ plus the variance of the rater $\sigma_0^{\,2}$. The intraclass correlation is thus defined as

$$\rho = \frac{\sigma_b^{\,2}}{\sigma_b^{\,2} + \sigma_0^{\,2}}.$$ If the rater variance is small relative to the total, then the

variation in measurements among different cases will be due largely to natural variation in the population and thus close to 1. Hence we can be confident in the rater's reliability.

In neuroimaging applications, inter- and intra-rater reliability studies based on volumetric measurements have become standard. Commonly accepted values range from 0.9 to 0.99 for volume assessments with manual tracing of simply shaped subcortical structures or organs like kidneys and liver, for example.

2 Visualization of Intra- and Inter-rater Reliability

Visualization of intra- and inter-rater reliability on 2D cross-sections with label overlay and by 3D surface renderings is shown in Fig. 1. The concept is as follows: We load a 3D volumetric gray level image dataset and a series of segmentation results either by different raters or as repeated measurements of one rater into the tool. The labels are overlaid onto the original image with variable opacity. The 3D rendering reconstructs the 3D surfaces and displays either intra-rater or inter-rater variability as color overlays. This tool has shown its usefulness to act as a training tool for manual rater's segmentation. The new capability to visually assess rater differences on 2D slices and 3D views is new and not available by other packages.

Fig. 2 shows the screen of VALMET applied to hippocampus segmentation. Repeated 3D manual segmentations of the hippocampus provided by several experts are compared to qualitatively and quantitatively assess the intra- and inter-rater reliability. The tool displays three orthogonal cuts with overlay of labeled regions and a 3D surface rendering of the object boundaries. The hue indicates the local surface direction either inwards (blue, see color bar in Fig. 2) and outwards (red, again see color bar in Fig. 2) relative to the reference object and the distance between the surfaces, according to the metric chosen.

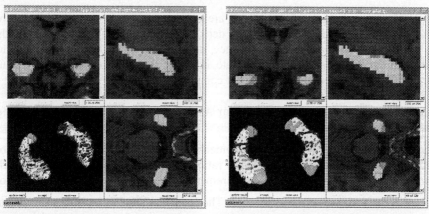

Fig. 1: Qualitative assessment of intra- and inter-rater reliability. The images show 2D orthogonal sections of a region of interest of the interior brain with segmentation of the left and the right hippocampal structures. Left: Intra-rater variability of 3 segmentations (observations) by one rater with yellow=3, green=2, and blue=1 votes per voxel. The 3D rendering displays the regional fuzziness of the boundary. Right: Inter-rater variability between two raters by comparison of two average segmentations. Yellow marks the region segmented by both, and blue and green regions segmented by only one of them. This displays clearly illustrates the agreement/disagreement between the raters, which is dominant in the hippocampus amygdala transition area (HATA) and the region of the hippocampal tail.

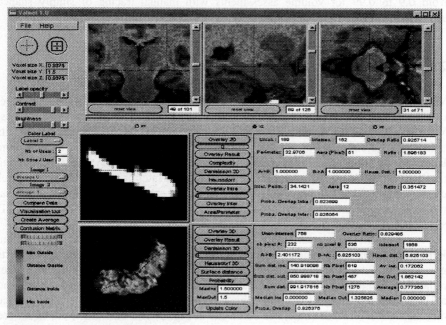

Fig. 2: User interface of VALMET. The tool calculates overlap measures, Hausdorff distance, mean absolute (and signed) surface distances, and probabilistic overlap. The 3D rendering provides a color display of both intersecting surfaces (green and red), showing regional differences between two surfaces. The application shows the result of a inter- and intra-rater hippocampus segmention study.

3. Segmentation Validation: Manual Hippocampus Segmentation

Unlike some anatomical structures the hippocampus as imaged through MRI has no clear boundaries, and it is very difficult to establish ground truth by manual segmentation. Hence it is very important to quantify variability in manual segmentations done by trained raters. As part of a large schizophrenia neuroimaging study, intra- and inter-rater reliability were tested with blind studies of series of 3D image data. For each series, we randomly selected 5 cases from an ongoing schizophrenia. The 5 cases were replicated 3 times and numbered randomly resulting in 15 image datasets, numbered differently for each rater. Trained raters go through all theses cases and segment left and right hippocampal structures using a new 3D segmentation tool IRIS [IRIS, 1999] developed by our group. The tool allows triplanar region editing and graphical 2D/3D interaction between image planes and segmented objects. We used an intraclass correlation program written in SAS (SAS Institute Inc.) to calculate intra- and inter-rater reliability.

Table 1 shows the reliability of two of the raters. We tested the reliability in two series, a first series after raters have been trained with the tools and became familiar with the instructions for hippocampus, and a second series after they evaluated and compared their results using the new tools described above. The results of the first series show that the reliability of raters A and B differs significantly between right and left hippocampus, each achieving a high reliability for one of the structures. The inter-rater reliability of 0.75 for the right and 0.62 for the left

Table 1: Reliability of manual hippocampus segmentation.

Intraclass Correlation: Manual Hippocampus Segmentation

Study design: 2 raters, 5 cases, 3 observations each
Analysis: Individual and pooled analysis

First reliability series

	individual analysis		pooled analysis	
	intra-rater rater A	intra-rater rater B	intra-rater A and B	inter-rater A vs. B
right hippocampus	0.89067	0.66422	0.77241	0.75062
left hippocampus	0.69061	0.85157	0.81391	0.61923

Second reliability series

	individual analysis		pooled analysis	
	intra-rater rater A	intra-rater rater B	intra-rater A and B	inter-rater A vs. B
right hippocampus	0.96073	0.88145	0.93229	0.67325
left hippocampus	0.95416	0.94822	0.96094	0.48218

522   G. Gerig, M. Jomier, and M. Chakos

hippocampus suggest that the left hippocampus is more difficult to segment than the right hippocampus. The second series was measured after the two raters visualized their segmentations using VALMET and revised the protocol. Interestingly, they both are becoming very reliable. This is reflected in reliabilities up to 0.95 and in the pooled intra-rater reliability of 0.93 and 0.96. However, the reliability between raters (inter-rater) became worse and dropped significantly from 0.75 to 0.67 for the right and from 0.61 to 0.48 for the left hippocampal structures. The second series used 5 different cases with 3 replications. In conclusion, we find that the intra-rater reliability for manual hippocampus segmentation was very high in comparison to studies done at other sites (Hogan 2000). A reliability of 0.95 for the manual segmentation of a structure as difficult as the hippocampus has to be considered excellent. We attribute this performance to the 2D/3D capabilities of the IRIS segmentation tool and VALMET. The inter-rater reliability is insufficient and reflects that both raters do excellent but different segmentations.

4. Discussion

No consensus exists regarding a necessary and sufficient set of measures to characterize segmentation performance. We plan to provide a suite comprising a reasonable variety of geometric and statistical methods. In addition to the measures already implemented in the prototype validation tool VALMET, we will consider providing a number of others including moments and volume of error voxels normalized by the surface area. Measures implemented in VALMET and other geometric measures reported in the literature tend to favor least squares measures. Measures in this class are intuitive and work well for noise-free data. However real medical images have structure noise and random noise that can lead to high spatial frequencies in segmented surfaces. Methods based on least-squares measures are very sensitive to even a small number of extreme data values in the sense that a small number of outlier voxels can disproportionately bias a measure and make an otherwise good segmentation appear to compare poorly with truth. Statistically robust methods include quantiles of distance, which are robust to extreme values. A next version of VALMET will include the calculation of a surface distance histogram and choice of arbitrary quantiles.

Bibliography

Bowyer, K.W., Phillips, P., Empirical Evaluation Techniques in Computer Vision, IEEE Computer Society, 1998
Chalana V and Kim Y: A methodology for evaluation of boundary detection algorithms on medical images, IEEE Trans. Med. Imaging 16: 642-652 (1997)
Hogan, R.E., Mark, K.E., Wang, L., Joshi, S., Miller, M.I. and Bucholz, R.D., Mesial Temporal Sclerosis and Temporal Lobe Epilepsy: MR Imaging Deformation-based Segmentation of the Hippocampus in Five Patients, Radiology 216, pp. 291-297, July 2000

IRIS (1999): Interactive Rendering and Image Segmentation, UNC student project spring 1999, Gregg, D., Larsen, E., Neelamkavil, A., Sthapit, S. and Wynn, Chris, Dave Stotts and Guido Gerig, supervisors, http://www.cs.unc.edu/~stotts/COMP145/homes/iris/

Kapur, T., Grimson, E.L., Wells, W.M., and Kikinis, R., Segmentation of brain tissue from magnetic resonance images, Medical Image Analysis, 1(2);109-127, 1996

Klette R, Stiehl SH, Viergever MA, and Vincken KL, eds: Performance Characterization in Computer Vision, Kluwer Academic Publishers (2000)

Niessen, W.J., Bouma, C.J., Vincken, K.L., Viergever, M.A., Error Metrics for Quantitative Evaluation of Medical Image Segmentation, in Performance Characterization in Computer Vision, Kluwer Academic Publishers, pp. 299-311, 2000

Remiejer P, Rasch C, Lebesque JV, and van Herk M: A general methodology for three-dimensional analysis of variation in target volume delineation. Med. Phys. 27: 1961-1970 (1999)

Vincken, K.L., Koster, A.S.E., De Graaf, C.N. and Viergever, M.A., Model-based evaluation of image segmentation methods, in Performance Characterization in Computer Vision, Kluwer Academic Publishers, pp. 299-311, 2000

A Dual Dynamic Programming Approach to the Detection of Spine Boundaries

Guo-Qing Wei[1], JianZhong Qian[1], and Helmuth Schramm[2]

[1] Imaging Department, Siemens Corporate Research, Inc.
755 College Road East, Princeton NJ 08536, USA
[2] Siemens AG, Medical Engineering
Erlangen, Germany

Abstract. Spine boundary is one of the key landmarks for quantifying deformities of pathological spines. In this paper, we propose a new approach to the detection of spine boundaries. We integrate two dynamic programming procedures into a single one to enable constraints between the left and right parts of the boundary to be enforced. This dual dynamic programming approach detects two boundary curves at the same time. Moreover we propose to use angular limits in a piecewise linear model as a new smoothness constraint. This leads to a computationally efficient way of introducing high order priors. Experimental results show a very robust performance of the method.

1 Introduction

Boundary or curve detection is a primary task in many computer vision and image processing applications. Currently, deformable models are the most popular ones used in the literature. Representative methods of this kind include the PDE (partial differential equation)-based active contour models [4,2], DP (dynamic programming) methods [1,3] and the level-set methods [5]. Since the level set methods are less flexible in incorporating prior knowledge, they will not be further pursued in this paper.

The active contour model [4] represents one major class of contour detection methods. In an active contour model, an object boundary is represented by a collection of points interacting with each other in a way to incorporate constraints from both physics and image data. Methods based on dynamic programming follows the same spirit of considerations, but use a different optimization method. Since both the active contour methods and the dynamic programming methods are based on the minimization of an energy function containing soft constraints (smoothness constraints), it is difficult, if not impossible, to explicitly control the shape of the final contour through any analytic forms for determining the smoothness weights. In addition, the dynamic programming method has a limitation that inclusion of higher order smoothness constraints will cause an exponential increase of the search space and of the computational complexity [1], limiting further the power of external control. Most distinctively, most previous

W. Niessen and M. Viergever (Eds.): MICCAI 2001, LNCS 2208, pp. 524–531, 2001.
© Springer-Verlag Berlin Heidelberg 2001

contour detection methods do not consider the simultaneous detection of two contours while maintaining constraints among them.

In this paper, we propose a new DP-based method to curve detection. We completely drop off the soft constraints and apply instead the limit constraints. This provides not only direct control over the final outcome of the detection, but also allows the use of high order shape constraints without sacrificing computational efficiency. Under this framework, we propose a dual-DP method that can detect two curves at the same time while maintaining constraints between them. The method is applied to the problem of spine boundary detection.

2   Dual Dynamic Programming Method

2.1   Problem Statement

A spine boundary consists of two special-property curves. They are the left and right boundaries of the spine, respectively. As a first property, both boundary curves are nearly vertical. Secondly, they are nearly parallel to each other. Figure 1 (a) depicts the left and right boundaries of a spine.

Properties delineating the spine boundaries from other anatomies are intensity edges, but what makes spine boundaries different from other boundaries or edges in other image processing tasks are that there are many anatomical structures interfering with the spine boundary. For example, there are ribs connecting to the spine, and between the left and right boundaries of the spine there are anatomies such as endplates or pedicles. These make both the boundary edge discontinuous and the region between the left and right boundaries inhomogeneous.

2.2   Piecewise Linear Model

To represent a spine boundary we propose a piecewise linear model. Since a spine is nearly vertical, we can parameterize the spine boundary by fixed, equally spaced points in the vertical direction. This is like to cut the image plane in vertical directions by a set of equally spaced cut lines. Suppose the y-coordinates of the cutting lines are $\{y_1, y_2, \dots, y_N\}$, where N is the number of cut lines. The left and right boundaries of the spine can be then represented by the nodal points $P_L = \{(x_{L,1}, y_1), (x_{L,2}, y_2), \dots, (x_{L,N}, y_N)\}$ and $P_R = \{(x_{R,1}, y_1), (x_{R,2}, y_2), \dots, (x_{R,N}, y_N)\}$, respectively. Since y_n's are fixed and predefined, the variables which control the shape of the boundaries are the x-coordinates $(x_{L,1}, x_{L,2}, \dots, x_{L,N})$ and $(x_{R,1}, x_{R,2}, \dots, x_{R,N})$. The spacing between the cut lines is chosen such that it reflects the shape scale of interest of the spine; we set it to approximately half of the average vertebra height. This parameter is either manually set or obtained from statistics. Figure 1 (b) shows a piecewise linear parameterization of the spine boundary of Figure 1 (a).

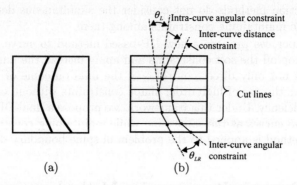

Fig. 1. The spine boundary model. (a) boundary curves; (b) piecewise linear model, with some geometric constraints illustrated.

2.3   Geometric Constraints

There are two kinds of shape constraints on a spine boundary: intra-curve and inter-curve. Intra-curve constraints describe shape constraints on individual boundary curves, whereas inter-curve constraints specify the correlations among them.

Under the piecewise linear model, intra-curve constraints place restrictions on **a)** the range of orientations of individual line segments, reflecting the fact that a spine is nearly vertical; **b)** the range of inter-segment angles for neighboring line segments, assuring that a smooth spine boundary is generated.

Denote the linear segments of the left and right boundaries by $S_L = \{\, s_{L,1}\,, s_{L,2}, ..., s_{L,N-1}\}$ and $S_R = \{s_{R,1}\,, s_{R,2}, ..., s_{R,N-1}\}$, respectively. The intra-curve constraints for the left boundary can be mathematically expressed as

$$O_{\min} < O(s_{L,n}) < O_{\max}; \quad n = 1, 2, ... N - 1 \tag{1}$$

and

$$\angle(s_{L,n}, s_{L,n+1}) < \gamma_{1,\max}; \quad n = 1, ... N - 2 \tag{2}$$

$$\angle(s_{L,n}, s_{L,n+1}) - \angle(s_{L,n-1}, s_{L,n}) < \gamma_{2,\max}; \quad n = 2, ... N - 2 \tag{3}$$

where $O_{\min}, O_{\max}, \gamma_{1,\max}$ and $\gamma_{2,\max}$ are threshold values, symbol $O()$ denotes the orientation of a segment, and $\angle(.,.)$ the angle between two segments. The same constraints can be written for the right boundary.

It is worthwhile mentioning that equations (2) and (3) represent the 1st order and 2nd order smoothness constraints expressed in angular measurements, respectively. There are two major differences between the smoothness constraint used here and those found in the conventional contour detection methods. The first obvious difference is that smoothness is measured in angles instead of the derivatives of the coordinates of nodal points. The advantage is that angles are rotational invariant, easier to understand and control: With bounds on the angles, we can explicitly control the space of admissible curves. On the contrary, in the conventional methods of using smoothness constraints, there is no explicit relationship between the values of smoothness weights and any wanted shape measurement in the final detection. The second difference is that our smoothness constraints will not appear in the cost function used for finding the boundary. This allows the use of high order constraints without causing exponential increase in the computational cost, as will be shown later.

To apply inter-curve constraints, limits are put on the angles between a segment in the left boundary and neighboring segments in the right boundary. As has already been noted, this constraint steams from the fact that the left and right boundaries of a spine are almost parallel. The 1st order inter-curve angular constraint can be written as

$$\angle(s_{L,n}, s_{R,n}) < \gamma_{LR,\max} \tag{4}$$

$$\angle(s_{L,n}, s_{R,n-1}) < \gamma_{LR,\max} \tag{5}$$

$$\angle(s_{L,n-1}, s_{R,n}) < \gamma_{LR,\max} \tag{6}$$

where $\gamma_{LR,\max}$ is the maximum angle allowed for local inter-curve segments.

Another inter-curve constraint specifies how vertebra width (or distances between nodal points) is allowed to change along the spine axis. Suppose W_n and W_{n+1} are the projections of the distances between corresponding nodal points onto directions orthogonal to the spine axis for the n-th and $(n+1)$-th cut lines, respectively. From the near-parallelism of the left and right boundaries, the inter-curve distance constraint can be written as

$$d_{\min} < W_{n+1}/W_n < d_{\max} \tag{7}$$

where $d_{\min}$ and $d_{\max}$ are predefined thresholds.

2.4 Hard Constraints

Hard constraints are external constraints specified by users as helps to the algorithm. One kind of such constraints are points on the boundary selected by users, e.g., per mouse click. The boundary curves are then required to pass through the given set of points. Suppose $Q_L = q_{L,i}, i = 1, .., K$ is a point set of this kind for the left boundary. Since the y-cutting lines are fixed, it is easy to determine which segment in the piecewise linear model should pass through which point. Suppose segment $s_{L,k}$ ought to pass through point $q_{L,i}$. The hard constraints for this condition can be written as

$$d(q_{L,i}, s_{L,k}) < \delta \tag{8}$$

where $d(q, s)$ denotes the distance from point q to segment s, and δ is a tolerance threshold close to zero. Similar hard constraints can be defined for the right boundary.

2.5   Optimization

Suppose $G(x,y)$ is the gradient magnitude of the spine image $I(x,y)$. The rule for finding the spine boundary is that it maximize the summed gradient magnitude along the path while satisfying all geometric and hard constraints. Formally, the segments $\{ s_{L,n} \}$ and $\{ s_{R,n} \}$ should maximize the following energy function

$$E = \sum_{n=1}^{N-1} (\sum_{(x,y)\in s_{L,n}} G(x,y) + \sum_{(x,y)\in s_{R,n}} G(x,y)) \qquad (9)$$

$$subject\ to : constraints\ (1) \sim (8) \qquad (10)$$

Note that in the above expression, all points on a segment, instead of only the nodal points, are contributing to the energy function. (This is usually not the case with many existing contour detection methods.) But since the pixels on a segment are completely determined by the nodal points, we can make it explicit the dependency of the above expression on the nodal coordinates by defining

$$S_G(x_{L,n}, x_{L,n+1}) = \sum_{(x,y)\in s_{L,n}} G(x,y) \qquad (11)$$

$$S_G(x_{R,n}, x_{R,n+1}) = \sum_{(x,y)\in s_{R,n}} G(x,y) \qquad (12)$$

Equation (9) can then be rewritten as

$$E = S_G(x_{L,1}, x_{L,2}) + S_G(x_{R,1}, x_{R,2}) + S_G(x_{L,2}, x_{L,3}) + S_G(x_{R,2}, x_{R,3}) + ...$$
$$+ S_G(x_{L,N-1}, x_{L,N}) + S_G(x_{R,N-1}, x_{R,N}) \qquad (13)$$

If there were no inter-curve constraints, the maximization of E in (13) could be obtained in two independent procedures, one for the left boundary, and the other for the right boundary:

$$E = E_L + E_R \qquad (14)$$

where E_L corresponds to the energy term of the left boundary:

$$E_L = S_G(x_{L,1}, x_{L,2}) + S_G(x_{L,2}, x_{L,3}) + ... + S_G(x_{L,N-1}, x_{L,N}) \qquad (15)$$

A similar form can be written for E_R of the right boundary. The maximization of a form like (15) can be attained by a standard 1-dimensional dynamic programming procedure.

In the presence of inter-curve constraints, however, the two boundaries must be considered collectively. If we define

$$X_{LR,n} = (x_{L,n}, x_{R,n}) \qquad (16)$$

$$S_G'(X_{LR,n}, X_{LR,n+1}) = S_G(x_{L,n}, x_{L,n+1}) + S_G(x_{R,n}, x_{R,n+1}) \qquad (17)$$

equation (13) can be arranged in a similar form to (15) and thus be maximized by the following recursive equations:

$$E'_2(X_{LR,2}) = \quad\quad \max_{X_{LR,1}} S'_G(X_{LR,1}, X_{LR,2}) \quad\quad (18)$$

$$E'_{n+1}(X_{LR,n+1}) = \max_{X_{L,n}}(S'_G(X_{LR,n}, X_{LR,n+1}) + E'_n(X_{LR,n})) \quad (19)$$

$$n = 2, ..., N-1$$

$$\max_{X_{L,1}, X_{L,2}, ..., X_{L,N}} E = \quad\quad \max_{X_{LR,N}}(E'_N(X_{LR,N})) \quad\quad (20)$$

This procedure is called *forward recursion* in this paper. We can think of it as the integration of two 1D DP's (thus the name *dual-DP*). The optimal path is obtained by *back-tracing* the maximum from the last cut-line.

In the recursive computation of the local optimal path for each point on cut-line $n + 1$ (refer to (19)), inter- and intra-curve constraints are enforced at the same time. For the orientation constraints (1), size constraints (7), and hard constraints (8), the variables $X_{LR,n+1}$ and $X_{LR,n}$ can be used directly to check whether these constraints are satisfied. If either of them is not, the path to $X_{LR,n+1}$ is made invalid. To exert the angular constraints (2)~(6), back-tracing is needed. For angular constraints of the k-th order it is necessary to trace back k steps from the maximum at $X_{LR,n}$. The locally traced segments are then checked to see whether the required constraints are satisfied. It is to note that in the conventional DP methods, back-tracing is used only in finding the final path when the last step of forward recursion has completed. In our approach, back-tracing is mixed with forward recursion. The computational cost of the extra backward tracing is negligible when compared with that of forward recursion, whereas in conventional DP methods the use of high order constraints will cause an exponential increase in the computational cost [1].

3   Experiments

3.1   Initialize the Search Area

To apply the piecewise linear model to spine boundary localization, the user needs to specify the first and last cut-lines in the image plane. We do this by manually selecting the beginning and ending points on the left and right spine boundaries. This provides also hard constraints on each boundary.

3.2   Examples

We first demonstrate how intra- and inter-curve constraints affect the detection results. Figure 2 (a) shows an original spine image. We set an orientation threshold at 60 degrees, and an inter-segment angular threshold at 50 degrees. Figure 2(b) shows the detected boundary curves with these intra-curve constraints applied, but without inter-curve ones. It can be seen that although the detected left boundary reflects well the true position of the spine's left boundary, the right boundary has serious errors due to the presence of a spurious strong edge

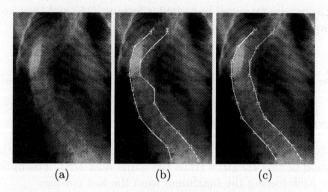

(a)   (b)   (c)

Fig. 2. The effects of inter-curve constraints. (a) the original spine image; (b) detected boundary without inter-curve constraints; (c) detected boundary by the dual-DP approach with inter-curve constraints.

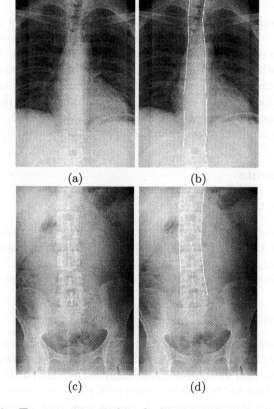

(a)   (b)

(c)   (d)

Fig. 3. Two more examples of spine boundary detection.

in the middle of the spine. With the inter-curve constraints, we get the detected curves shown in Fig. 2(c). By comparing Figs. 2 (b) and (c), we can see that the dual-DP method not only finds the correct position for the right boundary, but also improves the localization accuracy for the left boundary.

In the above example, the image size is 370× 520 pixels. It took 12 seconds on a Pentium III 500MHz PC to find the boundary.

Figure 3 shows two further examples of spine boundary detection by the dual-DP method. Even with gradual intensity changes (Fig.3(a)), a good localization can still be obtained.

The method has been tested on a small database of 14 images. The results are qualitatively evaluated by visual inspection. Except for one case which needs manual improvement, all other images give satisfactory and good localization results.

With the detected spine boundaries as reference positions, other anatomical landmarks can be searched for and used for quantifying the deformity of a pathological spine [6].

4   Conlusions

In this paper, we have presented a dual dynamic programming approach to the detection of spine boundaries. As a distinctive feature, the method is able to detect coupled curves simultaneously while keeping them constrained by each other by problem-specific priors.

We proposed a piecewise linear model for the representation of boundaries. Angular measurements between segments were used to replace the conventional coordinate-based smoothness constraint. Through bound limits, it is easier to control the final shape of the detected curves. High order priors can be imposed by the mixture of forward recursion and backward tracing, without causing extra computational burdens. Experiments show that reliable results have been achieved.

References

1. A. A. Amini, T.E. Weymouth, and R.C. Jain, "Using dynamic programming for solving variational problems in vision," *IEEE Trans PAMI*, Vol.12, No.9, 1990, pp.855-867.
2. L.D. Cohen, "Note: on active contour models and balloons," *CVGIP: Image Understanding*, Vol.53, no.2, pp.211-218, 1991.
3. D. Geiger, A. Gupta, L.A. Costa, and J. Vlontzos, "Dynamic programming for detecting, tracking, and matching deformable contours", *IEEE Trans PAMI*, Vol.17, No.3, 1995, pp.294-402.
4. M. Kass, A. Witkin, and D. Terzopoulos, "Snakes: Active contour models," *Proc. ICCV*, pp.321-331, 1988.
5. R. Malladi, J.A. Sethian, and B. C. Vemuri, "Shape modeling with front propagation", *IEEE Trans PAMI*, Vol.17, No.2, 1995, pp.158-175.
6. B. Verdon, et. al, "Computer Assisted Quantitative Analysis of Deformities of the Human Spine", *Proc. MICCAI* pp.822-831, 1998.

Geometrical Transformation Approximation for 2D/3D Intensity-Based Registration of Portal Images and CT Scan

David Sarrut[1] and Sébastien Clippe[2]

[1] ERIC laboratory
Université Lumière Lyon 2
5 Av. Pierre Mendès-France – 69676 Bron – FRANCE
dsarrut@univ-lyon2.fr
[2] Centre de Lutte Contre le Cancer Léon Bérard
28, rue Laënnec – 69008 Lyon – FRANCE
sclippe@univ-lyon2.fr

Abstract. Conformal radiotherapy treatments need accurate patient positioning in order to spare normal tissues. Patient pose can be evaluated by registering portal images (PI) with Digitally Reconstructed Radiographs (DRR). Several methods involve segmentation which is known to be a difficult task for noisy PI. In this paper, we study another approach by using a fully 3D intensity-based registration method, without segmentation. Our approach uses the correlation ratio as similarity measure and replace DRR generation with a treatment on pre-computed DRR. A specific geometrical transformation is applied to approximate a given projection by the composition of out-of-plane rotations and in-plane transformation. Some preliminary experiments on both simulated and real portal images, lead to good results (RMS error lower than 2 mm).

1 Medical Context

Introduction This work is done in collaboration with physicians from Lyon's Léon Bérard Institute (France) and concerns cancer treatment by conformal radiotherapy. The goal of radiotherapy is to accurately deliver a curative dose of X-rays (produced by linear accelerators) to the tumor while sparing surrounding normal tissues. With help of a computed tomography (CT) scan, physicians create a Radiotherapy Treatment Planning (RTP) which plans irradiation sessions, with one irradiation per day during several weeks. During each session, the patient must be in the same position as he was during CT acquisition.

However, it is a very difficult task to exactly position the patient in the same position each day and studies have shown that setup inaccuracies could lead to poorer local control or survival [1]. Numerous studies have evaluated displacements (see [2, 3]), they relate a mean setup error between 5.5 mm and 8 mm (the maximum could reach 18 mm). Even in recent series, displacements still remain important: 22 % of displacements are between 5 and 10 mm [2]

W. Niessen and M. Viergever (Eds.): MICCAI 2001, LNCS 2208, pp. 532–540, 2001.

and 57 % greater than 4 mm [3], despite the use of immobilization devices (such as polyurethan foam cast or thermoplastic mask). Such systems generally reduce setup errors but without eliminating all errors [4]. In order to control patient pose, a solution is to use images from EPID (Electronic Portal Imaging Devices) [5]. *Portal Images* (PI) are 2D projection images and are acquired with the irradiation device. By visual inspection, physicians have the possibility to roughly correct the position of the patient, but it is both inaccurate and time-consuming. Moreover, as conformal radiotherapy uses smaller margins around the target volume, high precision becomes more and more needed to be sure that no target is missed, with the risk of local recurrence.

We propose in this study an automatic method for setup errors evaluation. The next section presents related work, section 2 described the geometrical part of the registration and the intensity-based similarity measures. Experiments and results are in the section 3.

Related Works Several image registration methods have been used to compare control images (obtained from EPID or other modalities such as ultrasound images [6] or radiographic film [7]) with a reference image (CT scan). Most of the studies on this subject use a segmentation procedure: some features (bony structures) are extracted from the images and registered. Bijhold *et al.* [7] use a manual segmentation of bony outlines visible in both portal (a film) and reference images. Other methods [8, 3] use anatomical landmarks: several homologous points are determined in both images and then matched. Marker-based methods have also be proposed [9, 10]: they consist in the implantation of radio-opaque markers inside the body of the patient. However, the markers have to be fixed in the tumor volume, which is an important restriction for implantation. Fully 3D method was proposed in [11], and was based on the registration of a 3D surface extracted from the CT scan with several image contours, segmented from the PI. Numerous methods use digitally reconstructed radiographs (DRR). DRR are 2D projection images computed by a specific volume-rendering (pinhole projection model) from the CT-scan. Gilhuijs *et al.* [12] developed a 3D method with partial (segmented) DRR. However, the segmentation is a difficult task and often fails [13] because PI have very low contrast (due to the high energy, 5-20 Mega-volt). In order to avoid or help segmentation, some authors use intensity-based methods, based on a similarity measure computed with the value of (potentially) all the pixels (see section 2.3). Few works about 3D image registration using such techniques in this context have been published [14, 15, 16, 17].

2   Intensity-Based 2D/3D Registration

2.1   Overview of the Method

In this work, we focus on rigid transformation, denoted by T (3 translation and 3 rotation parameters). The CT scan is denoted by $\mathcal{V}$. In-plane (2D) registration of a single DRR with a single PI is known to be inaccurate in case of out-of-plane rotations or large translations [7, 18, 13]. Hence, we use *several* PI and *several* DRR. In practical situation, due to the limited amount of radiation received by the patient, two ($n = 2$) PI are acquired from orthogonal viewpoints. The ith PI is denoted by $\mathcal{I}_i$, and the corresponding projection matrices (obtained with a calibration procedure) are denoted by Q_i. Given a similarity measure $\mathcal{S}$, and $\mathcal{I}$ the vector of n PI's, the main 3D optimization procedure is:

$$\widehat{T} = \arg_T \max \mathcal{S}(\boldsymbol{QT}(\mathcal{V}), \boldsymbol{\mathcal{I}}) \tag{1}$$

In eq.(1), $\boldsymbol{QT}(\mathcal{V})$ denotes a vector of n DRR, according to the n projection Q_i and the patient displacement T. Each iteration of eq.(1) requires the (*on-line*) generation of n DRR. However, this is a too long process to be tractable. Several authors have study ways to speedup DRR generation [19, 12, 16], at the cost of DRR's quality (and thus the quality of the similarity criterion). We choose to study another solution which is to generate a set of DRR before the registration stage, when there is no time limitation.

2.2 Geometrical Transformation Approximation for DRR Generation

During an iteration of eq.(1), a DRR must be generated from a given projection QT (subscript i is omitted for clarity). It is obviously impossible to pre-generate DRR from all the possible orientations. Moreover, the space P of projections, even bounded to the space of plausible projections (*e.g.* rotations lower than 10 degrees, translations lower than 2 cm) has 6 dimensions, and it is difficult to efficiently sample this space. Our main idea is to reduce the dimensionality of P by only considering out-of-plane rotations (2 parameters) and using in-plane (2D) transformations to retrieve ideal projection QT. This decomposition assumes that the 3D displacements which make in-plane registration fail, are due to out-of-plane rotations. Obviously, this is not theoretically true because the projection model is a pinhole one. However, the distance between the camera and the patient is much more larger than the patient displacement amplitude, and our experiments show that this approximation is sufficient for our purpose. We are thus looking for a decomposition, described by out-of-plane rotations (apply before projection by Q) and by in-plane transformation (after Q), which is the closest to the projection of a given position QT.

We denote by Oz the projection direction. We decompose a 3D rotation into *out-of-plane* and *in-plane* rotations. In-plane rotation is around axe Oz. We denote by $R_{\alpha,\Delta}$ the out-of-plane rotation of angle α around the axe Δ. Axe Δ goes through the iso-center O, is orthogonal to the projection direction Oz, and Δ is parameterized with a single parameter, the angle β according to the Ox axe (see figure 1). Then, the objective projection QT is replaced by $LQR_{\alpha,\Delta}$, with L an in-plane transformation. In order to find α, β and L for a given T, we perform a least square optimization, see eq.(2).

$$\left.\begin{array}{c} L_T \\ R_T \end{array}\right\} = \arg_{L,\alpha,\Delta} \min \sum_{\boldsymbol{x} \in H} \left(QT(\boldsymbol{x}) - LQR_{\alpha,\Delta}(\boldsymbol{x}) \right)^2 \tag{2}$$

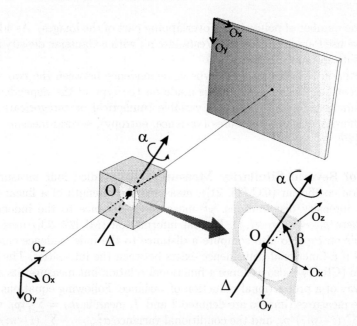

Fig. 1. Out-of-plane rotation according to a projection direction Oz, parameterized with angle α around axe Δ in the $OxOy$ plane.

In eq.(2), L can have 3 (2 translations and a rotation) or 4 parameters (with a scaling factor). The set H is composed of random points $x \in \mathbb{R}^3$. This optimization is performed with the Powell-Brent method described in [20]. The subspace of P, described with the two parameters α and β, can now be sampled. By bounding such space to plausible rotations and by choosing a sampling rate (for example 0.5 degrees), it is possible to generate a set DRR before patient treatment. In conclusion, we replace the expensive DRR generation required at each iteration of eq. (1) by a two-pass approach: optimization eq.(2) and application of the in-plane transformation L_T on the pre-computed DRR given by projection R_T.

2.3 Intensity-Based Similarity Measures

Joint Histograms. The relative position of two images is evaluated with an intensity-based similarity measure which requires no segmentation. Measures, such as correlation coefficient [21], mutual information [22, 23] or correlation ratio [24], are all based on joint histograms (even if we do not need to explicitly compute it). A joint histogram, denoted by H_L, is a 2D histogram computed according to a transformation L between the two images. Quantities $H_L(i,j) = n_{ij}$ are computed by summing for each couple of intensities (i,j), the number of co-occurrent pixels. Probabilities p_{ij} ($p_i = \sum_j p_{ij}$, $p_j = \sum_i p_{ij}$) must then be estimated from n_{ij}. Most authors used a frequential estimation ($p_{ij} = \frac{n_{ij}}{n}$, with n the number of points in the overlapping part of the images). As advocated in [23], we use Parzen windowing to estimate p_{ij} with a Gaussian density function (probabilities are locally averaged).

A criterion $\mathcal{S}$ measures some type of dependence between the two distributions: according to the assumptions made on the type of the dependence (*e.g.* linear, functional), on the type of variable (numerical or categorical), and by using different *diversity* measures (variance, entropy), several measures can be defined [25].

Study of Several Similarity Measures. We studied four measures. The correlation coefficient (CC [26, 21]), measures the strength of a linear relation between intensity distributions. χ^2 measures a distance to the independence case (where $p_{ij} = p_i\,p_j\ \forall i,j$). Mutual information (MI [22, 23]) uses relative Shannon's entropy to also compute a distance to the independence case. MI is maximal if a functional dependence exists between the intensities. The correlation ratio (CR [24]) also assumes a functional relation but measures its strength by the way of a proportional reduction of variance. Following equations express the three measures (images are denoted I and J, mean is $m_I = \sum_i ip_i$, variance is $\sigma_I^2 = \sum_i(i-m_I)^2 p_i$, and the conditional variance $\sigma_{I|j}^2 = \frac{1}{p_j}\sum_i(i-m_{I|j})^2 p_{ij}$):

$$CC(I,J) = \sum_{ij} \frac{(i-m_I)(j-m_J)}{\sigma_I\,\sigma_J} p_{ij} \qquad \chi^2(I,J) = \sum_{ij} \frac{(p_{ij}-p_ip_j)^2}{p_ip_j}$$

$$MI(I,J) = \sum_{ij} p_{ij}\log\frac{p_{ij}}{p_ip_j} \qquad CR(I|J) = 1 - \frac{1}{\sigma_I^2}\sum_j p_j\sigma_{I|j}^2$$

Interpolation is performed by *partial volume* [22]. CR is not a symmetric criterion (whereas the others are) and an image (I) must be chosen to estimate the other (J): the optimization eq.(1) compares the same PI with several DRR and CR is normalized according to I, so we decided to choose $I = DRR$ and $J = PI$. We do not discuss further the properties of such measures, interested reader could see [22, 23, 24, 25].

In eq.(1), $\mathcal{S}$ must quantify similarity between a *vector* of images couples. A solution can be to perform a linear combination of the similarity values between each couples $\sum_i^n \alpha_i\,\mathcal{S}(DRR_i,\mathcal{I}_i)$. However, it is not clear how to determine the weights α_i. So, we propose the following original solution: for each images couples, we update the same joint histogram. Then, a similarity measure (whatever it is) can be computed from the unique histogram. Moreover, this force the criterion to measure the same type of dependence for all the images couples.

3   Experiments

Materiel and Method A CT-scan of an anthropomorphic phantom was acquired (88 slices, thickness 3 mm, 512^2 pixels of size $0.87^2\ mm^2$). The artificial object was positioned on the irradiation table according to several random positions. For each position, two orthogonal PI were acquired (see figure 2). Size of irradiation field corresponds to realistic treatment (about $15^2\,cm$ at the isocenter, 280^2 pixels). We performed two sets of experiments: with simulated data and with real PI. Simulated PI are generated from DRR computed from known displacement. Noisy aspect is simulated by smoothing the DRR and adding large Gaussian noise. Quality of such images was assessed by physician (see figure 2).

Parameters of the initial projection matrices Q_i are obtained from a calibration procedure between CT and accelerator coordinate systems. For each position (with generated or real PI), we performed our method in order to obtain an estimation of the position. The set of pre-computed DRR is the following: out-of-plane rotations were taken between $-7°$ and $+7°$ with a sample step $k = 0.5°$, leading to $30 \times 30 = 900$ images. Each estimation was performed with the same set of parameters, the starting point of the optimization was randomly chosen.

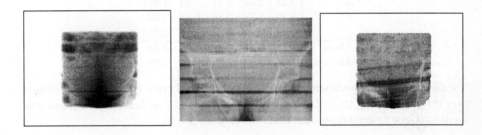

Fig. 2. Portal image, DRR and simulated PI.

Results For each position i we compute the RMS (Root Mean Square) error, denoted by ε_i, between the estimation found by our method and the reference position. The RMS error is the average distance (in millimeter) between points transformed by the two compared transformations. We used 1000 points spread inside a cube of $15^3\,cm^3$ centered at the target point (the tumor) in order to obtain a realistic error; a RMS error of $x\,mm$ means that, in average, each point is $x\,mm$ away from the desired position. ε_r denotes the RMS error of the displacement to be retrieve. Table 1 summarizes results on 100 positions from simulated images. It depicts mean, median and percentage of estimations which improve the initial position ($\varepsilon_r > \varepsilon_i$). Table 2 summarizes results of tests on 7 real couples of PI. For each position, it depicts the initial error ε_r and final error ε_i, obtained with different measures. Last lines depict mean and median RMS error. Estimations with RMS lower than $3\,mm$ are displayed in grey boxes.

In the first experiment, the four measures are significantly different (using mixed model two ways ANOVA[1]), $p < 10^{-6}$. Using least significant difference test, neither CR and MI, nor CC and χ^2 are significantly different (0.01 level). But, these two groups are significantly different. For CR and MI, RMS error

---

[1] Analyze of Variance

	ε_r	CC	χ^2	MI	CR
Mean	10.07	3.78	4.63	2.10	2.75
Median	10.24	2.83	4.39	0.85	1.20
$\varepsilon_r > \varepsilon$	—	92%	94%	99%	99%

Table 1. First experiment on simulated PI (100 positions): RMS error according to each similarity measure: mean, median, percentage of improvement.

Positions	ε_r	CC	χ^2	MI	CR
1	6.00	2.41	2.78	1.47	1.43
2	6.00	9.79	12.83	21.00	2.00
3	10.00	2.54	15.99	2.88	2.46
4	7.00	2.52	1.18	2.68	1.29
5	3.21	3.62	7.27	5.34	1.95
6	5.29	5.38	3.36	5.82	4.33
7	9.18	18.64	4.49	5.16	2.51
Mean	5.83	5.61	5.99	5.54	1.99
Median	5.34	2.65	2.73	2.75	1.62

Table 2. Second experiment on real PI: initial RMS error (ε_r) and final estimation error according to each similarity measure. Last two lines depict mean and median. Grey boxes emphasize RMS lower than 3 mm.

decreases from 10 mm to 1.2/0.85 mm (CR/MI). The second experiment shows weak results with CC and χ^2, but also with MI. However, estimations with CR manage to recover patient pose in almost every cases (only one RMS is greater than 3) and always improve incorrect pose.

4   Conclusion

We have presented in this paper an original method for patient pose estimation using 2D portal images and 3D CT scan. The method is fully 3D, avoids segmentation, uses several PI, uses pre-generated DRR and is an intensity-based registration procedure. In the experimental tests, we obtain good position estimations both for simulated and real PI (median RMS is about 1.2 mm with simulated images and 1.6 mm for real PI). Our approach can be used with any number of PI (thanks to the unique JH, updated for each couple of images) and with any types of PI (by use of different similarity measures based on JH, such as MI or CR). The overall procedure is very fast, less than 3-4 minutes to complete on a common workstation (Ultra Sparc 5, 333 Mhz). The presented method is fully automatic and does not require any user intervention. The sampling of the set of pre-computed DRR plays an important role in the accuracy of the estimation. Experimental results show that 0.5° is a good tradeoff between precision and volume storage.

Further works are ongoing to improve the optimization procedure, and experiments on larger set of images are planned. The presented method is only valid for rigid body transformation, but we plan to study non-rigid deformations and organs displacements with the same principles (DRR generation and 2D transformations).

Acknowledgments

This work is supported by the *Région Rhône-Alpes* under the grant *AdéMo* ("Modélisation et suivi spatio-temporel pour le diagnostique et la thérapie").

References

[1] C. Carrie, S. Hoffstetter, and F. Gomez et al. Impact of targeting deviations on outcome in medulloblastoma: study of the french society of pediatric oncology (SFOP). *Int. J. Radiat. Oncol. Biol. Phys.*, 45(2):435–9, September 1999.

[2] U. Mock, K. Dieckmann, U. Wolff, T.H. Knocke, and R. Potter. Portal imaging based definition of the planning target volume during pelvic irradiation for gynecological malignancies. *Int. J. Radiat. Oncol. Biol. Phys.*, 45(1):227–232, 1999.

[3] J.C. Stroom, M.J. Olofsen van Acht, and S. Quint et al. On-line set-up corrections during radiotherapy of patients with gynecologic tumors. *Int. J. Radiat. Oncol. Biol. Phys.*, 46(2):499–506, 2000.

[4] C.M. Nutting, V.S. Khoo, V. Walker, H. McNair, C. Beardmore, A. Norman, and D.P. Dearnaley. A randomized study of the use of a customized immobilization system in the treatment of prostate cancer with conformal radiotherapy. *Radiother. Oncol.*, 54(1):1–9, 2000.

[5] P. Munro. Portal imaging technology: past, present, and future. *Sem. Radiat. Oncol.*, 5(2):115–133, 1995.

[6] G. Ionescu, S. Lavalle, and J. Demongeot. Automated registration of ultrasound with ct images: Application to computer assisted prostate radiotherapy and orthopedics. In *MICCAI'99*, volume 1679 of *LNCS*, pages 768–777, Cambridge, England, September 1999.

[7] J. Bijhold, M. van Herk, R. Vijlbrief, and J.V. Lebesque. Fast evaluation of patient set-up during radiotherapy by aligning features in portal and simulator images. *Phys. Med. Biol.*, 36(12):1665–79, 1991.

[8] J. Van de Steene, F. Van den Heuvel, and A. Bel et al. Electronic portal imaging with on-line correction of setup error in thoracic irradiation: clinical evaluation. *Int. J. Radiat. Oncol. Biol. Phys.*, 40(4):967–976, 1998.

[9] K.L. Lam, R.K. Ten Haken, McShan DL, and Thornton AF Jr. Automated determination of patient setup errors in radiation therapy using spherical radioopaque markers. *Med Phys*, 20(4):1145–52, 1993.

[10] K.P. Gall, L.J. Verhey, and M. Wagner. Computer-assisted positioning of radiotherapy patients using implanted radiopaque fiducials. *Med. Phys.*, 20(4):1153–9, 1993.

[11] S. Lavallée and R. Szeliski. Recovering the Position and Orientation of Free-Form Objects from Image Contours Using 3D Distance Maps. *IEEE Transactions on Pattern Analysis and Machine Intelligence*, 17(4):378–390, April 1995.

[12] K.G. Gilhuijs, K. Drukker, A. Touw, P.J. van de Ven, and M. van Herk. Interactive three dimensional inspection of patient setup in radiation therapy using digital portal images and computed tomography data. *Int. J. Radiat. Oncol. Biol. Phys.*, 34(4):873–85, 1996.

[13] P. Remeijer, E. Geerlof, L. Ploeger, K. Gilhuijs, M. van Herk, and J.V. Lebesque. 3-D portal image analysis in clinical practice: an evaluation of 2-D and 3-D analysis techniques as applied to 30 prostate cancer patients. *Int. J. Radiat. Oncol. Biol. Phys.*, 46(5):1281–90, 2000.

[14] D. Plattard, G. Champleboux, P. Vassal, J. Troccaz, and M. Bolla. EPID for patient positioning in radiotherapy: calibration and image matching in the entroPID system. In H.U. Lemke, editor, *CARS'99*, pages 265–9. Elsevier science, 1999.

[15] R. Bansal, L. Staib, Z. Chen, A. Rangarajan, J. Knisely, R. Nath R, and J. Duncan. A minimax entropy registration framework for patient setup verification in radiotherapy. *Computer Aided Surgery*, 4(6):287–304, 1999.

[16] R. Goecke, J. Weese, and H. Schumann. Fast volume rendering methods for voxel-based 2d/3d registration - a comparative study. In *International Workshop on Biomedical Image Registration*, pages 89–102, Bled, Slovenia, August 1999.

[17] D. Sarrut and S. Clippe. Patient positioning in radiotherapy by registration of 2D portal to 3D CT images by a contend-based research with similarity measures. In *Computer Assisted Radiology and Surgery*, pages p 707–712, San Fransisco, USA, June 2000. Elsevier Science.

[18] J. Hanley, G.S. Mageras, J. Sun, and G.J. Kutcher. The effects of out-of-plane rotations on two dimensional portal image registration in conformal radiotherapy of the prostate. *Int. J. Radiat. Oncol. Biol. Phys.*, 33(5):1331–1343, 1995.

[19] G.P. Penney, J. Weese, J.A. Little, P. Desmedt, D.L.G. Hill, and D.J. Hawkes. A comparison of similarity measures for use in 2D-3D medical image registration. *IEEE Transaction on Medical Imaging*, 17:586–595, 1998.

[20] W.H. Press, B.P. Flannery, S.A. Teukolsky, and W.T. Vetterling. *Numerical Recipes in C: The Art of Scientific Computing*. Cambridge University Press, second edition, 1992.

[21] D.H. Hristov and B.G. Fallone. A grey-level image alignment algorithm for registration of portal images and digitally reconstructed radiographs. *Med Phys*, 23(1):75–84, 1996.

[22] F. Maes, A. Collignon, D. Vandermeulen, G. Marchal, and P. Suetens. Multimodality Image Registration by Maximization of Mutual Information. *IEEE Transaction On Medical Imaging*, 16(2):187–198, April 1997.

[23] W.M. Wells, P.A. Viola, H. Atsumi, S. Nakajima, and R. Kikinis. Multi-Modal Volume Registration by Maximization of Mutual Information. *Medical Image Analysis*, 1(1):35–51, 1996.

[24] A. Roche, G. Malandain, X. Pennec, and N. Ayache. The Correlation Ratio as a New Similarity Measure for Multimodal Image Registration. In *MICCAI'98*, pages 1115–1124, Cambridge Massachusetts (USA), October 1998.

[25] D. Sarrut. *Recalage multimodal et plate-forme d'imagerie médicale à accès distant.* PhD thesis, Université Lumière Lyon 2, January 2000. In french.

[26] L. Dong and A.L. Boyer. An image correlation procedure for digitally reconstructed radiographs and electronic portal images. *Int. J. Radiat. Oncol. Biol. Phys.*, 33(5):1053–60, 1995.

Elastic Matching Using a Deformation Sphere

J. Lötjönen[1] and T. Mäkelä[2,3,4]

[1] VTT Information Technology, P.O.B. 1206, FIN-33101 Tampere, Finland
{Jyrki.Lotjonen@vtt.fi}
[2] Laboratory of Biomedical Engineering, Helsinki University of Technology, P.O.B. 2200,
FIN-02015 HUT, Finland
[3] CREATIS, INSA, Batiment Blaise Pascal, 69621 Villeurbanne Cedex, France
[4] BioMag Laboratory, Helsinki University Central Hospital, P.O.B. 503,
FIN-00029 HUCS, Finland

Abstract. A novel method is proposed for elastic matching of two data volumes. A combination of mutual information, gradient information and smoothness of transformation is used to guide the deformation of another of the volumes. The deformation is accomplished in a multiresolution process by spheres containing a vector field. Position and radius of the spheres are varied. The feasibility of the method is demonstrated in two cases: matching inter-patient MR images of the head and intra-patient cardiac MR and PET images.

1 Introduction

Proper interpretation and comparison of medical volumes from different modalities can be accomplished by transforming all data into common spatial alignment, also referred to as registration [1]. In many cases, a satisfactory solution can be found by using rigid registration, i.e. a volume is only translated and rotated. The registration algorithms can be coarsely divided into three groups which register: 1) a set of landmark points, such as external markers and anatomic landmarks [2], 2) geometric image features, such as edges [3], and 3) image intensity based similarity measures, such as mutual information (MI) [4,5]. Algorithms combining these groups exist too, e.g. Pluim *et al.* [6] used geometric features and intensity based similarity measures.

Elastic registration or matching is required as inter-patient volumes or regions containing non-rigid objects are registered. The goal is to remove structural variation between the two volumes to be registered. Many approaches have been proposed for the problem in recent years [7,8,9,10,11,12]. In the method proposed by Christensen *et al.* [7], physical properties of either elastic solids or viscous fluids were simulated as the model was deformed. The criterion for the deformation was to minimize the difference in voxel gray values between two volumes while constraining the transformation to be smooth. Wang and Staib [8] used intensity similarity combined with statistical shape information. The formulation of the elastic model was similar to the one used by Christensen *et al.* but the information on typical deformations, derived from individuals, was incorporated to guide the deformation. Thirion [9] developed a fast 3D matching method based on Maxwellian demons. The displacement vectors for the model were derived from an optical flow equation and smoothed by Gaussian filtering. MI was utilized in non-rigid registration by Gaens *et al.* [10]. In their approach, neighborhood

W. Niessen and M. Viergever (Eds.): MICCAI 2001, LNCS 2208, pp. 541–548, 2001.
© Springer-Verlag Berlin Heidelberg 2001

regions around each point of a discrete lattice were locally translated so that MI was increased. Then, the calculated displacement, filtered by a Gaussian kernel, was applied to the points in the neighborhood. The process was iterated by decreasing gradually the size of the neighborhood and by using a multiresolution approach. Rueckert *et al.* [11] proposed a method where they applied MI and imposed the smoothness of the transformation to constrain the matching. The deformation of data was accomplished using a free-form deformation (FFD) deformation grid. Collins *et al.* [12] maximized a correlation between voxels in two volumes while simultaneously smoothing the transformation by the average displacement vector around each voxel of interest. FFD was used to deform the model. A multiresolution approach was applied.

If one volume to be registered is an atlas, i.e. a volume where the tissue classes of the voxels are known, the result of elastic matching provides also a segmentation. The use of elastic models or deformable models, such as snakes, in the segmentation is a widely studied field in medical image processing [13].

We propose a method by which a model volume with gray-scale information or an atlas consisting of gray-scale data and a set of triangulated surfaces is elastically matched to a data volume. In order to perform the registration, a weighted sum of three energy components is maximized. The first component is the MI between the images [4] while the second component is derived from the intensity gradients of the images [6]. The third component controls either the smoothness of the transformation [11] or the shape of the surfaces in the atlas [14]. The model is deformed using deformation spheres where the transformation is computed only for the model points inside the spheres. A high number of spheres with varying position and radius is used. In addition, a multiresolution approach is adopted.

2 Methods

In this study, the model used is a gray-scale volume taken from an individual. If the segmentation of the objects of interest is available, triangulated surfaces of these objects are incorporated in the model, i.e. the model is an atlas. In practice, the model contains also a gradient volume computed from the gray-scale data using a Canny-Deriche operator.

The multi-resolution approach is adopted. A low resolution volume is produced by Gaussian filtering and subsampling a high resolution volume. The matching is done first at the lowest resolution level. As the maximum energy is attained, the process is repeated for a higher resolution level.

Rigid registration is required before elastic transformation if the two volumes have significantly different initial positions. For reference, the mispositioning of the lungs by 5 cm was, however, recovered by the elastic matching in our tests.

In the following, the gray-scale volume of the model is referred to as a *volume M*, and the data volume taken from a patient, and to which the model is matched, *volume D*. Consequently, a sample point, i.e. a voxel, from the volume M is $\mathbf{m} = (m_1, m_2, m_3)$ and from the volume D $\mathbf{d} = (d_1, d_2, d_3)$. The transformation applied to the sample points in the model volume is denoted by $\mathbf{T} : (x, y, z) \mapsto (x', y', z')$.

2.1   Energy Function

The motivation in using more than one energy term is to create an energy function with less local minima and therefore to make matching more robust [6]. The energy components provide complementary information on the matching: the gradient component incorporates spatial information while the regularization of the transformation aims to preserve, in a way, the prior knowledge of the shape of the object.

Mutual information. MI measures the degree of dependence between the volumes M and D. MI is high if the gray-scale value of the voxel i in D can be estimated with a high accuracy as the gray-scale value of the corresponding voxel in M is known. If the gray-scale values of the volumes M and D are considered random variables A and B, respectively, the MI, proposed in [4] and denoted here by energy E_{MI}, is be computed from the equation:

$$E_{MI} = \sum_{a,b} p_{AB}(a,b) log \frac{p_{AB}(a,b)}{p_A(a)p_B(b)}, \tag{1}$$

where $p_A(a)$ and $p_B(b)$ are marginal probabilites and $p_{AB}(a,b)$ is the joint probability distribution. $p_A(a)$ is the probability that the gray-scale value of a voxel is a in volume M. $p_{AB}(a,b)$ is the probability that the corresponding voxels in the volumes M and D have the gray-scale values a and b.

Joint gradient information. The points in the model should match similarly oriented points in the data. The method used is a simplified version of [6]. The energy component E_{grad} derived from the gradients is computed as follows:

$$E_{grad} = \frac{1}{N} \sum_{(\mathbf{m},\mathbf{d}) \in (M \cap D)} \frac{\nabla \mathbf{m} \cdot \nabla \mathbf{d}}{|\nabla \mathbf{m}||\nabla \mathbf{d}|} min(|\nabla \mathbf{m}|, |\nabla \mathbf{d}|). \tag{2}$$

where N is the number of model points overlapping the volume D. Because a minimum of gradients is used in two volumes, the intensity ranges need to be set nearly similar in the both volumes.

Since the gray-scale value of a tissue depends on imaging sequence or imaging modality, the gradients on the edges of the tissue may have opposite directions in different volumes. If this is the case with volumes M and D, Eq. 2 is modified by taking an absolute value from the dot-product.

Regularization of transformation. The transformation $\mathbf{T}$ can be constrained to be smooth by incorporating the energy component $E_{model,1}$ [11]:

$$E_{model,1} = \frac{1}{N} \sum_{x,y,z} [(\frac{\partial^2 \mathbf{T}}{\partial x^2})^2 + (\frac{\partial^2 \mathbf{T}}{\partial y^2})^2 + (\frac{\partial^2 \mathbf{T}}{\partial z^2})^2 + 2(\frac{\partial^2 \mathbf{T}}{\partial x \partial y})^2 + 2(\frac{\partial^2 \mathbf{T}}{\partial x \partial z})^2 + 2(\frac{\partial^2 \mathbf{T}}{\partial y \partial z})^2], \tag{3}$$

where the sum is over all voxels in the model volume and N is the number of points summed. The energy term is the 3D counterpart of the 2D bending energy associated to a thin-plate metal. To speed up computations only three first terms are used in practice.

Alternatively, if the surface model is available, the smoothness of the transformation can be controlled by constraining the change in the shape of the model surfaces. In our study [14] where a boundary element template was matched to volume data, various regularization strategies were tested. The method with the aim of preserving the orientation of the model's surface normals was preferred. This method is applied also in this study. The energy component is computed as follows:

$$E_{model,2} = \frac{1}{N_{tr}} \sum_{i=1}^{N_{tr}} \mathbf{n}_i \cdot \mathbf{n}_i^o, \tag{4}$$

where N_{tr} is the total number of triangles in the model, $\mathbf{n}_i$ and $\mathbf{n}_i^o$ are the deformed and the original directions of the normal of the triangle i, respectively.

Total energy. The model is deformed by maximizing the following energy function:

$$E_{total} = E_{MI} + \alpha E_{grad} + \beta E_{model}, \tag{5}$$

where α and β are user-defined weight parameters for the energy components.

2.2   Model Deformation

In our earlier study [14], a boundary element template was deformed using a FFD grid. Since the relative positions of the control points and the model points can not be arbitrarily chosen, the opportunity to control the transformation is limited. In this work, a volumetric transformation is used but the transformation can be better focused on the regions of interest. The potential of the method to include statistical shape information on the deformation is discussed in Section 4.

All model points, including voxels and surface points, inside a deformation sphere are transformed. The center $c = (c_1, c_2, c_3)$ and the radius r of the sphere can be freely chosen. In practice, a high number of spheres (tens of thousands) are applied sequentially. The transformation vector $\mathbf{v}$ for a model point at (x, y, z) inside the sphere is computed as follows:

$$\mathbf{v} = \frac{e^{-k\frac{(x-c_1)^2+(y-c_2)^2+(z-c_3)^2}{r^2}} - e^{-k}}{1.0 - e^{-k}} \mathbf{V}, \tag{6}$$

where $\mathbf{V}$ is a movement vector posed to the center of the sphere and k is a parameter which specifies the sharpness of the weight function. A 2D version of the weight function with $k = 3$ is visualized in Fig. 1.a.

The vector $\mathbf{V}$ is chosen in such a way that it maximizes the energy in Eq. 5. In practice, the center of the sphere is displaced to several locations, the model is deformed and energy computed, and the location having the highest energy is chosen. The user can define the number of locations tested (N_{loc}) around the center as well as the maximum displacement for the center (s), e.g. $s = 0.3r$. The six closest neighbors in 3D are always included in the set of tested locations. In Fig. 1.b, the grid around the center of the sphere, shown by a circle in 2D, represents the search space and visualizes the possible new locations for the center. The locations tested are shown by gray squares and the center by a black square. The motivation for testing several locations is that the simple gradient descent method is known to attach relatively easily to local energy minima or maxima. In this strategy, the energy function is maximized more globally.

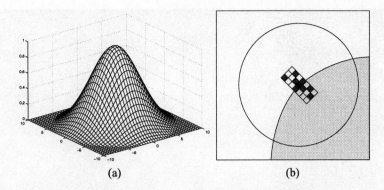

(a)   (b)

Fig. 1. *(a) A 2D weight function for the deformation ($r = 10$). (b) A 2D search space visualized in the center of the sphere ($N_{loc} = 8$).*

By default, the maximum displacement s is equal in all directions. In other words, the search space is cubic. However, many methods applying deformable models prefer deformations in the direction of the surface normals. This approach can be followed, if the surface is available in the model. The approach is accomplished as follows. First, define all surface points inside the sphere and compute the average of the surface normals by weighting each normal according to the weight in Eq. 6. Denote the length of the average vector by q. Then, define $s = s$ in the direction of the average and $s = (1 - q)s$ in orthogonal directions. In Fig. 1.b, the surface is represented in 2D by the contour around the light gray object. Since the average of the surface normals inside the sphere is approximately in the diagonal direction, the value of $q \approx 1$. Therefore, the search space is highly anisotropic and the diagonal displacements are privileged.

By default, the locations of the spheres are randomly chosen inside the model volume M. However, if the surface information is included in the model, the locations are randomly chosen at the positions of the surface points. The model should contain surfaces for the regions which are required to be well matched in the final result. For example, if the lung borders are to be segmented from the image, the transformation inside and outside the borders are not of great interest. The use of the surfaces locates the deformation to the most interesting regions, and it speeds up the process because a great part of the volume is excluded, such as background. However, the spheres used at the lowest resolutions levels contain usually the whole or the most of the model, and allow therefore global transformation also for the regions far from the edges.

In the beginning of the deformation, the radius of the spheres is high. As the energy does not change more than a user-specified limit ϵ during an iteration, the radius of the sphere is reduced. The user can set the maximum and minimum radius. The number of spheres used in one iteration is relative to the volume of the model divided by the volume of the sphere.

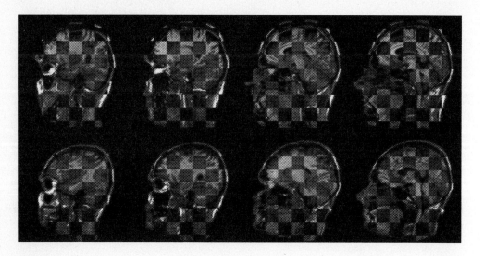

Fig. 2. *Matching of two T1-weighted MR volumes from the head. The top row shows the model and patient data interlaced before matching and the bottom row after elastic matching.*

3 Results

The method was developed for two purposes. 1) An automated method was needed by which individualized geometric models can be built for bioelectromagnetic inverse problems from magnetic resonance (MR) images. 2) Elastic matching of cardiac MR and positron emission tomography (PET) images taken from a patient was also needed.

In Fig. 2, the top row shows the original model and patient data interlaced using a chessboard visualization. The bottom row presents the same volumes after the model was elastically matched with the patient data. By visual inspection the edges of anatomic objects appear well aligned after elastic matching, i.e. edges are reasonably continuous between the chess-boxes. The typical run time of the program is 5–15 minutes using a 600 MHz Pentium as the size of the volumes is about $128 \times 128 \times 100$. In this case, the surface information was available and four resolution levels were used. The weights used in Eq. 5 were $\alpha = 2$ and $\beta = 10$. However, the result does not change appreciably as the weight values several times higher or lower are used. The radius of deformation spheres varied from 20 to 6 voxels.

Fig. 3 visualizes a result for cardiac MR-PET matching as the MR volume was the model. The top row shows the volume interlaced before elastic matching and the bottom row after matching. The left ventricle is matched reasonably well, e.g. the matching of the septum is indicated by the white arrows. In this case, the images were not rigidly registered before elastic matching. As the rigid registration is used, the images appear often well aligned already before the elastic transformation. The accurate assessment of the result is difficult because of highly blurred PET images. Therefore, the conditions for the use of elastic matching should be carefully evaluated in future studies.

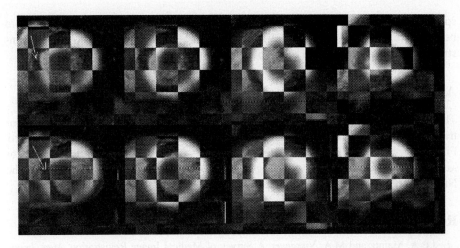

Fig. 3. *Matching of cardiac MR and PET volumes from the left ventricle. The top row shows the model and patient data interlaced before elastic matching and the bottom row after matching.*

4   Discussion

Elastic matching and segmentation of data volumes is often a pre-requisite for a successful diagnosis and treatment of a patient. This work proposes a method by which this image processing problem can be solved with a reasonable accuracy in a few minutes. So far, the method has been, however, tested only for a few volumes and the results are therefore preliminary.

Although the program allows several parameters to tune the matching, the values do not need to be often varied in practice. Proper parameter values for the energy components depend on imaging modality. If intra-modality anatomic images, such as MRI or computerized tomography (CT), are used, gradient information is weighted more in Eq. 5. However, mutual information should have a major impact on images which have very smooth gradients, such as PET images. The more pathologic the images are, i.e. the images to be matched are highly different or noisy, the more the transformation should be regulated.

Two methods to compute E_{model} was presented. If a surface is not included in the model, only the smoothness of the transformation can be controlled. If the surface is available, the method regulating the normal directions is recommended, because it makes the run time remarkably shorter.

The method will be further improved by including statistical shape information. This can be done by defining typical transformations for various positions of the model. In the current version of the method, the deformations in the direction of the surface normals are preferred. However, information could be incorporated from test data for which the typical transformations are known, and constrain deformations to typical orientations. In the current version, all transformation vectors inside the sphere are parallel. Typical transformations could be better simulated, if curved transformations inside the sphere were applied. In addition, more general shapes than a sphere could be used to bound deformation regions, such as a "banana-shaped" object. This would allow constraining the deformation to a more specific region if necessary.

Acknowledgements

The authors express thanks to The Department of Radiology, Helsinki University Central Hospital, Finland, INSERM Unité 280, Lyon, France, and Turku PET Centre, Turku, Finland for providing volume images. The authors thank also Dr Patrick Clarysse for his constructive comments concerning the manuscript. Research was supported by the National Technology Agency, Finland.

References

1. J.B.A. Maintz and M.A. Viergever. A Survey of Medical Image Registration. *Med. Image Anal.*, 2(1):1–36, 1998.
2. K.S. Arun, T.S. Huang and S.D. Blostein. Least-Squares Fitting of Two 3-D Point Sets. *IEEE Trans. Pattern Anal. Machine Intell.*, 9(5):698–700, 1987.
3. P.A. Van den Elsen, J.B.A. Maintz, E-J.D. Pol and M.A. Viergever. Automatic Registration of CT and MR Brain Images Using Correlation of Geometrical Features. *IEEE Trans. Med. Imag.*, 14(2):384–396, 1995.
4. F. Maes, A. Collignon, D. Vandermeulen, G. Marchal and P. Suetens. Multimodality Image Registration by Maximization of Mutual Information. *IEEE Trans. Med. Imag.*, 16(2):187–198, 1997.
5. P. Viola and W.M. Wells III. Alignment by Maximization of Mutual Information. *Int. J. Comp. Vision*, 24(2):137–154, 1997.
6. J.P.W. Pluim, J.B.A. Maintz and M.A. Viergever. Image Registration by Maximization of Combined Mutual Information and Gradient Information. *IEEE Trans. Med. Imag.*, 19(8):809–814, 2000.
7. G.E. Christensen, M.I. Miller, M.W. Vannier and U. Grenander. Individualizing Neuroanatomical Atlases Using a Massively Parallel Computer. *IEEE Computer*, January, 1996.
8. Y. Wang and L.H. Staib. Elastic Model Based Non-rigid Registration Incorporating Statistical Shape Information. *Lecture Notes in Computer Science 1496: Medical Image Computing and Computer-Assisted Intervention, MICCAI98, editors W.M. Wells, A. Colchester and S. Delp*, Springer, 1162–1173, 1998.
9. J-P. Thirion. Fast Non-Rigid Matching of 3D Medical Images. *INRIA Report 2547*, 1995.
10. T. Gaens, F. Maes, D. Vandermeulen and P. Suetens. *Lecture Notes in Computer Science 1496: Medical Image Computing and Computer-Assisted Intervention, MICCAI98, editors W.M. Wells, A. Colchester and S. Delp*, Springer, 1099–1106, 1998.
11. D. Rueckert, L.I. Sonoda, C. Hayes, D.L.G. Hill, M.O. Leach and D.J. Hawkes. Nonrigid Registration Using Free-Form Deformations: Application to Breast MR Images. *IEEE Trans. Med. Imag.*, 18(8):712–721, 1999.
12. D.L. Collins, C.J. Holmes, T.M. Peters and A.C. Evans. Automatic 3-D Model-Based Neuroanatomical Segmentation. *Human Brain Mapping*, 3:190-208, 1995.
13. T. McInerney and D. Terzopoulos. Deformable Models in Medical Image Analysis: a Survey. *Med. Image Anal.*, 1(2):91–108, 1996.
14. J. Lötjönen, P-J. Reissman, I. E. Magnin and T. Katila. Model Extraction from Magnetic Resonance Volume Data Using the Deformable Pyramid. *Med. Image Anal.*, 3(4):387–406, 1999.

Affine Registration with Feature Space Mutual Information

Torsten Butz and Jean-Philippe Thiran

Swiss Federal Institute of Technology (EPFL), Signal Processing Laboratory (LTS),
CH-1015 Lausanne, Switzerland
{torsten.butz, jp.thiran}@epfl.ch,
http://ltswww.epfl.ch/~brain, FAX: +41-21-693-7600

Abstract. This paper introduces two important issues of image registration. At first we want to recall the very general definition of mutual information that allows the choice of various feature spaces to perform image registration. Second we discuss the problem of finding the global maximum in an arbitrary feature space. We used a very general parallel, distributed memory, genetic optimization which turned out to be very robust. We restrict the examples to the context of multi-modal medical image registration but we want to point out that the approach is very general and therefore applicable to a wide range of other applications. The registration algorithm was analysed on a LINUX cluster.

1   Introduction

In the last years mutual information (MI) has had a large impact on multi-modal signal processing in general and on medical image processing in particular. Since the initial work of Viola et al. [1] and Maes et al. [2] several groups have analysed the modification of the optimization objective MI itself. The work is so rich, that a comprehensive overview would over-charge this paper. We still want to mention the work of Studholme et al. [3] who introduced normalized mutual information to rigidly register multi-modal images with different fields of view, Pluim et al. [4] who added a gradient-based term to the MI in order to decrease the number of local maxima and Rueckert et al. [5] who used second order entropy estimation to model the dependency of a voxel's gray value on the intensities of a local neighborhood around that voxel.

On the other hand, several papers discuss image registration with image features. Maintz et al. [6] studied different ridge detectors and used correlation for multi-modal image registration. In [7], Rangarajan et al. discussed feature point registration with MI. This direct combination of image features with MI is very interesting as it fuses two approaches that have mostly been treated independently in the literature. Our own work continues along this line and merges most of the approaches mentioned above in one single formalism. For this we simply used the fact that MI is defined on an arbitrary probability space, i.e. an arbitrary feature space (Figure 1).

W. Niessen and M. Viergever (Eds.): MICCAI 2001, LNCS 2208, pp. 549–556, 2001.
© Springer-Verlag Berlin Heidelberg 2001

Unfortunately the behavior of MI in an arbitrary feature space is very hard to predict. As a consequence, most optimization schemes would get stuck in local maxima. Viola et al. [1] proposed stochastic gradient descent in order to avoid local maxima. Nevertheless this approach avoids mainly maxima that are related to imaging noise but is still just locally convergent. For example the symmetry in brain images can cause stochastic gradient descent to fail (e.g. front/back and left/right symmetry). This might be a minor problem in the context of brain images, as a rough interactive registration can easily be performed in order to avoid these local optima. When passing to more complex feature spaces than the widely used intensity space, the number and positions of local maxima may make this approach impossible.

Therefore we used genetic optimization for maximization of MI in a general feature space. We propose a multi-scale genetic optimization and implemented a master/slave parallelization scheme [8]. The genetic optimization itself is based on the open source library written by Matthew Wall [9]. We added the communication utilities for distributed memory architectures using the MPICH implementation of the "Message Passing Interface" (MPI) [10], [11].

2   Methods

2.1   Feature Space Mutual Information

MI is a widely used information theoretical distance measure between probability densities [12]. Let's shortly recall its definition: Let X and Y be two random variables with marginal probability distributions $p(x)$ and $p(y)$, and joint probability distribution $p(x,y)$, then the MI between X and Y is:

$$I(X;Y) = H(Y) - H(Y|X) \tag{1}$$

$$\text{(evt. discretisation)} = \sum_{x,y} p(x,y) \cdot log(\frac{p(x,y)}{p(x) \cdot p(y)}) \tag{2}$$

where $H(.)$ stands for the Shannon-Wiener entropy of a continuous or discrete random variable. X and Y are arbitrary random variables and can therefore stand for discrete, continuous, single-variate or multi-variate variables. In order to calculate the MI between two signals, a representative observation of the signal has to be taken (choice of an adequate feature space). Then a probability estimation will create a probabilistic model of the signal from the observation. The sampling space is therefore arbitrary, but should be chosen to model the signal as accurately as possible. This is summarized in figure 1.

In [1], the measured features are simply the voxel intensities, in [5] the sampling space is defined by the intensities of two neighbored voxels (i.e. a two-dimensional feature space) and in [7] it is defined by the voxel being or not being a particular feature point (i.e. a discrete feature space). For the latter, the maximum entropy principle is used for density estimation [13].

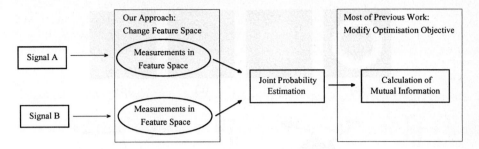

Fig. 1. We show the general pipeline to estimate the MI of two signals. Instead of modifying the MI itself, we analyse the choice of different sampling or feature spaces.

In this paper, we restrict the discussion to a feature space that can be represented by continuous variables, called edgeness. We never conclude from this measurement on whether a specific voxel is an edge or not. This fact allows us to use joint-histogramming to estimate the joint probability of the two images. The approach is very general and can easily be extended to other image features or to the combination of different feature types.

2.2   Edgeness Measure

We have tested two different edgeness measures. The first is simply the norm of the gradients. The second is slightly more complex, as it considers the intensity variance within a variable distance from the voxel. Let's call d a fixed radius and d_0 the coordinate vector of a voxel. It's edgeness is defined as:

$$c(d_0) = \sum_{|d_i - d_0| < d} |g(d_i) - g(d_0)| \tag{3}$$

where $g(.)$ stands for the image intensities. Figures 2 a) through d) show an output from this operator. Other edgeness operators are possible.

2.3   Parallel Genetic Optimization

So far, the presented approach is very similar to the well known maximization of MI, except that we recalled that MI is by far not restricted to the intensity space. The problem with other spaces is the presence of local maxima which will cause local optimization algorithms to fail. Let's underline the fact that stochastic gradient descent does not solve this problem, as the local maxima are effectively present in the feature space MI and are not due to imaging noise. Figure 2 should clarify the problem.

In order to find the global maximum, we have to use a globally convergent algorithm. We employed Matthew Wall's genetic algorithm library [9], but won't discuss genetic optimization in this text. [14] is a good introductory reference.

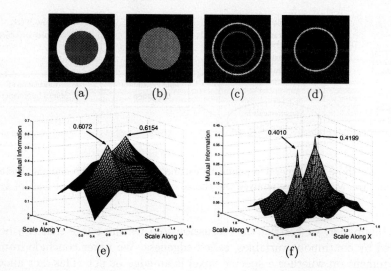

Fig. 2. To show the problem of feature space MI for affine registration, we present two template images of concentric circles (a and b) as well as their edgeness images (c and d) defined by equation 3 respectively. We see that both, the intensity based MI (e) as well as the edgeness MI (f) have local maxima. But the edgeness based measure has more and very pronounced local maxima, which underlines the necessity of a globally convergent optimization scheme.

We will neither discuss the parallelization scheme which we added on top of the genetic optimization. Let's just mention that it's known as a master/slave parallelization [8] with a SPMD (Single Program Multiple Data) model. The parallelization is independent of the objective function to be optimized and can therefore be used for any chosen feature space. For further speed-up we used a multi-scale genetic optimization.

3   Results

3.1   Affine, Multi-modal, Inter-patient Image Registration

Multi-modal affine registration is a very important task for image registration as it gives a good initialization for several non-rigid registration algorithms [15], [16]. In this study, we registered MR-scans onto a CT reference image of another patient (inter-patient) and compared the gradient based MI with the intensity based MI. The results for two MR-scans are shown in figure 3. Their interpretation, in particular of the images e/f) and l/m) resp., is presented in 4.

3.2   Angiograms of the Retinal Blood Vessels

In this study, we show that the presented feature space MI combined with the globally convergent genetic optimization can extend the MI based image registration to other medical applications.

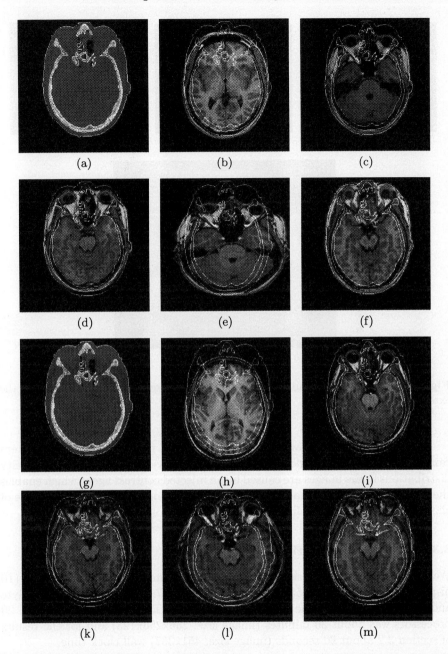

(a)   (b)   (c)

(d)   (e)   (f)

(g)   (h)   (i)

(k)   (l)   (m)

Fig. 3. a) is the CT-target image. In b), the contours of the target image are superposed on the floating MR-scan. In c) and d) we see the results after a rigid optimization, when using resp. the intensity based MI and the edgeness MI. In e) and f) we show the corresponding results for affine registration. Figures g) through m) show the results for a second MR-scan. In e) and f) (resp. l) and m)) we recognize a significant improvement with the edgeness based MI; resp. that the global maximum of intensity based MI doesn't correspond to good registration.

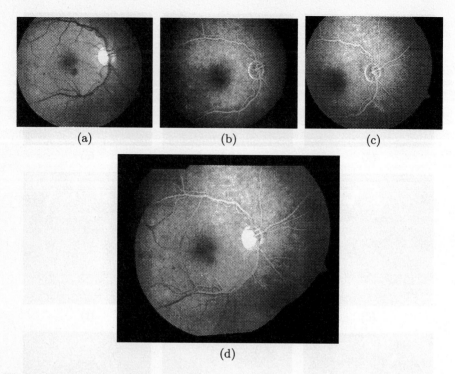

(a)   (b)   (c)

(d)

Fig. 4. The figures a), b) and c) had first to be registered in order to reconstruct the extended view shown in d).

In figure 4 we show how three partial views of the retinal vascular system can be combined to provide a virtually extended view. The different intensity distributions in the images are caused by an injected contrast agent which enables the study of the retinal blood flow for diabetic retinopathy. The feature space of choice was the edgeness defined in eq. 3 with an atom radius d of 5 pixels.

3.3 Genetic Optimization

We ran the parallel, genetic optimization algorithm on a LINUX cluster (10 bi-processor PCs: 2x PIII 550MHz each. Memory: 7x 512MByte, 2x 256MByte and 1x 384MByte). For the results of section 3.1, the execution time for all 20 processors was about 30 minutes (image size: 256x256x123) and for the results of section 3.2 about 90 seconds (image size: 451x367) wall clock time.

4 Discussion

In section 3.1 we have compared the gradient based MI with intensity based MI. For rigid registration the quality of the results is comparable, while for affine transformations the global maximum of intensity based MI might not correspond to good registration and the presented feature space defines a much better result. The edgeness defined by the gradient emphasizes contours in the medical images while the intensity based MI over-emphasizes the volumetric information in the scans and therefore risks to neglect finer but important features in the images. An example is the skull and the brain: The brain covers lots of volume while the human skull is a relatively fine but anatomically important structure. Therefore the intensity based registration favors the statistical matching of the brain. On the other hand the gradient based MI reflects the statistical presence of surfaces. As a result, the skull and the brain have about the same importance and a compromise for their fitting is obtained. Figure 3, in particular the images e/f) and l/m) resp., shows a significant improvement with this approach.

In section 3.2 we have shown an additional application of image registration where the chosen feature space has been adapted to the image contents. The example also underlines the importance of a globally convergent optimization scheme as the fine blood vessels in the retina give rise to local optima due to "accidental" partial matching of non-corresponding short vessel segments. The global optimization forces convergence to maximum matching and therefore towards correct registration of the entire vessels and not just vessel segments.

Finally the timing results showed that the genetic optimization can be competitive when a parallel implementation is used. From a practical point of view, optimal results can be obtained when a local optimization refines the output of the genetic optimization.

5   Conclusion

This paper shows that specifically designed feature space MI out-performs the widely used intensity based MI optimization for several medical registration tasks. The mathematical expression of MI itself doesn't constrain the choice of feature spaces and therefore incorporates the described approach.

The described drawback of local maxima in the optimization objective can be solved by globally convergent genetic optimization. A parallel implementation provides a powerful algorithm for a wide range of optimization tasks.

Future work will study and compare additional feature spaces (e.g. multi-dimensional spaces) and its applications to other registration tasks. It's important to note that the curse of dimensionality in multi-variate density estimation [17] limits the maximum possible dimension of the chosen feature space.

6   Acknowledgements

We want to thank Conor Heneghan, Ph.D., (Digital Signal Processing Laboratory, University College Dublin) for providing the fundus images of section 3.2.

References

[1] W.M. Wells III, P. Viola, H. Atsumi S. Nakajima, and R. Kikinis, "Multi-modal volume registration by maximization of mutual information," *Medical Image Analysis*, vol. 1, no. 1, pp. 35–51, March 1996.

[2] F. Maes, A. Collignon, D. Vandermeulen, G. Marchal, and P. Suetens, "Multimodality image registration by maximization of mutual information," *IEEE Transactions on Medical Imaging*, vol. 16, no. 2, pp. 187–198, April 1997.

[3] C. Studholme, D.J. Hawkes, and D.L.G. Hill, "An overlap invariant entropy measure of 3d medical image alignment," *Pattern Recognition*, vol. 32, pp. 71–86, 1999.

[4] Josien P.W. Pluim, J.B. Antoine Maintz, and Max A. Viergever, "Image registration by maximization of combined mutual information and gradient information," October 2000, vol. 1935, pp. 452–461.

[5] D. Rueckert, M.J.Clarkson, D.L.G. Hill, and D.J. Hawkes, "Non-rigid registration using higher-order mutual information," in *Proceedings of SPIE 2000*, February 2000, pp. 438–447.

[6] J.B. Maintz, Petra A. van den Elsen, and Max A. Viergever, "Evaluation of ridge seeking operators for multimodality medical image matching," *Transactions on Pattern Analysis and Machine Intelligence*, vol. 18, no. 4, pp. 353–365, April 1996.

[7] Anand Rangarajan, Haili Chui, and James S. Duncan, "Rigid point feature registration using mutual information," *Medical Image Analysis*, vol. 3, no. 4, pp. 425–440, 1999.

[8] Erick Cantú-Paz, "A survey of parallel genetic algorithms," Tech. Rep., The University of Illinois, 1997, IlliGAL Report No. 97003, ftp://ftp-illigal.ge.uiuc.edu/pub/papers/IlliGALs/97003.ps.Z.

[9] Matthew Wall, *GAlib 2.4.5: A C++ Library of Genetic Algorithm Components*, Massachusetts Institute of Technology, http://lancet.mit.edu/ga/.

[10] W. Gropp and E. Lusk, *User's Guide for mpich, a Portable Implementation of MPI Version 1.2.1*, http://www-unix.mcs.anl.gov/mpi/mpich/.

[11] W. Gropp, E. Lusk, and A. Skjellum, *Using MPI: Portable Parallel Programming With the Message-Passing Interface*, MIT Press, second edition, 1999.

[12] T.M. Cover and J.A. Thomas, *Elements of Information Theory*, John Wiley & Sons, Inc., 1991.

[13] E.T. Jaynes, "On the rationale of maximum-entropy methods," *Proceedings of the IEEE*, vol. 70, no. 9, pp. 939–952, 1982.

[14] David E. Goldberg, *Genetic Algorithms in Search, Optimization, and Machine Learning*, Addison-Wesley Publishing Company, Inc., 1989.

[15] A. Guimond, A. Roche, A. Ayache, and J. Meunier, "Multimodal brain warping using the demons algorithm and adaptative intensity corrections," Tech. Rep., Inst. National de Recherche en Informatique et en Automatique, Sophia Antipolis, 1999.

[16] Jean-Philippe Thiran and Torsten Butz, "Fast non-rigid registration and model-based segmentation of 3d images using mutual information," in *Medical Imaging*, 2000, pp. 1504–1515.

[17] L. Devroye, *A Course in Density Estimation*, Birkhäuser, 1987.

A New Method for the Registration of Cardiac PET and MR Images Using Deformable Model Based Segmentation of the Main Thorax Structures

Timo Mäkelä[1,2], Patrick Clarysse[2], Jyrki Lötjönen[3], Outi Sipilä[4], Kirsi Lauerma[4], Helena Hänninen[5,7], Esa-Pekka Pyökkimies[1], Jukka Nenonen[1], Juhani Knuuti[6], Toivo Katila[1,7], and Isabelle E. Magnin[2]

[1] Laboratory of Biomedical Engineering, Helsinki University of Technology, P.O.B. 2200, FIN-02015 HUT, Finland
{Timo.Makela, Toivo.Katila}@hut.fi
[2] CREATIS, INSA, Batiment Blaise Pascal, 69621 Villeurbanne Cedex, France
{Patrick.Clarysse, Isabelle.Magnin}@creatis.insa-lyon.fr
[3] VTT Information Technology, P.O.Box 1206, FIN-33101 Tampere, Finland
Jyrki.Lotjonen@vtt.fi
[4] Department of Radiology, Helsinki University Central Hospital, P.O.B. 340, FIN-00029 HUS, Finland
[5] Division of Cardiology, Helsinki University Central Hospital, P.O.B. 340, FIN-00029 HUS, Finland
[6] Turku PET Centre, c/o Turku University Central Hospital, Box 52, FIN-20521, Finland
[7] BioMag Laboratory, Helsinki University Central Hospital, P.O.B. 503, FIN-00029 HUS, Finland

Abstract. Integration of magnetic resonance (MR) and positron emission tomography (PET) images of the heart has proved its usefulness for the estimation of the myocardial viability. In this paper, a method for the rigid registration of cardiac MR and PET images is presented. It is based on the matching of the surfaces of thorax structures extracted by a deformable model from PET transmission and MR transaxial images. MR short axis registration with PET emission image is easily derived and allows the study viability in the proper anatomic conditions. The method has been evaluated on ten patients suffering from three vessel coronary artery disease. Qualitative results were good with 9 over the 10 available cases. A quantitative estimation of the registration quality confirmed the nice abilities of this approach.

1 Introduction

The combination of multiple cardiac image modalities like Magnetic Resonance Imaging (MRI) and Positron Emission Tomography (PET), has gained an increasing interest for physiologic understanding and diagnostic purposes, specially

W. Niessen and M. Viergever (Eds.): MICCAI 2001, LNCS 2208, pp. 557–564, 2001.

for viability studies. The combination requires the geometric alignment i.e. registration of multimodal images. This is a difficult problem mainly due to the continuous motion of the heart. Methods to correlate PET cardiac studies by using a surface based image registration technique of PET transmission images has been presented in [1] and [2]. In this work, we propose a new method for cardiac transaxial and short axis (SA) MR and PET image registration. A preliminary approach has been presented in [3]. Here, the method has been greatly improved by substituting the manual segmentation of the thorax structures by a deformable model based automatic segmentation. The data and the method are presented in section 2. The registration results are presented in section 3 and discussed in section 4.

2   Material and Method

2.1   Data

The data set is composed of MR and PET images of ten patients suffering from three vessel coronary artery disease [4]. Mean age was 69 (8 men, 2 women). All patients underwent MR and fluorine-18-deoxyglucose (FDG) PET imaging within 10 days. The MR imaging was performed at the Department of Radiology of Helsinki University Central Hospital with a 1.5 T Siemens Magnetom Vision imager (Siemens, Erlangen, Germany). A series of 39 ECG-gated contiguous transaxial images was acquired during free respiration using TurboFLASH sequence with the body array coil (Fig. 1a). The pixel size and the slice thickness were 1.95 x 1.95 mm and 10 mm, respectively. Five ECG-gated breath-hold cine SA slices covering the ventricles were also acquired. The pixel size for SA slices was 1.25 x 1.25 mm and the slice thickness 7 mm with a gap of 15 mm between slices (Fig. 1b).

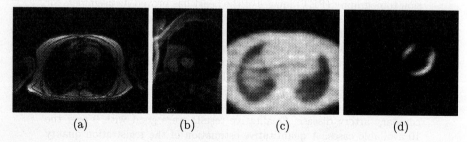

(a)   (b)   (c)   (d)

Fig. 1. (a) Transaxial and (b) SA MR images of the thorax and heart, (c) PET transmission and (d) emission images.

PET imaging was performed at the Turku PET Centre using a Siemens ECAT 931/08-12 (Siemens/CTI, Knoxville, USA) PET scanner. A series of 16 contiguous transmission and emission images was acquired. The pixel size and the slice thickness were 2.41 x 2.41 mm and 6.75 mm, respectively (Fig. 1c, d).

2.2   Registration Protocol

The proposed registration method is based on the matching of the thorax and lungs surfaces which are visible in both PET transmission and MR transaxial images. The registration protocol first matches PET transmission and transaxial MR images and then computes the SA PET slices that correspond to the SA MR slices. The main steps are:

1) Image resizing to get the same isotropic voxel dimensions. Tri-linear interpolation was used.

2) Segmentation of the thorax and lungs was performed for the transaxial MR and PET transmission images by a deformable model based method [5] which is summarized in subsection 2.3.

3) Selection of a set of points from the segmented surfaces of the thorax and lungs in the PET model. The uniformly distributed nodes of the deformable model were used.

4) Calculation of the rigid registration parameters (3 translations, 3 rotations) to find the best matching between the point set and the surface of the segmented MR image. The minimization algorithm is explained in subsection 2.4.

5) Registration of the PET emission image to the transaxial MR image using the computed registration parameters.

6) Registration of SA MR images with PET data. Slice position information contained in the MR image header provides the transformation between transaxial MR and SA MR slices. The SA PET slices corresponding to SA MR images are computed using the estimated parameters of the transformation.

2.3   Deformable Model Based Segmentation

The segmentation of the thorax structures is based on the elastic deformation of a topologic and geometric prior model using a multiresolution approach [5]. A thorax model including full triangulated thorax and lungs surfaces was used with transaxial MR images (Fig. 2a). With the transmission PET images, a truncated model with only a part of the thorax was used (Fig. 2b).

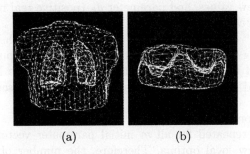

(a)   (b)

Fig. 2. Geometric and topologic prior model of the thorax for (a) transaxial MR and (b) transmission PET image segmentation.

The deformation algorithm adapts the prior model to locally fit the salient edges in the image within a minimization process. The energy to be minimized is

$$E_{total} = E_{image} + \gamma E_{model}, \tag{1}$$

where E_{image} represents the matching error between the prior model and the partial edges in the data volume. E_{model} tends to preserve the model's shape by restricting the deformation of the prior model. It describes the deviation of the model's surface normals from their original orientation. The image energy results from a distance map [6] built upon edges extracted either by a Canny-Deriche method [7] or image thresholding. In order to select corresponding edges with the model, oriented distance maps [5] were used. The parameter γ sets the contribution of the two energy components. A multiresolution process speeds up the minimization of the energy and improves the convergence.

2.4 Estimation of the Rigid Transformation

The 6 rigid registration parameters (3 translations, 3 rotations) result from the best match between the set of the nodes of the triangulated surfaces extracted from the PET transmission image and the surfaces of the segmented MR image. The optimal transformation minimizes the sum of the distances between the transformed points and a distance map built upon the segmented MR surfaces using the chamfer distance transformation [6].

For the sake of simplicity, the minimization algorithm is described here only for 2 parameters representing, for example, the translation in x- and y-directions on a 2-D plane. The extension to 6 parameters is straightforward. The parameters to be optimized form the parameter vector (t_1, t_2). The optimal parameter vector is iteratively searched in the discrete search space. The initial position for the parameter vector is (t_{1o}, t_{2o}) (Fig. 3). The iteration steps for the search of a new parameter vector are as follows:

1) Possible values for the parameter t_k, $k \in [1,2]$ are $t_k\text{-}gd_k$, $t_k\text{-}(g\text{-}1)d_k,.. t_k, ..,$ t_k+gd_k, where g is a user-defined positive integer parameter affecting the number of the possible new values, and parameter d_k (positive real number) represents the magnitude by which the parameter t_k is varied.
2) For all $(2g+1)^n$ combinations of the parameter vector, where n is the number of parameters (big dots in Fig. 3), the cost function is computed.
3) A user-defined number of combinations, m, having the lowest registration error, are selected for the new initial parameter vectors (selected positions of step 1, Fig. 3).
4) Each d_k-component is divided by 2.
5) Steps 1-2 are repeated for all m initial parameter vectors. Then, steps 3-4 provides an new local optima. Therefore, the number of initial parameter vectors remains constant during the iterations. Iterations are repeated until the cost function does not decrease more than a user-predefined value ϵ.

The algorithm does not necessarily converge to a global minimum of the cost function. However, the method samples the search-space more than a basic gradient descent method and allows find a minimum with a higher probability. The sampling of the search space is controlled by the parameters g and d_k. In addition, the computation time is only a few seconds, which is generally not the case with global optimization algorithms.

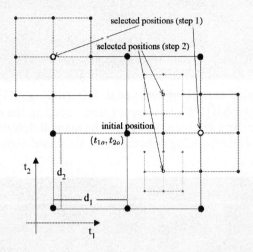

Fig. 3. Principle for the search of the optimal translation parameters.

3   Results

3.1   Segmentation Results

Three multiresolution levels were used (for image data, model and deformation grid). Canny-Deriche method or image thresholding were used for the edge extraction. Fig. 4 presents the segmentation results of case E1 for MR (top) and PET transmission image (down). Segmentation results (white contours) are compared to manual delineation (gray contours).

3.2   Registration Results

Fig. 5 presents the registration result obtained with the E1 case. SA PET images which correspond to the MR SA image planes are computed using the obtained registration parameters. In Figs. 6 and 7 registered end-diastolic MR and PET emission images are presented in the transaxial and SA planes, respectively.

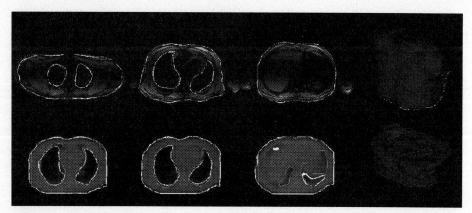

Fig. 4. Segmentation results of transaxial MR (top) and PET transmission (down) images for case E1. White contours correspond to the deformable model based segmentation and gray contours show the manual delineation. A 3-D visualization [8] of the corresponding deformable model based segmentation is shown on the right.

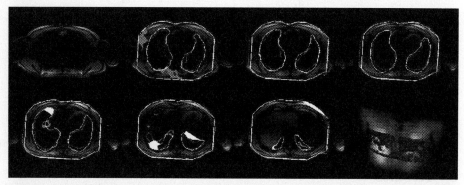

Fig. 5. Contours from registered PET images are superimposed onto the MR transaxial image plane. Automatically segmented contours are shown in white and manually delineated in gray. Bottom right corner: A 3D visualization illustrates the positioning of the registered PET transmission data relatively to the ray traced MR thorax image.

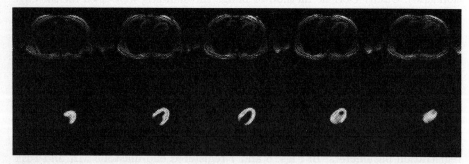

Fig. 6. Registered transaxial end-diastolic MR (top) and PET emission (bottom) image slices for the E1 case.

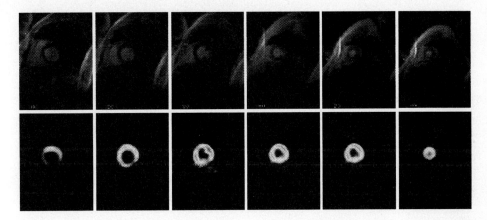

Fig. 7. Registered end-diastolic SA MR (top) and PET emission (bottom) image slices.

4   Discussion and Conclusion

The proposed method was applied to the 10 available cases. It did give visually good results for 9 cases out of the 10. In the failing case, there were unexpected artifacts in the FDG PET data. In order to quantitatively evaluate the algorithm, the statistics of the distance between registered PET surface points and segmented MR image surface were computed. When using deformable model based automatic segmentation, registration error was 2.8 ± 0.5 mm (minimum 1.9 and maximum 3.8 mm). With the manual delineation of the thorax structures, registration error was 2.4 ± 0.9 mm (minimum 0.5 and maximum 3.5 mm). Although this computed error term mainly quantify the difference between segmentation results of PET and MR thorax models, it gives a reasonable index of the quality of the registration in the absence of a reference data set.

Due to the presence of arms in MRI and their absence in PET, we did exclude points of the PET model located on the thorax sides for the calculation of the registration parameters. Initial parameter vector should also be close enough for the algorithm to converge to optimal result. This was the case in all of the studies since the positioning of the patient was identical in both imaging modalities, and as a result, the initial alignment of the MR distance map volume and the PET model was similar.

We did not observe major differences between registration based on manual delineation and automatic segmentation. In some cases, registration based on manual delineation performed better. One possible reason for this is that sometimes the automatic deformable model based segmentation locally fails to follow deep cavities. One additional segmentation step using a denser deformation grid could help to solve this problem.

The automatic segmentation of the MR and PET images with size 256 x 256 x 217 voxels takes less than 3 minutes on a PC workstation (PIII, 800 MHz). With the same image size, the execution time for registration was about 50 seconds when about 400 points were selected to compute the rigid transformation parameters. The speed of registration algorithm depends on factors like the need of the preprocessing, the complexity of the cost function and the number of the cost function evaluations performed by the optimization algorithm [10]. Compared to the iterative closest point (ICP) algorithm [9], our approach also requires the segmentation of the data. In our method, the distance map is computed once as a preprocessing step and after that the estimation of the distances between the model and the data points is immediate. On the contrary, in the ICP algorithm, distances are explicitly computed at every iteration. In our experiments the proposed registration parameter search strategy did provide a fast and reliable results. In future works, we will compare current method to other registration methods and also validate this method by using simulated images.

References

1. Pallotta S., Gilardi M. C., Bettinardi V., Landoni C., Striano G., Masi R. and Fazio F.: Application of a surface matching image registration technique to the correlation of cardiac studies in positron emission tomography (PET) by transmission images. Phys. Med. Biol., **40** (1995) 1695–1708.
2. Kim R., Aw T., Bacharach S., Bonow R.: Correlation of cardiac MRI and PET images using lung cavities as landmarks. Computers in Cardiology, (1991) 49–52.
3. Mäkelä T., Clarysse P., Lötjönen J., Sipilä O., Hänninen H., Nenonen J., Lauerma K., Knuuti J., Katila T. and Magnin I. E.: A method for registration of cardiac MR and PET images for the myocardial viability study. In: Marzullo, P. (ed.): NATO advanced research workshop - Understanding Cardiac Imaging Techniques From Basic Pathology to Image Fusion. NATO Science Series: Life and Behavioural Sciences. Vol. 332. IOS Press (2001) 155–165.
4. Lauerma K., Niemi P., Hänninen H., Janatuinen T., Voipio-Pulkki L., Knuuti J., Toivonen L., Mäkelä T., Mäkijärvi M. A. and Aronen H. J.: Multimodality MR imaging assessment of myocardial viability: combination of first-pass and late contrast enhancement to wall motion dynamics and comparison with FDG-PET. Radiology, **217** (2000) 729–736.
5. Lötjönen J., Reissman P.-J., Magnin I.E. and Katila T.: Model extraction from magnetic resonance volume data using the deformable pyramid. Medical Image Analysis, **4** (1999) 387–406.
6. Borgefors G.: Hierarchical chamfer matching: A parametric edge matching algorithm. IEEE Trans. Pattern Anal. Machine Intell., **6** (1988) 849–865.
7. Canny J.: A computational approach to edge detection. IEEE Trans. Pattern Anal. Machine Intell., **8** (1986) 679–698.
8. Pyökkimies E. P, Salli E. and Katila T. Fast image order volume rendering algorithm for multimodal image visualization. In: Nenonen J., Ilmoniemi R.J. and Katila T. (eds.): Biomag2000, Proc. 12th Int. Conf. on Biomagnetism, (2001) 1043–1045.
9. Besl P.J. and McKay N.D.: A method for regisration of 3-D shapes. IEEE Trans. Pattern Anal. Machine Intell., **14** (1992) 239–256.
10. Van Herk M.: Image registration using chamfer matching. In: Bankman I. N. (ed.): Handbook of medical imaging. Academic Press (2000) 515–527 .

Modeling Surgical Procedures for Multimodal Image-Guided Neurosurgery

P. Jannin[1], M. Raimbault[1], X. Morandi[1,2], and B. Gibaud[1]

[1] Laboratoire IDM, Faculté de Médecine, Université de Rennes 1, 2, avenue du Pr Léon Bernard, CS 34317, 35043 RENNES Cedex France
{pierre.jannin,melanie.raimbault,xavier.morandi,
bernard.gibaud}@univ rennes1.fr
http///idm.univ-rennes1.fr
[2] Department of Neurosurgery, Hôpital Universitaire de Rennes, Rue H. Le Guilloux, 35033 RENNES Cedex 9 France

Abstract. We present a model of surgical procedures that facilitates the management of multimodal information (i.e. anatomical and functional) in the context of multimodal image-guided craniotomies. We suggest that a surgical procedure be considered as a script consisting of a set of successive steps. Each step comprises a list of image entities extracted from multimodal images and relevant for the performance of this surgical step, and an action describing the purpose of the step. Each image entity has a role that may be different from step to step. This model is described by a UML class diagram and a textual description. We also present the results of a preliminary validation of the model performed on 15 clinical cases. The validation has shown the relevance of our model on the clinical cases studied and has confirmed the main assumptions we made to define the model. Even though further semantic validation is required, some benefits of this approach can be outlined: it improves management of multimodal information by describing when and why images are essential in the performance of the surgical act (e.g. place and role of images in the surgical script) and adapts visualization and interaction modes in neuronavigation. Our model should enhance preparation and guidance of surgery and lead to the development of simulation and even teaching tools.

1 Introduction

The development of new imaging devices providing multimodal information (e.g. anatomical and functional) with new image analysis tools (e.g. segmentation, registration and visualization) and localization systems that can match the patient in the operating room directly with his or her preoperative images has led to the growing clinical use of image-guided surgery systems (e.g. neuronavigation systems). Their intraoperative use requires a preliminary planning stage, which consists in extracting information that is relevant to the performance of the surgical act from preoperative images [1,6,8,9]. Information includes target areas (e.g. tumors, malformations), areas to be avoided (e.g. high risk functional areas, vessels) and reference areas (e.g. sulci, vessels, anterior and posterior commissures, basal ganglia). For example, contours of a tumor and sulci segmented from T1-weighted MR imaging, and functional data such as dipolar sources reconstructed from magnetoencephalography examination from

W. Niessen and M. Viergever (Eds.): MICCAI 2001, LNCS 2208, pp. 565–572, 2001.

motor stimulations may provide indices and references for the performance of the surgical act. Neuronavigation systems display these areas of interest during surgery as graphical overlays in a surgical microscope or as images or graphics in a companion computer workstation. Many authors have demonstrated the clinical added value of multimodal (anatomical and functional) neuronavigation [2,5,7,10,12,15].

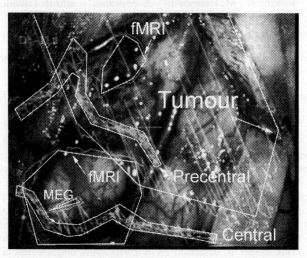

Fig. 1. Intraoperative view of graphical overlays representing anatomical information (precentral and central sulci), pathological information (oligo-astrocytoma) and functional information (MEG and fMRI for motor and somato-sensory activations) as seen through the ocular of a surgical microscope.

However, according to our experience [7], augmented reality in microscope-based multimodal neuronavigation, although it has proved to be clinically useful, is still hampered by hardware limitations (e.g. overlays are monochromic, monoscopic and consist of 2-D cut planes of 3-D surfaces) and functional limitations (e.g. the surgeon has to switch the overlays on and off to understand the graphics)[1]. Therefore, complex multimodal information may lead to a barely understandable scene, in which the surgeon may find it difficult to identify anatomical and functional features, as illustrated in Figure 1. This point may become crucial in exceptional cases where the person who did the planning is not the one actually performing surgery, although this may occur increasingly often, or if the surgical strategy has to be discussed between people located in different places. This paper focuses on the management of multimodal information in neuronavigation systems. We suggest that the management of multimodal information can be improved based on prior knowledge of surgical procedures. This includes two aspects: a « data management » aspect, enhancing when and why images are essential in the performance of the surgical act (e.g. place and role of images in the surgical script) and a « representation and interaction »

---

[1] Of course, another major issue of image-guided surgery is the possibility to update preoperative images according to intraoperative anatomical modifications due to the surgical procedure.

aspect focusing on selecting appropriate visualization and interaction features for image entities, according to their place and role in the surgical script.

More precisely, this paper introduces a model of surgical procedures that breaks them down into steps and associates a goal and relevant information with each step. The object of this research was not to define the surgical procedure with its every detail (e.g. taking into account surgical tools and bio-mechanical tissue properties) as it may be done for robotic purposes. Our primary concern was rather to manage multimodal information more ingeniously to improve and simplify multimodal image-guided craniotomies, especially when using microscope-based multimodal neuronavigation systems. We chose to build and validate our model with three kinds of surgical procedures in which multimodal image-guided surgery provides a real added value: surgery of supratentorial intra-parenchymatous tumors, surgery of supratentorial cavernomas, and selective amygdalo-hippocampectomy for medically intractable epilepsies. We present the results of a preliminary validation of the model performed on 15 clinical cases.

2 Methods

The basic idea was to break down the surgical procedure into steps defining the surgical script. Steps can be determined during the planning stage of the surgical procedure. A list of relevant image entities is assigned to each step (i.e. anatomical and/or functional entities extracted from preoperative images) and the role of each entity in the step is specified (i.e. target area, area to be avoided, reference area). One of our initial goals was to adapt interaction and visualization features according to this model. For instance, during surgery, only the relevant image entities belonging to the step currently being performed are displayed, and colors are related to their role. That way the neurosurgeon can focus his or her attention on the basic information of a given step of the surgical procedure.

We defined a generic information model describing the main concepts and relationships involved in our field of interest (i.e. multimodal image-guided craniotomies). We chose UML [11] (Unified Modeling Language) among the numerous techniques and formalisms available because it may now be considered as a standard. To produce a generic model, we studied three types of procedures, accounting for approximately 75% of supratentorial procedures in our neurosurgical department (excluding traumatology, shunts, and vascular procedures): surgery for supratentorial intra-parenchymatous tumors (67%), for supratentorial cavernomas (5%) and selective amygdalo-hippocampectomies for medically intractable epilepsies (3%). We selected these procedures because they can benefit significantly from multimodal neuronavigation. The design of the model started with the analysis of surgical procedures as described by neurosurgeons in both generic descriptions (i.e. referring to standardized procedures expressed as an abstraction of many concrete clinical cases) and specific clinical cases studied both during surgery and postoperatively from videotapes (6 tumours, 3 cavernomas and 3 amygdalo-hippocampectomies). This analysis was then formalized into UML object diagrams, describing instances of objects involved, and a UML class diagram, describing the corresponding classes. The final class diagram was iteratively obtained by assessing the model with the three types of procedures. We used a UML design tool (Visual UML 2.5, Boulder CO, USA) to design the model and validate the syntax of the scheme.

In order to demonstrate the relevance and the added value of this approach, we developed a software application to instantiate the model in clinical situations. The neurosurgeon defines a number of surgical steps and assigns to each of them relevant image entities selected from a list of available 3-D image entities previously segmented from preoperative data. Anatomical information may include skin and brain surfaces, ventricles, sulci, and lesions segmented from 3-D T1-weighted anatomical MRI and vessels segmented from MR Angiography. Functional information may include volumes of interest extracted from correlation volumes computed from functional MRI examinations, equivalent current dipoles reconstructed from MEG and epileptogenic areas segmented from ictal SPECT. A role is attributed to each image entity. Display parameters (color and transparency) can be independently assigned to each image entity associated with a surgical step. A 3-D VRML scene is generated for each step, including 3-D surfaces of the corresponding image entities. A viewpoint and a view direction (i.e. view trajectory) can be assigned to each scene. Display parameters and view features are stored along with the 3-D surfaces of the image entities in each VRML file. The surgeon can therefore visualize the procedure step by step by displaying the different 3-D scenes corresponding to the successive steps.

3 Results

Figure 2 presents a UML class diagram showing the major conceptual entities involved in our field of interest and their relations.

SurgicalProcedure is the basic entity of this model. A *SurgicalProcedure* concerns one or more *Targets* and comprises one or more ordered *Steps*. In multimodal image-guided surgery, the procedure may require several *ImageEntities* corresponding to image entities (points, surfaces or volumes) extracted from multimodal images (anatomical or functional). A *Target* may have an *ImageEntity* which is its graphical representation segmented from images. A *Target* has properties (e.g. size, orientation and amplitude) and is located within the right and/or left hemisphere (*Side*). A *Target* may concern several anatomical concepts (*AnatConcept*) such as a gyrus or a lobe in which it is located. A *Target* is also characterized by a pathological concept (*PathoConcept*) such as a cavernoma, a glioma or an epileptogenic focus. A *Concept* is an abstract class presenting the properties that are common to all of its specializations (*PathoConcept, AnatConcept, FunctConcept*). It may eventually refer to existing knowledge of these concepts through terminology such as Neuronames [3] included in UMLS since 1992. Each *ImageEntity* refers to one or more *Concepts*, representing anatomical, functional or pathological information.

A *Step* comprises a single *Action*, which is the goal of this step (e.g. incision of the dura mater). An *Action* acts upon one pathological, functional or anatomical entity (*Concept*). A *Step* may also have an *ImageEntityList*, listing the *ImageEntities* (anatomical and/or functional) relevant to this specific *Step*. Each *ImageEntity* belonging to a specific *ImageEntityList* has a *Role* representing the kind of use anticipated for that instance in that *Step*, such as target, area to be avoided, or reference areas. A *Step* may refer to an *ActionModel* and may be described by one or more *ActionAttributes*. An *ActionModel* may be for instance a graphical element representing the action to be performed, such as contours of the craniotomy or a segment representing an approach to a cavernoma. An *ActionAttribute* provides further details on the action to be completed. For example, the action of positioning the patient may be further described by the position to be used (right or left lateral positions, supine or prone positions).

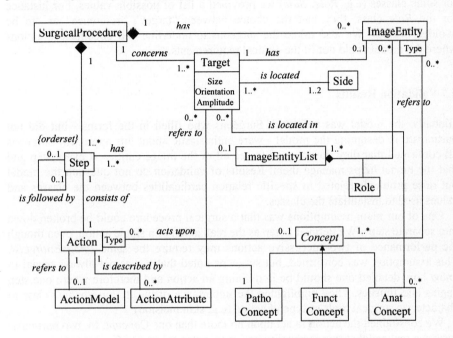

Fig. 2. UML class diagram of multimodal image-guided craniotomies

We instantiated our model with our software application for a few clinical cases, and verified that the 3-D display modes and the production of one 3-D virtual scene per surgical step - including the relevant image entities, viewpoint and a single trajectory - were well adapted to our requirements.

4 Validation

4.1 Validation Method

The semantics of the model were validated with a retrospective study. Forms listing the objects of our model were designed and filled in by three different neurosurgeons with the instances of the objects relative to real surgical procedures. Clinical cases were selected according to the scope of the model (9 supratentorial intra-parenchymatous tumors, 3 supratentorial cavernomas, and 3 selective amygdalo-hippocampectomies for medically intractable epilepsies). Naturally, these clinical cases were different from those used to design the model. The operator could define as many steps as required for the procedure and as many *ImageEntities* as ideally required for the action implemented in each step (i.e. what kind of image information should the graphical overlay display in the oculars of a surgical microscope to perform surgery?). Surgeons were relatively free to fill in forms with any values. But for some classes (e.g. *Role*, *Side*) we provided a list of possible values. For instance for the *Role* class, they had the choice between "target", "reference" or "to be avoided" values. We also asked the surgeons to underline and document situations where the model could not fit the clinical requirements.

4.2 Validation Results

Globally, the model was validated. Surgeons who filled in the forms - but did not participate in designing the model - were enthusiastic about this approach. Surgeons all confirmed that they do not need to see all of the image entities at every step and that the model helps manage them. Results of validation do not question the model but raise problems related to specific relation cardinalities between the classes and values used to instantiate the classes.

One of our main assumptions was that a surgical procedure could be broken down into separate steps. We defined a step as the realization of a single action, even though the performance of two successive actions may require the same *ImageEntityList*. This assumption was confirmed, but surgeons noted that it was not always trivial to know how detailed one should be in defining an action and therefore where one step begins and finishes. They highlighted the importance of the *ActionAttribute* class to characterize surgical tools or type of action (e.g. skin incision).

We constrained the action to act upon no more than one *Concept*. In two particular cases we realized that this cardinality had to be extended to one *Concept* or more. For a right-handed patient with a right temporal glioblastoma, the resection step concerned both tumor and adjacent cerebral tissue (partial temporal lobectomy) and consequently the *Step* acted upon two *Concepts*. One difficulty when filling the forms was related to the instance values to be used. For the *ActionModel* class, which concerns a graphical representation of the action, it was sometimes difficult to find a representation that was not an image entity and to differentiate the target from the action. For the resection of a deep cavernoma, the surgeon chose a trans-sulcal approach via the pre-central sulcus. Therefore the set of values proposed for the *Role* class has to be extended to take into account the "trajectory" value. A last remark concerns the *Concept* class and related *PathoConcept*, *FuncConcept* and *AnatConcept* classes. It was not easy for the surgeon to understand exactly what kind of information these concept classes involved and make the difference between information directly related to the patient (e.g. exact anatomical location of an image entity) and generic knowledge (e.g. the precentral gyrus is an anatomical part of the frontal lobe). Therefore, it may be relevant to distinguish two levels: one for instantiated knowledge and a second for canonical knowledge [14].

5 Discussion and Conclusions

In this paper we introduced a generic model of neurosurgical procedures to improve multimodal image-guided craniotomies. Few studies have described surgical procedures models. The closest existing work provides a common terminology of the surgical procedures names (the GALEN/GASP representation [13,17]) but without considering its dynamic aspect. Our model manages image information according to its place and role within the surgical script. During neuronavigation, it may contribute to adapt visualization and interaction modes. This model provides a framework to model knowledge involved in the performance of neurosurgical acts and therefore leads to the definition of an ontology [4] of our field of knowledge. In this approach, semantics (i.e. meaning) are assigned to image data (i.e. image entities) relatively to our context (multimodal image-guided craniotomies). Making this meaning explicit is a key aspect of successful information sharing between the different software components used for planning and surgery and between which a perfect inter-operability is required.

Validation has shown the relevance of our model on the clinical cases studied, confirmed our main assumptions and provided us with some leads to improve our model (e.g. modifying some cardinalities, refining possible values for classes, adding new features to the *Target* class, distinguishing instantiated knowledge from canonical knowledge). However, this validation has to be improved by involving a broader set of clinical cases and surgical procedures and a larger community of neurosurgeons.

The study of the different clinical cases emphasized the fact that there are few variations between cases requiring the same surgical procedure. The same steps are associated with the same actions and similar relevant image entities. Consequently, it may be worth defining models of these specific procedures, which would *a priori* include the expected steps and the image entities to assign.

This paper presents a work in progress. While further validation and modifications are required, the first benefits of this approach can already be outlined. It should confer real added value to the different levels of image-guided surgery, from preprocessing to planning, as well as during surgery. Models of surgical procedures can manage image data according to the surgical script, which should lead to better anticipation of surgery through the development of simulation tools. Furthermore, they may greatly improve the performance of surgery under microscope-based neuronavigation systems by optimizing both visualization and interaction features of multimodal preoperative images. Finally our approach may facilitate the decision-making process (e.g. choice between surgery, biopsy or radiotherapy), and may contribute to generate case reports and develop teaching tools.

We are convinced that our approach, in conjunction with other *a priori* knowledge such as anatomical and physiological models [16], will contribute to defining decision support systems to improve image-guided surgery.

Acknowledgements

We wish to thank E. Seigneuret and L. Riffaud from the Neurosurgical Department of the Hôpital Universitaire of Rennes (France) who participated in the design and validation of the model. We would also like to thank O. Dameron, from the Laboratoire IDM, for fruitful discussions to improve the model and Pr. J.M. Scarabin, from the Laboratoire IDM and the Neurosurgical Department, Rennes. This research program was supported in part by grants from the "Conseil Régional de Bretagne".

References

1. Apuzzo MJ: New dimensions of neurosurgery in the realm of high technology: possibilities, practicalities, realities. Neurosurgery, 38 (1996) 625-639
2. Alberstone CD, Skirboll SL, Benzel EC, et al.: Magnetic source imaging and brain surgery: presurgical and intraoperative planning in 26 patients. J Neurosurg 92 (2000) 79-90
3. Bowden DM, Martin RF: Neuronames Brain Hierarchy. Neuroimage, 2 (1995) 63-83
4. Chandrasekaran B, Josephson JR, and Benjamins VR: What are ontologies and why do we need them? IEEE Intelligent Systems January-February (1999) 20-26
5. Gallen CC, Bucholz R, Sobel DF: Intracranial neurosurgery guided by functional imaging. Surg Neurol, 42 (1994) 523-530
6. Hardenack M, Bucher N, Falk A, and Harders A: Preoperative planning and intraoperative navigation : status quo and perspectives. Computer Aided Surgery 3 (1998) 153-158
7. Jannin P, Fleig OJ, Seigneuret E, et al.: A data fusion environment for multimodal and multi-informational neuronavigation. Computer Aided Surgery 5 (2000) 1-10
8. Kikinis R, P. Langham Gleason, Moriarty TM, et al.: Computer-assisted three-dimensional planning for neurosurgical procedures. Neurosurgery 38 (1996) 640-651
9. Kockro RA, Serra L, Tseng-Tsai Y, et al.: Planning and simulation of neurosurgery in a virtual reality environment. Neurosurgery 46 (2000) 118-137
10. Maldjian JA, Schulder M, Liu WC, et al: Intraoperative functional MRI using a real-time neurosurgical navigation system. J Comput Assist Tomogr 21 (1997) 910-912
11. Muller PA. Modélisation objet avec UML. Eyrolles Eds (1999)
12. Nimsky C, Ganslandt O, Kober H, et al: Integration of functional magnetic resonance imaging supported by magnetoencephalography in functional neuronavigation. Neurosurgery 44 (1999) 1249-1256
13. Rector AL, Rogers JE, and Pole P: The GALEN High Level Ontology. Proceedings of Medical Informatics in Europe (MIE'96), IOS Press, Amsterdam (1996) 174-178
14. Rosse C, Mejino JL, Modayur BR, et al.: Motivation and Organizational Principles for Anatomical Knowledge Representation. JAMIA 5 (1998) 17-40
15. Schulder M, Maldjian JA, Liu WC, et al: Functional image-guided surgery of intracranial tumors in or near the sensorimotor cortex. J Neurosurg 89 (1998) 412-418
16. Taylor C, Draney MT, Ku JP, et al.: Predictive medicine: computational techniques in therapeutic decision making. Computer Aided Surgery 4 (1999) 231-247
17. Trombert-Paviot B, Rodrigues JM, Rogers JE, et al.: GALEN: a third generation terminology tool to support a multipurpose national coding system for surgical procedures. International Journal of Medical Informatics 58-59 (2000) 71-85

A Generic Framework for Non-rigid Registration Based on Non-uniform Multi-level Free-Form Deformations

Julia A. Schnabel[1], Daniel Rueckert[2], Marcel Quist[3], Jane M. Blackall[1],
Andy D. Castellano-Smith[1], Thomas Hartkens[1], Graeme P. Penney[1], Walter A. Hall[4],
Haiying Liu[5], Charles L. Truwit[5], Frans A. Gerritsen[3], Derek L. G. Hill[1], and
David J. Hawkes[1]

[1] Computational Imaging Science Group, Radiological Sciences and Medical Engineering,
Guy's Hospital, King's College London, UK
julia.schnabel@kcl.ac.uk
[2] Visual Information Processing, Dept. Computing, Imperial College of Science, Technology
and Medicine, London, UK
[3] EasyVision Advanced Development, Philips Medical Systems, Best, NL
[4] Dept. Neurosurgery, University of Minnesota, Minneapolis, MN, USA
[5] Dept. Radiology, University of Minnesota, Minneapolis, MN, USA

Abstract. This work presents a framework for non-rigid registration which extends and generalizes a previously developed technique by Rueckert et al. [1].
We combine multi-resolution optimization with free-form deformations (FFDs) based on multi-level B-splines to simulate a non-uniform control point distribution. We have applied this to a number of different medical registration tasks to demonstrate its wide applicability, including interventional MRI brain tissue deformation compensation, breathing motion compensation in liver MRI, intra-modality inter-modality registration of pre-operative brain MRI to CT electrode implant data, and inter-subject registration of brain MRI. Our results demonstrate that the new algorithm can successfully register images with an improved performance, while achieving a significant reduction in run-time.

1 Introduction

Non-rigid image registration is playing an increasingly important role in both clinical and research applications. Even though there is a large number of registration methods to be found in the literature [2,3], existing methods have usually been designed for or fine-tuned to specific, mostly single-modality applications. In this paper we propose a flexible framework for non-rigid registration which covers a range of deformation tasks in medical applications. This framework extends and generalizes a previously published method based on free-form deformations (FFDs) using B-splines which was developed for registration of contrast enhanced MR mammography images [1]. The original method was formulated as a two-stage process: first, the global motion is corrected using a rigid or affine transformation. The global motion then becomes the starting estimate for the second stage, where the local motion is further modelled using FFDs based on B-splines. Manipulating the underlying mesh of control points yields a

W. Niessen and M. Viergever (Eds.): MICCAI 2001, LNCS 2208, pp. 573–581, 2001.

smooth deformation of structures embedded in the image, where the control points act as parameters of the transformation. The combined motion model can be written as:

$$\mathbf{T}(x, y, z) = \mathbf{T}_{global}(x, y, z) + \mathbf{T}_{local}(x, y, z) \tag{1}$$

with the local motion at each point given by the 3D tensor product of the familiar 1D cubic B-splines [4]. The optimal transformation $\mathbf{T}$ is determined by minimizing a registration cost function:

$$\mathcal{C} = -\mathcal{C}_{similarity}(\mathcal{I}_A, \mathbf{T}(\mathcal{I}_B)) + \lambda \mathcal{C}_{deformation}(\mathbf{T}) \tag{2}$$

The similarity term maximizes the voxel similarity between the image pair, and is chosen to be normalized mutual information (NMI) [5]. The deformation cost term is defined as the 3D equivalent of a thin-plate bending energy in order to maximize the smoothness of the transformation, weighted by a factor λ.

The performance of this registration method is limited by the resolution of the control point mesh, which is linearly related to the computational complexity: more global and intrinsically smooth deformations can only be modelled using a coarse control point spacing, whereas more localized and intrinsically less smooth deformations require a finer spacing. If it is known *a priori* which magnitude of deformation is to be expected, the mesh resolution can be chosen accordingly, and folding can be penalized using a suitable deformation cost term. However, often a range of deformations needs to be modelled which cannot be captured by a single mesh resolution. More importantly, it may be desirable to have a non-uniform control point spacing to restrict deformation to localized regions in the image pair, while excluding regions where the images are already in alignment, form part of image background, or have been identified as rigid bodies. For many applications, non-uniform control point spacing may not be necessary, however the computational complexity can be decreased without compromising the registration performance. In the following, we present our multi-resolution non-rigid registration framework that can have a non-uniform control point distribution.

2   Framework

2.1   Multi-resolution Registration

To model a large range of deformations, a multi-resolution mesh representation is needed. This issue has been addressed in [1] in a coarse-to-fine fashion where the mesh is progressively refined by alternating between mesh deformation and mesh subdivision using suitable B-spline subdivision techniques [6]. As an alternative, Rueckert et al. [1] formulated an approach using multi-level B-splines to create a hierarchy of local deformation meshes [4] which will be presented in this work. Multi-resolution registration using this concept is then achieved by deforming a sequence of control point meshes $\Phi^1, \cdots, \Phi^H$ of arbitrarily increasing resolution using multi-level B-splines (each level corresponding to a single-resolution B-spline mesh). After registration, the local deformation of each point in the image volume domain is given by the sum of the local deformations across levels:

$$\mathbf{T}_{local}(x,y,z) = \sum_{h=1}^{H} \mathbf{T}_{local}^{h}(x,y,z) \tag{3}$$

where each $\mathbf{T}_{local}^{h}(x,y,z)$ is computed with respect to the B-spline of that level h. To avoid the overhead of recalculating previously recovered local deformations up to level $h-1$, these can be efficiently pre-computed for the deformation of level h.

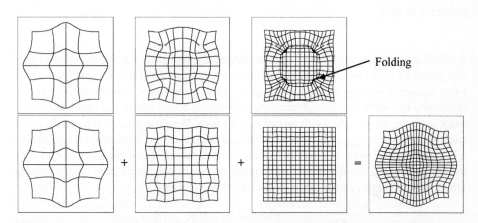

Fig. 1. 2D slices through 3D single- and multi-resolution FFDs for a synthetic reg-istration task. Top: Single-resolution FFDs are limited by low mesh resolutions, and may develop folding at high resolutions (see arrow). Bottom: Multi-resolution FFDs are modelling deformations of different magnitudes at the respective mesh resolution, without developing any folding. Note that at intermediate resolution, deformations of the preceding lower resolution are partially corrected.

Fig. 1 shows 2D slices through 3D single- and multi-resolution FFDs for the regis-tration of a synthetic cube and sphere. One can observe that multi-resolution FFDs can model large deformations without folding at higher resolution levels, whereas FFDs at a single mesh resolution are locally not flexible enough at low resolutions, and can be subject to folding at higher resolutions without any additional smoothness constraints. Hence, when using multi-resolution FFDs, the deformation cost term regularizing the smoothness of the deformation in Eq. 2 is no longer crucial and and we can set $\lambda = 0$.

2.2 Non-uniform Control Point Spacing

Non-uniform control point spacing for FFDs is a well known concept from computer graphics. For example, Non-Uniform Rational B-Splines (NURBS) [7] have been used for FFDs to represent and interactively manipulate object shapes. We propose to sim-ulate this concept by extending the multi-resolution registration presented in section 2.1, while avoiding the more complex lattice traversal and control point manipulation of NURBS. We introduce a control point status S associated with each control point at each level in the multi-resolution mesh hierarchy, marking it as either *active* or *passive*.

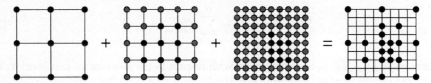

Fig. 2. Simulation of non-uniform control point spacing by combining multi-resolution registration with a control point status. Active control points are marked as black, passive ones as grey.

Active control points are allowed to move during the registration process, whereas passive control points remain fixed. Fig. 2 illustrates this concept. Prior knowledge derived from segmentation may be used to assign a control point status. Alternatively, we have developed two different, complementary approaches which derive the status automatically from the image data. Both investigate the local B-spline support regions $\Phi_{i,j,k}$ of each control point $\phi_{i,j,k}$, which provide natural bounds for the local support region that a B-spline control point at a certain resolution level has. Within these bounds, and over the whole image domain, a statistical measure $\mathcal{M}$ can be calculated from the underlying image data to determine the status of each control point as:

$$S(\phi_{i,j,k}) = \begin{cases} active & \text{if } \mathcal{M}(\Phi_{i,j,k}) > \epsilon \\ passive & \text{otherwise} \end{cases} \tag{4}$$

where ϵ is a selection threshold, which may be normalized by the global measure $\mathcal{M}$. In the following, we distinguish between measures computed over the reference image, and joint measures computed over the image pair.

Reference image measures characterize the reference image locally, and are applicable for serial registration to a baseline scan, inter-subject registration to a common reference subject, or registration to an atlas. They are computed prior to the registration process for all undeformed meshes in the B-spline hierarchy. One such measure which describes the information content of the image intensity distribution is the Shannon-Wiener entropy $H = -\sum p(a) \log p(a)$, where $p(a)$ is the probability that an image voxel has intensity a. Other local intensity measures include intensity variance σ, features based on higher order image differentials, or more complex noise estimators. Using such measures, image background regions can be naturally excluded without explicit segmentation, and local image structure is deformed with the appropriate mesh resolution. For the inter-subject registration application in this work, we have investigated both H and σ as suitable reference image measures.

Joint image pair measures describe the degree of local image alignment. They need to be recomputed for each level after the deformation of the preceding levels for progressive adaptation, and include local measures such as intensity or gradient differences, local correlation, and information-theoretic measures computed over local histograms. These measures should be normalized by the integration measure over the whole image domain. We propose a more consistent, generalized joint image pair measure which is based on the local gradient $\partial \mathcal{C}/\partial \phi_{i,j,k}$ of the global registration cost term of Eq. (2), which does not rely on potentially insufficient statistics defined over small local image regions or histograms. Computing the gradient of the cost functions to determine local adaptivity has also very recently been proposed in [8].

3   Applications

In the following, we present example results for the new framework for intra- and inter-modality, intra-subject and inter-subject registration tasks. Figs. 3-6 show example 2D slices through 3D volumes, where registration has been performed on 3D volume pairs.

Intra-subject intra-modality registration:

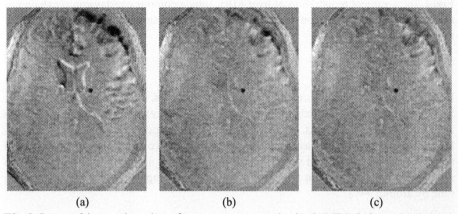

(a)   (b)   (c)

Fig. 3. Intra-subject registration of pre- to post-operative brain MRI. Subtraction images after registration: (a) rigid, and non-uniform non-rigid using joint image pair adaptation at (b) 15mm spacing, and (c) 15mm refined to 7.5mm spacing.

Fig. 3 shows an example slice through subtraction images after rigid and non-rigid registration of an MP-RAGE MR brain scan before dura puncture to an MP-RAGE MR brain scan after a functional surgical procedure where a unilateral thalamic stimulator was inserted stereotactically to suppress tremor. After rigid registration, a shift in the brain tissue can be observed which may have been caused by patient positioning on the operating table, loss of cerebral spinal fluid, and tissue deformation. It was previously shown that the non-rigid algorithm by Rueckert et al. [1] can correct for this shift [9]. The locality of the shift, and the expected magnitude of up to 15mm for this case can be used to adapt B-spline meshes of 15mm and refinement to 7.5mm control point spacing using the local similarity gradient as a joint image pair measure M ($\epsilon = 0.01$). Control points in areas where shift can be observed, and where $M > \epsilon$, are automatically marked as *active*, and as *passive* in remaining areas which are sufficiently aligned after rigid registration. This has reduced the number of active control points and the associated computing time by 60% (15mm) and 97% (7.5mm) for this case.

Fig. 4 shows an example for registration of liver MRI between exhale and inhale positions for a volunteer. To correct for the rigid, mostly translational movement of the

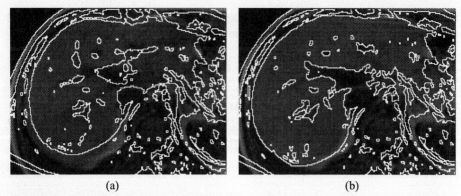

(a)	(b)

Fig. 4. Intra-subject registration of liver MRI. Inhale contour overlays onto exhale image after (a) rigid and (b) non-rigid registration. Deformation was restricted to the liver at exhale.

liver, and the additional deformation within the liver tissue, we have segmented the liver in the reference image (at exhale) prior to registration to exclude all external structure from the registration process. Non-rigid registration was performed using a mesh resolution of 23.12mm, chosen as a multiple of the in-plane voxel size. Note the improved alignment of the surface and vessels within the liver after non-rigid registration, shown as contour overlays. The non-uniform control point spacing has reduced the computing time by around 94%.

Intra-subject inter-modality registration:

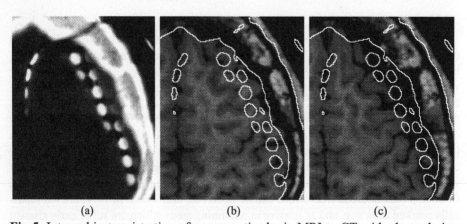

(a)	(b)	(c)

Fig. 5. Intra-subject registration of pre-operative brain MRI to CT with electrode implants. (a) CT, and CT contour overlays showing brain surface and electrodes onto MR after (b) rigid and (c) non-rigid registration. Deformation was restricted to the intra-cranial cavity.

Fig. 5 shows an example for inter-modality registration for a pre-operative MR brain scan to a post-operative CT scan of a patient with epilepsy after an electrode grid implantation to map electrical activity. Similar to the liver registration task, we have performed a segmentation prior to registration. The reason for this is that the high intensity values of the electrode grid would otherwise be mapped to the dura in the MR scan. Adapting the mesh with respect to setting only the control points within the intra-cranial cavity to *active* reduced the non-rigid registration time by 85%, and, more importantly, the shift of the brain surface caused by the grid implantation was recovered without deforming the dura. Another example for intra-subject inter-modality registration, which is not shown in this paper, is the registration of pre-contrast to contrast-enhanced MR mammographic images. In [1], B-spline subdivision was proposed to perform a coarse-to-fine deformation compensation for that application, which alternatively can be achieved using the multi-resolution scheme presented in this work.

Inter-subject intra-modality registration:

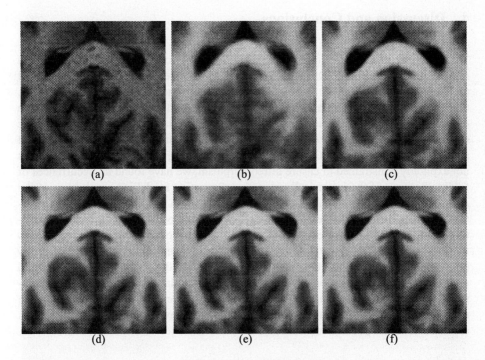

Fig. 6. Inter-subject registration of brain MRI of 7 healthy subjects. ROI of (a) reference subject and averages after registration: (b) affine, (c) uniform non-rigid at 20mm, (d) uniform non-rigid at 20mm, refined to 10mm and 5mm, and non-uniform non-rigid at 20mm, refined to 10mm and 5mm using (e) entropy H and (f) variance σ as reference image measures.

As an example for inter-subject, intra-modality registration, we have registered MR T1-weighted brain volumes of 6 control subjects to one reference control subject. After

580   J.A. Schnabel et al.

registration, averages of the aligned image volumes were generated. Fig. 6 shows an example region of the reference subject and averages after affine and non-rigid registration using uniform control point spacing of 20mm, and refinement via 10mm to 5mm spacing. One can visually perceive the improved alignment when going from affine to non-rigid registration using 20mm spacing, as well as an improved refinement to 5mm. We have also used non-uniform control point spacing on the basis of the local entropy ($\epsilon = 0.75H_{total}$) and variance ($\epsilon = 0.5\sigma_{total}$) as reference image measures. The result is comparable to the uniform mesh refinement, but needed considerably less computing time (reduction by 43-66% for $M = H$ and by 29-55% for $M = \sigma$, for increasing mesh resolutions, respectively). Using a 5mm control point spacing from the start was found to be computationally prohibitively expensive. Both reference image measures were found to be robust and well-behaved estimates with respect to the control point support regions and a measure-specific, but constant threshold ϵ across resolutions.

4   Discussion and Conclusions

We have presented a non-rigid image registration framework based on multi-resolution refinement of adaptable FFDs using B-splines, which extends the work of Rueckert et al. [1]. We have applied the framework to a variety of medical registration problems, demonstrating its flexibility and wide applicability. In particular, its ability to constrain deformation to selective regions, on the basis of segmentation, or automatically using reference or joint image pair measures provides a large gain in computing time without any apparent loss of registration quality. Although folding of the deformation field was not explicitly constrained to ensure diffeomorphism, we have found no occurrences of folding because of the intrinsically smooth deformation modelling capabilities of the multi-resolution FFD. Validation of non-rigid registration is a challenging task, and often limited to visual assessment. We have recently developed a biomechanical deformation simulator using finite element methods [10] which we have successfully applied to the registration algorithm by Rueckert et al. for contrast-enhanced MR mammography [1]. We are planning to use this method to validate and further improve the non-rigid registration framework presented in this paper. In particular, we will investigate the parameter selection for the adaptivity criteria, and the range and sampling values for the multi-level FFDs. For inter-subject registration, we are investigating target registration errors on the basis of anatomical landmarks which is subject to ongoing work.

Acknowledgements

JAS is funded by Philips Medical Systems EV-AD, DR is partially funded by EPSRC GR / N / 24919, GPP is funded by EPSRC GR / M53752, ADCS and TH are funded by EPSRC GR / M47294. The electrode data were provided by Prof. Charles Polkey from Dept. Healthcare, KCL, the brain control data by the Institute of Psychiatry, KCL, the interventional MRI data by the University of Minnesota, and the liver data were acquired at Guy's Hospital.

References

1. D. Rueckert, L. I. Sonoda, C. Hayes, D. L. G. Hill, M. O. Leach, and D. J. Hawkes. Non-rigid registration using Free-Form Deformations: Application to breast MR images. *IEEE Transactions on Medical Imaging*, 18(8):712–721, 1999.
2. H. Lester and S. R. Arridge. A survey of hierarchical non-linear medical image registration. *Pattern Recognition*, 32(1):129–149, 1999.
3. J. V. Hajnal, D. L. G. Hill, and D. J. Hawkes. *Medical image registration*. CRC Press, 2001.
4. S. Lee, G. Wolberg, and S. Y. Shin. Scattered data interpolation with multilevel B-splines. *IEEE Transactions on Visualization and Computer Graphics*, 3(3):228–244, 1997.
5. C. Studholme, D. L. G. Hill, and D. J. Hawkes. An overlap entropy measure of 3D medical image alignment. *Pattern Recognition*, 32:71–86, 1999.
6. D. R. Forsey and R. H. Bartels. Hierarchical B-spline refinement. *ACM Transactions on Computer Graphics*, 22(4):205–212, 1988.
7. L. Piegl and W. Tiller. *The NURBS Book*. Springer Verlag, 1997.
8. G. K. Rohde, A. Aldroubi, and B. M. Dawant. Adaptive free-form deformations for inter-patient medical image registration. In *Proc. Medical Imaging: Image Processing*. SPIE, 2001. In press.
9. C. R. Maurer Jr., D. L. G. Hill, A. J. Martin, H. Liu, M. McCue, D. Rueckert, D. Lloret, W. A. Hall, R. E. Maxwell, D. J. Hawkes, and C. L. Truwit. Investigation of intraoperative brain deformation using a 1.5T interventional MR system: preliminary results. *IEEE Transactions on Medical Imaging*, 17(5):817–825, 1998.
10. J. A. Schnabel, C. Tanner, A. Castellano Smith, M. O. Leach, C. Hayes, A. Degenhard, R. Hose, D. L. G. Hill, and D. J. Hawkes. Validation of non-rigid registration using Finite Element Methods. In *Proc. Information Processing in Medical Imaging (IPMI'01)*, volume 2082 of *Lecture Notes in Computer Science*, pages 344–357. Springer Verlag, 2001.

Improving the Robustness in Extracting 3D Point Landmarks from 3D Medical Images Using Parametric Deformable Models

Manfred Alker[1], Sönke Frantz[1], Karl Rohr[2], and H. Siegfried Stiehl[1]

[1] Universität Hamburg, FB Informatik, AB Kognitive Systeme,
Vogt-Kölln-Str. 30, D-22527 Hamburg,
{alker,frantz,stiehl}@kogs.informatik.uni-hamburg.de
[2] International University in Germany, D-76646 Bruchsal,
rohr@i-u.de

Abstract. Existing approaches to the extraction of 3D point landmarks based on parametric deformable models suffer from their dependence on a good model initialization to avoid local suboptima during model fitting. Our main contribution to increasing the robustness of model fitting against local suboptima is a *novel hybrid optimization algorithm* combining the advantages of both the conjugate gradient (cg-)optimization method (known for its time efficiency) and genetic algorithms (exhibiting robustness against local suboptima). It has to be stressed, however, that the scope of applicability of this nonlinear optimization method is not restricted to model fitting problems in medical image analysis. We apply our model fitting algorithm to 3D medical images depicting tip-like and saddle-like anatomical structures such as the horns of the lateral ventricles in the human brain or the zygomatic bone as part of the skull. Experimental results for 3D MR and CT images demonstrate that in comparison to a purely local cg-optimization method, the robustness of model fitting in the case of poorly initialized model parameters is significantly improved with a hybrid optimization strategy. Moreover, we compare an *edge strength-based fitting measure* with an *edge distance-based fitting measure* w.r.t. their suitability for model fitting.

1 Introduction

The extraction of 3D anatomical point landmarks from 3D tomographic images is a prerequisite for landmark-based approaches to 3D image registration, which is a fundamental problem in computer-assisted neurosurgery. While earlier approaches to 3D point landmark extraction exploit the local characteristics of the image data by applying differential operators (e.g, [16],[11]), an approach based on parametric deformable models has recently been proposed in [5]. The approach in [5] takes into account more global image information than existing differential approaches, allows to localize 3D point landmarks more accurately, and also reduces the number of false detections. However, since a local optimization method is employed, a drawback of this approach is the need of a good model initialization in order to avoid local suboptima during model fitting.

W. Niessen and M. Viergever (Eds.): MICCAI 2001, LNCS 2208, pp. 582–590, 2001.

For the purpose of increasing the robustness of model fitting in the case of poorly initialized model parameters, we propose a new *hybrid optimization algorithm* that is suitable for general poorly initialized nonlinear optimization problems and that combines the computational efficiency of the (local) conjugate gradient (cg-)optimization method with the robustness of (global) genetic algorithms against local suboptima. Existing optimization algorithms for fitting deformable models are either purely local (e.g., [13],[18],[1],[5]) or strictly global (e.g., [4],[17]). Moreover we compare an *edge strength-based fitting measure* based on the strength of the intensity gradient along the model surface (e.g., [18]) with an *edge distance-based fitting measure* (cf., e.g., [1]) w.r.t. their suitability for model fitting. The fitting algorithm proposed here is applied to the extraction of salient surface loci (curvature extrema) of *tip-* and *saddle-like structures* such as the ventricular horns in the human brain or the saddle points at the zygomatic bones being part of the skull (see Fig. 1(a),(b)). To represent the 3D shape of such

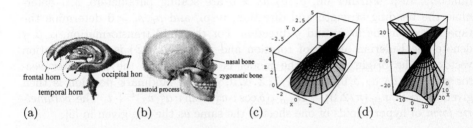

(a)   (b)   (c)   (d)

Fig. 1. (a),(b): Ventricular horns of the human brain (from [12]) and the human skull (from [2]). Examples of 3D point landmarks are indicated by black dots. **(c),(d)**: Quadric surfaces as parametric deformable models for tips ((c): bended and tapered half-ellipsoid) and for saddle structures ((d): undeformed half-hyperboloid of one sheet). The landmark positions are indicated by a black dot.

structures, we utilize quadric surfaces undergoing global deformations (Sect. 2). The fitting measures for model fitting are then described in Sect. 3, while our hybrid algorithm for optimizing a fitting measure w.r.t. the model parameters is outlined in Sect. 4. Experimental results of studying the robustness of model fitting for 3D tomographic images of the human head are presented in Sect. 5. In particular, we analyze the landmark localization accuracy of our new approach and compare it with that of a purely local cg-optimization algorithm.

2   Modeling Tip- and Saddle-like Structures with Quadrics

In the literature, a variety of 3D surface models has been used for different applications (e.g., [13],[15],[4],[18],[1]; see [9] for a survey). As geometric models for

tip- and saddle-like structures, we here use quadric surfaces ([5]) since they well
represent the anatomical structures of interest here, but still have few model parameters, and both a parametric and an implicit defining function. Bended and
tapered ellipsoids are utilized for representing 3D tip-like structures such as the
ventricular horns, whereas hyperboloids of one sheet are used for 3D saddle-like
structures such as the zygomatic bones (see Fig. 1(c),(d)). For tip-like structures,
the *parametric form* of our model is obtained by applying quadratic bending [4]
and linear tapering deformations [13],[4] as well as a rigid transformation allowing for arbitrary poses in 3D space to the parametric form of an ellipsoid:

$$\boldsymbol{x}_{tip}(\theta,\phi) = \boldsymbol{R}_{\alpha,\beta,\gamma} \begin{pmatrix} a_1 \cos\theta \cos\phi/(\rho_x \sin\theta+1)+\delta \cos\upsilon (a_3 \sin\theta)^2 \\ a_2 \cos\theta \sin\phi/(\rho_y \sin\theta+1)+\delta \sin\upsilon (a_3 \sin\theta)^2 \\ a_3 \sin\theta \end{pmatrix} + \boldsymbol{t}, \quad (1)$$

where $0 \le \theta \le \pi/2$ and $-\pi \le \phi < \pi$ are the latitude and longitude angle parameters, resp. Further on, $a_1, a_2, a_3 > 0$ are scaling parameters, δ, υ determine the bending strength and direction, resp., and $\rho_x, \rho_y \ge 0$ determine the
tapering strengths in x- and y-direction. For the rigid transformation, α, β, γ
denote the Eulerian angles of rotation and $\boldsymbol{t}^T = (X,Y,Z)$ is the translation
vector of the origin. Hence, the model is described by the parameter vec-
tor $\boldsymbol{p} = (a_1, a_2, a_3, \delta, \upsilon, \rho_x, \rho_y, X, Y, Z, \alpha, \beta, \gamma)$. The landmark position is then
given by $\boldsymbol{x}_l = \boldsymbol{x}_{tip}(\pi/2,0) = \boldsymbol{R}_{\alpha,\beta,\gamma}(\delta \cos\upsilon a_3^2, \delta \sin\upsilon a_3^2, a_3)^T + \boldsymbol{t}$. The *parametric form* of hyperboloids of one sheet is the same as the one given in [5].

3   Model Fitting with Edge-Based Fitting Measures

To fit the geometric models from Sect. 2 to the image data, a fitting measure is
optimized w.r.t. the model parameters. Here, we consider an edge strength-based
fitting measure and an edge distance-based fitting measure.
For the *edge strength-based fitting measure* M_{ES} (e.g., [18],[14]), the strength of
the intensity gradient e_g is integrated over the model surface M:

$$M_{ES}(\boldsymbol{p}) = -\int_M e_g(\boldsymbol{x})dF = -\iint_{\theta,\phi} e_g(\boldsymbol{x}(\theta,\phi)) \left\| \frac{\partial \boldsymbol{x}}{\partial \theta} \times \frac{\partial \boldsymbol{x}}{\partial \phi} \right\| d\theta d\phi \to \text{Min!}, \quad (2)$$

where $e_g(\boldsymbol{x}) = \|\nabla g(\boldsymbol{x})\|$ is the gradient magnitude of the intensity function g
and $\boldsymbol{x}$ is a point on the model surface M which is parameterized by θ, ϕ. To
emphasize small surfaces, we additionally apply a *surface weighting factor* to
the fitting measure (2) which then takes the form $M_{ES} = -\frac{\int_M e_g(\boldsymbol{x})dF}{\sqrt{\int_M dF}}$.
The *edge distance-based fitting measure* M_{ED} used here is written as (cf., e.g.,
[13],[1],[17])

$$M_{ED}(\boldsymbol{p}) = \sum_{i=1}^{N} e_g(\boldsymbol{\xi}_i) \; \rho \left(\frac{1-\hat{F}(\boldsymbol{\xi}_i,\boldsymbol{p})}{\|\nabla\hat{F}(\boldsymbol{\xi}_i,\boldsymbol{p})\|} \right) \to \text{Min!}. \quad (3)$$

The sum is taken over all N image voxels $\Xi = \{\boldsymbol{\xi}_1, \ldots, \boldsymbol{\xi}_N\}$ which – to diminish the influence of neighbouring structures – lie within a *region-of-interest (ROI)* and whose edge strength $e_g(\boldsymbol{\xi}_i)$ exceeds a certain threshold value. The vector of model parameters is denoted by $\boldsymbol{p}$. Further on, we use $\rho(x) = |x|^{1.2}$ for all $x \in \mathbb{R}$ as a distance weighting function to reduce the effect of outliers ([19]). The argument of ρ is a first order distance approximation between the image voxel with coordinates $\boldsymbol{\xi}_i$ and the model surface (cf., e.g., [17]). The inside-outside function of the tapered and bended quadric surface after applying a rigid transform is denoted by $\hat{\mathrm{F}}$ (cf., e.g., [13],[4],[1]). Also, a volume factor is used in conjunction with (3) to emphasize small volumes. This factor has been chosen as $1 + \frac{a_1 a_2 a_3}{a_{1,est} a_{2,est} a_{3,est}}$, where the weighting factor $a_{1,est} a_{2,est} a_{3,est}$ is coarsely estimated to a value of $10^3\ vox^3$ (vox denotes the spatial unit of an image voxel). For volume weighting factors (or size factors), see also, e.g., [13].

4   A Novel Hybrid Optimization Algorithm

Most optimization algorithms considered in the literature for fitting deformable models are local algorithms such as the *conjugate gradient (cg-)method* (e.g., [13],[18],[1],[5]). The cg-method combines problem specific search directions of the *method of steepest descent* with optimality properties of the method of *conjugate directions* (e.g., [6]). However, since it is a purely local method, it is prone to run into local suboptima. On the other hand, global optimization methods such as genetic algorithms (GAs; e.g., [7]) have been proposed to avoid running into local suboptima (e.g., [4],[17]). However, global methods are plagued with slow convergence rates. We here propose a *hybrid algorithm* which combines the advantages of a local optimization method such as the cg-method (computational efficiency) with a global method similar to a GA (robustness against local suboptima). Similar to GAs, we consider a whole *population* of parameter vectors which all compete for finding the *global optimum*. However, there are several differing features of our approach to traditional GAs such as the *mutation strategy*, which in our case is much better motivated and adapted to the specific optimization problem. Traditional GAs use *bit-flips* and *crossovers* to imitate natural mutation strategies ([7]). By contrast, our search strategy is to use not only the global optimum resulting from the *line search algorithm* at the end of each cg-step, but several most promising local optima resulting from line search in order to obtain a new population of parameter vectors. The search strategy may either draw upon only a few population members – calculating many cg-iterations per member (in-depth-search) – or it may incorporate many population members. Depending on the particular optimization problem at hand, either the former or the latter strategy may show better convergence behaviour. Because we want to have one strategy which is able to cope with a broad class of optimization problems, we dynamically adapt the population size to the complexity of the problem by increasing the maximal population size each time a candidate solution converges to a local optimum, i.e. when its objective function value does not improve for a given number of cg-iterations. Consequently, several parameters can be adapted to the specific optimization problem at hand:

- the maximum population size that must not be exceeded (here: 20),
- the number of cg-iterations after which the least successful population members (measured by their objective function values) are discarded (here: 5),
- the minimum number of population members that are retained after each such 'survival of the fittest' step (here: 5),
- the number of cg-iterations with no significant improvement of the objective function value after which a population member is marked convergent and not subject to further cg-iterations (here: 80), and
- a difference threshold for two parameter vectors of the deformable model below which they are considered as being equal.

The mentioned parameters have been used in all our experiments. Except for the need of adjusting these parameters, the optimization strategy presented here is a general-purpose method for poorly initialized nonlinear optimization problems and its applicability is not confined to model fitting problems in medical image analysis. Only one example of a *hybrid optimization algorithm* in image analysis is known to us: In [8], a visual reconstruction problem is described mathematically as a coupled (binary-real) nonconvex optimization problem. An informed genetic algorithm is applied to the binary variables, while an incomplete Cholesky preconditioned cg-method is applied to the remaining real variables for a given configuration of the binary variables visited by the GA. This is different to our approach, where the local and the global part cannot be separated.

5   Experimental Results for 3D Tomographic Images

Scope of Experiments In all our experiments, the deformable models were fitted to tip-like and saddle-like anatomical structures and our hybrid optimization algorithm has been compared to purely local cg-optimization w.r.t. poorly initialized model parameters using

- different *types of image data*: two 3D T1-weighted MR images and one 3D CT image of the human head
- different *types of landmarks*: frontal/occipital horn of the left/right lateral ventricle, left/right zygomatic bone as part of the skull,
- different *fitting measures*: edge distance-based, edge strength-based, and
- different sizes of the *region of interest (ROI)*: ROI radius of 10 *vox* and 15 *vox*.

Experimental Strategy For the different landmarks in the different images, an initial good fit is determined by visual inspection of the fitted deformable model with roughly estimated initial values and by repeating model fittings where necessary. To obtain poor initial estimates for model fitting, the parameter values that result from the initial good fit are varied by adding Gaussian distributed random numbers with zero expectation value and sufficiently large variances.

To assess the accuracy of landmark localization, the landmark positions calculated from the fitted deformable models are compared to ground truth positions that were manually determined in agreement with up to four persons (landmark localization error e). In addition, to measure the model fitting accuracy, we consider the root-mean-squared distance between the edge points of the image and the whole model surface, e_{RMS}, using a Euclidean distance map ([10]) from the image data after applying a 3D edge detection algorithm based on [3]. For each landmark and each image considered, the model fitting algorithm is repeated sufficiently often (here: 100 times) with random model initializations. The mean values and RMS estimates of the resulting values of e, e_{RMS} are tabulated then. For evaluating the strength of the intensity gradient, e_g, in (2),(3), cubic B-spline interpolation and Gaussian smoothing are used (see [5]).

General Results Common to all experiments is that the final objective function value is better by about 10-50% for hybrid optimization than for purely local cg-optimization. In most cases, the landmark localization and the model fitting accuracy also improve significantly. Thus, hybrid optimization turns out to be superior to purely local cg-optimization at the expense of an increase in computational costs of a factor of 5-10 (30s–90s for local cg-optimization and 150s–900s for hybrid optimization on a SUN SPARC Ultra 2 with 300MHz CPU).

The edge distance-based fitting measure in (3) turned out to be more suitable for 3D MR images of the ventricular horns with high signal-to-noise ratio since it incorporates *distance* approximations between the image data and the model surface (*long* range forces, cf. [15]). However, in comparison to (2), it is relatively sensitive to noise. Moreover, it is not suitable for hyperboloids of one sheet due to inaccuracies of the first order distance approximation associated with it.

Results for the Ventricular Horns The tips of the frontal and occipital horns of the lateral ventricles in both hemispheres are considered here. Typical examples of successful model fitting, which demonstrate the robustness of model fitting and of landmark localization in the case of poorly initialized model parameters, are given in Fig. 2. Here, contours of the model initialization are drawn in black and the results of model fitting using purely local cg-optimization are drawn in grey, while the results of model fitting using the hybrid optimization algorithm are drawn in white. The ground truth landmark positions are indicated by a ⊕-symbol. Figs. 2(a),(b) in particular demonstrate the increase of robustness of hybrid optimization in comparison to purely local cg-optimization. As can be seen from the averaged quantitative results in Table 1, hybrid optimization is superior to purely local cg-optimization and yields not only better objective function values, but in most cases also better model fitting (e_{RMS}) and landmark localization (e) results. Note that rather coarsely initialized model parameters have been used ($\overline{e}_{initial} \approx 7 \ldots 9 \, vox$), and thus some unsuccessful fitting results – particularly in the case of the less pronounced occipital horns – deteriorate the average accuracy of model fitting as shown in Table 1.

Fitting results for 3D MR images of the horns of the ventricles						
		Model initi- alization	Edge dist.-b. obj. func.		Edge strength-b. obj. func.	
			local cg-opt.	hybrid opt.	local cg-opt.	hybrid opt.
Frontal	e	7.71 ± 3.16	3.28 ± 2.99	1.40 ± 1.18	3.54 ± 2.18	2.49 ± 2.21
horn (left)	e_{RMS}	2.22 ± 1.10	1.00 ± 0.63	0.65 ± 0.22	1.04 ± 0.31	0.87 ± 0.35
Frontal	e	6.57 ± 3.18	3.87 ± 2.16	3.15 ± 2.18	6.55 ± 3.53	5.19 ± 3.70
horn (right)	e_{RMS}	2.12 ± 1.11	1.05 ± 0.60	0.78 ± 0.25	1.56 ± 1.26	1.28 ± 0.79
Occipital	e	9.08 ± 4.42	6.90 ± 3.89	6.68 ± 3.93	4.74 ± 4.33	4.61 ± 4.31
horn (right)	e_{RMS}	3.00 ± 1.40	2.06 ± 0.93	2.04 ± 0.87	1.34 ± 0.87	1.29 ± 0.78

Table 1. Fitting results averaged over 100 model fittings with poor model initializations for the *frontal/occipital* horns of the lateral ventricles from 3D MR images (e: landmark localization error (in vox), e_{RMS}: RMS distance between deformable model and image data within the region of interest (in vox), voxel size $= 0.86 \times 0.86 \times 1.2 \text{mm}^3$).

Results for the Zygomatic Bones All results for the zygomatic bones presented here are obtained with the edge strength-based fitting measure (2) from a 3D CT image. Model fitting and landmark localization for the saddle points at the zygomatic bones (e.g., Fig. 2(c)) are not as successful as they are for the tips of the ventricular horns since our geometric primitive, hyperboloids of one sheet, do not describe the anatomical structure at hand as accurately. However, the average landmark localization error e can be reduced from initially $\bar{e}_{initial} = 6.4 \ldots 6.9 \, vox$ to $\bar{e} = 2.5 \ldots 3.2 \, vox$ and the accuracy of model fitting is $\bar{e}_{RMS} = 1.5 \ldots 1.8 \, vox$ (voxel size $= 1.0 \text{mm}^3$).

6   Conclusion

In this paper, landmark extraction based on parametric deformable models has been investigated in order to improve the stability of model fitting as well as of landmark localization against poorly initialized model parameters. To this end, a novel hybrid optimization algorithm which can be applied to general nonlinear optimization problems has been introduced and edge strength- and edge distance-based fitting measures have been compared. Experimental results demonstrate the applicability of our hybrid optimization algorithm as well as the increased robustness in the case of poorly initialized parameters as compared to purely local cg-optimization. However, the experimental results do not clearly favour one fitting measure. For the frontal horns of the lateral ventricles, our edge distance-based fitting measure yields a more successful model fitting, while for the less pronounced occipital horns of the lateral ventricles and for the zygomatic bones, the edge strength-based fitting measure is more suitable.

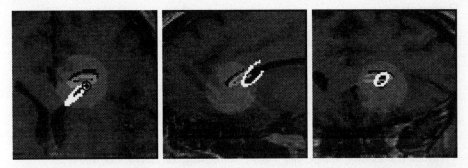

(a) 3D MR image of the *frontal* horn of the *left* lateral ventricle, edge *distance-*based fitting measure, ROI size 15.0 *vox*

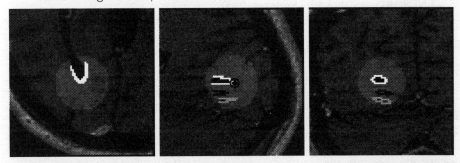

(b) 3D MR image of the *occipital* horn of the *right* lateral ventricle, edge *strength-*based fitting measure, ROI size 15.0 *vox*

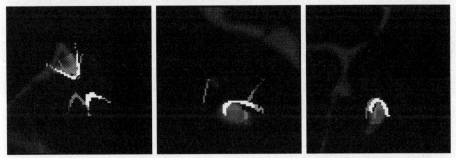

(c) 3D CT image of the *left* zygomatic bone, edge *strength*-based fitting measure, ROI size 15.0 *vox*

Fig. 2. Examples of successfully fitting tapered and bended half-ellipsoids to 3D MR images of the frontal and occipital horns of the lateral ventricles (Fig. 2(a-b)) as well as of fitting a half-hyperboloid with no further deformations to a 3D CT image of the zygomatic bone (Fig. 2(c)). Contours of the model surfaces in axial, sagittal, and coronal planes are depicted here (from left to right). *Black:* model initialization, *grey:* fitting result for local cg-optimization, and *white:* fitting result for our hybrid optimization algorithm. The ground truth landmark positions are indicated by a ⊕-sign here.

References

1. E. Bardinet, L.D. Cohen, and N. Ayache. Superquadrics and Free-Form Deformations: A Global Model to Fit and Track 3D Medical Data. *Proc. CVRMed'95*, LNCS 905, pp. 319–326. Springer, 1995.
2. R. Bertolini and G. Leutert. *Atlas der Anatomie des Menschen. Band 3: Kopf, Hals, Gehirn, Rückenmark und Sinnesorgane.* Springer, 1982.
3. J.F. Canny. A Computational Approach to Edge Detection. *PAMI*, 8(6):679–698, 1986.
4. K. Delibasis and P.E. Undrill. Anatomical object recognition using deformable geometric models. *Image and Vision Computing*, 12(7):423–433, 1994.
5. S. Frantz, K. Rohr, and H.S. Stiehl. Localization of 3D Anatomical Point Landmarks in 3D Tomographic Images Using Deformable Models. *Proc. MICCAI 2000*, LNCS 1935, pp. 492–501. Springer, 2000.
6. G.H. Golub and C.F. Van Loan. *Matrix Computations.* Johns Hopkins University Press, 1996.
7. D. Goldberg. Genetic Algorithms in Search, Optimization and Machine Learning. Addison Wesley, 1989.
8. S.H. Lai and B.C. Vemuri. Efficient hybrid-search for visual reconstruction problems. *Image and Vision Computing*, 17(1):37–49, 1999.
9. T. McInerney and D. Terzopoulos. Deformable Models in Medical Image Analysis: A Survey. *Medical Image Analysis*, 1(2):91–108, 1996.
10. D.W. Paglieroni. A Unified Distance Transform Algorithm and Architecture. *Machine Vision and Applications*, 5(1):47–55, 1992.
11. K. Rohr. On 3D differential operators for detecting point landmarks. *Image and Vision Computing*, 15(3):219–233, 1997.
12. J. Sobotta. *Atlas der Anatomie des Menschen. Band 1: Kopf, Hals, obere Extremität, Haut.* Urban & Schwarzenberg, 19th edition, 1988.
13. F. Solina and R. Bajcsy. Recovery of Parametric Models from Range Images: the Case for Superquadrics with Global Deformations. *PAMI*, 12(2):131–147, 1990.
14. L.H. Staib and J.S. Duncan. Model-Based Deformable Surface Finding for Medical Images. *IEEE Trans. Med. Imag.*, 15(5):720–731, 1996.
15. D. Terzopoulos and D. Metaxas. Dynamic 3D Models with Local and Global Deformations: Deformable Superquadrics. *PAMI*, 13(7):703–714, 1991.
16. J.-P. Thirion. New Feature Points based on Geometric Invariants for 3D Image Registration. *Internat. Journal of Computer Vision*, 18(2):121–137, 1996.
17. V. Vaerman, G. Menegaz, and J.-P. Thiran. A Parametric Hybrid Model used for Multidimensional Object Representation. *Proc. ICIP'99*, vol. 1, pp. 163–167, 1999.
18. B.C. Vemuri and A. Radisavljevic. Multiresolution Stochastic Hybrid Shape Models with Fractal Priors. *ACM Trans. on Graphics*, 13(2):177–207, 1994.
19. Z. Zhang. Parameter Estimation Techniques: A Tutorial with Application to Conic Fitting. *INRIA Rapport de recherche*, No. 2676, 1995.

Integration and Clinical Evaluation of an Interactive Controllable Robotic System for Anaplastology

Andreas Hein[1], Martin Klein[2], Tim C. Lueth[1], Jochen Queck[1], Malte Stien[1], Olaf Schermeier[1], Juergen Bier[2]

[1]Berlin Center for Mechatronic Medical Devices
Fraunhofer IPK – Charité • Campus Virchow, Clinic for Oral and Maxillofacial Surgery
Augustenburger Platz 1, 13353 Berlin
{andreas.hein, tim.lueth, jochen.queck, malte.stien, olaf.schermeier}@charite.de
http://www.charite.de/rv/mkg/srl/

[2]Clinic for Oral and Maxillofacial Surgery
Charité, Campus Virchow, D-13353 Berlin, Germany
{martin.klein, juergen.bier}@charite.de
http://www.charite.de/rv/mkg/

Abstract. In this paper the integration and evaluation of a robotics system developed at the Surgical Robotics Lab at the Charité, Berlin is presented. In the first clinical application the robotic system was used for the exact placement of implants to retain facial prostheses. In addition, the facial prostheses were fabricated using a rapid prototyping method and by mirroring the other side of the patient's face. In the paper the authors' experiences integrating the system into clinical routine are described. It became evident that only a careful optimization of each step of the intervention, starting with image acquisition and the patient fixation through the planning and the intraoperative execution by the robot leads to a significant advantage.

1 Introduction

Surgery is a relatively new and a rapidly growing field of application for robotics technology. Robots can be used to enhance the accuracy and the dexterity of a surgeon, decrease the factor of human tremble and amplify or reduce the movements and/or forces applied by the surgeon. Especially in fields of surgery where the human hand is the limiting factor for further optimization of surgical techniques – neurosurgery, orthopedic and maxillofacial surgery – robotics technology can be applied.

The drilling or shaping of bone structures is of great importance in surgery. In contrast to the situation with soft tissue, a static model of bone structures derived from CT images can be used. Currently, these operations are carried out by surgeons free hand. In the vicinity of sensitive regions, manual handling can lead to complications due to inaccuracies or shattering of the drill or shaper. Especially in maxillofacial surgery the accuracy of an intervention is of paramount importance due to the high social and aesthetic impact of the face. Therefore, a high accuracy is desirable when the surgeon

W. Niessen and M. Viergever (Eds.): MICCAI 2001, LNCS 2208, pp. 591-598, 2001.
© Springer-Verlag Berlin Heidelberg 2001

positions and moves drills or shapers. Additional difficulties in maxillofacial surgery
are the restricted access to the bone structures through small incisions, the swelling of
tissue during the intervention, and the close proximity of vital organs or structures.
In this paper the first clinical application and experiences in integrating this system
into the intervention process are described. It will be shown that the application of a
robotic system is only successful if a number of infrastructure problems such as fixation, image acquisition and planning have been solved.

2   State of the Art

The commercially available surgical robots can be distinguished by their different
control strategies:
- *Automatic systems*: are used for the autonomous performance of a preplanned intervention. Examples are the shaping of cavities for total hip replacement [1] and the
shaping of surfaces at the knee joint [2]. Because of the high safety requirements
for automatic systems, the application only makes sense for complex interventions
where the robot can carry out a part of the intervention without any interaction with
the surgeon. Commercial systems available are Robodoc by ISS and Caspar by
Orto Maquet.
- *Telemanipulation systems*: are used for minimally invasive interventions where the
surgeon has no direct access to the operation site. The systems reduce the human
tremble factor and allow movements or forces to be scaled up or down. Currently
systems are available for positioning cameras (Aesop by Computer Motion [3]) and
instrument-carrying telemanipulators (Zeus by Computer Motion and da Vinci by
Intuitive Surgical [4]).
- *Interactive controllable systems*: are a mixture of the two system approaches described above. The surgeon is not spatially separated from the patient. Additionally,
during the entire intervention the surgeon can intercept the course of the operation.
Apart from the systems developed by the authors [5][6] up to now only systems for
positioning operation microscopes have been developed (SurgiScope by Jojumarie
and MKM by Zeiss).
A direct human-machine coupling is the basis for the interactive control of a robot.
Methods are the attachment of input devices directly at the manipulator (e.g. the space
mouse at the MKM and joysticks at the SurgiScope) or the insertion of a force/torque
sensor between the hand axis and the instrument to guide a robot. In [7] this approach
is used for teaching positions and trajectories with industrial robots. A similar approach is used in [8] for the teaching of registration markers at the patient. This architecture does not allow the distinction between forces applied by the operator and
forces caused by interactions with the environment or the patient. Therefore in [9] and
[10] the manipulators have been supplied with two force/torque sensors – one between
tool and manipulator and one between manipulator and operator. Disadvantages of
this extension are increased costs and – especially inconvenient in surgery – the necessary modification of the mounted surgical instrument or a different use of the instrument.

The authors use an architecture with only one force/torque sensor. The main advantage for the surgeon is the use of unmodified surgical instruments in the usual manner. A similar approach has been used in [11] for an experimental system.

Apart from the authors' system, only two other systems are being developed currently in maxillofacial surgery. The system described in [12] consists of a passive manipulator used for positioning instruments. The disadvantage of passive systems is the time consuming positioning procedure required with them and the impossibility of moving along desired trajectories with force constraints. The other system [13] is an experimental automatic system that is not designed for interaction with the surgeon. Such systems seem unsuitable for actual application in maxillofacial surgery.

3 Description of the Treatment

An ear prosthesis is an alternative to plastic reconstructive surgery if the whole ear is involved. Ear anomalies can be congenital in origin or the result of tumor surgery or trauma. The best method for retaining the prosthesis is the insertion of implants to carry the ear prosthesis. Usually a two-stage surgical intervention is carried out. In the first stage the implants are inserted in the area of the outer helix of the artificial ear. The implants are covered by skin and after a three week healing phase are uncovered. A supraconstruction is then fixed through the skin. Using impressions of the supraconstruction the artificial ear is modeled out of silicon in a manual procedure. Usually it takes at least three months before the patient gets his facial prosthesis.

To shorten this procedure and to enhance the quality of the intervention, the authors have developed a robot-assisted procedure. Fig. 1 shows the workflow of the whole intervention. The following steps will be described in detail in this paper:

- **Image Acquisition and Fixation**: In contrast to navigation systems, robotic systems require stable fixation of the patient. An additional stabilization of the operating table, an individual head rest and an intermaxillary splint were used for this purpose. The patient's position was also fixated for the CT scan. In this way the quality of the image data was improved.
- **Planning and Fabrication of the Facial Prostheses**: The insertion of craniofacial implants for the secure retention for facial prostheses must be carried out according to functional and esthetic considerations. The amount of available bone and the soft tissue in the prospective implant position must be taken into consideration to preclude any damage to important anatomic structures. The prosthesis is manufactured from the planning data using rapid prototyping before the intervention.
- **Robot-Assisted Placement of the Implants**: At the end of the planning and fabrication process the robotic system is used for exact drilling at the preplanned positions and the insertion of the implants in a way that the implants are parallel and have the defined distance. Up to now, navigation techniques and operation templates have been used for this. The implant site can be located with navigation, but an exact freehand positioning of the implants is not possible. Templates are difficult to keep fixed and do not afford accurate guidance while drilling.

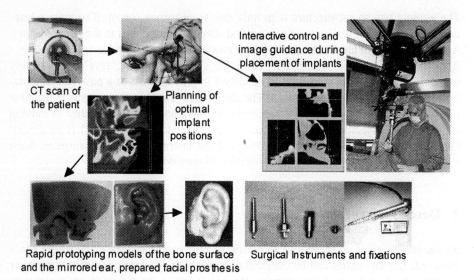

CT scan of the patient → Planning of optimal implant positions → Interactive control and image guidance during placement of implants

Rapid prototyping models of the bone surface and the mirrored ear, prepared facial prosthesis   Surgical Instruments and fixations

Fig. 1. Workflow for the fabrication of a facial prosthesis using rapid prototyping and implant insertion using a robot system.

3.1 Image Acquisition and Fixation

To achieve optimal image quality for the preoperative planning and near-to-identical conditions during data acquisition and the actual intervention, the patient's position was fixated during both steps with the same fixation system and at the same OR table. The fixation system consisted of an individual polyurethane foam dish and a custom intermaxillary splint (**Fig. 2**). The foam provided a large contact surface for the patient's soft tissue and allowed a rough positioning of the patient. The intermaxillary splint provided rigid contact between the patient's head and a lockable hydraulic arm. This arm held the patient rigidly to the OR table. A reference frame of the navigation system was also attached to the splint.

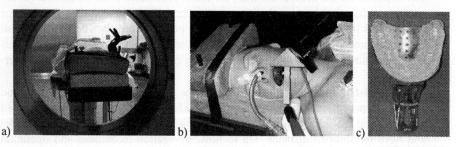

a)   b)   c)

Fig. 2. Fixation system for the robot assisted intervention. The system consists of a individual head rest and a arm rigidly holding the patient by means of an intermaxillary splint. a) Fixation during CT scan, b) during the intervention, and c) custom-made intermaxillary splint.

The registration was done via markers around the operation site. These markers were fixed within a mold of silicon and not on the patient's skin. In this way errors due to movement of markers on the skin were minimized. After the CT scan the positions of the markers relative to the reference frame of the navigation system were determined. Using the marker positions within the image coordinate system the registration matrix was calculated with a point matching algorithm. Because the repositioning accuracy achieved with the intermaxillary splint was sufficiently high, no further registration was necessary during the intervention, but rather the robot controller received the registration matrix from the planning tool.

3.2   Planning and Fabrication of the Facial Prostheses

In the planning tool (**Fig. 3**a) the implant positions and orientation were determined preoperatively according to available bone, soft tissue situation and esthetic considerations. Most important for high initial implant stability and to avoid infections is that the implants must not penetrate into mastoid cells (**Fig. 3**b). Bone thickness at the site must be adequate. Another problem is determining the aesthetically optimal position and orientation of the ear and therefore of the implants. Because only the necessary images are taken during the CT scan, the spatial orientation is very difficult. To solve this problem the anaplastologist preparing the facial prosthesis defined the optimal ear and implant positions before the CT scan. At these positions metal threads were fixed beneath the mold. During the planning the tool visualized these positions (**Fig. 3**c) and the surgeon could position the implants accordingly.

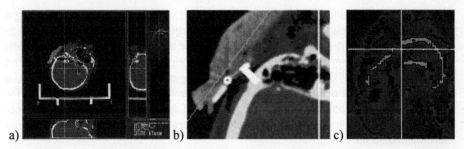

Fig. 3. a) Planning tool with three slices and a rendered 3D view right hand side. b) Operation area in the axial view with an inserted implant. On the right of the implant air-filled mastoid cells can be seen. c) Part of the 3D view with the position aids (aesthetically preferred implantation positions and outer helix of the ear).

After the implant and marker positions had been defined, the data together with a region of interest were exported to the robot controller for execution and the modified images were exported to a surface model in STL format (Standard Transformation Language). Rapid prototyping was used to fabricate a model of the operation area with the implants (**Fig. 4**a) and the mirror-image replica of the patient's healthy ear (**Fig. 4**b). These two pieces were to enable the anaplastologist to produce the silicone ear prosthesis prior to surgery. However, due to errors in the slice distance of the CT (slice distance of 2 mm can differ by up to 20%; [14]), errors during the segmentation of the skin, and metal artifacts from the fixation system and the patient's dental fillings, the quality of this first surface model (a and b) was too poor for use, and an alternative approach was necessary. An exact replica of the surface skin of the defect site was then made from a mold. This plaster model was registered, and two parallel implants and magnets were inserted into it in a robot assisted model operation (**Fig. 4c**). With this model and with the mirror-image replica of the healthy ear, the anaplastologist was able to manufacture the facial prosthesis before the intervention.

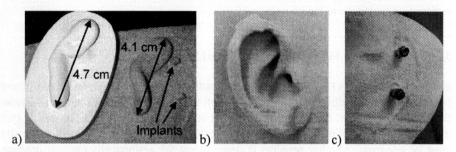

Fig. 4. a) Differences between the plaster cast of the replaced ear part and the stereolithographic model. The size of the ear parts deviate by 6 mm. b) Reconstruction errors caused by noise and artifacts in the image data. At the top of the ear an erroneous structure appeared. c) Successful plaster model with inserted implants.

3.3   Robot-Assisted Placement of the Implants

The SurgiScope (originally by Elekta IGS) was used as the basis for the developing a robotics system for maxillofacial surgery. The SurgiScope system was designed to position microscopes for neurosurgery. For invasive applications, the controller software and the tools were changed [5][6]. The robotics system consists of a parallel manipulator (Delta-3 kinematic), an infrared navigation system (IGT FP 3000), a control cabinet with a computer for the navigation system and a control computer for the manipulator. A tool system with a mechanism for changing tools and a force-torque sensor were constructed. For maxillofacial surgery, a standard drilling machine was mounted on the robot.

The robotic system differs from other systems through its completely interactive control. During the entire intervention the robot behaves passively, and moves only if the surgeon grasps and applies force to the drill. Through specially designed control schemes the surgeon can operate the instrument as usual except in cases where he/she wants to work with more precision (e.g. find a predefined position or drill along a defined axis). In these cases the robotic system controls the necessary position and orientation degrees and the surgeon can only interactively control the remaining degrees (e.g. rotations around the z-axis of the drill). Currently the system can be interactively moved to target positions along trajectories and within predefined volumes. The information from the planning system is transferred by a file which also contains the image information of a region of interest. This image information is used on the one hand for intraoperative visualization and on the other hand for autonomous derivations of control commands and to update the patient model.

4   Results and Conclusions

Initial phantom experiments with the system showed a positioning accuracy of 0.5 mm ± 0.4 mm (N=40). The relative accuracy was determined during the placement of implants in plaster bodies. The mean deviation from the defined distance was 0.2 mm ± 0.5 mm and the deviation from the parallel orientation was 0.6° ± 0.5° (N=9). The system's handling and accuracy under real conditions were assessed in the clinical evaluation.

Robot assisted implantation was carried out on 13 patients. In total 30 craniofacial implants (Entific Medical Systems) were inserted in out-patient surgery under general anesthesia. All patients had congenital ear defects which were rehabilitated with implant-anchored silicone ear prostheses. Three implants were inserted in the first four patients, with one serving in each case as a reserve. In the following nine patients, given the positive experience of the first operations, only two implants were inserted. No intraoperative injuries with opening of the mastoid cells or damage to the venous sinuses at the base of the cranium or dura mater encephali occurred. With the exception of one patient whose intermaxillary splint disconnected due to insufficiently deep anesthesia, all targeted positions were reached with an accuracy of about ±1 mm. For this single patient new implant positions were determined intraoperatively, but the preoperatively created prosthesis did not fit. In the other cases the preoperatively manufactured ear prostheses were fitted (**Fig. 5**), but these patients were advised not to wear the prosthesis constantly for the first three months to avoid disturbing the osseointegration.

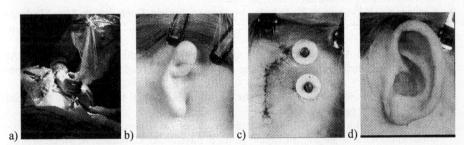

a)   b)   c)   d)

Fig. 5. Clinical application of the interactive controlled robot system (a) and result in a patient: b) preoperative, c) postoperative, d) facial prosthesis fixed by the implants.

The robot assisted implantation presented here and the new concept of preoperative manufacture of the prosthesis are as a whole more complex than manual implant insertion. They demand much more precise preoperative planning, intraoperative execution, and a careful integration into the usual course of the intervention. Nonetheless, a trained team which takes all potential sources of error into consideration can deliver

598   A. Hein et al.

excellent esthetic and functional results. Furthermore, the patient's rehabilitation time is shortened, because with the exception of one patient, all patients could wear the new prosthesis directly after the intervention. The new manufacturing process for the facial prosthesis saves the anaplastologist one day's modeling time, and the patient is spared hours in repeated fittings. The positive clinical experience and the accuracy attained in the insertion of craniofacial implants to retain ear prostheses is good cause to apply this robot system for insertion of implants in other areas of the head or as the next planned application to support the surgeon shaping and inserting pedicle screws in spinal surgery.

References

1. Taylor, R. H. *et al.*: An Image-Directed Robotic System for Precise Orthopaedic Surgery. IEEE Trans. o. Robotics and Automation, Vol.10, No.3 (1994), pp. 261-75.
2. Kaiser, C.: Einführung in die technischen Grundlagen des totalen Kniegelenkersatzes mit CASPAR. In Maßberg, W., G. Reinhart, M. Wehmöller (Ed.), Neue Technologien in der Medizin, Shaker Verlag (2000).
3. Jacobs LK, Shayani V, Sackier JM: Determination of the learning curve of the AESOP robot. Surg Endosc, Jan; 11(1) (1997), pp. 54-5.
4 Guthart, G.S., J.K. Salisbury: The Intuitive telesurgery system: overview and application. ICRA IEEE Int. Conf. on Robotics and Automation (2000).
5 Lueth, T.C. *et al.*: A Surgical Robot System for Maxillofacial Surgery. IEEE Int. Conf. on Industrial Electronics, Control, and Instrumentation (IECON), Aachen, Germany, Aug. 31-Sep. 4, (1998) 2470-2475.
6 Hein, A.: Eine interaktive Robotersteuerung für chirurgische Applikationen. Ph.D. Thesis. Fortschritt–Berichte, Nr. 195, VDI–Verlag, Düsseldorf (2000).
7 Hirzinger, G., K. Landzettel: Sensory feedback structures for robots with supervised learning. ICRA IEEE Int. Conf. on Robotics and Automation (1985), pp. 627-35.
8 Kazanzides, P. *et al.*: Force sensing and control for a surgical robot. ICRA IEEE Int. Conf. on Robotics and Automation (1992), pp. 612-7.
9 Kosuge, K., Y. Fujisawa, T. Fukuda: Mechanical System Control with Man-Machine-Environment Interactions. ICRA IEEE Int. Conf. on Robotics and Automation (1993), pp. 239-44.
10. Taylor, R. *et al.*: A steady-hand robotic system for microsurgical augmentation. MICCAI Int'l Conf. on Medical Image Computing and Computer-Assisted Intervention (1999), pp. 1031-41.
11. Ho, S. C. *et al.*: Force control for robotic surgery. ICAR IEEE Int'l. Conf. on Advanced Robotics (1995), pp. 21-31.
12. Cutting, C., F. Bookstein, R. Taylor: Applications of simulation, morphometrics and robotics in craniofacial surgery. In Taylor, R. H., S. Lavallee, G. C. Burdea, R. Mösges (eds.), Computer-integrated surgery: technology and clinical applications, MIT Press, (1996) 641-662.
13. Bohner, P. *et al.*: Operation planning in cranio-maxillo-facial surgery. Medicine Meets Virtual Reality 4 (MMVR4'96), San Diego, California, (1996).
14. Albrecht, J., T.C. Lueth , A. Hein, J. Bier: Measurement of the Slice Distance Accuracy of the Mobile CT Tomoscan. CARS 2000, Computer Assisted Radiology and Surgery, (2000). pp. 651-5.

Smart Alignment Tool for Knee MosaicPlasty Surgery

Albert W. Brzeczko[1], Randal P. Goldberg[2], Russell H. Taylor[2,3], Peter Evans[4]

1 Baltimore Polytechnic Institute High School, Baltimore, MD, USA
2 Mechanical Engineering Department, The Johns Hopkins University, Baltimore, MD, USA
3 Computer Science Department, The Johns Hopkins University, Baltimore, MD, USA
4 Department of Orthopedic Surgery, Johns Hopkins Hospital, Baltimore, MD, USA

Abstract. The Smart Alignment Tool for Knee MosaicPlasty Surgery is a device that aids in aligning the MosaicPlasty harvesting chisel with the cartilage surface of the knee. In the standard arthroscopic procedure, the angle at which the graft is harvested and inserted is determined visually by the surgeon through a single endoscopic view. The ability of the surgeon to obtain and place these grafts in an orientation perpendicular to the cartilage surface determines, in large part, the efficacy of the procedure. By instrumenting the tool, the angle of the tool relative to the surface is fed back to the surgeon. Preliminary experiments show this greatly increases the accuracy and consistency of this task.

1 Introduction

The MosaicPlasty procedure for knee osteochondral grafts, pioneered by Dr. Lazló Hangody describes a technique to repair articular cartilage degeneration onset by

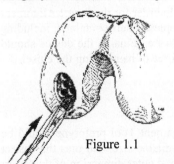

Figure 1.1

trauma or aging (1). The defects in the cartilage are replaced by cylindrical osteochondral grafts taken from a non-weight-bearing portion of the knee, such as the patellofemoral joint. The grafts fill the sections of the knee where the cartilage had been worn (Figure 1.1). Because these grafts are smaller than other autograft transplantation procedures, and because the procedure integrates transplanted cartilage with the adjacent hyaline cartilage via fibrocartilage, MosaicPlasty provides a smooth cartilage surface, mimicking closely the surface of the knee before it had suffered from defects. Another advantage of the MosaicPlasty procedure is the integration of the spongy element of the graft, which fuses with the spongy bed at the recipient site (2). The resulting cartilage surface is very stable because it has a strong foundation with the underlying bone.

W. Niessen and M. Viergever (Eds.): MICCAI 2001, LNCS 2208, pp. 599-605, 2001.
© Springer-Verlag Berlin Heidelberg 2001

A procedural aspect that greatly impacts the efficacy of the MosaicPlasty procedure is the harvesting and placement of the osteochondral graft. If the graft is not harvested and placed perpendicular to this surface, many of the advantages of the technique are lost, as the implanted cartilage does not line up properly with the surface. Additionally, the projecting element of the cartilage has very little support and behaves as cartilage placed on an osseous surface (2). The possibility also exists that the articular surface may be injured by the misaligned graft-harvesting tool (3). Presently when performing this procedure arthroscopically, the surgeon looks through an endoscope to estimate the perpendicularity of the chisel, a difficult task to perform from the single view present. This difficulty causes a majority of these procedures to be performed open.

The Smart Alignment Tool, an angle-sensing device that mounts on the MosaicPlasty graft-harvesting tool, is able to detect the angle between the bone surface and a vertical reference axis. The device uses three points, maintained by feelers placed on the cartilage surface and tracked by linear potentiometers, to locate the cartilage surface, and compare its normal to the axis of the tool. This gives a quantitative measurement of the vital angle independent of the surgeon's ability to perform visual inspection.

2 Prototype Design

2.1 Requirements

The first step of the project was determining the constraints the MosaicPlasty surgery would pose on the design. The device needed to fit within an arthroscopic portal, so size was a very important consideration. Ideally, the device's diameter should be within approximately 5 mm that of the grafting chisel so the size of the portal needed would not need to be increased significantly. The device should also allow the chisel to be hammered in approximately 15mm to the osteochondral surface. The device should provide angles accurate to approximately 1°. In order for the Smart Alignment Tool to become a useful surgical tool, it must be completely self-contained, including onboard signal processing and feedback display hardware. Finally, the device should be durable enough to withstand sterilization and the force of hammering the chisel.

2.2 Design

It was determined that the design of the Smart Alignment Tool prototype would be based on an 8.5 mm chisel, as this was the largest available size, and thus the easiest to build upon. The use of this size required that the total outer dimension of the Smart Alignment Tool be approximately 14 mm or less.

The device uses three "feelers" to contact the cartilage surface. These feelers are permitted to slide parallel to the axis of the tool as it is oriented, maintaining the surface of the knee. Motion of these feelers is tracked with BI Technologies Model 404 linear compact potentiometers with spring-returning sliders of approximately

15mm travel length, and midrange resistance values (~10 kΩ). Each potentiometer returns a voltage that corresponds to the feeler position.

The grafting chisel is rigidly mounted within the Smart Alignment Tool, locked in place with a setscrew. The potentiometers allow sufficient range of motion for the tool alignment and insertion to be performed.

2.3 Signal Processing

The next task was to create a data acquisition (DAQ) system for the tool so that the voltages output from the potentiometers could be processed into an angle. As a preliminary setup, a National Instruments Lab PC+ ISA DAQ card and LabVIEW software were used. However, this PC-dependent setup went against the requirement for the device to be as portable as possible. It was necessary to implement secondary signal processing setup allowing the Smart Alignment Tool to be free of a full-sized computer. The Handy Board, a C-programmable Motorola 68HC11-based controller board designed by MIT, is being used as an intermediate step.

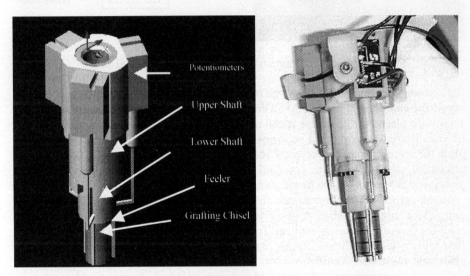

Figure 2.1: CAD Model and Photo of Prototype Alignment Tool

A program was written for the Handy Board that converts each potentiometer voltage output into a Z-coordinate (parallel to the axis of the tool). The X- and Y-coordinates are fixed per the construction of the device. The three resulting points define the surface of the cartilage. The normal of this surface is then compared to the Z-axis of the tool to obtain a measurement of the angle between them. This angle is then output to the Handy Board's LCD for viewing.

602   A.W. Brzeczko et al.

3 Experiments

To begin with, a simple validation experiment was performed. A calibrated Optotrack Rigid Body was mounted in the Smart Alignment Tool, and the angle measured by the Smart Alignment Tool was compared to the Optotrack reading. The experiment showed that the device was accurate to an average accuracy of 1.39°.

Next, two sets of experiments simulating the arthroscopic surgery were performed. In the first set of experiments, the operator's field of vision and range of motion were impaired in ways resembling the actual MosaicPlasty procedure. A box enclosing a

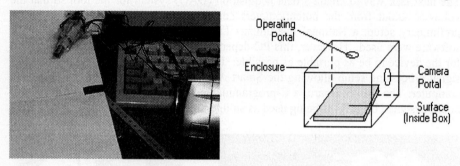

Figure 3.1: Diagram and Photo of Experimental Setup

flat surface at an arbitrary angle to the table was built, with access and view portals to mimic the endoscopy (Figure 3.1). The grafting chisel and inactive Smart Alignment Tool were placed in the access portal and a camera was placed in the vision portal. Eleven different subjects then performed five timed trials in which they attempted to place the chisel perpendicular to the surface, relying solely on eyesight. After chisel placement, the Smart Alignment Tool was activated and the angle between chisel placement and normal to the surface was recorded.

In the second set of experiments, the Smart Alignment Tool was active the entire time. Test subjects were thus given visual information from the camera and angle readouts from the Smart Alignment Tool. As was the case in the first experiment, five trials were conducted. After each chisel placement, elapsed time and the placement angle were recorded.

From these experiments, the time and accuracy of chisel placement without the aid of the Digitizer was compared to the time and accuracy with the Digitizer.

4 Results

Results of experiments were as follows. "Angle" denotes degrees divergence from perpendicularity to the test plane. "Time to place" denotes the elapsed time before perpendicularity was perceived and test instrument was driven.

4.1 Results of Experiment without Active Smart Alignment Tool:

Subject	Angle Placement (Degrees)		Time Elapsed (seconds)	
	Mean	Standard Deviation	Mean	Standard Deviation
1	2.6	1.1	21.8	12.5
2	3.2	1.6	11.0	2.5
3	5.8	1.8	29.4	14.5
4	9.8	3.4	30.0	9.4
5	3.4	2.1	8.6	4.6
6	11.8	7.4	6.2	1.8
7	6.0	5.7	13.0	13.3
8	7.8	3.8	14.8	8.8
9	8.0	3.7	16.0	11.8
10	11.4	2.7	14.6	5.5
11	5.2	2.5	14.8	4.1
Overall	6.8	4.5	16.4	11.0

4.2 Results of Experiment with Active Smart Alignment Tool:

Subject	Angle Placement (Degrees)		Time Elapsed (Seconds)	
	Mean	Standard Deviation	Mean	Standard Deviation
1	0.0	0	40.0	19.8
2	1.4	1.1	8.4	7.6
3	0.6	0.5	37.2	32.9
4	1.2	1.6	22.6	9.8
5	0.8	0.4	10.8	7.6
6	1.4	0.9	9.8	6.7
7	1.0	0.9	14.0	6.5
8	0.4	0.5	34.8	16.3
9	0.4	0.5	17.8	18.1
10	3.2	2.5	14.4	3.9
11	0.6	0.5	21.2	6.4
Overall	1.0	1.3	21.0	17.2

5 Discussion

5.1 Analysis of Results

The data show that the chisel was placed more accurately and with greater consistency when using the Smart Alignment Tool for feedback. The mean angle

604   A.W. Brzeczko et al.

from the normal was 1.0° with the aid of the Smart Alignment tool and 6.8° without it, including maximum angular error of 20°. The mean elapsed time increased in the Smart Alignment Tool trials. However, this can be attributed to the fact that the subjects had numeric angle readouts, and were willing to take extra time to ensure the angle was placed accurately. For the subjects using only eyesight, the overall standard deviation of angle placement was 4.5, versus 1.3 with the Smart Alignment Tool's angle readout.

It should be noted that the validation experiments indicated an average error of 1.4° and maximum errors of up to 3.4° after four outliers were removed due to drastic bending of the feelers. While this shows that the device is less accurate than the target 1° error, it does not change the qualitative conclusions that can be drawn from the simulated surgery experiments. Rather, it points at clear improvements to be made in forthcoming iterations of the design.

5.2 Future Plans/Experiments

A problem with the current prototype arises from the stiffness of the feelers, stemming from the feeler material and wear in the plastic body by which they are guided. In the next iteration of the Smart Alignment Tool, these features will be made of stiffer material, which will significantly improve the accuracy of the device.

Another feature to be added is a "footprint". The current feeler tips are likely to pierce the cartilage surface, rather than rest on them. In the next iteration, a ring will be mounted to the bottoms of the three feelers, increasing their footprint and distributing their force more evenly along the cartilage surface. This will further aid in stiffening the feelers, as well as reduce errors which may be introduced by the unevenness in the cartilage surface.

Other design refinements will be made to increase the overall functionality of the device. An onboard signal processor would contribute to the compactness and portability of the Smart Alignment Tool to directly display the angle readout. With this comes the ability to display additional information. Work is being done to determine the most effective way to indicate the direction and magnitude of the angle on such a display. From observation in the experiments, this extra information would likely have a significant positive impact on time it takes to align the tool. It will also be advantageous to modify the design such that the Smart Alignment Tool can accommodate a full range of chisel sizes.

Ultimately, cadaver experiments and clinical trials will be performed to further demonstrate the Smart Alignment Tool's effect on the results of the Knee MosaicPlasty procedure.

Acknowledgments

The authors gratefully acknowledge the support of the National Science Foundation Engineering Research Center Grant #EEC9731478.

References

1) Bobic, Vladimir. *The Utilisation of Osteochondral Autografts in the Treatment of Articular Cartilage Lesions*. 15 Sep. 2000 <http://www.isakos.com/innovations/oats.html>.

2) Christel, P., et al. *Osteochondral Grafting using the Mosaicplasty Technique*. 15 Sep. 2000 <http://www.maitrise-orthop.com/corpusmaitri/orthopaedic/mo76_mosaicplasty/index.shtml>.

3) Higgs, Geoffrey B, and Arthur L Boland. *Cartilage Regeneration and Repair*. 15 Sep. 2000 <http://www.mgh.harvard.edu/depts/hoj/html/cartilage_repair.html>.

Multi-DOF Forceps Manipulator System for Laparoscopic Surgery - Mechanism Miniaturized & Evaluation of New Interface -

Ryoichi Nakamura[1], Takeshi Oura[2], Etsuko Kobayashi[2], Ichiro Sakuma[2],
Takeyoshi Dohi[2], Naoki Yahagi[2], Takayuki Tsuji[2], Mitsuo Shimada[3],
Makoto Hashizume[4]

[1] Dept. of Precision Engineering, Graduate School of Engineering,
[2] Institute of Environmental Studies, Graduate school of Frontier Science,
the Univ. of Tokyo, 7-3-1, Hongo, Bunkyo-ku, Tokyo 113-8656 Japan
{ryoichi, takeshi, etsuko, sakuma, dohi, yahagi,
tsuji}@miki.pe.u-tokyo.ac.jp
[3] Department of Surgery and Science, Graduate School of Medical Sciences,
[4] Dept. of Disaster and Emergency Medicine, Grad. School of Medical Science,
Kyushu University, 3-1-1, Maidashi, Higashi-ku, Hukuoka 812-8582 Japan
mshimada@surg2.med.kyushu-u.ac.jp
mhashi@dem.med.kyushu-u.ac.jp

Abstract. The Multi-DOF forceps manipulator we developed has two additional DOF of bending on the tip of forceps, and provides new surgical fields and techniques for surgeons. The most remarkable characteristics of the prototype described in this paper are: **1)** the *small* diameter and the *small* radius of curvature of bending; **2)** the confirmation of *perfect cleanness and sterilization* of this manipulator. In this paper, we will show some new mechanisms of the forceps manipulator. Firstly, we made new mechanism of bending forceps. Using the mechanism, we made new prototype of forceps manipulator *which diameter is 5mm*. Secondly, we developed *new concept of man-machine interface for the system*. It will show the new control method and surgeons can operate surgeries with more dexterity and without confusion. We evaluated the system including new interface on typical laparosurgical procedure using simulator, and confirmed the effectiveness of this concepts.

1 Introduction

Laparoscopic surgery is now widely established as minimal invasive surgery (MIS). However, it has some problems and difficulties due to the "minimal invasive" method. The forceps and laparoscope are inserted into the visceral cavity through the trochars that are fixed on the abdominal wall. These tools have only four degrees of freedom of movement (DOF) and small working areas (Fig. 1).

Using conventional tools (forceps), surgeons can approach an operation point only through a single approach path. However, in some cases, various alternative approach paths for an operation area are needed. The tools thus require additional DOF to solve these problems (Fig. 2).

W. Niessen and M. Viergever (Eds.): MICCAI 2001, LNCS 2208, pp. 606-613, 2001.
© Springer-Verlag Berlin Heidelberg 2001

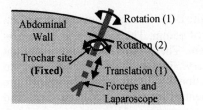

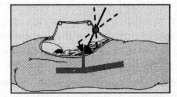

Fig. 1. Four DOF of surgical tools in laparoscopic surgery

Fig. 2. Approach path of surgical tools
← is approach path of conventional tools.
←‑ ‑ are approach paths of tools with additional DOF.

Surgical robots, which can help surgeons' manipulation such as steadier holding, more precise operating, and remote control, are being studied and developed. However, there are many problems in the use of robots in medical fields. The most important consideration must be safety, both in terms of engineering and medical effectiveness. Recently, forceps with additional DOF for MIS have been studied in many institutes and applied to many actual cases [1][2][3][4][5][8], but there is a problem with the following points;

● *Diameters of Forceps with additional DOF are still big*
   The major diameter of commercial forceps for laparoscopic surgery is 5mm and is gradually smaller, but the major diameter of the forceps with additional DOF that has been studied in many institutes is around 10mm.
● *Sizes of the whole system of Forceps with additional DOF are still big*
   Big space around the operation table in operation room is needed for the system and it cause the problems about the coexistence with doctor and safety.

Taking these problems into account, we developed Multi-DOF Forceps Manipulator System for laparoscopic surgery [6].

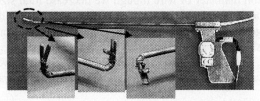

Fig. 3. First Prototype of Multi-DOF forceps manipulator

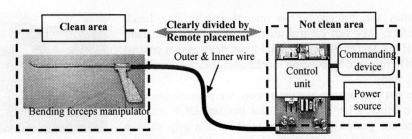

Fig. 4. Total system components of the Multi-DOF forceps manipulator.

This Forceps manipulator has 6mm diameter and the characteristic of less-space-consuming that is achieved by the divided architecture of forceps & actuators. In this paper, we present new two mechanisms of Multi-DOF forceps manipulator system. The first mechanism is the bending mechanism of φ5mm. The second one is the new man-machine interface of the manipulator system. These mechanisms are important features to realize the more evolutional surgery. The methods used in order to construct the mechanisms are presented in Section 2. The experimental results are presented in Section 3, including the measurement of mechanical characteristics and the performance of this manipulator in surgical environments. Using this manipulator, problems in laparoscopic surgery are clearly solved, and new standards with higher effectiveness and safety are achieved.

2   Method

2.1   Bending Mechanism

We developed the Multi-DOF forceps manipulator, which provides two additional DOF of bending. The bending mechanism is composed of four stainless steel rings with a coupling giving one DOF, stainless wire, and Teflon tubes (shown in Fig. 5 and 6). This mechanism is driven by four stainless steel wires. The ranges of bending motion are 0 to 90 degrees for each two DOF. [6]

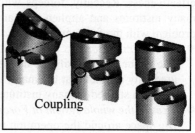

Fig. 5. Stainless steel ring joint

The important problem on miniaturizing mechanism is to have to maintain strength / hardness of joint and diameter of wire though we decrease total size. In this study we miniaturized the mechanism by detaching the wire conservation with a Teflon tube.

In addition, we got drive range in former φ6mm diameter Forceps Manipulator System by establishing two joints for each DOF (drive range of 1 joint: 45deg * 2 = 90 deg). However, I considered a fall of efficiency / outbreak power of the wire with mechanism miniaturized and produced the joint that had big drive range of 60 deg.

2.2   New Man-Machine Interface

Surgeons use forceps in an operation with one hand. Therefore, they can control all movement with one hand even if the degree of freedom and input devices that control the DOF increase by bending mechanism that we developed in this study.

In the last year system we developed, we possess the input device which a joy-stick button for bending DOF and two buttons for grasping DOF were built in to a grip as man machine interface to operate the 3 degree of freedom on the tip of Multi-DOF Forceps Manipulator System. (Fig. 6)

However, in this device, some problems were figured through tests and evaluations.

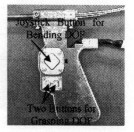

Fig. 6. Button Interface for Multi-DOF Forceps

(1) It is difficult to operate bending and grasping move quickly and without confusion because there are many buttons in small area.
(2) It is hard to do operation of intuitionally because the arrangement of direction of buttons and a direction of bending axes on the tip of forceps do not correspond.
(3) There are no correspondence between input value and output value. (Input value is time to push the button / Output value is degree of bending)
(4) It is difficult to use more than one DOF simultaneously and coordinatively (synchronized drive).

Development of better interface is much necessary in order to do complicated procedures in laparosurgery (e.g. suturing, ligation, etc.) using this Multi-DOF Forceps Manipulator. In addition, in this manipulator, it is different from major surgical robot systems (Master-slave manipulator) in the point that surgeons maintain forceps manipulator by their own hand and operate the DOF on the tip part as well. It offers the following advantage to surgeons;
1. Surgeon keeps his haptic sense during the surgery even if he uses manipulator. (In many cases, the lack of haptic sense is main consideration in developing surgical manipulator)
2. The time / spacial / economical cost of this manipulator is much more few than the cost of the surgical robot system which control the whole DOF for controlling forceps (7DOF or more)
Therefore, simple and small interface to reflect intention of surgeons at sight becomes necessary to establish the Multi-DOF Forceps Manipulator System which keeps these advantages.

In this study, we developed the new man-machine interface mechanism. On this interface, surgeons drive the two bending axes using the two bending axes of their first finger. (shown in Fig. 7)

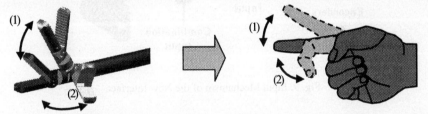

Fig. 7. DOF Comparison between the bending forceps and the first finger

This system is the technique that we paid its attention to bending movement of a first finger. Bending movement of a first finger corresponds to bending axis (2) of Forceps Manipulator, and up-and-down motion product of a first finger corresponds to bending axis (1) of Forceps Manipulator. We think that there is a little influence that operation with a first finger gives to a stability maintenance state of a grip, because the part, which is actually concerned with holding the grip, is three fingers (middle finger / third finger / little finger) and the part of the root of thumb. A first finger is not concerned greatly when I grasp a thing, hence the interface using it is appropriate for this manipulator.
The prototype of the new interface is shown in Fig.8.

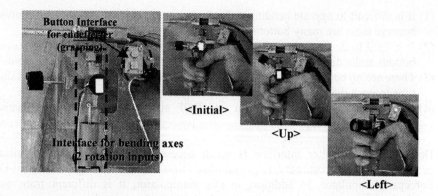

Fig. 8. The Prototype of New Interface for Multi-DOF Forceps Manipulator

The mechanism of the interface is explained in Fig. 9. The characteristics of the manipulator are presented in Table 1.

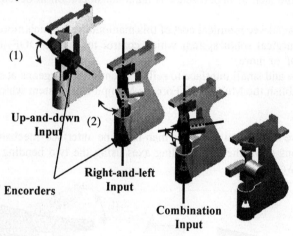

Fig. 9. Input Mechanism of the New Interface

Table 1. Specification of the bending forceps manipulator system

Range of actions (DOF)	2 bending and 1 grasping
Moving range	0-60 °(bending) / 0-60 °(grasping)
Diameter	5 mm
Size	345 mm (l) x 135 mm(h) x 15 mm(d)
Weight	250g (Multi-DOF forceps)
Material	Stainless (SUS304)

3   Experimental Results

3.1   Mechanical Characteristics

Firstly, we checked the characteristics of bending movements. The movement characteristics have hysteresis, with large backlash due to the stretching and friction of the wires. The difference between φ6mm drive and φ5mm drive is mainly caused by the efficiency fall of wire driving force and deterioration of a wire due to the mechanism miniaturized. The Teflon tube removal and the errors in manufacture and assembly are the biggest effect to the bending drive. Due to these problems, the characteristics of the bending drive (φ5mm) go little worse than that of φ6mm. But these problems will be solved through the reshaping the wire drive system and manufacture method and by using more appropriate materials.

3.2   Testing in *a Semi-clinical Situation*

We tested the clinical performance of this Multi-DOF forceps manipulator by using it in a semi-clinical situation. The surgeon carried out trial operations (grasping, bending, extension, and ligation, etc.). This test is carried out on the training tool set for laparoscopic surgery. (Fig. 12)

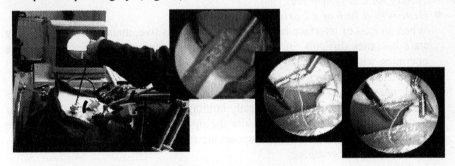

Fig. 12. Testing overviews of the Multi-DOF forceps manipulator system

As a result of having used Multi-DOF forceps, the advantages was recognized compared with a general forceps which was a straight, in the following points;
(1) *Turning thread around the total bile duct and detaining thread:*
    The surgeon can send thread easily without excessive force because the "circumference" operation can be carried out.
(2) *Winding thread around the forceps and catching another end of the thread and pulling it (ligation):*
    The surgeon can accomplish the ligation easier when the range between two forceps is nearly plumb. Multi-DOF forceps can control the range more easily than the commercial straight forceps. Using straight one, the ability of controlling the range depends on the positions of trochars.

In addition, it is easy to start an operation order and is hard to make a mistake in using 2 axes stick type interface compared with a button type, and the possibility of improvement of the surgeon's dexterity was recognized.

However, the poor responses of movement (due to the backlash of the wire drive system) become more serious than the case of 6mm forceps manipulator. We must solve this problem for the establishment of the total forceps manipulator system with additional DOF and which provide surgeons high performance of laparo-procedure (with high dexterity, high accuracy, etc).

In this experiment, although there were indeed problems, the basic functions of this Multi-DOF forceps manipulator with new mechanism were confirmed as sufficiently useful for laparoscopic surgery.

4   Discussion

4.1   Multi-DOF Forceps Manipulator with New Mechanisms

The new mechanism of ϕ5mm forceps manipulator has some problems in drive characteristics. Through the establishment of the high precision manufacturing and assembly of the small components and the adoption of the materials and design appropriate for the mechanism, we will develop the small Multi-DOF Forceps Manipulator System with high performances. The performance of new Interface is confirmed as useful basically in the evaluation. The improvement points considered to be necessary for this system are;

- *Heaviness & lash of a 2 axis stick interface*
  When an axis of interface is too light and too sensitive, maintenance of bending state becomes difficult. In opposite, when too heavy and too insensitive, the operation with high accuracy and high response cannot be carried out.
- *Optimization of the grip shape*
  It is necessary to drive the bending axes and the other DOF of forceps simultaneously. Therefore, the steady holding of forceps grip with three finger is very important. We must consider the optimization of the grip shape or the development of new holder that support the steady holding of this manipulator.
- *The Interface for grasping*
  In this paper, we only developed the new interface for bending axes. If pursuing the intuitional drive, it is desirable to establish the interface for grasping that imitated movement of "grasping" instead of using two buttons.
- *More convictive evaluation*
  In this experiment, we tested the system in very limited case and method. It's of course not enough to discriminate the effectiveness of this system in real surgery. We need some more quantitative evaluations and comparison of the system to conventional laparoscopic instruments and many existing active forceps research.

4.2   Future Work ~ from Additional DOF to Additional Function ~

This Multi-DOF Forceps Manipulator System is developed under the desire for additional DOF of surgical tools in MIS. And there is another strong desire for new surgical tools. That is the surgical tool with "Additional Function".

We are now planning and prototyping a Multi-DOF Bipolar Coagulator Manipulator. Using this manipulator, the surgeons can possess the wide surgical field, wide surgical approach pass, and wide surgical procedure, and they can be free from many limitations in laparoscopic surgery, e.g. due to the necessity of retaining the surgical fields, changing many forceps according as situations, and the difficulty in management of vessels and vascular (clipping or ligation).

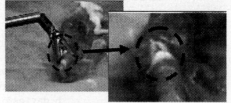

Fig. 13. Multi-DOF Bipolar Coagulator Manipulator System

5   Conclusion

We have developed a Multi-DOF forceps manipulator with new two mechanisms. Through the testing in a semi-clinical situation, although some problems were found, the effectiveness of this manipulator was clearly demonstrated. Especially, as for the stick type interface, the effectiveness of improvement of operability was recognized enough. With the improvement of the DOF arrangement and the stability of bending drive, the construction of the new interface for surgical tools will be possible.

6   Acknowledgements

This study was partly supported by the **Research for the Future Program JSPS-RFTF 96P00801 & JSPS-RFTF 99I00904,** and by **Grant-in-Aid for Scientific Research (JSPS Fellow).**

References

1. Rininsland H.: ARTEMIS. A telemanipulator for cardiac surgery, *European Journal of Cardio-Thoracic Surgery* 16(2) (1999) 106-111
2. Shennib H., Bastawisy A., McLoughlin J., Moll F.: Robotic computer-assisted telemanipulation enhances coronary artery bypass, *Journal of Thoracic & Cardiovascular Surgery* 117(2) Feb (1999) 310-313
3. Cohn, M., L. S. Crawford, J. M. Wendlandt, S. S. Sastry: Surgical Applications of Milli-Robots, *Journal of Robotic Systems* 12(6) (1995) 401-416
4. Steve Charles, Hari Das, Tim Ohm, Curtis Boswell, Guillermo Rodriguez, Robert Steele, Dan Istrate: Dexterity-enhanced Telerobotic Microsurgery *Proceedings of 8th International Conference on Advanced Robotics (ICAR '97)* (1997) 5-10
5. Ikuta K., Kato T., Nagata S.: Micro active forceps with optical fiber scope for intra-ocular microsurgery, *Proceedings of the IEEE Micro Electro Mechanical Systems (MEMS)* (1996) 456-461
6. Nakamura R. et al: Multi-DOF Forceps Manipulator System for Laparoscopic Surgery, *Proceeding of Medical Image Computing and Computer-Assisted Intervention - MICCAI 2000* ,Springer, LNCS, Vol.1935, (2000) 653-660
7. Hashimoto D.: *Gasless Laparoscopic Surgery* World Scientific Publishing (1995)
8. Breedveld P., Stassen H., Meijer D., Jakimowicz J.: Manipulation in Laparoscopic surgery: Overview of Impeding Effects and Supporting Aids, Journal of Laparoendoscopic & Advanced Surgical Techniques 9(6) (1999) 469-480

The Development of a Haptic Robot to Take Blood Samples from the Forearm

Aleksandar Zivanovic and Brian Davies

Mechatronics in Medicine Laboratory, Mechanical Engineering Dept,
Imperial College, Exhibition Road, South Kensington, London SW7 2BX
b.davies@ic.ac.uk,
http://www.me.ic.ac.uk/case/mim/index.html

Abstract. This paper presents the results of tests of a robotic mechanism constructed to take blood samples from the forearm. The system was designed to both identify the location of a vein and to insert a needle into the vein, using a single force sensor.

To locate the vein, a probe was pressed against the surface of the forearm in multiple locations across the width of the patient's arm. An algorithm was developed to analyse the force/position profiles obtained during this process to identify the presence of a vein.

An additional feature of the robot design was to insert a needle into the previously located vein, under force control. A control strategy was developed so that the robot would stop automatically and avoid overshoot of the needle.

Results are presented that indicate that the robot can both locate a vein and insert a needle.

1 Introduction

1.1 Palpation

The robot described in this paper finds the veins in a patient's arm by the use of palpation. Clearly, to (partially) automate palpation, a tactile sensor, as part of a haptic device, is required. Other researchers have recognized the usefulness of tactile sensing as a diagnostic tool and have proposed various electro-mechanical systems. Gentle [1] proposed using an array of pressure sensors to screen for breast cancer. Dario [2] proposed a robot driven probe to mimic palpation, intended for the diagnosis of cancer. Wellman and Howe [3,4,5] also investigated palpation, particularly for detecting tumors in breast tissue.

1.2 The Conventional Venepuncture Procedure

The following section briefly describes the conventional venepuncture procedure as described in [6] and [7]. It also identifies the problems faced by the human practitioner which may be overcome by the use of a mechatronic device.

The arm is palpated until a vein is found. The vein should be firm and slightly bouncy, rather like an underinflated balloon. Then the needle is inserted into the

W. Niessen and M. Viergever (Eds.): MICCAI 2001, LNCS 2208, pp. 614–620, 2001.

vessel at between a 30 and 45 degree angle at a speed estimated to be of the order of 20 mm per second. The deepest veins that can be found by a trained medic are generally between 5 mm and 7 mm deep.

The ability to find a suitable vein is is affected by factors such as the amount of subcutaneous fat, the size of the vein, scar tissue present on the arm and the age of the patient (particularly infants and the elderly). The difficulty in finding a suitable vein may lead to multiple needle insertions in an attempt to find a vein. This causes trauma to the patient. Also, when the needle is inserted, it may overshoot the vein and cause painful bruising. A mechatronic device that can find a vein more accurately than a human, and insert a needle without overshooting, would reduce the pain caused to many patients.

2 The Robot

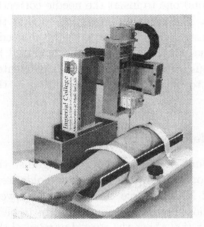
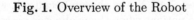
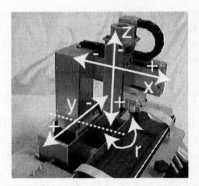

Fig. 1. Overview of the Robot   **Fig. 2.** Axes of the robot, as referred to in this thesis

The robot (see Fig. 1) was designed from specifications drawn up as a result of the feasibility tests described in [8]. It has three powered (linear motion) axes and one unpowered (rotational) axis (see Fig. 2):

The z-axis motor drives a carriage up and down, so that it goes towards and away from the arm that is strapped in under it. This carriage is used to hold either a blunt probe (for finding a vein) or a syringe and needle combination. A single axis piezo-resistive force sensor is mounted on the carriage to measure the force on the probe or needle.

The x-axis motor moves the carriage across the width of the arm. This enables the probe to press in a series of places along the width of the arm.

The r-axis, which is unpowered, enables a human operator to tilt the robot. This is so that, once a vein has been found, the needle can be inserted into the arm at the correct angle.

The y-axis motor moves the whole robot along the length of the arm. This was designed to compensate for the slight difference between where the probe has identified a vein, and where the needle enters the skin, once the robot has been tilted.

The motors used are all inexpensive, standard, stepper types, controlled by the parallel port of a PC, via driver cards. The output from the piezo-resistive force sensor is amplified and then read by a 12-bit analogue-to-digital card in the PC. Switches (read by the parallel port) at the ends of the travel of the x- and z-axes enable home positions to be established for these axes.

Software to control the robot was written in C++ on a PC running Windows 98. There were two major parts of the main control program. The first dealt with the graphical user interface. It checked for user input and plotted the graphs on the screen. The second part dealt with the time critical aspects of the system. This procedure implemented a state machine, which had two phases: one to identify the position of the vein and a second one to insert the needle correctly.

Safety issues were of high importance. The robot was designed so that the needle insertion motion was physically constrained so as not to push the needle beyond a maximum depth of 20 mm. Also, all the axes could be operated by hand in the event of a power failure. Various software devices were implemented to check the behaviour of the robot and to default to a safe condition in the event of an error.

2.1   Software for Automatic Vein Identification

The z-axis was controlled so that the blunt probe pressed down against the surface of the arm. The z-position was noted when two force thresholds were reached - one at 1.77 N and one at 3.82 N. The force threshold values were selected in the following way: 1.77 N was chosen to be sufficiently high as to be in the linear region of the force/position graph (i.e. above the curved portion of the graph that is typical of visco-elastic response). 3.82 N was chosen because it was the maximum force that felt comfortable to a patient when the probe was pressed against the surface of the skin. The thresholds were chosen empirically; further research is required to determine how to select threshold values for different patient types.

This probing process was repeated at multiple locations across the width of the arm. The z-position at the first threshold was taken to be a measure of the elasticity of the tissue beneath the probe and this was the criterion used to choose the location of the vein.

2.2   Software for Automatic Needle Insertion

The initial task was to position the needle above a vein, so that when the needle insertion motor was activated, the needle would enter the vein at the correct angle. The x-axis position was decremented until the x-position of the vein (as determined by the software described in the section above) was reached. The program then prompted the operator of the robot to manually loosen the locking screw and tilt the robot to its maximum position, away from the patient. This resulted in the needle insertion path being at an angle of 30° to the patient's arm, the angle recommended for conventional venepuncture. The operator was also prompted to change the probe for a needle. When this was complete, he/she clicked a button to allow the robot to continue.

The most critical software module was one to detect the moment of breakthrough of an elastic membrane. This could then be used to detect breakthrough of both the skin and the vein wall. The key force/position characteristics of penetration of an elastic membrane are a peak, followed by a drop in force level. The software detected these features by storing the current maximum value of the force. If the five following values were less than this maximum, membrane breakthrough was deemed to have occured. Thus, penetration was detected within 10 ms.

The software advanced the z-axis motor so that the needle moved downwards towards the skin surface. The algorithm detected the skin membrane breakthrough and then the vein wall breakthrough, at which point the z-axis motor was halted. The program then prompted the human operator of the robot to take the required blood samples by inserting a vacuum capsule. It did nothing else until the operator clicked on a 'continue' button, at which point the needle was withdrawn.

3 Results

3.1 Vein Identification Tests on a Human

The sample procedure was carried out 14 times on a single human arm (at which point the arm was too sore to continue). A tourniquet was used, as in the conventional venepuncture procedure. The results are shown in Fig. 3. Out of the 14 scans, the system chose position 6 to be the vein 3 times, and position 7, 11 times. The position of the vein was judged (visually) to be at 7. Thus, the system identified the position of the vein correctly 11 out of 14 attempts, a success rate of 78%. However, this figure is deceptive because the arm moved slightly between scans, so occasionally the vein would be shifted closer to position 6. Also, the distance between the samples was relatively large, so the probe did not always press against the centre of the vein. This could be improved by taking samples closer together, but then a scan would take too long, unless the cycle time per scan were improved.

Further tests are planned on a wide variety of patient types.

3.2 Needle Insertion Tests on Biological Specimens

The robot was first tested on a phantom and behaved well, with the needle being inserted into the artificial vein without overshooting. The next experiments had to be carried out on more biologically realistic subjects. Animal testing was impractical because of the difficulty in obtaining ethical permission. Also, the

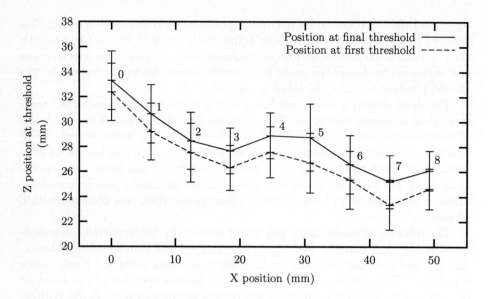

Fig. 3. Graphs obtained pressing on a human arm

force characteristics of animal tissue are different to human tissue, challenging the validity of such tests. Human cadavers were not suitable because of the change in characteristics of soft tissue soon after death, and the effects of the chemicals used to preserve the cadaver. Also, the veins in a cadaver would no longer be filled with blood and so would not behave in a realistic way.

The ideal situation would have been to test the device on live human subjects. However, the difficulty (and time) involved in obtaining permission from the appropriate authorities negated this possibility. Instead, tests were carried out on samples of lamb and chicken (obtained from the butchers). Although the behaviour of these tissues is not identical to human tissue, it was decided that these would be sufficient to test the system's efficacy on non-homogeneous material. The tissues did not have blood vessels, so an 'artificial vein' (a silicon rubber tube filled with liquid) was placed under the layer of skin and fat on the lamb and chicken. This artificial vein was taken from a phantom developed to train medical practitioners to take blood. The 'vein' and 'blood' were designed to mimic the physical behaviour of natural tissue in this procedure. Therefore, it was concluded that its response to needle insertion would be close to that experienced in humans patients.

The samples of lamb and chicken were cut with a scalpel in order that the tube could be inserted under the layer of skin and fat so that the top of the 'vein' was flush with the surface of the muscle. The samples were placed in the position where the patient's arm would normally lie, and the needle insertion software was run. During the run, the meat and 'vein' assembly were held firmly to avoid slippage. When the program paused to indicate that the needle was inside a vein, the chicken skin was manually peeled back to enable a visual inspection. The needle entered the vein and did not overshoot. The point of entry of the needle into the vein was marked on both the vein and the needle. When the needle was withdrawn, the distance of this mark from the tip was measured and found to be 5 mm. Thus, the distance the needle tip reached from the outer surface of the vein was (5.sin 30=) 2.5 mm, approximately half the diameter of the vein, the ideal position for taking a blood sample.

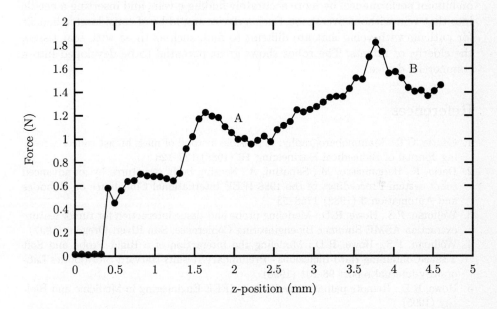

Fig. 4. Graph of force against position as the needle is inserted into chicken flesh. Points A and B are explained in the text

Fig. 4 shows the force/position profile as the needle was inserted into the chicken flesh. Point A on the graph indicates the moment when the program determines that skin breakthrough has occured and point B indicates the moment when the program determines that the vein wall has been penetrated.

4   Conclusion

This paper has presented research work on a device to take blood samples from the forearm. However, the approach taken dealt with generic issues such as feature identification using a single force control probe, automatic needle insertion that could be used in other procedures, and control strategies for soft tissue. It also gathered data about the physical characteristic of soft tissue, an area that has received scant attention.

Further tests are planned to be carried out on a wide range of patient types (infants, elderly, obese, etc.) to verify that the approach described in this paper is applicable. These tests would also ascertain the reliability of the device, its accuracy and its limitations (e.g. what is the minimum size of vein that can be found ?).

The blood sampling procedure involves considerable pain and discomfort to many people, and yet no devices are in common use to improve the performance of the nurses and doctors who carry it out. The novel device described in this paper was used to obtain results that show that the robotic device can improve on human performance, by more accurately finding a vein, and inserting a needle into that vein without overshoot. Such a device would be of considerable benefit for patients with veins that are difficult to find, such as those with scar tissue, the elderly, or infants. The robot shows great potential to be developed into a commercial device.

References

1. Gentle, C.R.: Mammobarography: A possible method of mass breast cancer screening Journal of Biomedical Engineering **10** (1988) 122–126
2. Dario, P., Bergamasco, M., Sabatini, A.: Sensing body structures by an advanced robot system Proceedings of the 1988 IEEE International Conference on Robotics and Automation **3** (1988) 1758–63
3. Wellman, P.S., Howe, R.D.: Modeling probe and tissue interaction for tumor feature extraction ASME Summer Bioengineering Conference, Sun River, Oregon, (1997)
4. Wellman, P.S., Howe, R.D.: Modeling the Interaction of a Rigid Probe and Soft Tissue Containing Hard Inclusions - Preliminary Results Harvard BioRobotics Laboratory internal report 98-101 (1998)
5. Howe, R.D.: Remote palpation technology IEEE Engineering in Medicine and Biology (1995)
6. Black, F., Hughes, J.: Venepuncture in A Guide to Intravenous Therapy, RCN Publishing Company (1999) 3–8
7. Dougherty, L.: Intravenous Cannulation in A Guide to Intravenous Therapy, RCN Publishing Company (1999) 11–16
8. Zivanovic, A., Davies, B.L.: A Robotic System for Blood Sampling IEEE Transactions on Information Technology in Biomedicine **4** 1 (2000)

Computer Aided Diagnosis for Virtual Colonography

Gabriel Kiss, Johan Van Cleynenbreugel, Maarten Thomeer,
Paul Suetens, Guy Marchal

Faculties of Medicine & Engineering
Medical Image Computing (Radiology - ESAT/PSI)
University Hospital Gasthuisberg
Herestraat 49
B-3000 Leuven, BELGIUM
Gabriel.Kiss@uz.kuleuven.ac.be

Abstract. The success of CT colonography (CTC) depends on
appropriate tools for quick and accurate diagnostic reading. Current
advancements in computer technology have the potential to bring
such tools even to the PC level. In this paper a technique for
Computed Aided Diagnosis (CAD) using CT colonography is
described. The method labels positions in the volume data, which
have a strong likelihood of being polyps and presents them in a user-
friendly way. This method will reduce the amount of time needed by
the radiologist to make a correct diagnosis. The method was tested on
a study group of 18 patients and the sensitivity for polyps of 10 mm
or larger was 100%, comparable to that of human readers. The price
paid for a high detection rate was a large number of approximately 8
false positive findings per case.

1 Introduction

Computed Tomographic Colonography (CTC) is a new non-invasive imaging tool
that employs advanced imaging software to CT data for producing both two and three
dimensional images of the colon [1]. The resulting images can be presented to a
radiologist under one of the following formats: 2D axial slices, multi-planar
reformatted 3D images (MPR), 3D endoluminal images or axial 3D images. The
images can be generated instantaneously using software or hardware renderers or can
be stored as digital movies.

The success of CTC depends on the applicability of the technique for large
population screenings. The main limitations of CTC at this moment are the lengthy
interpretation time and the possibility of perceptual errors.

Our experience [2] shows that the evaluation of 2D axial slices and axial 3D
movies for both forward and reverse directions in both supine and prone positions
takes about 30 minutes. The cost of CTC should be lower than the cost of
colonography in order to be usable for large-scale screening. One possibility for time
saving, and hence for cost saving is Computer Aided Diagnosis (CAD). Using CAD
the radiologist does not have to concentrate on the whole volume, instead his attention
will be focused only on small sub-volumes.

W. Niessen and M. Viergever (Eds.): MICCAI 2001, LNCS 2208, pp. 621-628, 2001.
© Springer-Verlag Berlin Heidelberg 2001

2 Short History of CAD

Probably the best-known application area for CAD is mammography on digital high-resolution radiographs [3]. With this technique breast calcifications are detected and classified, in order to prevent unnecessary surgical biopsies. Another area of applicability for CAD is the detection of lung cancer in CT images [4].

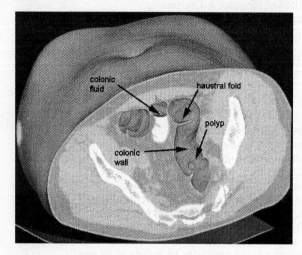

CAD for CTC is a relatively new research topic. The colon has a spatial extended and very complex structure (Figure 1), including smooth colonic wall, haustral folds, residual fluid and polyps. A direct implication of this fact is the huge amount of data that has to be inspected, resulting in time-consuming CAD algorithms. Only recent advances in computing speed make these algorithms usable.

Fig. 1. The complex nature of the human colon.

Some approaches have been already applied in CTC CAD [5][6][7][8]; the methods used can be based on surface curvature, on surface normal, on sphere fitting, on polypoid shape detection, or on graph methods. Summers et al. tried to apply methods form virtual bronchoscopy to solve the CAD problem [9].

Surface curvature methods are based on concepts from differential geometry: minimum and maximum principal curvatures, mean and Gaussian curvatures. A thresholding based on these curvature values is applied and the remaining regions are declared as polyp candidates.

Surface normal methods exploit the fact that normals to the colonic surface intersect with neighboring normals depending on the curvature features of the colon. The main problem is the differentiation between polyps and haustral folds, which have similar curvature properties; one observation usable in this case is that haustral folds have a lower tendency of surface normal convergence than polyps, due to their cylindrical nature.

Sphere fitting methods exploit the spherical nature of polyps. Polyps can not be modeled as simple spheres because usually they are more complex entities. An alternative is to model polyps as spherical patches, followed by the detection of sphere center clusters situated in close vicinity (applying graph methods).

3 Method

Our method uses a combination of the surface normal and sphere fitting methods and has the following steps: segmentation, polyp candidate generation, polyp center generation, polyp extraction and finally presentation. We preferred this alternative to an approach based on differential geometry due to its simplicity and computational efficiency.

To make the text easier to understand we start by presenting all of the threshold and predefined parameters used by our method. We also present their meaning and specify in which step they will appear. A visual summary of the method is shown in Figure 3.

Threshold parameters	Threshold symbol	Step	Short description
Colonic wall	$T_{segment}$	Segmentation	Differentiate between air, colonic wall and surrounding tissue
Bounding box size	T_{box}	Polyp candidate generation	Defines the 3D volume of interest we take into consideration for a colonic wall voxel
Convexity	T_{convex}	Polyp candidate generation	Distance between a neighbor point and the intersection point of the local gradient with the tangent plane
Hits/total ratio	T_{hits}	Polyp candidate generation	Minimum number of neighbors relative to the total number of neighbors that have to satisfy the convexity threshold
Sphere radius	T_{radius}	Polyp center generation	Distance between the current point and the center of an imaginary sphere
Extraction	$T_{extract}$	Polyp extraction	Minimal value in the center map to be considered as polyp candidate

Table 1. Threshold parameters, their name, symbol, appearance and meaning.

3.1 Segmentation

The goal of segmentation is to extract the colonic wall, in order to apply further processing on it. This step will reduce the amount of voxels we take into account as being candidates.

Our segmentation is based on a classical region-growing algorithm, as described in [10]. The user chooses a seed voxel and a region of connected voxels meeting the threshold criteria ($T_{segment}$) is grown outwards in a breadth first manner. $T_{segment}$ can be adjusted based on the intensity values of the structure of interest. Sometimes a simple region growing operation may not be able to fill the entire desired structure (an air filled colon with a collapsed segment or due to colonic fluid). Multiple seed points can be specified and then multiple regions are grown separately. Region growing will detect voxels (the set A) given by colonic air. Colonic wall is assumed to be the set C of all adjacent voxels to A, and having a value higher than $T_{segment}$. For each voxel belonging to A all its 26 neighbors are taken into consideration, this can lead to a wall thickness of 2 voxels.

The obtained result C is a subset of the colonic wall because in some patients where wet preparation was used, the air-fluid boundary was also classified as colonic wall, and the submerged parts of the colonic wall were not segmented. A solution to this problem is the use of digital cleansing prior to CAD [2].

3.2 Polyp Candidates Generation

Only a small number of elements belonging to C will turn into polyp candidates. At this step the main criteria for polyp candidate selection is the convexity or the concavity of the wall over a region of interest.

To find possible candidates for each voxel in C we compute its gradient. The gradient will be perpendicular to the wall and oriented from air towards tissue. A Zucker and Hummel operator (an extension of the two-dimensional gradient to three dimensions) [10] is applied. Basically this operator will give as output the surface normal in the considered point. Having the gradient and the current point we can find the equation of the plane tangent to the surface in the current point.

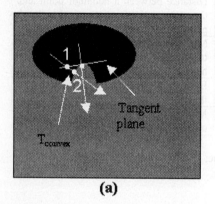 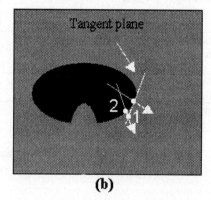

(a)   **(b)**

Fig. 2. Difference between convex and concave surfaces; notice the different relative positioning of point 1 and point 2. For convex surfaces (a) point 1 is situated in negative direction relative to point 2, while for concave surfaces (b) point 1 is situated in positive direction relative to point 2 on the line given by the local gradient. For convex surfaces we apply a threshold based on T_{convex}.

Suppose $v \in C$, B_v is the bounding box around v defined by T_{box} and P_v is the tangent plane in v. Then for each $w \in B_v \cap C$ we compute its gradient and the intersection of this gradient with P_v, say i_{vw}. The relative location of i_{vw} with regards to w can be exploited to assess convexity or concavity of the colon's surface in v. Furthermore if the surface is convex, T_{convex} can be applied to the distance d between w and i_{vw}.

For each $v \in C$ two values (V_c, V_t) are computed. V_c is the number of voxels situated in $B_v \cap C$ that satisfy T_{convex}, while V_t is the total number of voxels in $B_v \cap C$. All the voxels v for which V_c/V_t is higher than T_{hits} are declared candidates.

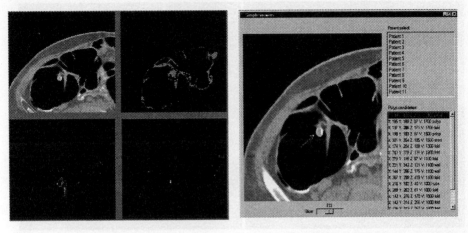

Fig. 3. The figure illustrates the four steps of our algorithm. Although our approach is truly 3D, we only show results on 2D slices. On the left a 2D region of interest is presented first as an original slice, then the results of segmentation, polyp candidate generation and polyp center generation are shown. On the right the user interface of the polyp presentation module is captured.

Due to the fact that haustral folds and polyps have similar convexity properties, this step will not only generate voxels that belong to polyps, but additionally voxels situated on haustral folds, and some voxels caused by irregularities on the colonic wall. Discrimination between voxels belonging to real polyps and those belonging to haustral folds is therefore a next step.

3.3 Polyp Center Generation

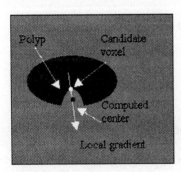

Fig. 4. Simplified illustration (2D example) of how the sphere centers are computed.

This discrimination is based on the fact that folds have a fairly cylindrical shape while polyps have mainly a spherical shape.

First for all of the previously selected candidates we compute a sphere center. The sphere has the point on its surface and the local gradient perpendicular to its surface. The radius (T_{radius}) of the sphere can be selected and has to be in close correspondence with the size of the polyps to be detected. Because folds have a cylindrical shape the centers given by such structures will be dispersed along a line. For polyps however these centers will converge towards a relatively small area. For polyps having the shape of a perfect sphere (semi-sphere) these centers would converge towards a single point.

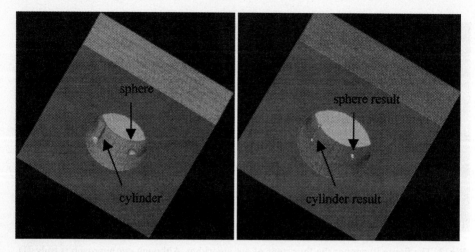

Fig. 5. The dispersion of centers for a cylinder, as opposed to a sphere. A 3D rendering of the original phantom (left) and of the results (right) are presented.

3.4 Polyp Extraction and Presentation

The previous step generates a map that represents the concentration of sphere centers in the data volume. As we want to present to the user polyp candidates on axial slices, given this map, we have to extract local maxima. To do this we look for values higher than $T_{extract}$. If we do not find any value higher than the threshold we declare the patient as negative. When searching for local maxima we have to take into account that centers are concentrated in small areas, so for each of these areas only one response is wanted. To solve this problem a non-maximum suppression technique is applied.

Finally, the local maxima thus obtained are pointed out to the reading radiologist as polyp candidates.

3.5 Initial Threshold Values Determination

To find initial values for thresholds (T_{box}, T_{convex}, T_{hits}, $T_{extract}$), we applied our method on a software phantom containing a perfect cylinder and a semi-sphere with a diameter of 10 mm, similar to the polyps of interest. The cylinder was mimicking a haustral fold while the semi-sphere was considered to be perfect polyp. Also we used this phantom to verify our presumption that on haustral folds centers will disperse whereas for polyps they will converge towards small regions (see Figure 5).

4 Results

The presented CAD method was applied to 18 different CT-volumes, belonging to eighteen patients that underwent both CT-colonography and standard colonoscopy.

Informed consent was obtained from all patients. CT was performed using a Multi Slice Helical CT (Siemens, Volume Zoom) using a 4x1 mm detector configuration, 7 mm table feet per 0.5 s tube rotation, 0.8mm reconstruction increment as well as 60 effective mAs and 120 kV. The average number of slices was 496.

Colonoscopy was taken as ground truth; results from CAD were compared with the results obtained by a radiologist using the CTC method of axial-3D [2]. Nine of the patients had polyps proven by colonoscopy, while the other nine were declared negative. The size of the polyps was ranging from 3 up to 20 mm and the total number of polyps was 20 (1 of 3mm, 3 of 5mm, 2 of 6 mm, 9 of 10 mm, 4 of 10mm flat lesions, and 1 of 20mm) (Table 2)

Our method detected all the nine polyps of 10mm or larger, 1 from 2 polyps of 6mm, 1 from 3 polyps of 5 mm and missed the polyp of 3mm and the four flat lesions of 10mm. The average computation time was 23.30 minutes, on an Intel Pentium III system running at 533MHz and having 512MB of RAM. The total number of false positives was 147, which gives us a mean value of 8.16 false positives per case. Additionally we can mention that an average of 3.22 seed points was needed to segment correctly the colonic wall. The causes of false positives were colonic wall (45.58%), haustral folds (31.97%), colonic stool or fluid (12.25%), the insuflation tube (7.48%), and the ileocecal valve (2.72%).

Polyps	Total	Detected	Sensitivity
Smaller than 5mm	1	0	0%
Between 5-9 mm	5	2	40%
Flat lesions	4	0	0%
Bigger than 10mm	10	10	100%
Overall	20	12	60%

Table 2. Total number of polyps, detected number of polyps and sensitivity overall and for each group of polyps.

5 Discussion and Conclusions

Although the size of significant polyp is a debate subject between different radiologists and also between radiologists and gastroenterologists, we assumed that 10mm polyps can be accepted as significant one's for virtual colonography. Therefore our primary goal was the detection of polyps bigger than 10 mm. A secondary goal was a reasonable number of false positives per case. Using the polyp presentation application the radiologist can quickly go through the polyp candidate list and discriminate between real and false positive findings.

From literature, we can deduce that there is a strong correlation between sensitivity and the number of false positives generated. For example Tomasi et al. [6] are using a graph method optimized for the detection of polyps larger than 10mm. They achieve a sensitivity of 100% with a number of false positives (FP) as high as 50 per data set. Yoshida et al. [7] reported a sensitivity of 90% for polyps between 7-12mm and 1 FP per case. To achieve a sensitivity of 100% they reported an increase towards 1.5 FP per case. Beaulieu et al. [5] developed three different methods for polyp detection. Their contour normal method has a sensitivity of 96.4% for polyps larger than 5 mm at the cost of 25 FP per data set. The sphere fit method returns a number of 47 FP, meanwhile the surface curvature method has a low number of FP only 4, but a decreased sensitivity as well (3 out of 7 polyps detected).

We have to stress that we are looking at CAD as a prospective tool and not as a retrospective one. We used the same parameter settings for all of our patients, positives or negatives. However if we would count only the number of false positives until all the polyps bigger than 10mm have been identified, then we would only have 17 FP findings in 9 cases, so an average of 1.88 FP per case comparable with results given by other authors. Of course this kind of evaluation can be done only for retrospective studies.

The results of our experiments are at least encouraging. CAD will probably become the most common way of doing CTC, improving on current accuracy, efficiency and costs. Many further improvements to our algorithm are possible:

1. Application of digital cleansing prior to CAD, in order to remove the colonic fluid and thus eliminating the necessity of multiple seed points
2. Introduction of a polyp database when labeling a polyp candidate and taking the decision based on previous knowledge.
3. From the implementation point of view changing our data structures will lead to a better balance between speed and memory requirements.

Acknowledgement

This work is part of the GOA/99/05 project: "Variability in Human Shape and Speech", financed by the Research Fund, K.U. Leuven, BELGIUM.

References

1. Johnson C.D. (2000) CT Colonography, Mayo Clinic Experience, Second International Symposium on Virtual Colonoscopy, Boston proceedings, October 2000, pp 16-18
2. Kiss G. et al. (2001) An Image Processing and Visualization System for Virtual Colonography, Technical Report: KUL/ESAT/PSI/0103, KU Leuven Belgium, June 2001
3. Nappi J., Dean P.B. (2000) A multiscale algorithm for segmenting calcifications from high-resolution mammographic specimen radiographs, J Digit Imaging, May 2000, 13(2 Suppl1):130-2
4. Ukai et al. (2000) Computer Aided Diagnosis System for Lung Cancer Based on Retrospective Helical CT Images, CARS proceedings, June 2000, pp 767-772
5. Beaulieu C.F. (2000) Computer Aided Detection of Colonic Polyps, Second International Symposium on Virtual Colonoscopy, Boston proceedings, October 2000, pp 73-77
6. Tomasi C., Gokturk S.B. (2000) A Graph Method for the Conservative Detection of Polyps in the Colon, Second International Symposium on Virtual Colonoscopy, Boston proceedings, October 2000, pp 105
7. Yoshida H. et al. (2000) Computer Aided Detection of Colonic Polyps in CT Colonography, Second International Symposium on Virtual Colonoscopy, Boston proceedings, October 2000, pp 104
8. Paik D.S. et al. (2000) Computer Aided Detection of Polyps in CT Colonography: Free Response ROC Evaluation of Performance, RSNA, Chicago, 2000.
9. Summers R.M. et al. (2000) Automated polyp detector in CT colonography: feasibility study, Radiology 2000 Jul;216(1):284-90
10. Ballard D.M., Brown C.M. (1982) Computer Vision, Prentice-Hall, pp 149-166

Filtering h_{int} Images for the Detection of Microcalcifications

Marius George Linguraru, Michael Brady, and Margaret Yam

University of Oxford, Medical Vision Laboratory,
Old Library, Parks Road, Oxford OX1 3PJ, UK
mglin@robots.ox.ac.uk

Abstract. Recent figures show that approximately 1 in 11 women in the western world will develop breast cancer during the course of their lives. Early detection greatly improves prognosis and considerable research has been undertaken to this end. Mammographic images are difficult to interpret even by radiologists and this makes their task error prone. One of the earliest non-palpable signs is the appearance of microcalcifications, typically 0.5 mm in diameter, representing small deposits of calcium salts in the breast. A novel approach to detecting microcalcifications in x-ray mammography has been explored. The method is based on the use of the physics-based image representation h_{int} [1] and use of anisotropic diffusion to filter h_{int} images. The diffusion process becomes a method of detecting both noise and microcalcifications in mammograms.

1 Theory

The h_{int} representation results from a model of the mammogram image formation process. The appearance of mammograms varies massively according to the specific conditions, though the object of interest, the breast anatomy, remains invariant. The h_{int} model offers an alternative quantitative representation of the breast tissue, where the h_{int} of a pixel represents the amount of non-fatty breast tissue at that point. Figure 1.a shows a depiction of the h_{int} surface of a breast. An h_{int} representation can be easily visualised as an image, since the h_{int} values are in float format, where brighter parts correspond to regions of the breast with more interesting (non-fatty) tissue or calcifications, as shown in Figure 1.b. While microcalcifications appear in about 14% of mammograms, they are typically small and sparse. For this reason, Highnam and Brady's algorithm for estimating h_{int} [1] assumes only two types of tissue: fat and non-fat (i.e. parenchymal, tumour). Since the attenuation coefficient of microcalcification is typically 26 times that of *interesting tissue*, microcalcifications appear in h_{int} images as tall thin towers, Figure 2.a.

One of the major characteristics that we use in detecting microcalcifications is the difference that should be visible in the shape of a microcalcification versus noise [1]. While microcalcifications are anatomical structures with slightly blurred edges which appear in mammograms due to the effect of x-ray beams passing through the breast anatomical structure, noise tends to have extremely

W. Niessen and M. Viergever (Eds.): MICCAI 2001, LNCS 2208, pp. 629–636, 2001.

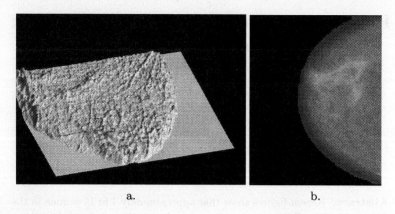

a.   b.

Fig. 1. (a) A depiction of the h_{int} surface of a breast, (b) an h_{int} representation visualised as an image.

sharp edges, as shown in Figure 2.b. Shot-noise may drastically influence the local image characteristics and represents the main source of false positives (FPs) in algorithms for microcalcification detection. We have previously demonstrated that the h_{int} representation can eradicate this type of noise [2], but since our method aims to detect shot noise as well, we did not remove shot noise from the images we tested. The appearance of h_{int} images would be extremely noisy, mainly due to the removal of the glare effect [2], extra-focal and scattered radiation [1] (which accounts for up to 40% of the total radiation exiting the breast). This would make the examination of the regions of interest difficult, making it harder to distinguish small structures in mammograms. Since microcalcifications correspond to high peaks in h_{int} images, only the most prominent spots of noise may lead towards FPs, the smaller ones being easily removed by the diffusion process. If glare is removed, facilitating the elimination of shot noise, the price to be paid is a massive decrease in the signal to noise ratio (SNR) in h_{int} [5]. Yam [6] attempts to overcome this visible increase in noise by Wiener filtering the original image before generating h_{int} surfaces, an approach that improves slightly the SNR. We prefer to work with the glare de-convolved (no shot noise removed) image and use anisotropic diffusion to differentiate edge sharpness of noise and microcalcifications.

2   Filter Model

We choose an anisotropic diffusion-based filter [3], [4] which aims to blur the input mammographic image while preserving some small regions of interest. The process relies on the use of a set of different parameters, e.g. time, contrast, size, and it is essential to determine the right choice of parameters. Figure 3 shows different output images after using anisotropic diffusion on a grey-level digital mammogram containing both a calcification and a large spot of noise.

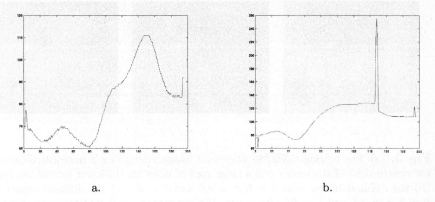

a.   b.

Fig. 2. (a) The plot of a filtered intensity image containing a microcalcification at position 150, (b) the plot of a filtered intensity image containing noise at position 147.

We found that Weickert's solution [4] for the diffusion tensor is best suited to our problem. We used a similar simplified tensor having eigenvalues (1), (2):

$$\lambda 1 = \begin{cases} 1 & |\nabla u_\sigma| = 0, \\ 1 - \exp\left(\frac{-1}{(|\nabla u_\sigma|/\lambda)^8}\right) & |\nabla u_\sigma| > 0 \end{cases} \qquad (1)$$

$$\lambda 2 = 1. \qquad (2)$$

Nonlinear anisotropic filtering proves to be highly flexible due to the variability of its parameters which help in covering a rather extensive set of possibilities in multi-scaling filtering with respect to the output one can get by filtering medical images, as Table 1 shows.

Table 1. Variation of anisotropic diffusion parameters: k - the contrast factor, σ - the scaling factor and t - the number of iterations; $\nearrow$ represents an increase, while $\searrow$ is a decrease of the parameter or feature.

	Blur in Image	Anatomical Features	Edges
$k \nearrow$	$\nearrow$	$\searrow$	$\searrow\searrow$
$\sigma \nearrow$	$\nearrow$	$\searrow$	$\searrow$
$t \nearrow$	$\nearrow$	$\searrow\searrow$	well preserved over a long time

Having obtained the anisotropically diffused image, we subtract it from the less blurred original. Some differences in the way microcalcifications, as opposed to noise, are diffused can be seen in Figure 4. Microcalcifications tend to be

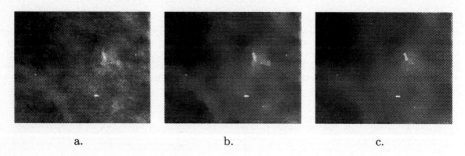

a.   b.   c.

Fig. 3. (a) The original 533x386 grey-level image containing a microcalcification in the centre-right of the image and a large spot of noise on the lower side of the image; (b) the diffused image with $k = 5, \sigma = 0.6$ and $t = 20$; (c) the diffused image with $k = 5, \sigma = 0.5$ and $t = 40$, where only the important small structures are kept and their edges enhanced.

smoothed faster than prominent noise spots, for an appropriate choice of parameters. After a certain number of iterations, the surface of the difference image contains significant changes for noise only.

3   Results

We first show some results of applying nonlinear anisotropic diffusion filtering to samples of real mammograms containing microcalcifications. We de-noise h_{int} images while preserving only calcifications and significant noise, Figure 5.a, .b, .e, .f.

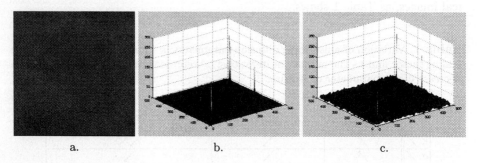

a.   b.   c.

Fig. 4. (a) The original preprocessed h_{int} 500x500 image containing a microcalcification on the left side, a large spot of noise on the lower right side and several other smaller noise structures; (b) the 3D plot of the difference image between the original image diffused with $k = 15, \sigma = 0.6$ and $t = 5$ and the same one diffused with $k = 15, \sigma = 0.6$ and $t = 10$; (c) the 3D plot of the difference image between the original image diffused with $k = 15, \sigma = 0.6$ and $t = 10$ and the same one diffused with $k = 15, \sigma = 0.6$ and $t = 15$.

In order to reduce processing time and the intervention of the operator in the filtering process, we chose a large value for the contrast factor k. We still chose a rather small value for the scaling factor σ for preserving tiny anatomical structures or noise over the first iterations in the process of diffusion. Due to the strong variability that exists in mammographic images (e.g. contrast, size of interesting tissue) a multi-scale approach would be preferable. Since the whole process should be robust and easy to use, we reduced the number of variable parameters to one, keeping constant the contrast and scale factors and varying only the number of iterations over a small range. We found that the time factor t gives optimal results for the filtering process over the whole set of h_{int} images when we used values between 3 and 7 iterations.

In demonstrating the efficiency of our method in increasing the number of true positives (TPs) we also considered images with high likelihood to present false positives. Such an example is presented in Figure 5.c, .d, .g, .h.

The detection method, of both calcifications and noise was based initially on the association one can make between the original h_{int} mammograms containing the structures of interest and the surface we built from the filtered images after just a few iterations. Since radiologists may have doubts when searching the original image for microcalcifications, the surface we present would show either hill-shaped structures for microcalcifications or sharp-edged formations for noise in the locations corresponding to the structures of interest. Moreover, we found the simple visual comparison of the two h_{int} images – the original noisy one and the filtered one – to be quite reliable in differentiating between microcalcifications and noise. While noisy structures tend to be better preserved by the filtering method applied with our final specific choice of parameters, microcalcifications fade faster and look like imploding structures.

3.1 Coarse Calcifications

The algorithm was initially tested on a set of 13 samples of average 32-float h_{int} mammograms containing 10 coarse calcifications pre-labeled by a radiologist and several artifacts. The size of the images varied between 124x180 and 251x251 at 50 μm resolution. The algorithm applied to the enhanced images gave a detection rate of 100%. No FPs were detected during our experiments. The free-response receiver operating characteristic (FROC) curve is shown in Figure 6.a.

3.2 Microcalcifications

The algorithm was then further tested on 20 samples of 32-float h_{int} mammograms containing 27 isolated microcalcifications pre-labeled by a radiologist and various pixels of noise. The size of the samples was 200x250 at a resolution of 50 μm. The set was meant to offer an overview of possible clinical aspects related to microcalcifications of different sizes, some of them clear while some other feint. The TPs fraction was 92.6 % for a number of 0.1 FPs per image.

We further applied an implementation of Yam *et al.*'s algorithm [5] to the same set of microcalcifications. The process differed slightly in this case. The

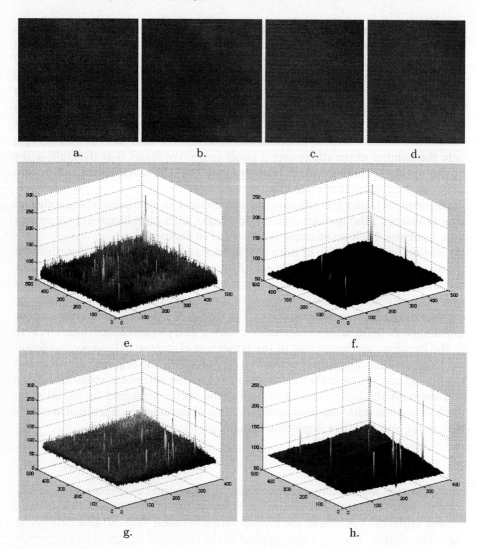

Fig. 5. (a) An original preprocessed h_{int} 500x500 image containing a microcalcification on the left side and a large spot of noise on the lower right side; (b) the diffused image from (a) with $k = 15, \sigma = 0.6$ and $t = 5$, we notice that the microcalcification has almost faded, while the noise is still preserved with high contrast; (c) an original preprocessed h_{int} 400x490 image containing only noise structures, the largest piece of noise on the upper right side could be easily considered of being a microcalcification since it does not present very high contrast from the surrounding tissue; (d) the diffused image from (c) with $k = 15, \sigma = 0.6$ and $t = 3$; (e) the 3D plot of the original h_{int} image in (a), we notice the extremely noisy appearance where the important structures can be hardly distinguished; (f) the surface of the diffused h_{int} image in (b), the microcalcification appears as a hill with smoother edges than those of the very sharp-edged noise structures in the same image; (g) the surface of the original h_{int} image in (c) with highly noisy appearance; (h) the surface of the diffused h_{int} image in (d) where all structures have very sharp edges and are labeled as noise.

original 32-float h_{int} mammograms were translated into tif images without contrast enhancement, in order to preserve a fixed scale for all mammogram samples. The algorithm developed by Yam *et al.* [5] was applied to the filtered versions of the original images. We obtained a 100% fraction of TPs with a number of 0.3 FPs per image. The FROC curve of the detection using the combination of the anisotropic diffusion filter and the algorithm implemented by Yam *et al.* is shown in Figure 6.b.

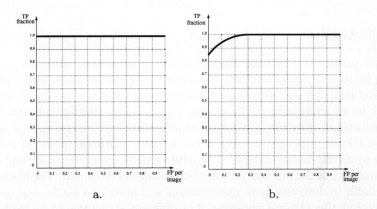

a.   b.

Fig. 6. (a) The FROC curve of the detection method for the set of 13 samples containing coarse calcifications; (b) the FROC curve of the combined detection method for the set of 20 samples containing different types of microcalcifications

4   Discussion

An important issue in the use of this new filtering method in x-ray mammography is the preservation of tiny anatomical structures over the diffusion process. Unlike most filters which actually blur the whole image and blend small regions together, our method preserves the anatomical independence of all small structures encountered in an image.

A major source of FPs in mammography corresponds to shot noise. The noise maps obtained after removing the glare-effect in the process of generating h_{int} images can be used as a further step to exclude this specific type of noise from mammograms and therefore reduce the number of FPs. We would therefore expect significantly improved results in the detection process presented in Section 3. As Yam *et al.*'s algorithm is built to use a combination of grey-level and h_{int} images, using its original implementation on h_{int}s only is expected to give poorer results. We believe that some changes in the algorithm, such as introducing a threshold that would remove shot noise or any other relevant bits of noise by means of detecting the small area change over the height of the structure, would eliminate most of the detected FPs and would not need to make use of the shot noise maps.

Time is important in the development of real-time clinical applications and filtering algorithms make use of a lot of it because of the subsequent application of kernels over one image. In order to reduce the necessary time for the diffusion process, we used a higher value for the contrast factor k. A higher k leads to faster diffusion over the image and fewer iterations are requested. The consistence of our choice is based on the high h_{int} values corresponding to both shot noise and calcifications. Both structures are preserving their characteristics for high contrast over a few number of iterations.

5   Conclusion

We have presented a filtering method based on anisotropic diffusion, a process known for its scale-space and edge detection properties. Our method implements such nonlinear diffusion filtering for the first time in digital mammography and aims to be an alternative to the Wiener filter used previously on breast images.

Our method uses the normalised representation of mammograms that the h_{int} generation provides, namely a robust and consistent physical-based approach to digital mammography. The initial results are encouraging and further improvements to the method promise better rates of detection. The algorithm is also reliable in detecting both calcifications and noise in a single step by taking into account the *physical* appearance of different structures of interest. While the term noise refers to shot noise only, as the main source of false positives, the term calcifications would include coarse calcifications as well as microcalcifications. Quantum mottle, an important source of errors in mammography, has little interference in our application as it is smoothed by our filter, with a right choice of the contrast and scaling factors. Furthermore, anisotropic diffusion is blurring the images in a more intelligent way than other more usual smoothing filters, making use of the edge enhancement property.

References

1. Highnam, R. Brady, J.M.: Mammographic Image Analysis. Kluwer Academic Publisher (1999)
2. Highnam, R. Brady, J.M., English, R.: Detecting Film-Screen Artifacts in Mammography using a Model-Based Approach. IEEE Transactions on Medical Imaging **18** (1999) 1016–1024
3. Perona, P. Malik, J.: Scale-space and Edge Detection using Anisotropic Diffusion. IEEE Transactions on Pattern Analysis and Machine Intelligence **12** (1990) 629–639
4. Weickert, J.: A Review of Nonlinear Diffusion Filtering. In: ter Haar Romeny, B. Florack, L. Koenderink, J. Viergever, M. (eds.): Scale-Space Theory in Computer Vision, Lecture Notes in Computer Science, Vol. 1252. Springer, Berlin (1997) 3–28
5. Yam, M. Brady, J.M. Highnam, R. English, R.: De-noising h_{int} Surfaces: a Physics-based Approach. In: Proc. Medical Image Computing and Computer-Assisted Intervention. Springer (1999) 227-234
6. Yam, M. Highnam, R. Brady, J.M.: Detecting Calcifications using the h_{int} Representation. In: Computer Assisted Radiology and Surgery. Elsevier (1999) 373-377

Using Optical Flow Fields for Polyp Detection in Virtual Colonoscopy

Burak Acar[1], Sandy Napel[1], David Paik[1], Burak Göktürk[2], Carlo Tomasi[3], and Christopher F. Beaulieu[1]

[1] Stanford University, Department of Radiology
LUCAS MRS Center, 3D Lab., Stanford, CA 94305-5488, USA
bacar, snapel@stanford.edu
paik@smi.stanford.edu, cfb@s-word.stanford.edu
www.3dradiology.org
[2] Stanford University, Electrical Engineering Department
Stanford, CA 94305, USA
[3] Stanford University, Computer Science Department
Stanford, CA 94305, USA

Abstract. Since the introduction of Computed Tomographic Colonography (CTC), research has mainly focused on visualization and navigation techniques. Recently, efforts have shifted towards computer aided detection (CAD) of polyps. We propose a new approach to CAD in CT images that attempts to model the way a radiologist recognizes a polyp using optical flow fields (OFF). Features extracted from OFFs are used by a linear classifier for polyp detection. An initial validation of our technique resulted in an average of 75% specificity at 100% sensitivity in a 10-fold cross validation study on a set of 220 polyp-like structures, 20 of which were true polyps.

1 Introduction

Computed Tomographic Colonography (CTC) was suggested in the early 1980's and realized in the 1990's as a minimally invasive method that would make mass screening of colorectal cancer feasible [1,2,3,4]. Since then several studies were conducted to assess the performance of CTC [5,6,7,8,9,10]. In almost all studies, CTC was based on the examination of CT images by an expert radiologist, using either the 2D images, 3D virtual colonoscopic views or both. Thus, until recently most efforts were directed towards developing better visualization and navigation techniques [4,11,12,13,14,15,16,17,18,19]. Lately, more effort has been put into computer aided detection (CAD), whose ultimate goal is to identify polyps in a 3D CT data efficiently, and with high sensitivity and specificity. Mir et al. reviews a set of techniques that can be used for shape description in CT images [20]. We are aware of two studies on CAD in CTC: Summers et al. reported a shape based polyp detector and concluded that CAD is feasible in CTC [21] and Paik et al. proposed a Hough Transform-based polyp detector [22,23]. However, these CADs suffer from low specificity, which would require radiologists to examine a large number of CAD hits to rule out false detections.

W. Niessen and M. Viergever (Eds.): MICCAI 2001, LNCS 2208, pp. 637–644, 2001.
© Springer-Verlag Berlin Heidelberg 2001

The goal of our research is to develop a highly sensitive and specific CAD for CTC. We attempted to model the way a radiologist recognizes a polyp by focusing on the changes in consecutive images as one views sequential cross-sections of the volumetric source CT data (3D CT data). We used Optical Flow Fields (OFF) to represent these changes, and a linear classifier acting on these features to recognize true polyps.

2   Method

2.1   Data Acquisition

Patients were imaged in the supine position after colon cleansing and air-insufflation of the colon on a GE HiSpeed Advantage single detector or GE LightSpeed multi-row detector scanner (GE Medical Systems, Milwaukee, WI). Typical acquisition parameters were 3 mm collimation, pitch 1.5-2.0, 1.5 mm reconstruction interval, 120 KVp, 200 MAs for the single detector scanner and 2.5 mm collimation, pitch 3.0, 1.0-1.5 mm reconstruction interval, 120 KVp, 56 MAs for the multi-row detector scanner. Data were stored as 2 byte unsigned integers. The size of the 3D data matrix was $512 \times 512 \times N$, N is the number of axial slices. N is typically around 350. The average voxel spacing was $0.74mm \times 0.74mm \times 1.31mm$.

2.2   Initial Detection

The data was preprocessed by a Hough Transform-based polyp detector (HTD) [22,23]. HTD basically computes the normals to an isointensity surface and searches for voxels at which a large number of normals intersect. Defining the number of normals that intersect in a given voxel as the HT score of that voxel, a threshold is applied for detection. Typically the voxels at the centers of spherical structures have high scores. The detected voxels mark the locations of polyps with high sensitivity but low specificity. We extracted a subvolume consisting of $21 \times 21 \times 21$ voxels centered on each detection with a score above a fixed threshold.

2.3   Optical Flow Field Computation

The aim of the OFF computation is to characterize the change in the location of the edges (tissue/air boundary) in the image plane while scrolling back and forth along the third dimension. This third dimension can be thought as the time axis [24]. If we name the image plane as the xy-plane then the basic optical flow equation is [25]:

$$\nabla I.\mathbf{v} + \frac{\partial I}{\partial t} = 0 \qquad (1)$$

where $\mathbf{v}(x,y)$ is the OFF and $I(x,y)$ is the image, i.e. the intensity function. Equation 1 allows only the computation of $\mathbf{v}_\perp$, the component along the local

∇I. This serves to our purpose and it is simple. We will refer to $\mathbf{v}_\perp$ as $\mathbf{v}$ in what follows.

Keeping in mind that the coordinates of the voxel detected by HTD (HT_hit) is $(0,0,0)$, $\mathbf{v}_t(x,y)$ is computed for $x,y,t \in [-10,10]$. t is first incremented from 0 to 10 and then from 0 to -10. This is equivalent to moving outwards from the center. This assures the consistency in the direction of motion of the edges of spherical structures. $\mathbf{v}_t(x,y)$ are summed and the resulting OFF is filtered with a moving average filter of window size of 3×3 *cells* as

$$\mathbf{v}_i(x,y) = Moving\_Average\left(\Sigma_t \mathbf{v}_t(x,y)\right) \ , i \subset X,Y,Z \tag{2}$$

Each $\mathbf{v}_i(x,y)$ corresponds to scrolling along the direction i.

2.4   Optical Flow Field Characterization

The OFF characterization starts with the detection of the parent and the child nodes. The parent node is defined to be the minimum divergence point in the vicinity (± 2 *cells*) of the HT_hit. This is the most likely location of the center of a polyp. The child nodes are defined to be the points on the incoming streamlines, 5 units away from the parent node. There are 8 child nodes, each corresponding to a streamline ending at a different immediate neighbor of the HT_hit.

A topology based quantitative characterization of the $\mathbf{v}_i(x,y) \ , i \in X,Y,Z$, at the parent node, is employed. It is represented as a point on the 2D $\alpha\beta$-plane, where α and β are defined as follows [26]. Let

$$\mathbf{J} = \begin{bmatrix} \frac{\partial v_x}{\partial x} & \frac{\partial v_x}{\partial y} \\ \frac{\partial v_y}{\partial x} & \frac{\partial v_y}{\partial y} \end{bmatrix}, \tag{3}$$

$$P = -trace(\mathbf{J}), \tag{4}$$

$$Q = |\mathbf{J}|, \tag{5}$$

then

$$\alpha = P, \tag{6}$$

$$\beta = sign(P^2 - 4Q)\sqrt{|P^2 - 4Q|}. \tag{7}$$

α and β essentially carry the information present in the eigenvalues of the characteristic equation

$$\lambda^2 + P\lambda + Q = 0 \tag{8}$$

They depend on the local divergence, curl and magnitude of the OFF. The origin of the $\alpha\beta$-plane corresponds to a uniform OFF.

As the third feature, the angular spread of the locations of child nodes around the parent node is defined as

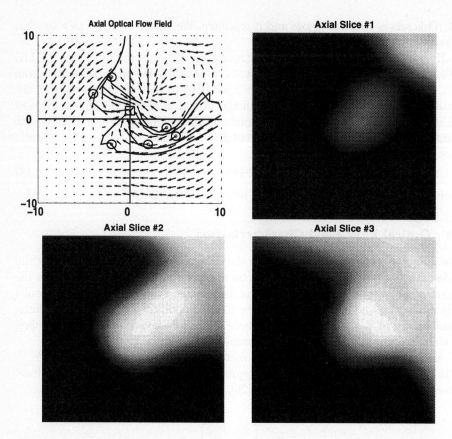

Fig. 1. 3 axial images (smoothed for visual purposes) and the axial OFF. The parent node is marked with a small square and the child nodes are marked with small circles. 3 of the 8 child nodes are coincident.

$$d = \frac{1}{8} \Sigma_i \left(\sqrt{\Sigma_j \theta_{ij}^2} \right) \ , \ \theta_{ij} = \angle(child_i, child_j) \in [0, \pi], \qquad (9)$$

taking the parent node as the origin. Larger d's indicate increased spread of the child nodes around the parent node.

The 3D feature vector, $[\alpha \ \beta \ d]$, is computed for all three $\mathbf{v}_i(x, y)$, $i \in X, Y, Z$. The median value for each feature is used in the final 3D feature vector used for classification. Figure 1 shows three axial images of a polyp, corresponding to three different t values (the image plane is the axial plane) and the computed OFF associated with this t-axis ($t \equiv z$).

3   Preliminary Analysis

Data were acquired from 8 patients (7 male and 1 female with age 41-85, mean age 63) as described in Section 2.1. Preprocessing with a HT score threshold of 10000 resulted in 220 HT_hits. Fiber optic colonoscopy results showed that 7 patients had a total of 20 polyps and that all polyps were detected by HTD. This means that the HTD, with the current threshold value, had 100% sensitivity and a high false positive rate. These 220 HT_hits were used as inputs to our algorithm.

We randomly divided the data set into 10 equal size mutually exclusive subsets, such that each subset contains 2 true positive and 20 false positive HT_hits. For each of 10 experiments, one of these subsets was used as the test set and the remaining nine subsets were used for training. We used a Mahalanobis distance based classifier. The Mahalanobis distance of a vector $\mathbf{f}$ to the mean vector, $\mathbf{m}_\Gamma$, of a population, Γ, is defined as [27],

$$r_{\mathbf{f},\mathbf{m}_\Gamma} = \sqrt{(\mathbf{f} - \mathbf{m}_\Gamma)^T \mathbf{C}_\Gamma^{-1} (\mathbf{f} - \mathbf{m}_\Gamma)} \tag{10}$$

where $\mathbf{C}_\Gamma$ is the covariance matrix of Γ. We added a bias term, b, to r that is used to trade off specificity and sensitivity of the classifier as

$$r_{\mathbf{f},\mathbf{m}_{\Gamma_1}} - r_{\mathbf{f},\mathbf{m}_{\Gamma_0}} + b \leq 0 \Rightarrow \mathbf{f} \in \Omega_1 \tag{11}$$
$$\text{otherwise} \Rightarrow \mathbf{f} \in \Omega_0$$

where, Γ represents the training set and $\mathbf{f}$ represents a sample from the test set, Ω. The subscript '1' refers to the subset of true positives, while the subscript '0' refers to the subset of true negatives.

In an attempt to assess the potential of OFFs in polyp identification, we measured the maximum specificity at 100% sensitivity, for each experiment, where the specificity was defined as the percentage of correctly identified non-polyp structures in each test set. The maximum specificity values at 100% sensitivity for each experiment was: 0.85, 0.85, 0.35, 0.90, 1.00, 0.15, 0.80, 0.80, 0.85, 0.95.

The analysis of an individual subvolume lasted 3.0 seconds using Matlab^{TM} 6.0 (The Mathworks Inc., MA, USA) on a PC with 1GHz Pentium III processor. The time measurements exclude the subvolume extractions.

4   Discussion

Our ultimate goal is to decrease the radiologists' reading time by directing them towards the true polyps. To do this, we model the way a radiologist recognizes a polyp in 3D CT data based on the motion of edges as one scrolls back and forth through parallel planes transecting a suspicious structure. It is obvious that the choice of scrolling direction affects the computed OFF. We tried to decrease this dependency by performing the analysis in three orthogonal directions and using the median values of each feature. A more robust approach would be to use multiple scrolling directions and construct a feature vector out of the histograms of measured feature values. Using additional features, like the homogeneity of the region of interest, might also improve performance.

We have observed that the divergence of the OFF at the parent node is of particular relevance for polyp identification. As such, the α and β parameters derived from the Jacobian of the OFF are very appropriate because they not only represent the information in the eigenvalues of the Jacobian matrix, but also the parameter α directly corresponds to the divergence of the OFF.

One of the two polyps in the test set of experiment 3 was completely hidden on the sagittal plane and could be seen properly only in the coronal plane. The median operation eliminated the measurements from the coronal plane, degrading the performance of the system (specificity was 0.35). The low specificity level of experiment 6 (0.15), on the other hand, is due to the large cancerous tumor (3.2cm in diameter) in the test set. Such big structures cannot be detected by OFFC with the current parameters, especially the subvolume size. These observations also suggest that increasing the number of scrolling directions would improve the performance.

The classifier we used performs linear discriminant analysis based on the minimization of the Mahalanobis distance between the learning and the test samples. The advantages of using the Mahalanobis distance are: *(i)* It automatically accounts for scaling, *(ii)* it takes care of the correlation between features and *(iii)* it can provide linear and curved decision boundaries. Another possible classifier would be the Support Vector Machines (SVM) [28]. SVMs are capable of trading off the training error with the generalization error. They can work practically in infinite dimensional feature spaces. The choice of the parameters and the feature space is critical for SVMs' performance and is the subject of future work. SVMs can even be used to learn directly from the computed OFFs, without extracting specific parameters, like α, β, d. This requires an appropriate kernel definition.

Our method is aimed to improve the HT-based CAD results by increasing the specificity without sacrificing sensitivity at a given operating point set by the HTD threshold. The specificity levels given in Section 3 show the achievable specificity levels at the operating point corresponding to the HTD threshold of 10000. It should be noted that in this data set HTD performs with high specificity levels (average of maximum specificity level over 10 experiments is $84 \pm 20\%$ at 100% sensitivity) at some other operating points. The improvement due to OFFC in specificity at those operating points would be different. Thus a direct comparison of this mean specificity level with that of OFFC post-processed data (mean specificity of $75\pm27.5\%$ at 100% sensitivity) is not possible. Moreover, the correlation coefficient between HT scores and the α, β, d parameters are -0.44, -0.05, 0.14, respectively. These results also support that the OFFC parameters assess different qualities of the CTC data. A more detailed analysis is given in [29,30].

The results presented here demonstrate the relevant information in OFFs for polyp detection in virtual colonography. However, higher specificity levels are required for practical clinical applications. Typically, the HTD threshold needs to be set low enough for 100% sensitivity, and that results in high false positive rates. Recent experiments that we conducted on a larger dataset that has low specificity at 100% sensitivity using HTD alone showed a significant increase in specificity without sacrificing the sensitivity set by HTD parameters [29,30].

It would also be possible to use the present method to detect polyps directly from the 3D CT data without the need for the HTD. The OFFs associated with different scrolling directions could be computed for the whole volume and then classification could be performed only in the vicinity of the colon, based on α, β and d values.

5 Conclusion

We showed that the idea of modeling the way a radiologist recognizes polyps in 3D CT data is feasible. Optical flow fields (OFF) provide a robust framework for quantitative analysis of inter-slice relations in the 2D CT images. Although many different features can be extracted from OFFs, we showed that α, β and d carry relevant information for polyp recognition. However, several other features may be useful to obtain better performance. Further research is required to optimize the feature space and the classifier.

References

1. Coin, C.G., Wollett, F.C., et al.: Computerized radiology of the colon: a potential screening technique. Comput. Radiol. **7(4)** (1983) 215–221
2. Chaoui, A.S., Blake, M.A., et al.: Virtual colonoscopy and colorectal cancer screening. Abdom. Imaging **25(2)** (2000) 361–367
3. Johnson, C.D., Dachman, A.H.: CT colonography: the next colon screening examination? Radiology **216(2)** (2000) 331–341
4. Vining, D.J.: Virtual colonoscopy. Gastrointest. Endosc. Clin. N. Am. **7(2)** (1997) 285–291
5. Hara, A.K., Johnson, C.D., et al.: Detection of colorectal polyps by computed tomographic colography: feasibility of a novel technique. Gastroenterology **110(1)** (1996) 284–290
6. Macari, M., Milano, A., et al.: Comparison of time-efficient CT colonography with two- and three-dimensional colonic evaluation for detecting colorectal polyps. Am. J. Roentgenol **174(6)** (2000) 1543–1549
7. Hara, A.K., Johnson, C.D., et al.: Detection of colorectal polyps with CT colography: initial assessment of sensitivity and specificity. Radiology **205(1)** (1997) 59–65
8. Rex, D.K., Vining, D., et al.: An initial experience with screening for colon polyps using spiral CT with and without CT colography. Gastrointest. Endosc. **50(3)** (1999) 309–313
9. ASGE, American Society for Gastrointestinal Endoscopy: Technology status evaluation: virtual colonoscopy: November 1997. Gastrointest. Endosc. **48(6)** (1998) 708–710
10. Dachman, A.H., Kuniyoshi, J.K., et al.: CT colonography with three-dimensional problem solving for detection of colonic polyps. Am. J. Roentgenol **171(4)** (1998) 989–995
11. Paik, D.S., Beaulieu, C.F., et al.: Visualization modes for CT colonography using cylindrical and planar map projections. J. Comput. Assist. Tomogr. **24(2)** (2000) 179–188

12. Kay, C.L., Kulling, D., et al.: Virtual endoscopy – comparison with colonoscopy in the detection of space-occupying lesions of the colon. Endoscopy **32(3)** (2000) 226–232

13. Lee, T.Y., Lin, P.H., et al.: Interactive 3D virtual colonoscopy system. IEEE Trans. Inf. Tech. Biomed. **3(2)** (1999) 139–150

14. Beaulieu, C.F., Jeffrey, Jr., R.B., et al.: Display modes for CT colonography. Part II. Blinded comparison of axial CT and virtual endoscopic and panoramic endoscopic volume-rendered studies. Radiology **212(1)** (1999) 203–212

15. Wang, G., McFarland, E.G., et al.: GI tract unraveling with curved cross sections. IEEE Trans. Med. Imaging **17(2)** (1998) 318–322

16. McFarland, E.G., Brink, J.A., et al. : Visualization of colorectal polyps with spiral CT colography: evaluation of processing parameters with perspective volume rendering. Radiology **205(3)** (1997) 701–707

17. Haker, S., Angenent, S., et al.: Nondistorting flattening maps and the 3D visualization of colon CT images. IEEE Trans. Med. Imaging **19** (2000) 665–670

18. Paik, D.S., Beaulieu, C.F., et al.: Automated flight path planning for virtual endoscopy. Med. Phys. **25(5)** (1998) 629–637

19. Samara, Y., Fiebich, M., et al.: Automated calculation of the centerline of the human colon on CT images. Acad Radiol. **6(6)** (1999) 352–359.

20. Mir, A.H., Hanmandlu, M., et al.: Description of shapes in CT images. IEEE EMBS Mag. **18(1)** (1999) 79–84

21. Summers, R.M., Beaulieu, C.F., et al.: Automated polyp detector for CT colonography: feasibility study. Radiology **216(1)** (2000) 284–290

22. Paik, D.S., Beaulieu, C.F., et al.: Computer aided detection of polyps in CT colonography: free response ROC evaluation of performance. Radiological Society of North America 86th Scientific Sessions, Chicago, IL, November, 2000.

23. Paik, D.S., Beaulieu, C.F., et al.: Detection of polyps in CT colonography: a comparison of a computer aided detection algorithm to 3D visualization methods. In: Proc. Radiological Society of North America 85th Scientific Sessions, Chicago, IL, November, 1999.

24. Yiu-Fai, W., Tsuhan, C.: Compression of medical volumetric data in a video-codec framework. ICASSP **4** (1996) 2128–2135

25. Beauchemin, S.S., Barron, J.L.: The computation of optical flow. ACM Computing Surveys **27(3)** (1995) 433–467

26. Lavin, Y., Batra, R., Hesselink, L.: Feature comparisons of vector fields using earth mover's distance. In: Proc. IEEE/ACM Visualization'98, North Carolina, October, 1998

27. Mahalanobis, P. C.: On the generalized distance in statistics Proc. Natl. Institute of Science of India, **12** (1936) 49-55

28. Vapnik, V.N.: The nature of statistical learning theory. New York : Springer, 1995

29. Acar, B., Beaulieu, C.F., et al.: Assessment of an optical flow field-based polyp detector for CT colonography. Submitted to the 23rd Annual Meeting of IEEE Engineering in Medicine and Biology Society, İstanbul, Turkey, 2001

30. Acar, B., Beaulieu, C.F., et al.: Optical flow field based-classification for improved detection of polyps in CT colonography. Submitted to IEEE Transaction on Medical Imaging

A New Visualization Method for Virtual Colonoscopy

F.M. Vos [1,2], I.W.O. Serlie [1,3], R.E. van Gelder [4], F.H. Post [3],
R. Truyen [5], F.A. Gerritsen [5], J. Stoker[4], A.M. Vossepoel [1]

[1] Pattern Recognition Group, Delft University of Technology
Lorentzweg 1, 2628 CJ Delft, The Netherlands
{frans,iwo,albert}@ph.tn.tudelft.nl

[2] Department of Radiology, University Hospital Rotterdam
Dr. Molewaterplein 40, 3015 GD Rotterdam, The Netherlands
frans@ph.tn.tudelft.nl

[3] Computer Graphics and CAD/CAM Group, Delft University of Technology
Zuidplantsoen 4, 2628 BJ Delft, The Netherlands
frits.post@cs.tudelft.nl

[4] Department of Radiology, Academic Medical Centre Amsterdam
P.O. Box 22700, 1100 DE Amsterdam, The Netherlands
r.e.vangelder@amc.uva.nl

[5] EasyVision Advanced Development Group, Philips Medical Systems Nederland B.V.
P.O. Box 10000, 5680 DA Best, The Netherlands
{roel.truyen,frans.gerritsen}@philips.com

Abstract. Virtual colonoscopy or 'colonography' is a patient-friendly, modern screening technique for polyps. Automatic detection of polyps can serve to assist the radiologist. This paper presents a method based on clustering the principal curvatures. Via automatic polyp detection 5/6 polyps (>5 mm) were detected at the expense of 9 false positive findings per case. For visualization, the bowel surface is presented to the physician in a 'panoramic' way as a sequence of unfolded cubes. Conventionally, only 93% of the colon surface is available for examination. In our approach the area in view is increased to 99.8%. The unfolded cube visualization is another step to optimize polyp detection by visual examination. Experiments show a sensitivity of 10/10 (on a per patient basis) for any polyp. The specificity was 7/10.

Keywords: radius of curvature, scientific visualization, virtual endoscopy.

1 Introduction

Colorectal polyps are considered important precursor of colon cancer [1]. Typically, such a benign tumour presents a sphere extending from the bowel wall on a small, thin stem (like a mushroom, see Figure 1). It may be distinguished from the physiologic surface structure by its isotropic curvature in the protruding direction (opposite to its surroundings). Commonly, only polyps larger than 5 mm are considered significant. This minimum polyp size is justified by a strong correlation between its size and the risk of

W. Niessen and M. Viergever (Eds.): MICCAI 2001, LNCS 2208, pp. 645-654, 2001.
© Springer-Verlag Berlin Heidelberg 2001

a malignant transformation [2]. Smaller polyps are nearly always benign, in which case an operation is unnecessary [3]. Not surprisingly, early detection of polyps has proven to lead to a decrease in incidence of colon cancer [4]. The interval before polyps develop into a malignancy is estimated to be in the order of 5 years [2]. Hence, screening seems an attractive possibility for prevention.

Until recently a barium enema and camera colonoscopy were the two procedures available for examining the colon [5][6]. Both techniques have serious drawbacks. The sensitivity of the barium enema is only 50-80% for polyps sized from 5 to 10 mm in diameter. Camera colonoscopy requires intravenous sedation to ease the discomfort. Consequently, many of those eligible for screening avoid the examination [7].

In the past few years, virtual colonoscopy (*'colonography'*) has been developed as a modern alternative [8]. Generally, the procedure comprises of the following steps. First, the patient's colon is cleansed and distended by transanal inflation with air. Subsequently, a 3D image volume is acquired of the abdomen by CT or MRI. Finally, the interior bowel surface is extracted and visualized, after which the physician virtually navigates through the colon and examines the surface for abnormalities (Figure 1, left).

Virtual colonoscopy relies heavily on a proper representation of geometric information. Important clues such as vascularization and wall texture are unavailable. Some authors suggest to support the exploitation of surface shape by automatic polyp detection. As yet, only preliminary results have been published, most in medical journals and not specifically focussed on technical details. Such detection was based on classification of the principal curvatures, local sphere fitting and orientation clustering of surface normals [9][10]. Although the development is still in an early stage, it is well recognized that automatic polyp detection may enhance the efficiency of the examination.

The current procedure is to explore the bowel in an interactive way. However, real-time visualization at a high frame-rate is not always possible due to the large data size and the inherent quality requirements. The latter problem is often solved by generating movies off-line. Typically, sequences are generated, with forward and backward viewing directions. In such a way, the observed part of the surface is maximized. Still, selective images on the colon wall are obtained. It may well be that important parts of the surface are missed, while insignificant parts are reviewed twice (Figure 1, right).

For a practical application, polyp detection must comply with requirements regarding

- scale dependency
- sensitivity/specificity
- effectiveness (in terms of area inspected)

The calculation of image features often introduces a scale parameter (e.g. the width of Gaussian derivatives). Special care must be taken to control the scale dependency of the outcome. In any case there must be a high sensitivity for detecting polyps larger than 0.5 cm in diameter, without introducing too many false positives. The previous claim is supported by making the complete surface accessible for inspection (hence the conventional dual sided view).

In this paper we will present a novel technique to detect polyps which comprises three steps:

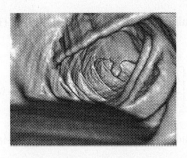 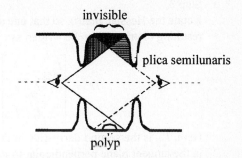

Fig. 1. Colonographic view on a polyp (left). The right picture shows which urface parts missed in two sided views.

- calculation of the principal isophote radii of curvature
- clustering
- visualization

The use of curvature information derives from the characteristic shape of polyps (see above). However, direct classification of the curvatures is insufficient for efficient detection (by yielding too many false positives). For that reason we introduced a clustering step to identify significant polyps and reject erroneous findings. The results serve to support the radiologist while he explores virtual endoscopic data. To that end, we integrated our method in a visualization environment presenting the bowel surface physician in a 'panoramic' way.

The paper is organized as follows. In Section 2, we will methodically describe the three stages of the technique. Results including a clinical evaluation will be presented in Section 3. The paper will finish by drawing conclusions and describe suggestions for future work.

2   Technique

2.1   Calculation of the Principal Normal Curvatures

A three step algorithm to calculate the principal curvatures from a 3D image volume is as follows [11]:

- Step 1
  Calculate the gradient vector (g) and the Hessian matrix (H) in each position. They are defined as:

$$ g = (I_x, I_y, I_z) \qquad H = \begin{bmatrix} I_{xx} & I_{xy} & I_{xz} \\ I_{xy} & I_{yy} & I_{yz} \\ I_{xz} & I_{yz} & I_{zz} \end{bmatrix} \qquad (1) $$

where each entry represents a partial derivative of the 3D image I. Each derivative is calculated through convolution with a Gaussian kernel at a specific width σ_{Gauss}.

- Step 2

  Rotate the Hessian matrix so that one axis aligns with the gradient direction. The resulting matrix H' can be written as:

$$H' = \begin{bmatrix} I_{gg} & - \\ - & \begin{matrix} I_{uu} & I_{uv} \\ I_{uv} & I_{vv} \end{matrix} \end{bmatrix} = \begin{bmatrix} I_{gg} & - \\ - & H_t' \end{bmatrix} \tag{2}$$

  Here, I_{gg} is the second derivative in the gradient direction and H'_t a 2D Hessian in the tangent plane perpendicular to g.

- Step 3

  Compute the eigenvalues of H'_t. These values λ_1 and λ_2 are respectively the maximum and the minimum second derivatives in the touching plane. The corresponding eigenvectors point in the direction of maximal and minimal curvature. It can be shown that the principal radii of curvatures are given by

$$\kappa_1 = \frac{\|g\|}{-\lambda_1} \qquad \kappa_2 = \frac{\|g\|}{-\lambda_2} \tag{3}$$

2.2   Clustering the Principal Curvatures and Visualization

Not surprisingly, a direct classification of the principal curvatures (e.g. by a direct threshold) yields imperfect results, mainly because voxels are individually addressed. Consequently, an isolated point may be identified as a polyp. The 'neighbourhood' aspect is incorporated by clustering the curvature values as follows. First, the colon's interior volume is obtained by thresholding the image, followed by a region growing from the centerline. Then, a dilation of the resulting object is performed, with the restriction of 6-connectivity. The contour added contains the surface voxels. Clearly, only those voxels are of interest that have a principal radius of curvature within a certain range of values ($R_{low} < \kappa_1 < R_{up}$ and $R_{low} < \kappa_2 < R_{up}$). Because such surface elements are expected to appear in clusters (due to the isotropy of polyps), a hierarchical clustering is performed by the single linkage method as described in [12]. At last, only those clusters are taken into account that contain a minimum number of voxels ($N_{curvatures}$). The location of such a cluster is determined by projecting the centre of gravity into the closest point on the colon wall.

For visualization, we designed an environment presenting the bowel surface in a 'panoramic' way. The polyp detector has been integrated in this environment to support the radiologist.

Let us first look into some general aspects of standard colonography. Conventionally, the virtual colon is inspected by an animated image sequence from coecum to rectum and vice versa. Increasing the viewing angle enlarges the amount of surface inspected. However, this approach goes at the expense of increased distortions towards the edges of the image. To avoid extreme deformations while showing the full visible field around a position, we present the physician with a series of 'unfolded cubic renderings' [13].

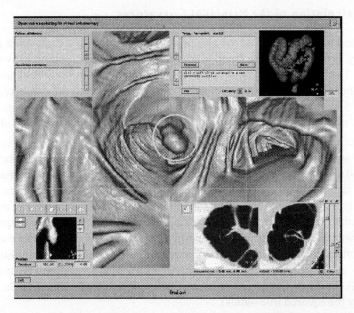

Fig. 2. A sequence of outfolded cubes is presented to improve efficiency

Consider a limited set of points sampled on the central path through the colon (for obtaining this central path we refer to [14]). Imagine that in each such position there is a cube of which the faces contain 90° views from the centre. Clearly, projection of the six images onto a single plane (the 'unfolded cubes) renders the complete field of view (see Figure 2 for an example). Additionally, discontinuities are restricted to the edges.

The interface for reviewing the unfolded cube data is shown in Figure 2. In the central part a sequence of images is displayed. The overview image depicts the current global position in the colon (top right). Two reformatted views allow exploration of the original CT data (bottom right). Both images are generated automatically when the user clicks in the unfolded cube. The centre of the two images is determined by projecting the selected point on the colon wall. The first image is perpendicular to the path where it is closest to the selected position. The second, orthogonal cross-section is parallel to the centerline tangent. The physician can scroll interactively through these images and rotate them for closer inspection of suspicious areas.

The top-left window contains a list of detected polyps. By clicking on any one item, the unfolded cube image is shown, rendered from the closest central path point. The position of such a polyp is always indicated by a circle.

3 Results

This section describes an evaluation of our approach, specifically in relation to requirements of scale dependency, sensitivity and effectivity (surface in view).

3.1   Calculation of the Principal Curvatures

We will test the calculation of the principal curvatures by its accuracy and precision. Obviously, both will vary as a function of σ_{Gauss} (width of the Gaussian derivatives, see Section 2.1). Clearly, σ_{Gauss} must be tuned to the size of the object under consideration (radius) and the noise level. At a typical CT image resolution of 0.5 mm/pixel, relevant polyps of 5-10 mm in diameter are approximated by spheres of 5 to 10 pixels in radius. In our CT images (see Section 3.2) we measured a contrast to noise ratio of about 0.05.

To monitor the effect of object size and noise we conducted the following experiments. A sphere with radius 5 pixels was generated (in the Fourier domain to obtain bandlimitedness). Those points were selected that were within 1 pixel from the true surface. Thus, the latter distance corresponds to positions 4 to 6 pixels from the centre. For each of these surface points the principal radii of curvature were calculated. The true values (gold standard) are given by the distance to the centre of the sphere. Consequently, the mean as well as the standard deviation were determined of the difference of ground truth and measured radius of Gaussian curvature ($= \kappa_1 \cdot \kappa_2$). Each of these two numbers (the 'bias' and standard deviation) were attained for varying σ_{Gauss} and an array of noise levels (Gaussian). The graphs in Figure 3 show normalized results (i.e. the outcome divided by the squared true radius).

As expected, a certain minimal filter width (σ_{Gauss}= 3-5 pixels) is required to obtain good accuracy and precision at any noise level. From the 'bias' it appears that the Gaussian curvature is increasingly overrated (note that the curves show gold standard - measured Gaussian curvature). Because the measurements involve a spherical object, the area outside the sphere relatively increases with larger σ. Consequently, the outcome is weighted with larger radii of curvature, yielding a biased result.

Previously (Section 1) we remarked that a distinguishing feature of polyps is that they jut out into the colon. While the *plicae semilunares* (or *haustral folds*, visible in Figure 1) have a protruding character in *one* principal direction, they have opposite curvature in the other. Because polyps present an smaller image structure than the colon surface, we propose to use the largest sigma that allows good measurement. Thus, to measure a polyp of 0.5 cm (diameter) at a resolution of 0.5 mm/pixel requires σ_{Gauss} = 5-9 (compare with Figure 3). In this way such a clinically relevant polyp is measured with good accuracy and precision. On the other hand irrelevant features (smaller protrusions) will be smoothed away as much as possible into the background (having opposite curvature).

3.2   Clustering and Visualization

For the evaluation of our work we collected data from 20 patients visiting the Academic Medical Centre Amsterdam. An informed-consent procedure was followed, in which the patient inclusion criterion was the referral for conventional colonoscopy. For each patient 3D image data were acquired by computed tomography (CT) in supine and prone position. The in-plane resolution of the images was approximately 0.6 mm/pixel at

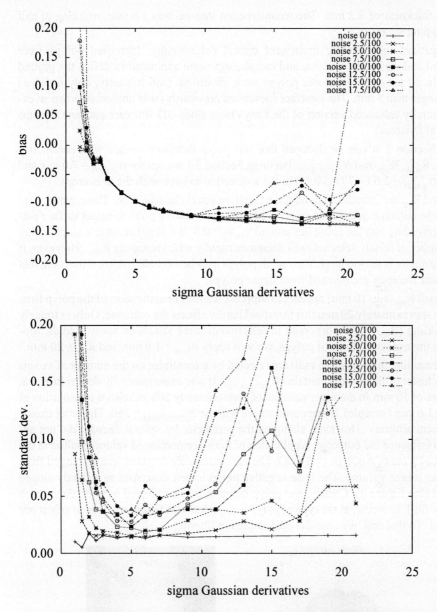

Fig. 3. A sphere with radius 5 pixels was generated. Those points were selected that were within 1 pixel from the true surface (i.e. 4 to 6 pixels from the centre). For each of these surface points the principal radii of curvature were calculated. The true values (gold standard) are given by the distance to the centre of the sphere. For all these points the mean as well as the standard deviation were determined of the difference of ground truth and measured radius of Gaussian curvature (= $\kappa_1 \cdot \kappa_2$). Each of these two numbers (the 'bias' and standard deviation) were attained for varying σ_{Gauss} and an array of noise levels. The graphs show normalized results

a slice thickness of 3.2 mm. The reconstruction interval was 1.6 mm, resulting in half overlapping slices.

Each patient subsequently underwent optical colonoscopy. Identified polyps were resected and their size, location and morphology were annotated to define the ground truth. In 10 patients 15 colonic polyps were identified. Unfortunately, only 6 polyps were larger than 5 mm. The interface (described previously) was implemented on an experimentally enhanced version of the EasyVision Endo-3D software package (Philips Medical Systems).

From Section 2 it can be deduced that our polyp detection comes with parameters σ_{Gauss}, R_{low}, R_{up}, and $N_{curvatures}$. Pursuing Section 3.1 we opt for $\sigma_{Gauss} = 7.0$ in x and y and $\sigma_{gauss} = 2.6 (= 7/(1.6/0.6))$ in the z-direction to cope with the anisotropy.

R_{low} and R_{up} are introduced to obtain a tentative voxel classification. These parameters affect the outcome in the next manner. Ideally, the breaking point to select surface patches protruding into the colon lies around κ_1, $\kappa_2 = 0.0$. It will not come as a surprise that the number of falsely selected radii decreases rapidly with increasing R_{low}. However, if this parameter is set too large, then small polyps may be excluded. Also, it turns out that radii near the apex are rejected from larger polyps.

Too small R_{up} (e.g. 10 mm) appears to suppress features near the stem of the polyp first. Above approximately 20 mm this threshold hardly affects the outcome. Only extremely large values ($R_{up} = 100$ mm) result in selection of some voxels on haustral folds. Modelling the expected shape of polyps, we will apply $R_{low} = 1.0$ mm and $R_{up} = 20$ mm.

Any remaining false positive radii are rejected by a constraint on the number of voxels that a cluster of them must contain ($N_{curvatures}$). It was experimentally determined that a sphere of 10 mm in diameter consists of approximately 500 voxels (at a resolution of 0.6^2 x 1.6 mm / sample). In concordance we will use $N_{curvatures} = 250$. The latter choice may seem arbitrary. However, changing the parameter by several decades did not appear to influence the outcome. Application of the aforementioned values resulted in detection of 5 out of 6 polyps (> 5 mm). The false positively detected lesions ranged from 5-15 per image volume. The false negative polyp is best described as a faintly sloped mound (see Figure 4). Clearly, our polyp detector is not designed to track down such shapes. Still, however, as the type of polyp is regarded significant, we need to adjust our method. To that end, we consider scale adaptive filtering.

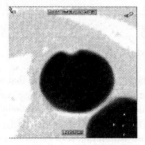 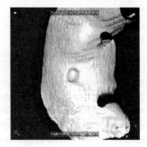

Fig. 4. An undetected polyp, on the left depicted in a reformatted CT image, on the right the virtual endoscopic view.

The effectiveness of the visualization was tested by calculating the surface area coming into view. Therefore, the wall voxels in each volume were identified in the same manner as described earlier (Section 2.2). Subsequently, it was determined which fraction of them was projected into the images upon navigation along the central path (as in [15]). The results are summarized in Table 1. The single plane entry is defined by considering the backward and forward views individually (n = 80). In a two sided view (the conventional approach) both sequences are considered simultaneously (n = 40).

Technique:	Single plane view	Two sided view	Unfolded cube
Surface in view (+ std. dev.):	73% (2.8)	93.8 (0.5)	99.5 (0.1)

Table 1: Effectiveness in terms of surface in view.

The 6.2% of the total area not seen using the two sided view corresponds to about 20000 voxels, the largest cluster of which contained 1200 elements. This is significantly more than the surface of a polyp, which is approximately 500 voxels (see above). The latter discrepancy clearly justifies the unfolded cube visualization.

The sensitivity and specificity (on a per patient basis) are collated in Table 2. The gold standard was obtained through retrospective examination of the image sets by one radiologist specialized in CT colonography. The evaluation times were 28 minutes for the

Technique:	Two sided view	Unfolded cube
Sensitivity (%):	7/10	10/10
Specificity (%):	8/10	7/10

Table 2: Sensitivity and specificity for the conventional and unfolded cube approaches.

two sided view technique and 12 minutes using the unfolded cubes (see also [13]. For the review, the 'conventional' virtual endoscopy system as well as the unfolded cube technique were used both supported by automatic polyp detection. As expected (due to the larger field of view), more polyps were retrieved using the outfolded cube than with the conventional approach (two sided view). Concurrently, however, the number of false positives increases, yielding slightly lower specificity. We acknowledge that the low number of cases does not reveal significant differences. Clearly, further study is required in this respect.

4 Conclusions

A modern technique to screen for colorectal polyps is by virtual endoscopy. Any such visualization relies heavily on a proper representation of the geometric information. For optimal exploitation of surface geometry, automatic detection of polyps can serve to assist the radiologist. We presented a method based on the local principal curvatures. It was shown that all round polyps could be detected at the expense of a limited number of false positives. However, flat and elongated specimens require a more sophisticated approach, e.g. by adaptive filtering. Still, we consider automatic detection a promising support for inspection.

The unfolded cube visualization is another step to optimize polyp detection by visual examination. The method imposes that the complete colon surface comes into view. The experiments showed a sensitivity of 10/10 for significant polyps.

Virtual endoscopy is rapidly becoming a state-of-the art tool for radiologists. The methods described in this paper aimed to contribute to its development.

5   References

[1]   B. Vogelstein, E.R. Fearon, S.R. Hamilton, 'Genetic alterations during colorectal-tumour development', *N. Engl. J. Med.*, vol. 319, pp. 525-532, 1988.

[2]   J.D. Potter, M.L. Slattery, R.M. Bostick, 'Colon cancer: a review of the epidemiology', *Epidemiol. Rev.*, vol. 15, pp. 499-545, 1993.

[3]   J.G. Fletcher, W. Luboldt, 'CT colonography and MR colonography: current status, research directions and comparison', *Eur.Radiol.*, vol. 10, pp. 786-801, 2000.

[4]   N.W. Toribrara, M.H. Sleisenger, 'Screening for colorectal cancer', *N Engl J Med*, vol. 332, pp. 332, pp. 861-867, 1995.

[5]   G.D.Dodd, 'Colon cancer and polyps imaging perspectives', *Proc. First International Symposium on Virtual Colonoscopy*, pp. 15-17, Boston University Press, 1998.

[6]   D.K. Rex, C.S. Cutler, G.T. Lemmel, 'Colonoscopy miss rates of adenomas determined by back-to-back colonooscopies', in *Gastroenterology*, vol. 112, pp. 24-28, 1997.

[7]   S.J. Winawer, R.H. Fletcher, L. Miller, 'Colorectal cancer screening: clinical guidelines and rationale', *Gastroenterology*, vol. 112, pp. 594-642, 1997.

[8]   L. Hong, S.Muraki, A. Kaufman, T. He, 'Virtual voyage: interactive navigation in the human colon', *Proc. ACM SIGGRAPH Conf.*, pp. 27-34, ACM Press, 1997.

[9]   C.F. Beaulieu, 'Computer aided detection of colonic polyps', *Second International Symposium on Virtual Colonoscopy*, pp. 73-77, Boston University Press, 2000.

[10]   R.M. Summers, C.F. Beaulieu, S.Napel, 'Automatic polyp detector for CT colonography: feasibility study', *Radiology*, vol. 216, pp. 284-290, 2000.

[11]   L.J. van Vliet and P.W. Verbeek, 'Curvature and bending energy in digitized 2D and 3D images', *Proc. 8th Scandinavian Conf. on Image Analysis*, pp. 1403- 1410, 1993.

[12]   M.R. Anderberg, 'Cluster analysis for applications', Academic Press Inc., 1973.

[13]   I.W.O. Serlie, F.M. Vos, R. van Gelder et al. 'Improved visualization in virtual colonoscopy using image-based rendering', accepted for publication in *Proc. ACM/Eurographics Vis Sym*, 2001.

[14]   R.Truyen, P.Lefere, S.Gryspeerdt, T.Deschamps, 'Speed and robustness of (semi-) automatic path tracking', *Proc. Second International Symposium on Virtual Colonoscopy*, p. 102, 2000.

[15]   D.S. Paik, C.F. Beaulieu, R.B. Jeffrey, C.A.. Karadi, S. Napel, 'Visualization modes for CT colonography using Cylindrical and planar map projections', *J Comput Assist Tomogr.*, vol. 24(2), pp. 179-188, 2000.

Classification-Driven Pathological Neuroimage Retrieval Using Statistical Asymmetry Measures*

Y. Liu[1], F. Dellaert[1], W.E. Rothfus[2], A. Moore[1], J. Schneider[1], and
T. Kanade[1]

[1] The Robotics Institute, Carnegie Mellon University, Pittsburgh 15213, USA
yanxi,dellaert,awm,schneide,tk@cs.cmu.edu
[2] University of Pittsburgh Medical Center, Pittsburgh, PA

Abstract. This paper reports our methodology and initial results on volumetric pathological neuroimage retrieval. A set of novel image features are computed to quantify the statistical distributions of approximate bilateral asymmetry of normal and pathological human brains. We apply memory-based learning method to find the most-discriminative feature subset through image classification according to predefined semantic categories. Finally, this selected feature subset is used as indexing features to retrieve medically similar images under a semantic-based image retrieval framework. Quantitative evaluations are provided.

1 Motivation

Medical images form an essential and inseparable component of diagnosis, intervention and patient follow-ups. In this work, we use a patient's image as an index to retrieve medically similar and relevant patient cases from a large multimedia database. Common practice in the image retrieval and pattern recognition community is to map each image into a set of numerical or symbolic attributes called *image indexing features*. Thus each image corresponds to a point in a multidimensional image feature space. Existing "content-based" image retrieval (CBIR) systems [6,13] depend on general visual properties such as color and texture to classify diverse, two-dimensional (2D) images. However, these general visual cues often fail to be effective discriminators for image sets taken within a single domain, where images have subtle, domain-specific differences. Furthermore, these global statistical color and texture measures do not necessarily reflect or have proven correspondence to the meaning of an image, i.e. the image semantics, nor are they suitable for handling three-dimensional (3D) volumetric images. Our objective is to go beyond the ill-defined, subjective visual feature indexing practiced in many current CBIR systems. Our approach is based on statistical learning, and contains the following components:

* This research is supported in part by an NIST grant #70NANB5H1183 and in part by the NIH/NCI research contract # N01-CO-07119.

W. Niessen and M. Viergever (Eds.): MICCAI 2001, LNCS 2208, pp. 655–665, 2001.
© Springer-Verlag Berlin Heidelberg 2001

1. **Feature extraction** maps each volumetric image into a multi-dimensional image feature space;
2. **Feature weighting and image similarity construction** imposes relative weights on the image feature space;
3. **Adaptive image retrieval** chooses image similarity best suited for the user intention.

The kind of medical database accessing capability we are developing will have many potential applications in clinical practice and medical education, including on-line consultation, differential diagnosis, surgical planning, recovery/outcome evaluation, and tele-medicine. As a realistic test-bed of our methodology, we choose a neuroimage database composed of volumetric CT image sets of hemorrhage (acute blood), bland infarct (stroke) and normal brains. Justifications for this endeavor are two-fold: first of all, a database composed of volumetric images and collateral information in a particular medical domain provides objective, semantically well-defined training sets and quantifiable results; second, due to the limitation of the popular color and texture image features used by many existing CBIR systems, finding novel image features and most discriminating feature subsets for medical image characterization become crucial.

As pointed out in [5]: "To date, all too often image analysis algorithm development ignores the analysis of different abnormal, pathological or disease states". Work on neuroimage analysis has been concentrated more on morphological variations of normal brains [2,7] or brains with mental disorders [15] using high resolution, high density MRI data. The image data used in this work, in contrast, is CT images obtained from clinical practice. The sparseness and incompleteness of the CT image data set pose more challenges in image understanding and indexing than does the complete, dense data used in other reported work. However, the database images we use more realistically reflect the type of query images that an end user will supply in practice.

Existing work on pathological medical image database retrieval deals mostly with 2D images and has not paid much attention to a systematic approach for image feature weighting. In the work of a dental radiography image database retrieval [17], the authors use a deformable shape contour selected by the system designer as the primary feature for image indexing. By selecting different modes in the finite element representation and eigen-decomposition of the contours (hand drawn by an expert dentist), the authors achieve classification rates between 87% (for normals) and 62% (for pathologies). What is missing in the image retrieval practice is an objective, quantitative evaluation of the extracted image features **before** they are used for image retrieval. The method we propose here directly addresses this issue.

2   Our Approach

A basic framework for classification-driven semantic based image retrieval is demonstrated in Figure 1, containing two stages with five essential components.

The two stages are an off-line stage for classification-driven image similarity metric learning (feature weighting), and an on-line stage for image retrieval. The five essential components are (1) image preprocessing, (2) image feature extraction, (3) feature subset weighting via image classification, (4) image retrieval, and (5) quantitative evaluation. Though the two stages share some common components, the goals and constraints differ. In the off-line stage the goal is to find the best and smallest subset of image features that capture image semantics. It requires an explicitly labeled image data set, and sufficient computer memory space to store a large feature attribute matrix and to support extensive search on this matrix. High computational speed is a plus but not necessary. During the on-line stage, on the other hand, the demands are fast retrieval speed and visualization of retrieved images given similarity metric and a query image.

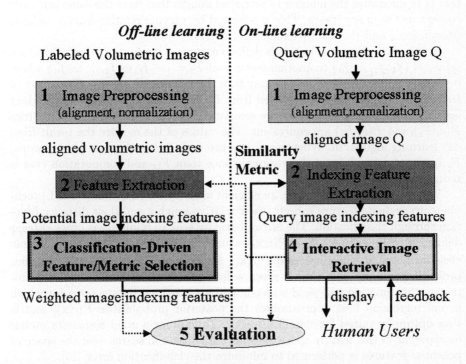

Fig. 1. Basic components for classification-driven semantic image retrieval

2.1 Novel Neuroimage Features

Human brains are approximately bilaterally symmetrical. In this work we have experimented with quantifying human brain asymmetry as a departure from an ideal midsagittal plane (Section 3.2).

2.2   Classification-Driven Feature Selection

We consider semantic-based image retrieval as a process of image classification by a k nearest neighbor classifier (kNN) [4]. As is well-known, the advantage of a kNN classifier is its non-linear, non-parametric nature and tolerance to arbitrary data distributions without the assumption that the forms of the underlying densities are known. It can therefore bypass probability estimation and go directly to decision functions [4]. However, a kNN classifier is suboptimal compared to Bayes error, **and** is sensitive to irrelevant, redundant, and noisy features. It can be proven that adding more features can increase the error rate for a kNN classifier [3]. To achieve a reasonable performance from a kNN classifier, therefore, it is *mandatory* to first go through a feature selection process. Given a query image and its k nearest neighbors, the goal of image retrieval under this context is to maximize the number of retrieved images that have the same semantic content as the query image. This is achieved by varying relative feature weights (dimension), and the distance function (metric).

In this work, feature selection is defined as a mapping from a potential feature set $F_1 = \{f_1, f_2, ..., f_n\}$ to another feature set $F_2 = \{w_1 f_1, w_2 f_2, ..., w_n f_n\}$ where $0 \leq w_i \leq 1$. Since some of the w_is may take the value 0, $|F_2| \leq |F_1|$. Two types of features are expected to be removed from F_1: irrelevant features and redundant features. As a result, for any image semantic class c_i the posterior probabilities $P(c_i|F_1)$ and $P(c_i|F_2)$ are equivalent. The values of the w_is are the result from our learning algorithm. When many w_is are zeros (as is the case in this work) F_2 becomes a much lower-dimensional space than F_1, and computation cost is reduced greatly.

We employ *kernel regression*, an efficient memory based learning (MBL) technique, to evaluate feature subsets, their relative weights and their distance function through classification. The error metric we seek to minimize is *cross entropy* defined as $E = -\sum_i \sum_c \delta_{ic} ln \hat{P}(c|\mathbf{x}_i)$ where δ_{ic} represents the 1-of-m multiple class membership encoding, and $\hat{P}(c|\mathbf{x}_i)$ is the approximation of the posterior probability $P(c|\mathbf{x})$ of a class c given a feature vector $\mathbf{x}$ via Bayes law. Minimizing this function will yield a metric and a smoothing parameter σ for which kernel regression best approximates the posterior probabilities $P(c|\mathbf{x})$, and is thus optimally suited for classification [1]. To look for a good *similarity metric* or *classifier* in this feature space, off-line, combinatorial search over the space of potential features is performed to minimize the classification error [14].

2.3   Image Retrieval and Evaluation

Once a locally optimal classifier is found, the associated image feature weights provide a proper scaling of the original feature space. The extracted image features form an N dimensional vector space, the overall distance function D of two images a, b is defined as $D(a, b) = \sqrt{(\mathbf{A} - \mathbf{B})^T \Sigma^{-1} (\mathbf{A} - \mathbf{B})}$ where $\mathbf{A} = f(a), \mathbf{B} = f(b)$ are the N dimensional image feature vectors of images a and b respectively, Σ is an $N \times N$ covariance matrix. When Σ is a diagonal matrix, D is a non-uniformly scaled Euclidean distance. Otherwise D is the Mahalanobis distance. Image retrieval is done using kNN with Euclidean distance. Evaluation of the retrieved images is measured by the *precision* rate $\mathbf{R_{P_k}} = N_{rp}/K$ and *recall* rate $\mathbf{R_{R_k}} = N_{rp}/N_p$ in the top K retrieved images, where N_{rp} is the number of correctly retrieved images with pathology class p in the top K retrieved images for the query, and N_p is the total number of instances in the database that have pathology class p and should be retrieved. When $K < N_p$, recall rate is identical to the precision rate.

3   Experiments

A study was performed using a data set of 48 volumetric CT brain scans containing normal (26), stroke (14) and blood cases (8). These are clinical CT images collected directly from a local hospital emergency room.

3.1   Image Alignment

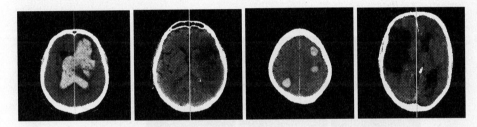

Fig. 2. The ideal symmetry axis is extracted as the intersection of a 3D brain image and its ideal midsagittal plane.

The first step is to align all 3D images such that the ideal midsagittal planes (iMSP) of different brain images are parallel and pitch angle is zero. 3D image intra- and inter-subject, multi-modality rigid and deformable registrations of normal brains have achieved excellent results [16,11]. However, no existing technology is readily available for registration of single or multi-modality, inter-subject, pathological brain images [8]. Matching two 3D pathological brains remains a difficult and controversial problem. This situation poses challenges to any 3D pathological neuroimage databases, especially for CT images. In our work, we have taken advantage of the approximate bilateral structure of human brains to develop a robust midsagittal plane (MSP) computation algorithm [9] for pathological brain alignment and comparison. The effect of the ideal midsagittal plane (iMSP) extraction algorithm [9] is not to find where the midsagittal plane is, but where it is supposed to be. This is especially useful for pathology brains since the anatomic midsagittal plane is often distorted (shifted or bent) due to large lesions. Figure 2 shows some 2D sample results after the midsagittal plane is extracted. The iMSP algorithm is robust under adverse conditions and has been evaluated extensively [9]. Axial and coronal slices are used simultaneously to handle large out-of-plane rotation angles effectively. No statistically significant difference is found between the iMSP algorithm and two experienced neuroradiologists.

3.2 Potential Indexing Feature Extraction

Though lesions are usually obvious to a trained eye, automatic image segmentation is a very hard problem in medical image analysis [5]. We take an alternative approach for image feature extraction which does not require precise segmentation of the image: human brains present an approximate bilateral symmetry, from which pathological brains often depart. Even the brains where pathology appears symmetrically present a different kind of symmetry from normal brains. Our intention is to quantify and capture the statistical distribution difference of various brain asymmetries. A set of relatively simple and computationally inexpensive statistical image features is collected (Figure 3). After the iMSP is

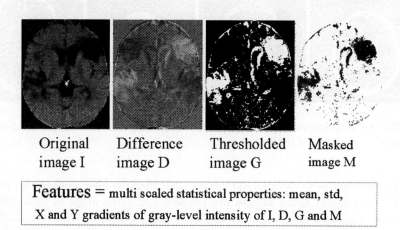

Original	Difference	Thresholded	Masked
image I	image D	image G	image M

Features = multi scaled statistical properties: mean, std,
X and Y gradients of gray-level intensity of I, D, G and M

Fig. 3. Image I: original image where its 3D MSP aligned and centered vertically. **Image D**: the intensity difference image between the original image I and its own vertical reflection. **Image G**: a thresholded image of image D. **Image M**: the product of image G with original image I (a masked image).

aligned in the middle of each 3D volumetric image (left most image in Figure 3), three types of asymmetry features are computed: 1) global statistical properties, 2) measures of asymmetry of halved and quartered brains, and 3) local asymmetrical region-based properties. These features are extracted from the original image (Fig. 3, image I) with its iMSP aligned, the difference image (Fig. 3, image D) of the original image and its mirror reflection with respect to iMSP, the thresholded difference image (image G^1), and the original image masked by the thresholded binary image (Figure 3, image M). The image features include: the means, variances, X and Y gradients of the intensity images at different regions and under various Gaussian smoothing, scaling and thresholding. A total of 48 image features are computed from each image.

3.3   Classification-Driven Feature Subset Evaluation

Now each image i becomes a vector V_i, and the length $N = |V_i|$ is the total dimension of the potential image feature space computed above. All the image data in the database form an $M \times N$ 2D sheet with M image points in the N dimensional feature space. A labeling, given by an experienced neuroradiologist, is added to the end of each row indicating the semantic class of the image, either simply the pathology type or pathology plus the anatomical location of the lesion(s).

We use a CMU proprietary combinatorial search engine called "Vizier" [14], to simultaneously find the image feature sub-dimensions and a proper kernel regression classifier that minimizes the leave-one-out cross-validation [12] on cross-entropy error of the training data given the classifier. The "Vizier" engine searches through a large set of possible classifiers within user specifications, and stops either when all possible choices are exhausted or a time limit given by the user is reached. Typically, we run a search between 20 minutes to a full hour on a standard PC. The output from Vizier is a specification of the best similarity metric found so far, consisting of the weight on each input feature attribute and a smoothing parameter σ.

Most physicians prefer using a 2D slice as a query to access digital databases. Though our framework and system design are for 3D volumetric images, 2D slices can be treated as basic image units as well. In this study, we have used three pathology types: blood,infarct and normal brain images, and used 2D slices as basic units. The total 3D image set S_{3D} is randomly divided (within each class) into a training set containing two thirds of S_{3D} (31) and a hold-out test set containing one third of S_{3D} (17), amounting to a total of 1250 2D slices. Care is taken to separate the test set and training set in such a way that there are no 2D slices from the same 3D brain belong to both training and testing sets.

3.4   Hierarchical Classifiers

An image classifier is simply a by-product of the process of feature subset evaluation through classification. The performance of the classifier may predict how well the selected feature subset will behave during image retrieval. For example, we can use a naive Bayes classifier as a 3D image classifier built on top of the 2D image classifiers, by using the ratios $r_S = n_S/n$ and $r_B = n_B/n$ as two 3D image features, where n_N, n_S, n_B are the numbers of predicted normal, stroke

---

[1] In our implementation, the absolute value of image G is used, whose value quantifies how asymmetrical the corresponding voxel regions are.

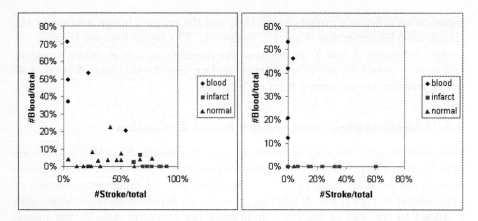

Fig. 4. The 3D image points are clustering in the two-ratio feature space while increasing the false negative penalty value of the 2D three-class classifier. The X-axis is r_S and Y-axis is r_B. The relative weights learned by Vizier are 0.5 and 1 respectively.

and blood 2D images from the same 3D image, and $n = n_N + n_S + n_B$. The image distribution in this two-dimensional feature space can be observed in Figure 4. From these feature spaces, one can observe that normal and blood cases are better separated than the normal and stroke cases. Using Bayes law, this probability can be expressed as $P(c|[r_S, r_B]) = \frac{P([r_S, r_B]|c)P(c)}{P([r_S, r_B])}$. A *cost matrix* can be imposed to bias the classifier. For example, a *false negative penalty $w > 1$* is incurred whenever a pathological image is classified as normal, whereas a unit cost or zero cost is incurred when a normal image is classified as pathological or when a class chosen is the correct class, respectively. The performance of such a 3D image classifier (when $w = 4$) is shown in the left of Figure 5.

3.5   Image Retrieval and Evaluation

Our approach is ideally suited to tuning an image similarity metric to the specific type of query that a user may submit to the system. As an example, one may simply want to know whether the query image is normal. In this case, the feature subset that is selected and optimally weighted for discriminating three different pathology types may not be optimal for a binary normal/abnormal discrimination. Thus we need to find an alternative feature subset. When we tried this, the locally optimal classifier found a different metric than the one from the ternary classification case. In both cases, Vizier finds a most discriminating feature subset containing 9-5 image features — a reduction in indexing feature dimension by nearly 5 to 10 fold. The similarity metric found in image classification can now serve as an image indexing vector for retrieving images in the reduced feature space. The right side of Figure 5 shows the mean retrieval precision rate for the hold out test images, one for the three-class case (normal, blood, infarct) and one for the two-class (normal, abnormal) case. One can observe a slightly better performance for the 2-class than for the 3-class image set.

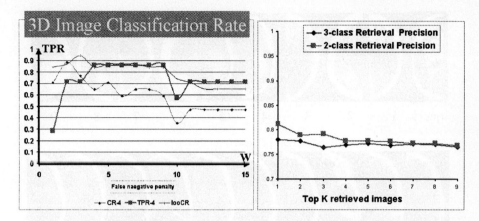

Fig. 5. Left (image classification, Bayes classifier): performance of a 3D image classifier on a randomly chosen, hold-out test-set when its false negative penalty $w = 4$. TPR-4: true positive rate. CR-4: classification rate. The horizontal axis is the 2D classifier false negative penalty value w. Right (image retrieval, kNN classifier): the mean value of retrieval precision as a function of the top K retrieved images. 2-class: normal, pathology. 3-class: normal, infarct, blood.

This is to be expected since 2-class classification leaves less space for errors to be made than the 3-class classification problem. However, in this problem the difficult class separation is between normals and strokes, which can be observed from the original image feature values and 2D classifier output (Figure 4), thus the improvement in 2-class is minimal.

Given near 80% precision rate on average for image retrieval, this result implies that in average 8 out of 10 top ranked retrieved images have the same pathology as the query image. Figure 6 shows two retrieval results for pathology cases: top – blood, bottom – infarct.

4 Conclusion and Future Work

In this work, we have demonstrated quantitatively the discriminating power of the statistical measurements of human brain asymmetry. One novelty of our approach in comparison to others in the medical image retrieval domain is to let the computer learn an image similarity metric suited for the given image semantics, instead of imposing such a metric by a human system designer subjectively. The main computational tools used in our study include memory based learning, Bayesian classification, and an effective search engine Vizier [14]. We have extended the basic framework of semantic-based image retrieval to image datasets other than pathology neuroimages, for example, multispectrum biology images [10].

Future work includes the study of a more comprehensive feature set, different weighted feature subsets for different query contents, and dynamic switching

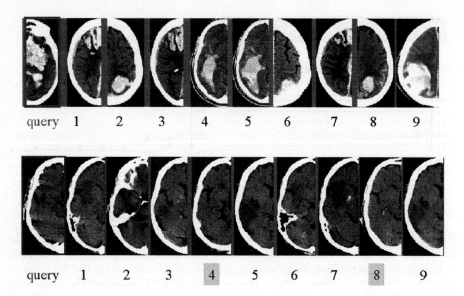

Fig. 6. Top left most: query image with acute blood, bottom left most: query image with bland infarct. The first nine retrieved half slices follow, from left to right in descending order of similarity. The pathologies on the top row retrieved images are all acute blood. The pathologies on the bottom row retrieved images are: infarct, infarct, infarct, normal, infarct, infarct, infarct, normal, infarct.

among them according to user feedback. We would also like to combine image features with collateral information such as age, gender and medical history of the patient to obtain a better retrieval rate. The basic framework presented here has provided us with such an *information fusion* capability.

References

1. C. M. Bishop. *Neural Networks for Pattern Recognition.* Clarendon Press, 1995. ISBN:0198538499.
2. C. Davatzikos, M. Vaillant, S. Resnick, J.L. Prince, S. Letovsky, and R.N. Bryan. A computerized approach for morphological analysis of the corpus callosum. *Comp. Ass. Tomography.*, 20:88–97, Jan./Feb. 1996.
3. L. Devroye, L. Györfi, and G. Lugosi. *A Probabilistic Theory of Pattern Recognition.* Springer-Verlag, London, Paris, Tokyo, 1997.
4. R.O. Duda, P.E. Hart, and D.G. Stork. *Pattern Classification.* John Wiley & Sons, New York, 2001.
5. J.S. Duncan and N. Ayache. Medical image analysis: Progress over two decades and the challenges ahead. *IEEE Transactions on Pattern Analysis and Machine Intelligence*, 22(1):85,106, 2000.
6. D. Faloutsos, R. Barber, M. Flickner, J. Hafner, W. Niblack, D. Petkovic, and W. Equitz. Efficient and effective querying by image content. *Journal of Intelligent Information Systems*, 1994.

7. R. Guillemaud, M. Sakuma, P. Marais, J. Feldmar, R. Crow, L. DeLisi, A. Zisserman, and M. Brady. Cerebral symmetry analysis from mri scans. *Submitted to Psychiatry Research Neuroimaging*, 1998.
8. D. L. G. Hill, P.G. Batchelor, M. Holden, and D. J. Hawkes. Medical image registration. *Physics in Medicine and Biology*, 46:1–45, 2001.
9. Y. Liu, R.T. Collins, and W.E. Rothfus. Robust Midsagittal Plane Extraction from Normal and Pathological 3D Neuroradiology Images. *IEEE Transactions on Medical Imaging*, 20(3), March 2001.
10. Y. Liu, T. Zhao, E.S. Wachman, D.L. Farkas, and T. Kanade. Learning discriminant features in multispectrual biological images. In *Mathematical Methods in Biomedical Image Analysis*. submitted, 2001.
11. F. Maes, A. Collignon, D. Vandermeulun, G. Marchal, and P. Suetens. Multimodality image registration by maximization of mutual information. *IEEE Transactions on Medical Imaging*, 16(2):187,198, 1997.
12. A. W. Moore, D. J. Hill, and M. P. Johnson. An Empirical Investigation of Brute Force to choose Features, Smoothers and Function Approximators. In S. Hanson, S. Judd, and T. Petsche, editors, *Computational Learning Theory and Natural Learning Systems, Volume 3*. MIT Press, 1994.
13. A. Pentland, R.W. Picard, and S. Sclaroff. Photobook: Content-based manipulation of image databases. *IJCV*, 18(3):233–254, June 1996.
14. J. Schneider and A.W. Moore. A locally weighted learning tutorial using vizier 1.0. *tech. report CMU-RI-TR-00-18, Robotics Institute, Carnegie Mellon*, 1997.
15. P.M. Thompson, C. Schwartz, and A.W. Toga. High-resolution random mesh algorithms for creating a probabilistic 3d surface atlas of the human brain. *Neuroimage*, 3(1):19–34, Feb 1996.
16. J. West, M. Fitzpatrick, and et al. Comparison and evaluation of retrospective intermodality brain image registration techniques. *Journal of Computer Assisted Tomography*, 21:554–566, July/August 1997.
17. W. Zhang, S. Sclaroff, S. Dickinson, J. Feldman, and S. Dunn. Shape-based indexing in a medical image database. *Workshop on Biomedical Image Analysis*, pages 221–230, June 1998.

Classification of SPECT Images of Normal Subjects versus Images of Alzheimer's Disease Patients

Jonathan Stoeckel[1], Grégoire Malandain[1], Octave Migneco[2,3],
Pierre Malick Koulibaly[3], Philippe Robert[4], Nicholas Ayache[1], and
Jacques Darcourt[2,3]

[1] EPIDAURE - Project, INRIA,
2004 route des Lucioles - 06 902 Sophia Antipolis, France
{Jonathan.Stoeckel,Gregoire.Malandain,Nicholas.Ayache}@sophia.inria.fr
http://www-sop.inria.fr/epidaure/
[2] Service de Médecine Nucléaire - Centre Antoine Lacassagne
33 avenue de Valombrose - 06 189 NICE cedex 2, France
[3] Laboratoire de Biophysique - Facult de Mdecine
28 avenue de Valombrose - 06 107 NICE cedex 2, France
[4] Service de Psychiatrie - CHU Pasteur
30, voie Romaine, B.P 69 - 06 000 NICE cedex, France

Abstract. This work aims at providing a tool to assist the interpretation of SPECT images for the diagnosis of Alzheimer's Disease (AD). Our approach is to test classifiers, which uses the intensity values of the images, without any prior information. Such a classifier is built upon a training set, containing images with two different labels (AD patients and normal subjects). It will then provide a classification for any new unknown image. The main problem to be handled is the small number of available images compared to the large number of features (here the image's voxels): the so-called *small sample size* problem. We evaluate here the ability of two linear classifiers to correctly label a set of 79 images. Our experiments show promising results. They also show that image classification based on intensity values only is possible and might be used for other applications as well.

Clinical Context: Alzheimer's Disease

Alzheimer's disease (AD) is a neuro-degenerative disease that produces among others memory loss, behavioural changes and cognitive impairment. Mainly elderly are affected by this disease. Because of the aging populations the number of patients will probably rise in the coming years.

Single photon emission computed tomography (SPECT) is being largely used for the study of cerebral blood flow (CBF). These studies provide unique information for the identification of functional abnormalities relevant to Alzheimer's disease.

The process of diagnosing AD is based on a qualitative evaluation of neuro-psychologic tests, combined with the analysis of SPECT images in case of serious

W. Niessen and M. Viergever (Eds.): MICCAI 2001, LNCS 2208, pp. 666–674, 2001.
© Springer-Verlag Berlin Heidelberg 2001

suspicion. The aim of this work is to provide a tool which will assist the interpretation of these images and, we hope, clarify the ambiguous cases. This is especially important in the early stages of the disease, when the patient can benefit most from drugs that may have an impact on the progression of the disease, and to be able to support the development of such drugs.

1 Introduction

In the recent past a lot of research has been done on comparing *groups* to find the areas where differences exist in the regional cerebral blood flow between groups of AD and normal subjects. These results show on average significant abnormalities in the parietotemporal regions between AD an normal subjects [1]. But these typical patterns do not occur within all patients with probable AD [2]. The majority of these results were obtained using techniques based on statistical parametric mapping (SPM) [3] or on principal component analysis (PCA)/singular value decomposition (SVD) [4,5,6]. However these methods only give us a tool to find significant differences between groups of images. They were not developed to give us information about individual subjects.

However, in this article we will explore the possibility to develop a classifier that can classify a *single* SPECT image as being an image of a normal subject or of a probable Alzheimer patient. As described in the previous section, defining clear features on which a classification can be based is extremely hard. Therefore we choose not to use any prior knowledge about AD in SPECT images. We directly use the intensity values of the image as input to our classifier.

Yet, the number of available images to train such a classifier compared to the number of voxels in the image is very small. This most often leads to very poor classification performance. It is called the *small sample size* problem (see section 2.2) in the pattern recognition literature [7].

In this article we will present and test two classifiers that are able to circumvent the small sample size problem. Herewith we will show that it is possible to classify 3D images only using the intensity values. In our particular case this provides us with a valuable tool for assisting the interpretation of SPECT images for Alzheimer's Disease diagnosis.

In the following section we first introduce the notations used throughout this article and introduce briefly the concept of classification. This is followed by a description and analysis of the small sample size problem (section 2.2). In section 2.3 two classifiers well adapted to our problem are presented.

Results based on the data described in section 3.1 are shown in section 3.3. Finally we discuss our approach and give some directions for further research.

2 Methods

2.1 Classifiers

As pointed out in the introduction, we are looking for a classifier that will assign one of the two possible class labels (AD or normal) to an image given as an input. This can be written as a function $g(x)$, which returns a positive value for one class and a negative value for the other class. x is a feature vector of length n describing the object we want to classify. Our images (objects) are described by simply putting the values of the n voxels in the feature vector. The objects can thus be seen as points in $\mathbb{R}^n$ (the feature space), and $g(x)$ as implicitly defining a surface in $\mathbb{R}^n$ discriminating the two classes.

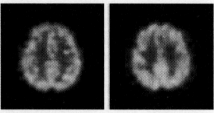

Fig. 1. *Example of a normal (left) and an AD (right) image shows the difficulty of visual interpretation.*

To define this surface a classifier needs to be trained. The training method is provided with a training set consisting of m example objects and their class labels. Once the classifier has been trained, it can be tested by comparing its results on a test set with the known labels of each object of this set. To make an unbiased estimation of the error rate of the classifier, the test set and the training set should be totally independent. In the ideal case, both sets are created by taking randomly objects out of the N objects with known class labels which form the total available object population. As might be expected the accuracy of the classification error depends not only on the independence of the test set but also on its size.

A classifier is said to have a good generalisation capability if it performs well on previously unknown objects. In this case, it does not model the noise of the learning set but the real structure of the data with respect to the class differences.

In practice the number of available objects is often too small to select large enough independent training *and* test sets. A number of alternative methods have been proposed for estimating the classification error [8]. The most well known method is the *re-substitution* method: both the training set and the test set contain exactly the same objects and this method is therefore optimistically biased. This measure does not say anything at all about the generalisation capabilities of a classifier. In this work, we will use the *leave one out* error estimate as described in section 3.2.

2.2   Small Sample Size Problem

Until recently it was believed that for classifiers trained with a number of training objects m smaller or around the dimensionality n of the feature space, no generalisation capability could be expected. This was based on the idea that the feature space needs to be *well filled* (curse of dimensionality). It principally came from the statistical point of view of needing many samples for being able to get good distribution estimates (see preface of [9]).

Logically it would seem that adding features to objects, and thus having relatively more information for classification of the objects, should lead to better results. The fact that it is often not the case, therefore leading to the small sample size problem, might be explained by the idea that a higher dimensional feature space provides a classifier with more degrees of freedom, which can then exactly model the training set. In this case, it does mainly model the objects of the learning set and its associated noise but not the real structure of the data.

One way to solve the small sample size problem is to reduce the number of features. On the contrary, modern approaches, that are aimed at finding the inherent structure of the data instead of the parameters of an a-priori distribution, seem to be able to overcome the small sample size problem. An excellent overview of this problem and several related classifiers are found in [7]. Some classifiers which are proposed in the literature are the nearest mean classifior (NMC) [10], several variants of the Fisher Linear Discriminant (FLD) [11,12], and even highly nonlinear classifiers like the Parzen classifier [13] or the Support Vector Classifier (SVC) [9].

2.3 Nearest Mean Classifier (NMC) and Pseudo Fisher Linear Discriminant (PFLD)

Because of the extremely high number of features compared to the number of available objects we chose to use classifiers with a low complexity. This leads to linear discriminant classifiers, in other words classifiers defining one single hyperplane in feature space which separates the two classes. The most basic approach is the nearest mean classifier (NMC), it classifies the object to the nearest class mean:

$$g_{\mathrm{NMC}}(x) = \left(x - \bar{x}^{(2)}\right)^T \left(x - \bar{x}^{(2)}\right) - \left(x - \bar{x}^{(1)}\right)^T \left(x - \bar{x}^{(1)}\right) \qquad (1)$$

where x is the object to be classified, $\bar{x}^{(1)}$ and $\bar{x}^{(2)}$ are the means of the feature vectors in the training set for the classes one and two respectively. It spans up an equidistant hyperplane between both class means.

The probably most used classification rule is the Fisher Linear Discriminant (FLD), it not only takes the class means into account but also the sample covariance S (assumed to be common to both classes):

$$g_{\mathrm{FLD}}(x) = \left[x - \frac{1}{2}\left(\bar{x}^{(1)} + \bar{x}^{(2)}\right)\right]^T S^{-1} \left(\bar{x}^{(1)} - \bar{x}^{(2)}\right) \qquad (2)$$

Please note that the NMC is a special case of the FLD, when S is the identity matrix the two classifiers are equivalent (Eq.(1)=Eq.(2) when $S = \lambda I$).

When the number of training samples is smaller than the number of features ($m < n$) the covariance matrix yields a singular matrix that cannot be inverted. The Pseudo Fisher Linear Discriminant (PFLD) [11] is formed by replacing the inverse of the covariance matrix by its pseudo inverse, $(S^T S)^{-1} S^T$. The pseudo inverse relies on the singular value decomposition of S and it becomes equal to the inverse of S when $m \geq n$. In this case, the PFLD is equivalent to the FLD.

Even though the FLD is seen in the classical way as designed for two multivariate Gaussian populations with equal prior probabilities differing in mean vectors, but sharing the same covariance matrix, the PFLD has also a more general geometric interpretation [14]. It defines a hyper-plane that maximises the distances to all given training objects. If $m < n$ all the training objects are in a linear subspace, and the discriminant is perpendicular to that subspace. This makes sense as it corresponds with an indifference to directions for which no training objects are given.

The PFLD is known to have very bad generalisation capabilities when $m \approx n$ [11]. In this application, we assume this problem will not play a role because we have $m \ll n$.

2.4 Preprocessing

This section describes the necessary pre-processing steps before using the images as input to a classifier: the two first points consists in spatial and intensity normalisation, while the third one is only necessary from a computational point of view.

Spatial Normalisation: Registration Due to different positions of the subjects in the scanner as well as differences of brain size and morphology between subjects, the same voxel location in two images may not correspond to the same anatomical position. Therefore image registration is necessary. Because global intensity variations exist (see below) a robust approach is needed. We searched for the affine transformations which maximise the correlation coefficient [15] using Powell's optimisation method. We have also tested a non-rigid [16] approach, but this did not improve classifier performance.

Intensity Normalisation A basic problem in the use of SPECT HMPAO images is the lack of an absolute signal level. There are several sources of variation of the measures signal among SPECT images. *Global* variations: they may be caused by differences in the dose of the radioactive tracer being present at the time of the image acquisition, scanner sensitivity, or the positioning of the patient with respect to the detectors. *Local* variations: differences occur normally between different subjects as well as within the same subject over time. Of course pathologies as AD do cause differences as well. Before analysis of the images global variations have to be corrected whereas local variations, especially those due to a pathology, should be preserved. The standard approach is to assume the global CBF to be the same for all subjects. This leads to simply dividing the intensities by the sum of the intensities in the brain. This approach is not very robust in the case of strong local variations. Saxena [17] proposed to divide by the mean of the top one percent intensities. Here, the assumption is that the voxels with the highest intensities (denoting highest levels of perfusion) would be in those areas that are relatively unaffected by AD. In our application choosing either one of these two methods did not influence the classification results.

Subsampling by Mean Filtering All images were subsampled by a certain factor in each dimension by simply taking the mean of the implicated voxels. This was done for the following reasons: firstly to obtain acceptable memory and calculation time requirements; secondly to eliminate noise and compensate for eventual registration imprecision. Misregistration can lead to two voxels at the same position for different subjects not to represent exactly the same anatomical position; this effect may be suppressed by the averaging of the voxels. Of course only the image voxels being part of the brain were used for the classification.

3   Results

3.1   Materials

A set of 29 images of probable AD patients (mean Mini Mental Test score 23.5), with clinically confirmed diagnosis were acquired as well as a set of 50 images of normal subjects. This last set of images was made available by The Society of Nuclear Medicine Brain Imaging Council (http://brainscans.med.yale.edu/). The rCBF was assessed with technetium-99m-D L-hexamethyl-propylene amine oxime (Tc-99m HMPAO), a tracer that is trapped inside the brain in proportion to the regional blood flow. All images were acquired using triple-head camera systems (Picker Prism 3000 series). The cameras were equipped with fan beam collimators.

Raw projection images were acquired in a 128×128 matrix. They were reconstructed using a ramp filter and the resulting slices post-filtered using a low-pass filter (Butterworth, order=6, cutoff=0.26). Chang attenuation correction [18] (cutoff=0.07) was applied to the filtered data. After registration and reslicing all images had 1.8 mm cubic voxels and 93 axial slices.

3.2   Leave One Out Method

A widely used classification error estimate when the number of objects is very small, is the *leave one out* method [8]. In this method all N available objects are used. The classifier is trained N times on a training set of $m = N - 1$ objects leaving out a different object each time. This object is used to test the classifier. This provides us with an unbiased error estimate if the observations of the objects are statistically independent.

3.3   Experiments

Table 1 show results using the 79 images described in section 3.1. The success rates were calculated using the leave one out method (see previous section). Note, that due to roundoff effects when selecting the voxels being part of the brain, the number of resulting features 4819 and 618 are not exactly 8 times more between subsampling factors 4 and 8. The results show a little improvement when using more features, probably some information is lost by too much subsampling. The

Table 1. Percentages of successfully classified images obtained using the leave one out method. Results are shown for all 79 images and for the two classes individually (AD = Alzheimer's Disease, NO = normal). Both the NMC and PFLD were tested for subsampling factors 4 and 8, corresponding respectively to 4819 and 618 features (i.e. voxels).

subsampling factor	NMC			PFLD		
	Total	AD	NO	Total	AD	NO
4	84.8%	79.3%	88.0%	89.9%	82.8%	94.0%
8	81.0%	72.4%	86.0%	88.6%	82.8%	92.0%

PFLD outperforms the NMC, this can be explained by the fact that it also takes the covariance into account, and thus the shape of the classes in feature space. The differences in success rates between normal and AD images might be explained by the presence of nearly two times more normal images than AD images. We also investigated if using less training objects would increase the performance of the PFLD. This was not the case and shows the assumption made (number of features is sufficently different from the number of training images) at the end of section 2.3 to hold for our data. Please note that four highly experimented observers, who were presented the 29 AD images amidst other images, classified on average only 66.4% of the AD images correctly (PFLD and subsampling factor 4 resulted in 82.8% for AD images, see table 1).

4   Discussion and Conclusion

In this article, we have presented a general framework for using classifiers directly on 3D volumetric images without using prior knowledge based on recent findings in the pattern recognition literature for the small sample size problem. Promising results for use in AD were shown in the previous section, especially when considering the difficulty human observers have in classifying this type of images. Of course feature extraction (e.g. symmetry features, texture features) may improve the results. But we have shown it feasible to do without. Our further research will explore the possibilities for feature extraction as well as using other well behaving classifiers in the small sample size problem. Another important point will be to compare the performance of our classifiers to that of human observers who do normally analyse this type of images. A classifier that not only gives a binary result but also a rating which indicates a degree of class-membership might provide an even more useful tool. It is important to notice that this type of classification methods could be applied to a lot of different applications in medical imaging. They can help to solve the problems related to the often complex diagnosis making in 3D volumetric images.

5   Acknowledgements

We would like to thank P. Cachier and A. Roche for fruitful discussions, and R.P.W. Duin for making PrTools [19] available. This work was partially supported by the Conseil Régional Provences-Alpes-Côte d'Azur and by a grant from the European Community *SPECT in Dementia BIOMED2*.

References

1. Jagust W.J. Functional imaging patterns in Alzheimer's disease. *Annals of the New York Academy of Sciences*, 777:30-36, 1996.
2. Nitrini R., Buchpiguel C.A., Caramelli P., Bahia V.S., Mathias S.C., Nascimento C.M.R., Degenszajn J., and Caixeta L. SPECT in Alzheimer's disease: features associated with bilateral parietotemporal hypoperfusion. *Acta Neurologica Scandinavica*, 101:172-176, 2000.
3. Frackowiak R.S.J., Friston K.J., Frith C.D., and Dolan R. *Human Brain Function*. Academic Press, 1997.
4. Jones K., Johnson K.A., Becker J.A., Spiers P.A., Albert M.S., and Holman B.L. Use of singular value decomposition to characterize age and gender differences in SPECT cerebral perfusion. *Journal of Nuclear Medicine*, 39:965-973, 1998.
5. Houston A.S., Kemp P.M., and Macleod M.A. A method for asseing the significance of abnormalities in HMPAO brain spect images. *Journal of Nuclear Medicine*, 35:239-244, 1994.
6. Johnson K.A., Jones K., Holman B.L, Becker J.A., Spiers P.A., Satlin A., and Albert M.S. Preclinical prediction of Alzheimer's disease using SPECT. *Neurology*, 50:1563-1571, 1998.
7. Duin R.P.W. Classifiers in almost empty spaces. In *Proceedings of the 15th International Conference on Pattern Recognition (ICPR2000), Vol. 2*, pages 1-7, Las Alamitos (CA), 2000. IAPR, IEEE Computer Society.
8. Raudys S.J. and Jain A.K. Small sample size effects in statistical pattern recognition: Recommendations for practitioners. *IEEE Transactions on Pattern Recognition and Machine Intelligence*, 13(3):252-264, March 1991.
9. Vapnik V.N. *Statistical learning theory*. John Wiley & Sons, 1998.
10. Skurichina M. and Duin R.P.W. Stabilizing classifiers for very small sample sizes. In *Proceedings of the 13th International Conference on Pattern Recognition (ICPR1996), Vol. 2*, pages 891-896. IAPR, IEEE Computer Society, 1996.
11. Raudys S.J. and Duin R.P.W. Expected classification error of the Fisher linear classifier with pseudo-inverse covariance matrix. *Pattern Recognition Letters*, 19:385-392, 1998.
12. Chen L.F., Liao H.Y.M., Ko M.T., Lin J.C., and Yu G.J. A new LDA-based face recognition which can solve the small sample size problem. *Pattern Recognition*, 33:1713-1726, 2000.
13. Hamamoto Y., Fujimoto Y., and Tomita S. On the estimation of a covariance matrix in designing Parzen classifiers. *Pattern Recognition*, 29(10):1751-1759, 1996.
14. Duin R.P.W. Small Sample Size Generalization. In *Proceedings of the 9th Scandinavian Conference on Image Analysis (SCIA95)*, pages 957-964, 1995.
15. Roche A., Malandain G., and Ayache N. Unifying Maximum Likelihood Approaches in Medical Image Registration. *International Journal of Imaging Systems and Technology*, 11:71-80, 2000.

16. P. Cachier and X. Pennec. 3D Non-Rigid Registration by Gradient Descent on a Gaussian-Windowed Similarity Measure using Convolutions. In *Proc. of MM-BIA'00*, pages 182-189, Hilton Head Island, USA, June 2000.
17. Saxena P., Pavel D.G., Quintana J.C., and Horwitz B. An automatic threshold-based scaling method for enhancing the usefulness of Tc-HMPAO SPECT in the diagnosis of Alzheimer's disease. In *Proceedings of the 1st international conference on Medical Imaging Computing and Computer-Assisted Intervention (MICCAI'98)*, volume 1496 of *Lecture Notes in Computer Science*, pages 623-630. Springer, 1996.
18. Chang L.T. A method for attenuation correction in radionuclide computed tomography. *IEEE Transactions on Nuclear Science*, 25:638643, 1978.
19. Duin R.P.W. *PRTools 3.1, A Matlab Toolbox for Pattern Recognition*. Delft University of Technology, Januray 2000.

Technologies for Augmented Reality: Calibration for Real-Time Superimposition on Rigid and Simple-Deformable Real Objects

Yann Argotti[1], Valerie Outters[2], Larry Davis[1], Ami Sun[2], and
Jannick P. Rolland[1,2]

[1] School of Electrical Engineering and Computer Science
[2] School of Optics
University of Central Florida
4000 Central Florida Boulevard
Orlando, Florida 32816-2700, USA
jannick@odalab.ucf.edu

Abstract. A current challenge in augmented reality applications is the
ability to superimpose synthetic objects on real objects within the environment. This challenge is heightened when the real objects are in motion and/or are non-rigid. Yet even more challenging is the case when the
moving real objects involved are deformable. In this article, we present a
robust method for calibrating marker-based augmented reality applications to allow real-time, optical superimposition of synthetic objects on
dynamic rigid and simple-deformable real objects. Moreover, we illustrate
this general method with the VRDA Tool, a medical education application related to the visualization of internal human knee joint anatomy
on a real human knee.

1 Introduction

In a large range of fields, the ability to enhance reality with synthetic information is an exciting alternative to traditional methods of acquiring information.
Applications where computer-generated objects are employed to augment user
perception of the real environment are referred to as augmented reality (AR)
applications.

A current challenge in AR applications is the ability to superimpose synthetic
objects on real objects within the environment. To overcome this challenge,
objects in the environment must be accurately tracked and the relationships
between real and synthetic objects must be precisely determined. When dealing
with medical AR applications, the real and synthetic objects in the environment
are often human anatomical structures.

Accurately tracking human motion is a difficult task. However, there have
been attempts to understand and quantify human motion. Spoor and Veldpaus
published a method for calculating rigid body motion from the spatial coordinates of markers that has been adapted to tracking skeletal motion [13]. In

W. Niessen and M. Viergever (Eds.): MICCAI 2001, LNCS 2208, pp. 675–682, 2001.
© Springer-Verlag Berlin Heidelberg 2001

addition, techniques have been devised that address the problems associated with accurately tracking anatomical motion [1][6][12]. In fact, much is known about the motion of anatomical structures, but they still pose a significant challenge to inclusion within AR systems. Aside from the fact that markers cannot be directly positioned on bones in daily settings, anatomical structures are not rigid. Moreover, attempting to track anatomical structures at interactive speed while maintaining registration of synthetic objects is especially challenging.

Thus, as a contribution to the body of virtual environment research, we examine the problem of tracking simple-deformable bodies within an AR application and present a general method for calibrating marker-based AR systems, which may result in accurate dynamic superimposition of synthetic objects on real objects at interactive speeds. In the following paragraphs, we present a marker-based calibration method for AR applications. In conjunction with a dynamic superimposition method found in [2], the method is applied to the Virtual Reality Dynamic Anatomy (VRDA) Tool, a visualization system developed for the study of complex anatomical joint motions [14].

2   Calibration Process

In the calibration process, the AR system is prepared for accurate superimposition. This includes computing the local coordinate system, or local frame of reference, for each real object in the environment, determining the transformations between real objects and their respective synthetic counterparts, and characterizing the stereoscopic display device. We treat the tracker coordinate system as the global frame of reference, or frame for short. In addition, we define simple-deformable objects as objects that are slightly changing in shape compared to an equivalent rigid object, which we show can be quantified by the change in the eigenvalues of the dispersion matrix associated with a cluster of markers.

2.1   Computing Local Frames for Real Objects

To determine the location and orientation of a real object, we choose to adopt a marker-based method because it offers a more accurate way to determine the position and orientation of real objects. Each real object is defined by a set of markers placed on its surface. Whatever type of marker-based tracking system is selected, we assume the system can provide the three-dimensional (3D) location of each marker in its frame of reference. However, this information is not sufficient to link real and synthetic objects; each marker location must be computed in a local frame defined for each real object.

For a rigid object, we compute the fixed marker locations in the local frame. Similarly, in the case of a simple-deformable object, we first make the assumption that the markers do not move significantly during the calibration phase. The relative motion of each marker in its local frame will be assessed in a later step and accounted for. In both scenarios, we can establish a local coordinate frame using eigenvalues and eigenvectors obtained from the locations of the markers on the object [1][6]. For rigid objects, the eigenvalues of a matrix characterizing the marker distribution are invariant, even though its eigenvectors vary according to the position and orientation of the object in the global frame or any other frame. This extends to simple-deformable objects under the previous assumption.

Thus, we take advantage of this invariance property to build a local marker frame, defined with the eigenvectors of a matrix that characterizes the marker set. A matrix that meets this criterion is the dispersion matrix, which is a form of the spatial covariance matrix over the marker distribution. We denote the coordinates of the centroid of the marker distribution y, the total number of markers n, and the coordinates of the ith marker in the global frame y_i. We also define $y'_i = y_i - y, i \in [1; n]$. Thus, the 3 x 3 symmetrical dispersion matrix, K, is given by

$$K = \sum_{i=1}^{n} y'_i y'_i{}^T .$$ (1)

We define the local frame as the eigenvectors of K, which will allow direct computation of the required transformation for the local frame to the global frame as now detailed. To determine the eigenvectors, we first diagonalize K, given that K is real and symmetric. The diagonalized K can be written as

$$diag(k_1, k_2, k_3) = V^{-1} K V$$ (2)

where k_1, k_2, and k_3 are the eigenvalues of K and V is the matrix of eigenvectors. Provided that V has an inverse, the relationship described in (2) is a similarity transform. An important property of similarity transforms is that eigenvalues are preserved, meaning K and its diagonalized version can be related to one another using an eigenvector basis. In this case, V is the eigenvector basis between K and its diagonalized version. The frame where K is diagonal is unique. We then sort the eigenvalues such that $k_1 > k_2 > k_3 > 0$ and recompute K using (2). V is the orthonormal matrix that transforms the frame where K is diagonal to the frame where K was first computed, meaning that V is the transformation from the local frame to the global frame. In addition, the inverse of V is equal to its transpose because V is an orthonormal matrix. Thus, we can express the local coordinates, $x_i, i \in [1; n]$, of the markers in a frame whose origin is the centroid, y, of the marker set and whose axes are given by the eigenvectors of the matrix K, with the relationship expressed as

$$x_i = V^T y'_i, \ i \in [i; n] .$$ (3)

The process previously described is valid when the tracking system detects all the markers on an object simultaneously. However, all the object markers may not be visible simultaneously, a situation that occurs when tracking systems are subject to occlusion.

We now present an extension of the method to compute the local coordinates of all markers, whether simultaneously visible or not. First, a local frame is built from the coordinates of the visible markers. At least three markers must be first detected. Then, the transformation from the local frame to the global frame, V, is determined. Once V is computed with a limited number of visible markers, we determine the coordinates of all the visible markers in the local frame, which we refer to as a partial local frame.

Next, the real object is slowly rotated. This allows previously undetected makers to be detected with at least three markers that were previously detected. We call these previously undetected markers, new markers, and the markers that were detected previously, old markers. When the new markers are detected, the rotation matrix, R_{ro_o}, and translation vector, T_{ro_o}, from a partial local frame to the global frame are calculated. A scaling transformation is unnecessary at this stage because we are using normalized coordinate systems.

The technique used for finding the rotation matrix and translation vector is Singular-Value Decomposition (SVD) [4]. We chose this method because it is a robust optimization method that always gives a solution, and, moreover, it is the best solution by projection on the solution space. The computation of the rotation matrix and translation vector, as well as a modification to the SVD method to account for hidden markers and simple-deformable objects, can be found in [2]. The inputs to the SVD are the computed marker coordinates x_i in the local frame and the measured marker coordinates y_i in the global frame. After the rotation matrix R_{ro_o} and the translation vector T_{ro_o}, are determined from the optimization procedure, we compute the local coordinates of the new markers in the current local frame as

$$x_i = R_{ro\_o}{}^T \left(y_i' - T_{ro\_o} \right) \ . \tag{4}$$

Finally, with all the new and old markers expressed in the current local coordinate system, we again compute the dispersion matrix and eigenvalues (see equations 1–3) to find an estimate of the new local frame and then compute the new local coordinates of the markers. We repeat this process as the real object is rotated until all the markers have been visible. This technique allows us to build a local frame for any kind of marker set and quickly calculate the local coordinates of the markers.

2.2   Determining Transformations Between Synthetic and Real Objects

After computing the local frames of real objects, we then associate the synthetic representation of an object to its corresponding real object. To link a real object and its synthetic representation, the transformation matrix from the synthetic object frame to the real object frame is computed. Because the definition of a synthetic object frame can be arbitrary, extra data must be provided to build the transformation matrix. To supply the additional information needed, landmarks are defined. These landmarks are corresponding points of significance on the real and synthetic objects. By utilizing landmarks and decomposing the transformation matrix to a rotation, scaling, and translation component, we can specify a relationship between the real and synthetic worlds as $y = RSx + T$.

We shall describe how we first solve for the scaling, S, due to the possibility of system noise and/or measurement errors distorting the size of the objects, and apply it to the entire synthetic object. Then, the rotation, R, and translation, T, are computed using a modified SVD method, with the real and synthetic landmark coordinates as input. The solution of R and T is detailed in [2].

Solving for S consists of computing the mean scaling, S_{mean}, for all the landmarks and deciding if uniform scaling by S_{mean} is appropriate. The mean scaling is determined by calculating the ratio of the distance between two landmarks in the real object frame and the distance between two landmarks in the synthetic object frame for all two- landmark combinations. The ratios are summed for each corresponding pair of landmarks and averaged as

$$S_{mean} = \frac{\sum_{i=1}^{n-1} \sum_{j=i+1}^{n} \left(\frac{d(y_i, y_j)}{d(x_i, x_j)} \right)}{C_2^n}, i \neq j \qquad (5)$$

where, y_i is the ith landmark in the real object frame, x_i is the corresponding i^{th} landmark in the synthetic object frame, and n is the total number of landmarks. It is important to note that the equation for finding the mean scaling is independent of any rotation and translation transformation of the landmarks. We also compute the standard deviation of the mean scaling, S_{sd}. If the value of S_{sd} is under a particular threshold level, the variations in scale are small enough to conclude that the scaling is uniform in three dimensions. The calculation of the threshold level is explained in [3]. If uniform scaling is sufficient, then $S = S_{mean} \cdot I$, where I is the identity matrix. If uniform scaling is insufficient, then scale parameters must be computed for the x, y, and z directions, respectively.

2.3 Characterizing the Display Device

The goal in characterizing the stereoscopic display device is to determine the correct viewpoint locations for each eye, the field of view of the optics, as well as account for optical distortions in order to correctly display synthetic objects. The stereo display device for AR applications is typically a Head-Mounted Display (HMD), of which there are three types: optical see-through, video see-through, and projective [9][7]. The display configuration is fixed and markers are placed upon the HMD to compute the changing location and orientation of the head of the user.

The choice of the local frame for the head of the user is not arbitrary. We set the head frame origin, O_h, at the middle of the line segment between the eyes of the user. The x-axis of the head frame, X_h, is along the segment, with +x oriented toward the right eye of the user. The y-axis, Y_h, is oriented along the line segment perpendicular to X_h , with +y oriented in the direction of the view of the user. Finally, the z- axis, Z_h, is obtained from X_h and Y_h with a cross product: $Z_h = X_h \times Y_h$.

To create a stereoscopic view, we must also define a transformation to the points from which the scene is rendered, referred to as the eyepoints. The choice of eyepoint location is important in minimizing depth perception errors [10]. The location of the eyepoints can be calculated as a translation from O_h of half of the inter-pupilary distance (IPD) along the X_h axis in the +x and -x directions (right and left eye, respectively). Thus, the transformations from the head frame to the left and right eyepoints are a translation of $-IPD/2$ and $IPD/2$, respectively. In addition to transformation matrices, we also define a perspective transform for each eye based upon the display device field of view [8].

Display devices with large fields of view are subject to optical distortion. This distortion is a warping of the image that can be calculated and then corrected optically, electronically, or within the rendering software. Optical correction and electronic correction may not be feasible for a given display device. Thus, we quantify the optical distortion within a system using either a theoretical model or a metrology approach and correct for it within the rendering process [8].

3   An Application: Dynamic Superimposition of a Knee Joint on a Patient Leg

When combined with the dynamic superimposition method found in [2], the calibration method described is well suited for implementation in complex AR systems. The Virtual Reality Dynamic Anatomy (VRDA) Tool is a system that allows medical practitioners to visualize anatomical structures superimposed on their real counterparts. To realize this effect, the medical practitioner wears a HMD to view a computer graphics model of the knee superimposed on the real leg of a model patient. In the following paragraphs, we demonstrate how the method is integrated within the VRDA Tool.

We treat the leg as two separate objects; the first object is associated with the thigh and the second object is associated with the shank. Each part of the leg is tracked independently. To find the best location of the markers, we considered the shape of the leg and chose the marker locations where they would probably move the least [6]. We defined the landmarks in places where there is less flesh, allowing the landmarks to be closer to the bones to reduce scaling or location errors. The landmark locations are shown in Fig 1. To avoid collisions between the synthetic objects, we refer to a precomputed look-up table that encodes the correct location of the femur relative to the tibia [5]. The entry to the table is the transformation between the two synthetic objects. The table returns the real-time location of the objects, allowing smooth, realistic motion without collisions.

We also evaluated the scaling threshold to determine if uniform or non-uniform scaling between real objects and synthetic objects is appropriate. To determine the relative motion of the markers on the leg, we made 1000 measurements of the global 3D location of the markers over a 10 second interval of standard motion for the leg. We found that the maximum standard deviation of the motion of markers is less than 15 mm. The tracking system is accurate to within 0.1 mm.

For the eyepoints, we chose the center of rotation of the eye because rendering is applied in near field visualization [11]. The field of view of the HMD is 26.11 degrees and the display resolution is 640 x 480 pixels. We also applied a coating to the LCD displays to minimize the pixelization of our synthetic objects.

The 3D models that represent the knee joint anatomy are high-resolution models from Viewpoint Corporation. The tracking system we employ is a NDI OPTOTRAK 3020, which uses active, infrared LEDs as markers. The choice of this system is based upon its resolution, robustness against common perturbations, and speed. The display device is a prototype see-through head mounted display. We perform both computations and stereoscopic rendering a SGI Onyx2. The complete implementation of this method allows superimposition at interactive-speed. We are currently able to achieve stereo frame rates of up to 26.6 Hz. Furthermore, because of the choice of the SVD method and the enhancement of noise attenuation, the superimposition process is robust and accurate.

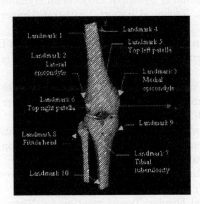

Fig. 1. Landmark locations

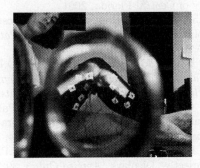

Fig. 2. The dynamic superimposition

4   Future Work

Future work with the VRDA tool will demonstrate deformable structures such as ligaments and muscles with respect to the bones as well. However, such demonstration is not required in quantifying the methods presented here. Furthermore, methods of non-uniform scaling of synthetic objects will be implemented in future developments. This is especially important in working with generic models that must be registered with specific real objects. Applications of augmented reality methods presented here will further be extended to perform full body motion capture.

682   Y. Argotti et al.

5   Acknowledgements

The work is supported by the National Institute of Health under grant 1-R29-LM06322-01A1, the National Science Foundation under grant EIA-99-86051, the Florida Education Fund, and the Lockheed-Martin Aeronautics Company. Videotapes may be requested at jannick@odalab.ucf.edu .

References

[1] T.P. Andriacchi, G. Alexander, M.K. Toney, C. Dyrby, and J. Sum. A Point Cluster Method for In Vivo Motion Analysis: Applied to a Study of Knee Kinematics. *Journal of Biomechanics*, 1999.

[2] Y. Argotti, L. Davis, V. Outters, and J.P. Rolland. Dynamic Superimposition of Synthetic Objects on Rigid and Simple-Deformable Real Objects. In *The Second IEEE and ACM International Symposium on Augmented Reality (ISAR '01), New York, NY*. IEEE Computer Society, IEEE Press, October 2001.

[3] Y. Argotti, V. Outters, L. Davis, A. Sun, and J.P. Rolland. Technologies for Augmented Reality: Real-time Superimposition of Synthetic Objects on Dynamic Rigid and Simple-deformable Real Objects. Technical Report TR01-004, University of Central Florida, 2001.

[4] K.S. Arun, T.S. Huang, and S.D. Blostein. Least-Squares Fitting of Two 3-D Point Sets. *IEEE Transactions on Pattern Analysis and Machine Intelligence*, PAMI-9(5):698–700, 1987.

[5] Y. Baillot, J.P. Rolland, K. Lin, and D.L. Wright. Automatic Modeling of Knee-Joint Motion for the Virtual Reality Dynamic Anatomy (VRDA) Tool. *Presence: Teleoperators and Virtual Environments*, 9(3):223–235, 2000.

[6] A. Cappello, A. Cappozzo, P.F. La Palombara, L. Lucchetti, and A. Leardini. Multiple Anatomical Landmark Calibration for Optimal Bone Pose Estimation. *Human Movement Science*, 16:259–274, 1997.

[7] H. Hua, A. Girardot, C.Y. Gao, and J.P. Rolland. Engineering of Head-Mounted Projective Displays. *Applied Optics*, 39(22):3814–3824, 2000.

[8] W. Robinett and R. Holloway. The Visual Display Transformation for Virtual Reality. *Presence: Teleoperators and Virtual Environments*, 4(1):1–23, 1995.

[9] J.P. Rolland and H. Fuchs. Optical Versus Video See-Through Head-Mounted Displays in Medical Visualization. *Presence: Teleoperators and Virtual Environments*, 9(3):287–309, 2000.

[10] J.P. Rolland, W. Gibson, and D. Ariely. Towards Quantifying Depth and Size Perception in Virtual Environments. *Presence: Teleoperators and Virtual Environments*, 4(1):24–49, 1995.

[11] J.P. Rolland and L. Vaissie. Albertian Errors in Head-Mounted Displays: Choice of Eyepoint Location. Technical Report TR01-001, University of Central Florida, 2001.

[12] I. Söedrkvist and P.Å. Wedin. Determining the Movement of the Skeleton Using Well-Configured Markers. *Journal of Biomechanics*, 26(12):1473–1477, 1993.

[13] C.W. Spoor and F.E. Veldpaus. Technical Note: Rigid Body Motion Calculated from Spatial Coordinates of Markers. *Journal of Biomechanics*, 13:391–393, 1980.

[14] D.L. Wright, J.P. Rolland, and A.R. Kancherla. Using Virtual Reality to Teach Radiographic Positioning. *Radiologic Technology*, 66(4):167–172, 1995.

Magnified Real-Time Tomographic Reflection

George Stetten and Vikram Chib

Department of Bioengineering, University of Pittsburgh,
Robotics Institute, Carnegie Mellon University.
www.stetten.com

Abstract. Real Time Tomographic Reflection (RTTR) permits *in situ* visualization of ultrasound images so that direct hand-eye coordination can be employed during invasive procedures. The method merges the visual outer surface of a patient with a simultaneous ultrasound scan of the patient's interior. It combines a flat-panel monitor with a half-silvered mirror such that the image on the monitor is reflected precisely into the proper location within the patient. The ultrasound image is superimposed in real time on the patient merging with the operator's hands and any invasive tools in the field of view. We aim to extend this method to remote procedures at different scales, in particular to real-time *in vivo* tomographic microscopic imaging modalities such as optical coherence tomography (OCT) and ultrasound backscatter microscopy (USB). This paper reports our first working prototype using a mechanically linked system to magnify ultrasound-guided manipulation by a factor of four.

1   Introduction

In the practice of medicine, the standard method of viewing an image is still to examine it on a film or screen rather than to look directly into the patient. A number of researchers have worked to develop more natural ways to visually merge images with the perceptual real world [1-7]. We have previously reported the concept of *real time tomographic reflection* (RTTR) and applied it successfully to ultrasound [8-11]. Ultrasound produces a *tomographic* slice within the patient representing a set of 3D locations that lie in a plane. The image of that tomographic slice, displayed at its correct size on a flat panel display, may be reflected to occupy the same physical space as the actual slice within the patient. If a half-silvered mirror is used, the patient may be viewed through the mirror with the reflected image of the slice superimposed on the patient, independent of viewer location. The reflected image is truly occupying its correct location within the patient and does not require any particular perspective to be rendered correctly.

To accomplish RTTR, certain geometric relationships must exist between the slice being scanned, the monitor displaying the slice, and the mirror. As shown in Fig. 1, the mirror must bisect the angle between the slice and the monitor. On the monitor, the image must be correctly translated and rotated so that each point in the image is paired with a corresponding point in the slice to define a line segment perpendicular to, and bisected by, the mirror. By fundamental laws of optics, the

W. Niessen and M. Viergever (Eds.): MICCAI 2001, LNCS 2208, pp. 683-690, 2001.

ultrasound image will thus appear at its physical location, independent of viewer position. The actual apparatus we have constructed is sketched in Fig. 2.

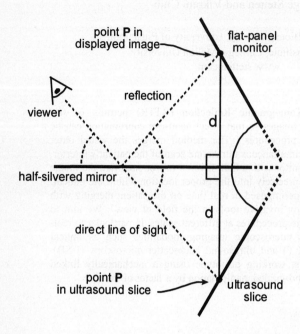

Fig. 1 The half-silvered mirror bisects the angle between the ultrasound slice (within the target) and the flat-panel monitor. Point P in the ultrasound slice and its corresponding location on the monitor are equidistant from the mirror along a line perpendicular to the mirror (distance = d). Because the angle of incidence equals the angle of reflectance (angle = α) the viewer (shown as an eye) sees each point in the reflection precisely at its corresponding physical 3D location.

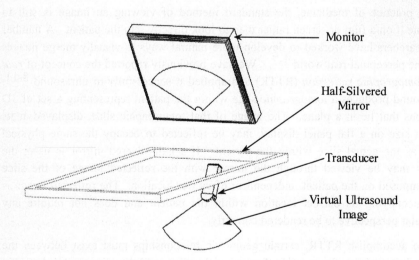

Fig. 2 Schematic representation of the apparatus. A flat-panel monitor and an ultrasound transducer are placed on opposite sides of a half-silvered mirror such that the mirror bisects the angle between them.

Superimposing ultrasound images on human vision using RTTR may improve an operator's ability to find targets while avoiding damage to neighboring structures, while generally facilitating interpretation of ultrasound images by relating them spatially to external anatomy. As such, it holds promise for increasing accuracy, ease, and safety during percutaneous biopsy of suspected tumors, amniocentesis, fetal surgery, brain surgery, insertion of catheters, and many other interventional procedures.

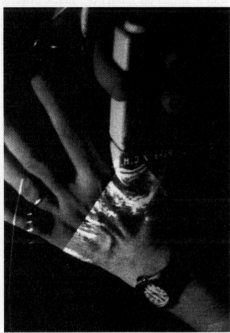

Fig. 3 Photograph, from the viewpoint of the operator, showing a scan of a hand using the apparatus in Fig. 2. The reflected ultrasound image is merged with the direct visual image.

In Fig 3, a human hand is seen with the transducer pressed against the soft tissue between the thumb and index finger. While not a common target for clinical ultrasound, the hand was chosen because it clearly demonstrates successful alignment. The external surfaces of the hand are located consistent with structures within the ultrasound image. The photograph cannot convey the strong sense, derived from stereoscopic vision, that the reflected image is located within the hand. This sense is intensified with head motion because the image remains properly aligned from different viewpoints. To one experiencing the technique in person, ultrasound targets within the hand would clearly be accessible to direct percutaneous injection, biopsy or excision.

2   Ultrasound Magnification Experiment

In the present work we intend to develop systems that provide hand-eye coordination for interventional procedures on patients and research animals *in vivo* at mesoscopic and microscopic scales. A number of other researchers are presently involved in this pursuit [12-14], but none has applied tomographic reflection. We have demonstrated an adaptation of RTTR, described below, in which the target is remote from the display and may be at a different scale. Interventional procedures could be carried out using a robotic linkage between the actual remote effector (such as a micropipette) and a hand-held "mock effector" constructed at a magnified scale.

We envision that real-time *in vivo* tomographic microscopy will be an important application of RTTR. This can be achieved by removing the actual target from the operator's field of view, enabling procedures at different scales and/or remote locations. Interventional procedures could be carried out remotely and at different scales by controlling a remote effector with a scaled-up model or "mock effector" held in the operator's hand. The mock effector would interact spatially in the operator's field of view with the virtual image of a magnified tomographic image from the remote operation.

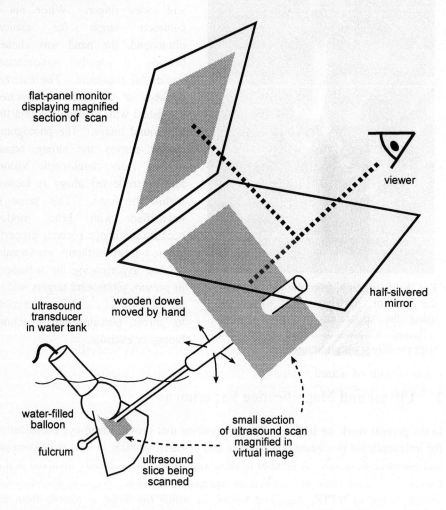

Fig. 4 Apparatus demonstrating magnified RTTR using a lever to control a remote effector at a magnified scale.

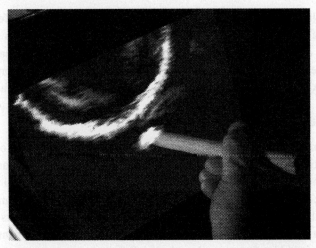

Fig 5 *Mock effector* (3/4" wooden dowel) interacting with the virtual image of a magnified ultrasound scan of the balloon, seen through the half-silvered mirror.

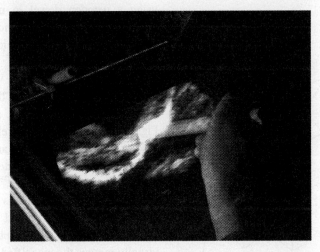

Fig 6 Result of *actual effector* (3/16" dowel) pressing into balloon visualized by merging *mock effector* (3/4" dowel) with virtual image.

This concept has been put into practice using the apparatus shown in Fig. 4, as a proof of concept. Starting with the previous floor-standing apparatus, the ultrasound transducer was removed from the operator's field of view, and a small water-filled balloon placed before the transducer in a water tank. A lever consisting of two sections of wooden dowel, 3/4" and 3/16" in diameter, was attached by the small end to one side of the water tank. The fulcrum was 4 times as far from the virtual image as it was from the actual ultrasound slice. This resulted in a mechanical magnification of four, which matched the magnification between the actual 3/16" effector and the 3/4" "mock effector". The operator held the mock effector, as shown in Fig. 5 and 6, moving it to control the actual effector remotely with two translational degrees of freedom. The small dowel produced an indentation in the balloon visible by ultrasound. A small section of the ultrasound slice was magnified by a factor of 4 and displayed on the flat-panel monitor so that virtual image was reflected to merge visually with the mock effector.

Figs. 5 and 6 show images captured with a camera from the point of view of an operator looking through the half-silvered mirror. The operator's hand is shown holding the mock effector (i.e., the 3/4" end of the dowel). The actual effector (the 3/16" cross-section of the dowel being scanned in the water tank) is magnified to 3/4" in the virtual image and accurately tracks the mock effector as it appears to cause the indentation in the magnified image of the balloon. The extension of the dowel into the water bath is hidden from view by selective lighting.

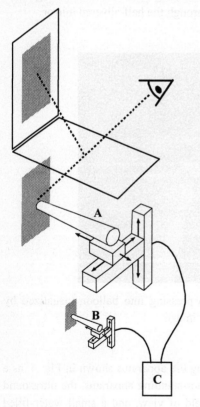

The preliminary work already described has demonstrated remote RTTR using a wooden dowel to mechanically link the actual effector and the mock effector. Clearly, mechanical linkages have severe limitations for real microscopic manipulation. We plan to develop electro-mechanical linkages that work on the same principle, as shown in Fig. 7. System **C** is shown electronically linking mock effector **A** to actual micro-effector **B** (e.g. a micropipette). **A** and **C** are both capable of 3 degrees of translational freedom in this illustration, although rotations could also be incorporated. A semitransparent mirror visually merges the magnified image from an *in vivo* tomographic microscope at the site of the micro-effector with the mock effector using RTTR. System **C** acts as a servo controller, so that the operator manually controls the mock effector using hand-eye coordination, and the actual micro-effector moves accordingly. At present, we are planning to implement this system using several imaging modalities as described in the following section.

Fig. 7 Apparatus demonstrating magnified RTTR using an electro mechanical linkage to control remote effector at a magnified scale (see text).

3   Magnified Remote RTTR for *in Vivo* Microscopy

A number of appropriate mesoscopic/microscopic (10-20 μ resolution) imaging modalities have recently become available that scan from an *in vivo* surface to produce tomographic slices at depths of 1-2 mm. We intend to use two of these as test-beds to develop remote RTTR.

The first of these modalities is *ultrasound backscatter microscopy* (UBM), which operates similarly to conventional ultrasound, except at higher frequencies (50-100 MHz) and has been shown capable of differentiating normal lymph nodes *in vivo* from those containing metastatic melanoma cells [15]. The other *in vivo* microscopic imaging modality that we propose to use for remote RTTR is *optical coherence tomography* (OCT). This relatively new modality uses reflected coherent infrared light in a manner similar to ultrasound. OCT has proven capable of producing real time tomographic images *in vivo* of the epidermis [16].

The mesoscopic/microscopic scale of resolution of UBM and OCT may prove very important for diagnosis, biopsy, and therapy, being able to delimit the extent of multi-cellular structures of differing types. Operating *in vivo* at these scales is an exciting frontier where remote RTTR may play an important role. We have demonstrated the first step towards these applications.

References

1.   Azuma, R., A Survey of Augmented Reality. *A Survey of Augmented Reality, in Presence: Teleoperators and Virtual Environments* **6**, 355-385 (1997).

2.   State, A., Livingston, M., Garret, W., Hirota, G., Whitton, M., Pisano, E. & Fuchs, H., Technologies for Augmented Reality Systems: Realizing Ultrasound-Guided Needle Biopsies. (*ACM SIGGRAPH,* New Orleans, LA,) 439-446 (1996).

3.   Fuchs, H., State, A., Pisano, E., Garret, W., Hirota, G., Livingston, M., Whitton, M. & Pizer, S., Towards Performing Ultrasound-Guided Needle Biopsies from within a Head-Mounted Display. (*Visualization in Biomedical Computing,*   Hamburg, Germany) 591-600 (1996).

4.   Fuchs, H., Livingston, M., Raskar, R., Colucci, D., Keller, K. & State, A., Augmented Reality Visualization for Laproscopic Surgery. (*MICCAI,* Massachusetts Institute of Technology, Cambridge, MA, USA) (1998).

5.   DiGioia, A., Colgan, B. & Koerbel, N., in *Cybersurgery* (ed. Satava, R.) 121-139 (Wiley, New York, 1998).

6.   Blackwell, M., Morgan, F. & DiGioia, A., Augmented Reality and Its Future in Orthopaedics. *Clinical Orthopaedic and Related Research* **345**, 111-122 (1998).

7.   Masamune, K., Masutani, Y., Nakajima, S., Sakuma, I., Dohi, T., Iseki, H. & Takakura, K., Three-dimensional slice image overlay system with accurate depth perception for surgery. (*Medical image Computing and Computer-Assisted Intervention (MICCAI),* Springer, Pittsburgh) **1935** 395-402 (2000).

8.   Stetten, G., Chib, V. & Tamburo, R., System for Location-Merging Ultrasound Images with Human Vision. (*Applied Imagery Pattern Recognition (AIPR) Workshop*, IEEE Computer Society, Washington, DC) 200-205 (2000).

9.   Stetten, G. & Chib, V., Real Time Tomographic Reflection with ultrasound: Stationary and hand-held implementations. (CMU Robotics Insititute Technical Report # CMU-RI-TR-00-28, 2000).

10. Stetten, G. & Chib, V., Overlaying ultrasound images on direct vision. *Journal of Ultrasound in Medicine* **20**, 235-240 (2001).

11. Stetten, G., U.S. Patent Pending: System and Method for Location-Merging of Real-Time Tomographic Slice Images with Human Vision. .

12. Birkfellner, W., Figl, M., Huber, K., Watzinger, F., Wanschitz, F., hanel, R., Wagner, A., Rafolt, D., Ewers, R. & Bergmann, H., The Varioscope AR - A head-mounted operating microscope for augmented reality. (*Medical image Computing and Computer-Assisted Intervention (MICCAI)*, Springer, Pittsburgh) Lecture Notes in Computer Science, **1935** 869-877 (2000).

13. Edwards, P. J., Hawkes, D. J. & Hill, D. L., Augmentation of reality using an operating microscope for otolaryngology and neurosurgical guidance. *J Image Guid Surg* **1**, 172-178 (1995).

14. Nelson, B. J. & Vikramaditya, B., Visually servoed micropositioning for robotic micromanipulation. *Microcomputer Applications* **18**, 23-31 (1999).

15. Uren, R. F., R.Howman-Giles, Thompson, J. F., Shaw, H. M., Roberts, J. M., Bernard, E. & McCarthy, W. H., High-resolution ultrasound to diagnose melanoma metastases in patients with clinically palpable lymph nodes. *Diagnostic Radiology* **43**, 148-152 (1999).

16. Pan, Y. T. & Farkas, D. L., Non-invasive imaging of living human skin with dual-wavelength optical coherence tomography in two and three dimenstions. *Journal of Biomedical Optics* **3**, 446-455 (1998).

A System to Support Laparoscopic Surgery by Augmented Reality Visualization

Stijn De Buck[1], Johan Van Cleynenbreugel[1], Indra Geys[1], Thomas Koninckx[1], Philippe R. Koninck[2], and Paul Suetens[1]

[1] Faculties of Medicine and Engineering
Medical Image Computing (ESAT and Radiology)
[2] Department of Gyncacology
University Hospital Gasthuisberg
Herestraat 49
B-3000 Leuven
stijn.debuck@uz.kuleuven.ac.be

Abstract. This paper describes the development of an augmented reality system for intra-operative laparoscopic surgery support.
The goal of this system is to reveal structures, otherwise hidden within the laparoscope view. To allow flexible movement of the laparoscope we use optical tracking to track both patient and laparoscope.
The necessary calibration and registration procedures were developed and bundled where possible in order to facilitate integration in a current laparoscopic procedure. Care was taken to achieve high accuracy by including radial distortion components without compromising real time speed.
Finally a visual error assessment is performed, the usefulness is demonstrated within a test setup and some preliminary quantitative evaluation is done.

1   Introduction

A laparoscopic surgery consists of making tiny holes into the peritoneum through which subsequently a camera and surgical tools are inserted. The camera view is in fact the only view on the surgery scene. Because this viewpoint is constantly changing to meet the surgeons need and because it is very different from the exoscopic view of the surgeon, the latter has to be very well trained and be able to interpret the laparoscopic images well. Due to its minimal invasive approach, laparoscopic surgery is able to reduce both the time of surgery and the recovery time of a patient.

The laparoscopic view though does not reveal all the structures the surgeon needs to see in order to complete the surgical procedure with success. These structures can for instance be hidden behind the peritoneal wall, like the ureter. This limitation can not only lead to a less efficiently performed surgery but also to further complications for the patient.

Often such structures can be extracted from pre-operative CT/MR-images. However the surgeon needs to interpret and to fuse these images mentally with

W. Niessen and M. Viergever (Eds.): MICCAI 2001, LNCS 2208, pp. 691–698, 2001.

the laparoscopic view. To alleviate this problem we propose an augmented reality approach in which the pre-operative images or at least the structures of interest deduced from these are visualized within the laparoscopic view. In this paper we describe the development of such a system and show our initial testing environment.

Previous work on augmented reality in the context of laparoscopic/endoscopic surgery has been concentrating on extracting 3D depth information from several images taken from different intra-operative positions. The resulting information can than be used to measure intra-operatively or display the 3D information over the endoscopic images [1]. Another application constructs a view of the intra-operative scene similar to conventional laparotomy [2]. Although these approaches also use an optical tracker for system and patient registration, they differ in a number of aspects. We augment the laparoscopic view, with which the surgeons are acquainted already. Since our approach can display structures totally invisible in the laparoscopic view, we believe it can be more versatile and holds potential to provide a considerable amount of added value to the surgeon.

2   System Overview

We use an optical tracker (Flashpoint 5000 of Image Guided Technologies), a laparoscope (Storz9050), and an Octane workstation (SGI) with Octane video card.

The tracker computes position and orientation of both patient and laparoscopic camera. In this way the flexibility the surgeon experiences today and which is necessary for proper navigation is preserved, while still providing an integrated visualization at real time rates.

The integrated visualization of *virtual* pre-operative objects, extracted from CT/MR-images, and the laparoscope view implies an accurate calibration of optical camera parameters. This algorithm should be as transparent as possible to the surgeon.

The combination of camera, optical tracker, together with pre-operative images requires registration procedures between at least three coordinate systems. Finally, visualization of integrated images should be realized at real time rates.

In the following we discuss the issues of calibration, registration and visualization more thoroughly.

2.1   Camera Calibration and Registration

We treat the camera calibration and registration problems together since they are closely related. The solution we propose integrates both thereby reducing the number of registration/calibration steps necessary to perform before surgery.

We attach a coordinate system to the laparoscopic camera (C_c), one to the tracker (C_t) and one to the pre-operative images (C_i). If we register C_c and C_t –which can be done pre-operatively–, only one patient-dependent registration operation has to be performed. Next, we show how to combine the camera calibration step and the registration of C_c and C_t.

Camera Calibration and C_c-C_t Registration As shown by [1] the calibration of a laparoscopic/endoscopic camera demands a camera model that incorporates radial distortion. The calibration procedure by Tsai [3] satisfies this condition. Therefore we apply this procedure through the free-ware implementation of Willson [4]. In this model projection can be described mathematically as:

$$w_i = K(R^t W_i + T) \tag{1}$$

where w_i is an image point $\left[\mu u_i \; \mu v_i \; \mu\right]^t$, W_i a 3D point, K an upper triangle projection matrix, R a rotation matrix and T a translation vector. The radial distortion in the images is modeled by:

$$\begin{bmatrix} u_i^{(rd)} \\ v_i^{(rd)} \end{bmatrix} + \begin{bmatrix} \delta u_i^{(r)} \\ \delta v_i^{(r)} \end{bmatrix} = \begin{bmatrix} u_i \\ v_i \end{bmatrix} \tag{2}$$

$$\begin{bmatrix} \delta u_i^{(r)} \\ \delta v_i^{(r)} \end{bmatrix} = \begin{bmatrix} u_i^{(rd)}(k_1 r_i^2 + k_2 r_i^4 + \ldots) \\ v_i^{(rd)}(k_1 r_i^2 + k_2 r_i^4 + \ldots) \end{bmatrix} \tag{3}$$

with

$r_i \quad = \sqrt{u_i^2 + v_i^2}$

$k_1, k_2 = $ the radial distortion coefficients

$u_i^{(rd)} \quad = $ the radial distorted image x-coordinate

$v_i^{(rd)} \quad = $ the radial distorted image y-coordinate

In order to automate the calibration, we designed a new calibration jig (cfr fig 1). The calibration procedure consists of three steps:

- First an endoscope image is taken by our camera of the calibration jig. The discs on the jig will project as ellipses in the image. The centroids of these ellipses can be extracted by iteratively applying the method described in [5] and taking into account the radial distortion. This results in a 2D image coordinate for each disc.
- Next, we correspond these 2D coordinates to their 3D locations. By attaching LED's to the calibration jig, we can compute the 3D coordinates of the black discs with respect to the C_t reference frame. This way an extra C_c-C_t registration step is made obsolete. A detailed description of the correspondence algorithm can also be found in [5].
- Finally these 2D-3D pairs are fed to the calibration algorithm of Tsai which returns the camera's intrinsic and extrinsic parameters.

Since in laparoscopic surgery the lens is changed before each surgery, it is an advantage for ergonomic reasons to combine both registration and optical camera calibration.

Tracker-Pre-operative Image Registration The goal of this procedure is to determine the C_t-C_i relation. Markers are attached to the patient, which are visible in the pre-operative images. The same markers are indicated on the patient before surgery. Next, the 2 point sets are registered by means of the method of Arun et al. [6].

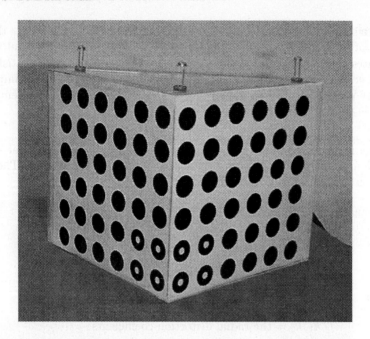

Fig. 1. The calibration/registration object by which the optical calibration and the registration of the laparoscope in the reference frame of the optical tracker are performed.

2.2 Visualization

In this section we treat two main issues in constructing an integrated visualization, namely:

- Visualizing the radial distortion at real time rate.
- Rendering the augmented view in a stable way.

Visualizing the Radial Distortion The result of our calibration are the extrinsic and intrinsic parameters describing how the laparoscopic camera perceives the world. Apart from the radial distortion component k_1, all the projection effects of the camera can be simulated by the pinhole model commonly used in computer graphics.

Implementing the radial distortion in the projection of the virtual objects would slow down the rendering [7], which in turn can compromise the real-time visualization constraint. In the case of laparoscopic surgery radial distortion can not be neglected (cfr section 2.1).

Therefore we propose a solution to render integrated images by rectification or de-distortion of the laparoscopic images. This is done by loading the laparoscopic video frames immediately into texture memory and warping this texture over a nurbssurface. The latter models the inverse radial distortion. A real-time visualization is obtained this way.

Rendering the Pre-operative Images Once the real laparoscope images are rectified, the virtual objects can be rendered by the standard pinhole model. Virtual objects are extracted from pre-operative images by segmentation and surface extraction. Their position and orientation is modified by the position of the probe attached to the patient. Also the position and orientation of the virtual laparoscope is changed by the probe attached to the real one. The data coming from the tracker is filtered first in order to reduce the noise present in the measurement.

3   A Setup for Error Evaluation

To evaluate our system qualitatively, we have constructed a setup (cfr fig 2) to visually inspect the accuracy of calibration/registration and the efficiency of our visualization .

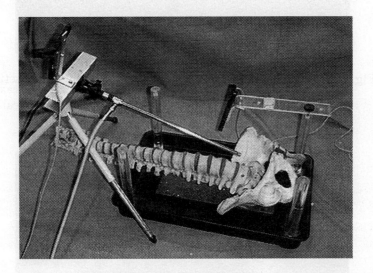

Fig. 2. The test setup we used to evaluate the system. Both camera and phantom are tracked.

The patient under surgery is represented by a phantom pelvis. To this phantom a number of radio-opaque markers were glued. The phantom was CT-scanned and a surface model was generated. After calibration and registration, we can verify the accuracy by comparing the alignment of our model with the real images when using our system (cfr figure 3 en 4).

To illustrate the clinical usefulness a copper wire was attached to the phantom (before CT-scan), representing the ureter. In real laparoscopic surgery locating the ureter is a common problem. Under the assumption the ureter is not moved or deformed with respect to the pelvis, this problem can be solved by the system

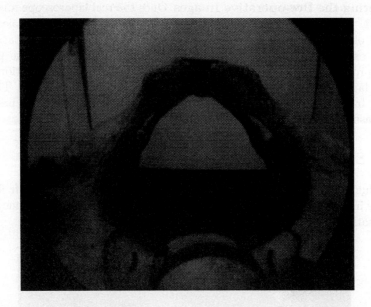

Fig. 3. A rectified laparoscope view constructed with the test setup

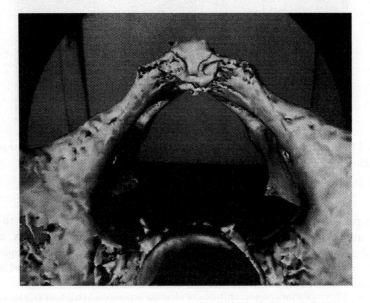

Fig. 4. Evaluation of the system by visual inspection

by generating an integrated view of the real phantom (the surgery view) and of the segmented ureter (the pre-operative images) as in figure 5.

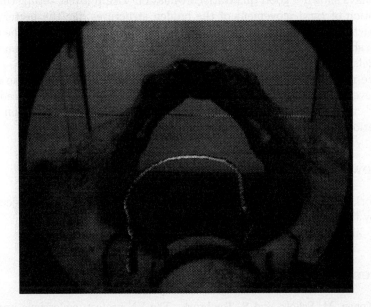

Fig. 5. Illustration of a possible application: although the ureter is invisible in the real view, it can be shown by augmented visualization.

We also include some preliminary quantitative evaluation results here. To assess a measure for the accuracy of the system as a whole, we displaced the calibration jig with respect to the calibration position. We than used our system to create a view without virtual objects and computed the image coordinates of the discs on the jig. Next, we compared these coordinates with the ones detected in the view. This resulted in an error ranging from 3.07 to 4.9 pixels for a displacement of 0 to 5 cm. Since the displacement is not very large and the camera position did not change after calibration, more extensive testing has to be done here.

4   Discussion

In this paper we presented a system for intra-operative laparoscopic surgery support by augmented reality visualization. This system holds a large potential in gynaecological laparoscopy.

Several subproblems were solved which arise in a typical laparoscopic environment. First of all, a single calibration procedure was developed to solve both the optical calibration of the laparoscope and its registration with respect to the optical tracker. Second, a real time visualization method was implemented,

taking into account the radial distortion of the laparoscope. Finally, tracker data
was filtered and a stable augmented view was created.

We have shown a good qualitative evaluation within a test setup. Under the
assumption of rigid movement of the hidden structures like the ureter –which
will have to be validated–, we demonstrated the clinical usefulness of the system.
We also showed some preliminary quantitative results which indicate an error of
± 4 pixels.

Since no more than two extra procedures are necessary to use the system,
we believe it can be easily integrated into a laparoscopic surgical procedure.

Our current work concentrates on further numerical quantification for the
registration, calibration and tracking errors in the system.

Acknowledgements

This work is part of SuperVisie, ITA-II/980302, an IWT ITA-II project sponsored by the Flemish Government.
We also like to thank Storz for providing the laparoscope.

References

1. W. Konen, M. Scholz, and S. Tombrock. The VN project: endoscopic image processing for neurosurgery. *Computer Aided Surgery*, 3(3):145–148, December 1998.
2. H. Fuchs, M.A. Livingston, R. Raskar, D. Colucci, K. Keller, A. State, J.R. Crawford, P. Rademacher, S.H. Drake, and M.H. Meyer. Augmented reality visualization
for laparoscopic surgery. In *MICCAI*, pages 934–943, October 1998.
3. R.Y. Tsai. An efficient and accurate camera calibration technique for 3D machine
vision. In *CVPR86*, pages 364–374, 1986.
4. R.G. Willson. Freeware implementation of R. Tsai's camera calibration algorithm.
http://www.cs.cmu.edu/afs/cs.cmu.edu/user/rgw/www/TsaiCode.html.
5. S. De Buck, J. Van Cleynenbreugel, G. Marchal, and P. Suetens. Towards visual
matching as a way of transferring pre-operative surgery planning. In W. de Leeuw
& R. Van Liere, editor, *Data Visualization 2000*, pages 249–258, May 2000.
6. K.S. Arun, T.S. Huang, and S.D. Blostein. Least-squares fitting of two 3-d point
sets. *PAMI*, 9(5):698–700, September 1987.
7. P.J. Edwards, A.P. King, C.R. Maurer Jr, D.A. de Cunha, D.J. Hawkes, D.L.G.
Hill, R.P. Gaston, M.R. Fenlon, A. Jusczyzck, A.J. Strong, C.L. Chandler, and
M.J. Gleeson. Design and evaluation of a system for microscope-assisted guided
interventions (magi). *IEEE Transactions on Medical Imaging*, 19(11):1082–1093,
November 2000.

Blood Pool Agent CE-MRA: Improved Arterial Visualization of the Aortoiliac Vasculature in the Steady-State Using First-Pass Data

C.M. van Bemmel[1]*, W.J. Niessen[1], O. Wink[1], B. Verdonck[2], and
M.A. Viergever[1]

[1] Image Sciences Institute, Room E 01.334, University Medical Center Utrecht,
Heidelberglaan 100, 3584 CX Utrecht, the Netherlands,
{kees,wiro,onno,max}@isi.uu.nl
[2] EasyVision Advanced Development, Philips Medical Systems,
Postbus 10000, Best, the Netherlands
bert.verdonck@philips.com

Abstract. Blood pool agent (BPA) contrast-enhanced magnetic resonance angiography (CE-MRA) images have been acquired during the
first-pass of the contrast agent and in the steady-state. Arterial visualization, which is hampered in the steady-state owing to simultaneous
enhancement of arteries and veins, can be improved if the central arterial
axis (CAA) is known. A method is presented that utilizes the first-pass
data to find the CAA in the steady-state data with minimum user interaction. The accuracy of the resulting CAA is compared to tracings
of two observers in three datasets. It was found that the average error
of the method is 0.73 mm in the first-pass data and 1.54 mm in the
steady-state data.

1 Introduction

Blood pool agents for CE-MRA have a prolonged intravascular halflife and provide strong T_1-relaxation even at low resolution [1]. Therefore, these agents allow
imaging in the steady-state, thus providing longer time windows for image acquisition, which can be advantageous if high contrast and/or resolution is required.
However, an important drawback is the simultaneous enhancement of arteries
and veins, which hampers the interpretation of the steady-state data (see Fig. 2).

In this paper it is investigated whether information from the arteriogram
acquired in the first-pass of the contrast agent can be used for improved arterial
visualization of the steady-state images. Hereto a path tracking tool is utilized,
which automatically outlines the central arterial axes (CAA) of the aortoiliac
region in the first-pass images based on four user defined points. Subsequently,
by registering the first-pass and steady-state data, the path is transferred to the
steady-state. A number of visualization techniques can be utilized once the CAA
is known in the steady-state images.

---

* This work is funded by Philips Medical Systems, Best, The Netherlands.

W. Niessen and M. Viergever (Eds.): MICCAI 2001, LNCS 2208, pp. 699–706, 2001.
© Springer-Verlag Berlin Heidelberg 2001

In order to evaluate the accuracy of the method, the obtained paths are compared with manual tracings of two observers.

2   Method

The CAA can be used to improve arterial visualization in steady-state BPA CE-MRA. Owing to the proximity of arteries and veins in the steady-state dataset, and the possible presence of pathologies, which mainly occur in the arteries, the CAA cannot readily be obtained from the steady-state data. Therefore, a method is introduced that utilizes images acquired during the first-pass of the contrast agent, in which only the arterial phase is enhanced, to estimate the CAA in the steady-state data. Hereto, first the CAA is determined in the first-pass image by finding a minimum cost path between user-defined points in an image where vessel-like structures are enhanced. Subsequently, this axis is transformed to the steady-stated data. The different steps are detailed below.

2.1   Vesselness Filter

A filter is employed which analyzes the local second-order image structure to determine the likeliness of a voxel to be part of a tubular structure [2]. The local image structure of an image L in the neighbourhood of a point $\mathbf{x}_0$ can be described with the Taylor-expansion:

$$L(\mathbf{x}_0 + \delta\mathbf{x}_0, \sigma) \approx L(\mathbf{x}_0, \sigma) + \delta\mathbf{x}_0^T \nabla_{0,\sigma} + \delta\mathbf{x}_0^T H_{0,\sigma} \delta\mathbf{x}_0 \tag{1}$$

where $\nabla_{0,\sigma}$ and $H_{0,\sigma}$ are the gradient vector and Hessian matrix of the image computed in $\mathbf{x}_0$ at scale σ, respectively.

The Hessian matrix at a given voxel $\mathbf{x}$ is defined as:

$$H(\mathbf{x}, \sigma) = \begin{bmatrix} L_{xx}(\mathbf{x}, \sigma) & L_{xy}(\mathbf{x}, \sigma) & L_{xz}(\mathbf{x}, \sigma) \\ L_{yx}(\mathbf{x}, \sigma) & L_{yy}(\mathbf{x}, \sigma) & L_{yz}(\mathbf{x}, \sigma) \\ L_{zx}(\mathbf{x}, \sigma) & L_{zy}(\mathbf{x}, \sigma) & L_{zz}(\mathbf{x}, \sigma) \end{bmatrix} \tag{2}$$

where $L_{\xi_1\xi_2}(\mathbf{x}, \sigma)$ denote regularized derivatives of the image $L(\mathbf{x})$, which are obtained by convolving the image with the derivatives of the Gaussian kernel at scale σ:

$$L_{\xi_1\xi_2}(\mathbf{x}, \sigma) \triangleq \sigma^2 \frac{\partial^2 G(\mathbf{x}, \sigma)}{\partial\xi_1\partial\xi_2} * L(\mathbf{x}) \tag{3}$$

$$G(\mathbf{x}, \sigma) \triangleq \frac{1}{\sqrt{(2\pi\sigma^2)^3}} e^{-\frac{\|\mathbf{x}\|^2}{2\sigma^2}} \tag{4}$$

The principal directions in which the local second-order structure of the image can be decomposed are obtained by eigenvalue analysis of the Hessian matrix. Let $\lambda_{\sigma,k}$ denote the ordered eigenvalues corresponding to the k-th normalized eigenvector $\hat{\mathbf{u}}_{\sigma,k}$, i.e. $|\lambda_{\sigma,1}| \leq |\lambda_{\sigma,2}| \leq |\lambda_{\sigma,3}|$. The eigenvectors $\hat{\mathbf{u}}_{\sigma,k}$ compose three orthonormal directions: $\hat{u}_1$ indicates the direction along the vessel (minimum intensity variation), $\hat{u}_2$, and $\hat{u}_3$ form a base of the orthogonal plane. For an ideal tubular structure in 3D images we have:

$$|\lambda_1| = 0, |\lambda_1| \ll |\lambda_2|, \lambda_2 = \lambda_3 \tag{5}$$

where the sign of λ_2 and λ_3 determines whether it concerns a bright or a dark vessel.

This approach has an intuitive justification (see Fig. 1); the second-order derivative of a Gaussian kernel at scale σ generates a kernel that measures the contrast between the regions inside and outside the range $(-\sigma, \sigma)$. In regions with bright vessels, λ_2 and λ_3 will be large and negative.

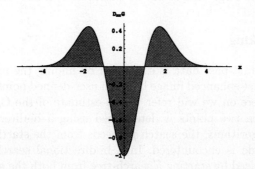

Fig. 1. Second-order derivative of a Gaussian kernel, with $\sigma = 1$.

In order to estimate the likeliness of a voxel to belong to a vessel based on analysis of the eigenvalues, two geometric ratios ($\mathcal{R}_A$ and $\mathcal{R}_B$), and one ratio ($\mathcal{S}$) for distinguishing background voxels from vessel voxels are introduced:

$$\mathcal{R}_A \triangleq \frac{|\lambda_2|}{|\lambda_3|}, \mathcal{R}_B \triangleq \frac{|\lambda_1|}{\sqrt{|\lambda_2 \lambda_3|}}, \mathcal{S} \triangleq \|\mathcal{H}\|_F = \sqrt{\sum_j \lambda_j^2} \tag{6}$$

The ratio $\mathcal{R}_A$ is essential for distinguishing between plate-like and line-like structures. The ratio $\mathcal{R}_B$ accounts for the deviation from a blob-like structure. $\mathcal{S}$ is a measure of "second-order structuredness", and will be low in the background where no structure is present. In regions with high contrast compared to the background, the norm will become larger since at least one of the eigenvalues will be large.

Since in CE-MRA vessels give higher signal than the background, the output of the vessel enhancement filter at a single scale, σ, is therefore defined as:

$$\mathcal{V}(\sigma) \triangleq \begin{cases} 0 & \text{if } \lambda_2 > 0 \text{ or } \lambda_3 > 0, \\ (1 - e^{-\frac{\mathcal{R}_A^2}{2\alpha^2}})e^{-\frac{\mathcal{R}_B^2}{2\beta^2}}(1 - e^{-\frac{\mathcal{S}^2}{2\gamma^2}}) & \text{otherwise} \end{cases} \tag{7}$$

The parameters α, β and γ tune the sensitivity of the filter to deviations in $\mathcal{R}_A$, $\mathcal{R}_B$ and $\mathcal{S}$ relative to the ideal behaviour for a line structure. Equation 7 explicitly states that the filter response is a function of the scale at which the Gaussian derivatives are computed. The filter is applied at multiple scales that span the range of expected vessel widths according to the imaged anatomy. In order to provide a unique filter output for each voxel, the multiple scale outputs undergo a *scale selection* procedure, *i.e.*, the maximum filter response across the scales is selected:

$$\mathcal{V}(\mathbf{x}) = \max_{\sigma_{min} \leq \sigma \leq \sigma_{max}} \mathcal{V}(\mathbf{x}, \sigma) \tag{8}$$

This way, different vessel sizes will be detected at their corresponding scales and both small and large vessels will be captured with the same scheme.

2.2   Path Tracking

The CAA in the first-pass data is estimated by finding the minimal cost path (MCP) in the vessel-enhanced image between user-defined points [3]. For reasons of clarity, from here on we will refer to the estimate of the CAA as the MCP. The MCP between two points is determined using a bi-directional search. In uni-directional algorithms, the search proceeds from the starting node forward until the goal node is encountered. In a bi-directional search the number of evaluations is reduced by starting a search-tree from both the starting node and the goal node simultaneously. The evolutions of the search tree are continued until the two fronts meet. The MCP is calculated using a feature image, in which the reciprocal vessel image as determined by Equation 7 represented the costs. Costs are normalized with respect to the length in order to cope with diagonal transitions and (possible) anisotropic voxels.

2.3   Registration

To correct for possible patient motion between acquisition of the first-pass and steady-state datasets, the first-pass dataset is rigidly registered to the steady-state dataset. Alignment is achieved by maximizing the mutual information [4,5]. The MI registration criterion states that two images are geometrically aligned by the transformation T^* for which $I(u(\mathbf{x}), v(T(\mathbf{x})))$ is maximal:

$$T^* = \arg\max_T I(u(\mathbf{x}), v(T(\mathbf{x}))) \tag{9}$$

where mutual information, I, is defined in terms of entropy and is a measure of the variability:

$$I(u(\mathbf{x}), v(T(\mathbf{x}))) \triangleq h(u(\mathbf{x})) + h(v(T(\mathbf{x}))) - h(u(\mathbf{x}), v(T(\mathbf{x}))) \tag{10}$$

$h(.)$ is the entropy and is defined for one variable $\mathbf{x}$ as:

$$h(\mathbf{x}) \triangleq - \int p(\mathbf{x}) \ln p(\mathbf{x}) dx \tag{11}$$

The obtained transformation matrix T^* is applied to the MCP found in the first-pass dataset to obtain an estimate of the CAA in the steady-state dataset.

3   Experiments

In this section the experiments to obtain the automatic MCP and the way to compare it with manually drawn paths are described.

3.1   Image Acquisition

For this study three datasets are examined. The images are obtained with blood pool agent MS-325 (EPIX Medical, Cambridge, Mass.). The images are obtained both during the first-pass and steady-state of the contrast. The voxel size of the reconstructed images is $0.86 \times 0.86 \times 1.50$ mm^3, and $0.86 \times 0.86 \times 0.95$ [0.90 - 0.98] mm^3, respectively.

3.2   Path Tracking

For the automatic path tracking, the vesselness image is computed at two scale ranges, depending on the anatomical region: above the aortic bifurcation $\sigma = 10.0$ - 20.0 mm (11 scales, equal step sizes) is used, while below the aortic bifurcation $\sigma = 1.0$ - 20.0 mm (20 scales, equal step sizes) is applied. The MCP is initialized at four points: at the height of the renal arteries (ra), approximately 20 mm above the aortic bifurcation (ab), in the left and right femoral artery (lf and rf, respectively). The MCP for the left (right) side of the vasculature is determined from ra, via ab, to lf (rf). For the evaluation of the MCP, two observers outlined the CAA twice, both in the first-pass and the steady-state datasets using a clinical workstation (EasyVision, Philips Medical Systems) with an interval of approximately two weeks.

3.3   Path Comparison

To determine the distance between two paths, $\mathbf{C_1}$ and $\mathbf{C_2}$, first the corresponding parts are determined and resampled in N points. Subsequently, a symmetric mean path, $\bar{\mathbf{C}}$ is constructed by averaging all corresponding path points. For all sample points i the distance $D(\mathbf{C_1}, \mathbf{C_2}, i)$ between the two paths is determined as:

$$D(\mathbf{C_1}, \mathbf{C_2}, i) = d(\mathbf{C_1}, \bar{\mathbf{C}}(i)) + d(\mathbf{C_2}, \bar{\mathbf{C}}(i)) \tag{12}$$

where $d(\mathbf{C_1}, \bar{\mathbf{C}}(i))$ is the smallest distance between the i-th sample point of $\bar{\mathbf{C}}$ and a densely resampled (sample rate 0.01 mm) version of $\mathbf{C_1}$. From these measurements the maximal distance (D_{max}), and mean distance (D_{mean}) are calculated. This procedure is performed to find the mean path of each observer ($\bar{C}_1$ and $\bar{C}_2$, respectively), as well as the mean path of the two observers ($\bar{C}_{\bar{12}}$, the mean of $\bar{C}_1$ and $\bar{C}_2$). The intra-observer variability is defined as the distance of individual tracings of an observer to the observers' mean path. The inter-observer variability is defined by using the averaged path, computed from all individual paths, yielding a gold standard. The gold standard is also used for testing the accuracy of the automatically determined CAA.

4   Results

In this section the intra-observer and inter-observer differences, and the error of the automated method are shown for the first-pass data in Table 1 and for the steady-state data in Table 2. The results are averaged over the three datasets and both legs. The average mean and maximum value and the corresponding ranges are listed.

Table 1. Mean intra-observer difference and mean inter-observer difference, and the average result of the automated method (MCP) in the first-pass data.

	Mean error (mm)	Maximum error (mm)
Intra observer (I) variability	0.41 [0.30-0.55]	1.72 [0.87-2.45]
Intra observer (II) variability	0.34 [0.31-0.40]	1.31 [0.95-1.53]
Inter observer variability	0.46 [0.34-0.71]	1.60 [0.96-2.83]
MCP vs $\bar{C}_{\bar{12}}$	0.73 [0.64-0.79]	2.18 [1.66-3.08]

Table 2.   Mean intra-observer difference and mean inter-observer difference, and the average results of the automated methods, without (MCP) and with registration (MCP_{reg}).

	Mean error (mm)	Maximum error (mm)
Intra observer (I) variability	0.43 [0.35-0.51]	1.89 [1.40-2.73]
Intra observer (II) variability	0.41 [0.36-0.53]	1.21 [0.92-1.52]
Inter observer variability	0.53 [0.40-0.77]	1.91 [0.94-3.69]
MCP vs $\bar{C}_{\bar{12}}$	1.55 [0.95-2.44]	3.46 [2.54-5.46]
MCP_{reg} vs $\bar{C}_{\bar{12}}$	1.54 [0.86-2.21]	3.49 [2.36-5.43]

From the Tables it can be observed that the differences between the observers (0.46 and 0.53 mm, respectively) and average differences between two tracings of one observer (0.37 and 0.42 mm, respectively) are smaller than the in-plane resolution for both the first-pass and steady-state data. The error of the automated method is almost similar in the first-pass data (0.73 mm), but it was observed that when placing different initialization points, the same path is found except at the initialization points. Therefore, the automated method has a better reproducibility. The error increased in the steady-state data (1.55 mm). This increase is expected, since the error is composed of an error in obtaining the MCP and an error in the registration. However, obtaining the central vessel axis manually from the steady-state data is a tedious procedure. By registering the first-pass and steady-state data using maximization of mutual information, the error in the steady-state data could not significantly be reduced. In all situations, the MCP is located inside the arterial vessel.

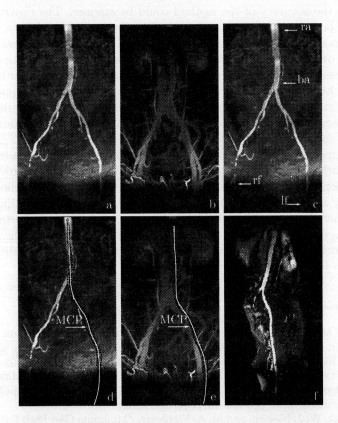

Fig. 2. Images acquired during the first-pass (a) and steady-state (b). The simultaneous enhancement of arteries and veins hampers arterial interpretation in the steady-state. After initializing four points (c, see Section 3.2) the arterial axis is estimated in first-pass data (d) and transformed, after registration to the steady-state (e). It can subsequently be used for improved arterial visualization. Here a curved reformat shows the artery over the entire segment (f), clearly displaying the path to be situated inside the artery.

The maximum errors for the method are larger in the first-pass data and larger in the steady-state. However, closer inspection of the paths reveals that these errors occur primarily at the bifurcation, where the CAA is ill-defined. Here the observers interpolate the path differently than the automated method.

5   Discussion

Arterial visualization in steady-state blood pool agent CE-MRA can be improved if the CAA is known. Moreover, the CAA can be used for further analysis of the steady-state data. A method has been presented which estimates the CAA with minimum user interaction, by utilizing an arteriogram acquired during the first-pass of the contrast agent. By comparing the method with two tracings of two observers, the accuracy of the method could be assessed. The observers traced the CAA both in the first-pass data and in the steady-state data, such that the influence of (i) errors in determining the MCP in the first-pass data, and (ii) errors owing to the misregistration of first-pass and steady-state data could both be assessed. The average error of the estimated CAA is similar in the first-pass data, but reproducibility is improved. The error is larger in the steady-state data. Registration using maximization of mutual information did not improve the accuracy of the automated method, therefore, other registration methods should be considered.

Acquiring the CAA in the steady-state by a manual observer is a tedious procedure which cannot be used in clinical practice. Moreover, for improved arterial visualization and further postprocessing it is more important that the method is sufficiently accurate. In the three datasets it is checked that the estimated CAA is everywhere located within the arterial system, which is an important prerequisite, *e.g.*, as a preprocessing step for segmentation algorithms. The evaluation carried out in this paper needs to be extended to determine whether this still holds for a larger number of datasets.

References

1. Grist TM, Korosec FR, Peters DC, Walovitch RC, Dolan RP, Bridson WE, Yucel EK, and Mistretta CA, "SteadyState and Dynamic MR Angiography with MS325: Initial Experience in Humans," *Radiology*, vol. 207, pp. 539–544, 1998.
2. A. F. Frangi, W. J. Niessen, K. L. Vincken, and M. A. Viergever, "Multiscale Vessel Enhancement Filtering," in *Medical Image Conference and Computer Assisted Interventions*. 1998, pp. 130–137, SpringerVerlag.
3. O. Wink, W. J. Niessen, and M. A. Viergever, "Minimum Cost Path Determination Using a Simple Heuristic Function," in *Proc. International Conference on Pattern Recognition - 4*, September 2000, pp. 1010–1013.
4. P. Viola and W.M. Wells, "Alignment by Maximization of Mutual Information," *Proc. 5th Int. Conf. on Computer Vision*, pp. 26–23, June 1995.
5. F. Maes, A. Collignon, D. Vandermeulen, G. Marchal, and P. Suetens, "Multimodality Image Registration by Maximization of Mutual Information," *IEEE Transactions on Medical Imaging*, vol. 16, pp. 187–198, 1997.

A Head-Mounted Display System for Augmented Reality Image Guidance: Towards Clinical Evaluation for iMRI-guided Neurosurgery

F. Sauer, PhD[1], A. Khamene, PhD[1], B. Bascle, PhD[1], and G.J. Rubino, MD[2]

[1] Imaging & Visualization Dept, Siemens Corporate Research, 755 College Road East, Princeton, NJ 08540, USA
{sauer, khamene, bascle}@scr.siemens.com

[2] UCLA, Division of Neurosurgery, Box 957039, Los Angeles, California 90095-7039, USA
rubino@surgery.medsch.ucla.edu

Abstract. We developed an augmented reality system targeting image guidance for surgical procedures. The surgeon wears a video-see-through head mounted display that provides him with a stereo video view of the patient. The live video images are augmented with graphical representations of anatomical structures that are segmented from medical image data. The surgeon can see e.g. a tumor in its actual location inside the patient. This *in-situ* visualization, where the computer maps the image information onto the patient, promises the most direct, intuitive guidance for surgical procedures. In this paper, we discuss technical details of the system and describe a first pre-clinical evaluation. This first evaluation is very positive and encourages us to get our system ready for installation in UCLA's iMRI operating room to perform clinical trials.

1 Introduction

Image guidance systems help the physician to establish a mapping between a patient's medical images and the physical body. In conventional systems, a pointer or an instrument is tracked and the location visualized in the medical images. The physician observes on a screen where the pointer or the instrument is positioned with respect to the internal anatomical structures. Hence, the conventional image guidance system maps the instrument into the medical data set and displays the relationship on a screen separate from the patient.

In contrast, augmented reality (AR) image guidance maps the medical data onto the patient's body. We propose the term "*in-situ*" visualization: anatomical structures are being displayed at the location where they actually are. The physician can see beyond the surface, the patient's body becomes transparent for him. This is the most direct and intuitive way of presenting the medical image information. Our work is concerned with exploring and realizing practical benefits of this *in-situ* visualization for image-guided procedures.

AR visualization in the medical field has first been suggested and investigated at UNC for ultrasound-guided procedures [1]. Further development of UNC's ultrasound

W. Niessen and M. Viergever (Eds.): MICCAI 2001, LNCS 2208, pp. 707–716, 2001.

AR system is reported in [2], another AR system for laparoscopic surgery is described in [3]. A large image guidance program is ongoing at Harvard/MIT that includes research on augmented reality. [4] reports on a system for interventional MRI where the surgeon is provided with an augmented video image, taken with a single, fixed video camera and displayed on a monitor above the patient. At Guy's and St Thomas's Hospitals in London, stereo augmented reality has been implemented on a surgical microscope [5,6]. Various other AR projects are being pursued as the interest in AR technology is growing. Faster computers and better displays are making AR more practical and affordable.

We developed an AR system around a stereo head-mounted display (HMD) of the video-see-through variety. Two miniature color video cameras are mounted on the HMD as the user's artificial eyes. The two live video streams are augmented with computer graphics and displayed on the HMD's two screens in realtime. With the HMD, the user can move around and explore the augmented scene from a variety of viewpoints. The user's spatial perception is based on stereo depth cues, and also on the kinetic depth cues that he receives with the viewpoint variations.

We gave a first general description of our system in [8]. A copy of that system was built at the University of Rochester in the course of a collaboration that put the system in a neurosurgical context [9]. In this paper, we report on a pre-clinical evaluation at UCLA that encourages us to move our system towards clinical trials. Section 2 presents technical details of our AR system. Section 3 describes our pre-clinical experience and section 4 concludes with an outlook to the work we are planning.

2   System Overview

Designing an AR system requires at least three fundamental choices. The first is the choice of the display. We chose a stereo head-mounted display over a monitor, which is externally mounted. An HMD ultimately promises the most intuitive and natural experience of the augmented world. The user can move around and observe the scene dynamically from various viewpoints. His 3D perception is based on stereo and kinetic depth cues.

Closely linked to the display choice is the choice of whether to combine the computer graphics with an optical view of the real scene in an optical way (optical-see-through AR) or with a video view in an electronic way (video-see-through AR). Reference [10] reviews some medical AR systems of both types. Optical-see-through systems require less computing power and provide unmatched resolution of the "real part" of the augmented scene. The conventional optical-see-through systems are, however, based on semitransparent displays through which the user observes the real scene. The real view and the augmenting graphics are merged ultimately only in the user's eye, and their registration depends critically on the position of the user's eye behind the optical-see-through HMD. Correct registration is a subjective experience, which makes the system calibration imprecise and an external monitoring of the calibration impossible. Optical microscopes equipped for augmented reality visualization get around this problem by combining real and graphic views in an intermediate image plane (see e.g. [6-8]). Here the registration is fixed in an objective way, independent of the user. We chose to work with video-see-through AR, where the combination of real and graphic views takes place in the computer. Registration is performed in an objective way. Moreover, video-see-through AR allows one the most control over the augmented image. Not only the graphics part but also the real part can now be manipulated for complete control over the final augmented visualization. This becomes essential when the surgical field contains textures and highlights that would interfere with the clear perception of the graphics information, unless one "cleans up" the video images (e.g. cuts out parts of them [2]).

The third choice concerns the tracking system. The tracking system is responsible for measuring the viewer's pose, i.e. position and orientation of the video cameras in the case of a video-see-through system. The pose information allows one to render the graphics from exactly the same vantage point and make it appear firmly anchored with respect to the real scene. Optical tracking technology achieves the highest precision. Most image guidance systems use optical tracking in the form of a stereo pair of video cameras. Instead of mounting such a commercial system next to our workspace, we employ a single tracking camera that we rigidly attach to the two other cameras on our HMD. The requirement that there be an unobstructed line-of-sight between tracker camera and optical markers is least restrictive in this head-mounted configuration. The user does not accidentally step in the way of the tracking system.

2.1 Hardware

The centerpiece of the system is a head-mounted display that provides the user with the augmented vision. Fig. 1 shows how three miniature cameras are rigidly mounted on top of the HMD. A stereo pair of color cameras captures live images of the scene. They are focused to about arm's length distance and are tilted downward so that the user can keep his head in a comfortable straight pose. A black-and-white camera, equipped with a wide-angle lens and a ring of infrared LEDs, detects retroreflective markers in the scene and is used for headtracking.

The combination of HMD and cameras weighs over 2kg, and one would not find it comfortable to wear it over extended periods of time. But with a resolution of 1024x768 (XGA) for each eye our system represents the highest resolution realtime AR system that we know of. In that respect it is well suited to investigate the potential benefits of AR visualization for image guided procedures. A fully integrated video-see-through head-mounted display weighing only 340g is described in [11]. We tested a prototype and found that its 640x480 resolution is not adequate for surgical application. The protoype makes it easy, however, to envision lightweight, comfortable, and high-resolution camera/HMD combinations for the future.

Fig. 2 shows how display and cameras are connected to two PCs. One SGI 540 processes the tracker camera images and renders the augmented view for the left eye, an SGI 320 renders the augmented view for the right eye. Both PCs communicate over an Ethernet connection to exchange information concerning camera pose, synchronization, and choice of graphics objects to be used for augmentation. Table 1 lists the particular hardware components that we are using.

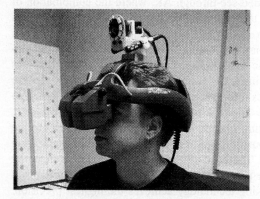

Fig. 1. Video-see-through HMD with head-mounted tracker camera.

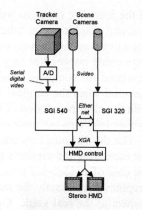

Fig. 2. System block diagram

Table 1. Hardware Components

HMD	Kaiser Proview XL35, XGA resolution, 35° diagonal FOV
Scene cameras	Panasonic GP-KS1000 with 15mm lens, 30°diagonal FOV
Tracker camera	Sony XC-77RR with 3.8mm fisheyelens, 178° FOV
A/D converter	Miranda ASD-101i
Computers	SGI 540 and 320 with Windows 2000

2.2 System Calibration

For correct registration between graphics and patient, we need to calibrate the system. We need to determine the transformation that maps the medical data onto the patient, and we need to determine the internal parameters and relative poses of the three video cameras in order to show the mapping correctly in the augmented view.

Camera calibration and camera – patient transformation. Fig. 3 shows the calibration object we fabricated for the calibration of our camera triplet (which also doubles as a stage for AR experiments [8]). We determine the 3D coordinates of the markers with an Optotrak®, measure the 2D coordinates of the markers in the images, and calibrate the cameras based on 3D-2D point correspondences with Tsai's algorithm [12,13]. For realtime tracking, we rigidly attach a set of markers with known 3D coordinates to the patient (resp. a head frame) defining the patient coordinate system.

MR data – patient transformation. We are currently preparing our AR system for use in UCLA's neurosurgical iMR operating room [14]. The patient's bed can be placed in the magnet's fringe field for the surgical procedure or swiveled into the magnet for MR scanning. The bed with the head clamp, and therefore also the patient's head, are reproducibly positioned in the magnet with a specified accuracy of ±1mm. We pre-determine the transformation between the MR volume set and the head clamp with a phantom and then re-apply the same transformation when mapping the scan data to the patient's head. Fig. 4 shows the planar phantom that consists of a set of markers visible in the MR data set and a set of optical markers visible to the tracker camera. We track the optical markers, and – with the knowledge of the phantom's geometry – determine the 3D locations of the MR markers in the patient coordinate system. We also determine the 3D locations of the MR markers in the MR data set, and calculate the transformation between the two coordinate systems based on the 3D-3D point correspondences.

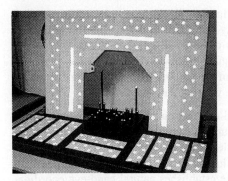 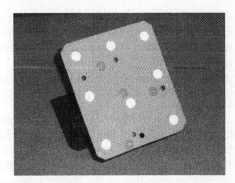

Fig. 3. Camera calibration object. The markers retroreflect the light of the camera's flash.

Fig. 4. Calibration phantom with MR and optical markers.

2.3 System Performance

Timing. Our AR video system is running at the full standard video rate of 30 frames per second. We synchronize video and graphics, eliminating any time lag between the real and the virtual objects. The virtual objects do not lag behind, neither does one see them swim or jitter with respect to the real scene. As the augmented view shows the graphics firmly anchored in the real scene, the user can assess the information in a comfortable way. Overall, there is a time delay of about 0.1seconds between an actual event and its display to the user (see also section 3.2).

Registration accuracy. We initially performed an accuracy test of our AR system with the calibration setup shown in Fig. 3. The calibrated system was used to augment video images of the central marker configuration with a graphics model of the same marker configuration. The mismatches between the real markers and their virtual counterparts were recorded as errors. We found the errors to be typically below 1mm, going up to 2mm at the borders of the scene. We do not have any measurements yet with the head frame marker arrangement from Fig. 5. But the first application that we target, skin flap and craniotomy planning, does not require a high accuracy. For this application, our system's accuracy is well sufficient, even if the mapping between MR and patient space introduces additional errors in the range of a few millimeters.

3 Pre-clinical Experience

3.1 Plain Video View

The first natural concern with a video-see-through HMD is certainly this: to what extent does the video view diminish the ability to see fine details and perform delicate manual tasks? We summarize the subjective experience with our system in the following list. We gained this experience in a qualitative way through simple pick-and-place and point-and-touch experiments. One of the authors (Rubino) also tried out the use of surgical instruments on a cadaver while wearing the HMD.

Artificial eyes above head. Does the hand-eye coordination suffer when the artificial eye-point is displaced from the user's natural eye-point? When the user inserts his hand into the field-of-view, the hand does indeed appear at an unexpected position at first. But in our experience, by watching the hand's movement one is quickly able to adapt. Concentration on the limited workspace establishes natural hand-eye coordination. This situation may be similar to working under a microscope where the user can also adapt to a view that is different from what he is used to see with his naked eye. While it is possible to construct a video-see-through HMD with the camera viewpoints matching the user's eyepoints [11], it may not be necessary for surgical applications.

Video resolution. We capture the video images with a resolution of 720x648 and display them scaled to a size of 1024x768. Of course, the upscaling of the images does not increase their actual resolution, but the appearance of the graphics benefits from the use of the XGA display. A sharper video image (HDTV in the future?) would be welcome, but – again from a subjective perspective – the present video resolution seems to be adequate to perform at least the planning for the surgical work. We find a digital zoom helpful. Even though no new details are created in the video images, the magnification gives one an easier grasp of the details that are present.

Limited depth perception cues. Our pair of cameras has a fixed convergence, and the user looks at fixed screens where he does not adjust his focus according to the distance of the objects that he is observing. The main depth cue comes from the stereo disparity of the two video images. This stereo depth cue alone provides a good depth perception for people with normal stereo vision ability. With the HMD, the user can furthermore vary his viewpoint, and as close objects appear to move faster than more distant objects, he receives additional kinetic depth cues about the structure of the scene. We found the ability to freely vary the viewpoint very helpful to understand scenes where the 3D structure was not immediately apparent.

Fixed focus lenses. The lenses on our cameras are focused to about 60cm, the arm's length distance where the user performs manual work in a comfortable way. We roughly estimate the depth of field as ten centimeters. The user has to move his head into the right distance from the object to see it sharp. Yet, for the work on the surgical field the fixed focus may not be experienced as a limitation, especially for surgeons who are used to wearing magnifying binoculars with an even smaller depth of focus. Our HMD is also not completely immersive. The user can look past the miniature displays to the right and left and in particular to the bottom and have some direct view of the surroundings. The surgeon may take advantage of this direct view for example when he has to reach out for an instrument that is being handed to him.

Time delayed visual feedback. There is an intrinsic time delay between an actual event and its display on the HMD. The CCD chip in the video camera has to be exposed, the image data read out, converted to digital format, written into computer memory, transferred to texture memory, written into the framebuffer, and finally being displayed at the monitor's next refresh cycle. This whole process may take about 0.1 s, only a small, but noticeable delay. This time delay in the visual feedback makes precise control of fast movements difficult. In testing the use of surgical instruments guided by video vision, our surgeon collaborator (Rubino) saw the time delay as a most critical feature. He feels, though, that a surgeon can learn to adapt his technique to the slight time delay in the visual feedback.

3.2 Augmented Video View

Augmentation is the value we are adding to the video view, which alone would be inferior to the direct optical view. The usefulness of the augmented video view determines the usefulness of the system. Visualization and perception issues become important, as the goal is to provide the user with intuitive, task-oriented guidance. We list here some relevant issues.

Time lag between video and graphics. The user gets easily disturbed when, by moving his head, he sees the graphics lagging behind the real objects in the scene. Such a time lag is unavoidable in optical-see-through AR. Here the real scene changes instantaneously with the movement, but tracking the movement and rendering the graphics always takes a finite time. In our video-see-through system we delay the display of a video frame until the corresponding graphics is ready and thereby avoid the time lag completely. The graphics appears firmly anchored with respect to the real objects, what makes it easier for the user to follow the guidance.

Increased time delay of visual feedback. As we synchronize video and graphics to avoid time lag, we are adding the time required for tracking and graphics rendering to the overall delay of the visual feedback. Our tracking software takes only about 10ms to provide the pose information given the tracker camera image, which is not significant. However, when we rendered complex graphics we easily ended up delaying the final augmented image unacceptably long. Fortunately, the need to work with simple graphics matches well with the goal of providing intuitive guidance. The concentration on relevant information helps the user, whereas too much unnecessary detail may only confuse him.

Depth perception and occlusion depth cues. We have a simple experiment where the user is asked to touch the wick of a virtual candle with the tip of a (real) wooden wand. After getting used to the augmented view, most test persons are easily able to touch the correct point in space and light up a virtual fire.

The depth perception becomes more difficult, when real and virtual objects are overlapping in a way that does not reflect their correct spatial relationship. We know the viewer's vantagepoint and can make the graphics objects appear at the desired 3D locations. A correct visual interaction between real and graphics objects, however, would require 3D information about the real objects as well. This 3D information is usually not available, the graphics objects are simply superimposed onto the 2D image of the real scene. Real objects can be hidden by virtual objects, but not vice versa. This is the well-known occlusion problem in AR. It is very critical for applications like surgical guidance where the user needs to interact with the augmented scene.

For correct occlusion, one needs to obtain some 3D information of the real scene. We find, however, that one can reduce the disturbing effect of wrong occlusion cues significantly with appropriate rendering of the graphics. We show segmented structures not as solids, but as wire frames, not with thick lines but with thin lines, not opaque but semitransparent, not finely structured but coarsely structured where details are not important. Overall, we show only the relevant structures in a sparse representation.

3.3 Head Phantom Augmented with MR Data

Fig. 5 shows our styrofoam head phantom as it is inserted into a mock-up head frame. The head frame is equipped with a bridge of retroreflective markers. We can detect these markers with our head-mounted tracker camera and calculate the user's viewpoint with respect to the head frame. That enables us to show an augmented view of the head phantom with the video-see-through HMD.

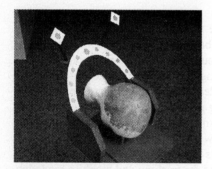
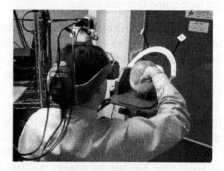

Fig. 5. Head phantom   **Fig. 6.** Testing the AR system.

For the augmentation, we segmented an MR data set that was taken with the Siemens OpenViva 0.2T magnet in UCLA's iMRI operating room. Figs 7 (a) and (b) are examples of two augmented views. In (a), the user sees - overlaid onto the head phantom - a set of yellow contour lines describing part of the skull, a blue wire frame model of the tumor, and one of the original MR slices. This view is helpful for studying the anatomy. In (b), the MR slice is omitted. This view is appropriate when the user wants to take action and, e.g., mark onto the head the outlines for a skin flap or craniotomy. Less graphics means less disturbance by the occlusion problem. One could even omit the skull contour lines, or at least limit their extent even further. The contour lines do not present essential anatomical information; they do support, though, the user's spatial perception of the scene. When looking at the pictures, one needs to bear in mind that the monoscopic images presented here cannot convey the user's actual experience. This experience is strongly determined and enhanced by the stereo vision.

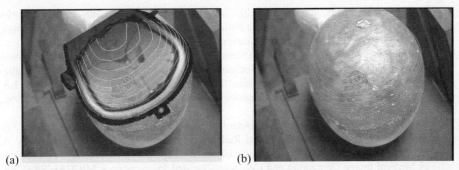

(a)   (b)

Fig. 7. Augmented views of the head phantom, showing skull contours and tumor. (a) with original MR slice, (b) without MR slice

Fig. 6 shows one of the authors examining the head phantom's augmented view. Seeing a model of the tumor in the tumor's actual location makes it very straightforward to plan appropriate access. The augmented vision supports craniotomy planning in a very intuitive and efficient way. From these initial experiences we feel strongly encouraged to move on to clinical tests. For critical cases, augmented reality guidance has the potential to become an important tool.

4   Conclusion and Future Plans

The initial evaluation of our AR system is very positive and encouraging. The head-mounted display – even though heavy and not very comfortable at present – gives the surgeon intuitive access to the structure of the anatomy. In a natural way he can explore the anatomy from various angles. Stereo and kinetic depth cues provide good 3D perception. Features that make our system particularly suited for medical applications are the high (XGA) resolution of the display, the elimination of time lag between video and graphics, and the low latency of the visual feedback of only about 0.1s.

We are currently preparing our system for use in UCLA's neurosurgical iMRI operating room [14]. Advanced augmented reality image guidance seems to be a good match with interventional MRI, where the surgical progress is monitored with a series of interoperative MR scans and the surgeon repeatedly has to map the new images onto his patient. We want to enable the surgeon to look at the surgical field and directly see e.g. the remaining parts of a tumor that still need to be resected. At first, we intend to use our system for skin flap and craniotomy planning, and then continue to explore further, more critical procedures.

References

1. M. Bajura, H. Fuchs, and R. Ohbuchi. "Merging Virtual Objects with the Real World: Seeing Ultrasound Imagery within the Patient." Proceedings of SIGGRAPH '92 (Chicago, IL, July 26-31, 1992). In Computer Graphics 26, #2 (July 1992): 203-210.
2. Andrei State, Mark A. Livingston, Gentaro Hirota, William F. Garrett, Mary C. Whitton, Henry Fuchs, and Etta D. Pisano, "Technologies for Augmented Reality Systems: realizing Ultrasound-Guided Needle Biopsies, " Proceed. of SIGGRAPH (New Orleans, LA, August 4-9, 1996), in Computer Graphics Proceedings, Annual Conference Series 1996, ACM SIGGRAPH, 439-446.
3. Henry Fuchs, Mark A. Livingston, Ramesh Raskar, D'nardo Colucci, Kurtis Keller, Andrei State, Jessica R. Crawford, Paul Rademacher, Samual H. Drake, and Anthony A. Meyer, MD, "Augmented Reality Visualization for Laparoscopic Surgery, " Proceedings of Medical Image Computing and Computer-Assisted Intervention – MICCAI '98 (Cambridge, MA, USA, October 11-13, 1998), 934-943.
4. W. Eric L. Grimson, Ron Kikinis, Ferenc A. Jolesz, and Peter McL. Black, "Image-Guided Surgery," Scientific American, June, 1999, 62-69.
5. P.J. Edwards, D.J. Hawkes, DLG Hill, D. Jewell, R. Spink, A. Strong, and M. Gleeson, "Augmentation of Reality in the Stereo Operating Microscope for Otolaryngology and Neurosurgical Guidance," Computer Aided Surgery 1:172-178, 1995.
6. King AP, Edwards PJ, Maurer CR, de Cunha DA, Gaston RP, Clarkson M, Hill DLG, Hawkes DJ, Fenlon MR, Strong AJ, Cox TCS, Gleeson, MJ, "Stereo augmented reality in the surgical microscope," Presence: Teleoperators and virtual environments 9:360-368 2000.
7. W. Birkfellner, K. Huber, F. Watzinger, M. Figl, F. Wanschitz, R. Hanel, D. Rafolt, R. Ewers, and H. Bergmann, "Development of the Varisocope AR, a See-through HMD for Computer-Aided Surgery," IEEE and ACM Int. Symp. On Augmented Reality – ISAR 2000 (Munich, Germany, October 5-6, 2000), pages 54-59.
8. F. Sauer, F. Wenzel, S. Vogt, Y.Tao, Y. Genc, and A. Bani-Hashemi, "Augmented Workspace: Designing an AR Testbed," IEEE and ACM Int. Symp. On Augmented Reality – ISAR 2000 (Munich, Germany, October 5-6, 2000), pages 47-53.
9. C. Maurer, F. Sauer, C. Brown, B. Hu, B. Bascle, B. Geiger, F. Wenzel, R. Maciunas, R. Bakos, A. Bani-Hashemi, "Augmented Reality Visualization of Brain Structures with Stereo and Kinetic Depth Cues: System Description and Initial Evaluation with Head Phantom," SPIE Int. Symp. on Medical Imaging 2001 (San Diego, CA, February 2001).
10. J.P.Rolland and H. Fuchs, "Optical versus Video See-Through Head-Mounted Displays in Medical Visualization," Presence (Massachusetts Institute of Technology), Vol. 9, No. 3, June 2000, pages 287-309.
11. A. Takagai, S. Yamazaki, Y. Saito, and N. Taniguchi, "Development of a Stereo Video-See-Though HMD for AR Systems," IEEE and ACM Int. Symp. On Augmented Reality – ISAR 2000 (Munich, Germany, October 5-6, 2000), pages 68-77.
12. Roger Y. Tsai, "A versatile Camera Calibration Technique for High-Accuracy 3D Machine Vision Metrology Using Off-the-Shelf TV Cameras and Lenses", IEEE Journal of Robotics and Automation, Vol. RA-3, No. 4, August 1987, pages 323-344.
13. http://www.cs.cmu.edu/~cil/v-source.html: freeware implementation of the Tsai algorithm.
14. G.J. Rubino, K. Farahani, D. McGill, B. Van de Wiele, J.P. Villablanca, A. Wang-Mathieson, "Magnetic resonce imaging-guided neurosurgery in the magnetic fringe fields: the next step in neuronavigation," Neurosurgery 2000; 46: 643-654.

Novel Algorithms for Robust Registration of Fiducials in CT and MRI

Sangyoon Lee[1], Gabor Fichtinger[2], and Gregory S. Chirikjian[1]

[1] Department of Mechanical Engineering
Johns Hopkins University, Baltimore, MD 21218, USA
{sanglee, gregc}@jhu.edu
[2] Center for Computer-Integrated Surgical Systems and Technology
Johns Hopkins University, Baltimore, MD 21218, USA
gabor@cs.jhu.edu

Abstract. In this paper we present several numerical algorithms for registering fiducials in planar CT or MRI images to their corresponding three-dimensional locations. The unique strength of these methods is their ability to robustly handle incomplete fiducials patterns, even in extreme cases when as much as one third of the fiducial data is missing from the images. We compare the effectiveness of these algorithms in terms of flops and robustness on actual CT data sets.

1 Introduction

Our primary objective in this paper is to present robust numerical methods for registration of rigid-body fiducials to the CT/MRI image space with the use of a single image slice. A key feature of our methods is that they guarantee reliable registration in situations when conventional methods commonly fail. Our secondary objective is to make these methods applicable to a plurality of conceivable fiducial patterns, without the need for algorithmic refinement or modification.

The primary cause of a failure to register an image slice is a situation when only part of the rigid body fiducial shows up in the resulting image, thus not providing sufficient input data for the registration algorithm. This problem occurs quite frequently during frame-based radiosurgery and neurosurgical planning, when an image slice does not cut across the entire headframe. Thus, only some, but not all, of the fiducial rods are visible in the image. In robotically assisted surgery the end-effector of a robot can be registered to the scanner from a single image slice using a small rigid body fiducial. Most intuitively, a miniature version of a stereotactic head frame is used [8]. Incomplete data tend to be a chronic problem in these systems because it is common for the robot to accidentally move the fiducial frame out of the field of view, causing the image slice to become incomplete for registration. Traditional methods cannot handle this problem without taking extra images, which is not an acceptable solution.

Image guided robots must often work in tight spaces like inside the gantry of a CT or even inside the patient's body, where there is no room for a conventional

W. Niessen and M. Viergever (Eds.): MICCAI 2001, LNCS 2208, pp. 717–724, 2001.
© Springer-Verlag Berlin Heidelberg 2001

fiducial device composed from a triplet of V-or N-shaped planar motifs. Worse yet, every time when a new fiducial design is introduced, a new registration algorithm and new image processing software has to be developed. Our goal was to devise a method that can cope with an arbitrary pattern of fiducial lines. In this generic scenario, conventional fiducial devices like the BRW [1] or Kelly [2] headframes are uniformly handled, and incomplete scans also fit in the framework. As a byproduct of our robustness analysis, we obtained practical limits for the incompleteness of images (see Section 4).

Stereotactic head frames have been in use for over two decades. Initial applications were intra-cranial neurosurgery and radiosurgery [1, 2, 3]. The methodology has been further extended for extra-cranial radiotherapy applications [4, 5, 6, 7], and then recently for robotically assisted surgery [8]. Popular registration algorithms follow the theme described by Brown [1] and many years later by Susil [8]. Those authors calculate one corresponding point of the image plane from each of the three N-shaped motifs, and reconstruct the image plane from those three calculated points. The main weaknesses of this approach are (1) the inability to handle incomplete patterns when not all fiducial rods leave marks in the image and (2) the inconvenience that the computer software has to be "reinvented" every time the geometry and/or shape of fiducial motifs are modified. Zylka et al. [9] assumed all the image slices have been computed without motion of the head frame between image slices (all slices were parallel), and they registered the lines from the 3D chunk of image data to the head-frame. They, however, did not solve the problem of registering planar point patterns to lines in space, therefore their approach is not applicable to single sliced based registration.

The mathematical problem in this paper is basically to register a planar image in space, given a set of n known lines in space, given a pattern of n points in a plane, and given a correspondence between the lines and points. The geometrical configuration of lines and image plane is displayed in Figure 1.

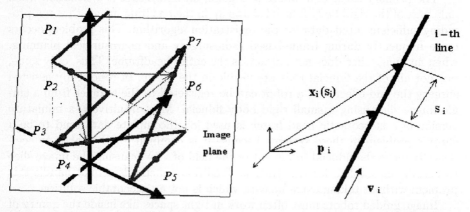

Figure 1: Intersection of image plane.   Figure 2: Parameters of a line.

While the problem of registering one set of points to another has received a lot of attention (see [10] and references therein), the general problem of registering points to lines has not been studied as extensively.

There are two variants on this problem that are addressed here. In the first, we are interested in finding the equation of the plane. If we know this, then the planar registration of one planar set of points to the other can be performed afterwards. In the second formulation of the problem, a frame of reference is attached to the intersecting plane, and we solve for the position and orientation of this frame in three-dimensional space. Hence, in the first approach two three-parameter problems are solved sequentially, while in the second approach one six-parameter problem is solved. We refer to these as the 3×2 and 6×1 approaches, respectively. We present several algorithms for each of these approaches.

2   Algorithms for the 3×2 Approach

2.1   Algorithm 1: Solving a System of Polynomials

The problem can be solved by simultaneously satisfying $n(n-1)/2$ constraint equations (n is the number of lines) of the form in (1)

$$\|\mathbf{x}_i(s_i) - \mathbf{x}_j(s_j)\|^2 = d_{ij}^2. \tag{1}$$

In general, this problem is overdetermined, so only an approximate solution is possible. As shown in Figure 2, $\mathbf{x}_i(s_i)$ is a position vector of a point on the i-th line which is defined by the position $\mathbf{p_i}$ and unit direction of $\mathbf{v_i}$. s_i is the arc length from $\mathbf{p_i}$ to $\mathbf{x}_i(s_i)$ and d_{ij} is the Euclidean distance between $\mathbf{x}_i(s_i)$ and $\mathbf{x}_j(s_j)$.

This set of equations will in general be a second-order polynomial in s_i and s_j of the form:

$$s_i^2 - 2s_i s_j \cos\theta_{ij} + s_j^2 + a_{ij}s_i + b_{ij}s_j = d_{ij}^2 + c_{ij}.$$

The constants a_{ij}, b_{ij}, θ_{ij}, and c_{ij} all come from the geometry of the problem and $\cos\theta_{ij} = \mathbf{v_i} \cdot \mathbf{v_j}$.

The approach we take to solve the system of polynomials is to iteratively solve the system by assuming that each of the parameters can vary with "artificial" time. We make an initial guess $s_i(0)$ (in practice this guess corresponds to the plane whose normal is the axis of the head frame with value of c_{ij} that causes this plane to cut the head frame in half).

Then we take the time derivative to get

$$2s_i\dot{s}_i - 2(\dot{s}_i s_j + s_i\dot{s}_j)\cos\theta_{ij} + 2s_j\dot{s}_j + a_{ij}\dot{s}_i + b_{ij}\dot{s}_j = 2d_{ij}\dot{d}_{ij}. \tag{2}$$

The right-hand-side follows from the fact that c_{ij} is a constant.

We can assemble the $n(n-1)/2$ equations of the form in (2) as

$$J(\mathbf{s})\dot{\mathbf{s}} = \mathbf{w}. \tag{3}$$

The problem does not dictate the behavior of $\dot{d}_{ij}$ in the mathematical model. However, if we specify

$$\dot{d}_{ij} = (d_{ij})_{measured} - d_{ij},$$

where $(d_{ij})_{measured}$ denotes the Euclidean distance between the i-th and j-th fiducial points on image plane, then iterating (3) with the simple update rule

$$\mathbf{s}(t + \Delta t) = \mathbf{s}(t) + \Delta t (J^T J)^{-1} J^T \mathbf{w}(t),$$

converges to the solution as long as $\det(J^T J) \neq 0$ for all values of $\mathbf{s}$ encountered during the iterations. Since s_i values determine $\mathbf{x}_i(s_i)$, we can establish the equation of the plane.

2.2   Algorithm 2: Look Up Table

Of course in practice, there is no need to perform the computations described in Algorithm 1 in real time. This algorithm can be used off line to define a look-up table. Given a table of s_i values defined on equally spaced values of d_{ij}, the corresponding values of s_i can be interpolated from the look-up table and the measured values of d_{ij}.

3   Algorithms for the 6×1 Approach

3.1   Algorithm 1: Rate-Linearization of Position and Orientation

Given the line defined by the position $\mathbf{p_i}$ and unit direction vector $\mathbf{v_i}$, and a point in space $\mathbf{x_i}$, we calculate the Euclidean distance between the line and point by minimizing the cost function

$$c(s) = \|(\mathbf{p} + s\mathbf{v}) - \mathbf{x}\|^2 = \|\mathbf{p} - \mathbf{x}\|^2 + 2s\mathbf{v} \cdot (\mathbf{p} - \mathbf{x}) + s^2.$$

Setting $dc/ds = 0$, we see that the minimizing value of s is $s_{min} = -\mathbf{v} \cdot (\mathbf{p} - \mathbf{x})$, and so the vector pointing from $\mathbf{x}$ to the closest point on the line is

$$\mathbf{h} = (\mathbf{p} - \mathbf{x}) - [\mathbf{v} \cdot (\mathbf{p} - \mathbf{x})]\mathbf{v},$$

which we can write as $\mathbf{h} = (\mathbf{p} - \mathbf{x}) - \mathbf{v}\mathbf{v}^T(\mathbf{p} - \mathbf{x}) = [\mathbb{1} - \mathbf{v}\mathbf{v}^T](\mathbf{p} - \mathbf{x})$.

We can formulate the problem as finding the rigid-body trajectory $(R(t), \mathbf{b}(t))$ such that $\mathbf{x}_i(t) = R(t)\mathbf{y}_i + \mathbf{b}(t)$ drives each of the vectors

$$[\mathbb{1} - \mathbf{v_i}\mathbf{v_i^T}](\mathbf{p_i} - \mathbf{x_i}(t)) = \boldsymbol{\delta}(t) \tag{4}$$

to zero, where $\mathbf{y}_i$ denotes the coordinates of i-th fiducial in the image plane. If this can be accomplished, it means that each of the fiducials is driven to its corresponding element of the three-dimensional cage.

Note that the matrix $[\mathbb{1} - \mathbf{v}\mathbf{v}^T]$ is not invertible since $\|\mathbf{v}\| = 1$ implies that the matrix $\mathbf{v}\mathbf{v}^T$ has an eigenvalue equal to one corresponding to eigenvector $\mathbf{v}$.

Making the substitution $\mathbf{x}_i(t) = R(t)\mathbf{y}_i + \mathbf{b}(t)$ in (4) and rearranging terms we see that

$$[\mathbb{1} - \mathbf{v}_i\mathbf{v}_i^T]\mathbf{p}_i - [\mathbb{1} - \mathbf{v}_i\mathbf{v}_i^T](R\mathbf{y}_i + \mathbf{b}) = \boldsymbol{\delta}_i(t).$$

We now take the derivative of both sides with respect to artificial time, and observe that $\mathbf{p}_i$ and $\mathbf{v}_i$ are constant vectors. If in addition we observe that

$$\dot{R}\mathbf{y}_i = \dot{R}R^T R\mathbf{y}_i = \boldsymbol{\omega} \times (R\mathbf{y}_i) = -(R\mathbf{y}_i) \times \boldsymbol{\omega}$$

where $\boldsymbol{\omega} = \text{vect}(\dot{R}R^T)$, then we can write

$$[\mathbb{1} - \mathbf{v}_i\mathbf{v}_i^T][\text{matr}(R\mathbf{y}_i), -\mathbb{1}][\boldsymbol{\omega}^T, \dot{\mathbf{b}}^T]^T = \dot{\boldsymbol{\delta}}_i. \qquad (5)$$

Here matr( ) denotes that for a vector $\mathbf{z}$, matr($\mathbf{z}$) is the skew symmetric matrix such that matr($\mathbf{z}$)$\mathbf{x} = (\mathbf{z}) \times \mathbf{x}$. In other words, vect(matr($\mathbf{z}$)) = ($\mathbf{z}$).

If we force $\dot{\boldsymbol{\delta}}_i$ to zero by defining

$$\dot{\boldsymbol{\delta}}_i = -\alpha\boldsymbol{\delta}_i$$

for some positive constant α, then $\boldsymbol{\omega}$ and $\dot{\mathbf{b}}$ can be solved for at each value of time along the way by inverting the over constrained system resulting from concatenating (5) for $i = 1, 2, ..., n$. Once this is done, the values of $\mathbf{b}(t)$ and $R(t)$ can be updated using the rules

$$\mathbf{b}(t + \Delta t) = \mathbf{b}(t) + \Delta t\dot{\mathbf{b}}(t)$$

and

$$R(t + \Delta t) = [\mathbb{1} + \Delta t\,\text{matr}(\boldsymbol{\omega})(t))]R(t).$$

Since the rotational updates have the potential to cause $R(t)$ to stray from being a rotation matrix, the occasional renormalization

$$R(t) \rightarrow R(t)(R^T(t)R(t))^{-1}$$

may be required. This step could be replaced by finding the Euler angles or Cayley parameters that best approximate $R(t)$, then replace $R(t)$ with the resulting rotation matrix.

We note that if the actual rotation matrix is close to being the identity matrix (as will be the case when the image plane is close to cutting the cage straight on), then only one iteration may be required.

3.2   Algorithm 2: Minimization over Position, Orientation, and Arc Lengths

Given the coordinates $\{\mathbf{y}_i\}$ of fiducials in the image plane, we can simultaneously solve for the position and orientation of a reference frame attached to the image plane and the arc lengths $\{s_i\}$ as follows.

We observe that

$$\mathbf{p}_i + s_i\mathbf{v}_i = R\mathbf{y}_i + \mathbf{b}. \qquad (6)$$

Let us assume that we have an initial guess of the orientation of the frame attached to the image plane, and that the actual orientation is not very different than this initial guess. Then we write

$$R = R_0(\mathbb{1} + \Omega).$$

Here $\Omega = -\Omega^T$ has entries that are small. The vector $\boldsymbol{\omega}$ is defined such that

$$\boldsymbol{\omega} \times \mathbf{x} = \Omega \mathbf{x}$$

for any $\mathbf{x} \in \mathbb{R}^3$, This means we can rewrite (6) as

$$\mathbf{p}_i = -s_i \mathbf{v}_i + R_0 \mathbf{y}_i - R_0(\mathbf{y}_i \times \boldsymbol{\omega}) + \mathbf{b}.$$

By defining Y_i to be the matrix such that $Y_i \mathbf{x} = \mathbf{y}_i \times \mathbf{x}$ for every $\mathbf{x} \in \mathbb{R}^3$, it follows that we can write the following linear equation:

$$\mathbf{p}_i - R_0 \mathbf{y}_i = [\mathbf{0}, ..., \mathbf{0}, -\mathbf{v}_i, \mathbf{0}, ..., \mathbf{0}, -R_0 Y_i, \mathbb{1}] \begin{bmatrix} \mathbf{s} \\ \boldsymbol{\omega} \\ \mathbf{b} \end{bmatrix}$$

where

$$\mathbf{s} = [0, ..., 0, s_i, 0, ..., 0]^T.$$

Stacking these equations on top of each other for $i = 1, ..., n$ results in a system of $(3n) \times (n + 6)$ scalar equations in $n + 6$ parameters (n arc lengths and 6 rigid-body motion parameters). This can be solved in the least-squares sense using a pseudo-inverse.

4   Numerical Results and Experimental Data

The algorithms that are described in the previous sections are applied to real CT data. Among commonly used stereotactic devices, the BRW and Kelly frames are used. The comparison of the algorithms is made in terms of the number of flops and the robustness. We use 44 and 9 image slices which are acquired from the BRW frame and the Kelly frame, respectively.

It is observed that the application of algorithm 1 for the 3×2 approach generates convergent s_i values. Figure 3 demonstrates the convergence of s_i values for an image slice from the Kelly frame. It is also observed that the error converges to zero as the number of iterations increases in algorithm 1 for the 3×2 approach and algorithms 1 and 2 for the 6×1 approach. Figure 4 displays the convergence of error to zero for an image slice from the BRW frame in the application of the algorithm 1 for the 6×1 approach.

The numbers in Table 1 are the average value of the results for all the tested image slices. It is observed that algorithm 1 for the 3×2 approach is superior to the other algorithms in terms of flops. Table 1 also demonstrates the comparison of algorithms 1 and 2 for the 3×2 approach. Three-dimensional linear interpolation is used in the look-up table algorithm. Interestingly, $1mm$ and $0.1mm$

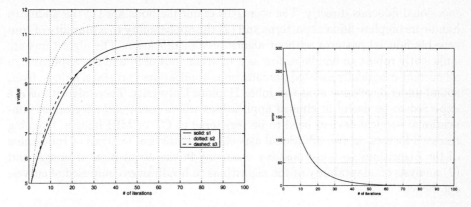

Figure 3: s_i **values vs. No. of iterations.   Figure 4: error vs No. of iterations.**

Table 1. Comparison of algorithms in terms of flops end error

algorithms	flops	comparison to 9 rod case (100 %)			
		8 rods	7 rods	6 rods	5 rods
algorithm 1 for 3×2	24126	99.8617	99.7742	99.5636	99.0888
algorithm 2 for 3×2	61504				
algorithm 1 for 6×1	332113	99.8997	99.8963	99.3482	98.4203
algorithm 2 for 6×1	455384	99.8640	99.8529	99.6326	98.6278

increments in d_{ij} result nearly the same accuracy. Due to limited disk space and time for the generation of the table, a $50 \times 50 \times 50$ table is used. The look-up table algorithm does not show advantage in flops despite a small size of table, thus we omitted this method from further testing.

We tested the robustness of three algorithms to missing fiducial marks. Theoretically, as few as 3 slanted rods for the Kelly frame and 4 rods for the BRW frame are necessary to reach convergence. However, in real surgical cases we have never observed less than 6 marks when using such frames. All those three algorithms are found stable with 8,7,6 and even 5 markers. Table 1 shows that less than 1.6 % difference in parameter values is found between cases where all 9 markers are used and only 5 markers are used. The best performing method in this aspect too was algorithm 1 for the 3×2 approach.

5 Summary and Conclusions

In this paper we have presented a number of different techniques for determining the spatial location of fiducial features in planar images. The two broad categories of algorithms that we developed are classified according to (1) whether they first seek the parameters describing the image plane, and then register within that plane or (2) whether they register the planar points to the three di-

724   S. Lee, G. Fichtinger, and G.S. Chirikjian

mensional fiducials directly. The strengths of our methods are (1) the ability to handle incomplete fiducial patterns and (2) the applicability to a plurality of conceivable fiducial patterns without algorithmic modification. The algorithms are sufficiently robust to handle as few as 6 fiducials (out of 9) and are applicable in all current robotically assisted percutaneous applications (prostate, kidney, liver, spine) under development at the Johns Hopkins University. These algorithms are expected to be useful in clinical applications where robot end-effectors or conventional surgical devices need to be registered to CT or MRI images. Ongoing research focuses on two additional aspects: (1) statistical analysis of robustness of the algorithms to noise possibly occurring in the acquisition of image; and (2) analysis of adaptability of the algorithms to headframes composed of curves, e.g. helices.

References

[1] Brown R. A., Roberts T. S., and Osborne A. G., "Stereotactic frame and computer software for CT-directed neurosurgical localization," *Invest. Radiol.*, Vol. 15, pp. 308-312, 1980.
[2] Goers S., et al, "A computed tomographic stereotactic adaptation system," *Neurosurgery*, Vol. 10, pp. 375-379, 1982.
[3] Leksell L. and Jerenberg B., "Stereotaxis and tomography: a technical note," *Acta Neurochir*, Vol. 52, pp. 1-7, 1980.
[4] Lax I, et al. "Stereotactic radiotherapy of malignancies in the abdomen. Methodological aspects.," *Acta Oncol.*, Vol. 33, No. 6, pp.677-83, 1994.
[5] Takacs I and Hamilton AJ, "Extracranial stereotactic radiosurgery: applications for the spine and beyond," *Neurosurg Clin N Am*, Vol. 10, No. 2, pp.257-70, April 1999.
[6] Lohr F, et al., "Noninvasive patient fixation for extracranial stereotactic radiotherapy," *Int J Radiat Oncol Biol Phys*, Vol. 45, No. 2, pp. 521-7, September 1999.
[7] Erdi Y., Wessels B., DeJager R., Erdi A., et al., "A new fiducial alignment system to overlay abdominal CT or MR images with radiolabeled antibody SPECT scans," *Cancer*, 73 (3 Suppl), pp. 923-931, 1994.
[8] R. Susil, J. Anderson, R. Taylor, " A single image registration method for CT guided interventions," *Proceedings to MICCAI'99, Lecture notes in Computer Science*, Vol. 1679, pp 798-808, Springer 1999.
[9] Zylka W, Sabczynski J, Schmitz G, "A Gaussian approach for the calculation of the accuracy of stereotactic frame systems," *Medical Physics*, Vol. 26, No. 3, pp. 381-391, March 1999.
[10] Chirikjian, G.S., Kyatkin, A.B., *Engineering Applications of Noncommutative Harmonic Analysis*, CRC Press, October 2000.

Automatic 3D Registration of Lung Surfaces in Computed Tomography Scans

Margrit Betke, PhD[1], Harrison Hong, BA[1], and Jane P. Ko, MD[2]

[1] Computer Science Department
Boston University,
Boston, MA 02215, USA
betke@cs.bu.edu
http://www.cs.bu.edu/faculty/betke
[2] Department of Radiology
New York University Medical School
New York, NY 10016, USA

Abstract. We developed an automated system that registers chest CT images temporally. Our registration method matches corresponding anatomical landmarks to obtain initial registration parameters. The initial point-to-point registration is then generalized to an iterative surface-to-surface registration method. Our "goodness-of-fit" measure is evaluated at each step in the iterative scheme until the registration performance is sufficient. We applied our method to register the 3D lung surfaces of 10 pairs of chest CT scans and report a promising registration performance.[1]

1 Introduction

Chest computed tomography (CT) has become a well-established means of diagnosing pulmonary metastasis of oncology patients and evaluating response to treatment regimens. Since diagnosis and prognosis of cancer generally depend upon growth assessment, repeated CT studies are used to determine growth rates of pulmonary nodules. Chest CT is currently being evaluated as a method for screening for lung cancer. Lung cancer remains the leading cause of cancer death in the United States, killing 160,000 people a year. The overall 5-year survival rate is 15%, but early detection and resection can improve the prognosis significantly. For example, the 5-year survival rate for Stage I cancer is 67% [13].

Our long-term objective is to develop an image analysis system that assists the radiologist in detecting and comparing pulmonary nodules in repeated CT studies in a clinical setting. Such a system must solve the classical problems in medical image analysis – segmentation, detection, and registration – for the important domain of chest CT images. References [4] and [10] describe our preliminary system. It automatically segments the thorax, lungs, and structures

---

[1] The support of the Office of Naval Research, National Science Foundation, Radiological Society of North America, and the Whitaker Foundation is gratefully acknowledged.

within the lungs, and detects nodules in axial chest CT images. Human intervention is needed to match up the studies. In the current paper, we focus on automating the registration task. In particular, we describe a method for automatic three-dimensional (3D) alignment of lung surfaces in repeated CT scans.

A large body of literature has been published on registration techniques [1, 2, 3, 6, 7, 8, 9, 11, 14, 15]. Here we can only point to some approaches that are most closely related to our work, e.g., approaches that use anatomical landmarks for registration [7], register points to points [8] or surfaces [2, 11], and correlate subimages [1]. Often only a small misalignment of the images is assumed [1]. Other registration methods require some manual input to compensate for rotational and translational differences between two studies [14]. Earlier surveys on registration are [6, 15].

Medical registration techniques have primarily been developed for the brain. Registration of chest radiographs has been addressed by Kano et al. [9]. To the best of our knowledge, an automated system to register chest CT images temporally has not been developed yet. Registration of thoracic CT studies is challenging, since patient position varies each time a study is taken in terms of differences in torso rotation and translation. Differences in inspiratory volumes between two studies are other obstacles to registration.

In this work, the lung surfaces of two CT scans were segmented and registered for 10 patients. We first describe an automatic landmark-based registration method, then generalize it to surface-to-surface registration, and improve it with an iterative algorithm, which extends Besl's registration scheme [2]. Finally, we report and discuss the registration results for the 10 pairs of chest CT scans.

2   Methods

Registration of Anatomical Landmarks. Registration techniques determine the *absolute orientation* of one data set with respect to the other. The 3D coordinates of corresponding points in the two different data sets are known. For our 3D data sets, it is difficult to establish the anatomical correspondence of voxels, even for a human observer. We therefore use the voxels that make up anatomical landmarks for our initial registration method. We do not use external fiduciary markers, which would be impractical in a clinical setting.

Bones are rigid anatomical features that can be registered reliably. In particular, the sternum and vertebrae are excellent anatomical landmarks, because their positions are relatively fixed within the chest. We also use the trachea as an anatomical landmark. Although the position and shape of the trachea change with respiration, the trachea centroid serves as a reliable landmark for registration of our data sets. Finally, we also tested the use of structures within the lungs, for example nodules, for registration. Figure 1 shows how the centroids of sternum, trachea, and a nodule in the left lung are registered in corresponding axial images of two CT data sets.

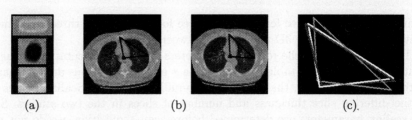

(a)   (b)   (c).

Fig. 1. (a) Template images of the sternum, trachea, and spine. (b) Corresponding CT images in two studies. The landmarks are the centroids of the sternum, trachea, and a nodule in the left lung. (c) The light grey test points in study 2 must be matched to the white model points in study 1. The best transformation of the test points is shown in dark grey.

Correlation-Based Recognition of Anatomical Features. We use template images of anatomical landmarks, such as sternum, vertebra, and trachea shown in Fig. 1, to detect these landmarks in our test data. The template images are created offline by manually cropping subimages of the features out of a training data set. Although the features look slightly different in the test data, training and test data generally match well. This is particularly true if we use a deformable template that can be scaled or rotated.

Let $\mathbf{a}$ describe the affine parameters position, scale, and rotation of the template. We use the normalized correlation coefficient to find the best estimate of the affine parameters. In our previous work [5], we showed when the statistically optimal estimator for the affine parameters takes the form of the normalized correlation coefficient. It quantifies how well the measured data in subimage $I_q(x, y)$ matches the template feature in $q(x, y; \mathbf{a})$. The normalized correlation coefficient is defined by $r(\mathbf{a}) = 1/(\sigma_I(\mathbf{a})\sigma_q(\mathbf{a})(A(\mathbf{a})\sum_{(x,y)\in O} I_q(x,y)q(x,y;\mathbf{a}) - m_I(\mathbf{a})m_q(\mathbf{a}))$, where $m_I(\mathbf{a}) = \sum I_q(x,y)$ and $m_q(\mathbf{a}) = \sum q(x,y;\mathbf{a})$ are the respective local image means, $\sigma_I^2(\mathbf{a}) = A(\mathbf{a})\sum I_q(x,y)^2 - (\sum I_q(x,y))^2$ and $\sigma_q^2(\mathbf{a}) = A(\mathbf{a})\sum q(x,y;\mathbf{a})^2 - (\sum q(x,y;\mathbf{a}))^2$ are the respective local variances, and where the sums are computed over a region O that is the union of all pixels that contain the expected feature and $A = |O|$ is the number of pixels in O.

The ambiguity surfaces for the position estimates of anatomical features have global peaks with correlations of at least 0.8, which lie far above the expected correlation $E[r(\mathbf{a})] = 0$. In addition, once a feature, such as the trachea, is found in some axial image, the search space for the same feature in subsequent images can be reduced significantly. In addition, we update the template feature q automatically online with the cropped image of the detected feature in the previous slice. This results in high correlations (≥ 0.9) and reliable estimates of feature position and size.

Three-Dimensional Affine Point-to-Point Registration. Given a voxel $\mathbf{x}$ in study 1 and a voxel $\mathbf{p}$ in study 2, the general 3D affine transformation $\mathbf{x} = \mathbf{Ap} + \mathbf{x_0}$ maps $\mathbf{p}$ into $\mathbf{x}$, where the 3×3 matrix $\mathbf{A}$ can be expressed in terms

of nine parameters, three for rotation, three for scaling, and three for skewing.
Vector $\mathbf{x_0}$ describes the 3D translation between $\mathbf{x}$ and $\mathbf{p}$.

In our application, the rotation parameters model the orientation of the patient's body on the CT table. Scaling in the x and y dimensions models changes in the field-of-view, i.e., the pixel-width-to-millimeter ratio. Scaling in z is due to the differing slice thickness and number of slices in the two studies. Since the scaling parameters are determined before scan acquisition, we do not need to invert for the scaling parameters. We assume that the CT scanner does not introduce skewing and preserves the Cartesian coordinates of 3D points. Then the problem of finding the general affine transformation reduces to finding the rigid-body transformation after the 2 studies have been adjusted for scaling differences. The rigid-body transformation $\mathcal{T}$ maps $\mathbf{p}$ into $\mathbf{x}$,

$$\mathbf{x} = \mathcal{T}(\mathbf{p}) = \mathbf{R}\mathbf{p} + \mathbf{x_0}, \tag{1}$$

where the orthonormal 3×3 matrix $\mathbf{R}$ rotates $\mathbf{p}$ into vector $\mathbf{R}\mathbf{p}$, which is then shifted into $\mathbf{x}$ by translation vector $\mathbf{x_0}$. We have 12 unknowns (9 matrix coefficients and 3 translation parameters) and only 3 linear equations. So we need at least 4 corresponding points to compute the unknown transformation parameters. If we impose the orthonormality condition, we obtain an additional equation and therefore only need 3 corresponding points.

Since there may be errors in the measurement of the points or in the corresponding landmark detection algorithm, a greater accuracy in determining the transformation parameters can be obtained if more than three points are used. Given a set X of n points $\mathbf{x_1}, \ldots, \mathbf{x_n}$ in study 1 and a set P of corresponding points $\mathbf{p_1}, \ldots, \mathbf{p_n}$ in study 2, we minimize the sum of square residual errors

$$\sum_{i=1}^{n} \|\mathbf{e}_i\|^2 = \sum_{i=1}^{n} \|\mathbf{x}_i - \mathcal{T}(\mathbf{p}_i)\|^2 = \sum_{i=1}^{n} \|\mathbf{x}_i - \mathbf{R}\mathbf{p}_i - \mathbf{x_0}\|^2 \tag{2}$$

with respect to the unknowns $\mathbf{R}$ and $\mathbf{x_0}$. A closed-form optimal solution to this least-squares problem was given by Horn [8]. The best translation vector $\hat{\mathbf{x}}_0$ is the difference between the centroid $\bar{\mathbf{x}} = 1/n \sum_{i=1}^{n} \mathbf{x}_i$ of point set X and the centroid $\bar{\mathbf{p}} = 1/n \sum_{i=1}^{n} \mathbf{p}_i$ of point set P rotated by rotation $\mathbf{R}$:

$$\mathbf{x_0} = \bar{\mathbf{x}} - \mathbf{R}(\bar{\mathbf{p}}). \tag{3}$$

Therefore, the translation can be computed easily once the rotation is found. To find the rotation, the coordinates of voxels in X and P are converted into coordinates of voxels in X' and P' of coordinate systems that are originated at the respective centroids, e.g., $\mathbf{x_i'} = \mathbf{x_i} - \bar{\mathbf{x}}$ for all $\mathbf{x_i} \in X$. This reduces the least-squares problem of Eq. 2 to a minimization of $\sum_{i=1}^{n} \|\mathbf{x}_i' - \mathbf{R}\mathbf{p}_i'\|^2 = \sum_{i=1}^{n} \|\mathbf{x}_i'\|^2 - 2\sum_{i=1}^{n} \mathbf{x}_i'^T \mathbf{R}\mathbf{p}_i' + \sum_{i=1}^{n} \|\mathbf{p}_i'\|^2$ with respect to rotation $\mathbf{R}$ only, or $\max_{\mathbf{R}} \sum_{i=1}^{n} \mathbf{x}_i'^T \mathbf{R}\mathbf{p}_i'$. The solution of this maximization problem is given by a unit quaternion (see details in [8, 3]). In Fig. 1, the centroids of the sternum, trachea, and a nodule in study 1, shown in white, are registered to the corresponding centroids in study 2, shown in light grey. The registration results are shown in dark grey.

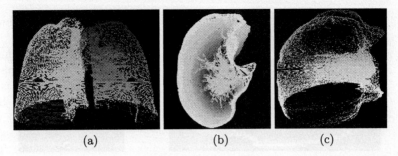

(a)   (b)   (c)

Fig. 2. 3D visualization of the lung. (a) Coronal view of both lungs, (b) top-down axial view of the right lung, and (c) wire-frame visualization of the right lung.

Three-Dimensional Affine Shape Registration. In this paper, we focus on lung border surfaces that are segmented from the full 3D data set using the method described in our ealier work [10, 4]. Figure 2 visualizes lung surfaces segmented from a low-dose CT scan. Our goal is to register such a surface to the lung surface of the same patient that is imaged at a later time.

The point-to-point registration algorithm described above assumes that the correspondence between points has been established. For certain points, e.g., the centroids of the sternum in corresponding axial slices, correspondence can be determined with relatively high confidence, but the correspondences of other point pairs are not as easily established. For example, a lung border point in the apex of study 1 corresponds to *some* border point in the apex of study 2, but *which* point generally cannot be determined, even by a human observer. We therefore define the correspondence C of two points on different surfaces by their distance. In particular, test point $\mathbf{p}_i$ corresponds to model point $\mathbf{x}_j = C(\mathbf{p}_i)$, if their Euclidean distance is the shortest among all distances between $\mathbf{p}_i$ and any point in X, i.e., $C(\mathbf{p}_i) = \mathbf{x}_j$, for which $\|\mathbf{x}_j - \mathbf{p}_i\| = \min_{\mathbf{x}_k \in X} \|\mathbf{x}_k - \mathbf{p}_i\|$. With this definition, we can match two surfaces that contain a different number of voxels.

The computed correspondences are reliable if the two data sets are close to each other, in particular, if they have been registered. This creates a paradoxical situation: we would like to register corresponding points, but need to register them first in order to establish their correspondences. To resolve this situation, we solve the registration and correspondence problems concurrently, an approach proposed by Besl [2]. We first detect anatomical landmarks in studies 1 and 2 and compute the 3D affine transformation that registers them optimally. We then segment the lungs [10, 4] and register them with the transformation parameters computed for the landmark registration. We establish correspondences by computing the Euclidean distances between all point pairs of the two data sets, register the transformed lung borders in study 2 to the lung borders in study 1, compute the new correspondences and error, and then iterate. Once the error is sufficiently small, the process is terminated. Note that this process does not guarantee that corresponding points are the same physical point.

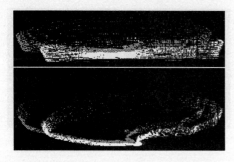
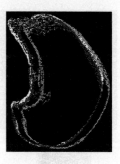

Fig. 3. Visualization of the 3D registration of 10 left lung border curves with views from the lung's side (top left), bottom (bottom left), and top (right). Points in study 2 (light grey) are registered to points in study 1 (white) by a transformation that maps them into points shown in dark grey. The registration error is minimal.

Function `LungRegistration` takes as inputs 3D voxel data sets `CTstudy1` and `CTstudy1` that have been adjusted for field-of-view differences, and a parameter `threshold` that is used to decide when the function can terminate with a sufficient registration result. It outputs the transformation parameters for translation and rotation. For its function calls, we use C-style notation to distinguish input parameters, e.g., in line 5, `lung1`, from parameters that change during the function call, e.g., `&lungR`, `&translation`.

```
1 Function LungRegistration (CTstudy1, CTstudy2, threshold) {
2    DetectLandmarks(&landmarks1, &landmarks2);
3    RegisterLandmarks(landmarks1, landmarks2, &translation, &rotation);
4    SegmentLungs(CTstudy1, CTstudy2, &lung1, &lung2);
5    RegisterLungsInitially(lung1, lung2, translation, rotation, &lungR);
6    ComputeCorrespondencesAndError(lung1, lungR, &error);
7    while (error > threshold) {
8       RegisterLungs(lung1, &lungR, &translation, &rotation);
9       ComputeCorrespondencesAndError(lung1, lungR, &error); }
10   OutputResults(translation, rotation); }
```

3   Results

Ten patients with cancer diagnoses and pulmonary nodules were selected, who had two thoracic CT scans for clinical indications between 1993 and 2001. A total of 20 CT studies was evaluated. Fourteen chest CT scans had been performed helically on GE HiSpeed Advantage machines. The scans were obtained from the lung apices through the adrenal glands using a 1:1 pitch either with $5mm$ collimation for the entire study or $10mm$ collimation with $5mm$ collimation through the hila. Six studies were taken on a multi-helical Siemens Somatom Volume Zoom CT and reconstructed in 1.0 mm intervals. The landmarks used for the

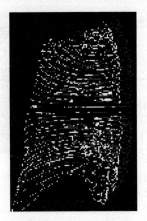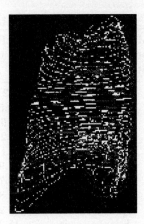

Fig. 4. On the left, wire models of the right lung for study 1 (grey) and study 2 (white). On the right, the transformed lung surface of study 2 (white). It matches well with the lung surface of study 1 (grey).

initial registration are the centroids of the trachea at the apex and just above the carina, and of the sternum and vertebra also in the slice above the carina. We evaluated the results quantitatively with the sum-squared-differences (SSD) measure (Eq. 2) and qualitatively by visual inspection. Table 1 summarizes the results. Using a fixed length of 25 iterations, the registration error was reduced up to 86% of the initial error. We also registered CT scans based on corresponding vessel landmarks that a radiologist identified and report the differences in registration results between human and computer. Visual inspection of the 3D lung registration results in Figs. 3 and 4 shows that the measured and computed points match well and confirms the results of our quantitative error analysis.

4   Discussion and Conclusions

To overcome the need of human intervention in our preliminary system [10, 4], we developed an automatic 3D registration method that matches the lung surfaces in repeated CT studies. Our results for 10 pairs of CT scans are very promising. In the future, we will also test if our system can reliably register corresponding nodules in repeated chest CT scans and thus become a clinically useful tool for nodule growth assessment.

We presented a *global* registration method – any change in a transformation parameter influences the transformation of the 3D data set as a whole [15]. In the future, we will design deformable surface models [12] to describe local transformations that are due to differences in patient respiration. We will then address the difficult task of registering structures within the lung. This will require modeling of nodule shape and position as a function of lung surface deformation, since nodules may move within the lung due to the patient's respiration.

Table 1: Registration Results

Patient	Months between Studies	Reconstruction interv. in mm	Rotation in Euler Angles	Translation in mm	SSD Error Reduction after 25 it.	Transl. Error Comp. vs. Radiol. mm
1	2	10/5/10	(2.3, 0, 9.3)	15	21%	10
2	$4\frac{1}{2}$	10/5/10	(-0.5, 0.3, -2.4)	26	34%	8
3	$1\frac{1}{2}$	5	(3.6, 1.2, -8.6)	6	86%	9
4	$1\frac{1}{2}$	10/5/10	(0.2, -0.6, 3.7)	142	7%	–
5	4	1	(0.1, -4.0, 1.9)	5	20%	2
6	7	1	(-1.9, -1.4, 1.8)	3	51%	3
7	$6\frac{1}{2}$	1	(-6.7, -5.5, 4.4)	27	78%	8
8	2	5	(-1.8, 3.6, -9.8)	21	75%	4
9	$1\frac{1}{4}$	5	(0.2, 0.1, 4.5)	58	8%	6
10	1	5	(5.2, 1.5, 3.3)	14	81%	4

Landmark detection and registration significantly improve the speed of the registration process. Since there is a tradeoff between speed and precision of registration, we will test the impact of resolution reduction on registration performance. We will also investigate whether initial registration of a larger set of landmarks will improve registration precision and speed.

In summary, we have developed a 3D method for registration of lung surfaces in repeated chest CT scans and shown a promising registration performance for 10 patients.

Acknowledgements

The authors thank David Naidich, MD, Marilyn Noz, PhD, and Chekema Prince for their support.

References

[1] R. J. Althof, M. G. J. Wind, and J. T. Dobbins III. A rapid and automatic image registration algorithm with subpixel accuracy. *IEEE Trans Med Imag*, 16(3):308–316, 1997.

[2] P. J. Besl and N. D. McKay. A method for registration of 3-D shapes. *IEEE Trans Pattern Anal Mach Intell*, 14(2):239–256, 1992.

[3] M. Betke, H. Hong, and J. P. Ko. Automatic 3D registration of lung surfaces in computed tomography scans. http://www.cs.bu.edu/techreports, 2001.

[4] M. Betke and J. P. Ko. Detection of pulmonary nodules on CT and volumetric assessment of change over time. In *Medical Image Computing and Computer-Assisted Intervention – MICCAI'99*, pages 245–252. Springer-Verlag, Berlin, 1999.

[5] M. Betke and N. C. Makris. Recognition, resolution and complexity of objects subject to affine transformation. *Int J Comput Vis*, 44(1), 2001.

[6] L. G. Brown. A survey of image registration techniques. *ACM Computing Surveys*, 24(4):325–375, December 1992.

[7] W. R. Fright and A. D. Linney. Registration of 3-D head surfaces using multiple landmarks. *IEEE Trans Med Imag*, 12(3):515–520, 1993.

[8] B. K. P. Horn. Closed-form solution of absolute orientation using unit quaternions. *J Opt Soc Am*, 4(4):629–642, 1987.

[9] A. Kano, K. Doi, H. MacMahon, D. D. Hassell, and M. L. Giger. Digital image subtraction of temporally sequential chest imagers for detection of interval change. *Med Phys*, 21(3):453–461, 1994.

[10] J. P. Ko and M. Betke. Chest CT: Automated nodule detection and assessment of change over time – preliminary experience. *Radiology*, 218(1):267–273, 2001.

[11] C. R. Maurer, G. B. Aboutanos, B. M. Dawant, R. J. Maciunas, and J. M. Fitzpatrick. Registration of 3-D images using weighted geometrical features. *IEEE Trans Med Imag*, 15(6):836–849, 1996.

[12] D. N. Metaxas. *Physics-Based Deformable Models: Applications to Computer Vision, Graphics, and Medical Imaging*. Kluwer Academic Press, Boston, 1997.

[13] C. F. Mountain. Revisions in the international system for staging lung cancer. *Chest*, 111(6):1710–1717, June 1997.

[14] C. A. Pelizzari, G. T. Chen, D. R. Spelbring, R. R. Weichselbaum, and C. T. Chen. Accurate three-dimensional registration of CT, PET and/or MR images of the brain. *J Comput Assist Tomogr*, 13:20–26, 1989.

[15] P. A. Van den Elsen, E.-J. D. Pol, and M. A. Viergever. Medical image matching – A review with classification. *IEEE Eng Med Biol Mag*, pages 26–39, March 1993.

Multisubject Non-rigid Registration of Brain MRI Using Intensity and Geometric Features

Pascal Cachier[1], Jean-François Mangin[2], Xavier Pennec[1], Denis Rivière[2], Dimitri Papadopoulos-Orfanos[2], Jean Régis[3], and Nicholas Ayache[1]

[1] Projet Epidaure, INRIA, Sophia-Antipolis, France
{Pascal.Cachier, Xavier.Pennec, Nicholas.Ayache}@inria.fr
[2] Service Hospitalier Frédéric Joliot, CEA, Orsay, France
mangin@shfj.cea.fr
[3] Service de Neurochirurgie Fonctionnelle, CHU La Timone, Marseille, France

Abstract. In this article we merge point feature and intensity-based registration in a single algorithm to tackle the problem of multiple brain registration. Because of the high variability of the shape of the cortex across individuals, there exist geometrical ambiguities in the registration process that an intensity measure alone is unable to solve. This problem can be tackled using anatomical knowledge. First, we automatically segment and label the whole set of the cortical sulci, with a non-parametric approach that enables the capture of their highly variable shape and topology. Then, we develop a registration energy that merges intensity and feature point matching. Its minimization leads to a linear combination of a dense smooth vector field and radial basis functions. We use and process differently the bottom line of the sulci from its upper border, whose localization is even more variable across individuals. We show that the additional sulcal energy improves the registration of the cortical sulci, while still keeping the transformation smooth and one-to-one.

1 Introduction

While the goal of monosubject registration is somewhat clear and corresponds intuitively to the retrieval of motion, multisubject brain registration is an ill-posed problem because the topology of the brain, and especially the cortex, varies strongly from one individual to another. Geometrically, there is an ambiguity on which feature should be matched to a given feature. Therefore, intensity-based registration algorithms are expected to fail at least on some pathological cases.

These geometrical ambiguities can be partially resolved when using higher-level, anatomical knowledge. Indeed, the sulci of the cortex can be labelled, and for a number of labels (e.g. the central sulcus) we know that the associated sulcus has roughly the same position and topology for all brains, and are therefore landmarks that should be registered in any cases. Collins [3] extracts 2×16 (16 for each hemisphere) parametric sulcal ribbons, and adds a chamfer matching step in his intensity registration algorithm. Hellier [4] extracts 2×6 parametric sulcal ribbons, and adds the distance between homologous control points of these

W. Niessen and M. Viergever (Eds.): MICCAI 2001, LNCS 2208, pp. 734–742, 2001.
© Springer-Verlag Berlin Heidelberg 2001

active surfaces to his registration energy, which underlies a strong assumption about the segmentation. Vaillant [13] inflates each cortex into a sphere, and then matches both spheres using the trace of a few sulci on the spheres as a constraint. Thompson [12] segments the cortex using balloon surfaces and 2×7 interactively outlined sulcal ribbons which are then matched together with the cortical surface. Chui [2] semi-automatically extracts 2×5 sulci of both hemispheres before matching them with a piecewise affine robust point-matching algorithm.

While the role of some major sulci as anatomical and even functional landmarks can be admitted [14, 15], some research still has to be done on the role of other minor sulci. Moreover, even the reliable manual or automatic identification of standard sulci for any brain is still an open issue, because of the variability of sulcus interruptions.

In this article, we present a new non-rigid matching algorithm using both intensity and sulcus matching. The whole set of the cortical sulci is first automatically extracted with a non-parametric approach, which enables the capture of the complex and variable topology of the sulci. They are then automatically labelled by a neural network using a set of 45 labels per hemisphere. We construct a registration energy made up of an intensity similarity measure, a geometric distance between sulcal points of the same label, and a regularization energy. The minimization of this energy leads to a transformation that is a combination of a dense smooth vector field and radial basis functions. We show that the introduction of the sulcal energy helps to better match the sulci, especially when the initial affine registration cannot match them well in the first place: this may happens because of the variability of the topology and the position of the sulci across individuals. Furthermore, we show that this improvement of matching does not deteriorate the smoothness and the bijectivity of the transformation.

2 Methodology

Intensity-based non-rigid registration algorithms have proven to be a fast and accurate way to achieve registration of volumetric images, at least in the case where the organs to be registered have approximately the same geometry. Our intensity-based algorithm uses the following generic registration energy:

$$E(C,T) = E_{sim}(I, J, C) + \sigma||C - T||^2 + \sigma\lambda E_{reg}(T) \qquad (1)$$

where I and J are two images to register, C and T are non-parametric transformations (C pairs homologous points according to the similarity measure, T is the smooth estimate of the non-rigid transformation), E_{sim} is an intensity similarity energy and E_{reg} a regularization energy or physical model. The attractive behavior and properties of this form of registration energy is extensively discussed in [1].

In the case of the registration of two different brains, the intensity constraint is not sufficient anymore, especially if we are interested in the cortex, because there is an ambiguity on which sulci should be matched to a given sulcus. These anatomical decisions are far beyond the capacity of an intensity similarity measure.

To resolve these ambiguities, we introduce geometric features in the images and mix geometric and intensity matching. The geometric features are labelled segmentations of the bottom and border lines of sulci, which contain a strong anatomical *a priori* knowledge.

2.1   Sulci Extraction

The sulci are first automatically extracted from an MRI. The main steps of the process segmenting the sulci are [8]: ① Non-uniform bias correction; ② Segmentation of grey matter/CSF; ③ Homotopic skeletonization; ④ Splitting into simple surfaces.

These surfaces are then automatically labelled with the algorithm of Rivière [10], using a set of 90 labels. This algorithm uses a neural network trained on a manually-labelled set. The informations used by the neural network to label a sulcus is both intrinsic (size, depth, localization, etc. of the sulcus) and relational (number of neighbors, minimal distance, etc. with neighboring sulci).

The computed error rate of the algorithm is about 24%. However, errors are partly due to an actual ambiguity of the labelization on some areas of the cortex, and to errors of the manual labelization done by the expert to build the training data set. Sometimes, the result found by the neural network actually seems more coherent than the labels found manually by the expert.

From these surfaces, we then extract two one-dimensional features (fig. 1), defined from discrete topology [6]:

- The sulcal bottom, which is the edge of the sulcus deep in the brain;
- The sulcal border, which is the outside edge of the sulcus and correspond to its junction with the hull of the brain.

Note that because we use non-parametric sulci, and also because several cortical folds may have the same label, a sulcus may have a very complex topology.

The use of the sulcal bottom lines as a geometrical feature for registration is driven by anatomical and computational considerations.

On an anatomical point of view, a theory has risen that the sulcal bottom lines are more stable anatomical landmarks than the sulci themselves. These lines, indeed, correspond to the shallow creases that appear on the foetal brain during the beginning of the cortical folding process. These lines are very stable across individuals because they delimit the main functional areas of the human brain [15, 9]. The rest of the sulci, however, is more difficult to match across individuals, because the sulcus border localization on the cortical surface depends on the local extent of the folding process, which varies with the subjects. This interpretation also explains the presence or absence of secondary folds or branches around the main sulcus.

On a computational point of view, the use of one-dimensional features drastically reduces the number of points to be processed and hence improves the speed of the algorithm.

The use of the sulcal borders helps the intensity-based algorithm to match the entire sulcus, not only its bottom. However, to follow the anatomical understanding of the folding process mentioned above, we want them to help the registration only if they are distant. Hence, the matching of sulcal borders is looser than for sulcal bottoms.

Given a label ℓ, $1 \le \ell \le 90$, we note $\mathcal{S}_\ell(I)$ the set of points of the image I classified as belonging to the sulcus ℓ. We note $\mathcal{S}_\ell^\downarrow(I)$ the subset of points of $\mathcal{S}_\ell(I)$ making up its sulcal bottom, and $\mathcal{S}_\ell^\uparrow(I)$ those belonging to the sulcal border. Finally, we note $\mathcal{S}(I) = \bigcup_\ell \mathcal{S}_\ell^\downarrow(I) \cup \mathcal{S}_\ell^\uparrow(I)$.

2.2   Registration Using Intensity and Geometric Features

Given two brain MR images I and J, we do not want to perfectly register the sulci $\mathcal{S}_\ell^\downarrow(I)$ and $\mathcal{S}_\ell^\downarrow(J)$ (or sulcal borders $\mathcal{S}_\ell^\uparrow(I)$ and $\mathcal{S}_\ell^\uparrow(J)$) because:

1. $\mathcal{S}_\ell^\downarrow(I)$ and $\mathcal{S}_\ell^\downarrow(J)$ may have very different topologies, e.g. the number of creases or branches. Sometimes, the same sulcus can even be made of one part in one brain, and two parts in the other: an exact matching would require the creation of an additional fold, which implies discontinuities in the deformation field on the cortex. Therefore, we want to get them as close as possible without actually totally map one onto the other. A partial matching is often the intuitive solution, as if one of the sulcus has grown further than the other.
2. The neighbors of a given sulci are not always the same for all brains. Matching two sulci that do not have the same neighboring relation in both brains would also lead to discontinuities in the deformation field on the cortex. Look at labelled brains in [10] for an illustration of these two first points.
3. On top of that, there exits a problem of robustness due to the errors in the automatic labelization. Therefore $\mathcal{S}_\ell^\downarrow(J)$ might not be the corresponding feature of $\mathcal{S}_\ell^\downarrow(I)$.

To integrate sulcus matching in our algorithm, we generalize the registration energy (1) by introducing a second set of correspondences C_2 between points of both images located on a landmark with the same label ℓ, i.e. $\forall \mathbf{x} \in \mathcal{S}_\ell^\downarrow(I)$, $C_2(\mathbf{x}) \in \mathcal{S}_\ell^\downarrow(J)$ (and similarly for $\mathbf{x} \in \mathcal{S}_\ell^\uparrow(I)$). We now set

$$E(C_1, C_2, T) = E_{sim}(I, J, C_1) + \sigma \|C_1 - T\|^2 + \sigma\gamma\|C_2 - T\|^2 + \sigma\lambda E_{reg}(T) \ (2)$$

where in the following $E_{sim}(I, J, C_1) = \int (I - J \circ C_1)^2$, $E_{reg}(T)$ is a quadratic energy whose impulse response is a Gaussian, and γ is a trade-off coefficient between intensity matching and sulcal matching. The minimization of this energy with respect to C_1, C_2 and T leads to a 3-step algorithm:

1. Minimize $E_{sim}(I, J, C_1) + \sigma.\|C_1 - T\|^2$ w.r. to C_1, i.e. find dense correspondences C_1 between voxels according to the intensity information.
2. Minimize $\|C_2 - T\|^2$ w.r. to C_2, i.e. find corresponding points C_2 between sulci with the same label ℓ closest to T with a closest point algorithm.

3. Fit T to C_1 and C_2 by minimizing $||C_1 - T||^2 + \gamma.||C_2 - T||^2 + \lambda.E_{reg}(T)$ w.r. to T. T is thus of the form

$$T(\mathbf{x}) = \alpha G * C_1(\mathbf{x}) + \sum\nolimits_{\mathbf{x}_i \in \mathcal{S}(I)} \boldsymbol{\alpha}_i G(\mathbf{x} - \mathbf{x}_i)$$

where G is the impulse response of the filter associated to E_{reg}, in our case a Gaussian, $\alpha \in \mathbb{R}$ and $\boldsymbol{\alpha}_i \in \mathbb{R}^3$, $\forall i$. (See [1] for technical details).

4. Go back to the first step until convergence.

We will however slightly modify this third step, as it would need the fitting of radial basis functions (RBF) at typically 2000 points at each iteration, which implies the inversion of a consequently huge matrix, and also because the errors of labelization and the topology variability, as previously discussed, imply the use of a robust fitting. A sulcal point $\mathbf{x}_i \in \mathcal{S}_\ell^{\{\downarrow,\uparrow\}}(I)$ being associated to another sulcal point $C_2(\mathbf{x}_i) \in \mathcal{S}_\ell^{\{\downarrow,\uparrow\}}(J)$, we associate to $\mathbf{x}_i$ the RBF $\alpha_i[C_2(\mathbf{x}_i)-T(\mathbf{x}_i)]G(\mathbf{x}-\mathbf{x}_i)$, where $\alpha_i \in \mathbb{R}$ a multiplicative coefficient which is equal to

- 1 if $\mathbf{x}_i$ belongs to a small set of 30 sulci for which we have a confident labelization for all brains,
- $\exp(-||C_2(\mathbf{x}_i)-T(\mathbf{x}_i)||^2/\beta)$ otherwise, β being a cut-off distance above which we decide that two points cannot be homologous, which may help both for labelization and topological problems.

We furthermore multiply α_i by $1 - \exp(-||C_2(\mathbf{x}_i) - T(\mathbf{x}_i)||^2/\beta_2)$, $\beta_2 < \beta$, if $\mathbf{x}_i$ belongs to a sulcal border, because the localization of these features on the cortical surface are not as accurate as for the sulcal bottom.

The final estimate transformation is then a weighted average of the fitting of intensity and feature points:

$$T(\mathbf{x}) = \lambda G * C_1(\mathbf{x}) + (1 - \lambda).\frac{\sum_i \alpha_i.[C_2(\mathbf{x}_i) - T(\mathbf{x}_i)].G(\mathbf{x} - \mathbf{x}_i)^2}{\sum_i G(\mathbf{x} - \mathbf{x}_i)}$$

where λ is a trade-off coefficient between intensity and feature matching. All the parameters λ, β, β_2 are chosen *a priori*. Before registration, we applied an anisotropic diffusion to the images, and carefully removed their bias [7] to use the SSD. The whole registration process is also set in a multiresolution scheme which helps preventing from local minima.

3   Experiments

We have run our multisubject registration on a set of 5 labelled brains. One of the brains have been arbitrarily chosen as the reference brain, and we have registered the other brains on it, using a robust affine registration [11] (also used as an initial alignment for non-rigid registration), and our non-rigid algorithm without and with the sulcus matching.

The results of the registrations, for a manually-chosen set of registration parameters, is given in fig. 2. The intensity-based method is able to match the sulci

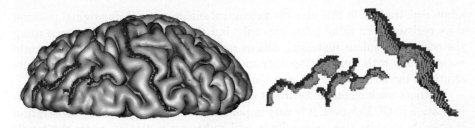

Fig. 1. *Three segmented sulci S in green, and their associated sulcal bottom $S^{\downarrow}$ in red and sulcal border $S^{\uparrow}$ in blue.*

when their topology is simple (i.e. mostly linear) and the initial affine registration is good. For example, the central sulci in red are generally matched; however, for one the brain, the central sulcus is relatively backwards, and a part of the precentral sulcus initially matches the central sulcus of the reference brain after

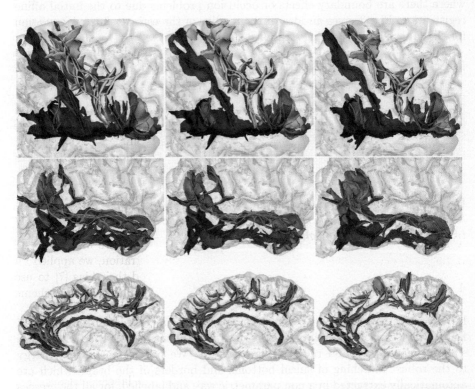

Fig. 2. *Position of the sulci after affine registration (left column), and after non-rigid registration without (middle column) and with (right column) sulcus matching. The sulcus matching helps to pair homologous sulci when they are initially far apart, and also improves the precision of the matching especially when the topology of the sulci is complex.*

affine registration: in this case the precentral sulcus stays at its original position if we register them using intensities only, but they are correctly registered using the additional sulcus matching. Sulcus matching also helps to more efficiently register sulci with complex topology such as the precentral sulcus, and generally improves the accuracy of the matching of all sulci.

Authors working on multisubject registration often omit to present the transformation itself. However, it is very important to make sure that the registration is smooth and bijective, especially in multisubject registration where the topology preservation is more than ever in competition with the matching of sulci. Presenting the position of the registered sulci is only one aspect of the non-rigid registration; the other is the smoothness of the transformation, and it is always possible to have a better sulci registration by deteriorating the smoothness and the topology. Here, the sulcal matching is done without deteriorating the smoothness and the bijectivity of the transformation: the Jacobian of the transformation is always positive, except for some points outside of the brain where there are boundary effects or occlusion problems due to the initial affine registration. Fig. 3 gives an idea of the quality of the estimated transformation for the four multisubject registrations.

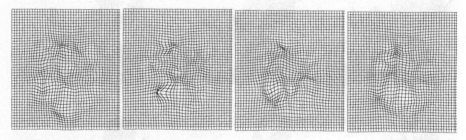

Fig. 3. *Estimate of the transformation at an arbitrary axial slice, for the 4 multisubject brain registration. Despite the additional sulcus matching, the recovered transformation is still smooth and one-to-one.*

4   Conclusion

In this work, we presented a registration energy that merges intensity and point feature registration. Its minimization leads to a linear combination of a dense smooth vector field and radial basis functions. We have adapted this energy to the robust matching of sulcal bottoms and borders of the brain, which are automatically extracted in a non parametric way and labelled, for all the creases of the cortex. We show that this additional information helps the algorithm to register homologous sulci while keeping the estimated transformation very smooth and one-to-one.

An extension of this work will consist in using a more detailed labelling of the sulcal patterns using the sulcal root model [9, 5]. Sulcal roots correspond to elementary creases always appearing on the foetal brain as only one connected component. Several studies tend to prove that sulcal roots may be identified in adult brains using variations of depth or curvature properties along sulcus bottoms. The simpler topology of these roots relative to standard sulci could allow us to use more stringent sulcal constraints in order to achieve a perfect matching of the folding patterns.

Another application of this work is the study of secondary folds after registration in order to discover stable patterns across individuals that could improve the description of the human cortex.

References

[1] P. Cachier and N. Ayache. Regularization in Image Non-Rigid Registration: I. Trade-Off between Smoothness and Similarity. Technical report, INRIA, 2001.

[2] H. Chui, J. Rambo, J. Duncan, R. Schultz, and A. Rangarajan. Registration of Cortical Anatomical Structures via Robust 3D Point Matching. In *Proc. of IPMI'99*, number 1613 in LNCS, pages 168 – 181, Visegrád, Hungary, June 1999.

[3] D. L. Collins, G. Le Goualher, and A. C. Evans. Non-Linear Cerebral Registration with Sulcal Constraints. In *Proc. of MICCAI'98*, volume 1496 of *LNCS*, pages 974 – 984, Cambridge, USA, October 1998. Springer.

[4] P. Hellier and C. Barillot. Coupling Dense and Landmark-Based approaches for Non Rigid Registration. Technical Report 1368, IRISA, November 2000.

[5] G. Lohmann and D. Y. von Cramon. Automatic Labelling of the Human Cortical Surface using Sulcal Basins. *Medical Image Analysis*, 4(3):179 – 188, 2000.

[6] G. Malandain, G. Bertrand, and N. Ayache. Topological Segmentation of Discrete Surfaces. *Int. J. of Comp. Vision*, 10(2):158 – 183, 1993.

[7] J.-F. Mangin. Entropy minimization for automatic correction of intensity nonuniformity. In *Proc. of MMBIA'00*, pages 162 – 169, 2000.

[8] J.-F. Mangin, V. Frouin, I. Bloch, J. Regis, and J. López-Krahe. From 3D MR images to structural representations of the cortex topography using topology preserving deformations. *J. of Math. Imaging and Vision*, 5(4):297 – 318, 1995.

[9] J. Régis, J.-F. Mangin, V. Frouin, F. Sastre, J. C. Peragut, and Y. Samson. Generic Model for the Localization of the Cerebral Cortex and Preoperative Multimodal Integration in Epilepsy Surgery. *Stereotactic Functional Neurosurgery*, 65:72 – 80, 1995.

[10] D. Rivière, J.-F. Mangin, D. Papadopoulos, J.-M. Martinez, V. Frouin, and J. Régis. Automatic Recognition of Cortical Sulci using a Congregation of Neural Networks. In *Proc. of MICCAI'00*, volume 1935 of *LNCS*, pages 40 – 49, Pittsburgh, USA, October 2000. Springer.

[11] A. Roche, G. Malandain, and N. Ayache. Unifying Maximum Likelihood Approaches in Medical Image Registration. *Int. J. of Imaging Systems and Technology*, 11:71–80, 2000.

[12] P. Thompson and A. W. Toga. A Surface-Based Technique for Warping 3-Dimensional Images of the Brain. *IEEE Trans. on Medical Imaging*, 15(4):402–417, 1996.

[13] M. Vaillant and C. Davatzikos. Hierarchical Matching of Cortical Features for Deformable Brain Image Registration. In *Proc. of IPMI'99*, volume 1613 of *LNCS*, pages 182 – 195, Visegrád, Hungary, June/July 1999. Springer.

742   P. Cachier et al.

[14] J. D. G. Watson, R. Myers, and R. Frackowiak *et al.* Area (V5) of the human cortex: evidence from a combined study using positron emission tomography and magnetic resonnance imaging. *Cerebral Cortex*, 3:79–94, 1993.

[15] W. Welker. Why does the cerebral cortex fissure and fold. *Cerebral Cortex*, 8B:3 – 135, 1989.

Fusion of Histological Sections and MR Images: Towards the Construction of an Atlas of the Human Basal Ganglia

S. Ourselin[1], E. Bardinet[1], D. Dormont[3], G. Malandain[1], A. Roche[1],
N. Ayache[1], D. Tandé[2], K. Parain[2], and J. Yelnik[2]

[1] INRIA, Epidaure Project, Sophia Antipolis, France
[2] INSERM U289, Salpêtrière Hospital, France
[3] Neuroradiology Dept and LENA UPR 640-CNRS, Salpêtrière Hospital, France

Abstract. In neurosurgery, localisation of deep brain structures is a crucial issue, which can be assisted by a 3-dimensional brain atlases. Our goal is to build such an atlas by fusing histological data with a 3D MR image of the same subject. This requires two steps: first a 2D realignment of the histological sections in order to obtain a three-dimensional block, then a 3D registration between this reconstructed block and the MR image. Both steps are based on the same robust registration algorithm.

1 Introduction

Accurate localisation of brain structures is a crucial issue for neuro-scientists. Recently, a new surgical treatment of Parkinson's disease consisting of deep brain stimulation (DBS) has been developed. In the first attempts, the target was in the thalamus [2], then moved to the internal globus pallidus, and finally to the sub-thalamic nucleus [5]. In this procedure, the surgical success depends primarily on the localisation of the target. Up to now, the target has been localised using ventriculographic landmarks [1] or MR images [3] in stereotactic conditions, and a statistical estimation based on an anatomical atlas, usually the Schaltenbrand and Wahren [13] or Talairach and Tournoux atlases [15].

However, for such a purpose, information provided by such atlases present several drawbacks: 3-dimensional alignment of contiguous sections has not been verified; the atlas resolution (from 1 to 4 mm in Z direction) is not sufficient for a precise localisation (e.g. the sub-thalamic nucleus is viewed in very few slices of the Schaltenbrand atlas); cerebral contours are not in a form suitable for automatic registration with digital MR images of individual patients.

Using interpolation, it is possible to generate an isotropic (with a constant inter-slice distance of 0.5 mm) Schaltenbrand atlas [18]. This improves the consistency of the atlas for visualisation and manipulation purposes, but not from an anatomical point of view as the necessary information is still missing. Moreover, interpolation is sensitive to wrong alignment between the original sections.

Therefore, to determine with accuracy the DBS target localisation, the key issue appears to be the construction of a 3D atlas of the human basal ganglia,

W. Niessen and M. Viergever (Eds.): MICCAI 2001, LNCS 2208, pp. 743–751, 2001.
© Springer-Verlag Berlin Heidelberg 2001

designed for further propagation onto the MR acquisition of a given patient, to allow a precise surgery planning.

We present here the first steps of the construction of an atlas of the human basal ganglia designed for our purpose, built by fusing a *post mortem* MR T1-weighted 3D image with a series of 2D histological sections. Superimposition onto the MR acquisition of a given patient could then be achieved by elastic matching (e.g. [?]). Data acquisition is detailed in section 2. Fusion methods and results are given in section 3.

2   Data Acquisition and Preprocessing

2.1   MR Images

The MR study was conducted 36 hours after death, before extraction of the brain. It consisted of a T1-weighted acquisition in the axial plane ($256 \times 256 \times 124$, $0.9375 \times 0.9375 \times 1.3$ mm^3). A T2-weighted image in the coronal plane is acquired too, but was not used in this study.

2.2   Histological Sections

After MR acquisition, the brain was processed for histology.

- The brain was stored in 4% paraformaldehyde for 8 days and in phosphate buffer with sucrose for 7 days. In this process, the brain, and especially the ventricles, were submitted to a global compression.
- One hemisphere was sectioned into 4 blocks (1.5 cm thick) in order to favour a better fixation, and stored frozen at -40°C, which causes a global shrinkage.
- The blocks were cut into $70\,\mu$m thick sections which were collected serially. Sectioning was done on a Tetrander Jung freezing microtome.

During the two first steps of the procedure, global distortions of the histological block with respect to the *ground truth* occur, and the ventricles almost collapse, while the third step caused slight uncorrelated local non-linear distortions on each section.

Sections were treated according to different immunohistochemical procedures. One out of ten sections (thus every $700\,\mu$m) was stained using the Nissl technique (Figure 1) to reveal cytoarchitectonic contours of cerebral regions. Another series was processed using Calbindin immunoreactivity. After staining, histological sections were scanned. Manipulations of the section during this last part of the procedure may also cause uncorrelated non-linear distortions on each section.

We segmented for each section the foreground from the background, using a threshold computed on each slice's histogram. In the course of the staining process, intensity differences occurred among histological sections. To correct this, we normalise all intensity histograms by centering the principal peak (representing the principal organic tissue) of each section.

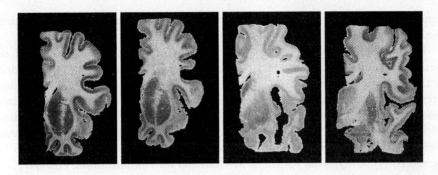

Fig. 1. *Four digitised sections after Nissl staining and background removal.*

3   Fusion of Histology and MR Images

Among the available data (MR T1, MR T2, Nissl and Calbindin), we choose
to fuse the T1-weighted MR image with the Nissl histological series because of
three reasons: the T1-weighted MR image is less distorted than the MR T2; the
Nissl dataset is more similar to the MR T1; Calbindin staining, which needs
more intermediate steps than Nissl, produces more distortions.

We choose a twofold approach: 1) construction of a 3D histological block, by
2D realignment of the histological sections; 2) 3D registration of this block with
the MR image. Both steps are conducted with the same registration algorithm,
which will be presented after a short review of the literature.

3.1   Fusion of Histology and MR Images in the Literature

Image registration is often a key step for biomedical imaging applications. In
brain mapping [17], the quality of the atlas construction depends of the quality
of the image registration, and in our case the quality of the histology-MR registration. Up to now, only a reduced number of papers have been published on
this particular registration problem.

Most of the approaches proposed so far are based on surface matching, i.e.
registration of the same anatomical surfaces extracted from both data sets.

In [7], for an Alzheimer's disease study, a 3D elastic warping algorithm is
used to deform the contours of the stained sections to the rigid shape imaged in
the cryomacrotome. Then, the digital cryovolume is registered to a pre-mortem
[18F]fluorodeoxyglucose (FDG) PET using a rigid intensity-based registration algorithm. This way, the authors obtain a 3D correspondence between the stained
sections and the FDG-PET. More recently, Jacobs *et al* [4] proposed a methodology for a 2D warping of MRI with rat's brain histological sections. The authors
use a surface matching technique for the rigid registration. With the resulting
contours, the 2D warping procedure is done using thin-plate splines.

In these first two studies, the authors used the external contours of the
brain (cortical surface, ventricles, ...), visible on all the modalities (cryomacro-

tome-stained sections [7], MRI-brain sections [4]) to register the histological sections together and with the 3D image.

In another approach, Schormann *et al* [14] proposed a method based on correlated landmarks. In this article, the authors assume that the histological sections are already aligned. For the histology/MR registration, the user defines interactively a set of reference points in the MR (a sub-volume is defined around these points) and the algorithm finds correspondences using the correlation coefficient criterion. This particular similarity criterion implicitly assumes that there exists a affine relationship between the intensities in sub-volumes to be registered [?]. Only small rotations are handled for computational efficiency.

In our application, it was not possible to use contours to register histological sections with the MR. Indeed, the basal ganglia, which are the structures of interest, can hardly be distinguished in the MR. Other structures do not provide enough contours. On the other hand, there is a fairly good functional relationship between the intensities of the MR T1 and the Nissl stained sections. These reasons make us prefer an intensity-based registration method.

We present in section 3.2 a local intensity-based algorithm, which will be used to perform both the reconstruction of the 3D block from histological sections (section 3.3) and the registration of the MR image with the reconstructed block (section 3.4).

3.2   Registration: An Intensity-Based Robust Algorithm

The method is based on a block-matching strategy. First, for each block in the first image, we compute its best corresponding block in the second image, by minimising a local similarity criterion. This criterion can be chosen with respect to the assumed relationship between both images' intensities [?]. Processing all blocks yield a set of correspondences, with which a global parametric transformation (e.g. rigid or affine) can then be estimated with a least trimmed squares (LTS) minimisation, which is more robust with respect to outliers than the classical least squares. These two steps are iterated and integrated into a multi-scale scheme.

Within this approach, two choices have to be made: the similarity measure and the class of transformations. We justify our choices for each registration case in sections 3.3 and 3.4.

3.3   Reconstruction of a 3D Block from the Histological Sections

This first registration step consists in reconstructing a 3D histological block from a set of 2D histological sections.

Usually, this step is presented as a trivial preprocessing task (see section 3.1). The main difficulty arises from the fact that two consecutive slices represent two different anatomical sections. Thus, two kinds of shape difference may appear: the first one is related to anatomical changes from section to section, while the second one is due to local distortions induced by the sectioning process. Thanks to its robustness, our algorithm will exploit only the coherent correspondences, due to local similarities, to find the best transformation, and reject the ones due to large changes or local distortions.

For the 3D alignment of consecutive 2D slices, such as histological sections, we use a 2D version [9] of the block matching algorithm presented in section 3.2. By computing a transformation between each two consecutive sections, we can collect all of them in a single 3D block. Our particular choices for these registrations are the correlation coefficient as similarity measure, and 2D rigid transformations as global parametric transformation.

The correlation coefficient assumes that there exists a affine relationship between the intensities of corresponding blocks of two successive sections. This choice seems to be reasonable for histological data (see Figure 1).

There is a gap of $700\,\mu$m between two consecutive histological sections: assuming that anatomy from one slice to the next differs only slightly seems to be reasonable, yielding to the choice of rigid transformations.

Elastic transformations (e.g. affine) may correct some of the observed morphological changes from section to section. However, as we can not distinguish between anatomical changes and local distortions to the histological process, searching such transformations may introduce false deformations and can therefore compromise the next step of the data fusion.

Results In Figure 2, we present the reconstructed 3D block obtained from the histological sections. First, we simply show the stack obtained by putting each digitised original Nissl section on top of the previous one. Then, we see the same block after alignment. Precisely, starting from the slice in the middle of the original stack, we computed rigid transforms from this slice to the next ones, and then, by combining the resulting slice-to-slice transforms, we obtained the reconstructed block. As can be seen, the continuity of both sulci and structures of the basal ganglia has been improved, compared to the original stack. Nevertheless, one can also observe intensity variations between slices, especially on the sagittal and axial views. This is the reason why an intensity normalisation is needed, and it yields the third block, where both misalignments and intensity variations have been corrected. This block is going to be used for the registration of MR and histology images.

3.4   Registration of the Reconstructed Histological Block with the MR Images

Once the 3D histological block has been reconstructed, we have to register it with the 3D MR image, which will be done with a 3D version [?] of the block matching algorithm presented in section 3.2.

As the MR T1 acquisition is larger and presents less distortions than the histological 3D image, we will compute a transformation from the block *towards* the MR image, which we consider as a reliable anatomical reference.

As previously explained, the choice of the similarity measure depends on the expected relationship between the intensities of the images to be registered [?].

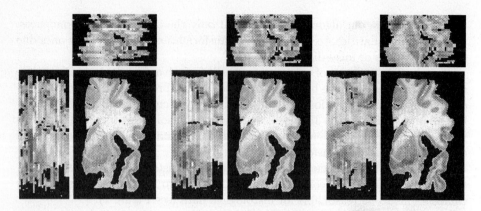

Fig. 2. *Reconstructed 3D block from histological sections; left block: stack of digitised original Nissl sections; middle block: same block after alignment; right block: same block after alignment and intensity normalisation. For each block: bottom left: sagittal view; bottom right: coronal view; top right: axial view.*

In the case of histology and MR images, a reasonable assumption is a functional relationship, and thus we choose the correlation ratio.

Concerning the choice of the transformation to be looking for, we choose affine transformations. Indeed, the histological procedure (section 2.2) has caused global shape changes, that may be captured by such transformations. Unfortunately, the additional uncorrelated in-slice distortions can not be modelized by a 3D transformation, and thus can not be corrected at this point. Nevertheless, we have to point out that the robustness of the estimation procedure allows us to treat them as outliers: thus they will not perturb the estimation of the 3D transformation.

To avoid some local minima during estimation, we perform a *hierarchical global registration*: we first compute a 3D rigid transformation; after convergence, we use it as initialisation for the estimation of the 3D affine registration.

Results We present in Figure 3 results of the affine registration between the reconstructed block obtained in the previous section and the MR T1-weighted image. The registered images have been superimposed and are shown with increasing opacity factors. Each row corresponds to different cuts through the volumes, and shows three slices (sagittal, coronal and axial).

First, the overall impression is that the affine registration provides a fairly good solution. Correspondence of the sulci and the cortex is consistent, see first row (axial and coronal slices), and third row (sagittal slice). Correspondence of the caudate nucleus and putamen is also consistent, see first row (axial slice), and third row (axial and coronal slices). The first (coronal slice) and the second (sagittal slice) rows illustrate that histology / MR registration allows to localise areas that were almost undetectable directly on the MR image.

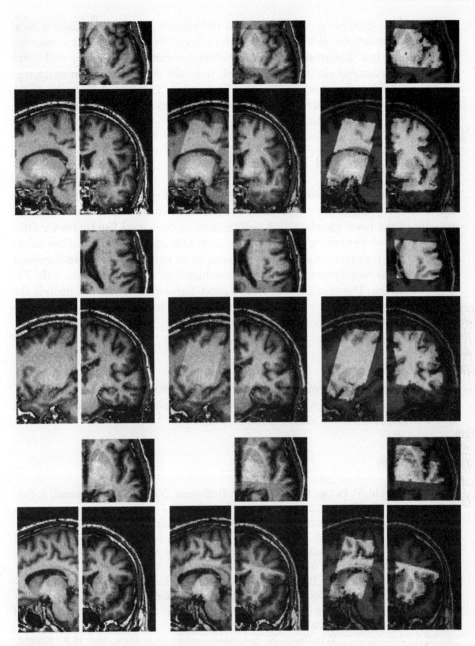

Fig. 3. *Affine registration of reconstructed histological block with MR T1 image. From left to right: MR and histological block are superimposed with increasing opacity factors (left column: MR:1, Histo.: 0; middle: MR:0.5, Histo.: 0.5; right: MR: 0.2, Histo.: 0.8) The three rows show three different cuts through the volumes (see text for details). For each block: bottom left: sagittal view; bottom right: coronal view; top right: axial view.*

750   S. Ourselin et al.

Finally, a ventricle collapse occurred during histology, which caused local non-linear distortions. Here again, the affine registration provided a consistent solution, see first (sagittal and coronal slices), second (axial slice) and third (sagittal and coronal slices) rows. Indeed, only the corpus callosum is misregistered (it lies in the ventricle in the MR image). This shows that the slight non-linear distortions were considered as outliers and rejected during the affine transformation computation.

4   Conclusion and Future Work

In this article, we have presented a methodology to fuse 2D histological sections and a 3D MR image. This represents the first step towards the construction of an atlas of the basal ganglia which will be used to determine the target for DBS of parkinsonian patients with higher accuracy. Our method, using an intensity-based robust registration algorithm, allowed us to get, after a first realignment step, an affine correspondence between the histological block and the MR T1-weighted image. The results looked fairly good. Subsequent steps will include the fusion of anatomical contours and the treatment of local non linear distortions by using elastic registration algorithms.

Acknowledgements

This work was partly supported by Medtronic (Research agreement no. 97506). We thank Johan Montagnat for providing the intensity normalisation tool, and Hervé Delingette for the visualisation software.

References

1. A.L. Benabid, P. Pollak, C. Gervason, D. Hoffmann, D.M. Gao, M. Hommel, J. Perret, and J. De Rougemont. Long-term suppression of tremors by chronic stimulation of the ventral intermediate thalamic nucleus. *Lancet*, 337:403–406, 1991.
2. A.L. Benabid, P. Pollak, A. Louveau, S. Henry, and J. De Rougemont. Combined (thalamotomy and stimulation) stereotactic surgery of the vim thalamic nucleus for bilateral parkinson disease. *Appl. Neurophysiol.*, 50:1–6, 1987.
3. D. Dormont, P. Cornu, B. Pidoux, A.M. Bonnet, A. Biondi, C. Oppenheim, D. Hasboun, P. Damier, E. Cuchet, J. Philipon, Y. Agid, and C. Marsault. Chronic thalamic stimulation using 3-dimensional mr stereotaxic imaging. *American Journal of Neuroradiology*, 8:1093–1107, 1997.
4. M.A. Jacobs, J.P. Windham, H. Soltanian-Zadeh, D.J. Peck, and R.A. Knight. Registration and Warping of Magnetic Resonnance Images to Histological Sections. *Med. Phys.*, 26(8):1568–1578, 1999.
5. P. Limousin, P. Pollak, D. Benazzouz, D. Hoffmann, J.F. Le Bas, E. Broussolle, J.E. Perret, and A.L Benabid. Effect of parkinsonian signs and symptoms of bilateral subthalamic nucleus stimulatiom. *Lancet*, 345, 1995.
6. J. B. A. Maintz and M. A. Viergever. A survey of medical image registration. *Medical Image Analysis*, 2(1):1–36, 1998.

7. M.S. Mega, S.S. Chen, P.M. Thompson, R.P. Woods, T.J. Karaca, A. Tiwari, H.V. Vinters, G.W. Small, and A.W. Toga. Mapping Histology to Metabolism: Coregistration of Stained Whole-Brain Sections to Premortem PET in Alzheimer's Disease. *Neuroimage*, 5:147–153, 1997.

8. S. Ourselin, A. Roche, S. Prima, and N. Ayache. Block Matching: A General Gramework to Improve Robustness of Rigid Registration of Medical Images. In A.M. DiGioia and S. Delp, editors, *Third International Conference on Medical Robotics, Imaging And Computer Assisted Surgery (MICCAI 2000)*, pages 557–566, Pittsburgh, Pennsylvania USA, October 11-14 2000.

9. S. Ourselin, A. Roche, G. Subsol, X. Pennec, and N. Ayache. Reconstructing a 3D Structure from Serial Histological Sections. *Image and Vision Computing*, 19(1-2):25–31, January 2001.

10. A. Roche, G. Malandain, N. Ayache, and S. Prima. Towards a Better Comprehension of Similarity Measures used in Medical Image Registration. In *Proc. MICCAI'99*, volume 1679 of *LNCS*, pages 555–566, Cambridge (UK), October 1999.

11. A. Roche, G. Malandain, X. Pennec, and N. Ayache. The Correlation Ratio as a New Similarity Measure for Multimodal Image Registration. In *First International Conference on Medical Image Computing and Computer-Assisted Intervention*, volume 1496 of *Lecture Notes in Computer Science*, pages 1115–1124, Cambridge (USA), October 1998. Springer.

12. Peter J. Rousseeuw and Annick M. Leroy. *Robust Regression and Outlier Detection*. Wiley Series in Probability and Mathematical Statistics, first edition, 1987.

13. G. Schaltenbrand and W. Wharen. *Atlas for Stereotaxy of the Human Brain*. Stuttgart: Georg Thieme Verlag, 1977.

14. T. Schormann, M. Von Matthey, A. Dabringhaus, and K. Zilles. Alignment of 3-D Brain Data Sets Originating From MR and Histology. *Bioimaging*, 1:119–128, 1993.

15. J. Talairach and P. Tournoux. *Co-planar Stereotaxic Atlas of the Human Brain*. New York: Thieme Medical Publishers, Inc., 1988.

16. P.M. Thompson and A. Toga. A Surface-Based Technique for Warping Three Dimensional Images of the Brain. *IEEE Transaction on Medical Imaging*, 15:1–16, 1993.

17. A.W. Toga and P.M. Thompson. The Role of Image Registration in Brain Mapping. *Image and Vision Computing*, 19(1-2):3–24, January 2001.

18. M. Yoshida. Creation of a Three-Dimensional Atlas by Interpolation from Schaltenbrand-Bailey's Atlas. *Appl. Neurophysiol*, 50:45–48, 1987.

Rigid Point-Surface Registration Using an EM Variant of ICP for Computer Guided Oral Implantology

Sébastien Granger[1,2], Xavier Pennec[1], and Alexis Roche[1]

[1] INRIA, Epidaure Project, Sophia Antipolis, France
[2] AREALL, Neuilly-sur-Seine, France
{Sebastien.Granger, Xavier.Pennec, Alexis.Roche}@sophia.inria.fr

Abstract. We investigate the rigid registration of a set of points onto a surface for computer-guided oral implants surgery. We first formulate the Iterative Closest Point (ICP) algorithm as a Maximum Likelihood (ML) estimation of the transformation and the matches. Then, considering matches as a hidden random variable, we show that the ML estimation of the transformation alone leads to a criterion efficiently solved using an Expectation-Maximisation (EM) algorithm. The experimental section provides evidences that this new algorithm is more robust and accurate than ICP and reaches a global accuracy of 0.2 mm with computation times compatible with a peroperative system.

1 Introduction

Oral implantology is a domain where computer guided surgery can lead to drastic improvements in safety and quality of the operation for the patient. The operation is planned on a preoperative CT-Scan and the purpose of such a system is to help the dentist to drill the implant in the predefined position and orientation. The *DentalNavigator* system (patent pending), developed by AREALL [5], is a peroperative system based on surface registration. In the CT-Scan image, the teeth and jaw bone surfaces are segmented using a Marching-Cube algorithm resulting in about 100000 triangulated points. Points on the same structures are measured on the patient using an ultrasound sensor mounted on a passive robotic arm. This time we get between 50 and 1000 unstructured points. After the registration, the US sensor is replaced by the drill on the robot arm and the system visually guides the surgeon to the planned position and orientation for drilling. In this article, which is a short version of research report [15], we investigate the registration step of this system.

The registration of two sets of points is usually performed using one of the multiple variations around the ICP algorithm [9,14]. Many variants and improvements of this algorithm have been proposed: features more complex than points, Mahalanobis distance to take heteroscedastic (non isotropic, non-homogeneous) noise into account, use of robust estimators for outliers rejection, etc [14,13,11]. In almost all these variants, each scene point is matched with only one model

W. Niessen and M. Viergever (Eds.): MICCAI 2001, LNCS 2208, pp. 752–761, 2001.

point with an implicit constant weight. Moreover, sudden changes in the closest-point function lead to a highly non-convex energy function, full of local minima. An improvement consists in using multiple weighted matches for each scene point: Rangarajan et al. introduced a probabilistic vision of the matching problem, and developed smooth point-matching models based on Gaussian weight (SoftAssign [1]) and Mutual Information [2], leading to a smaller number of local minima and thus presenting a better accuracy and robustness.

Starting from ICP, our main motivation was to improve the accuracy and the robustness in scope of a real-time system. We experimentally observed that Rangarajan's algorithms [1,2] were only efficient for registering two comparable sets of points (e.g. landmarks or surface equally sampled). Our problem is slightly different because the peroperative set of points is highly sub-sampled compared to the segmented surface and scene points are sparse enough to be considered as independent. Following Rangarajan's probabilistic approach, we develop in section 2 a registration criterion based on EM principles. The same criterion, inspired from [12], was independently developed in [7], but the derivation and use of our algorithm is original. Moreover, in section 3, we demonstrate new important properties leading to an efficient implementation of the algorithm. Finally, we discuss in section 4 the experimental results on our oral implantology application in terms of robustness, internal and global accuracy.

2 Maximum Likelihood Estimations of the Transformation

In this section, we model the scene as a random process, and we show that a maximum likelihood estimation of the transformation and the matches leads to the ICP algorithm using the Mahalanobis distance. Then, we consider the matches as a random matrix (or the model as a mixture of Gaussians) and we search for the ML estimate knowing only the transformation. Finally, we show how to solve efficiently this last criterion using an EM algorithm. This framework can be easily robustified by adding a probability to match a scene feature to the background [12, pp.78], which amounts to thresholding the Mahalanobis distance.

2.1 Maximum Likelihood and Standard ICP

Let s_i be the features of the scene $\mathcal{S}$, m_j the features of the model $\mathcal{M}$, μ^2 the Mahalanobis distance between features and T a rigid transformation from the model to the scene. Assuming that s_i *is homologous to* m_j (a measure of $T \star m_j$) with an additive Gaussian noise, its density probability function is:

$$p(s_i|m_j, T) = k^{-1} \cdot \exp(-\mu^2(s_i, T \star m_j)/2) \tag{1}$$

Because we deal later on with multiple and weighted matches, we use a matrix A to represent matches estimation where $A_{ij} = 1$ if s_i matches m_j and

0 otherwise. Since each scene point s_i is assumed to correspond exactly to one model point with index say $j^\star$, we have $A_{ij} = \delta_{jj^\star}$ and $\sum_j A_{ij} = 1$ for all scene index i. As $\alpha^1 = \alpha$ and $\alpha^0 = 1$, we can write the conditional pdf of s_i as: $p(s_i|A, \mathcal{M}, T) = \prod_j (p(s_i|m_j, T))^{A_{ij}} = p(s_i|m_{j^\star}, T)$. Now, assuming that *all scene points are conditionally independent*, the scene likelihood is:

$$p(\mathcal{S}|A, \mathcal{M}, T) = \prod_i p(s_i|A, \mathcal{M}, T) = \prod_{ij} (p(s_i|m_j, T))^{A_{ij}} \qquad (2)$$

Taking the negative log, we obtain the following criterion to be maximised:

$$C(T, A) = \tfrac{1}{2} \sum_{ij} A_{ij}.\mu^2(s_i, T \star m_j) + N_{\mathcal{S}}.\log k$$

One recognises here the standard ICP criterion using the Mahalanobis distance. This proves that ICP maximises the scene likelihood under a Gaussian noise with exact correspondences. Moreover, [8] showed that this is the best (minimal variance) estimator. Here, the criterion is invariant w.r.t a global scaling of the noise variance. This property will not hold for the following EM formulation.

2.2   Maximum Likelihood with Uncertain Matches

In the previous section, the transformation and the matches were both estimated by directly maximising the scene likelihood knowing these variables. In fact, we only need to determine the transformation for our application, and the matching matrix is an auxiliary variable. Moreover, there can be ambiguities in the matching estimation and considering multiple matches amounts to seeing the scene points as measurements of a mixture of Gaussians around the model points. This interpretation is specially adapted for our case since the model is a surface and not a collection of landmarks. Thus, the idea is to take into account these multiples matches in the criterion but weighted by their a posteriori probability. In fact, the proper way to do this is to search for the transformation that maximises the likelihood of the scene knowing only the transformation.

Consider now a random matching matrix $\mathbf{A}$. Each possible matching matrix A has a probability $p(A) = P(\mathbf{A} = A)$ and verifies the previous constraints: $\overline{A_{ij}} = E(\mathbf{A}_{ij}) = P(\mathbf{A}_{ij} = 1) \in [0, 1]$ and $\sum_j \overline{A_{ij}} = 1$. Finally, since scene points are assumed to be independent: $p(A) = \prod_{ij/A_{ij}=1} P(\mathbf{A}_{ij} = 1) = \prod_{ij} (\overline{A_{ij}})^{A_{ij}}$.

Let us start from an a priori probability law given by $p(A) = \prod_{ij} (\overline{\pi_{ij}})^{A_{ij}}$ (a relevant choice is the uniform law $\overline{\pi_{ij}} = \frac{1}{N_\mathcal{M}}$). Using Bayes rule and Eq. 2, we can deduce the joint scene and matching matrix likelihood:

$$p(\mathcal{S}, A|\mathcal{M}, T) = p(\mathcal{S}|A, \mathcal{M}, T).P(A|\mathcal{M}, T) = \prod_{ij} (\overline{\pi_{ij}}.p(s_i|m_j, T))^{A_{ij}}$$

Thus, the likelihood of the scene knowing only the transformation is $p(\mathcal{S}|\mathcal{M}, T) = \sum_{\{A\}} p(\mathcal{S}, A|\mathcal{M}, T)$. Taking the negative log, we obtain the registration criterion:

$$C(T) = -\log (p(\mathcal{S}|\mathcal{M}, T)) = -\sum_i \log \left(\sum_k \overline{\pi_{ik}}.p(s_i|m_k, T) \right) \qquad (3)$$

2.3 From the Maximum Likelihood to the EM Criterion

This criterion, like the first ICP criterion, has no closed form solution. We construct in this section an auxiliary criterion, depending explicitly on the matching matrix, and we use an alternated optimisation scheme. This construction follows EM principles [3,10] and the auxiliary variables framework of [4].

Designing the Auxiliary Criterion For any matching matrix A, we can write the criterion using Bayes rule: $C(T) = -\log p(A, \mathcal{S}|\mathcal{M}, T) + \log p(A|\mathcal{S}, \mathcal{M}, T)$. Since this is valid for any matching matrix A, it is still for the expectation w.r.t. *any* random matching matrix $\mathbf{A}$:

$$C(T) = -E_\mathbf{A}(\log p(A, \mathcal{S}|\mathcal{M}, T)) + E_\mathbf{A}(\log p(A|\mathcal{S}, \mathcal{M}, T))$$

To introduce an explicit dependence on the matching matrix, we add to this criterion the Kullback-Leibler distance $E_\mathbf{A}(\log p(A) - \log p(A|\mathcal{S}, \mathcal{M}, T))$ between the random variable $\mathbf{A}$ and the random variable $\mathbf{A}_T$ defined by $P(\mathbf{A}_T = A) = p(A|\mathcal{S}, \mathcal{M}, T)$. This distance is null for $\mathbf{A}_T$, positive otherwise. Thus, we have:

$$C(T, \mathbf{A}) = -E_\mathbf{A}(\log p(A, \mathcal{S}|\mathcal{M}, T)) + E_\mathbf{A}(\log p(A)) \qquad (4)$$

with $C(T) = \min_\mathbf{A} C(T, \mathbf{A}) = C(T, \mathbf{A}_T)$. A natural optimisation scheme for this new criterion is then to alternate an Expectation step to estimate the matching matrix and a Minimization step to solve for the transformation.

E-Step: Estimation of Matches In this step, we want to compute the optimal values $\overline{A_{ij}}$. By definition of our auxiliary criterion, the optimal $\mathbf{A}$ has the pdf:

$$p(A_T) = p(A|\mathcal{S}, \mathcal{M}, T) = \frac{p(A, \mathcal{S}|\mathcal{M}, T)}{p(\mathcal{S}|\mathcal{M}, T)} = \prod_{ij}\left(\frac{\overline{\pi_{ij}}.p(s_i|m_j, T)}{\sum_k \overline{\pi_{ik}}.p(s_i|m_k, T)}\right)^{A_{ij}}$$

Since we have $p(A_T) = \prod_{ij}((A_T)_{ij})^{A_{ij}}$, we obtain by identification:

$$\overline{(A_T)_{ij}} = \frac{\overline{\pi_{ij}}.p(s_i|m_j, T)}{\sum_k \overline{\pi_{ik}}.p(s_i|m_k, T)} = \frac{\overline{\pi_{ij}}.\exp(-\mu^2(s_i, T \star m_j)/2)}{\sum_k \overline{\pi_{ik}}.\exp(-\mu^2(s_i, T \star m_k)/2)} \qquad (5)$$

Contrary to the ICP (see remark at end of 2.1), these values are not invariant w.r.t a global scaling of the noise variance. Hence, the noise variance is an effective parameter of the EM algorithm (see section 3).

M-Step: Registration Now that we have an estimation of the matching matrix, we can optimize the criterion w.r.t. the transformation. In Eq. 4, only the first term depends on the transformation. Therefore we have to minimise $-E_\mathbf{A}(\log p(A, \mathcal{S}|\mathcal{M}, T)) = -\sum_{ij} \overline{A_{ij}} \log(\overline{\pi_{ij}}.p(s_i|m_j, T))$ Discarding constant and normalisation factors, we are left with the minimization of:

$$\sum_{ij} \overline{A_{ij}}.\mu^2(s_i, T \star m_j) = \sum_{ij} \overline{A_{ij}}.\|s_i - T \star m_j\|^2 / \sigma_s^2 \qquad (6)$$

758   S. Granger, X. Pennec, and A. Roche

degrees), used it as initialisation of the ICP and EM algorithms and plot in figure 2 (top) the distance of the estimated to the "exact" transformation. For ICP, (upper left), we observe many local minima, and it is difficult to differentiate a clear structure around 0 from a uniform distribution elsewhere. As rotation and translation are well correlated under 1 mm and 1 deg, we arbitrarily decided that these transformations were representative of the internal accuracy. For the EM algorithm (upper right), the number of local minima has significantly decreased and there is a clear separation between transformations very close to zero and other local minima. Propagating the transformation covariance on test points in the area of interest (the jaw) gives us a measure of the internal accuracy: 0.2 mm for ICP, and 0.007 mm for EM.

Now, to determine the size of the attraction basin, we have to look for the smallest initial translation for which the result is classified as bad. We plot in Fig. 2 (bottom left) the percentage of convergence to the global minimum w.r.t. the initial transformation: an initial translation of 2 mm can lead to bad results with ICP, whereas this limit is shifted to 9 mm for the EM. Last but not least, we present in Fig. 2 (bottom right) the distributions of the criterion values for both algorithms: there is a clear threshold distinguishing good from bad results with EM, whereas there is no such clustering for ICP. Numerous experiments with various number of points and surface shapes showed that this threshold on EM strongly depends on the noise variance but only slightly on the data shape. Thus, it can be estimated only once for a given application.

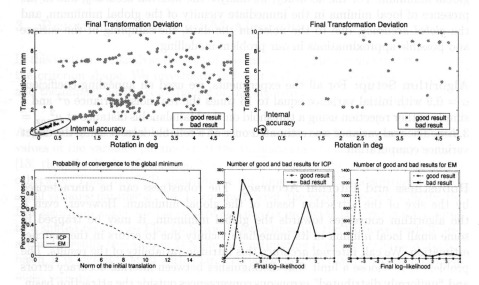

Fig. 2. Top: *Final transformations distribution for ICP (on the left) and EM (right).* **Bottom:** *probability of convergence to the global minimum with respect to the norm of the initial translation (left), and distribution of the criterion value (right).*

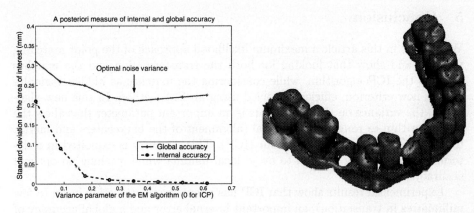

Fig. 3. Left: *global and internal accuracy of the EM with respect to the variance. ICP (at σ = 0) exhibits internal and global accuracies of 0.22 mm and 0.31 mm, while EM presents at the optimal variance internal and global accuracies of 0.007 mm and 0.22 mm.* **Right:** *A view a the points-surface registration for the optimal variance.*

Global Accuracy Evaluation To evaluate the global accuracy (i.e. the difference between the "exact" and estimated transformation) of the algorithms in real conditions, ten sets of 50 scene points, each time randomly placed on the fixed jaw, were acquired and registered onto the same model, segmented from a CT-Scan. Thus, the model variability was not taken into account, but all other sources of errors (segmentation error, scene points measurement error, and especially effect of surface sampling) were realistic. The "exact" registration was determined by the registration of all sets of points together to the model surface: this transformation should have a variance 10 times smaller than individual registrations, but hides a possible bias. Figure 3 presents the standard deviation of test points on the jaw for different values of the variance in the EM algorithm: underestimating this parameter appears to be much more penalising in terms of accuracy than overestimating it.

Registration Time In scope of a peroperative system, the computation time is a key parameter. In both algorithms, this time depends strongly on the number of scene points and iterations, and the distance threshold. Thanks to efficient space-partitioning structures, it only slightly depends on the number of model points. For each iteration (with the same data and distance threshold), EM only adds a 30% overhead to the ICP time, but it usually needs much more iterations to converge. Typically, it took 50 iterations (including 20 for deterministic annealing) on the above experiment, against 20 for ICP. The final time comparison is four to one in favour of ICP. However, the total computation time of EM is about 30 s in our case, which is still reasonable for our peroperative system.

5   Conclusion

We present in this article a maximum likelihood approach of the point matching problem and show that looking for both the transformation and the matches leads to the ICP algorithm, while considering the matches as hidden variables gives a new criterion, efficiently solved using an EM method. In this new algorithm, the variance on the data points is an important parameter that allow the EM algorithm to range from a global (alignment of the barycenters and inertia tensors) to a purely local behaviour (ICP). This property is exploited in a deterministic annealing method to avoid local minima while reaching an optimal accuracy.

Experimental results show that ICP has a very small attraction basin (a few millimetres in translation), an important internal error and a global accuracy of 0.31 mm in the jaw area. The EM algorithm exhibits a much wider attraction basin (around 1 cm) with a negligible internal error and a better global accuracy (0.22 mm). This gain in robustness and accuracy is counterbalanced by a larger computation time (a factor 4), which remains however compatible with our peroperative system.

Future work will include the parallelisation of the algorithm, the study of the surface sampling influence on the accuracy, the use of oriented points (position + normal to the surface) and the online prediction of the registration uncertainty.

Acknowledgements This work was supported by a CIFFRE Ph.D fellowship from AREALL, who also provided all the data used in this study.

References

1. A. Rangarajan and al. A Robust Point-Matching Algorithm for Autoradiograph Alignment. *Medical Image Analysis*, 1(4):379–398, 1997.
2. A. Rangarajan, H. Chui and J.S. Duncan. Rigid Point Feature Registration Using Mutual Information. *Medical Image Analysis*, 3(4):425–440, 1999.
3. C. Couvreur. The EM Algorithm: A Guided Tour. In *Proc. of CMP'96*, pp.115–120, Pragues, Czech Republik, August 1996.
4. L. Cohen. Auxiliary Variables and Two-Step Iterative Algorithms in Computer Vision Problems. *J. of Mathematical Imaging and Vision (JMIV)*, (6):59–83, 1996.
5. D. Etienne, A. Stankoff, X. Pennec, S. Granger, A. Lacan and R. Derycke. A New Approach for Dental Implant Aided Surgery. *CARS'2000*, pp.927–931, 2000.
6. D.W. Eggert, A. Lorusso and R. Fisher. Estimating 3D rigid body transformations: A comparison of four major algorithms. *Mach. Vis. & App.*, 9:272–290, 1997.
7. H. Chui and A. Rangarajan. A Feature Registration Framework using Mixture Models. In *Proc. MMBIA'2000*, pages 190–197, 2000.
8. K. Kanatani. *Statistical Optimization for Geometric Computation : Theory and Practice.* Elsevier Science (Amsterdam), 1996.
9. P.J. Besl and N.D. McKay. A Method for Registration of 3D Shapes. *IEEE Transactions on Pattern Analysis and Machine Intelligence*, 14(2):239–256, 1992.
10. R. M. Neal and G. E. Hinton. A View of the EM Algorithm that Justifies Incremental, Sparse, and other Variants. *Learning in Graphical Models*, 1998.

11. T. Masuda, K. Sakaue, and N. Yokoya. Registration and Integration of Multiple Range Images for 3D Model Construction. In *Proc. ICPR'96*, pages 879–883, 1996.
12. W. Wells. Statistical Approaches to Feature-Based Object Recognition. *IJCV*, 21(1):63–98, 1997.
13. X. Pennec and J.P. Thirion. A Framework for Uncertainty and Validation of 3D Registration Methods based on Points and Frames. *IJCV*, 25(3):203–229, 1997.
14. Z. Zhang. Iterative Point Matching for Registration of Free-Form Surfaces. *IJCV*, 13(2):119–152, 1994.
15. Granger et al.. Rigid Point-Surface Registration using Oriented Points and an EM Variant of ICP for Computer Guided Oral Implantology. *RR-4169 INRIA*, 2001.

A Stochastic Iterative Closest Point Algorithm (stochastICP)

G.P. Penney, P.J. Edwards, A.P. King, J.M. Blackall, P.G. Batchelor, and D.J. Hawkes

Division of Radiological Sciences and Medical Engineering, The Guy's, King's and St. Thomas' Schools of Medicine and Dentistry, Guy's Hospital, London, SE1 9RT, UK.

Abstract. We present a modification to the iterative closest point algorithm which improves the algorithm's robustness and precision. At the start of each iteration, before point correspondence is calculated between the two feature sets, the algorithm randomly perturbs the point positions in one feature set. These perturbations allow the algorithm to move out of some local minima to find a minimum with a lower residual error. The size of this perturbation is reduced during the registration process. The algorithm has been tested using multiple starting positions to register three sets of data: a surface of a femur, a skull surface and a registration to hepatic vessels and a liver surface. Our results show that, if local minima are present, the stochastic ICP algorithm is more robust and is more precise than the standard ICP algorithm.

1 Introduction

The iterative closest point (ICP) algorithm [1] has been used for a wide variety of applications both in the field of medical imaging [2,3] and engineering. We are primarily concerned with using the ICP algorithm to register intraoperative ultrasound data to preoperative 3D modalities for use in image-guided surgery or interventions. This can enable surgeons or interventionists to navigate towards their surgical targets by viewing preoperative images which are spatially aligned with either the physical coordinate system of the patient or the intraoperative modality.

The ICP algorithm is usually an efficient method to minimise the root mean square (RMS) distance between two feature sets. However, it can be prone to finding local minima, especially in noisy feature sets. Previous attempts have been made to increase the robustness of the ICP algorithm. Masuda and Yokoyo [4] improve robustness by using a random sample of points (rather than the whole dataset) which are altered at each iteration. In Luck *et al.* [5] robustness is improved by using both a simulated annealing and an ICP algorithm. Essentially the simulated annealing algorithm is used to produce "good" starting points for the ICP algorithm.

We propose a novel approach to increase the robustness of the ICP algorithm by adding random Gaussian noise to perturb the position of the features in one feature set. The magnitude of the noise is reduced during the registration process until finally it is set to zero when the algorithm reverts back to standard ICP.

The structure of our paper is as follows. We initially outline the standard ICP algorithm and detail our modifications. We then describe our experiments to register three sets of data: a femur, a skull and a liver dataset.

W. Niessen and M. Viergever (Eds.): MICCAI 2001, LNCS 2208, pp. 762–769, 2001.

2   Method

2.1   Outline of ICP Algorithm

The iterative closest point algorithm is widely used and well known, and so only a very brief summary is given in this paper. Our description will concentrate on the case where the source dataset consists of n points $\mathbf{p}_j, j = 1, \ldots, n$, whereas the target feature set can consist of points, lines or surfaces.

The algorithm registers two sets of features by repeating the following steps.

1. For each source point, calculate the closest point, or position on a line or surface in the target dataset.
2. Calculate the transformation matrix $\mathbf{T}$ which minimises the RMS distance between the two sets of corresponding points.
3. Repeat the above steps until a suitable stopping criterion is met.

2.2   Modifications to the Algorithm

We have modified the algorithm in two significant but related ways. The first is to introduce an extra step to be carried out before point correspondence is calculated i.e. step 0 in the framework shown in section 2.1.

0. Add a random Gaussian perturbation to the position of the source points: $\mathbf{p}'_j = \mathbf{p}_j + \mathbf{s}_j, j = 1, \ldots, n$, where $\mathbf{s}_j$ represents a vector in a random direction, with a magnitude which has standard deviation σ.

Steps 1 and 2 are now carried out using the perturbed $\mathbf{p}'_j$ rather than the original $\mathbf{p}_j$ source points.

The second alteration to the algorithm is to change the stopping criterion (step 3) to be a set of criteria which define when the noise σ should be reduced. We would like to reduce σ when the algorithm has reached an optimum position. In most cases the algorithm tends to move towards the optimum position and then fluctuates about this position. In our stochastICP algorithm, due to the random perturbations, the residual error can both increase and decrease. Therefore, it is not obvious how the residual error value can be used to define the noise reduction criterion. Instead we have used the following criterion which is based on the rigid body parameters $\mathbf{E} = (\theta_x, \theta_y, \theta_z, X, Y, Z)$. These parameters can be calculated by decomposing the transformation matrix $\mathbf{T}$. The values of these parameters are logged after each iteration and if the current set of parameters $\mathbf{E}_N$ are within a certain threshold t of a previous set of parameters $\mathbf{E}_i$ then the algorithm reduces the size of σ,

$$\exists\, i_0 \in \{1, \ldots, N-5\} : \max_{k=1,\ldots,6} |E_{i_0}^k - E_N^k| < t \tag{1}$$

where E^k represents the individual elements in the 6-tuple $\mathbf{E}$, i_0 represents a particular iteration and N equals the current number of iterations. The last five sets of parameters are not included in the search i.e. only $\mathbf{E}_i, i = 1, \ldots, N-5$ are used for the following reason. By excluding the last five iterations we aim to distinguish between the following two cases. Firstly, where the algorithm is simply moving slowly through the search space; in this case the algorithm is still moving towards the optimum position and so we do not want to alter σ. Secondly, where the algorithm has revisited a position in the 6-dimensional parameter space; this should indicate that the algorithm is fluctuating about an optimum position and so σ should be reduced. The exclusion of the last five parameters was empirically chosen.

For the experiments described in this paper we begin with $\sigma = 16$mm. When the noise reduction criterion is met σ is reduced by a factor of $1/\sqrt{2}$ and the algorithm continues until $\sigma < 0.25$mm. At this point the noise is set to zero. The final stopping criterion for the algorithm is a standard stopping criterion i.e. where the change in the residual error falls below a threshold (10^{-4}mm for the experiments described in this paper).

The parameter t was set equal to $\sigma/5$ for the experiments using the femur and liver datasets and was set equal to $\sigma/50$ for the experiments using the skull dataset. These ratios were chosen empirically. Our reasons for choosing these values for t are as follows. The parameter t defines how precisely the algorithm must revisit a position for the noise reduction criterion to be met. Our choice for the size of t depends on the size of the variations in the values of the rigid body parameters $\mathbf{E}$ between different iterations. If these parameters vary by a large amount, then t must also be fairly large, otherwise the algorithm may take an extremely large number of iterations to reach registration. However, if $\mathbf{E}$ varies by only a small amount, then t should also be small to prevent the noise reduction criterion being met before the algorithm has reached an optimum position. The rigid body parameters $\mathbf{E}$ vary due to two factors, the size of the noise σ and the speed with which the algorithm moves towards the optimum position. We account for the first of these factors by setting t to be a fraction of σ, therefore, the size of t is reduced as the noise decreases. The two different values for this ratio were necessary because the parameters $\mathbf{E}$ varied by a much smaller amounts between successive iterations when registering the skull dataset, compared to the femur and liver datasets. This is probably due to the almost constant curvature of the upper part of the cranium.

2.3   Experiments

Experiments have been carried out using three sets of data. We are primarily concerned with the registration of intraoperative ultrasound data with preoperative 3D modalities for use in image guided surgery or interventions. Consequently each dataset used in this paper simulates ultrasound to CT or MR registration. However, our modifications do not detract from the generic nature of the ICP algorithm and so it should be useful for a wide range of registration problems.

The three target datasets were: a CT scan of a phantom femur (see figure 1), a MR scan of a volunteer's head and a MR scan of a volunteer's liver. In each case the source modality was freehand 3D ultrasound. The datasets are summarised in table 1. The 3D surfaces were extracted using a marching cubes algorithm [6] implemented in VTK [7] which was applied to binary images segmented from the 3D volumes. The binary volumes were produced by applying a threshold to segment the femur surface from the CT volume and by manual segmentation for the two MR volumes using the ANALYZE software package (Biomedical Imaging Resource, Mayo Foundation, Rochester, MN,

USA). The line features in the liver dataset were created from a number of manually picked points which define the centrelines of blood vessels.

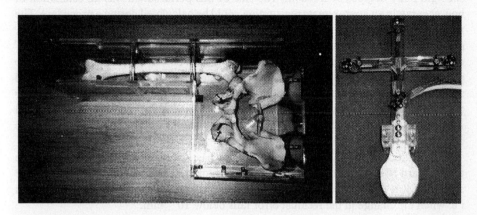

Fig. 1. Femur phantom (left) and a 10.5MHz ultrasound probe with infra-red LEDs attached (right).

The source points were manually picked from sets of freehand 3D ultrasound images. A 10.5MHz ultrasound probe (see figure 1), tracked using an Optotrak 3020 optical tracking system from Northern Digital Inc., was used to acquire source bone points for the femur and volunteer skull datasets. A 3.5MHz probe, tracked using a Polaris optical tracking system from Northern Digital Inc., was used to acquire the liver surface and midline of hepatic vessels for the liver dataset. The approximate 3D spatial accuracy of the Optotrak and Polaris are 0.2mm and 0.35mm respectively.

For the phantom femur dataset a "gold-standard" registration was calculated using fiducial markers attached to the box which contained the femur. For the volunteer head data a "gold-standard" registration was calculated by attaching a locking acrylic dental stent (LADS) [8] to the volunteer. Markers attached to the LADS were used to calculate a point based image to physical registration. No "gold-standard" was available for the liver dataset.

Target Modality	Target Feature	Source Feature
CT 320×320×177 voxels 1.094×1.094×3mm	femur surface 11484 facets	835 ultrasound bone points
MR 256×256×200 voxels 0.898×0.898×1.2mm	skull surface 12146 facets	375 ultrasound bone points
MR 256×256×26 voxels 1.328×1.328×10mm	liver surface (3044 facets) + hepatic vessels (175 line segments)	71 ultrasound liver surface 46 ultrasound vessel points

Table 1. Summary of the datasets showing voxel sizes, image dimensions, type of target feature and number of source points.

One hundred registrations were carried out using each dataset. The starting positions were the "gold-standard" registration position with random noise added to each of the six rigid body degrees of freedom. The size of this perturbation was an estimation of how accurately an approximate registration could be calculated during a procedure. The random noise used was 15mm or degrees for the femur and skull datasets and 30mm or degrees for the liver dataset. When registering using the liver dataset no "gold-standard" registration was available. Instead an initial registration was estimated by placing the probe on the inferior end of the volunteer's sternum and acquiring an axial ultrasound slice. This ultrasound slice was approximately registered to the MR volume by making the following assumptions: that the x and y axes of the ultrasound image are parallel to the x and y axes in the MR volume and that the centre of the ultrasound image corresponds to the centre of the MR volume.

Registrations were carried out using our stochastICP algorithm and for comparison the standard ICP algorithm was also used. The stopping criterion for the standard ICP algorithm was identical to the final stopping criterion using the stochastICP algorithm i.e. when the change in the residual error falls below 10^{-4}mm.

3   Results

The registration results were analysed in the following ways. Firstly, failed registrations were removed. A registration was deemed to be a failure if its mean target registration error (TRE) [3] was greater than five times the minimum value of mean TRE over the set of 100 registrations. It was not possible to calculate a TRE for the liver dataset as there was no "gold-standard" registration, instead a registration was deemed to be a failure if the residual error was more than 25% larger than the minimum residual error for the set of 100 registrations.

A mean TRE was calculated by transforming a number of points, one for each voxel within a region of interest, firstly by the "gold-standard" matrix and secondly by the final registration matrices and calculating the RMS distance between the two positions. The regions of interest chosen for the three datasets were all the voxels within either the femur, the skull or the liver.

A RMS distance measure was also calculated to indicate the spread of the final registration positions (i.e. a measure of precision). This was calculated using the following method. Each point within the region of interest was taken in turn and transformed using each of the successful final registration matrices. For a given point the mean transformation position was determined and then the RMS distance to the mean position was calculated. The RMS distance quoted is the RMS value of these RMS distances calculated over the entire region of interest.

The registration results are given in table 2. This table shows the mean residual error, RMS distance, mean TRE and mean number of iterations for the successful registrations. It also shows the algorithm failure rate. Renderings, showing the target features and the final position of the source points for a typical successful registration, are shown in figure 2.

The results for all three datasets showed that the algorithms produced very similar residual error values. The stochastICP algorithm recorded lower RMS distance values

Feature	Algorithm	Mean Residual (mm)	RMS Distance (mm) (precision measure)	Mean TRE (mm) (accuracy measure)	Mean No. Iter.	Fail Rate (%)
Femur	ICP	0.72	0.15	1.18	81	36
	stochastICP	0.72	0.03	1.17	122	0
Skull	ICP	0.86	1.98	2.89	357	1
	stochastICP	0.86	1.57	2.65	479	1
Liver	ICP	6.14	2.60	-	102	24
	stochastICP	6.12	1.10	-	140	7

Table 2. Registration results, showing the mean residual, RMS distance, mean TRE and mean number of iterations for the successful registrations. Failure rate is also shown.

and mean TRE values for all three datasets, in particular when using the liver dataset where the RMS distance value was less than half that recorded using the standard ICP algorithm.

The largest differences between the two algorithms occurred in terms of the number of iterations required to reach registration and the failure rate. The stochastICP algorithm produced a much lower failure rate when using the femur and liver datasets, however, it required between 34% – 51% more iterations to reach registration.

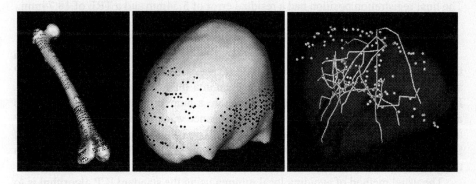

Fig. 2. Registration results from a typical successful registration position showing the source points overlaid onto the target surface and line features.

4 Discussion

The results using both the femur and the liver datasets show that the stochastICP algorithm is more robust than the standard ICP algorithm. The likely reason for this improvement is the presence of local minima in these datasets. It is clear that the standard ICP algorithm is not able to manoeuvre out of a local minimum, whereas the stochastICP algorithm, due to the random perturbations added to the point positions, can escape from some local minima. In the case of the femur data the standard ICP algorithm resulted in solutions which were a long way from the "gold-standard" position. Figure 3 shows a rendering of the source points and target surface for one of the failed registrations using the standard ICP algorithm. This local minimum is caused by the points from the ultrasound images, which were mainly acquired from the anterior surface of the femur (as the posterior surface can be more difficult to image in a patient), crossing over to register to opposite sides of the femur surface. Because the femur is a long thin structure a very small rotational misalignment can place the feature sets in such a local minimum.

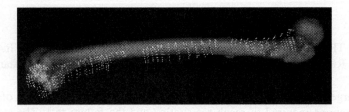

Fig. 3. A rendering of the source points and target surface femur dataset showing a misregistration position found using the standard ICP algorithm. The opacity of the femur surface has been reduced to show target points within the centre of the femur. The final registration position had a residual error of 5.54mm and a TRE of 18.74mm.

In the case of the liver data there are some local minima a long distance away from the registration position which caused some registrations to fail. Again the stochastICP algorithm was less affected by these local minima than the standard ICP algorithm. In both the liver and the skull datasets there are a number of local minima clustered around the global minimum. The lower RMS distance value when using the stochastICP algorithm is believed to be because this algorithm was able to skip over or climb out of these local minima, whereas the standard ICP algorithm tended to become trapped in the first local minimum which was encountered.

The usual method of avoiding local minima using the standard ICP algorithm is to use a number of starting positions. Therefore, although the stochastICP algorithm requires more iterations, its increased robustness should mean that fewer starting positions are required and so the stochastICP algorithm may be ultimately more computationally efficient.

Our stochastICP method could be thought of as combining a simulated annealing optimisation method [9] with the ICP algorithm, where the size of perturbation is analogous to the temperature parameter. This is a much more integrated combination of the two types of algorithm than the method proposed by Luck *et al.* [5], where a simulated annealing algorithm is used to provide good starting estimates for an ICP algorithm. Our method could also be thought of as combining a multi-scale or multi-resolution optimisation method (which have been found to be robust methods for voxel based registration [10]) with the ICP algorithm. In this case the size of the perturbation is analogous to the size of the blurring kernel used.

Future work on the stochastICP algorithm will include an investigation into the factors affecting the values of the additional parameters, in particular, σ and t. The values of these parameters are expected to be influenced by factors such as the shape of the object being registered and also the amount of noise in the source and target datasets. Work is also required to investigate the robustness of the algorithm to changes in these parameters. We also intend to extend our validation of the algorithm by greatly increasing the number of datasets used in our investigation and to compare the algorithm with other, more robust, ICP algorithms [4,5].

5   Conclusions

We have developed a stochastic ICP algorithm. From our results using three datasets it appears that, although our stochastICP algorithm requires more iterations, in the presence of local minima it is more robust (i.e. yields fewer failures) and more precise than the standard ICP algorithm.

6   Acknowledgements

The authors would like to thank the EPSRC (grant numbers GR/M53752, GR/L62221 (via the MedLINK programme), GR/N04867 and PhD studentship for J.M. Blackall). We would also like to thank Depuy for providing the femur phantom.

References

1. P.J. Besl and N.D. McKay. A method for registration of 3-D shapes. *IEEE Trans. on Pattern Analysis and Machine Intelligence*, 14(2):239–256, 1992.
2. J. Feldmar, N. Ayache, and F. Betting. 3D-2D projective registration of free-form curves and surfaces. *Comput. Vision Image Understanding*, 65(3):403–424, 1997.
3. C.R. Maurer, Jr., G.B. Aboutanos, B.M. Dawant, Maciunas R.J., and J.M. Fitzpatrick. Registration of 3-D images using weighted geometrical features. *IEEE Trans. Med. Imaging*, 15(6):836–849, 1996.
4. T. Masuda and N. Yokoya. A robust method for registration and segmentation of multiple range images. *Comput. Vision Image Understanding*, 61(3):295–307, 1995.
5. J.P. Luck, W.A. Hoff, R.G. Underwood, and C.Q. Little. Registration of range data using a hybrid simulated annealing and iterative closest point algorithm. submitted to IEEE PAMI. available at http://egweb.mines.edu/whoff/publications/2000/pami2000.pdf
6. W. E. Lorensen and H. E. Cline. Marching cubes: A high resolution 3-D surface reconstruction algorithm. *Computer Graphics*, 21(4):163–169, 1987.
7. W. Schroeder, K. Martin, B. Lorensen, L. Avila, R. Avila, and C. Law. *The Visualization Toolkit: An Object-Oriented Approach to 3-D Graphics*. Prentice-Hall, 1997.
8. M.R. Fenlon, A.S. Jusczyzck, P.J. Edwards, and A.P. King. Acrylic resin dental stent for image guided surgery. *J. of Prosthetic Dentistry*, 83(4):482–485, 2000.
9. S. Kirkpatrick, C.D. Gelatt, Jr., and M.P. Vecchi. Optimization by simulated annealing. *Science*, 220(4598), 1983.
10. C. Studholme, D.L.G. Hill, and D.J. Hawkes. Automated 3D registration of MR and CT images of the head. *Medical Image Analysis*, 1(2):163–175, 1996.

Shape Preserving Filament Enhancement Filtering

Michael H.F. Wilkinson and Michel A. Westenberg

Institute for Mathematics and Computing Science,
University of Groningen, P.O. Box 800,
9700 AV Groningen, The Netherlands,
(michael, michel)@cs.rug.nl
http://www.cs.rug.nl/~michael/

Abstract. Morphological connected set filters for extraction of filamentous details from medical images are developed. The advantages of these filters are that they are shape preserving and do not amplify noise. Two approaches are compared: (i) multi-scale filtering (ii) single-step shape filtering using connected set (or attribute) thinnings. The latter method highlights all filamentous structure in a single filtering stage, regardless of the scale. The second approach is an order of magnitude faster than the first, filtering a 256^3 volume in 41.65 s on a 400 MHz Pentium II.

1   Introduction

Enhancement of curvi-linear, dendritic or other filamentous details has many applications in medical image analysis. Examples include computer analysed microscopy of filamentous microorganisms [9], confocal laser scanning microscopy of neurons, and various forms of angiography [4, 13]. Many methods have been proposed to enhance such details (for a review see e.g. [6]). Many of these methods have shortcomings, either in amplifying noise, or distorting certain important details, such as aneurisms or stenoses which may not be classified as filamentous features in some filters [6]. In particular, the use of linear scale spaces using Gaussian filters in multi-scale analysis can lead to distortion, merger, and movement of features in the image as more and more blurring is applied.

An entirely different issue is that of computational cost. Some of the more successful multi-scale approaches can be computationally very costly. For example, the multi-scale method of Sato et al. [8] requires 10 minutes of computations using eight 168 MHz Sun Ultrasparc processors for an image of $256 \times 256 \times 102$ voxels, even when using just three scales. A similar method by Frangi et al. [4] is also done off-line due to the computational burden [13]. Even if the approaches are not multi-scale, they often require repeated filtering with kernels sensitive to filaments running in different directions, which may mean combining 13 different directional filters [3].

The aim of this paper is to explore the possibilities offered by connected-set morphological filters in this context. Connected-set filters [5] have the distinguishing characteristic that they can enhance or remove an existing edge in an

W. Niessen and M. Viergever (Eds.): MICCAI 2001, LNCS 2208, pp. 770–777, 2001.
© Springer-Verlag Berlin Heidelberg 2001

image, but never move it or introduce new edges. It is this edge, and therefore *shape preserving* property which offers the promise of vessel enhancement without changing vessel shapes, which is a prevalent problem in existing methods. Furthermore, because a great deal of progress has been made in the development of fast algorithms for these filters [1, 7, 12], filament extraction by connected filters is now a viable option.

We will first discuss the use of multi-scale morphological approaches, comparing classical morphological openings with their connected set counterparts: openings-by-reconstruction. One problem with these multi-scale methods is the repeated use of often costly filters: at least one for each scale. We therefore compare this approach with the use of shape based filters [10], which can extract all features of a given shape, regardless of their scale. These could find e.g. all filamentous structures in an angiogram in a single filtering stage, rather than by repeated operations as is done classically. It will be shown that operators with these characteristics can be found in the class of attribute operators [1, 7]. The discussion will focus on enhancing bright filamentous details only, because extension to dark details is trivial.

This paper mainly aims to show the speed gains of shape filters. A full-blown comparison with existing techniques will be performed later.

2   Multi-scale Mathematical Morphology

2.1   Openings

Extracting details at a particular scale using mathematical morphology can be done in a variety of ways, but the simplest is through the use of openings. An opening is a filter that removes bright or foreground details smaller than some particular scale from an image. A straightforward way to do this is by using grey scale erosions and dilations, also known as minimum and maximum filters, respectively. To perform an opening we first erode the image by assigning to each voxel the minimum grey value in a given neighbourhood (called *structuring element*). Next, the eroded image is dilated by assigning to each voxel the maximum grey value in the same neighbourhood. The size of the structuring element determines the scale of the details removed. In the following discussion, openings with spherical or cubic structuring elements of radius r will be denoted by γ_r^B. In these openings the scale is determined by the local width of structures in the image.

Openings by structuring elements are not connected set filters, and therefore not shape preserving. An adaptation of these openings, called openings-by-reconstruction [11] are connected set filters, and therefore shape preserving. An opening-by-reconstruction is performed by first eroding the image with a structuring element, and then reconstructing all details not completely removed by the erosion. In this way they remove image details completely, or leave them unaffected, but never change their shapes. Using structuring elements as above, the scale is again defined by width, but in this case it is the maximum width of a feature which determines the scale.

A different class of openings, which use different scale parameters is the class of attribute openings [1]. The earliest of these was the area opening [2], which in 3-D becomes a volume opening. In the binary case, a volume opening removes all connected foreground components with a volume smaller than some given threshold λ. If $T_h(f)$ denotes a binary image obtained by thresholding f at grey level h, and Γ_λ^V denotes the binary volume opening with scale parameter λ, the grey scale volume opening γ_λ^V for image f is given by:

$$(\gamma_\lambda^V(f))(x) = \sup\{h | x \in \Gamma_r^V(T_h(f))\}. \tag{1}$$

The interpretation of this equation is that the volume opening of an image assigns each point the highest threshold at which it still belongs to a connected foreground component C with $V(C) \geq \lambda$, with $V(C)$ denoting the volume of C. This removes details in much the same way as the opening-by-reconstruction, but it uses the volume, rather than width as criterion.

In the following subsection we will introduce sets of openings called *size distributions* which can be used for filament extraction.

2.2 Size Distributions

A set of openings $\{\gamma_r\}$, in which r is from some totally ordered set, with the property that

$$\gamma_r(\gamma_s(f)) = \gamma_{\max(r,s)}(f) \tag{2}$$

is called a size distribution or granulometry. All the openings described previously can be used to construct size distributions.

Suppose $r < s$. Obtaining an image g containing all details from image f within scale range $[r \ldots s)$ boils down to

$$g = \gamma_r(f) - \gamma_s(f) \equiv \gamma_r(f) - \gamma_s(\gamma_r(f)). \tag{3}$$

In words: remove everything smaller than r from f, then remove all details smaller than s, and deduct the result from the opening at scale r. It does not matter whether we remove the details smaller than s from the original image or from $\gamma_r(f)$.

2.3 Multi-scale Filament Extraction

If the scale parameter used is based on the width of the details, which is the case if we use $\{\gamma_r^B\}$ as size distribution, we can extract elongated details by removing all details with a volume smaller than some given threshold from g. If the scale r defines the radius of the neighbourhood used in γ_r^B, objects with volumes larger than $\epsilon 8 r^3$, with $\epsilon \gg 1$ a measure of eccentricity of the object, are likely to be filamentous. Thin slabs of sufficient size will also be retained. Thus, the image $\gamma_{\epsilon 8 r^3}^V(g)$ will contain the filamentous details at scale r. It will retain straight, curved and forked filaments equally.

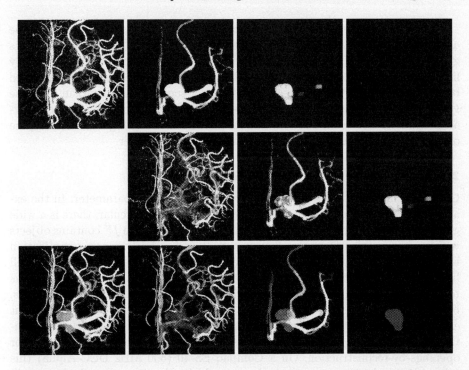

Fig. 1. Multiscale extractions of filamentous details using openings γ_r^B at scales 1, 3 and 9, using $\epsilon = 4$. The leftmost column shows the original image (top) and final result (bottom). Each of the columns to the right show the process of extracting filamentous details at each of the scales. The top row contains the openings $\gamma_{r_i}^B$; the centre row the difference images with the opening at the previous scale (or original image at scale 1); the bottom row contains the volume opening $\gamma_{32r_i}^V$ of the difference image.

We are now in a position to extract the filamentous details, starting at the thinnest, at N different scales $r_1, r_2, \ldots, r_N$. The basic method is shown in Figure 1, which shows maximum intensity projections (MIP) of a $256 \times 256 \times 256$ rotational b-plane CT-angiogram (CTA) of the arteries of the right half of a human head. A contrast agent was used and an aneurism is present. In the first step, the original image f_0 (top left) is opened by $\gamma_{r_1}^B$ (second column, topmost). This image is subtracted from the original to extract the details at scales smaller than r_1 (second column, middle row), yielding an image we will denote as f_1^B. After this, we apply a volume opening $\gamma_{\epsilon 8 r_1}^V$ (second column, bottom row) to this image to obtain the filamentous detail at scale r_1. This image is denoted f_1^V.

At the next scales, we compute the opening $\gamma_{r_i}^B$, subtract this from $\gamma_{r_{i-1}}^B(f_0)$, to obtain detail image f_i^B, open that using $\gamma_{\epsilon 8 r_i}^V$ to obtain filament image f_i^V. This is shown for two higher scales in the third and fourth column. Once all f_i^V are obtained, we sum them to obtain the output image (bottom left).

Figure 1 shows that filamentous details are indeed extracted, but that the aneurism is processed *after* it has been separated from the vessels, and that its grey level is greatly reduced. In other words, it is not recognized as a clearly filamentous structure by this version of the algorithm. This is easily corrected by the use of connected set filters, which cannot separate the aneurism from the vessels. The multi-scale algorithm can be modified by replacing γ_r^B by the equivalent openings-by-reconstruction. The result can be seen in Figure 2. Clearly, the opening-by-reconstruction retains the aneurism much better.

2.4   Problems with the Multi-scale Approach

One problem which arises is the quantization of the scale parameter. In the example shown in Figure 1 only three scales are used. In particular, there is a wide gap between scale $r_2 = 3$ and $r_3 = 9$. This means that image f_3^B contains objects with widths ranging from $r = 3$ to $r = 8$. If such a fairly coarse quantization is used, elongated structures at the lower end of the range within one bin will be removed sooner than the thicker ones. This means that there will be a bias towards thicker structures in f_3^V. Ideally, we would want to filter at all scales, but this would be prohibitively costly. As it stands, performing a 3-scale filament extraction of a $256 \times 256 \times 256$ volume takes about 168 s on a 400 MHz Pentium II processor (640 MB RAM) for the structural openings γ_r^B, and 192 s for openings-by-reconstruction. On a Compaq ES-40 (500 MHz DEC-Alpha) this takes 146 s and 131 s respectively. In general, the algorithm described here will have a computational cost proportional to the number of scales N. In the next section we will introduce a single step, connected set filtering approach, which effectively processes the image at all scales, without the computational cost.

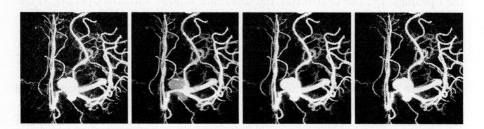

Fig. 2. A comparison of connected set filters and non-connected-set filters for filament extraction: from left to right: MIP of original image; result of multi-scale method using γ_r^B; result of multi-scale method using openings-by-reconstruction; result using attribute thinning $\phi_{2.0}^S$ as shape filter (see Section 3).

3   Shape Filters

A shape filter allows filtering based strictly on shape criteria, regardless of scale. As is shown in [10] attribute thinnings using the so-called subtractive rule provide such shape filters. This type of attribute thinning can be thought of as thresholding the original image at all possible grey levels, removing all connected foreground components of the wrong shape in each of the resulting binary images, and adding the resulting binary images up again. Selection of a particular shape category can be done by computing some shape number of each connected foreground component, and comparing it to some threshold value. The action of such an attribute thinning is shown in Figure 3. As can be seen, the thinning removes those features in the image which do not meet some shape criterion, whilst retaining all others. These filters can be computed efficiently for a variety of shape criteria using an adaptation of the Max-tree algorithm by Salembier et al. [7]. The only problem that remains is that of obtaining a shape criterion which can distinguish filamentous objects from all others.

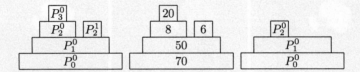

Fig. 3. The components P_j^i of a grey level image f (left), the corresponding attributes (middle) and the attribute thinning with a threshold $t = 10$ (right).

The shape filter we propose is based on two different size criteria: the volume V discussed above, and the moment of inertia I. For a given volume, the moment of inertia is minimal for a sphere, and increases rapidly as the object becomes more elongated. It can also be computed efficiently in the context of the Max-tree algorithm. For a connected set of pixels C it is defined as

$$I(C) = \frac{V(C)}{4} + \sum_{\mathbf{x} \in C} (\mathbf{x} - \bar{\mathbf{x}})^2, \tag{4}$$

in which $V(C)$ denotes the volume of C. The first term is required to account for the moment of inertia of individual voxels (which are assumed to be cubes). For a given 3-D shape, the moment of inertia scales with the size to the fifth power, whereas the the volume scales with the third power of the size. Therefore the ratio $S = \frac{I}{V^{5/3}}$ is a purely shape dependent number, i.e. it is scaling invariant, which has a minimum for a sphere (0.23) and increases rapidly with elongation. A thinning which extracts only components in which S is larger than some threshold t is denoted as ϕ_t^S. An example of applying $\phi_{2.0}^S$ to the CTA used before is shown rightmost in Figure 2. The results are difficult to distinguish from the multi-scale connected set filter approach, but the thinning takes only 41.65 s to compute on a 400 MHz Pentium II, and 33.15 s on a 500 MHz DEC Alpha.

4   Discussion

Traditional structured openings such as γ_r^B have a number of drawbacks for vessel extraction. Figure 4 shows a slice from the CTA cut through the aneurism, after filtering using the structured openings γ_r^B, and with the connected set shape filter $\phi_{2.0}^S$. The former method "hollows out" both the aneurism and thicker vessels: the central grey level is distinctly lower than that at the edge. This could pose severe problems for subsequent segmentation algorithms. By contrast, the connected set method does not suffer from this problem.

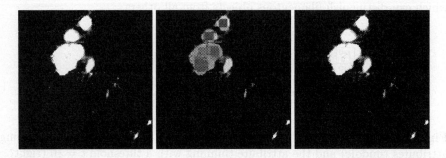

Fig. 4. Slice through CTA containing aneurism: (left) original; (middle) filtered using multi-scale approach with γ_r^B; (right) filtered using $\phi_{2.0}^S$. The middle image clearly shows a reduced grey level in the centre of the aneurism and some of the larger vessels. The connected filter approach does not suffer from this problem.

Figure 5 shows the results for $\phi_{2.0}^S$ applied to a phase contrast magnetic resonance angiogram (MRA) of $256 \times 256 \times 124$. The background is clearly suppressed, and the vessels are retained without distortion.

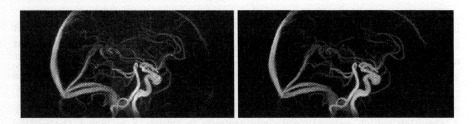

Fig. 5. MIP of MRA of a human brain: (left) original; (right) filtered using $\phi_{2.0}^S$. Filamentous detail is retained, whereas the background is suppressed.

It has been shown that connected-set filters can be used to extract filamentous details from images, either by a multi-scale approach, or by connected set shape filters. The latter approach is far faster, especially if many scales are needed.

The great advantage of connected-set filters is their inability to move edges. This allows extraction of filamentous details without distortion, and without increasing noise. Of course, these filters are not perfect. There are many instances in which edges should be moved, e.g., to suppress boundary noise. This could be achieved by post-processing. It also remains to be seen whether connected-set shape filters improve segmentation. Finally, the attribute and threshold used in this shape filter may not be optimal, even though the performance in the images tested is encouraging. In the near future we intend to address these issues, and test shape filters against other methods systematically.

References

[1] E. J. Breen and R. Jones. Attribute openings, thinnings and granulometries. *Computer Vision and Image Understanding*, 64(3):377–389, 1996.

[2] F. Cheng and A. N. Venetsanopoulos. An adaptive morphological filter for image processing. *IEEE Trans. Image Proc.*, 1:533–539, 1992.

[3] Y. P. Du and D. L. Parker. Vessel enhancement filtering in three-dimensional MR angiograms using long-range signal correlation. *J. Magn. Reson. Imag.*, 7:447–450, 1997.

[4] A. F. Frangi, W. J. Niessen, K. L. Vincken, and M. A. Viergever. Multiscale vessel enhancement filtering. In W. M. Wells, A. Colchester, and S. Delp, editors, *Medical Image Computing and Computer-Assisted Intervention – MICCAI'98*, volume 1496 of *Lecture Notes in Computer Science*, pages 130–137. Springer, 1998.

[5] H. J. A. M. Heijmans. Connected morphological operators for binary images. *Comput. Vis. Image Understand.*, 73:99–120, 1999.

[6] M. Orkisz, M. Hernández-Hoyos, P. Douek, and I. Magnin. Advances of blood vessel morphology analysis in 3D magnetic resonance images. *Mach. Vis. Graph.*, 9:463–471, 2000.

[7] P. Salembier, A. Oliveras, and L. Garrido. Anti-extensive connected operators for image and sequence processing. *IEEE Transactions on Image Processing*, 7:555–570, 1998.

[8] Y. Sato, S. Nakajima, N. Shiraga, H. Atsumi, S. Yoshida, T. Koller, G. Gerig, and R. Kinikis. 3D multi-scale line filter for segmentation and visualization of curvilinear structures in medical images. *Medical Image Analysis*, 2:143–168, 1998.

[9] A. Spohr, T. Agger, M. Carlsen, and J. Nielsen. Quantitative morphology of filamentous micro-organisms. In M. H. F. Wilkinson and F. Schut, editors, *Digital Image Analysis of Microbes*, pages 373–410. John Wiley and Sons, Ltd, Chichester, UK, 1998.

[10] E. R. Urbach and M. H. F. Wilkinson. Shape distributions and decomposition of grey scale images. IWI-report 2000-9-15, Institute for Mathematics and Computing Science, University of Groningen, 2001.

[11] L. Vincent. Morphological grayscale reconstruction in image analysis: application and efficient algorithm. *IEEE Transactions on Image Processing*, 2:176–201, 1993.

[12] M. H. F. Wilkinson and J. B. T. M. Roerdink. Fast morphological attribute operations using Tarjan's union-find algorithm. In *Proceedings of the ISMM2000*, pages 311–320, Palo Alto, CA, June 2000.

[13] O. Wink, W. J. Niessen, and M. A. Viergever. Fast delineation and visualization of vessels in 3-D angiographic images. *IEEE Transactions on Medical Imaging*, 19:337–346, 2000.

3D Freehand Echocardiography for Automatic Left Ventricle Reconstruction and Analysis Based on Multiple Acoustic Windows

Xujiong Ye, J. Alison Noble, and Jerome Declerck

Medical Vision Laboratory, Department of Engineering Science, University of Oxford,
Parks Road, Oxford OX1 3PJ, UK.
{xujiong, noble, jdecler}@robots.ox.ac.uk

Abstract. A new method is proposed to reconstruct and analyse the left ventricle (LV) from multiple acoustic windows 3D ultrasound acquired using a 3D rotational probe. Prior research in this area has been based on one acoustic window acquisition. However, the data suffers from several limitations that degrade the 3D reconstruction, such as motion of the probe during the acquisition and the presence of shadow due to bone (ribs) and air (in the lungs). In this paper we aim to overcome these limitations by automatically fusing information from multiple acoustic windows sparse-view acquisitions and using a position sensor to track the probe in real time. Geometric constraints of the object shape, and spatio-temporal information relating to the image acquisition process are used to propose new algorithms for (1) grouping endocardial edge cues from an initial image segmentation and (2) defining a novel reconstruction method that utilises information from multiple acoustic windows. We illustrate our new method on phantom and real heart data and compare its performance against our previous approach that is based on a single acoustic window.

1 Introduction

Advances in both acquisition technology and computing power have meant that three dimensional (3D) cardiac image analysis has become an active area of research. In particular, 3D cardiac ultrasound offers potential advantages over X-ray angiography and nuclear medicine methods in terms of its lack of ionising radiation and, with respect to cardiac MR, better spatial resolution.

The state-of-the-art method for 3D cardiac ultrasound acquisition uses a 3D rotational scanning configuration, in which the transducer rotates about a central axis of the probe at a fixed angle increment. This generates a series of 2D sequences with a common axis of rotation for different cardiac cycles.

Most prior research on 3D ultrasound left ventricle (LV) analysis has focused on one acoustic window [1][2][3]. However, in this case, the data suffers from several limitations that degrade the reconstruction and reduce the clinical value. Most notably: 1) The presence of bone (ribs) and air (in the lungs) makes integration of 2D slices from one acoustic window particularly difficult, as large parts of the field of view are shadowed. 2) Respiration gating is employed to obtain "optimal" image acquisition quality. The net effect is that acquisition times can be long (several miniutes) and this inevitably results in slight motion of the probe during the scanning.

In this paper we aim to overcome these limitations by using a position sensor to track the probe in real time and fusing automatically detected image features from multiple acoustic window sparse-view acquisitions. We use geometric constraints of the object shape and image acquisition process to propose new algorithms for (1) grouping endocardial edge cues from an initial image segmentation and (2) defining a novel reconstruction method that utilises information from multiple acoustic windows. We illustrate our new method on phantom and real heart data and compare its performance to our previous approach that was based on a single acoustic window.

The most closely related research to our own is the work by Legget et al [4]. The major differences are that they used 2D scanning rather than 3D rotational scanning and 3D reconstruction was based on manually delineated feature points.

2 Proposed Method and Algorithms

Figure 1 shows a flow-diagram outlining the key steps in our approach. In the following section each step is described.

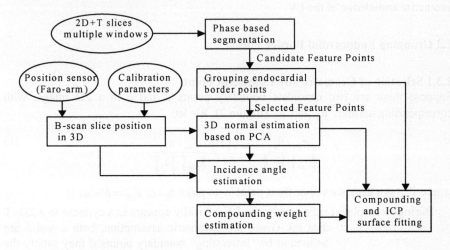

Fig. 1. Overall block diagram of the proposed method.

2.1 Image Acquisition

Digital 3D+T data was acquired on a HP SONOS 5500 ultrasound machine (Agilent Technologies) using a 3-5MHZ 3D rotating transducer with the Faro-arm position sensor (FARO Technologies) attached to enable real-time recording of probe position. The angle increment of the rotational probe was set to 6 degrees, so that for each acoustic window 30 co-axial slices were obtained. The Faro-arm was calibrated using an in-house calibration routine based on a ping-pong ball calibration object [5].

Scanning was performed using ECG and respiration gating on two acoustic windows: apical long-axis view and parasternal short-axis view. Subjects were asked to remain as still as possible during data acquisition so that there was a good spatial alignment between the different views. Data was acquired at a rate of 25 frames per second.

2.2 Phase Congruency Based Segmentation

A phase congruency (PC) based feature detection method is used to find candidate endocardial points [6]. Briefly, this algorithm involves calculating a measure of feature asymmetry (edgeness) using a band of log-Gabor wavelet filter pairs spread in a 2D or 3D space. The measure values vary from a maximum of 1, indicating a very significant feature, down to 0, indicating no significance. This provides an intensity invariant feature detection method. The normal to the features can also be estimated and the direction of the normal is defined as a negative edge (from bright to dark).

This segmentation method provides accurate localisation of endocardial borders in situations of changing image contrast and poor signal-to-noise ratio. But one of the disadvantages of this method is that it produces a large number of "spurious" noisy points at the same time (Figure 3(a)). To reject these points, the following grouping method has been developed which exploits spatio-temporal information and geometric knowledge of the LV.

2.3 Grouping Endocardial Border Points

2.3.1 Selection of Geometrically Consistent Points

Suppose there are two candidate boundary points a and b in a 2D image, with corresponding normals $\vec{n}_a$ and $\vec{n}_b$ (Figure 2). We let:

$$f_1 = \frac{\vec{c}_{ab} \cdot \vec{n}_a}{\|\vec{c}_{ab}\| \cdot \|\vec{n}_a\|} \quad , \quad f_2 = \frac{\vec{c}_{ba} \cdot \vec{n}_b}{\|\vec{c}_{ba}\| \cdot \|\vec{n}_b\|} \tag{1}$$

where $\vec{c}_{ab}$ is a distance vector from point a to point b. i.e, $\vec{c}_{ab} = b - a$.

During a complete cardiac cycle, the LV basically appears as a cylinder in a 2D+T data set. Given this geometric assumption, both a and b are defined to be "interesting" boundary points if they satisfy the following three criteria:

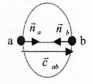

(1) The endocardial boundary points must have sufficient face-to-faceness [7] F defined as $F(a,b) = f_1 \cdot f_2$. Values for F near +1 occur when both boundary points face inward (or outward). An error threshold ε is set for acceptable face-to-faceness, namely, $F(a,b) > 1 - \varepsilon$.

Fig.2. A definition of face-to-faceness for two points.

(2) The normals of endocardial points are inward, namely, $f_1 > 0$ and $f_2 > 0$.

(3) The distance from one boundary point to the other must lie between $c_{\min}$ and $c_{\max}$, the parameters are determined by the structure of LV.

Figure 3(b) shows the result of applying the above three criteria on an initial PC based segmentation end-diastole image (Figure 3(a)). A low error threshold for acceptable face-to-faceness was set (ε =0.05). Referring to this figure, note that the output of this shows that most of the noisy points are filtered, but some spurious boundary points are still present. Further, some real boundary points have been filtered due to shadow on one part of image. To further recover the endocardial feature points and reject the spurious points the following refinement step is adopted.

2.3.2 Refinement of Edge Points Grouping

The refinement process involves fitting a cubic parametric B spline curve to the selected candidate feature data points that is represented as:

$$p(u) = \sum_{i=0}^{n} d_i B_{i,3}(u) \quad , \quad u \in [u_3, u_{n+1}] \tag{2}$$

where d_i represents the i-th control point (of n control points), B is the B-spline basis function attached to the parameterisation u, defined on a regular knot distribution u_i.

There are two advantages in using this step. First, we can define more accurately region of interest (ROI) around the endocardial boundary. This is useful for automatically defining a processing ROI that can speed up the analysis on the following time frames, as the endocardial boundary on the following frames is inside the boundary region of the first time frame (end-diastole). Second, the normal at each point on the fitting curve can be calculated by its tangent vector that is defined as:

$$p^{(1)}(u) = \sum_{i=0}^{n} d_i^{(1)} B_{i,2}(u) \quad , \quad d_i^{(1)} = 3 \cdot \frac{d_i - d_{i-1}}{u_{i+3} - u_i} \tag{3}$$

here $p^{(1)}(u)$ is the first differential. The other parameters are the same as in Eq. (2).

Both the location and normal vector are considered in the distance measurement to recover the missing endocardial feature points and reject further spurious points. Figure 3(c) shows a fitting result on the selected feature points; Figure 3 (d) shows the final result of grouped endocardial boundary points.

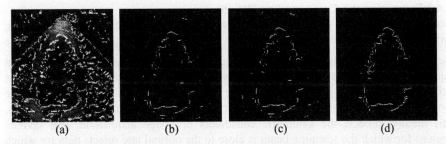

(a)   (b)   (c)   (d)

Fig. 3. (a) Initial PC based candidate boundary points overlaid on the end-diastole data slice. (b) Selection of endocardial feature points using face-to-faceness method. (c) A cubic B-spline fitting on feature points. (d) Final result of grouped endocardial features with the fitting curve.

2.4 3D Reconstruction from Multiple Acoustic Windows

We now turn to the problem of how to recover a 3D endocardial surface. The first step is to reconstruct a 3D data volume from a series of grouped endocardial feature points obtained from multiple acoustic windows. In our freehand imaging system the real 3D location of every feature point in every B-scan slice can be computed and combined into a 3D data volume after the calibration process. The "nearest neighbour" approach is used in this step, which means for each pixel, the nearest voxel is filled with the value of that pixel. For overlapping data from different views, rather than using the maximum or average intensity method, we adopt a weighted compounding approach in which the weight of each point is determined by the incidence angle of the ultrasound beam that is defined between the scanning beam and the 3D normal to the surface at the given point [8].

2.4.1 Estimating the 3D Normal Based on Principal Components Analysis
The 3D feature point normal can be estimated from the neighbouring data points using principal components analysis (PCA), which is described as follows:

For each 3D data point x_i, k points which are closest to x_i are found. This set is denoted by Nbhd(x_i). Our purpose is to find a 3D vector n_i that is most orthogonal to the k-neighbourhood set as a whole by solving the eigenvalue equation:

$$Rq = \lambda q \qquad (4)$$

where $R = \sum_{x \in Nbhd(x_i)} (x - o_i) \otimes (x - o_i)$, and o_i is the centroid of Nbhd(x_i).

If $\lambda_i^1 \geq \lambda_i^2 \geq \lambda_i^3$ denote the eigenvalues of R associated with unit eigenvectors $\vec{q}_i^1$, $\vec{q}_i^2$, $\vec{q}_i^3$ respectively, n_i is chosen to be either $\vec{q}_i^3$ or $-\vec{q}_i^3$. In our case, the selection of the correct sign is determined by using the point's 2D in-plane component normal $\vec{n}_{2d}$, which is obtained by the PC based segmentation. If $\vec{n}_{2d} \cdot \vec{q}_i^3 > 0$, $\vec{q}_i^3$ is chosen as the 3D normal of the point x_i, while $-\vec{q}_i^3$ is for the condition of $\vec{n}_{2d} \cdot \vec{q}_i^3 < 0$.

2.4.2 Estimating the Compounding Weight
For overlapping data from the multiple views, we use a weighted compounding approach. The compounding weight α is defined as $\alpha = |\cos(\theta)|$, where θ is the incidence angle at each point that is defined as an angle between the scanning beam and the 3D normal to the surface at a given point. The position sensor provides information about the probe's direction, or the direction of the scanning beam. The smaller the incidence angle θ is, the bigger the weight α assigns to this point. Thus, this method reflects the geometric constraints of image acquisition, and favours regions for which the scanning beam is close to the normal and rejects data for which the scanning beam is far away from the normal.

In the final step, as in our previous work, an Iterative Closest Point (ICP) based surface fitting algorithm is used to recover the endocardial surface [9][10].

3. Experimental Results

3.1 Study on Glove Phantom

One finger of a latex glove was fully filled with tap water as a phantom, and securely fixed in a small box containing water.

Data sets were acquired from two acoustic windows on this phantom. Figure 4(a) is the feature points in 3D selected using our method for one acoustic window and for second window in (b). The incidence angle weighted 3D feature points reconstruction from two windows is shown in (c) and the results of the ICP based surface fitting on each window and combined windows are shown in (d), (e) and (f), respectively.

The phantom volume measurement was calculated to be 230ml for the true volume while 220.73ml for the fitting result from two windows (Figure (f)), 194.22ml and 165.63 ml from each window (Figure (d) and (e)). This demonstrates the two views method has better performance for recovery object shape than from a single window.

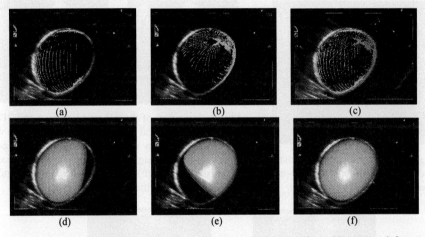

Fig. 4. Results on a glove phantom overlaid on one image slice. 3D grouped feature points on each acoustic window (a and b), and combined windows (c). ICP surface fitting on each window points (d and e) and combined window points (f).

3.2 Study on Real Heart Data

In this experiment, data sets were acquired from two acoustic windows: apical long-axis view and parasternal short-axis view. For each view (30 co-axial slices), scanning lasted 3-4 minutes during which there was slight motion of the probe. Figure 5 shows the true positions of the probe on each slice during two acoustic windows scanning. The maximum motion of the probe during each view acquisition is about 2mm. Figure 6 shows the 3D reconstruction of slices from two acoustic window acquisitions.

Figure 7 and Figure 8 show results using the new method. Figure 7 shows the projection of the 3D surfaces and grouped endocardial feature points onto one image slice. Figure 7(a) is from the apical long-axis view only, (a conventional view used in

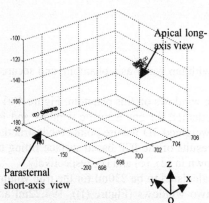

Fig. 5. Probe positions of two acoustic window scanning

LV volume analysis from ultrasound), while (b) is to combine feature points from both the apical long-axis view and parasternal short-axis view. Note that, the gap between the grouped endocardial feature points in (a) can be connected using the feature points from the short-axis view in (b).

In Figure 8, the 3D endocardial surfaces from the long-axis view, short-axis view and combined views can be seen in (c), (d) and (e), respectively. Due to the large area of shadowing in the apical long-axis scanning, there is a big hole in the 3D features reconstruction

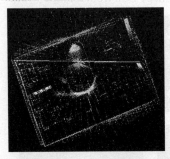

Fig. 6. 3D reconstruction of image slices from long-axis window and short-axis window acquisitions.

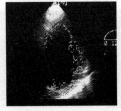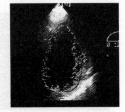

Fig. 7. Projection of the 3D fitted surface and 3D grouped endocardical feature points, lying within a clipped slab (2 mm width) centred on one image slice. Surface fitting on one apical endocardial boundary points (left) and on combined apical and parasternal endocardial boundary points (right).

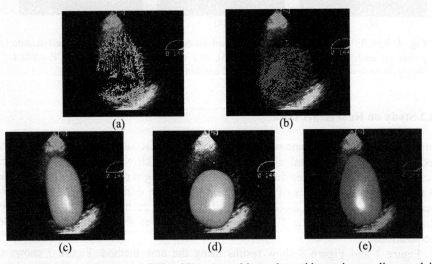

Fig. 8. Results of the proposed algorithms on real heart data with one image slice overlaid on; (a)~(b) 3D endocardial feature points from long-axis window and short-axis window; (c)~(e) ICP surface fitting on each window and combined acoustic windows, respectively.

(left of the 3D points in Figure 8(a)). Using the new method this is filled using information from the parasternal short-axis view (see (b)). Note that, in this experiment, apart from the presence of the shadow in the short-axis window, we just acquired one part of the LV data during the short-axis window scanning.

4. Conclusions and Future Work

In this paper we have proposed and performed initially testing on a new method for automatically fusing information from multiple 3D echocardiographic windows. The approach is novel in the way that it works on the automatically detected feature points and information is fused based on the use of geometric constraints of image acquisition and knowledge of the object. Our experimental results show that fusing information from multiple acoustic windows can fill in data points in shadow regions of other windows and improve the quality of 3D reconstruction relative to those based on a single acoustic window. Future plans include looking more closely at how the denseness of data affects the method, and evaluating against a reference such as cardiac MR imaging.

Acknowledgments: The authors gratefully acknowledge the financial support of the UK Medical Research Council (grant G9802587), and Dr Nigel Clarke at the Oxford John Radcliffe Hospital for assistance in acquiring experimental data. We would also like to thank Guofang Xiao and David Atkinson for spending time discussing some of this work with us.

References

1. Giachetti.A. Online analysis of echocardiographic image sequences. Medical Image Analysis, 2(3), 261-284, 1998.
2. Sanchez-Ortiz, G.I., Noble. J.A. et al. Automating LV motion analysis from three dimensional echocardiography. Proceedings of MIUA, Oxford. UK, 85-88, 1999.
3. Sanchez-Ortiz,G.I., Declerck,J. et al. Automating 3D echocardiographic image analysis. Proceedings of MICCAI. Pittsburg, PA, USA, 687-696, 2000.
4. Legget, M.E., Leotta, D.F. et al. System for quantitative 3D echocardiography of the left ventricle based on a magnetic-field position and orientation sensing system. IEEE Trans. Biomedical Engineering, 45(4), 495-504, 1998.
5. Xiao, G.F. 3D freehand ultrasound imaging of breast. PhD thesis, University of Oxford, 2001.
6. Mulet-Parada,M. and Noble,J.A. 2D+T boundary detection in Echocardiography. Proceedings of MICCAI. Cambridge, Mass. U.S.A, 186-196, 1998.
7. Stetten, G.D. and Pizer, S.M. Medial-Node Models to Identify and Measure Objects in Real-Time 3D Echocardiography. IEEE Trans. Medical Imaging, 18(10), 1025-1034, 1999.
8. Leotta, D.F. et al. 3D ultrasound imaging of the rotator cuff: spatial compounding and tendon thickness measurement. Ultrasound in Med. & Biol., 26(4), 509-525, 2000.
9. Besl, P. and McKay, N. A method for registration of 3-D shapes. IEEE Trans. Pattern Analysis and Machine Intelligence, 14(2), 239-256, 1992.
10.Declerck, J. et al. Automatic registration and alignment on a template of cardiac stress and rest reoriented SPECT images. IEEE Trans. Medical Imaging, 16(6), 727-737, 1997.

A Quantitative Vascular Analysis System for Evaluation of Atherosclerotic Lesions by MRI

William Kerwin[1], Chao Han[1], Baocheng Chu[1], Dongxiang Xu[2], Ying Luo[2], Jenq-Neng Hwang[2], Thomas Hatsukami[3], and Chun Yuan[1]

[1] University of Washington, Department of Radiology, Box 357115, 1959 NE Pacific St., Seattle, WA 98195, USA
{bkerwin,chaohan,chubc,cyuan}@u.washington.edu
http://vil.rad.washington.edu
[2] University of Washington, Department of Electrical Engineering, Box 352500, Seattle, WA 98195-2500, USA
{xdx,luoying,hwang}@ee.washington.edu
[3] University of Washington, Department of Surgery, Box 358280, 1660 S Columbia Way, Seattle, WA 98108, USA
tomhat@u.washington.edu

Abstract. An analysis package called QVAS (quantitative vascular analysis system) is presented for the evaluation of atherosclerotic arterial lesions visualized in vivo by magnetic resonance imaging. QVAS permits interactive identification of vessel and lesion boundaries, segmentation of tissue classes within the lesion, quantitative analysis of lesion features, and three dimensional display of lesion structure. The performance of QVAS is demonstrated using images of carotid artery lesions.

1   Introduction

Cardiovascular disease is the leading cause of death in the West and most heart attacks and strokes result when an atherosclerotic lesion ruptures, which leads to local formation of a thrombus or release of emboli that block distal vessels [1]. The structural features that predispose lesions to rupture can now be resolved in vivo using high resolution magnetic resonance (MR) imaging, at least for large vessels such as the carotid arteries [2,3]. From MR images, quantitative measurements of the lesion size, composition, and distribution can be made, which may allow researchers to study lesion progression, pharmacologists to evaluate the response to drug therapy, or clinicians to assess the risk associated with a particular lesion [4,5]. Such analyses would be facilitated by a computer-based package for the evaluation of vascular MR images.

A number of general purpose packages for the evaluation of medical images exist, including NIH Image (National Institutes of Health, Bethesda, MD) and ANALYZE (Mayo Clinic, Rochester, MN). For specialized applications, however, these packages are often insufficient. As a result, tailored image analysis packages have been proposed, including MASS and FLOW (MEDIS, Danbury, CT), which are used for quantitative measurement of cardiac function. A similar package

W. Niessen and M. Viergever (Eds.): MICCAI 2001, LNCS 2208, pp. 786–794, 2001.

specifically designed for analysis of atherosclerotic lesions is warranted by several challenging aspects of the lesions. First, the lesions are small, with diameters on the order of 1-2 cm at the largest. Within this small space, lesions often exhibit a highly complicated morphology with rapid transitions between tissue types. Finally, any of a large number of clinically significant tissue types may or may not be present in a given lesion.

In this paper we present a comprehensive, tailored analysis package for evaluating atherosclerotic lesions as visualized by MR imaging. The package is called the Quantitative Vascular Analysis System (QVAS) and addresses three primary goals. Foremost, QVAS enables computer assisted identification of lesion boundaries, constituent tissue types, and distribution of tissues. Second, the information extracted via QVAS can be converted into quantitative measurements of lesion severity. Third, QVAS permits the construction of a three dimensional model of the lesion for use in an interactive display.

The current version of QVAS is capable of processing a single set of MR images that span the length of a lesion and have a single contrast weighting. Individual images are serially processed to identify relevant boundaries and tissue types. Extracted information is then propagated from one image to the next to increase automation.

This paper is organized as follows. In Section 2, we describe the pathology of atherosclerotic lesions and their visualization by MR imaging. Then, in Section 3, we provide a synopsis of the image processing algorithms utilized by QVAS. In Section 4, we discuss data flow and demonstrate it with results from carotid artery lesions. Finally, we conclude in Section 5 with a discussion of QVAS applications and planned improvements to QVAS.

2   Background on Atherosclerosis

Pathology. A typical advanced atherosclerotic lesion surgically removed from a carotid artery is shown in Fig. 1a. At the center is the lumen, which is the normal passageway for blood. Separating the lumen from the bulk of the lesion is an encapsulating fibrous layer (fibrous cap). Behind the cap lies the core of the lesion, which may include lipid-rich necrotic material, cholesterol crystals, calcifications, intraplaque hemorrhage, and/or microvessels.

Culprit lesions, implicated in heart attacks, are characterized by erosion and rupture of the fibrous cap exposing the thrombogenic core [6]. Traditionally, the risk of rupture is determined by percent narrowing of the artery (stenosis), but lesions with only moderate stenosis often rupture as well [7]. Studies show that the fibrous cap may be prone to rupture if it is markedly thinned, overlies a predominantly lipid core, is adjacent to substantial amounts of microvessels, or has adjacent calcifications [1,6,8]. Identification of these lesion features may therefore provide the best risk assessment.

Imaging. Magnetic resonance imaging has been shown to be sensitive to the different tissues present in atherosclerotic lesions and therefore can be used to

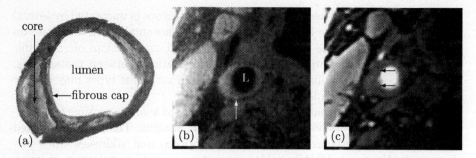

Fig. 1. Atherosclerotic lesion: (a) surgically removed from a carotid artery and stained (H&E), with tissue regions labeled; (b) imaged in vivo (vessel indicated by arrow, lumen by "L") using a black-blood double inversion recovery T1 weighted sequence (TR/TI/TE = 800/650/9 msec); (c) imaged in vivo using a time-of-flight sequence (TR/TE = 23/4 msec) that generates a bright lumen and dark fibrous cap (arrows).

assess risk of rupture [3]. Most in vivo studies have involved the relatively large carotid artery, which is commonly implicated in strokes and can be imaged in high detail because its location in the neck permits the use of highly sensitive surface coils [2,9]. Other studies have shown the potential for MR imaging of aorta lesions and coronary lesions [10,11].

Typical in vivo images of a carotid lesion are shown in Fig. 1 with T1 and time-of-flight (TOF) contrast weightings. The T1 weighted image provides the best contrast for the lumen and outer wall boundaries. The TOF weighting provides the best visualization of the fibrous cap, which is characterized by low intensity [4]. Lipid-rich core and hemorrhage are both characterized by moderate to high intensities on T1 and TOF weighted images. Calcifications are characterized by low intensity on all contrast weightings.

3   Image Processing Methods

The fundamental processing goal for quantitative analysis of lesion structure is to divide the MR images into regions of known tissue type. Our framework for this division is a "coupled contour mesh" as illustrated in Fig. 2. The coupled contour mesh consists of "nodes," denoted by the asterisks, and "paths" that connect the nodes. A region is delineated by a closed sequence of nodes and the paths connecting them. Finally, each region may have a corresponding tissue type if it is known. Generating such a coupled contour mesh is accomplished interactively with the assistance of several basic image processing tools: segmentation, boundary identification, and tissue classification.

Segmentation. The first image processing tool we employ segments the image pixels into clusters with similar brightness characteristics. The segmentation

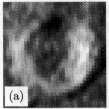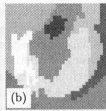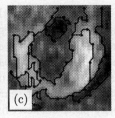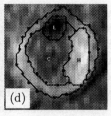

Fig. 2. Processing of a coupled contour mesh: (a) Region of interest around an atherosclerotic lesion; (b) Segmented image with different regions shown as different gray scales; (c) Coupled contours that divide the image into the segmented regions; (d) Coupled contours after editing with the active contour algorithm and tissue classification (L = lumen, C = core, H = hemorrhage).

algorithm is a two step Markov random field (MRF) approach called quadtree highest confidence first (QHCF) [12]. The first step in QHCF is to identify m seed pixels as initial estimates of cluster means and locations. This is done by quadtree division of an image into rectangular subregions until the variance of all pixel intensities within each subregion falls below a user-specified threshold T. Then, the one pixel in each subregion that is closest to the mean intensity is extracted and used as an initial cluster, while all other pixels are left unassigned.

The final clusters are identified by seeking the maximum of an MRF probability function or, equivalently, by minimizing

$$E = \sum \left[(y_i - \mu_i)^2 + V_N(y_i) + V_E(y_i) \right] , \tag{1}$$

where y_i is the intensity of the ith pixel, μ_i is the mean of the region to which the ith pixel has been assigned, and V_N and V_E are additional energies based on neighborhoods and edges, respectively. The term $(y_i - \mu_i)^2$ forces pixels to be assigned to a region with similar intensities. The term V_N favors assignments to the dominant region in a 3×3 neighborhood N and is given by

$$V_N(y_i) = \beta_1 \sum_{j \in N} U(i,j) ,$$

where $U(i,j)$ is 1 if y_i and y_j are in different regions and -1 if they are in the same region; β_1 is a user-specified weight. The term V_E adds an additional penalty if pixels on opposite sides of a Canny-detected edge are assigned to the same region. Finally, the assignments to regions are performed by iteratively finding the pixel assignment that will provide the greatest reduction in (1) until no further reductions are possible, an approach known as "highest confidence first." An example of a segmented image is shown in Fig. 2b.

Active Contour Boundary Identification. From the segmentation, a coupled contour mesh can be generated, as in Fig. 2c, by placing nodes at intersections of three or more regions and at intervals along boundaries between two regions,

and then connecting the nodes with paths running along region boundaries. To
correctly identify tissue regions, however, this mesh requires further editing, including insertion of nodes and paths to define or split regions, removal of nodes
and paths to combine regions, and repositioning of existing nodes. After manually editing node positions, new paths between connected nodes are generated
with an active contour method that searches for a minimal energy path [13].

The minimal energy path between fixed nodes is defined as the curve $C(v)$
that minimizes

$$E = \int_{\Omega} g(|\nabla I(C(v))|)|C'(v)|dv \qquad (2)$$

where ∇I is the gradient of the image, g is a strictly decreasing potential and
$\Omega \in [0, 1]$ is the parameterization interval for the contour segment. Based on this
formulation, the minimal path will follow high gradient boundaries in the image
and will be smoothly varying so that the first derivative is near zero. In practice,
this minimal path is approximated by selecting a sequence of points from one
node to the other, where the optimal sequence of points is found using graph
search techniques over a finite grid. An example of the end result of boundary
identification is shown in Fig. 2d.

The search for a minimal path does not address the fact that the original
nodes may not have been placed at minimal energy positions. The QVAS package
therefore also includes two optional contour evolution modes in which selected
node positions are updated. The first is known as "wriggling," which progressively refines overlapping subsegments of a contour that may include nodes [13].
The second mode is "rule-based wriggling," which seeks a specific tissue type
within a closed contour. In this mode, a contour segment will balloon outward if
the adjacent pixels on either side have a mean intensity that is similar to the desired tissue (i.e. the segment lies within the tissue). The segment shrinks inward
if the adjacent pixels on either side have a mean intensity that is not similar (i.e.
the segment is outside the tissue). Finally, the standard minimal path search
is employed if only the pixels on the inner side of the segment are similar in
mean intensity to the desired tissue (i.e. the segment is near the boundary). If
the initial boundary contains any portion of the desired tissue within it, then
rule-based wriggling will converge to the correct boundary, even if the initial
estimate of contour position is poor.

Tissue Classification Once the tissue regions have been identified, a tissue label
such as fibrous cap, lipid core, or calcification must be associated with each. In
general, tissue labeling must be done manually by a trained expert. We have,
however, developed an adaptive algorithm that facilitates labeling. For each contrast weighting, we have compiled a library of regional brightness values and associated tissue types. To assign a label to an unknown region we find the tissue
type from the library with the nearest mean brightness value. To account for
absolute signal differences, we perform histogram equalization before computing
means or making comparisons.

Initially, this labeling scheme is highly prone to errors because of the variation
between patients. As the QVAS user corrects mislabeled regions by hand, the

program enters an adaptive mode, wherein the mean intensities from the library are adjusted to better match the current lesion. The adjustment is performed along the first two principle components of variation, seeking to minimize the total squared difference between the adjusted means and the brightness values observed in the current lesion. As QVAS adapts in this manner, fewer and fewer user interventions are necessary.

4   Image Analysis Results

Building a Coupled Contour Typical steps by which a QVAS user employs the image processing tools to construct a coupled contour mesh are illustrated in Fig. 3. First, a region of interest is identified around the artery (Fig. 3a) and the segmentation algorithm is applied. The threshold T is interactively adjusted until a small number of regions approximately covers the vessel lumen and an additional set covers the entire vessel wall (Fig. 3b). Then the sets of nodes that define the lumen and outer wall boundaries are chosen (Fig. 3c), which provides an initial delineation of the lesion boundaries. Next, refinement of the lesion boundaries is performed using the active contour algorithm (Fig. 3d). Ordinarily, the wriggle procedure is used to automatically adjust the boundaries to minimum energy positions. If, however, the boundary is partially obscured or otherwise poorly defined, the user may be required to manually adjust the nodes of one or both contours. Once the lesion boundaries have been finalized, the segmentation algorithm is reapplied, this time only to the pixels contained within the contours. Again, the user interactively controls the segmentation threshold, selecting a level that best delineates the observed regions in the lesion (Fig. 3e). Finally, the subregions are manually edited using the active contour tools and semi-automated tissue classification is performed (Fig. 3f).

Feed Forward To characterize an entire lesion volume, coupled contour meshes must be built for each of a stack of images spanning the lesion. Although each image could be treated independently, significant time savings are possible if information is fed forward from one image to the next using the following hierarchy. First, the lumen and outer wall boundaries from the previous image are mapped to the next image and allowed to evolve by wriggling, specifically using rule-based wriggling for the more homogeneous lumen. If either boundary search fails, user adjustment is necessary. Next, the segmentation algorithm is applied seeking initial quadtree regions with intensities similar to the previous regions. After application of the segmentation algorithm, the user may manually adjust the delineated regions. Alternatively, if the segmentation results are poor, the algorithm may be reapplied using the standard quadtree initialization scheme. Finally, for tissue classification, the adapted tissue means from the previous image are used in the current one. The end result is a complete 3D segmentation of the lesion, an example of which is rendered in Fig 4.

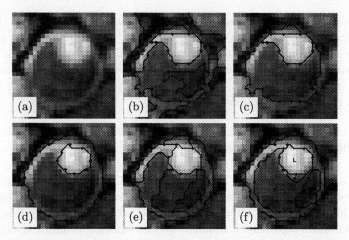

Fig. 3. Processing steps in lesion analysis: (a) region of interest is selected; (b) segmentation algorithm is applied; (c) contours that best correspond to the lumen and outer wall boundaries are chosen; (d) boundaries are refined using the active contour algorithm; (e) regions between the boundaries are segmented; (f) regions are edited and assigned tissue types: lumen (L), fibrous (F), core (C), calcium (CA).

5 Discussion

The QVAS package is an interactive environment for rapid processing of MR images of atherosclerotic lesions to identify tissue regions and types for clinical and investigative applications. Specifically, QVAS facilitates quantitative measurements such as total volume, percent lipid content, or fibrous cap thickness. Such measurements may be formulated as a "lesion index" for monitoring response to therapy or assessing risk of heart attack or stroke [14].

Additionally, the regions identified by QVAS can be used for volumetric reconstruction of the lesion, which may be used to study disease progression or for surgical planning. For example, the artery reconstructed in Fig. 4 was imaged prior to endarterectomy. The lumen size (Fig. 4c) is ordinarily the only information available to the surgeon via angiography. While this clearly indicates the presence of a large lesion impinging on the internal carotid artery, it does not show that significant calcifications exist in the vicinity of the bifurcation, as seen in Fig. 4b. QVAS thus provides important information for surgical planning.

Finally, although QVAS incorporates a number of automatic and semiautomatic tools for the user, further automation would be necessary for routine clinical use. Also, simultaneous analysis of multiple images taken at the same position is necessary for applications such as the study of contrast agent dynamics. For these reasons, we are developing an advanced version of QVAS that simultaneously operates on multiple images of the same slice obtained with different contrast weightings. The package will include a registration module, a multispectral segmentation algorithm, and an active contour model that com-

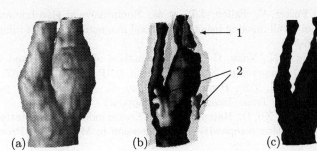

Fig. 4. Reconstructed carotid arteries rendered using OpenDX (IBM, Armonk, NY): (a) Outer wall of the carotid arteries showing the common carotid artery bifurcating into the external carotid artery (in front) and internal carotid artery (in back); (b) Within the wall, a lipid core (1) and several calcifications (2) are present; (c) The severely stenosed (arrow) vessel lumen shows evidence of the lipid core, but no indication of the calcifications.

bines boundary information from multiple images. The details of the new version will be reported in the future.

Acknowledgement. This work was supported by NIH grant R01-HL61816 and by AstraZeneca pharmaceuticals.

References

1. Fuster, V., Stein, B., Ambrose, J.A., et al.: Atherosclerotic plaque rupture and thrombosis. Evolving concepts. Circ. **82**(3 Suppl) (1990) II47–59
2. Fayad, Z.A., Fuster, V.: Characterization of atherosclerotic plaques by magnetic resonance imaging. Ann. N.Y. Acad. Sci. **902** (2000) 173–186
3. Ingersleben, G.V., Schmiedl, U.P., Hatsukami, T.S., et al.: Characterization of atherosclerotic plaques at the carotid bifurcation: Correlation of high resolution MR with histology. RadioGraphics **17** (1997) 1417-1423
4. Hatsukami, T., Ross, R., Polissar, N., Yuan, C.: Visualization of fibrous cap thickness and rupture in human atherosclerotic carotid plaque in vivo with high resolution magnetic resonance imaging. Circ. **102** (2000) 959-964
5. Yuan, C., Beach, K.W., Smith, H.L., Hatsukami, T.: In vivo measurements of maximum plaque area based on high resolution MRI. Circ. **98** (1998) 2666–2671
6. Falk, E.: Why do plaques rupture? Circ. **86** (6 Suppl) (1992) III30–42
7. Libby, P.: The interface of atherosclerosis and thrombosis: Basic mechanisms. Vasc. Med. **3** (1998) 225-229
8. Virmani, R., Kolodgie, F.D., Burke, A.P., et al.: Lessons from sudden coronary death. A comprehensive morphological classification scheme for atherosclerotic lesions. Aterioscler. Thromb. Vasc. Biol. **20** (2000) 1262-1275
9. Hayes, C.E., Mathis, C.M., Yuan, C.: Surface coil phased arrays for high resolution imaging of the carotid arteries. JMRI **1** (1996) 109-112
10. Fayad, Z.A., Nahar, T., Fallon, J.T., et al.: In vivo magnetic resonance evaluation of atherosclerotic plaques in the human thoracic aorta. Circ. **101** (2000) 2503-2509

11. Fayad, Z.A., Fuster, V., Fallon, J.T., et al.: Noninvasive in vivo human coronary artery lumen and wall imaging using black-blood magnetic resonance imaging. Circ. **102** (2000) 506-510
12. Xu, D., Hwang, J.N., Yuan, C.; A robust method of identifying and measuring fibrous cap in 3D time-of-flight MR image. Proc. ICIP **2** (1999) 164-167
13. Han, C., Hatsukami, T.S., Hwang, J.N., Yuan, C. A fast minimal path active contour model. IEEE Trans. Image Proc. (to appear)
14. Yuan, C., Kang, X., Xu, D., Hatsukami, T.S.: Lesion index: A quantitative measure of atherosclerotic lesion complexity and progression in MR images. Proc. ISMRM (1999) #85

Imaging Metabolism with Light: Quantifying Local Fluorescence Lifetime Perturbation in Tissue-like Turbid Media

David Hattery[1,2], Victor Chernomordik[1], Amir Gandjbakhche[1], and
Murray Loew[2]

[1] Laboratory of Integrative and Medical Biophysics,
National Institutes of Health, Bethesda, MD 20892-5626
hattery@ieee.org, {vchern, amir}@helix.nih.gov
[2] Dept. of Electrical and Computer Engineering, Institute for Medical Imaging and
Image Analysis, George Washington University, Washington, DC 20052
loew@seas.gwu.edu

Abstract. Fluorescence lifetime imaging creates a map of spatial differences in local lifetime. These lifetime differences can be correlated with local metabolic levels which makes this a valuable biomedical imaging modality. We examine the ability to localize a fluorescence signal from deeply embedded sites in highly scattering, turbid, tissue-like media. We show how a specific point-spread-like function may be used to quantify an isolated lifetime perturbation between two sites in tissue. This new minimally invasive method offers the opportunity to infer near-real-time estimates of metabolic activity.

1 Introduction

Optical techniques are among the most valuable diagnostic tools available in medicine. Microscopy-based histology, for example, is the definitive diagnostic tool for cancer. Optical contrast agents, such as the stains used in histology, improve the ability to distinguish tissue types. Fluorescence contrast agents also have proven useful in biomedical research; for example, in examining cellular functions. Fluorophores may be linked to selectively binding molecules and inserted into tissue. Then, localization of those fluorophores indicates the presence of specific receptor molecules. Alternatively, fluorescence lifetime may be used as specific contrast. Fluorescence lifetime techniques have an advantage over intensity-based fluorescence techniques where pharmacokinetics are very non-uniform; differences in intensity must be weighed against non-uniform distribution and washout of the fluorophore. In contrast, lifetime techniques rely upon a change in the fluorophore behavior, not the concentration, and thus will provide good results as long as a sufficient signal exists.

The characteristic fluorescence lifetime is the mean time that a specific type of fluorophore spends in an excited state before emitting a photon. Intensity at the fluorophore emission wavelength falls off exponentially, $I_f = I_0 exp(-t/\tau)$,

W. Niessen and M. Viergever (Eds.): MICCAI 2001, LNCS 2208, pp. 795–802, 2001.

where I_0 is the initial intensity after the fluorophores receive a brief pulse of light at the exciting wavelength, t is the time after the pulse and τ is the lifetime. Thus, lifetime may be estimated by fitting time-resolved measurements of intensity to the exponential model.

The lifetime may be dependent on environmental factors such as pH, temperature, or the presence of specific molecules such as oxygen [1]. When the relationship between lifetime and a specific environmental factor is known, the local environment may be quantified by measuring the lifetime of fluorophores at the site. Thus, fluorescence lifetime methods may be used as remote probes; for example, metabolic processes indicated by changes in pH. This technique has been applied in transparent media, such as cells under a microscope. Extending this technique to probe deep into tissue is made difficult by multiple scattering of light. After traveling one millimeter in tissue, photons enter a diffusion-like state in which there is large dispersion in the path lengths of photons traveling between two points. This path length dispersion introduces variability in times-of-arrival of photons at a detector, making it impossible to measure lifetime by an inverse exponential-based method.

For fluorescence lifetime imaging in tissue, the inverse method must reconstruct the optical parameters of the tissue, as well as the fluorescence properties at each site of interest in the tissue. The minimum required number of intensity measurements on the surface of the tissue is determined by the number of unknown parameters. Several researchers [2, 3, 4, 5, 6] have developed frequency-domain methods for extracting a lifetime map that are based on the diffusion approximation to transport theory. For time-resolved measurements, those methods require large data memory space and complicated numerical methods to solve. We have taken a different approach and used a random-walk-based method to arrive at analytical solutions for fluorescence intensity that suggest a much simpler method for quantifying fluorescence lifetime at sites in highly turbid media [7].

Our method uses a unique linearizing function both to quantify lifetime and to spatially localize the source of particular lifetime differences in tissue-like media. In this paper, we will show how this function is able to extract lifetime from a specific site in the tissue using just two sets of intensity measurements. We will look only at the performance obtained from single measurements of contrast. We believe that the additional information present in multiple contrast measurements may be used to obtain better localization and lifetime quantification and still have lower data memory requirements than approaches based on the diffusion approximation. Those enhancements will be necessary before this technique may be used to obtain useful information about metabolic activity from tissue sites deep in the body.

2   Results

To quantify lifetime in highly scattering tissue, one must have a model that describes photon transit properties. Subtracting the characteristics of photon transit will leave only those aspects related to fluorescence; for example, lifetime, concentration, and quantum efficiency. We begin by examining the case of a single fluorophore site in the tissue and then extend the problem to account for many fluorophore sites.

For a single isolated fluorophore as shown in Fig. 1, the probability of a detected fluorescent photon is the product of the probabilities of three events: a source photon reaches the fluorophore site; the source photon has a fluorescent encounter that results in the emission of a photon; the emitted photon reaches the detector. For time-resolved measurements, there is a duration associated with each of those three probabilities. The product of the three probabilities yields a time-of-flight plot that provides the probability of photon arrival at a detector for each point in time.

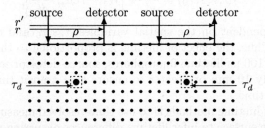

Fig. 1. For a single fluorescent lifetime contrast measurement, two isolated fluorophore sites are required (fluorophore isolated to dashed box regions), contrast is obtained from two measurements (at locations r and r') where the fluorophore site at depth d is centered between a source and detector separated by ρ and contrast is a function of difference in lifetime, $\tau_d - \tau_d'$, between the two sites

The problem may be separated into a transport component and a fluorescent component. The transport part includes only the first and third events as described above. The probability of a photon starting at the source, passing through the fluorophore site and arriving at the detector may be expressed in the frequency domain as the product of two Green's functions [8, 9], one describing the probability of motion from the source to the fluorophore site, $\hat{G}_1$, and the other the motion from the fluorophore site to the detector, $\hat{G}_2$. In the time-domain, we will define the inverse Laplace transform of the product as W_t:

$$W_t \equiv L^{-1}\{\hat{G}_1 \hat{G}_2\} \tag{1}$$

where W_t may be shown to be analogous to the point-spread-function (PSF) of an imaging system [10, 11]. W_t is dependent on the source-detector separation, fluorophore site, and separate absorption coefficients, μ_{ai} for the source wavelength and μ_{ae} for the fluorescence emission wavelength, as well as the respective scattering coefficients μ_{si}' and μ_{se}'.

There are three probabilities in step two that describe fluorescence at the fluorophore site. First is the probability that a photon at the fluorophore site will interact with the fluorophore. This probability, μ_{af}/μ_{si}', is a function of fluorophore concentration, μ_{af}, also known as the fluorescence absorption coefficient.

Next is the probability of a fluorescent emission given the interaction, Φ, which is the quantum efficiency of the fluorophore. The third component quantifies the mean delay while the fluorophore is in the excited state which is the fluorescent lifetime τ. The lifetime of fluorophores that emit in the near-infrared, where tissue has low absorption and a lifetime probe may be used to quantify deep tissue properties, is typically 10 to 1000 ps. Making the assumption that fluorescence lifetime is small compared to typical transit times, which is appropriate for deep sites [7], we may write the probability of a fluorescent photon from an isolated fluorophore located at s, reaching a detector located at r given a source at r_0 as as a function of time, t:

$$\gamma(t, r, s, r_0) = \frac{\mu_{af}}{\mu'_{si}} \Phi \left[W_t - \tau c \mu'_{si} \frac{dW_t}{dt} \right] \qquad (2)$$

where W_t is dependent on the spatial variables, r, s, r_0 and c is the speed of light in tissue. Thus, the effect of lifetime is proportional to the time derivative of the PSF. For 100 ps lifetime fluorophores, source-detector separations should be approximately 10 mm or greater to ensure that transit times remain short compared to lifetime.

The intent of lifetime methods is to use time-resolved measurements of intensity on the tissue surface to infer lifetime differences occurring within the tissue. To extend Eq. 2 to the case where the fluorophores are uniformly distributed throughout the tissue, fluorescence-based absorption, μ_{af}, must be added to the μ_{ai} absorption term used in W_t to account for increased absorption during photon transit through the tissue. With this change, the intensity from a collection of fluorophores may be expressed as the sum of contributions from each fluorophore site, s, in the tissue. If measurements are made at two or more locations with the same source-detector distance, ρ, we may define contrast as the difference in intensity between two detector locations, r and r' as shown in Fig. 1, as

$$C(t, r, r') = \sum_s \gamma(t, r, s, r_0) - \sum_{s'} \gamma(t, r', s', r'_0) \qquad (3)$$

where contrast is also a function of time. We will examine in detail the case where the optical and fluorescent characteristics of the tissue at two locations are identical except for two sites, s_d and s'_d, each located at depth d below a point midway between their respective sources and detectors. The lifetimes at those sites are different: τ_d and τ'_d respectively. Given only the intensity measurements from the two detector positions, we would like to quantify both the lifetime perturbation, $\tau_d - \tau'_d$ and the fluorophore location. From Eqs. 2 and 3, we may now write

$$C(t, r, r') = \mu_{af} \Phi (\tau_d - \tau'_d) c \frac{dW_t}{dt} \qquad (4)$$

If contrast is plotted as a function of dW_t/dt, the result will be linear with a slope of $\mu_{af}\Phi(\tau_d - \tau'_d)c$. Since W_t is a function of position, including depth, one may try numerous positions until the result is linear, yielding the actual position. In practice, this requires prior knowledge of tissue scattering and absorption coefficients. These values may be estimated using diffuse reflectance measurements at the source and emission wavelengths concurrently with the fluorescence contrast measurements. Given typical tissue optical properties [12] where $\mu'_{si} = \mu'_{se} = 1/mm$ and $\tilde{\mu}_a = 0.005/mm$, Fig. 2 shows how the function yields various curves for estimated positions other than the correct one corresponding to 10 mm depth. Lateral offsets, as well as offsets in depth, will produce non-linear plots. Since small lateral offsets in detector position may be used to determine the lateral position of a fluorophore site and are required to image, we will consider the more difficult problem of estimating the site's depth.

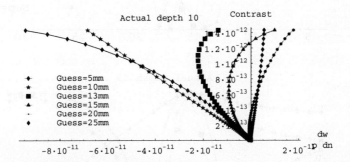

Fig. 2. Contrast plotted as a function of dW_t/dt for estimated depths of 5, 10, 13, 15, 20, and 25 mm. At the actual fluorophore depth of 10 mm, the plot is linear and passes through the origin

Using linear regression, the coefficient of regression, R^2, may be used as a measure of linearity. An R^2 value near 1.0 will indicate a good estimate of fluorophore depth. For a number of source-detector separations, R^2 is plotted as a function of estimated depth for a fluorophore at actual depths of 10, 15 and 20 mm in Fig. 3. The R^2 values for all source-detector separations peak at the actual fluorophore depth. In addition, there are secondary peaks at depths both greater and smaller than the actual fluorophore depth. These secondary peaks, however, correspond to negative differences in lifetime; the sign indicates whether the lifetime at the site is shorter, or longer than the reference site. Under the assumption of uniform fluorophore concentration (which was used to obtain Eq. 4), however, the line should pass through the origin. At the secondary peaks, the y intercept is much larger than at the primary peak as may be seen in Fig. 2. For example, the line with a positive slope at an estimated depth of 25 mm has has a larger y intercept than the line corresponding to the correct depth of 15 mm (which passes through the origin as expected). Thus, the actual fluorophore depth is unambiguous despite the presence of secondary local peaks in R^2.

Since intensity measurements may be obtained using a variety of source-detector separations, we would like to know the optimum separation given a fluorophore site at a particular depth. It may be seen in Fig. 3 that some source-

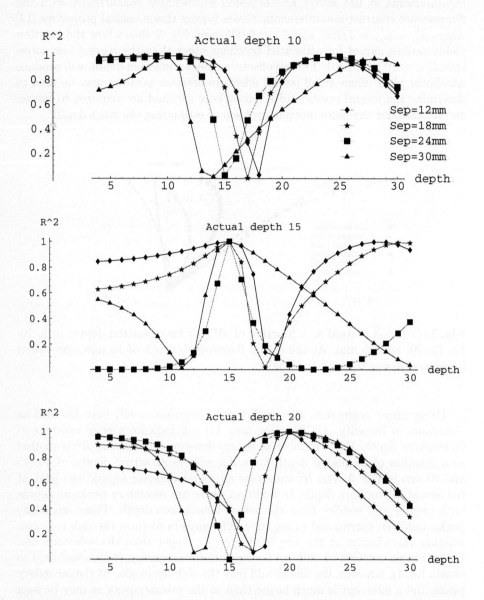

Fig. 3. Linear regression R^2 as a function of estimated fluorophore depth for source-detector separations of 12, 18, 24 and 30 mm and actual fluorophore depths of 10, 15 and 20 mm. Peak R^2 values occur when the estimated depth is the fluorophore's actual depth. An optimum source-detector separation exists for each fluorophore depth which yields a sharp and narrow peak in R^2 when the estimated and actual fluorophore depth are in agreement

detector separation curves peak more sharply at the actual fluorophore depth than others. For a fluorophore at 15 mm depth, a source detector separation of 24 mm has a very sharp peak at the fluorophore depth of 15 mm. This implies that the PSF is able to filter very selectively for the lifetime of a fluorophore at 15 mm depth which may be useful given noisy data. By contrast, the much broader 30 mm source-detector separation curve implies that the PSF is less selective for the 15 mm deep fluorophore site. As may be seen in Fig. 3, for fluorophores at greater depths, the most selective source-detector distance is smaller and for shallower depths, the optimum source-detector distance is larger.

3 Conclusion

We have presented a method for obtaining localized fluorescence lifetime differences from sites deep within highly scattering, tissue-like media. Both scattering and fluorescence lifetime create a spread in photon times-of-arrival at a detector. This spread precludes the use of simple measures of fluorescence lifetime. Instead, one must first model the spread that results from photon transit to and from the fluorophore site. The analytical method we have used is based on random walk theory and starts by showing the effect on photon times-of-arrival from a single isolated fluorophore. For media with fluorophores distributed throughout, the effect of each site would be added after first adjusting absorption in the tissue to account for fluorescence-based absorption. This method quantifies differences in lifetime at two sites from intensity measurements made near each site. The time-dependent difference in the two intensity measurements is the contrast.

To localize the site within the tissue, we use the time derivative of a specific PSF-like function. Values of this PSF are calculated for each point in the tissue which requires knowledge of the tissue scattering and absorption properties at the source and emission wavelengths. In practice, those values may be obtained from diffuse reflectance measurements at the two wavelengths. Contrast, when plotted versus the time-derivative of the PSF, will be linear for the case of a difference in lifetime at a single site. The value of the slope is a function of the local fluorescence concentration and the difference in lifetime at two sites in the same position relative to the two intensity measurements making up the contrast measurement.

In the presence of multiple fluorophores, each with small differences in lifetime, performance of the method may be shown to degrade. The differences in lifetime at sites other than the one of interest may be considered noise and make small contributions to contrast. Due to the excellent spatial selectivity of the PSF, this noise results in small errors in localization and lifetime quantification; less than 13 percent error with lifetime noise $\sigma = 10$ ps as will be presented in a paper currently being prepared for publication. The ability of the PSF to resolve a lifetime difference at a particular depth is a function of source-detector separation. For each fluorophore depth, there is an optimal source-detector separation.

These results were obtained from single measures of contrast. To construct a lifetime map of the tissue, many measurements will be required. The non-linearity of the PSF indicates that there may be additional information to be obtained by using multiple measurements, such as the measurements at adjacent points on the tissue surface and measurements at multiple source-detector separations, that may improve the quantification of both location and fluorescence lifetime. Localization of the lifetime perturbation is already impressive and further improvement will make this method a potentially valuable tool for utilizing fluorescence lifetime as a probe of metabolic status in living tissue.

References

[1] D. Y. Paithankar, A. U. Chen, B. W. Pogue, M. S. Patterson, and E. M. Sevick-Muraca. Imaging of fluorescent yield and lifetime from multiply scattered light reemitted from random media. *Applied Optics*, 36(10):2260–2272, Apr 1997.

[2] C. L. Hutchinson, J. R. Lakowicz, and E. M. Sevick-Muraca. Fluorescence lifetime-based sensing in tissues: a computational study. *Biophysical Journal*, 68(4):1574–1582, Apr 1995.

[3] D. Y Paithankar and E. M. Sevick-Muraca. Fluorescence lifetime imaging with frequency-domain photon migration measurement. In E. Sevick-Muraca and D. Benaron, editors, *Trends in Optics and Photonics on Biomedical Optical Spectroscopy and Diagnosis*, volume 3, pages 184–194. Optical Society of America, 1996.

[4] Huabei Jiang. Frequency-domain fluorescent diffusion tomography: a finite-element-based algorithm and simulations. *Applied Optics*, 37(22):5337–5343, Aug 1998.

[5] J. S. Reynolds, T. L. Troy, R. H. Mayer, A. B. Thompson, D. J. Waters, K. K. Cornell, P. W. Snyder, and E. M. Sevick-Muraca. Imaging of spontaneous canine mammary tumors using fluorescent contrast agents. *Journal of Photochemistry, Photobiology B-Biology*, 70(1):87–94, Jul 1999.

[6] Ralf H. Mayer, Jeffery S. Reynolds, and Eva M. Sevick-Muraca. Measurement of the fluorescence lifetime in scattering media by frequency-domain photon migration. *Applied Optics*, 38(22):4930–4938, Aug 1999.

[7] David W. Hattery, Victor V. Chernomordik, Murray Loew, Israel Gannot, and Amir H. Gandjbakhche. Analytical Solutions for Time-Resolved Fluorescence Lifetime Imaging in a Turbid Medium Such as Tissue. *Journal of the Optical Society of America JOSA-A*, 18(7):In press, Jul 2001.

[8] M. S. Patterson and B. Pogue. A mathematical model of time-resolved and frequency-domain fluorescence spectroscopy in biological tissue. *Applied Optics*, 33:1963, 1994.

[9] Eva M. Sevick-Muraca and Christina L. Burch. Origin of phosphorescence signals reemitted from tissues. *Optics Letters*, 19(23):1928–1930, Dec 1994.

[10] A. H. Gandjbakhche, R. F. Bonner, R. Nossal, and G. H. Weiss. Effects of multiple passage probability on fluorescent signals from biological media. *Applied Optics*, 36:4613–4619, 1997.

[11] A. H. Gandjbakhche, V. Chernomordik, J. C. Hebden, and R. Nossal. Time-dependent contrast functions for quantitative imaging in time-resolved transillumination experiments. *Applied Optics*, 37:1937–1981, 1999.

[12] S. L. Jacques. Time-Resolved Reflectance Spectroscopy in Turbid Tissues. *IEEE Transactions on Biomedical Engineering*, 36(12):1155–1160, 1989.

Limits to the Accuracy of 3D Thickness Measurement in Magnetic Resonance Images

Yoshinobu Sato[1], Katsuyuki Nakanishi[2], Hisashi Tanaka[2], Takashi Nishii[3],
Nobuhiko Sugano[3], Hironobu Nakamura[2], Takahiro Ochi[4], Shinichi Tamura[1]

[1] Division of Interdisciplinary Image Analysis
[2] Department of Radiology
[3] Department of Orthopaedic Surgery
[4] Division of Computer Integrated Orthopaedic Surgery
Osaka University Graduate School of Medicine
yoshi@image.med.osaka-u.ac.jp, http://www.image.med.osaka-u.ac.jp/yoshi

Abstract. Measuring the thickness of sheet-like (or plate-like) anatomical structures, such as articular cartilages and brain cortex, in 3D magnetic resonance (MR) images is often an important diagnostic procedure. The purpose of this paper is to investigate the fundamental limits to the accuracy of thickness determination in MR images. Given imaging and postprocessing parameters, the characteristics of thickness determination accuracy are derived by means of a theoretical simulation method, focusing especially on the effect of sheet structure orientation on accuracy in the case of noncubic (anisotropic) voxels. The theoretical simulation was validated by *in vitro* experiments.

1 Introduction

Thickness measurement of sheet-like (or plate-like) anatomical structures in magnetic resonance (MR) images is an important diagnostic procedure in, for example, the diagnosis of joint diseases by evaluating the distribution of articular cartilage thicknesses [1], [2], [3], [4], [5], [6], [7], [8], or of specific neuropsychiatric disorders by assessing cortical thicknesses in the brain [9], [10]. While several methods for thickness quantification have been proposed [5],[6],[9],[8], accuracy limits arising from finite resolution have not been evaluated. Although Sato et al. examined accuracy limits due to partial volume averaging, especially the effect of anisotropic voxels, by software simulation [8], the modeling of MR image acquisition was insufficient and validation with actual MR images was not demonstrated.

The goal of the work described here is to provide a theoretical procedure for ascertaining the inherent limits to the accuracy of thickness determination in MR images. We especially address the manner in which how the accuracy depends on the orientation of sheet structures when a voxel shape is anisotropic. Sheet structures of interest are often distributed within specific orientation ranges – for example, on an approximately cylindrical surface. In this case, the resolution in the plane orthogonal to the axis of the approximated cylinder should be higher

W. Niessen and M. Viergever (Eds.): MICCAI 2001, LNCS 2208, pp. 803–810, 2001.

than that along the axis to maximize the accuracy of thickness measurement. Given the orientation distribution of sheet structures and the fixed volume of a voxel – which is directly related to the signal-to-noise ratio – the voxel shape can be optimized. In this paper, we define thickness as the distance between the outer and inner boundaries measured at subvoxel resolution, which are the zero-crossings of directional second derivatives along the normal directions of the sheet surface. We establish a method for evaluating the accuracy of thickness measurement by numerical simulation, and validate the method through *in vitro* experiments.

2   Materials and Methods

2.1   Numerical Simulation

Modeling a Sheet Structure A three-dimensional (3D) sheet structure orthogonal to the x-axis is modeled as

$$S(\mathbf{x}; t) = B(x; t) \tag{1}$$

where $\mathbf{x} = (x, y, z)$.

$$B(x; t) = \begin{cases} 1, & -\frac{1}{2}t \leq x \leq \frac{1}{2}t \\ 0, & \text{otherwise,} \end{cases} \tag{2}$$

in which t represents the thickness of the sheet.

Let θ be the rotation angle of the sheet structure around the y-axis. The 3D sheet structure with rotation θ is written as

$$S(\mathbf{x}; t, \theta) = S_0(\mathbf{x}'; t), \tag{3}$$

where $\mathbf{x}' = R_\theta \mathbf{x}$, in which R_θ detnotes a 3×3 matrix representing rotation θ around the y-axis.

Modeling MR Image Acquisition The one-dimensional (1D) point spread function (PSF) of MR images [11] is given by

$$M(x; \Delta_x) = \frac{1}{N_x} \frac{\sin(\pi \frac{x}{\Delta_x})}{\sin(\pi \frac{x}{N_x \Delta_x})}, \tag{4}$$

where N_x is the number of samples in the frequency domain, and Δ_x represents the sampling interval in the spatial domain. Eq. (4) is well-approximated [12] by

$$M(x; \Delta_x) = \frac{1}{N_x} \frac{\sin(\pi \frac{x}{\Delta_x})}{\pi \frac{x}{\Delta_x}}. \tag{5}$$

The 3D PSF is given by

$$M(\mathbf{x}; \Delta_x, \Delta_y, \Delta_z) = M(x; \Delta_x) M(y; \Delta_y) M(z; \Delta_z) \tag{6}$$

The MR image of the sheet structure with rotation θ and thickness t is given by

$$I(\mathbf{x}) = S(\mathbf{x}; t, \theta) * M(\mathbf{x}; \Delta_x, \Delta_y, \Delta_z), \tag{7}$$

where $*$ denotes the convolution operation.

Theoretical Methods for Thickness Determination Thickness is determined by measuring the distance between boundaries corresponding to the inner and outer edges of a sheet structure, which are the zero-crossings of directional second derivatives along the normal vector of the sheet. The directional second derivatives are combined with Gaussian blurring. In actual situations, Gaussian blurring is typically employed to reduce the effect of noise. The partial second derivative combined with Gaussian blurring for the MR image $I(\mathbf{x})$, for example, is given by

$$I_{xx}(\mathbf{x}; \sigma) - \frac{\partial^2}{\partial x^2} G(\mathbf{x}; \sigma) * I(\mathbf{x}), \tag{8}$$

where $G(\mathbf{x}; \sigma)$ is the isotropic 3D Gaussian function with the standard deviation σ.

Let $\nabla^2 I(\mathbf{x}; \sigma)$ be the Hessian matrix of $I(\mathbf{x}; \sigma)$, which is given by

$$\nabla^2 I(\mathbf{x}; \sigma) = \begin{bmatrix} I_{xx}(\mathbf{x}; \sigma) & I_{xy}(\mathbf{x}; \sigma) & I_{xz}(\mathbf{x}; \sigma) \\ I_{yx}(\mathbf{x}; \sigma) & I_{yy}(\mathbf{x}; \sigma) & I_{yz}(\mathbf{x}; \sigma) \\ I_{zx}(\mathbf{x}; \sigma) & I_{zy}(\mathbf{x}; \sigma) & I_{zz}(\mathbf{x}; \sigma) \end{bmatrix}. \tag{9}$$

The directional second derivative along the normal direction of the sheet structure is given by

$$D_2(\mathbf{x}; \sigma, \mathbf{r}) = \mathbf{r}^\top \nabla^2 I(\mathbf{x}; \sigma) \mathbf{r}, \tag{10}$$

in which $\mathbf{r} = (\cos\theta, 0, \sin\theta)$.

Similarly, the directional first derivative along the sheet normal is given by

$$D_1(\mathbf{x}; \sigma, \mathbf{r}) = \mathbf{r}^\top \nabla I(\mathbf{x}; \sigma), \tag{11}$$

in which $\mathbf{r} = (\cos\theta, 0, \sin\theta)$ and $\nabla I(\mathbf{x}; \sigma)$ is the gradient vector given by

$$\nabla I(\mathbf{x}; \sigma) = (I_x(\mathbf{x}; \sigma), I_y(\mathbf{x}; \sigma), I_z(\mathbf{x}; \sigma)). \tag{12}$$

Both sides of the boundaries for sheet structures can be defined as the points having the maximum and minimum values of $D_1(\mathbf{x}; \sigma, \mathbf{r})$ among those satisfying the condition given by $D_2(\mathbf{x}; \sigma, \mathbf{r}) = 0$, where $\mathbf{r} = (\cos\theta, 0, \sin\theta)$. The distance between the two detected boundary points along the direction $\mathbf{r}$ is defined as the measured thickness, T.

Simulation Method Voxels in MR volume data are typically anisotropic since they usually have lower resolution along the third direction (orthogonal to the slice plane) than within slices. Hence, we assume that the resolution along the z-axis is lower than that in the xy-plane and that pixels in the xy-plane are square. Let $\Delta_{xy}(= \Delta_x = \Delta_y)$ be the pixel size within the slices and $\Delta_{xy} \leq \Delta_z$. We then determine the measured thickness, T, by the above-described numerical simulation under different combinations of t, θ, Δ_{xy}, Δ_z, and σ.

2.2 *In Vitro* Experiments

Materials and MR Image Acquisition To validate the numerical simulation
method, we used a resected femoral head, approximately spherical in shape, with
articular cartilages distributed on its surface. The cartilages were used as the
material for the experiments, in which we assumed they were distributed on a
spherical surface. The cartilage thickness was then measured along the normal
direction of the spherical surface approximating the femoral head.

3-D MR images of sagittal sections were obtained using 3-D-spoiled gradient-
echo sequences (SPGR) [7] under the following two conditions.

- MR imaging with cubic voxels: $\Delta_{xy} = \Delta_z = 0.7$ (mm).
- Routinely performed MR imaging with noncubic voxels (routine imaging):
  $\Delta_{xy} = 0.625$ (mm), $\Delta_z = 1.5$ (mm).

To obtain an acceptable signal-to-noise ratio, the imaging time with cubic voxels
was three times as long as that employed in routine imaging with noncubic voxels.
In each 3-D MR image, the matrix size was 256×256.

Procedures for Segmentation and Quantification

Interpolation: 3-D MR images were trimmed and then interpolated using
sinc interpolation [13],[14] such that (i) the signal sampling was isotropic in all
three directions and (ii) the image size was doubled. The sampling interval in
the interpolated data was 0.35 (mm) in the imaging with cubic voxels and 0.3125
(mm) in the routine imaging. Note, however, that the volume ndata obtained
using the routine imaging were inherently more blurred in the z direction than
in the xy-plane even though the signal sampling was isotropic.

Cartilage Segmentation: In the real MR images, cartilage region segmentation was needed before thickness quantification. To facilitate segmentation,
cartilage enhancement filtering was performed according to the following equation:

$$I_{cartilage}(\mathbf{x}) = \max_i \{-\sigma_i^2 D_2(\mathbf{x}; \sigma_i, \mathbf{r})\}, \qquad (13)$$

where $\sigma_i = 2^{(i-1)/2}$ (voxels) (in which $i = 1, 2, 3$) and $\mathbf{r} = \frac{\mathbf{x}-\mathbf{c}}{|\mathbf{x}-\mathbf{c}|}$ (in which $\mathbf{c}$ is the
center position of the sphere approximating the femoral head). In the multiscale
integration of Eq.(13), σ_i^2 was multiplied for the normalization of each scale σ_i
[15],[16].

The filtered images $I_{cartilage}(\mathbf{x})$ were thresholded, with the threshold values
being determined through operator interaction. Using connectivity analysis, the
approximated segmented regions of the cartilage, $S_{cartilage}$, were extracted.

Thickness Quantification: The extracted 3-D cartilage regions were thinned to a width of one voxel by non-maximum suppression along the radial directions of the filter-enhanced cartilage images. A cartilage thickness was assigned
to each point of the thinned cartilage regions.

For each point of the thinned regions, the profile of the directional second derivative $D_2(\mathbf{x}; \sigma, \mathbf{c})$ was reconstructed along the radial directional line that passed through this point and originated from the center point, $\mathbf{c}$, of the sphere approximating the femoral head. Here, σ was the standard deviation of the Gaussian blurring combined with the second derivative computation. Similarly, binary profiles were reconstructed along the same radial directional line for the binary images of the segmented cartilage $S_{cartilage}$.

Profile reconstruction was performed at subvoxel resolution by using a tri-linear interpolation for the directional second derivative and a nearest-neighbor interpolation for the segmented cartilage. Let $D_2(r)$ be the profile of the radial directional second derivative, and $S_{cartilage}(r)$ be the profile of the segmented binary cartilage images (here, r denotes the distance from the center of the sphere approximation, $\mathbf{c}$). Cartilage edges were localized in two steps: finding the initial point for the subsequent search using $S_{cartilage}(r)$, and then searching for the zero-crossing of $D_2(r)$. The initial point of the outer edge, p_{out_0}, was given by the maximum value of r that satisfied $S_{cartilage}(r) = 1$ if it existed. Otherwise, the edge localization process terminated. The initial point of the inner edge, p_{in_0}, was given by the minimum value of r that satisfied $S_{cartilage}(r) = 1$.

Given the initial point of the search, if $D_2(p_{out_0}) < 0$, search inbound (the direction in which r decreases) toward the center along the profile for the zero-crossing position p_{out}. Otherwise search outbound. Similarly, if $D_2(p_{in_0}) < 0$, search outbound along the profile for the zero-crossing position p_{in}. Otherwise search inbound. The thickness, T, was given by $|p_{in} - p_{out}|$.

3   Results

3.1   Numerical Simulations

Sheet structures with thickness $t = 1.2, 1.6, 2.0,$ and 2.4 (mm) were modeled. Each sheet model had orientations, θ, from 0 to 90 degrees. The MR imaging numerical simulations were performed using the following parameters.

- Simulating MR imaging with cubic voxels: $\Delta_{xy} = \Delta_z = 0.7$ (mm).
- Simulating routine MR imaging with noncubic voxels: $\Delta_{xy} = 0.625$ (mm), $\Delta_z = 1.5$ (mm).

For σ, used in postprocessing for thickness determination, the following three parameter values were employed: 0, $\frac{1}{2}\Delta_{xy}$, and Δ_{xy}.

Figure 1 shows the variations in the estimated thicknesses against the angles, θ, of the sheet structures in simulations of MR imaging with cubic voxels. While cubic voxels have the same resolution in the three orthogonal directions along the coordinate axes, they are still not isotropic for all directions. When $\sigma = 0$, considerable differences in the estimated thicknesses were observed between the directions along the coordinate axes ($\theta = 0°, 90°$) and the diagonal directions ($\theta = 45°$). When $\sigma = \Delta_{xy}$, the angle dependency was reduced and the true and estimated thicknesses were well-correlated. However, when $\sigma = 2\Delta_{xy}$, although the angle dependency was further reduced, considerable overestimation was observed as the sheet structures became thinner. Appropriate Gaussian smoothing ($\sigma = \Delta_{xy}$) was thus effective in reducing the angle dependency as well as in improving accuracy.

Figure 2 shows the variations in the estimated thicknesses against the angles, θ, of sheet structures in simulations of MR imaging with noncubic voxels. The angle dependency was significantly large while the accuracy was sufficiently good when $\theta < 25°$. Appropriate Gaussian smoothing ($\sigma = \Delta_{xy}$) was also effective in the case of noncubic voxels.

3.2   Validating the Numerical Simulation by *In Vitro* Experiments

Figure 3 shows the variations in the estimated cartilage thicknesses against θ, which is the angular difference between the xy-plane of the 3-D MR image and the surface normal direction of the sphere approximating the femoral head. Figure 3(a) shows an MR slice image of the resected femoral head. The articular cartilages are imaged as bright sheet structures distributed on the spherical head surface. We used $\sigma = 0.5\Delta_{xy}$ in the thickness determination. In Fig. 3(b), thicknesses estimated in imaging with cubic voxels ($\Delta_{xy} = \Delta_z = 0.7$ (mm)) were used as reference thicknesses. The accuracy of these thicknesses was confirmed to be sufficiently high for every angle of the sheet structures from the simulation results shown in Fig. 1. The experimental results in Fig. 3 correlate well with the theoretical ones in Fig. 2.

4   Conclusions

The fundamental limits to the accuracy of thickness determination in MR images were investigated. A simulation method was established to derive the characteristics of thickness determination accuracy, given both imaging and postprocessing parameters. The effect of sheet structure orientation on accuracy in the case of noncubic (anisotropic) voxels was clarified through the simulation. It was also found that postprocessing (Gaussian) blurring plays an important role in realizing accurate and well-behaved thickness determination. The simulations were validated by comparison with results obtained in *in vitro* experiments using the cartilages of a resected femoral head.

Future work will include the formulation of a method for automatically estimating the orientation of a sheet structure and determining its thickness with a theoretically derived confidence measure. When thickness quantification is applied to *in vivo* MR images, the segmentation of sheet structures of interest becomes important as well as the quantification itself. We are planning to develop a unified framework for both segmentation and quantification based on multi-scale and multi-orientation 3D image analysis.

Acknowledgment This work was partly supported by JSPS Research for the Future Program JSPS-RFTF99I00903 and JSPS Grant-in-Aid for Scientific Research (C)(2) 11680389.

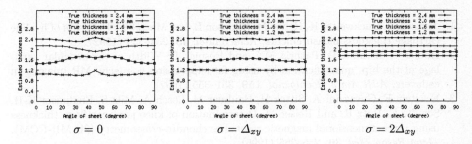

Fig. 1. Numerical simulations for thickness determination from images with cubic voxels. Variations in the estimated thicknesses against the angles (θ) of the sheet structures are shown. $\Delta_{xy} = \Delta_z = 0.7$ (mm).

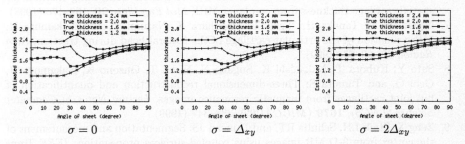

Fig. 2. Numerical simulations for thickness determination from routine MR images with noncubic voxels. $\Delta_{xy} = 0.625$ (mm), $\Delta_z = 1.5$ (mm).

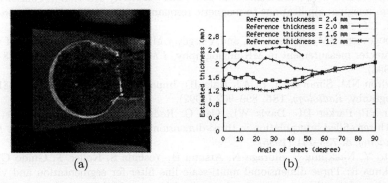

(a)   (b)

Fig. 3. *In vitro* experiments for thickness determination. (a) MR slice image of resected femoral head. (b) Variations in the estimated thicknesses with routine MR imaging against the angles of sheet structures. The thicknesses estimated in imaging with cubic voxels were used as reference thicknesses.

References

1. Jonsson K, Buckwalter K, Helvie M, Niklason L, and Martel W: Precision of hyaline cartilage thickness measurements, *Acta Radiol*, **33**, 234–239 (1992).
2. Hodler J, Trundell D, Pathria MN, and Resnick D: Width of the articular cartilage of the hip: quantification by using fat-suppression spin-echo MR imaging in cadavers, *AJR Am J Roentgenol*, **159**, 351–355 (1992).
3. Eckstein F, Gavazzini A, Sittek H, Haubner M, Losch A, Milz S, Englmeier K-H, Schulte E, Putz R, and Reiser M: Determination of knee joint cartilage thickness using three-dimensional magnetic resonance chondro-crassometry (3D MR-CCM), *Magn Reson Med*, **36**, 256–265 (1996).
4. Solloway S, Hutchinson CE, Waterton JG, Taylor CJ, The use of active shape models for making thickness measurements of articular cartilage from MR images, *Magn Reson Med*, **37**, 943–952 (1997).
5. McGibbon CA, Dupuy DE, Palmer WE, and Krebs D.: Cartilage and subchondral bone thickness distribution with MR imaging, *Acad Radiol*, **5**, 20–25 (1998).
6. McGibbon CA, Palmer WE, and Krebs DE: A general computing method for spatial cartilage thickness from co-planar MRI, *Med Eng Phys*, **20**, 169–176 (1998).
7. Nakanishi N, Tanaka H, Nishii T, Masuhara K, Narumi Y, and Nakamura H: MR evaluation of the articular cartilage of the femoral head during traction, *Acta Radiol*, **40**, 60–63 (1999).
8. Sato Y, Kubota T, Nakanishi K, Sugano N, Nishii T, Ohzono K, Nakamura H, Ochi O, and Tamura S: Three-dimensional reconstruction and quantification of hip joint cartilages from magnetic resonance images, *Lecture Notes in Computer Science (LNCS)*, **1679** (*MICCAI'99*), 338–347 (1999).
9. Zeng X, Staib LH, Schults RT, and Duncan JS: Segmentation and measurement of the cortex from 3-D MR images using coupled-surfaces propagation, *IEEE Trans Med Imaging*, **18**, 927–937 (1999).
10. Magnotta VA, Andreasen NC, Schultz SK, Harris G, Cizadlo T, Heckel D, Nopoulos P, Flaum M: Quantitative *in vivo* measurement of gyrification in the human brain: changes associated with aging, *Cereb Cortex*, **9**, 151–160, 1999.
11. Parker DL, Du YP, and Davis WL: The voxel sensitivity function in Fourier transform imaging: applications to magnetic resonance angiography, *Magn Reson Med*, **33**, 156–162 (1995).
12. Hoogeveen, RM, Bakker CJG, and Viergever MA: Limits to the accuracy of vessel diameter measurement in MR angiography, *J Magn Reson Imaging*, **8**, 1228–1235 (1998).
13. Hylton NM, Simovsky I, Li AJ, Hale JD: Impact of section doubling on MR angiography, *Radiology*, **185**, 899–902 (1992).
14. Du YP, Parker DL, Davis WL, Cao G: Reduction of partial-volume artifacts with zero-filled interpolation in three-dimensional MR angiography, *J Magn Reson Imaging*, **4**, 733–741 (1995).
15. Sato Y, Nakajima S, Shiraga N, Atsumi H, Yoshida S, Koller T, Guido G, and Kikinis R: Three dimensional multi-scale line filter for segmentation and visualization of curvilinear structures in medical images, *Med Image Anal*, **2**, 143–168 (1998).
16. Sato Y, Westin C-F, Bhalerao A, Nakajima S, Shiraga N, Tamura S, and Kikinis R: Tissue classification based on 3D local intensity structures for volume rendering, *IEEE Transactions on Visualization and Computer Graphics*, **6**, 160–180 (2000).

Maximum Likelihood Estimation of the Bias Field in MR Brain Images: Investigating Different Modelings of the Imaging Process

Sylvain Prima[1], Nicholas Ayache[1], Tom Barrick[2], and Neil Roberts[2]

[1] INRIA Sophia Antipolis, EPIDAURE Project, France
[2] MARIARC, University of Liverpool, United Kingdom

Abstract. This article is about bias field correction in MR brain images. In the literature, most of the methods consist in modeling the imaging process before identifying its unknown parameters. After identifying two of the most widely used such models, we propose a third one and show that for these three models, it is possible to use a common estimation framework, based on the Maximum Likelihood principle. This scheme partly rests on a functional modeling of the bias field. The optimization is performed by an ECM algorithm, in which we have included a procedure of outliers rejection. In this way, we derive three algorithms and compare them on a set of simulated images. We also provide results on real MR images exhibiting a bias field with a typical "diagonal" pattern.

1 Introduction

Imperfections of the RF coil and patient-dependent electrodynamic interactions (often referred to as RF penetration and standing-wave effects [20]) systematically cause smooth, biologically meaningless, variations of the tissue intensities across MR images, which can amount to as much as 30% of the signal amplitudes. Generally, this "bias field" has little effect on visual interpretation, but the artificial intra-tissue variability it causes can significantly affect the outputs of image processing tools (segmentation, rigid or non-rigid registration, *etc.*) and subsequent quantitative analyses. Classical methods are routinely used to improve the intensity uniformity during the acquisition process [13]; they are generally able to correct most of the gross nonuniformities due to the coil defects, but unable to eliminate those due the patient anatomy. As an alternative, numerous retrospective methods have been devised to estimate and correct intensity variations after the image has been acquired. The common general approach consists in modeling the imaging process that connects the true emitted signal (uncorrupted by the bias field effects and the random noise due to the measuring device) with the observed data (*i.e.*, the MR image), and then estimating the parameters of the model best fitting the data. More precisely, given a voxel i with coordinates v_i in a MR image, its intensity y_i is widely considered to be related to the true emitted signal x_i according to:

$$y_i = b_i x_i + \varepsilon_i^{mea}$$

W. Niessen and M. Viergever (Eds.): MICCAI 2001, LNCS 2208, pp. 811–819, 2001.

Throughout the paper, given there are n voxels in the 3D volume, we note the bias field $b = (b_i)_{i=1...n}$, the MR image $y = (y_i)_{i=1...n}$, and the "ideal", uncorrupted, brain image $x = (x_i)_{i=1...n}$. The bias field is generally considered to be a slowly spatially varying function of the coordinates (*i.e.*, $b_i = b(v_i)$), and assumed to be multiplicative, consistently with the intrinsic nature of the corrupting physical processes [21]. In MR magnitude images, the random noise ε_i^{mea} due to the measuring device is known to have a Rician p.d.f. [19], which is shown to be quasi-Gaussian at high signal-to-noise ratio (SNR ¿ 3). Thus, the assumption of an additive, stationary, spatially white and Gaussian noise with a low standard deviation σ in the intracranial cavity is generally made: $\varepsilon_i^{mea} = \varepsilon^{mea} \sim N(0, \sigma^2)$. A commonly used and convenient modeling is to consider that every head voxel reflects the biological properties of one single underlying structure. In the following, the brain segmentation is noted $c = (c_i)_{i=1...n}$, c_i being the label of voxel i. A simple assumption is to model the intracranial cavity as composed of a reduced set of m tissues of interest. Considering cerebro-spinal fluid, grey matter and white matter, which generally exhibit distinct average grey levels in magnitude MR images, is a usual choice. Within a given neuroanatomical structure ω_k, natural intensity variations are always observed, due to changes in its composition across the head volume. Thus, the signal emitted by a particular structure is often assumed to be distributed around a mean value μ_k, which can be simply written $x_i = \mu_k + \varepsilon_i^{bio}$ if the voxel i belongs to ω_k. This "biological noise" ε_i^{bio}, due to a natural variability, is observed to be spatially correlated, but in many works related to brain segmentation, it is widely modeled as spatially white, with a stationary tissue-conditional Gaussian p.d.f. of low variance σ_k^2: $\varepsilon_i^{bio} = \varepsilon^{bio} \sim N(0, \sigma_k^2)$ [1,5,10,18]. This leads to rewrite the general model:

$$y_i = b_i(\mu_k + \varepsilon_i^{bio}) + \varepsilon^{mea}, \ \varepsilon^{mea} \sim N(0, \sigma^2) \text{ and } \varepsilon_i^{bio} \sim N(0, \sigma_k^2) \text{ if } c_i = \omega_k \quad (1)$$

Following this very general model, many authors have proposed additional hypotheses and subsequent algorithms for estimation of the bias field and correction of the intensity nonuniformities in brain MR images. Most of these algorithms are based on two simplified versions of (1), that we call Models 1 and 2. What motivates this article is the observation that the variety of the algorithms proposed so far makes it difficult to compare the models they rest on.

In this paper, we suggest a third simplification of (1), which we call Model 3 (Section 2). Then, we propose to compare these three models, apart from the conceptually very different methods of the literature that has been developed so far to identify their underlying parameters (in particular, the bias field) ; our aim is to know which model is best suited to real data. For this purpose, we adopt a common estimation strategy, already proposed in [23,24] for Model 2. It consists in a probabilistic interpretation of these models, a functional modeling of the bias field, and a Maximum Likelihood estimation of the unknown parameters (tissue characteristics and bias field coefficients) by way of an Expectation/Conditional Maximization algorithm (Section 3). This estimation approach leads to simple iterative schemes, extensively described in a research report available on the web (http://www.inria.fr/rrrt/index.en.html). Moreover, we propose to include in the three such derived algorithms a procedure of outliers rejection, inspired by the LTS estimation [16]. In particular, this technique allows to eliminate voxels affected by partial volume effects. We present results on simulated and real MR images (Section 4).

2   Three Different Models

In some works [2,12,15,14,22], x is supposed to be (at least locally) piecewise constant, depending on the underlying tissue ω_k: $x_i = \mu_k$ if $c_i = \omega_k$. This amounts to neglect the intensity variations due to the biological intra-tissue variability with respect to those due to the measurement noise ε^{mea} ($\varepsilon_i^{bio} \ll \varepsilon^{mes}$). Then the general model (1) becomes:

$$y_i = b_i\mu_k + \varepsilon^{mea} \text{ if } c_i = \omega_k, \text{ with } \varepsilon^{mea} \sim N(0,\sigma^2) \qquad \textbf{(Model 1)}$$

In other works [23,24,25], it is supposed that the measurement noise can be at least partially removed by a low-pass prefiltering of the data (for instance, anisotropic diffusion [5]). A risk is to suppress also the relevant biological information conveyed by the intra-tissue natural variability [7]. However, as this latter is spatially correlated, it is less likely to be removed by such a filtering than the spatially white ε^{mea}. Then, (1) simply reduces to $y_i = b_i x_i$. In [25,7,23,24], mainly for reasons of computational simplicity, a logarithmic transform is applied to this model, which turns the multiplicative bias field b into an additive one. Then, it is particularily convenient to suppose that (within a given anatomical structure ω_k) the intensities x_i fluctuate around a mean value μ_k', these fluctuations conveying a "biological noise" $\varepsilon_i^{'bio}$ following a Gaussian noise $N(0,\sigma_k'^2)$. This hypothesis is contradictory to the traditional assumption done in algorithms of MR images segmentation, which suppose that ε_i^{bio} is Gaussian [1,5,10,18]; in this case, $\varepsilon_i^{'bio}$ is not. This point is not evoked in the concerned papers [25,7,23,24]. However, following this hypothesis, (1) becomes:

$$\log y_i = \log b_i + \mu_k' + \varepsilon_i^{'bio}, \text{ with } \varepsilon_i^{'bio} \sim N(0,\sigma_k'^2) \text{ if } c_i = \omega_k \qquad \textbf{(Model 2)}$$

If, contrary to Model 2, we choose to keep the hypothesis of a Gaussian law for ε_i^{bio}, which seems more natural, we get a third model, defined as follows:

$$y_i = b_i(\mu_k + \varepsilon_i^{bio}), \text{ with } \varepsilon_i^{bio} \sim N(0,\sigma_k^2) \text{ if } c_i = \omega_k \qquad \textbf{(Model 3)}$$

3   Three Algorithms for Bias Field Correction

3.1   Maximum Likelihood Formulation

In the following, we consider that there are $m = 3$ tissues of interest (cerebro-spinal fluid, grey matter, white matter) and n voxels in the intracranial volume. We propose to make a functional parameterization of the bias field (detailed in Section 3.3), represented by a low number of coefficients $\alpha_1, \ldots, \alpha_d$. The objective is to estimate the optimal parameters of the three models according to the Maximum Likelihood principle. These parameters are gathered in the vector $\Theta = (\mu_1, \ldots, \mu_m, \sigma_1, \ldots, \sigma_m, \alpha_1, \ldots, \alpha_d)$ (or $\Theta = (\mu_1, \ldots, \mu_m, \sigma, \alpha_1, \ldots, \alpha_d)$ for Model 1). The optimal vector Θ maximizes the likelihood L of the image y, which can be written, using the theorem of total probabilities:

$$L(y;\Theta) = L(y_1, ..., y_n; \Theta) = \prod_{i=1}^{n} p(y_i; \Theta) = \prod_{i=1}^{n} \sum_{k=1}^{m} p(y_i | c_i = \omega_k; \Theta) P(c_i = \omega_k; \Theta)$$

Practically, we consider that the *a priori* probabilities $P(c_i = \omega_k; \Theta)$ are independent of the model parameters: $P(c_i = \omega_k; \Theta) = P(c_i = \omega_k)$. As suggested in [8,23,24], these probabilities $P(c_i = \omega_j)$ are obtained by affine registration of a probabilistic brain atlas for the three tissues of interest and give a rough *a priori*, fixed and spatially varying, knowledge of the tissue parameters and locations in the MR volume. We use the atlas from the Montral Neurological Institute [4].

3.2   Maximization of the Criterion

Analytical maximization of L is impossible. Given an initial estimate $\Theta^{(0)}$ of the parameters, the algorithm Expectation/Maximization (EM) [3] consists in building a series of vectors $(\Theta^{(p)})$ such that L converges towards a (at least local) maximum. This iterative process is composed of one "M-step" and one "E-step" defined as follows:

$$\nabla_\Theta Q(\Theta, \Theta^{(p)}) = \sum_{i=1}^{n} \sum_{k=1}^{m} P(c_i = \omega_k | y; \Theta^{(p)}) \nabla_\Theta [\log p(y_i | c_i = \omega_k; \Theta)] = 0 \ \textbf{(M-step)},$$

$$\text{where } P(c_i = \omega_k | y; \Theta^{(p)}) \propto p(y_i | c_i = \omega_k; \Theta^{(p)}) P(c_i = \omega_k) \ \textbf{(E-step)}$$

After choosing a functional parametrization of the bias field as described in Section 3.3, the M-step yields a system of $(2m + d)$ non-linear equations with $(2m + d)$ unknown parameters (or $(m + d + 1)$ for Model 1). This non-linearity makes it impossible to maximize the likelihood by a classical EM algorithm; a generalization is proposed in Section 3.4 to tackle this problem.

3.3   Modeling the Bias Field

As suggested in [23,24] for Model 2, an adapted functional parameterization of the bias field allows to characterize it with a limited number of parameters, while ensuring its spatial smoothness. We propose three functional modelings of the bias field adapted to each of the three models of the imaging process presented in Section 1. The objective is to obtain simple formulae for the p.d.f. of y_i (or $\log y_i$ for Model 2), such that the ML estimation of the whole set of parameters is made possible. Given the monomials ϕ_j, $j = 1, \ldots, d$, where $\phi_1 : (x, y, z) \mapsto (x - tx/2)$, $\phi_2 : (x, y, z) \mapsto (y - ty/2)$, $\ldots, \phi_7 : (x, y, z) \mapsto (x - tx/2)(y - ty/2)$, etc., where tx, ty, tz are the sizes of the 3D image in the x, y and z directions, we make the following choices:

- **Bias Field Model 1**: $b_i = b(v_i) = 1 + \sum_{j=1}^{d} \alpha_j \phi_j(v_i)$
- **Bias Field Model 2**: $b_i = b(v_i) = \exp(\sum_{j=1}^{d} \alpha_j \phi_j(v_i))$
- **Bias Field Model 3**: $b_i = b(v_i) = 1/(1 + \sum_{j=1}^{d} \alpha_j \phi_j(v_i))$

3.4   The ECM Algorithm

Practically, the M-step of the classical EM algorithm yields intractable equations (see the research report): the optimal tissue or noise parameters (means and variances) explicitly depend on the optimal bias field coefficients in a non-linear fashion. To tackle this problem, a variant of the EM algorithm has been proposed in [11], that consists in partitioning the parameters vector as $\Theta = (\Theta_1, ..., \Theta_N)$, and replacing the original M-step by N successive Conditional Maximization steps (CM-steps) as described below. As the original EM approach, this Expectation/Conditional Maximization (ECM) algorithm provides a series of vectors $(\Theta^{(p)})$ such that L converges towards a (at least local) minimum [11].

- **CM-step 1:** $\Theta_1^{(p+1)} = \max_{\Theta_1} Q((\Theta_1, ..., \Theta_N), \Theta^{(p)})$
  $(\Theta_2, ..., \Theta_N) = (\Theta_2^{(p)}, ..., \Theta_N^{(p)})$ are held fixed.
- **CM-step 2:** $\Theta_2^{(p+1)} = \max_{\Theta_2} Q((\Theta_1^{(p+1)}, \Theta_2, ..., \Theta_N), \Theta^{(p)})$
  $(\Theta_1, \Theta_3, ..., \Theta_N) = (\Theta_1^{(p+1)}, \Theta_3^{(p)}, ..., \Theta_N^{(p)})$ are held fixed.
- And so on...
- After the last **CM-step** N, the estimated vector $\Theta^{(p+1)} = (\Theta_1^{(p+1)}, ..., \Theta_N^{(p+1)})$ is the input of the following E-step.

We consider the partition $\Theta = (\Theta_1, \Theta_2)$ with $\Theta_1 = (\mu_1, \ldots, \mu_m, \sigma_1, \ldots, \sigma_m)$ (or $\Theta_1 = (\mu_1, \ldots, \mu_m, \sigma)$ for Model 1), and $\Theta_2 = (\alpha_1, \ldots, \alpha_d)$. The equations for the mean and variance parameters constitute the first CM-step, which yields a straightforward explicit solution $\Theta_1^{(p+1)}$, the bias field coefficients being held fixed at the value $\Theta_2^{(p)}$. Then, given the estimated $\Theta_1^{(p+1)}$, the second CM-step amounts to solve a linear system of d equations, for Models 1 and 2.

In case of Model 3, the second CM-step is still a non-linear system of d equations, and is analytically intractable. Thus, we use an approximation, called

One-Step-Late (OSL), and proposed in [6] for reconstruction from SPECT data. The idea is to replace the non-linear terms of the CM-Step 2 of iteration $(p+1)$ of the ECM algorithm by their values estimated at the previous iteration (p), i.e., to replace $1/(1 + \sum_{j=1}^{d} \alpha_j^{(p+1)} \phi_j(v_i))$ by $1/(1 + \sum_{j=1}^{d} \alpha_j^{(p)} \phi_j(v_i))$. Then the system becomes linear as in Models 1 and 2. An heuristic justification is to say that the ECM algorithm, as the original EM, is known to converge slowly, and this non linear term will not be much different between iterations (p) and $(p+1)$. We call the three such derived schemes Algorithms 1, 2 and 3.

3.5 Outliers Rejection Scheme

So far, we have proposed to minimize $\sum_{i=1}^{n} s_i$ with respect to Θ, where $s_i = -\log p(y_i; \Theta)$, and $\Theta = (\mu_1, \ldots, \mu_m, \sigma_1, \ldots, \sigma_m, \alpha_1, \ldots, \alpha_d)$. Typically, s_i is large when the intensity y_i fits the presumed underlying mixture model badly. In particular, this is the case for voxels affected by partial volume effects, and thus far from the m classes of interest. These voxels can severely offset the ML estimation. By an analogy with the LTS estimation [16], to eliminate these meaningless voxels and thus achieve a better robustness, we propose to minimize $\sum_{i=1}^{h}(s)_{i:n}$, where $(s)_{1:n} \leq \ldots \leq (s)_{n:n}$ are the ordered "residuals" and h is an integer superior to $\lfloor n/2 \rfloor$. In [17], an iterative scheme is proposed to compute a (at least) local minimum of the LTS criterion, which amounts to successive simple LS computations; following the same idea, we propose the following scheme (we do not give proof of convergence of this heuristic procedure, which practically gives good results, see Fig. 1) to minimize $\sum_{i=1}^{h}(s)_{i:n}$:

- Step 1: compute the ML estimate $\tilde{\Theta}$ of Θ on the whole dataset $(y_1, \ldots, y_n)$ by an ECM algorithm
- Step 2: compute the residuals $s_i = -\log p(y_i; \tilde{\Theta})$ on the whole dataset
- Step 3: sort out the residuals s_i
- Step 4: recompute the ML estimate $\tilde{\Theta}'$ on the data that exhibit the h lowest residuals, likely to be best suited to the model, by an ECM algorithm
- Step 5: go back to Step 2, set $\tilde{\Theta} = \tilde{\Theta}'$, and iterate until convergence

4 Validation

4.1 Experiments on Synthetic MR Images

Which of these three models is best suited to real MR data? As there is no ground truth for this latter, we propose a validation and comparison of the three models based on the MR simulator of the Montreal Neurological Institute [9], incorporating realistic models for bias field, measurement noise, uncorrupted intra-tissue intensity distributions and partial volume effects. Practically, we simulated 6 isotropic T1-weighted MR volumes (of voxel size $1mm^3$) with different levels of noise (0%, 3%, 7%) and bias (20%, 40%). We use the RMS difference

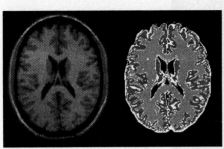

Fig. 1. Robust estimation of the parameters. Left: synthetic T1-weighted MR image, generated by the MNI simulator [9], with noise level 0% and bias field level 40%. Right: intensity-corrected MR image (by Algorithm 3); the voxels in white have been rejected from the estimation. Most of these voxels are close to the tissue boundaries, and are affected by partial volume effects.

between the applied and the computed bias field as a measure of error to evaluate the precision of the three algorithms. Figure 2 shows the results of these 6 experiments. When the noise is weak (0 or 3%), Algorithm 3 performs slightly better than Algorithm 2, and both of them are largely better than Algorithm 1. When the noise level is higher (7%), Algorithm 2 performs largely better than Algorithms 1 and 3. On average, Algorithm 2, and thus the underlying Model 2, seems to be the best.

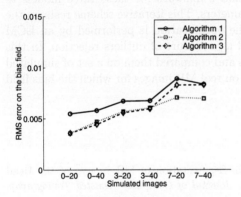

Fig. 2. RMS errors on the bias field for the three algorithms applied to the six simulated images. The degree of the three polynomials of the bias field models is $D = 2$. In average, Algorithm 2 performs better than the two others.

4.2 Experiments on Real MR Images

We applied Algorithm 3 on 10 images of healthy subjects, provided by the MARI-ARC, University of Liverpool, UK. Acquired by a MR scanner GE SIGNA 1,5 T using a circularly polarized coil, they are of size $256 \times 256 \times 124$ (voxel size $0.78125 \times 0.78125 \times 1.6$). In Figure 3, we display 10 axial slices of the original MR images and the estimated bias fields, which have a characteristic "diagonal" structure. For each subject, the voxels in the right temporal and frontal lobes have higher intensities than their counterparts in the other hemisphere; this pattern is inverted in the occipital lobes. This result confirms works of other authors [20], who link this bias field asymmetry with the elliptical shape of the head.

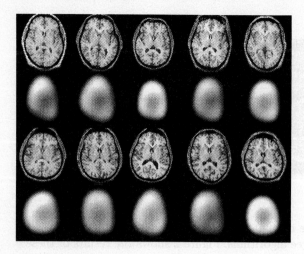

Fig. 3. Bias field estimation on 10 MR brain images. These images are in neurological conventions. $D = 4$. The voxels in the temporal and frontal lobes have higher intensities than their counterparts in the other hemisphere; this pattern is inverted in the occipital lobes.

5   Conclusion

In this article, we have identified two widely used models of the imaging process for bias field estimation. We have proposed a third model, and shown that it is possible to use a common estimation framework for these three models to identify the set of their unknown parameters. This iterative scheme rests on the principle of Maximum Likelihood. The optimization is performed by an ECM algorithm, in which we have included a procedure of outliers rejection. In this way, we have derived three algorithms and compared them on a set of simulated images. We have given a set of results on real MR images for which the bias field has a typical diagonal pattern.

References

1. H.E. Cline *et al.* Three-Dimensional Segmentation of MR Images of the Head Using Probability and Connectivity. *Journal of Computer Assisted Tomography,* 14(6):1037–1045, 1990.
2. B.M. Dawant *et al.* Correction of Intensity Variations in MR Images for Computer-Aided Tissue Classification. *IEEE TMI,* 12(4):770–781, December 1993.
3. A. P. Dempster *et al.* Maximum likelihood from incomplete data via the EM algorithm. *Journal of the Royal Statistical Society,* 39:1–38, 1977.
4. A.C. Evans *et al.* 3D statistical neuroanatomical models from 305 MRI volumes. In *IEEE Nuclear Science Symposium and Medical Imaging Conference,* pages 1813–1817, San Francisco, USA, October 1993.
5. G. Gerig *et al.* Nonlinear Anisotropic Filtering of MRI Data. *IEEE TMI,* 11(2):221–232, June 1992.
6. P.J. Green. Bayesian Reconstructions From Emission Tomography Data Using a Modified EM Algorithm. *IEEE TMI,* 9(1):84–93, March 1990.
7. R. Guillemaud and M. Brady. Estimating the Bias Field of MR Images. *IEEE TMI,* 16(3):238–251, June 1997.

8. M. Kamber *et al.* Model-based 3D segmentation of multiple sclerosis lesions in dual-echo MRI data. In *VBC'92*, volume 1808 of *SPIE*, pages 590–600, Chapel Hill, USA, October 1992.

9. R.K.-S. Kwan *et al.* An Extensible MRI Simulator for Post-Processing Evaluation. In *VBC'96*, volume 1131 of *LNCS*, pages 135–140, Hamburg, Germany, September 1996. Springer-Verlag. MRI simulator: http://www.bic.mni.mcgill.ca/brainweb/.

10. Z. Liang *et al.* Parameter estimation and tissue segmentation from multispectral MR images. *IEEE TMI*, 13:441–449, September 1994.

11. X.L. Meng and D.B. Rubin. Maximum likelihood estimation via the ECM algorithm: A general framework. *Biometrika*, 80(2):267–278, 1993.

12. C.R. Meyer *et al.* Retrospective Correction of Intensity Inhomogeneities in MRI. *IEEE TMI*, 14(1):36–41, March 1995.

13. P.A. Narayana *et al.* Compensation for surface coil sensitivity variation in magnetic resonance imaging. *Magnetic Resonance Imaging*, 6(3):271–274, 1988.

14. D.L. Pham and J.L. Prince. A Generalized EM Algorithm for Robust Segmentation of Magnetic Resonance Images. In *33rd Annual Conference on Information Sciences and Systems , CISS'99*, pages 558–563, Baltimore, USA, March 1999.

15. J.C. Rajapakse and F. Kruggel. Segmentation of MR images with intensity inhomogeneities. *Image and Vision Computing*, 16(3):165–180, 1998.

16. P.J. Rousseeuw and A.M. Leroy. *Robust Regression and Outlier Detection.* Wiley Series in Probability and Mathematical Statistics, 1987.

17. P.J. Rousseeuw and K. Van Driessen. Computing LTS Regression for Large Data Sets. Technical report, Statistics Group, University of Antwerp, 1999. submitted.

18. P. Schroeter *et al.* Robust Parameter Estimation of Intensity Distributions for Brain Magnetic Resonance Images. *IEEE TMI*, 17(2):172–186, April 1998.

19. J. Sijbers *et al.* Maximum Likelihood estimation of Rician distribution parameters. *IEEE TMI*, 17(3):357–361, 1998.

20. J.G. Sled and G.B. Pike. Magnetic Resonance Imaging - Standing-Wave and RF Penetration Artifacts Caused by Elliptic Geometry: An Electrodynamic Analysis of MRI. *IEEE TMI*, 17(4):653–662, August 1998.

21. J.G. Sled and A.P. Zijdenbos. A Nonparametric Method for Automatic Correction of Intensity Nonuniformity in MRI Data. *IEEE TMI*, 17(1):87–97, February 1998.

22. M. Styner *et al.* Parametric estimate of intensity inhomogeneities applied to MRI. *IEEE TMI*, 19(3):153–165, March 2000.

23. K. Van Leemput *et al.* Automated Model-Based Bias Field Correction of MR Images of the Brain. *IEEE TMI*, 18(10):885–896, October 1999.

24. K. Van Leemput *et al.* Automated Model-Based Tissue Classification of MR Images of the Brain. *IEEE TMI*, 18(10):897–908, October 1999.

25. W. M. Wells III *et al.* Adaptive Segmentation of MRI Data. *IEEE TMI*, 15(4):429–442, August 1996.

Inferring Vascular Structure from 2D and 3D Imagery

Abhir Bhalerao[1], Elke Thönnes[2], Wilfrid Kendall[2], and Roland Wilson[1]

[1] Department of Computer Science
[2] Department of Statistics
University of Warwick, UK
{abhir|elke|wsk|rgw}@{dcs|stats}.warwick.ac.uk

Abstract. We describe a method for inferring vascular (tree-like) structures from 2D and 3D imagery. A Bayesian formulation is used to make effective use of prior knowledge of likely tree structures with the observed being modelled locally with intensity profiles as being Gaussian. The local feature models are estimated by combination of a multiresolution, windowed Fourier approach followed by an iterative, minimum mean-square estimation, which is both computationally efficient and robust. A Markov Chain Monte Carlo (MCMC) algorithm is employed to produce approximate samples from the posterior distribution given the feature model estimates. We present results of the multiresolution parameter estimation on representative 2D and 3D data, and show preliminary results of our implementation of the MCMC algorithm [1].

1 Introduction

The problem of inferring vascular structure from two and three dimensional image data is an important one, especially in the area of surgical planning, which requires a combination of efficient computation and a method of using prior knowledge. Previous work in the area has tended to focus on the modelling of specific vascular features, using deformable templates [7,3] or to use heuristic approaches such as adaptive thresholding or level sets [4,6].

The aim of the work described here is to formulate a general method for the inference, which can be applied in two or three dimensions and makes effective use of prior knowledge, yet which is sufficiently general to be applied to a wide range of problems. The common statistical methods for such medical image analysis have typically used likelihood techniques, such as Expectation-Maximisation [11,9]. Although iterative, EM methods can be efficient computationally, but provide only a limited way of incorporating prior knowledge. A general and powerful way of including further prior information is to use a Bayesian method, such as *maximum a posteriori* (MAP) estimation. The difficulty with Bayesian techniques is essentially a computational one: they typically require the use of Markov chain Monte Carlo (MCMC) algorithms, which may

---

[1] This project is funded by UK EPSRC

W. Niessen and M. Viergever (Eds.): MICCAI 2001, LNCS 2208, pp. 820–828, 2001.
© Springer-Verlag Berlin Heidelberg 2001

run for hundreds of thousands of iterations to yield reliable results [5]. This
has restricted their use in applications involving large data sets such as medical
images.

The method we have adopted is grounded in statistical inference, combining
local likelihood maximisation using a Gaussian model of the spatial intensity profile, and global structure determination using a Bayesian technique derived from
a general model of vasculature as a collection of tree structures. By approaching the problem in this way, we can keep the efficiency of likelihood techniques,
while exploiting the power and generality of a Bayesian approach. To improve
the efficiency and robustness of the computation, we have adopted a multiresolution method, similar to that described in [12]. After a brief description of the
estimation algorithms, we present results of two and three dimensional structure
inference on real data. The paper is concluded with some observations on the
technique.

2   Local Structure Estimation

We approximate the local shape of a vessel as being linear (lines and cylinders)
and employ an iterative fitting technique to minimise the sum of squared residuals between the data f and our model g. The global shape of an object, in
general, cannot be modelled by a single such primitive structure, hence the need
to localise the model to a small neighbourhood.

In the continuous spatial domain, if a feature such as a line (or cylinder)
is windowed by a smooth function $w()$, then it can be approximated by a n-
dimensional Gaussian function:

$$g(\boldsymbol{x}|\Theta) = A\exp(-(\boldsymbol{x} - \boldsymbol{\mu})^T C^{-1}(\boldsymbol{x} - \boldsymbol{\mu})/2) \qquad (1)$$

parameterised by $\Theta = \{A, \boldsymbol{\mu}, C\}$ with amplitude A, centred on $\boldsymbol{\mu}$ and the covariance matrix $C = R^T C' R$, where C' is the diagonal matrix of variances
representing the extent of the function in the major axes and R is the matrix of
rotation from the feature orientation vector, to the x-axis.

To obtain maximum likelihood (ML) estimates of the parameters, the win-
dowed image data, $f_w(\boldsymbol{x}) = w(\boldsymbol{x})f(\boldsymbol{x})$, are modelled as conditionally normal,
given the local model $f_w(\boldsymbol{x}) \sim N(g(\boldsymbol{x}|\Theta), \sigma^2)$. To maximise the likelihood, we
minimise the sum of squared residuals between the windowed data in an image
block of size B^n and the model:

$$\chi^2 = \frac{1}{B^n} \sum_{\boldsymbol{x}}^{B^n} (g(\boldsymbol{x}|\Theta) - f_w(\boldsymbol{x}))^2 \qquad (2)$$

From an initial estimate of $\Theta_0 = \{A_0, \boldsymbol{\mu}_0, C_0\}$ at iteration $t = 0$, we calculate
the sample estimates for Θ weighted by the inner product of f_w and g using the
iterative scheme (dropping the position subscript $\boldsymbol{x}$ for clarity):

$$A_{t+1} = \sum_{x} f_w g(\Theta_t) / \sum_{x} g(\Theta_t) g(\Theta_t) \tag{3}$$

$$\mu_{t+1} = \sum_{x} x f_w g(\Theta_t) / \sum_{x} f_w g(\Theta_t) \tag{4}$$

$$C_{t+1} = 2 \sum_{x} (x - \mu_t)(x - \mu_t)^T f_w g(\Theta_t) / \sum_{x} f_w g(\Theta_t) \tag{5}$$

The initial estimate Θ_0 is obtained by using the multiresolution Fourier Transform (MFT) [12]. The windowed Fourier transform of $f_w(x) \leftrightarrow \hat{f}_w(u)$ is also a Gaussian with the spectral energy distribution dependent on the type of feature (see [10]). The principal components of the moment of inertia tensor I of the spectral energy:

$$I = \frac{1}{B^n} \sum_{u} u u^T |\hat{f}_w(u)|^2 \tag{6}$$

where B is the block size, gives n eigenvalues $\lambda_1 \geq .. \geq \lambda_n$, which are inversely related to the covariance, C, and the spatial orientation of a linear feature is that of the eigenvector associated with the largest eigenvalue λ_1.

The first derivative of the phase spectrum, $\phi(u)$, will be related to the position or centroid μ of the spatial function if the window function for the image block is real and even, via the Fourier shift theorem [8]:

$$\phi'(u) = arg(\hat{f}'_w(u)) = -\mu.u \tag{7}$$

The feature centroid μ can therefore be estimated by taking average pairwise correlations between neighbouring coefficients along each of the n axes

$$\mu_{0i} = \frac{1}{2\pi B^n} \sum_{u} \hat{f}_w(u_i - 1) \hat{f}_w(u_i)^* \tag{8}$$

If $f_w(x)$ is locally Gaussian and noise free, then Θ_0 will be close to Θ_{ML}. In general, the iterative estimation greatly improves the MFT estimate, converging rapidly (5-10 iterations) to a stable solution. Furthermore, the resulting χ^2 provides a useful measure of goodness of fit of the model to the data.

3   Inferring the Global Structure

To draw inferences about the global structure, we employ a Bayesian formalism: the data are modelled as a random tree-like structure and we then use an MCMC algorithm [2] to sample from the posterior distribution, which is conditioned on the data. The sampling distribution is an approximate equilibrium of a random process whose configuration space is the space of tree-like structures and whose equilibrium is designed to be the target conditional distribution. As well as gaining information about the global structure, variation in the posterior samples enables us to quantify uncertainties about the image interpretation.

The prior distribution is that the global structure is a *forest* of a random number of trees. Each such tree is a binary tree: branches divide only into two sub-branches at a time. A physical realisation of such a tree needs each node to be located in space. Unfortunately, the simplistic approach of displacing each node from its parent by a Gaussian displacement of zero mean (a "random-walk" tree) leads to a tangled local structure (left hand figure 1). We therefore introduce a correlation by allowing the mean displacement to be a small linear multiple of the displacement of the parent node from the grandparent node (an "AR(1)" tree) (right hand of figure 1). To each node we then associate a Gaussian kernel that represents the corresponding vessel segment.

The posterior distribution for a random number N of trees $\tau_1, \ldots, \tau_N$ is given by

$$\pi(\tau_1, \ldots, \tau_n | \Theta) \propto \mathbb{P}(N = n) \prod_{i=1}^{n} \prod_{\nu \in \tau_i} p_{v(\nu)} \phi(x_\nu | x_\eta, \eta \in \mathcal{A}(\nu)) \psi(\theta_\nu | \theta_{\text{parent}(\nu)})$$
$$\times L(\tau_1, \ldots, \tau_n | \Theta), \tag{9}$$

where p_0, p_1, p_2 are the family size probabilities of the branching process and $v(\nu)$ is the valence of the node ν. Moreover, $\phi(x_\nu | x_\eta, \eta \in \mathcal{A}(\nu))$ is the location distribution of x_ν which depends on the location of its parent and grandparent (if any) given by the ancestor set $\mathcal{A}(\nu)$. The distribution $\psi(\theta_\nu | \theta_{\text{parent}(\nu)})$ of the Gaussian kernel parameters θ_ν associated to each node ν depends on the parameters of the Gaussian kernel associated to its parent node. Finally, $L(\tau_1, \ldots, \tau_n | \Theta)$ denotes the likelihood of the forest given the local structure estimates Θ assuming pixelwise iid white Gaussian noise. The simulation, whose configuration at any

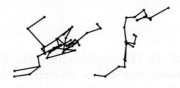

Fig. 1. Illustration of a random-walk tree and an AR(1) tree

one time is a collection of random trees, is designed to have *moves* which take it from one configuration to the next. These moves, some of which are illustrated in Figure 2, are: adding or deleting a tree, adding or deleting a twig at the end of a branch; displacing a node; splitting a tree into two or grafting two trees together into one; changing the parameters of the Gaussian kernel associated with a node. As long as each move has an 'opposite' (e.g. add versus delete, split versus graft) and the chances of each move are balanced against its opposite, it is straightforward to compute the required equilibrium distribution and to design the move probabilities to give the required posterior as equilibrium, using the Metropolis-Hastings technique (MH) [5]. The MH method iterates in two steps:

Adding versus deleting a twig   Displacement of a node   Grafting two trees versus splitting a tree

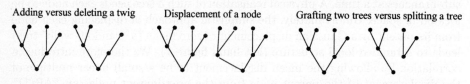

Fig. 2. Illustration of some moves

the first proposes a move from the collection of moves and the second accepts or rejects the move so as to ensure that the equilibrium coincides with the desired posterior. Generally, the decision whether to accept or reject a move depends on whether the resulting new tree will be a more adequate representation from the posterior than the current tree.

The efficiency of the algorithm depends crucially on the proposed moves. As all moves influence the likelihood only locally, the likelihood evaluation can be implemented efficiently. Moreover, to avoid inefficiencies due to a large number of moves being rejected, our moves are guided by likelihood considerations: the locality of a move is dependent on the amount of unexplained data in the surrounding spatial region and the mean direction of a proposed branch segment resembles the direction of the data in the vicinity of the segment. This approach is reminiscent of the Langevin Hastings algorithm, where proposals are influenced by the gradient of the posterior, see [1]. Global structure that can be inferred with high certainty locally will lead to a tree structure that is stable over time, while low local certainty results in a volatile tree-structure that alternates between different explanations for the global structure.

4   Experiments

Figure 3 illustrates results of the ML model estimation. We have used part of a 2D retinal angiographic image size 404×404 pixels (fig. 3(a)) for our 2D experiments. The background is first modelled as locally piece-wise linear and subtracted from the original data prior to the estimating the Gaussian feature parameter estimates. The orientation and position of the MFT feature estimates which form the initial block parameter estimates, Θ_0 are shown in the centre (fig. 3(b) and (c)), where the feature intensity is modulated by the goodness of fit of the model to the data. Despite the noise, there is good correspondence of the large scale arterial structure at block size $B = 64$. The background noise becomes insignificant at block size $B = 16$ (fig. 3(c)). The right hand column (fig. 3(d)-(e)) shows a data reconstruction of the 2D Gaussians in each block (at corresponding block sizes) after the iterative ML estimation. Note that the thickness of the vessels (the standard deviation of the model orthogonal to the feature) are accurately modelled at both large and small block sizes. Clearly, at lower spatial resolutions, the model cannot easily describe the presence of multiple vessels within the window, such as at vessel bifurcations, and the resulting low-amplitude, isotropic Gaussians are locally the 'best' description of these regions. However, these blocks can be identified from higher residual errors, χ^2 in equation (2).

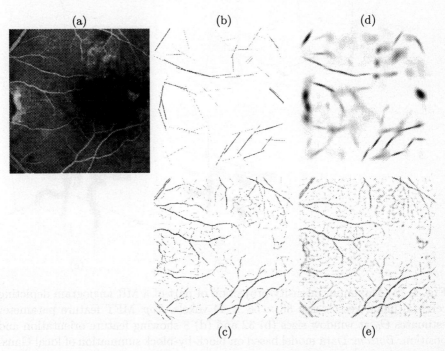

Fig. 3. *Left*: (a) 2D retinal angiogram size 404×404 pixels. *Centre*: MFT feature estimates Θ_0 for block sizes (b) 64 and, (c) 16. *Right*: Reconstruction of data from model parameters estimates Θ_{ML} for block sizes (d) 64 and, (e) 16.

The 3D implementation of the ML model estimator is demonstrated in figure 4(a)-(e). The local structure estimator was run on the *speed* image of part of a phase contrast MRA with cerebral blood vessels size $88 \times 58 \times 44$ voxels (fig. 4(a)). Illustrations of the MFT feature estimates and data reconstructions using 3D Gaussians are shown at two (cubic) window sizes: $B = 32$ and $B = 8$ (fig. 4: top and bottom rows respectively). The major vessels are captured at the lower resolution (fig. 4(b)-(c)) while the finer vessels can be seen in figure 4(d)-(e). Note that at both scales, as with the 2D retinal example, the vessel diameters are correctly estimated.

To demonstrate the utility of the use multiple window sizes, we generated a a multi-level data reconstruction after a simple top-down scale selection based on the normalised block residual errors, figure 5. In this reconstruction, we used 4.4% of the parameters sets, Θ_{ML}, from a total of 13596 across 4 block sizes. This reconstruction is able to capture both large and small local structures in the data.

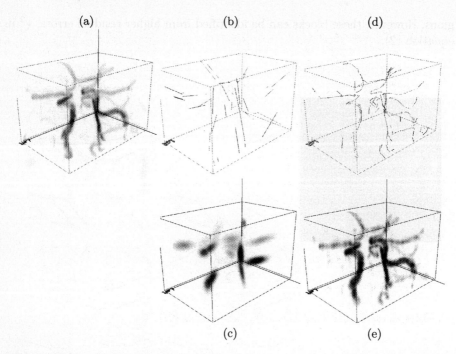

Fig. 4. (a) Maximum intensity projection of part of a MR angiogram depicting cerebral blood vessels size $88 \times 58 \times 44$ voxels. *Top*: MFT feature parameter estimates Θ_0 at window sizes (b) 32 and (d) 8 showing feature orientation and position. *Bottom*: Data model based on block-by-block summation of local Gaussian models Θ_{ML} at window sizes (c) 32 and, (e) 8. The Gaussian amplitude has been made proportional to the goodness of fit between the data and the model.

To infer global structure we have used an MCMC algorithm on the 2D retinal data to sample the posterior distribution in (9) using the Gaussian estimates (figure 6). These show that the method does indeed capture significant global structure.

5   Conclusions

Some encouraging preliminary results have been achieved using the approach described in section 3, demonstrating its potential for modelling vascular structure globally in a computationally efficient way. Fine-tuning the algorithm will lead to significant improvements. These will include, for example, the use of the local estimates to produce initial configurations for the MCMC algorithm, using a posterior based on the multiresolution representation, such as shown in figure 5. Such improvements are currently being implemented.

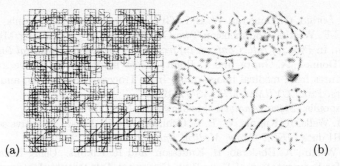

Fig. 5. (a) Multiresolution scale selection based on thresholding goodness of fit between model and data across levels with overlapping block sizes 64, 32, 16 and 8. (b) Multiresolution data reconstruction using parameter set depicted in (a).

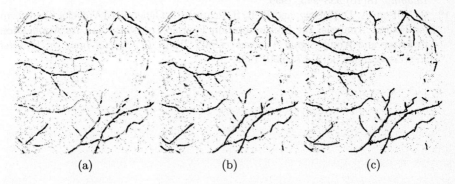

Fig. 6. (a) Iteration 2000 of the MCMC simulation based on posterior derived from block sizes $B = 8$ on the 2D retinal image. (b) Iteration 10000. (c) Iteration 50000.

References

1. J.E. Besag. Contribution to the discussion paper "Representation of knowledge in complex systems" by U. Grenander and M.I. Miller. *Journal of the Royal Statistical Society Series B*, 56:591 – 592, 1994.
2. S.P. Brooks. The Markov Chain Monte Carlo Method and its Application. *The Statistician*, 47:69 – 100, 1998.
3. A. F. Frangi, W. J. Niessen, R. M. Hoogeveen, Th. van Walsum, and M. A. Viergever. Model-based Quantitation of 3D Magnetic Resonance Angiographic Image. *IEEE Trans. Medical Imaging*, 18(10):946–956, 1999.
4. G. Gerig, T. Koller, G. Székely, Ch. Brechbühler, and O. Kübler. Symbolic description of 3-D structures applied to cerebral vessel tree obtained from MR angiography volume data. In H. H. Barrett and A. F. Gmitro, editors, *Information Processing in Medical Imaging IPMI'93, Lecture Notes in Computer Science*, volume 687, pages 94–111, 1993.
5. W. R. Gilks, S. Richardson, and D. J. Spiegelhalter. *Markov Chain Monte Carlo in Practice*. Chapman & Hall, 1996.

6. L. M. Lorigo, O. Faugeras, W. E. L. Grimson, R. Keriven, R. Kikinis, A. Nabavia, and C-F. Westin. Codimension-Two Geodesic Active Contours for MRA Segmentation. In *Proc. of Intl. Conf. on Information Processing in Medical Imaging*, 1999.
7. T. O'Donnell, A. Gupta, and T. Boult. A new model for the recover of cylindrical structures from medical image data. In J. Troccaz, E. Grimson, and R. Mösges, editors, *Proc. CVRMed-MRCAS'97*, 1997.
8. A. Papoulis. *Signal Analysis*. McGraw-Hill, New York, 1977.
9. W. M. Wells, R. Kikinis, W. E. L. Grimson, and R. Jolesz. Adaptive segmentation of MRI data. *IEEE Trans. Medical Imaging*, 15:429–442, 1996.
10. C-F. Westin, A. Bhalerao, H. Knutsson, and R. Kikinis. Using Local 3D Structure for Segmentation of Bone from Computer Tomography Images. In *Proc. of Computer Vision and Pattern Recognition '97*, Puerto Rico, 1997.
11. D. L. Wilson and J. A. Noble. An adaptive segmentation algorithm for extracting arteries and aneurysms from time-of-flight MRA data. *IEEE Trans. Medical Imaging*, 18(10):938–945, 1999.
12. R. Wilson, A. D. Calway, and E. R. S. Pearson. A Generalized Wavelet Transform for Fourier Analysis: the Multiresolution Fourier Transform and its Application to Image and Audio Signal Analysis. *IEEE Trans. IT, Special Issue on Wavelet Representations*, 38(2):674–690, 1992.

Statistical and Deformable Model Approaches to the Segmentation of MR Imagery and Volume Estimation of Stroke Lesions

Benjamin Stein[1], Dimitri Lisin[2], Joseph Horowitz[1], Edward Riseman[2], and Gary Whitten[2]

[1] Dept. of Mathematics and Statistics, Univ. of Massachusetts, Amherst, MA
http://www.math.umass.edu
[2] Dept. of Computer Science, Univ. of Massachusetts
http://vis-www.cs.umass.edu

Abstract. We propose two 3D methods to segment magnetic resonance imagery (MRI) of ischemic stroke patients into lesion and background, and hence to estimate lesion volumes. The first is a hierarchical, regularized method based on classical statistics that produces a rigorous confidence interval for lesion volume. This approach requires a limited amount of user interaction to initialize, but this step can be time-consuming. The second method integrates the first into the deformable models framework. This hybrid approach combines intensity-based information provided by the statistical method and shape-based information given by the deformable model. It also requires less initialization than the statistical method. Both procedures have been tested on real MR data, with volume estimates within 20% of those derived from doctors' hand segmentations. According to the physicians with whom we are working, these results are clinically useful to evaluate stroke therapies.

1 Introduction

In evaluating therapies for ischemic stroke patients, many physicians are interested in finding consistent, reliable estimates of lesion volume from MR images. We introduce two new methods to segment three-dimensional (3D) images into lesion and background, and thus to estimate lesion volumes. In section 2 we present the first procedure, called "packing," which is a hierarchical, regularized method based on classical statistics. Several other research groups have used statistical approaches to segment tissue types in MRI (see [1,8,12,13], e.g.), with varying degrees of user interaction, but with no single method emerging as superior. As in those methods, we are concerned with producing consistent estimates with limited user interaction, but our procedure goes beyond them in producing an assessment of the *error* of our estimate, in the form of a rigorous confidence interval for lesion volume. While this idea has been explored in [11] for near-infrared imaging, we do not know of any such results for MRI.

The packing method requires sometimes time-consuming user interaction to initialize, and uses only the statistical information in the image. By integrating

W. Niessen and M. Viergever (Eds.): MICCAI 2001, LNCS 2208, pp. 829–836, 2001.
© Springer-Verlag Berlin Heidelberg 2001

packing with the well-known deformable models ("snakes") framework [6], we reduce user interaction and take advantage of of geometric as well as statistical information in the image. Our second procedure (see section 3) is therefore a 3D "hybrid" method that uses a version of packing as an additional external energy term. Also, the addition of statistical information into the deformable models framework helps to suppress some of the limitations of snakes, including sensitivity to strong gradients produced by other nearby objects and the inability to adjust to large changes in lesion size from one slice to another.

We have tested the new procedures on actual MRI, and found that both methods are consistently estimating lesion volumes to within 20% of those derived from doctors' hand segmentations. According to the doctors, these results (see section 4) are clinically useful.

2   The Packing Method

We assume the lesion is imaged as a "bright spot" lesion, which means that the mean lesion intensity μ_L is higher than the mean of the intensities of any other tissue type in the region of interest (ROI). The diffusion-weighted pulse sequence shows an ischemic stroke lesion as the only bright object, so that the ROI can be the entire set of imagery. However, for pulse sequences such as T_2 and FLAIR, the user must extract the ROI manually.

Aside from choosing a ROI, the only other manual step necessary to initialize the process is to sample the data. The user chooses a "base slice" from the stack of two-dimensional images, and two regions bounded by closed contours in that slice: one region completely inside the lesion and the other in the background. The pixels inside these contours constitute the lesion and background samples that our statistical analysis will be based upon. This step tupically requires less than a minute of user interaction.

2.1   Coarse-Grid Segmentation

The method continues with no more outside assistance. We will describe this multi-step procedure by first explaining the mechanics of it at step $i, i = 1, ..., D$ (usually $D = 2$ or 3), with L_{i-1} the set of voxels classified as lesion in previous steps, and L_0 the lesion sample. We cover the ROI by a grid of cubes of edge length d_i, so that each cube contains d_i^3 voxels. In the initial steps of the method, we use large cubes, typically $d_1 = 8$ or 4, and decrease the size for later steps, making this a hierarchial procedure. We will discuss this further in section 2.2.

At step i, for each such cube C that borders but does not intersect L_{i-1}, we consider the following hypothesis test:

$$H_0 : C \text{ is entirely inside the lesion}$$
$$H_A : C \text{ is not entirely inside the lesion.}$$

More precisely, H_A says that at least one voxel in C is not completely inside the lesion. We write these qualitative hypotheses more precisely as follows:

$$H_0 : \mu_C \geq \mu_L - k_{i,L} \tag{1}$$

$$H_A : \mu_C < \mu_L - k_{i,L}, \tag{2}$$

where μ_C is the mean intensity of the cube being tested, and $k_{i,L}$ is a pre-set parameter that depends on i and the pulse sequence used to acquire the imagery.

Assuming that intensity follows a normal distribution [9], we use the standard two-sample t-test of size $\frac{\alpha}{DN_i}$ [5] to test H_0 vs. H_A, where α is a fixed constant between 0 and 1, and N_i is the number of cubes being tested at step i. A type I error occurs if C is actually inside the lesion, but is not accepted into it.

Using Bonferroni's inequality [5], it can be shown that the *overall* probability of a type I error can be controlled when all the cubes in the grid are tested. That is, let $C_{im}, m = 1, ..., N_i$, denote the cubes in the covering of the ROI at step i that border but do not intersect L_{i-1}, and let $\mathcal{L}_i$ denote the set of cubes C_{im} that are actually in the lesion. Then

$$P(\text{all } C_{im} \in \mathcal{L}_i \text{ are accepted into the lesion}) \geq 1 - \frac{\alpha}{D}. \tag{3}$$

2.2   Coarse-to-Fine Aspect

After step i is completed, we have L_i, the set of voxels classified as lesion in steps $1, ..., i$, and we now use it as the lesion sample for step $i + 1$, yielding the sample statistics $\overline{x}_{L_i}$ and $s_{L_i}^2$. In step $i + 1$, we cover the ROI with (smaller) cubes of edge $d_{i+1} < d_i$. This coarse-to-fine aspect of the method allows us to update our coarse segmentation from the previous steps into a more accurate one by "packing" it with smaller cubes.

At step $i + 1$, we test each cube $C_{(i+1)m}, m = 1, ..., N_{i+1}$, that borders but does not intersect L_i, for acceptance into the lesion via the two-sample t-test. We repeat for all steps $i = 1, ..., D$, so that L_D is the final segmentation of the lesion. Equation 3 says that we can control the overall probability of a type I error at each step; similarly we can also show that we can control the type I error for the entire multi-step procedure, namely,

$$P(\bigcap_{i=1}^{D} [\text{all } C_{im} \in \mathcal{L}_i \text{ are accepted into the lesion}]) \geq 1 - \alpha. \tag{4}$$

Proofs of the results (3) and (4) are in [10]. We could continue the procedure to the finest resolution, so that $d_D = 1$. However, in practice we stop before this finest level to diminish the effect of the high variability present in individual voxels; this helps us to regularize the segmentation.

2.3   One-Sided Confidence Bound for Volume

A lesion volume can be estimated by counting the number of voxels that are accepted into the lesion. From (4), we know (with $(1 - \alpha)100\%$ confidence) that

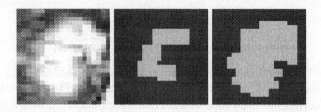

Fig. 1. Coarse-to-fine aspect of packing. Left: Sample slice (restricted to a ROI). Center: Lesion segmentation after $4 \times 4 \times 4$ boxes are tested. Right: Final segmentation after $2 \times 2 \times 2$ boxes are tested, which overestimates the lesion (see section 2.3).

we will admit all cubes that actually belong in the lesion. In terms of the volume estimate V_L and the actual volume V, we have that

$$P(V_L \geq V) \geq 1 - \alpha. \tag{5}$$

However, we do not control the possibility of admitting cubes that do not belong in the lesion. Cubes with a mixture of lesion and background voxels are especially susceptible of being incorrectly admitted. Thus V_L is not an unbiased estimator of the lesion volume, but rather an upper confidence bound of V.

2.4 Two-Sided Confidence Interval and Point Estimate for Volume

Using the same method as above to pack the *background*, we obtain another segmentation of the image. The resulting lesion volume V_B provides a lower confidence bound for V: $P(V_B \leq V) \geq 1 - \alpha$. Combining this with (5), we have

$$P(V_B \leq V \leq V_L) \geq 1 - 2\alpha. \tag{6}$$

Therefore, the interval (V_B, V_L) is a $(1 - 2\alpha)100\%$ confidence interval for the lesion volume. Any combination of V_B and V_L (the average, e.g.) is a valid point estimate for V. We will apply this method to real MRI in section 4.

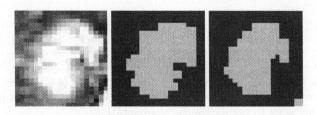

Fig. 2. Results for the packing method. Left: Sample slice. Center: Lesion segmentation via forward packing (an overestimate). Right: Lesion segmentation using background packing (an underestimate).

3 Hybrid Method

3.1 Deformable Models

A modeling techinique known as "active contours" or "snakes," is a semi-automatic approach to segmentation, originally proposed in [6]. It belongs to a class of methods known as deformable models. The idea is that a contour may be placed near some image feature and then deformed to optimally fit the feature.

The contour, or snake, is deformed automatically by minimizing an "energy functional," given by

$$E_{total} = E_{int} + E_{ext} = \int F_{int} + \int F_{ext}. \tag{7}$$

The internal energy, E_{int}, is typically defined as a smoothness constraint on the contour, E_{ext}, the external energy, is commonly defined as the negative of the gradient of the image, which pushes each portion of the snake to the strongest and nearest edge. F_{int} and F_{ext} are the corresponding forces, which we integrate over the contour.

External forces other than the image gradient have been proposed (see [4], e.g.). In section 3.2 we propose a new force, based on statistical packing, to help regularize the model. When the snake has converged to a minimal energy state, we classify the area inside it as lesion; see [6] for the computational details.

To go from a two-dimensional model to a three-dimensional one we use an approach similar to that of [2] and [14]. We propagate a final contour from one slice to serve as the initial contour in the next slice. Contours in adjacent slices are then connected with an additional force, imposing an overall smoothness constraint on the model. This 3D force assumes that only small changes in lesion shape and size occur in neighboring slices.

3.2 The Hybrid Algorithm

The approaches in sections 2 and 3.1 each have some limitations. Packing sometimes requires a large amount of user interaction, since the user must manually select the 3D ROI and the lesion and background samples. It is also sensitive to the quality of the initial samples. Meanwhile, the snake approach can be affected by other nearby objects creating strong edges, and it can perform poorly if there are significant changes in the size of the lesion in adjacent slices. It also can get stuck in a local energy minimum.

To minimize the problems of the two approaches, as well as to reinforce their strengths, we have combined them into a "hybrid" method: use a 2D version of packing described in [7] to produce a single lesion estimate, and use the gradient of the resulting binary image to define an additional external energy. The full algorithm is outlined as follows:

1. Manually initialize a snake in the base slice (Fig. 3A), and let it deform until it converges (Fig. 3B).

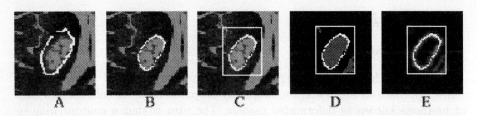

Fig. 3. Steps of the hybrid method (see text). A: Manual initialization of the contour. B: Converged contour. C: ROI. D: Statistical segmentation. E: Statistical energy.

2. Define a bounding box around the resulting contour, which will serve as the ROI in the current slice (Fig. 3C). The interior of the contour is used as the lesion sample, and the remainder of the box is the background sample.
3. Run the packing method and make the result into a binary image (Fig. 3D).
4. Define the negative of the gradient of the image as an additional external energy term (Fig. 3E).
5. Run the snake with this added energy to produce a segmentation of the slice.
6. Use the finished contour as the initialization for the adjacent slice. Repeat steps 2–5 until the number of pixels classified as lesion in a slice is less than some threshold. This will result in a 3D model of the lesion (Fig. 4).

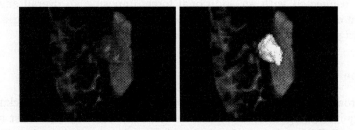

Fig. 4. Result of the hybrid method. Left: A portion of a 3D MR scan. Right: The lesion estimate superimposed (in white) onto the original image. 3D visualization software courtesy of Biomedical Imaging Group, UMass Medical Center, Worcester, MA.

With this approach we greatly reduce the amount of user interaction that the statistical procedure normally requires. All the user must do is draw a contour in the base slice; the ROI and the samples will then be obtained automatically. It also helps deal with the limitations of snakes, by adding the intensity-based statistical information to the snake model. This helps to keep it from being distracted by nearby normal, bright structures, and also helps to keep it on track in case of a non-incremental change from one slice to another. For implementation details see [7].

4   Results

We have tested the above methods on lesions in axial MRI. We obtained all of our data sets from Baystate Medical Center (West Springfield, MA) using a 1.5 T Picker Edge machine. One patient was imaged using a T_2 sequence with 1 mm slice thickness and no gaps. A FLAIR sequence with 2.5 mm slice thickness and no gaps was used for the other five.

To evaluate our results, we obtained two hand segmentations from each of two physicians at Baystate for each data set. We compare the volumes derived from these segmentations to the results for five different initializations of the packing and hybrid methods. All results are in Table 1.

	Hand Segmentation				Packing				Hybrid	
	Doctor 1		Doctor 2		Lower CB		Upper CB			
Patient	mean	sd	mean	sd	mean	sd	mean	sd	mean	sd
1	2069	120	1947.5	24.5	1914.6	56.3	2337	108.6	1927.6	49.3
2	3416	139.7	3617.5	183.8	2608	310.1	4709	142.7	3841.5	277.8
3	23555	762.3	21359	618.7	20019	1020	25891	760	21821.9	617.7
4	9962.5	67.2	10787.5	449.0	9434.5	320.4	11524.5	633.7	10031	906.8
5	10131	740.7	9377.5	1064.2	8603.5	320.2	11443.5	294.4	9536.9	251.8
6	3452.5	35.3	3504	160.9	2699.5	94.5	4205	476.2	3525	117.9

Table 1. Results for six MRI scans (in mm^3), including the means and standard deviations of lesion volumes from two physicians, those for the packing method (CB stands for a 90% confidence bound), using five different initializations, and for the hybrid method, also using five initializations.

The results show that the methods are consistently estimating lesion volume to within 20% of the physicians. The results from packing give only the lower and upper 90% confidence bounds for lesion volume; we use the average of the bounds to compare with the other estimates. The worst error, compared to the overall average of the doctors' estimates, was 6% for packing and 9% for the hybrid method, well within the 20% threshold that the physicians required. Comparing standard deviations, we see that the two methods generally are as consistent as the doctors, and more so in some cases. All pre-set parameters in the methods were the same for data imaged with the same pulse sequence; changes were necessary for packing between T_2 and FLAIR imagery, whereas no adjustments were necessary for the hybrid method. We have also tested the procedures on synthetic imagery, to evaluate them in the situation when the volume is known. Similar to real MRI, the error of our volume estimates did not, on average, exceed 5% in all cases.

5   Conclusion

We have introduced two new methods to segment MR imagery and estimate lesion volumes, one statistical and another that incorporates the statistical approach into a deformable models framework. Both methods are working well for actual patient data. The first procedure gives a rigorous confidence interval for lesion volume, but requires manual ROI extraction. The hybrid method reduces the user interaction, and generates a model of the lesion, insuring connectivity and smoothness, but a confidence interval has not yet been derived.

In the next step of our research we plan to integrate a full 3D version of packing into the snake framework, as well as to utilize the confidence interval to bound the error of the hybrid method. These steps will further increase the reliability and robustness of the hybrid method.

References

1. R. Adams and L. Bischof. Seeded region growing. *IEEE Trans on Pattern Analysis and Machine Intelligence*, 16:641–647, 1994.
2. I. Carlbom, D. Terzopoulos, K. Harris. Computer-assisted registration, segmentation, and 3D reconstruction from images of neuronal tissue sections, *IEEE Transactions on Medical Imaging*, 13(2), 351-362, 1994
3. H. Cline, W.E. Lorenson, R. Kikinis, F. Jolesz. Three-dimensional segmentation of MR images of the head using probability and connectivity. *Journal of Computer Assisted Tomography*, 14(6):1037–1045, 1990.
4. L.D. Cohen. On active contour models and balloons. *CVGIP: Image Understanding*, 53(2):211–218, 1991.
5. R. Johnson and D. Wichern. *Applied Multivariate Statistical Analysis*. Prentice-Hall, New Jersey, 1992.
6. M. Kass, A. Witkin and D. Terzopoulos. Snakes: Active contour models. *Intl. Journal of Computer Vision*, 1:321–331, 1987.
7. D. Lisin, B. Stein, J. Horowitz, G. Whitten, E. Riseman, D. Geman, R. Hicks, and B. Pleet. Statistical and computer vision techniques to support the clinical study of ischemic stroke treatment. Technical Report. UM-CS-2001-019. UMass, 2001.
8. A. Martel, S. Allder, G. Delay, P. Morgan, and A.R. Moody. Measurement of infarct volume in stroke patients using adaptive segmentation of diffusion weighted MR images. *Proc MICCAI Conference*, 1999.
9. J. Sijbers, A.J. Den Dekker, P. Scheunders, and D. Van Dyck. ML estimation of Rician distribution parameters. *IEEE Trans on Medical Imaging*, 17:357–361, 1998.
10. B. Stein. *Signal formation, segmentation, and lesion volume estimation in magnetic resonance imagery*. Ph.D. dissertation, University of Massachusetts, 2001.
11. T. Tosteson, B. Pogue, E. Demidenko, T. McBride, and K. Paulsen. Confidence maps and confidence intervals for near infrared images in breast cancer. *IEEE Trans on Medical Imaging*, 18:1188–1193, 1999.
12. C. Watson, C. Jack Jr., and F. Cendes. Volumetric magnetic resonance imaging. *Archives of Neurology*, 54:1521–1531, 1997.
13. W. Wells, R. Kikinis, W. Grimson, and F. Jolesz. Adaptive segmentation of MRI data. *IEEE Trans on Medical Imaging*, 15:429–442, 1996.
14. J. M. Whitaker and M. Braun. 3D image segmentation using active contours with interslice energy. *Proc APRS/CBT Image Segmentation Workshop*, 47–51, 1996.

Q–MAF Shape Decomposition

Rasmus Larsen, Hrafnkell Eiriksson, and Mikkel B. Stegmann

Informatics and Mathematical Modelling, Technical University of Denmark
Richard Petersens Plads, Building 321, DK-2800 Kgs. Lyngby, Denmark
{rl, he, mbs}@imm.dtu.dk, http://www.imm.dtu.dk/

Abstract. This paper address the problems of generating a low dimensional representation of the shape variation present in a set of shapes represented by a number of landmark points. First, we will present alternatives to the featured Least-Squares Procrustes alignment based on the L_∞-norm and the L_1-norm. Second, we will define a new shape decomposition based on the Maximum Autocorrelation Factor (MAF) analysis, and investigate and compare its properties to the Principal Components Analysis (PCA). It is shown that Molgedey-Schuster algorithm for Independent Component Analysis (ICA) is equivalent to the MAF analysis. The shape MAF analysis utilises the natural order of landmark points along shape contours.

1 Introduction

The Point Distribution Model (PDM) based on PCA of the Active Shape Model (ASM) [1,2] has been succesfully applied to the modelling of the shape of biological objects based on training sets represented by corresponding points. For use for simulation, prediction, or segmentation [3,4,1] a fair number of landmarks are necessary in order to achieve sufficiently good or realistic models. Landmarks are often distributed along outlines or on surfaces equi-distantly or using some other scheme.

Given their representation the objects are aligned wrt. translation, rotation, and scale (e.g. bmo. a Procrustes analysis [5]). Finally, the residual variation is decomposed into latent variables and a low dimensional representation is obtained by retaining only the most important of these. The decomposition of the variation has been based on a number of transformations, most importantly PCA [1,4]. The use of Fourier modes and wavelets are also reported [6,7].

We propose that the choice of landmarks carries important implications for the alignment when using the L_2-norm based Procrustes analysis and thereby for the resulting shape models. In order to lessen this effect we investigate the use of the L_∞-norm and the L_1-norm for aligning the shapes.

Furthermore, we propose an extension to the PCA PDM using the MAF analysis. The MAF by Paul Switzer [8] analysis was originally proposed as an alternative transformation of multivariate spatial imagery to the celebrated PCA transform. In the MAF analysis we seek a transformation that maximises the

W. Niessen and M. Viergever (Eds.): MICCAI 2001, LNCS 2208, pp. 837–844, 2001.
© Springer-Verlag Berlin Heidelberg 2001

autocorrelation between neighbouring observations (e.g. pixels). The basic assumption of the MAF analysis is that the interesting signal exhibits high autocorrelation, whereas the noise exhibits low autocorrelation. By building the additional information of the structure of the observations into the model, application examples (cf. [9,10]) result in a better separation between signal components in one end of the eigenvalue spectrum and noise components in the other end. This is particularly the case when some noise components have higher variance than some signal components. Because the PCA PDM is based on the first say t modes of variation MAF will in this case result in better models than PCA.

The MAF analysis requires estimation of the covariance matrix of the data as well as the covariance matrix of the difference between the original data and a spatially shifted version of the data. Preliminary results are presented in [11]. In an Appendix A we will show that the Molgedey-Schuster algorithm for ICA is equivalent to MAF analysis.

2   Metacarpal Data Set

The proposed methods are illustrated on annotated outlines of 24 metacarpals. The annotations are based on 2-D wrist radiographs, an example is shown in the background of Fig. 3(c). The annotations are prone to errors in the distal and especially in the proximal ends due to the bones being overlaid in the 2-D projection of the radiograph and thus difficult to discern. The annotation variation is therefore point dependent. We believe this to be a common problem to manual annotation. In order to be able to quantify this in the analyses we have simulated two metacarpal datasets. These datasets are generated by first fitting a B-spline to each of the metacarpal outlines after alignment, and second by adding independent Gaussian noise. The noise variance varies smoothly along the contours. It is small along the sides of the metacarpals and high at the ends.

3   Shape Alignment and Choice of Landmarks

Let there be given p training examples for a given shape class, and let each example be represented by a set of n landmark points (x_{ij}, y_{ij}), $i = 1, \ldots, p$ and $j = 1, \ldots, n$. The alignment problem in 2D consists of estimating an average shape, μ, and pose parameters for each shape. Let the pose parameters be scale: $\beta_i \in \mathbb{R}_+$, rotation: $\psi \in [0; 2\pi[$, and translation: $\gamma_i \in \mathbb{R}^2$. Then using a multiple linear regression formulation as described in [5] the alignment problem consists of a minimisation of a vector function

$$
F = \begin{bmatrix} \mu - Z_1\theta_1 \\ \vdots \\ \mu - Z_{p-1}\theta_{p-1} \\ \mu - Z_p \begin{bmatrix} 1\,0\,0\,0 \end{bmatrix}^T \end{bmatrix}, \text{ where } Z_i = \begin{bmatrix} x_{i1} & -y_{i1} & 1 & 0 \\ \vdots & \vdots & \vdots & \vdots \\ x_{in} & -y_{in} & 1 & 0 \\ y_{i1} & x_{i1} & 0 & 1 \\ \vdots & \vdots & \vdots & \vdots \\ y_{in} & x_{in} & 0 & 1 \end{bmatrix},
$$

wrt. $\theta_i = [\beta_i \cos \psi_i, \beta_i \sin \psi_i, \gamma_i^T]^T$. Note, that the average shape is constrained wrt. to size, rotation, and translation by alignment with the last shape. The ith aligned shape is given by $Z_i \theta_i$. Generalised Procrustes analysis is obtained by minimising the L_2-norm of this vector function. We will investigate the use of the L_1-norm and the L_∞-norm.

Different choices of landmarks for a given class of objects will result in differences in alignment. Consider a set of 10 triangles generated by adding i.i.d. Gaussian noise to an equi-lateral prototype. We will represent these triangles by (1) the coordinates of the corner points, and (2) the coordinates of the corner points and 19 points placed equi-distantly on the lower side. The triangles are shown in Fig. 1(a). The L_2 Procrustes alignment results in the aligned shapes shown in Figs. 1(b) and 1(e). Here the dense sampling of the lower side results in more emphasis being put on the alignment of this side In the aligned dataset the variation of the points on the densely sampled side exhibit smaller variation, whereas the third corner point exhibit larger variation than we observed in the 3 point representation. By using the L_∞–norm as shown in Figs. 1(c) and 1(f) we achieve independence of the representation. The L_1–norm (Figs. 1(d) and 1(d)) increases the effect of putting emphasis on densely sampled shape segments. The L_1–norm on the other hand aligns the lower side perfectly, and places all variation on the top point. In effect the top point is regarded (wrongly) as an outlier.

4   Maximum Autocorrelation Factor Analysis

Let the spatial (or temporal) covariance function of a multivariate stochastic variable, Y_k, where k denotes spatial position and Δ a spatial shift, be $\Pi(\Delta) = \text{Cov}\{Y_k, Y_{k+\Delta}\}$. Then by letting the covariance matrix of Y_k be Σ and defining the covariance matrix of the difference proces $\Sigma_\Delta = \text{Cov}\{Y_k - Y_{k+\Delta}\}$, we find

$$\Sigma_\Delta = 2\Sigma - \Pi(\Delta) - \Pi(-\Delta) \qquad (1)$$

Then the autocorrelation in shift Δ of a linear combination of Y_k is

$$\text{Corr}\{w_i^T Y_k, w_i^T Y_{k+\Delta}\} = 1 - \frac{1}{2} \frac{w_i^T \Sigma_\Delta w_i}{w_i^T \Sigma w_i}. \qquad (2)$$

This quantity is maximised by minimisation of the Rayleigh coeeficient in the second term. Therefore, the MAF transform is given by the set of conjugate eigenvectors of Σ_Δ wrt. Σ, $W = [w_1, \ldots, w_m]$, corresponding to the eigenvalues $\kappa_1 \leq \cdots \leq \kappa_m$ [8]. The resulting new variables are ordered so that the first MAF is the linear combination that exhibits maximum autocorrelation. The ith MAF is the linear combination that exhibits the highest autocorrelation subject to it being uncorrelated to the previous MAFs. The autocorrelation of the ith component is $1 - \frac{1}{2}\kappa_i$.

Let the tangent space coordinates of the aligned shapes with the origin placed at the mean shape be the rows of a data matrix, X. The PCA decomposition

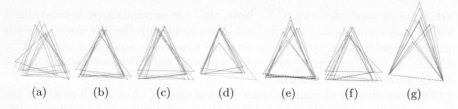

Fig. 1. (a) 10 unaligned triangles, (b-d) alignment based on the L_2, L_∞, and the L_1 norms, respectively. (e-g) aligned as (b-d) but with an additional 19 landmarks included distributed equidistantly on the lower side.

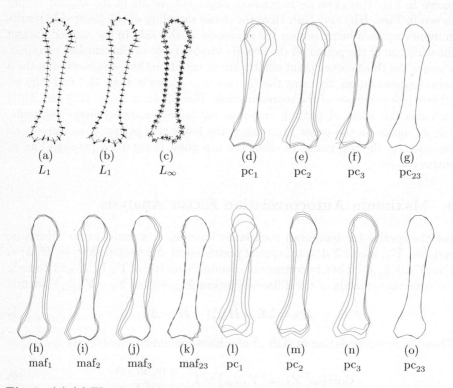

Fig. 2. (a)-(c) The metacarpal dataset aligned and projected into tangent space using the L_1-norm, L_2-norm, and L_∞-norm, respectively. (d)-(g) Principal components of the tangent space coordinates aligned using the L_2-norm. (h)-(k) Maximum autocorrelation factors of the tangent space coordinates aligned using the L_2-norm. (l)-(o) Principal components of the tangent space coordinates aligned using the L_∞-norm. The blue curve is the mean shape the red and green curves correspond to ± 5 standard deviations. The distal end is up and the proximal end is down.

of the dataset can be implemented by extraction of the right singular vectors of a singular value decomposition of X (cf. [12]). These eigen vectors can also be extracted by an eigenvalue decomposition of the symmetric matrix $X^T X$. In statistical terms this is called an R-mode analysis.

Now, let X_Δ be a matrix where the x and the y coordinates of each row of X have been cyclicly rotated Δ shifts to the right. Consider a stochastic variable consisting of the coordinates of a point across the shape training examples, observations of which are given by the columns of X. Then estimators for the covariance matrices in the MAF eigen problem in Eq. (2) are given by[1]

$$\hat{\Sigma} = \tfrac{1}{2n} X X^T \qquad \hat{\Sigma}_\Delta = \tfrac{1}{2n}(X - X_\Delta)(X - X_\Delta)^T \qquad (3)$$

It can be noted that we solve the MAF problem in Q-mode. Therefore we will denote the resulting transform Shape Q-MAF. The modes of variation from the average shape are given by $X^T W$. The low number of MAF components will exhibit variations where neighbouring landmark points deform similarly.

5   Analysis of the Metacarpal Data Set

The alignment of the dataset consisting of 24 annotated metacarpals using three different norms is shown in Figs. 2(a)–2(c). The alignments are computed using an optimisation software described in [13].

In Figs. 2(d)–2(g) and 2(h)–2(k), the variations of four (3 first and the last) principal components and Q-MAFs are shown. It turns out that the Q-MAF modes constitute a decomposition of (localised) spatial frequency along the contour with frequency increasing with mode number. Furthermore, the first two modes are easily interpreted as thickness of the cortical bone/aspect ratio, mode three as bending. In the high order number modes variations composed of neighbouring points deforming in opposite directions are concentrated.

The PCA eigen modes are less easily interpreted and it seems that many low number modes are devoted to descriptions of variations of the proximal end. These are variations that may partially stem from annotation arbitrariness. We would normally expect the most important variation in a dataset like this to be variations in aspect ratio. However, because the L_2–norm alignment has resulted in all shapes having the same length, this effect is transformed into thickness variation, which may lead to mis-interpretations. In Figs. 2(l)–2(o) 4 principal components calculated from the dataset aligned using the L_∞–norm are shown. Where the L_2 assigns high weight to alignment of the ends of the bone (i.e. favoring many small deviations on the sides to larger deviations in the ends), the L_∞ norm is insensitive to the sampling density. We therefore in some sense arrive at a more natural alignment. As we would expect, the first mode is aspect ratio varying from long and slender to short and stocky.

The more general variant of ASM, Active Appearance Models (AAM) [14] is based upon a PCA decomposition of a set of L_2 Procrustes aligned shapes. An AAM also includes a pixel-wise texture model. This is built by sampling object pixel intensities in each training example followed by a PCA. Consequently,

---

[1] The variables are corrected for ensemble means so $\hat{\Sigma}$ is a sums-of-squares matrix.

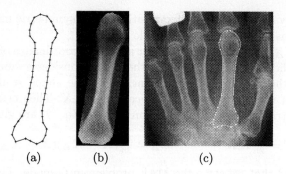

(a)   (b)   (c)

Fig. 3. (a) Metacarpal annotation. (b) Synthesised AAM metacarpal image. (c) AAM segmentation result.

AAMs can synthesise images of the object class in question, see Fig. 3(b). For segmentation purposes the model parameters are adjusted until the synthesised image best matches the unknown image, i.e. under some similarity measure.

Upon the 24 metacarpal shapes and their corresponding radiographs, a leave-one-out performance analysis has been carried out. Texture models consisted of ~10 000 pixels. The AAM was initialised using a search-based initialisation method [15], that failed once in each of the three models due to an overlapping metacarpal-1. These were discarded prior to assessment. An example segmentation is shown in Fig. 3(c). The average point to border distance for the L_1–,L_2–, and L_∞–norm AAMs were $1.06 \pm .25$, $1.04 \pm .21$ and $1.09 \pm .25$ pixels, respectively.

In order to evaluate the use of PCA vs. MAF and of the L_2–norm vs. the L_∞–norm for building shape models we have tested on the simulated dataset. The models are trained on 24 shapes, and validated on another 24 shapes with independent noise. For all numbers of modes included in the models we have computed the weighted root-mean-square (RMS) error between the fitted model, and the shape without noise. The weights used are the inverse standard deviations of the annotation noise. From plots of the RMS values shown in Fig. 4 we see that the optimal model size is approx. 10, and that the performance is very similar for the tested methods. L_∞-norm alignment results in RMS errors that are higher than for L_2–norm alignment.

6   Conclusion

In this paper we have described the use of the infinity norm for shape alignment. This resolves the problem of areas with densely sampled landmarks receiving high weight in the alignment. Furthermore, we have presented the Q-MAF tranformation – a novel method for shape decomposition. In applying L_∞–norm Procrustes alignment as well as the Q-MAF transform to modelling of the outline of metacarpal bones we have achieved better interpretability of the modes of variation at no cost wrt. precision.

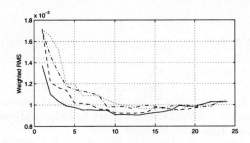

Fig. 4. RMS–error weigthed by the annotation noioc for an independent validation set. Solid: L_2, PCA; dashed: L_2, MAF; dotted: L_∞, PCA; dash-dotted: L_∞, MAF.

Acknowledgments

We thank M.D. Lars Hyldstrup, Dept. of Endocrinology, H:S Hvidovre University Hospital, Copenhagen for providing the metacarpal radiographs, and Hans Henrik Thodberg, Ph.D., Pronosco A/S for annotations. Hans Bruun Nielsen, Ph.D., IMM, DTU is thanked for programming B-spline routines.

A   Equivalence of ICA and MAF

It turns out that Molgedey-Schusters algorithm for performing ICA [16] is the same as the MAF analysis [8]. Assuming the linear mixing model of independent components analysis $X = AS$, where X is the $(P \times N)$ data matrix with each row consituting a signal, S is a matrix of the same form as X containing independent signals in the rows, and A is a linear mixing matrix. Furthermore, let X_Δ and S_Δ be X and S cyclicly shifted Δ steps rowwise. Then the solution is found by forming

$$Q = \frac{1}{2}\left[X_\Delta X^T + X X_\Delta^T\right](XX^T)^{-1} = A\left[\frac{1}{2}(S_\Delta S^T + S S_\Delta^T)(SS^T)^{-1}\right]A^{-1} \quad (4)$$

Due to the independence of the source signals the latter bracketed parenthesis is diagonal. Therefore the mixing matrix can be determined by an eigenvalue decomposition of the matrix Q, and the source signals up to a scale factor are estimated by $S = A^{-1}X$. Using Eq. (3) we find

$$Q = \frac{1}{2}[2\Sigma - \Sigma_\Delta]\Sigma^{-1} = \left[I - \frac{1}{2}\Sigma_\Delta\Sigma^{-1}\right]$$

The unity matrix I has no effect on the eigenvectors, so A simply consists of the conjugate eigenvectors of Σ_Δ wrt. Σ, i.e. the MAF problem given in Eq. (2).

It is easily shown that the MAF transform is invariant to affine transformations. Therefore we may execute a prewhitening beforehand, thus obtaining $\Sigma = I$. Then Q becomes symmetric yielding $A^{-1} = A^T$, and the MAF factors become $A^T X_{\text{prewhitened}}$, i.e. the independent components.

844   R. Larsen, H. Eiriksson, and M.B. Stegmann

References

1. T. F. Cootes, C. J. Taylor, D. H. Cooper, and J. Graham, "Active shape models –
   their training and application," *Computer Vision, Graphics and Image Processing*,
   vol. 61, no. 1, pp. 38–59, Jan. 1995.
2. A. D. Brett and C. J. Taylor, "Construction of 3D shape models of femoral articular
   cartilage using harmonic maps," in *Medical Image Computing and Computer-
   Assisted Intervention - MICCAI 2000*, Scott L. Delp, Anthony M. DiGioia, and
   Branislav Jaramaz, Eds. 2000, Springer.
3. D. C. Hogg, N. Johnson, R. Morris, D. Buesching, and A. Galata, "Visual modes
   of interaction," in *2nd International Workshop on Cooperative Distributed Vision*,
   Kyoto, Japan, 1998.
4. P. R. Andresen, F.. L. Bookstein, K. Conradsen, B. K. Ersbøll, J. L. Marsh, and
   S. Kreiborg, "Surface-bounded growth modeling applied to human mandibles,"
   IEEE Transactions on Medical Imaging, vol. 19, no. 11, Nov. 2000, 1053–1063.
5. C. Goodall, "Procrustes methods in the statistical analysis of shape," *Journal of
   the Royal Statistical Society, Series B*, vol. 53, no. 2, pp. 285–339, 1991.
6. L. H. Staib and J. S. Duncan, "Boundary finding with parametrically deformable
   models," *IEEE Transactions on Pattern Analysis and Machine Intelligence*, vol.
   14, no. 11, pp. 1061–1075, 1992.
7. A. Neuman and C. Lorenz, "Statistical shape model based segmentation of medical
   images," *Computerized Medical Imaging and Graphics*, vol. 22, pp. 133–143, 1998.
8. Paul Switzer, "Min/max autocorrelation factors for multivariate spatial imagery,"
   in *Computer Science and Statistics*, L. Billard, Ed. 1985, pp. 13–16, Elsevier Science
   Publishers B.V. (North Holland).
9. A. A. Green, M. Berman, P. Switzer, and M. D. Craig, "A transformation for
   ordering multispectral data in terms of image quality with implications for noise
   removal," *IEEE Transactions on Geoscience and Remote Sensing*, vol. 26, no. 1,
   pp. 65–74, Jan. 1988.
10. A. A. Nielsen and R. Larsen, "Restoration of GERIS data using the maximum noise
    fractions transform," in *Proceedings of the First International Airborne Remote
    Sensing Conference and Exhibition*, Strasbourg, France, 1994, vol. 2, pp. 557–568.
11. R. Larsen, "Shape modelling using maximum autocorrelation factors," in *Proceed-
    ings of the Scandinavian Image Analysis Conference, SCIA'01, Bergen, Norway,
    11-14 June 2001*, 2001, 98–103.
12. R. M. Johnson, "On a theorem stated by Eckart and Young," *Psychometrika*, vol.
    28, pp. 259–263, 1963.
13. P. C. Hansen and O. Tingleff, "Robust subroutines for non-linear optimization,"
    Tech. Rep. NI-90-06, Institute for Numerical Analysis, Technical University of Den-
    mark, 1990, 54 pp.
14. T. F. Cootes, G. J. Edwards, and C. J. Taylor, "Active appearance models,"
    in *Proceedings of the European Conf. On Computer Vision*. 1998, pp. 484–498,
    Springer.
15. M. B. Stegmann, R. Fisker, and B. K. Ersbøll, "Extending and applying active
    appearance models for automated, high precision segmentation in different im-
    age modalities," in *Proceedings of the Scandinavian Image Analysis Conference,
    SCIA'01, Bergen, Norway, 11-14 June 2001*, 2001, 90–97.
16. L. Molgedey and H. G. Schuster, "Separation of a mixture of independent signals
    using time delayed correlations," *Physical Review Letters*, vol. 72, no. 23, pp.
    3634–3637, 1994.

Vessel Axis Determination Using Wave Front Propagation Analysis

O. Wink[1]*, W.J. Niessen[1], B. Verdonck[2] and M.A. Viergever[1]

[1] Image Sciences Institute, Room E 01.334, University Medical Center Utrecht,
Heidelberglaan 100, 3584 CX Utrecht, The Netherlands,
{onno,wiro,max}@isi.uu.nl
[2] EasyVision Advanced Development, Philips Medical Systems,
Postbus 10000, Best, The Netherlands
bert.verdonck@best.ms.philips.com

Abstract. A method is presented that aims at finding the central vessel axis in two and three dimensional angiographic images based on a single user defined point. After the vessels in the image are enhanced using a special purpose filter, the operator is asked to point out the vessel of interest. Subsequently, a wave front propagation is started based on the response of the filter. By analyzing the evolution of the wave front, points are retrieved that are very likely to be part of the vessel of interest. These points can either be combined to form a connected structure or to retrieve the minimum cost path to the user defined point. In this paper examples of this approach are given that illustrate the performance of this method in different types of images and in situations where there is no or hardly any image evidence of the vessel at hand.

1 Introduction

A vast number of approaches have been proposed to facilitate the diagnosis of vessel segments requiring a different types of user interaction and empirical parameter settings. Iterative tracking or region growing procedures are frequently used, but these experience difficulties in the presence of severely stenoted regions or imaging artifacts where there is hardly any image evidence of the vessel to guide the algorithm. Figure 1a illustrates the use of an iterative approach, where the direction of the tracked axis depends merely on local information.

Several approaches have emerged that are based on the determination of a minimum cost path, which can handle these kind of situations, *e.g.* [1, 2, 3, 4, 5, 6]. In these approaches a wave front is propagated from a source node until a target node is reached, thus forming a path of minimum cost. In this paper an approach is suggested to determine the vessel axis based on the source node alone, by analyzing the propagation of the wave front. It is assumed that the nodes that make up the vessel are visited prior to its non-vessel neighbours in the propagation of the front. These nodes are used to form the central vessel axis which can serve as input in a subsequential visualization and quantification procedure. In Section 2 the method will be described in more detail.

---

* This work is funded by Philips Medical Systems, Best, The Netherlands.

W. Niessen and M. Viergever (Eds.): MICCAI 2001, LNCS 2208, pp. 845–853, 2001.

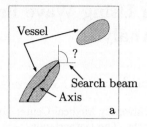 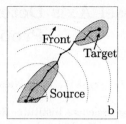

Fig. 1. Situation where an iterative line tracker, based on local information does not know how to proceed in case of a severe stenosis (**a**). The use of wave propagation to find a minimum cost path between a source and a target node that succeeds in determining an estimate of the vessel axis (**b**).

2   Description of the Method

In Fig. 2, different phases of the method are shown. First (section 2.1) tubular structures are enhanced in the image using a special-purpose multi-scale filter (Fig. 2b). The output of this filter is used to propagate the waves of minimum cumulative costs (section 2.2) from a user defined starting position. By analyzing the propagation of the wave front, points are selected that are very likely to be part of the vessel (section 2.3).

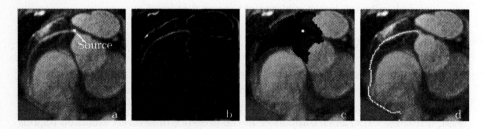

Fig. 2. A part of a slice in a MRA image containing the right coronary artery (RCA) and the user provided source point (**a**). The result of the eigenvalue filter (**b**). An instance of the wave front that is propagated (**c**). The "pioneer" nodes obtained (**d**).

Based on these "pioneer" nodes an estimate of the central vessel axis can be obtained (section 2.6).

2.1   Vessel Enhancement

First, the original data is filtered with a special-purpose multi-scale filter based on the eigenvalue analysis of the Hessian matrix [7, 8, 9]. This filter is designed to highlight tubular structures in the image and is capable of coping with anisotropic voxels and vessels with varying width. The idea behind the eigen-value analysis of the Hessian is to extract the principal directions in which the local second order structure of the image can be decomposed. Since this directly gives the direction of smallest curvature (along the vessel), application of several filters in multiple orientations is avoided. The latter approach is computationally more expensive and requires a discretization of the orientation space.

The second order derivative of a Gaussian used to construct the Hessian can be represented as a probe kernel that measures the contrast between the regions inside and outside the range $(-\sigma, \sigma)$ in the direction of the derivative (see the left frame of Fig. 3). The anisotropy of the dataset is handled by adjusting the

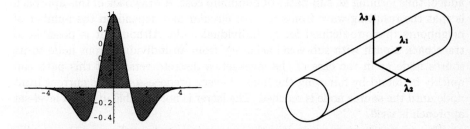

Fig. 3. Second order derivative of a Gaussian (inverse "Mexican Hat") at scale $\sigma = 1$ (left) and the orientation of the three eigenvectors of the Hessian matrix when the corresponding eigenvalues are sorted in increasing magnitude (right).

parameter vector σ in each direction. For a tubular structure, the eigenvalues, when sorted in increasing magnitude, will obey the following rules:

$$|\lambda_1| \approx 0 \tag{1}$$
$$|\lambda_1| \ll |\lambda_2| \tag{2}$$
$$\lambda_2 \approx \lambda_3 \tag{3}$$

The corresponding eigenvectors are given in the right frame of Fig. 3. The eigen-vector in the direction of the vessel corresponds to the smallest eigenvalue λ_1, while the eigenvectors that correspond to the larger eigenvalues λ_2 and λ_3, span a plane orthogonal to the vessel. Based on these observations, Lorenz *et al.* [9] proposed a filter $R(\sigma)$:

$$\mathcal{R}(\sigma) = \begin{cases} 0 & \text{if } \lambda_2 > 0 \text{ or } \lambda_3 > 0, \\ |\lambda_2 + \lambda_3| \end{cases} \tag{4}$$

The response of the filter is expected to be maximum at a scale that approximates the radius of the vessel. The response at different scales can be combined by taking the maximum response over a range of scales. In Fig. 2b an example is given of the output of the multi-scale filter.

2.2   Wave Front Propagation

There are two main approaches that can be taken to simulate the propagation of a wave front with minimum cumulative costs over a discrete grid *viz.* level-sets and graph-search. In the level-set approach [6] a path from one of the front nodes to the source node is determined using a backtracking procedure resulting in a sub-voxel accurate path with a true Euclidean measure. In case of the graph-search [10], the image is treated as a grid of nodes, where every node voxel is connected to its direct neighbours. The cost of traveling from a node n to its neighbour n' is given by the intensity of the voxel corresponding with n'. In every iteration the neighbours of the front node having the least cumulative costs are added, thus forming all sub-paths of minimum cost. A drawback of this approach is that the resulting wave fronts are not circular and depend on the number of neighbours that are defined for an individual node. Although it is possible to trace back a path with sub-voxel accuracy from an individual front node to its source node as in the case of the level-set, a discrete version of this path can quickly be found by following the links of every predecessor of the current front node until the source node is reached. The latter is not possible in case a level-set approach is used.

The approach as suggested in this paper is not depending on the specific method used as long as for every front node, a path to its origin can be retrieved. In the remainder of the paper the graph-search method is used.

2.3   Propagation Analysis

From Fig. 2c it can be observed that the wave front is stretched in the direction of the vessel. In principle, the nodes in the vessels will be visited before its surrounding non-vessel nodes. This phenomenon can be used to find a path based on a single initialization , or to extrapolate a path beyond the user defined points as will be discussed in the next section. During the evolution of the front it can be monitored which nodes are the first to be expanded at a given distance from its source. The distance is defined as the length of the path from the front node to its source. These "pioneer" nodes (see Fig. 2d) are likely to be positioned in the vessel if the tortuosity of the vessel segment is not too high and the discriminative power of the filter is large. Figure 4 shows an example where the proposed method is applied on an artificially created image where a "stenosis" is introduced. From the source node as depicted in 4a, the wave front is propagated based on the response of the filter (see Fig. 4b). If no maximum is set to the length of the minimum cost paths, every node in the image will contain the minimum costs that are needed to arrive at this node starting from the source node (see Fig. 4c). It can be appreciated that in between two adjacent vessel segments the cumulative cost are highest. As a result the pioneer nodes are first to be found inside the vessel and eventually able to overcome the loss of local information caused by the stenosis (see Fig. 4d) whereas a classical snake or connected structure will probably fail to bridge the gap.

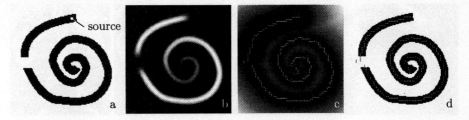

Fig. 4. Example of applying the method to an artificial image (128 x 128 pixels) where a "stenosis" is created and a source node is defined (**a**). The output of the eigenvalue-filter at the scale of 10 pixels(**b**). The image where every node contains the cost of the path back to the source node and where the "pioneer" nodes are overlayed (**c**). The ability of the method to overcome the stenoted region is clearly visible when the "pioneer" nodes are displayed at their corresponding position (**d**).

2.4 Initialization

If the source node is positioned in the middle of a vessel, the wave front will propagate in either direction of the vessel. As a result, the "pioneer" nodes will generally not be as close to each other as in the example of Fig. 4d. In this section three approaches are suggested which can be used to reduce this effect. In all three approaches two independent *bounded* search processes are started where the acceptance of a "pioneer" node depends on the relative position to its source node.

1. Start one bounded search process in the direction of the eigenvector corresponding to the lowest absolute eigenvector λ_1 which is assumed to point in the direction of the vessel (see right frame of Fig. 3). Start a second bounded search process in the opposite direction. An example is given in Fig. 5a.
2. Start a search process for only a limited number of iterations. Find the "pioneer" node that corresponds to the largest path from the source node and use this to determine the direction of the two bounded search processes.
3. Let the user provide at least one additional node inside the vessel of interest, and use this to determine the direction of the two bounded search processes (see Fig. 5b). A traditional minimum cost path approach can be used to obtain the axis between the user provided points.

In all cases the search area can be further restricted by defining an additional angle α (see Fig. 5b). In Fig. 5c and Fig. 5d the second initialization method is used.

2.5 Termination

Since the vessels generally make up only a small portion of the scanned volume, it is very time consuming to wait until all the voxels in the image (or in the allowed

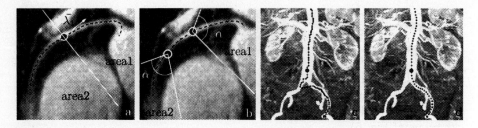

Fig. 5. Examples of bounded wave front propagation analysis. The source nodes are given by the black dots. Two areas are defined where the "pioneer" nodes of a single search process are allowed to be located. This area is based on the direction of the eigenvector $\bar{\lambda}_1$ in **a** and on user provided points in **b**. In case of the three dimensional Contrast Enhanced MRA of the abdomen (**c**) the image is filtered at a wide range of scales. The "pioneer" nodes are connected and subsequently resampled to create a smooth curve which is displayed on a MIP of the original image. It is shown that the "pioneer" nodes jump from the right iliac artery to the left, a situation which can solved by computing the minimum cost paths from the last "pioneer" nodes to the source node (**d**). Here the entire aorto-iliac trajectory has been outlined using a single initialization point.

areas) have been visited by the wave front. Moreover, the distances between the "pioneer" nodes will start to increase with the growing distance from its source, reducing its predictive value. It may therefore be advantageous to define one or more end-conditions which will terminate the propagation of the wave front. The most obvious end condition is to limit the maximum distance of the path to the "pioneer" nodes. Other options are *e.g.* to set a minimum to the required filter response, to stop the search process until the "pioneer" nodes have reached a maximum cumulative cost or the border of the image has been reached.

2.6   "Pioneer" Nodes or Minimum Cost Path

After the termination of the search process a list of "pioneer" nodes are retrieved. Each of these pioneer node are likely to be located in the vessel of interest. The pioneer nodes can be connected or interpolated to estimate the central vessel axis although they are not necessarily connected (see Fig. 5c). Another option is to use a specific "pioneer" node as an end point and start a traditional minimum cost path approach to estimate the central vessel axis (see Fig. 5d). If this "pioneer" node is very likely to be positioned in the vessel, the minimum cost path approach is the preferred method since it is guaranteed to result in a connected path which is able to cope with a stenoted region.

3   Evaluation

In this section the performance of the automated method using a 26-neighbour-hood is compared with the performance of two observers in a task to find the central coronary axis from three-dimensional MRA datasets. The data is filtered with the eigenvalue filter (see Eq. 4) at a scale of 1.0 mm. For every dataset the central coronary axis is manually determined starting from the trunk of the ascending aorta (t). A total of 14 Right Coronary Arteries (RCA) are manually delineated. The process is repeated after two weeks. The manually drawn paths are averaged to form a golden standard g for every dataset. This path is subsequently resampled every milimetre to form a set of sample nodes n (see also the left frame of Fig. 6). For every combination between the origin (t) and a sam-

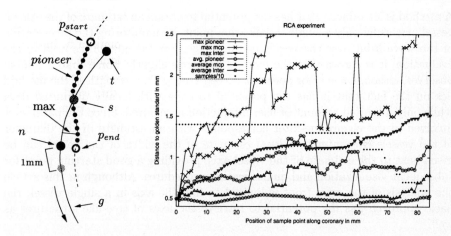

Fig. 6. Computing the maximum distance between a set of pioneer nodes originating from the source node s halfway between the trunk of the ascending aorta t and a sample node n (left frame). The results of the evaluation (right frame).

ple node n, a source node s is defined which is located halfway along the path between t and n. From this source a search process is started until 10 "pioneer" nodes are found. Based on the most distant "pioneer" node the orientation of the vessel is estimated and two independent bounded search processes are started with an angle α of 180 degrees. The "pioneer" nodes are connected into a single axis. The subset of this axis between the "pioneer" nodes p_{start} and p_{end} that are closest to the nodes t and n make up the *pioneer* axis. Based on p_{start}, the source node s and p_{end}, a minimum cost path *mcp* is subsequently computed. The nodes in the axes *pioneer* and *mcp* are used to compute the maximum -and average distance to the golden standard g. The average of these measurements over all the datasets are displayed in the right frame of Fig. 6. The differences between the two observers is given as a reference.

From the right frame of Fig. 6 it can be observed that the minimum cost path based on the last "pioneer" nodes performs consistently better than the collection of "pioneer" nodes itself. However the distances between the two observers is consistently lower than that of the automated approaches. The average distance between *mcp* and the golden standard does not exceed 0.93 mm, whereas the average in plane resolution is 0.71 mm., and the distances between the slices is 1.5 mm. The reason for the sudden increase of the error in the automated methods is due to the fact that in some datasets a structure close to the RCA has a higher filter output. The "pioneer" nodes are attracted to this other vessel which results in a larger error, especially if the other vessel is not running parallel to the coronary axis.

4 Discussion and Conclusions

A method is introduced that has the potential to obtain an estimate of the central vessel axis using only a single intialization point, by monitoring the propagation of the wave front over the voxels in the image. For the coronaries used in the evaluation, it is shown that the method performs slightly worse than a human observer, although the error does not exceed 1 mm. The strength of the method lies on the fact that it has the potential to cope with locally disrupted data while only a limited amount of user interaction is required. Since the parameter involved in the eigenvalue-filter corresponds with an estimate of the diameter of the vessels encountered, a local estimate of the width of the vessel can be given next to the estimate of the vessel axis, providing a good starting point for subsequent visualization and quantification procedures. Although in this article the analysis of the wave front is limited to find the axis in a single vessel, the basic approach has the potential to retrieve the axes of tree-like structures as well.

References

[1] T. Y. Law and P. A. Heng, "Automatic centerline extraction for 3D virtual bronchoscopy," in *Proc. Medical Image Computing and Computer-Assisted Intervention.* 2000, pp. 786–795, Springer-Verlag.

[2] B. B. Avants and J. P. Williams, "An adaptive minimal path generation technique for vessel tracking in CTA/CE-MRA volume image," in *Proc. Medical Image Computing and Computer-Assisted Intervention.* 2000, pp. 707–715, Springer-Verlag.

[3] O. Wink, W. J. Niessen, and M. A. Viergever, "Minimum cost path determination using a simple heuristic function," in *Proc. International Conference on Pattern Recognition - 4*, Barcelona, 2000, pp. 1010–1013, IEEE Computer Society.

[4] A. X. Falcão, J. K. Udupa, and F. K. Miyazawa, "An ultra-fast user-steered image segmentation paradigm: Live wire on the fly," *IEEE Transactions on Medical Imaging*, vol. 19, no. 1, pp. 946–956, 2000.

[5] T. Deschamps, J. M. Létang, B. Verdonck, and L. D. Cohen, "Automatic construction of minimal pahts in 3D images: An application to virtual endoscopy," in *Proc. Computer Assisted Radiology and Surgery,.* 1999, pp. 151–155, Elsevier Publishers, Amsterdam.

[6] J. A. Sethian, *Level Set Methods and Fast Marching Methods*, Cambridge University Press, second edition, 1999.

[7] A. F. Frangi, W. J. Niessen, K. L. Vincken, and M. A. Viergever, "Vessel enhancement filtering," in *Proc. Medical Image Computing and Computer-Assisted Intervention.* 1998, pp. 130–137, Springer-Verlag.

[8] Y. Sato *et. al*, "Three-dimensional multi-scale line filter for segmentation and visualization of curvilinear structures in medical images," *Medical Image Analysis*, vol. 2, no. 2, pp. 143–168, 1998.

[9] C. Lorenz, I. C Carlsen, T. M. Buzug, C. Fassnacht, and J. Weese, "Multi-scale line segmentation with automatic estimation of width, contrast and tangential direction in 2D and 3D medical images," in *Proc. CVRMed and MRCAS*, 1997, number 1205 in Lecture Notes in Computer Science, pp. 233–242.

[10] E. Dijkstra, "A note on two problems in connexion with graphs," *Numerische Mathematic*, vol. 1, pp. 269–271, 1959.

Size Independent Active Contour Model for Blood Vessel Lumen Quantification in High-Resolution Magnetic Resonance Images

Catherine Desbleds-Mansard[1], Alfred Anwander[1], Linda Chaabane[2],
Maciej Orkisz[1], Bruno Neyran[1], Philippe C. Douek[1], Isabelle E. Magnin[1]

[1]CREATIS, CNRS Research Unit (UMR 5515) affiliated to INSERM, Lyon, France
[2]Laboratory RMN, CNRS Research Unit (UMR 5012), Lyon, France
Correspondence address: CREATIS, INSA de Lyon, bât. Blaise Pascal,
7 rue J. Capelle, 69621 Villeurbanne cedex, France
catherine.mansard@creatis.insa-lyon.fr

Abstract. Atherosclerosis is the most common cause of myocardial infarction. To study the atherosclerotic plaque in high resolution Magnetic Resonance images we developed a software tool called ATHER. An active contour model is used for segmentation and quantification of blood vessel lumen. Its implementation, based on a dynamic scaling process, presents two interesting features: 1) independence of the influence of the inflating force from the current size of the contour, 2) strong reduction of the computational cost. Therefore the contour converges very quickly even when initialized by a single point. This paper reports a validation of the model in *ex vivo* vascular images from Watanabe heritable hyperlipidaemic rabbits. Results of automatic quantification were compared to measurements performed by experts. Average difference of the area measurements between ATHER and the experts was equal to the inter-observer variability, but intra-variability of the automatic measurements was significantly smaller than the intra-observer variability.

1   Introduction

Atherosclerosis is the most common cause of myocardial infarction and stroke. To prevent these acute accidents due to severe lumen obstruction and/or to the atherosclerotic plaque rupture, there is a growing number of investigations dealing with the plaque identification, evolution and characterization both in humans and in animal models [1-5]. In particular, Watanabe heritable hyperlipidaemic (WHHL) rabbit was described as a well suited model for the atherosclerosis. The studies of the plaque evolution require quantification of the vascular lumen and of the plaque in numerous images. This tedious task needs to be computer-assisted [6]. To do this, one can use a general-purpose software such as Osiris (University Hospital Geneva Switzerland). However, a specific application-tailored software is expected to provide better ergonomics and more precise results. The objective of the hereafter presented work was to realize such a software tool with a user-friendly graphical interface. It will be hereafter referred to as ATHER.

W. Niessen and M. Viergever (Eds.): MICCAI 2001, LNCS 2208, pp. 854-861, 2001.
© Springer-Verlag Berlin Heidelberg 2001

The quantification of the vascular lumen is based on an automatic extraction of its boundary. It is well known that simple edge detection often leads to discontinuous lines with gaps and protrusions, because of noise and of contrast variations, especially in the medical images context. In this context, techniques based on minimum-cost path search [7], on deformable models [8] or on deformable templates [9] are usually applied to extract smooth closed boundaries as expected in most cases, in particular in the case of the vascular lumen. A deformable model (curve, surface ...) is defined by the expected shape properties, by some "mechanical" properties (flexibility, elasticity) and by forces which gradually deform it to make it coincide with the actual boundaries in the image. External forces attract the initial form towards the points likely to belong to a boundary (*e.g.* maximum of the gradient), while internal forces attract it towards the expected reference shape. Many improvements of the very first implementation of planar deformable models, named active contours or snakes [10], were proposed in order to make the result initialization-independent.

Our original implementation, called Dynamic Active Contour (DAC), needs a single initialization point inside the lumen [11] and can propagate on a whole sequence of images representing contiguous vascular cross-sections. This paper describes a validation of its application to vascular lumen quantification in *ex vivo* high resolution magnetic resonance (MR) images from WHHL rabbits. Preliminary results of this validation were presented in [12]. The sequel of the paper will be organized as follows: short description of the animals and of the image acquisition protocol, presentation of the DAC model, summary of the characteristics of the graphical interface, explanation of the validation method and discussion of the obtained results.

2   Animals and Images

Six WHHL rabbits have been included in the entire study: three homozygous and three heterozygous, two of which had a lipid-rich diet. First, two kinds of *in vivo* MR images were acquired: one set of images focused on the vascular wall, the other one used a contrast agent in order to highlight the vessel lumen. Then the animals were sacrificed at age between 13 and 18 months. The entire aorta, heart and kidneys were removed after fixation under perfusion with paraformaldehyde. *In vitro* images of arteries thus obtained were used for the purpose of our validation.

The *in vitro* high resolution MR imaging was performed with a 2 T horizontal Oxford magnet and a SMIS console. The specimens were placed in a half-birdcage RF coil of 25 mm diameter working at 85.13 MHz. High resolution axial images of the thoracic and abdominal aorta were taken using a multi-slice 2D spin-echo sequence with a 256×128 matrix. The slice thickness was 1-0.8 mm and the pixel size was from 58 to 78 μm. T_1 and T_2 weighted images were obtained with TR/TE = 600/21 ms and 1800/50 ms respectively. Six territories of exploration have been studied from the aortic arch down to the iliac bifurcation. The acquired images were organized into series of contiguous slices, one series per territory.

3   Dynamic Active Contour Model

A planar closed active contour (snake) is approximated by a set of points defined in terms of the x and y coordinates, which are parameterized by i, a curvilinear parameter, and k a time parameter:

$$\mathbf{v}(i,k)=(x(i,k),y(i,k))^T.$$ (1)

These points are vertices of a polygon which alters its shape and size in an iterative process while seeking the state corresponding to an energy minimum. The energy of the snake is made up of internal and external energy terms :

$$E(\mathbf{v})=E_{int}(\mathbf{v})+E_{ext}(\mathbf{v}).$$ (2)

The internal energy depends solely on the shape of the contour and controls the elasticity and flexibility of the snake. It is computed from the first and second derivatives of the curve defined by the vertices. This energy prevents irregular deformations of the contour. The external energy depends on the image intensity values on the vertices. A balloon pressure [13] is added to the external energy so as to inflate the contour outwards. Differential calculus minimizes the two energy terms and aligns the regularized snake with boundaries in the image. The deformation in the plane is done in discrete time steps according to the following evolution equation:

$$\mathbf{v}(i,k)=[\gamma\mathbf{I}+\mathbf{A}]^{-1}[\gamma\mathbf{v}(i,(k-1))+F_{ext}(\mathbf{v}(i,(k-1)))].$$ (3)

The matrix $\mathbf{A}$ represents a discretized formulation of the internal energy. The derivatives of the contour are computed by finite differences using a curvilinear sampling distance h. The damping parameter γ controls the snake deformation magnitude per iteration.

In the conventional active contour implementation, after deformation, the active contour changes its size and shape, and the initial discretization step h does not correspond to the real distance between the snake points. Numerical computations of the derivatives of the contour are sensitive to the sampling distance and the evolution equation is only valid if the snake points are equally distanced and the step h is unchanged. If the actual distance between the points differs from the initial step h, the internal energy is mis-evaluated and the growth of the snake stops before the boundary is reached. Hence, in the usual implementations, the snake has to be re-sampled and a new model with a different sampling distance and a different number of snake points has to be set. This requires the inversion of the system matrix $[\gamma\mathbf{I}+\mathbf{A}]^{-1}$, which is a time-consuming task.

In our Dynamic Active Contour model, instead of the rediscretization of the model, the actual size of the contour is scaled to a reference size. The model is set once with a reference size fixed and with a contour length equal to the number of points (sampling distance $h=1$). The same model is used at each iteration step. The actual snake is scaled to this normalized size:

$$\mathbf{v}'(i,(k-1))=\mathbf{v}(i,(k-1))/h_{k-1},$$ (4)

where h_{k-1} is the sampling distance of the actual contour. This only modifies the coordinates of the snake points, but each point keeps the external-force vector calculated before the scaling. The reference model is used to compute the regularized deformation vector according to this external force vector. This deformation vector

$$\Delta \mathbf{v}'(i,k) = \mathbf{v}'(i,k) - \mathbf{v}'(i,(k-1)) \tag{5}$$

is directly applied on the non-scaled snake to compute the new contour:

$$\mathbf{v}(i,k) = \mathbf{v}(i,(k-1)) + \Delta \mathbf{v}'(i,k). \tag{6}$$

Since the deformation modifies the snake's shape, the distances between the vertices are unequal. The fixed number of snake points is redistributed on the polygonal contour. The perimeter of the polygon is computed and divided by the number of points. This new distribution step is applied to the polygon by sampling the outline at fixed distances h_k and by defining new vertices for the next iteration. The deformation is scale-independent, and the final outline is independent from the initialization. The dynamic scaling allows an initialization with a small circle of the size of only one pixel. Regular sampling distributes a sufficient number of N snake-points on the circle. The number N is about the length of the final contour.

The deformation speed of the dynamic active contour does not change with the size of the contour and can be fixed to a speed of one pixel per iteration by the damping parameter γ. The scaling and redistribution of the snake-points are computationally very fast and simple tasks and do not slow down the snake deformation speed. The snake does not need to be reinitialized with a varying number of points. This is a big advantage compared to traditional snake implementations which need a setup of the system matrix at each iteration.

4   Graphical Interface : ATHER

ATHER is our custom software for atherosclerosis MR image visualization and quantification. It displays one entire image series at a time. Each slice can be zoomed, its histogram can be interactively stretched and signal to noise ratio as well as the standard deviation of noise can be measured in user-selected regions. Vessel lumen contours can both be manually drawn and automatically extracted, with a possibility of interactive refinement if necessary. The automatic contour extraction needs no parameter tuning, since the parameters of the DAC model have been experimentally optimized for this application. Hence, the only necessary user interaction is a double-click in the vessel lumen in the selected slice. For further speed-up, the contour extraction can be performed in the entire series. The extracted contour's gravity center become the starting point for the contour extraction in the next slice. This method is applicable because each series represents a short, approximately straight, portion of the aorta (fig. 1a). Quantitative results (area, perimeter and diameter) are displayed and stored in a computer file. ATHER also features such additional functionalities as automatic extraction of the external contour of the vessel wall, as well as semi-automatic plaque quantification (fig 1b). They will not be detailed in this paper, because their validation is still ongoing.

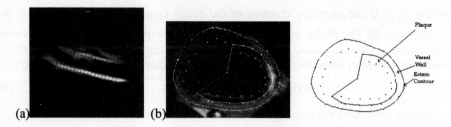

Fig. 1. Longitudinal section of a rabbit artery with lines showing the positions of cross sections from the corresponding series (a). Cross-section with internal and external contours of the vessel wall superimposed, and plaque delineated (b)

5   Measurement Protocol

Images from a subset of three amongst six rabbits were used for the purpose of validation of the DAC model. For these rabbits, expert-done measurements of the lumen area were already available for 121 slices. Indeed, these contours have been traced six months earlier, by an expert using Osiris software (University Hospital Geneva Swizterland). Let us note that Osiris also offers the possibility of an automatic contour extraction. However, it needs to be done in each slice separately. In practice, the expert used this automatic extraction and stored the result when, in her opinion, the contour perfectly fit the boundary. Otherwise she drew it manually. Only the area measurements have been stored, while the contour points themselves were lost.

Therefore, the first quantitative validation was based on area measurements. The areas of the contours traced by the expert were compared with the areas of the contours automatically extracted by ATHER in all the 121 slices. Average absolute difference was calculated as:

$$\mu = \underset{i}{\text{mean}} \left(\frac{\left| Area(i)_{ATHER} - Area(i)_{EXPERT} \right|}{Area(i)_{EXPERT}} \right) * 100 \cdot \tag{7}$$

ATHER's variability was calculated according to a similar formula, after applying the automatic contour extraction twice to all the data set. The users were authorized to change the initialization point in single image within a series but not to modify the resulting contours. Then, in order to quantify the operator-dependence of the non-automatic measurements, the same expert re-traced the contours in 45 slices (5 series) and a second expert also traced them twice in the same 45 slices. For the first expert the time interval between two measurements was six months, while for the second one it was one month and half.

For a qualitative comparison between ATHER and the experts, contours' forms were visually inspected. However, area measurements combined with qualitative appreciation might appear relatively forgiving. Hence the points of the contours traced by the second expert were stored and distances between these contours and the automatically extracted contours were measured. Moreover, these measurement sessions were an occasion to evaluate the speed-up achieved by our software compared to fully manual and semi-automatic procedure using Osiris.

6   Results

The contours automatically extracted using the DAC model fit very well the actual vessel lumen boundaries (fig. 2). This qualitative result agrees with the quantitative comparisons. Average absolute difference between the first expert's measurements of area and ATHER measurements, was equal to 4% for the entire set of data. It is to be compared with the variability of the expert-performed measurements. The experts' intra-observer variability respectively was 6,4% and 2,3%. The high value for the first expert can be explained by a longer time interval between the two measurements and by the fact that they were done on different screens. The inter-observer variability was as large as 4%. It was calculated using a formula similar to (7), where $Area(i)_{ATHER}$ was replaced by the average of the two values measured by one expert for the slice i. Similarly, $Area(i)_{EXPERT}$ in the numerator was replaced by the average of the two values measured by the other expert, while in the denominator it was replaced by the average of both experts' measurements. The variability of ATHER's measurements was not more than 1,2%. When the images are of good quality, the automatic contour gives very good results and is very insensitive to the position of the initialization point. In poor quality images, the initialization point may have more importance.

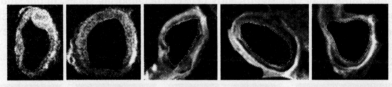

Fig. 2. Examples of results obtained with the DAC model in different territories. Note the variable quality (signal to noise ratio) of the images.

However, the maximum difference between ATHER and the first expert was as large as 19%. Such large errors occurred in a few images of particularly poor quality (high level of noise) and in the case of images with residual quantities of formol in the vessel lumen. In the latter case, even an experienced human eye can hardly distinguish the boundary between these residues and the vessel wall. Hence the second expert judged these images not exploitable and they were not included in the subset of 45 slices for which the distance between the hand-made and automatically detected contours was also measured. For this subset, the maximum distance was less than 2 pixels (fig. 3) and the average distance varied from 1/3 to 1/2 pixel according to the spatial resolution of the images.

Lastly, let us underline the time savings obtained with ATHER. The expert used approximately 2 hours to obtain the measurements for 45 slices, with her usual operating mode. All the operations, from image file opening to 3D surface rendering of the contours automatically extracted by ATHER, took 30 seconds per series on the same PC. Adding visual inspection of each result and correction of the starting point in one series, all the data subset was analyzed within less than 15 minutes.

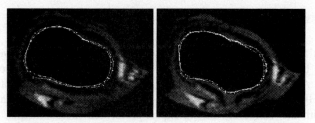

Fig. 3. Maximum distance between the contours drawn by ATHER and by the expert is less than 2 pixels. The curves' thickness, in this picture, is 1/3 of the pixel size.

7   Discussion and Conclusions

The main characteristics of our active contour implementation are fast computation and results stability with different starting points within the vessel lumen. The latter characteristic reduces to minimum the user intervention. In particular, when propagating the boundary extraction from one slice to another, the previous contour's center can be used as starting point. This is very useful when slice spacing is large and the contour forms may vary significantly between neighboring slices. In our study the slice spacing is large so as to coincide with the thickness of histological slices. However, with smaller spacing, the current contour can be initialized by the previous contour, slightly reduced. In this case, the contour extraction is even faster and more robust.

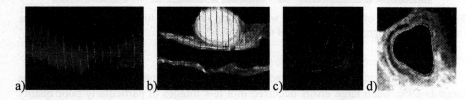

Fig. 4. 3D rendering of the internal surface of a vessel wall (a,c), generated from the extracted boundary points. Corresponding longitudinal (b) and cross-sectional 2D images (d).

The extracted planar contours are not only used for the purpose of quantification. They are also exploited for the sake of 3D visualization. From the detected boundary points, ATHER generates a shaded surface display (fig.4) which can be interactively animated. This is of great interest for visual assessment of the overall intraluminal morphology of the plaque.

The herein presented work is a part of a wider project. In the next task, ATHER will be applied to in vivo images from the same rabbits. This should give rise to a validation of our model also for the external boundaries of the vessels. In parallel, the same model was implemented in another graphical interface, named MARACAS, specially designed for the study of MR angiography images, *i.e.* images of the vascular lumen obtained after a contrast agent injection. It was already validated on images from phantoms [11]. Now, it is applied to images from our rabbits and from patients.

Acknowledgements

This work is supported by Rhône-Alpes region within AdeMo project. It is in the scope of the scientific topics of the GDR-PRC ISIS research group of the French National Center for Scientific Research (CNRS). The authors are grateful to Marcela Hernández-Hoyos and Éric Boix for their help in software implementation and to Emmanuelle Canet for her contribution in image acquisition and analysis.

References

1. Asdente M., *et al.* Evaluation of atherosclerotic lesions using NMR microimaging. *Atherosclerosis*, 1990. **80**(3): 243-53
2. Yuan C., *et al.* Techniques for high-resolution MR imaging of atherosclerotic plaque. *J Magn Reson Imaging*, 1994. **4**(1): 43-49.
3. Toussaint J.F., *et al.* Magnetic resonance images lipid, fibrous, calcified, hemorrhagic, and thrombotic components of human atherosclerosis in vivo. *Circulation*, 1996. **94**(5): 932-338.
4. Serfaty J.M., Chaabane L., *et al.* The value of T2-Weighted High Spatial Resolution Magnetic Resonance Imaging in Classifying and Characterizing Atherosclerotic Plaques: An In Vitro Study. *Radiology*, 2001, in press.
5. Chaabane L, Canet E, Serfaty JM, *et al.* Microimaging of atherosclerotic plaque in animal models. Magnetic Resonance Materials in Physics, Biology and Medicine 2000. **11**: 58-60.
6. Kang X.J., *et al.* Analysis of the measurement precision of arterial lumen and wall areas using high resolution magnetic resonance imaging, MRM, 44:968-972, 2000.
7. Wink, O., *et al.* Semi-automated quantification and segmentation of abdominal aorta aneurysins from CTA volumes. in CARS Paris (France) 1999. 208-212.
8. Mc Inerney, T. and Terzopoulos D., Deformable models in medical image analysis : a survey. *Med. Image Analysis*, 1996. **1**(2): 91-108.
9. Rueckert, D., *et al.* Automatic tracking of the aorta in cardiovascular MR images using deformable models. *IEEE Trans. Med. Imaging*, 1997. **16**(5): 581-590
10. M. Kass, A. Witkin, D. Terzopoulos, Active contour models, *Int J Comp Vision*, 1988. **1**: 321-331.
11. Hernández-Hoyos M., *et al.* A Deformable Vessel Model with Single Point Initialization for Segmentation, Quantification and Visualization of Blood Vessels in 3D MRA. MICCAI, Pittsburgh, Oct. 9-13, 2000. 735-745.
12. Desbleds-Mansard C. *et al.* Dynamic Active Contour Model for Size Independent Blood Vessel Lumen Segmentation and Quantification in High-Resolution Magnetic Resonance Images. Accepted for communication in Int. IAPR Conf. CAIP 2001, Warsaw (PL), Sept. 2001.
13. L. D. Cohen, On Active Contour Models and Balloons, *Computer Vision, Graphics and Image Processing: Image Understanding* 1991. **53**(2): 211-218.

Segmentation of Single-Figure Objects
by Deformable M-reps

Stephen M. Pizer, Sarang Joshi, P. Thomas Fletcher, Martin Styner,
Gregg Tracton, James Z. Chen

Medical Image Display & Analysis Group, University of North Carolina, Chapel Hill

Abstract. This paper describes the basis and behavior of segmentation of single figures in 3D by deformable m-reps models. Results are given for the segmentation of kidneys from CT and of hippocampi from MR images. Special focus is made on multi-scale-level stages of segmentation, on intrinsic correspondences under deformation that are provided by m-reps, and on the match against model-relative templates provided by both theoretical edge strength templates and templates derived from training images.

1. Introduction

A variety of authors have described methods of segmentation of anantomic objects from medical images by the single scale deformation of boundary models [Casseles 1997, Cootes 1999, Montagnat &. Delingette 1998, Kelemen 1999, Staib 1996] In [Joshi 2001] we have described a method of multi-scale segmentation by deformation of models using an m-reps representation. The focus of this paper is not the method itself but its basis and results. In this section we sketch the method, for the restricted case where the object to be found can be well modeled by a single medial mesh, i.e., as a single *figure*, leaving the details to [Joshi 2001]. In section 2 we discuss the theoretical advantages of m-reps models for deformable model segmentation. Sections 3 and 4 cover the areas of emphasis of this paper, with section 3 focusing on one particular advantage of m-reps, that of providing an object-intrinsic coordinate system to give positional, orientational, and scale correspondence between deformed versions of an object. We explain how this correspondence is used in both the geometric typicality term and geometry to image match term in the objective function being optimized to accomplish the model deformation. Section 4 discusses the results of this segmentation approach on the segmentation of two single-figure objects: the union of the kidney parenchyma and renal pelvis as it appears in CT images and the hippocampus as it appears in MR images. Quantitative comparisons between the results and those of manual segmentation are given for the kidney. Because this segmentation method is only a step along the way to the final method that we anticipate, section 5 discusses directions in which anticipated further developments will be made.

    The method. The deformable m-reps method operates from large to small scale levels, at each level deforming the represented object $\underline{m}$ by optimizing an objective function $F(\underline{m}, I_{target})$ over the set of geometric transformations available at that scale level. As with many deformable model based segmentation methods, the objective function F is the sum of two terms, one measuring the geometric typicality of $\underline{m}$ and

W. Niessen and M. Viergever (Eds.): MICCAI 2001, LNCS 2208, pp. 862–871, 2001.
© Springer-Verlag Berlin Heidelberg 2001

the other measuring the match of **m** to the target image I_{target}. The algorithm for single figure objects is as follows. At each stage of this algorithm the geometric typicality measures deviation from the deformed model that is the result of the previous stage.

Algorithm

1a. Manually place the model in the 3D image, thereby choosing a similarity transform

1b. Find and apply the similarity transform which optimizes $F(\mathbf{m}, I_{target})$

2. Until convergence, do

{For each medial atom in **m** {Transform the atom to optimize $F(\mathbf{m}, I_{target})$}

3. For each boundary tile implied by **m**

{Shift the position of the tile along the tile's normal to optimize $F(\mathbf{m}, I_{target})$}

The initial models $\mathbf{m_0}$ used in this work (Figs. 1 & 4) were developed in one of two ways:

By analysis of the geometry of a training set of hand segmented instances of the object over a variety of patients. This automatic analysis uses a method described in [Styner 2001].

By manual construction on a single training image according to set of rules determined by the mathematics of medial geometry [Pizer et al 2001].

Space limitations do not permit us to detail these model building methods here.

2. Theoretical Advantages of M-reps Based Segmentation

We desire successful segmentation performance that is linear in the number of the smallest scale geometric primitives, for example the boundary tiles defining the segmented object's surface or the voxels making up the object. We argue elsewhere that a) such behavior is achievable only by multi-scale-level segmentation with rather closely spaced scale levels, and b) at each level the diameter of the area or volume summarized by the geometric primitives (*atoms*) at that level and the distance of communication used at each geometric transformation of an atom or group of atoms are comparable. Either of these two distances can be taken as the measure of the scale at that level.

In our method the scale levels are indicated by the numbered steps in the algorithm above: [1] the figural scale levels, [2] the medial atom or figural section scale level, [3] the boundary atom scale level. In steps 1 and 2 the object is represented by medial atoms, and at step 3 it is represented by boundary atoms. A representation of a figure by medial atoms is called an *m-rep*.

An m-rep for a generic figure in our system is a quad-mesh of medial atoms (Fig. 1), where an interior medial atom is a medial position at which two vectors (called *port* and *starboard sails*) of equal length r share a sail and a mesh-edge medial atom in addition is equipped with a bisector vector of the two sails of length greater or equal to the common sail length. To allow shape representation and thus magnification invariance not only globally but locally, the spacing of the atoms in an m-rep is approximately proportional to the sail lengths r of the atom.

An m-rep represents a continuous 2-manifold of medial atoms. Thall and Yushkevich have developed two methods for interpolation of this manifold from the m-rep that are consistent with first order medial geometry [Fletcher et al. 2001]. The method of Thall is used in the results described here. The manifold of medial atoms defines a continuous m-rep implied boundary obtained from the union of all the sail-end positions, together with an interpolation of the crest between the sail tips and through the bisector vector tips of each mesh-edge atom. At each such boundary position the corresponding medial atom sail is normal to the implied boundary.

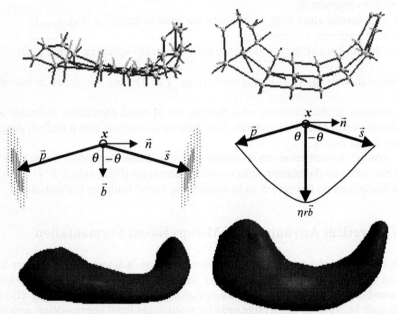

Figure 1. Top: an m-rep for a hippocampus, viewed from two directions. Each ball with two line segment sails forms a medial atom. Center: an internal medial atom and a mesh-edge medial atom, each with their implied boundaries. Bottom: The boundary implied by the m-rep, viewed from two directions.

M-reps have four advantages for representing objects to be segmented by deformable models.

1. Each medial atom represents an interior section of a figure, leading to a special capability for deformation of the interior.
2. Since figures typically have anatomic names and each medial atom in the m-rep corresponds to an interior slab of the figure bounded by its immediately neighboring medial atoms, the geometric transformations involved in the deformation can be described with medical relevance and with appropriate locality.
3. An m-rep lends itself directly to representation at multiple scale levels. There are additional important scale levels besides those already mentioned (figural, figural section, boundary). For objects consisting of more than one figure or for sets of objects, situations not described in this paper, there are the larger scale multi-

object and object scale levels. Also described elsewhere [Yushkevich 2001], there are opportunities for multiple levels of meshing of each figure.

4. Figures yield an intrinsic coordinate system with space varying frame and distance metric. Indeed, multi-figure complexes also yield an intrinsic coordinate system, not described in this paper due to lack of space. As described in section 3, this leads to correspondences under deformation that are important with deformable models.

3. Intrinsic Figural Coordinates and Their Use in Geometric Typicality and in Geometry to Image Match

Geometric typicality functions measure the closeness of a deformed model for a figure to a mean or most typical form of the figure. Since sensing of the figure is typically at the boundary, it is natural for this geometric typicality measure to involve the distances of corresponding boundary points between the deformed state of the figure and the typical state (Fig. 2). In a medial geometry, allowing shape to be characterized at all levels of scale (locality), the distances must be taken in multiples of r (the length of the relevant medial sail). In our method as it presently stands, the geometric typicality is measured by the mean squared r-proportional offset of the boundary. This mean is taken over the section of boundary appropriate for the present level of scale, and it is measured between the version of the deformed model produced at the next larger level of scale and the newly deformed candidate $\underline{m}$.

As is common, our method measures the match of $\underline{m}$ to the target image in a region near the object boundary that we we call a boundary *collar* (Fig. 2). A fruitful way of looking at matching $\underline{m}$ to I_{target} is that at corresponding positions in the collar, before and after deformation of the model into $\underline{m}$, a template defined on the model must match as closely as possible a template image defined with respect to the model. The template can be an ideal image, e.g., defined by directional derivatives of a Gaussian, the training image from which the model was built, or the statistics of a set of training images from which the model was built.

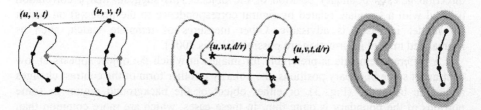

Fig. 2. Medially implied correspondences between a typical figure and a deformed figure for figural boundary positions (leftmost), for positions interior and exterior to the boundary (center), and for the boundary collar (right).

The boundary and collar position correspondences required by geometric typicality and the image match, respectively, are well provided by the medially based intrinsic coordinate system for a figure, as follows. Let the two dimensions of the quad mesh forming the m-rep be called u and v. Let the atom positions be taken as integer values of u and v. Let the interpolated medial sheet be parametrized by its (u,v) "figural" coordinate system in which distances are r-proportional along the medial manifold.

The medially implied boundary is parametrized via the medial coordinates, but in addition a parameter t is needed to select the side of the medial sheet. We let $t=1$ for boundary points touched by port sails and let $t=-1$ for boundary points touched by starboard sails. At the crest, where the boundary switches from the port side to the starboard side, t varies smoothly from $+1$ to -1 such that $t=0$ at the crest. Then every boundary point is parametrized by its figural coordinates (u,v,t). Each boundary point thereby carries a normal in the direction of the sail abutting there and a ruler $r(u,v)$. The (u,v,t) values are used to produce correspondences for boundary points to measure the geometric typicality between the state before and that after deformation and are also used in the boundary displacement final stage of the segmentation.

Points inside the figure and outside it but inside the caustic surface can also be put into correspondence in a figurally relative manner. Correspondences outside the caustic surface have also been defined [Crouch 2001], but this is beyond the scope of this paper. In the medial framework distances are measured in an r-proportional fashion along the sails, i.e., along boundary normals. Thus if d is the Euclidean distance from the medially implied boundary to a point in space, with points interior to the figure having negative distances and points exterior to the figure having positive distances, $(u,v,t,d/r)$ provides a shape-respecting figural coordinate for a point. Correspondences between the collars of a figure and its deformed version used in computing geometry to image match are then done according to equal values of the these figural coordinates for space. More precisely, at model building time a boundary sampling defined by equally spaced samples of u, v, and t is determined and an equally spaced sampling of d/r between $-k$ and $+k$ is specified ($k = 0.33$ is a typical value). These sample positions for the part of the boundary that can be shifted at the respective level of scale are used in producing the geometry to image match measure.

Many segmentation systems use directional derivatives of a Gaussian at some scale as a measure of contrast, which is expected to be high at a boundary. This is equivalent to correlation with a derivative of Gaussian template in the normal direction at each boundary position of the object. This suggests that a correlation method with a template related by figural correspondence to the image(s) on which the model is based is advisable. Other measures of template match, such as normalized mutual information are possible [Willis 2001].

A different template is preferable for images in which the object appears at low contrast at some boundary positions, the polarity or other form of the contrast changes along the boundary (Fig. 3), or either object or the background region in some portions of the boundary is quite thin. In these cases, which are more common than not, a template made from a training image or the mean of a set of training images is quite attractive. Such a template can avoid having the deformation be attracted by a high contrast nearby boundary in a region along which the object sought bounds an object with similar intensity and thus is known to provide no contrast.

We have implemented such a training image template for collars of half-width $r/3$. For certain kidneys they provide improved segmentation, and for the hippocampus they are essential.

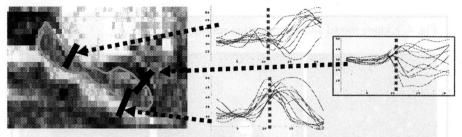

Fig 3. Intensity profiles for a set of patient's normal to the boundary at three separate locations. Compliments of G. Gerig.

4. Results on Single Figure Objects

We have tested this method for the extraction of three anatomic objects well modeled by a single figure: the lateral cerebral ventricle, the kidney parenchyma + pelvis, and the hippocampus. Extracting the lateral ventricle from MR images is not very challenging because the ventricle appears with high contrast, so our successful results are not shown. Extracting the kidney from CT has some challenge because in certain sections of the kidney, where it abuts the liver, there is essentially no contrast and the high contrast spine is nearby. Results of a kidney segmentation are visualized in Figs. 4 & 5. As laid out in Table 1, for 30 kidneys (18 right kidneys and 12 left kidneys, with the model having been built on a right kidney) we were able to extract the kidney with an median accuracy of boundary position of 1 voxel (2.0 mm) as compared to a human manual segmentation. All of the measurements in Table 1are made relative to a human segmentation that classified each voxel as in or not in the object and did not take anatomic understanding well into account when segmenting the renal pelvis from the ureter and other background. Moreover, the measurement tool measures offsets and overlaps only to the closest voxel. Therefore, our real median boundary accuracy is subvoxel, and the overlap percentatges are understated. Human to human agreement is of the same order.

5. Conclusions

Extracting the hippocampus from MRI is very challenging for humans and has great variability across human segmenters. This provides a major challenge for automatic segmentation, but so far we have achieved 8 successful, reproducible segmentations. Fig. 6 shows comparison for our deformable m-reps segmentation based on a training template to human manual segmentation.

Median boundary offset:	**Median case: 2.0* mm.**	**Worst case: 2.0* mm**
3rd quartile boundary offset:	**Median case: 2.0* mm.**	**Worst case: 3.4† mm**
Percent volume overlap:	**Median case: 89%**	**Worst case: 81%**

Table 1. Comparison of deformable m-reps segmentation to manual segmentation of four kidneys from CT, using a Gaussian derivative template. *distance between face-adjacent voxels, †distance between corner-adjacent voxels

training intensity template for the more difficult cases. While we have only a few cases of the kidney and all (but still only a few) cases of the hippocampus where we have used this training image template, we have found that success with the training image template in all cases if the match was successively made against a highly blurred version of the target image, then a moderately blurred version of the target image, and then the target image.

The method described here is by no means fully developed. The metrics, the segmentation algorithm, and the visualizations and user interface, and the program code have already been extended to deal with objects made up of multiple attached figures which must be kept in the correct geometric relations as they deform. Examples are the cerebral ventricle, the vertebra, and the kidney parenchyma. Extension has also been made to deal with multiple nonoverlapping figures which must be kept in the right geometric relations and to remain noninterpenetrating. Examples are the pubic bones, bladder, prostate, and rectum in the male pelvis and the full set of cerebral ventricles. Early, incomplete trials of the extended versions of the code suggest that m-reps have particular advantages also with multiple attached figures and multiple nonoverlapping figures.

Two important directions to improve deformable m-reps based segmentation are the following. Applying the segmentation at multiple levels of medial meshing, in coarse to fine order, is expected to speed the method for any level of effectiveness. This multiscale approach will overcome the question of what is the best level of meshing and replace it by the question of the spacing between the scale levels.

The replacement of the geometric distance measures for geometric typicality and average intensity correlation or mutual information for the geometry to image match measure by log probability measures [Cootes & Taylor 1999] has two important advantages. First, the probabilities reflect the modes of variability in the respective population. Second, the arbitrary, manually selected weight between geometric typicality and geometry to image match is no longer necessary. We will soon begin work on methods for measuring these probabilities from training sets, at each of the relevant scale levels based on a Markov random field model, and for using them in the model deformation process.

Acknowledgements

We are grateful to conceptual, geometric, algorithmic, or code contributions from Andrew Thall, Graham Gash, and Paul Yushkevich. We thank Edward Chaney and Guido Gerig for providing driving problems for this segmentation and images to segment. We appreciate the contributions of Daniel Fritsch and John Glotzer to earlier versions of this method. This work was done under the partial support of NCI Grant P01 CA47982 and NSF grant CCR SGER 9910419.

References

1. Casselles, V, R Kimmel and G Sapiro (1997). Geodesic Active Contours. *IJCV* **22**(1): 61-79.
2. Cootes, TF, C Beeston, GJ Edwards, CJ Taylor, A Unified Framework for Atlas Matching Using Active Appearance Models. *Information Processing in Medical Imaging* (IPMI 1999), A Kuba, M Samal, A Todd-Pokropek eds., Springer LNCS **1613**: 322-333.
3. Crouch, JR, SM Pizer, EL Chaney, M Zaider, Elastic registration of prostate images using the finite element method with m-rep models. Poster, 2nd Int. Conf. On Innovative Solutions for Prostate Cancer Care 2001. Also at website http://www.cs.unc.edu/Research/Image/MIDAG/pubs/presentations/prostate-mrep-Crouch2001_files/frame.htm.
4. Joshi, S, SM Pizer, PT Fletcher, A Thall, G Tracton, Multi-Scale 3-D Deformable Model Segmentation Based on Medical Description. *Information Processing in Medical Imaging* (IPMI 2001), MF Insana, RM Leahy, eds., Springer LNCS **2082**: 64-77.
5. Kelemen, A, G Szekely and G Gerig (1999). Elastic Model-Based Segmentation of 3D Neuroradiological Data Sets. *IEEE Transactions On Medical Imaging* **18**: 828-839.
6. Montagnat, J, H Delingette (1998). Globally Constrained Deformable Models for 3D Object Reconstruction. *Signal Processing* **71**: 173-186
7. Pizer, SM, PT Fletcher, Y Fridman, D Fritsch, AG Gash, J Glotzer, S Joshi, A Thall, G Tracton, P Yushkevich, EL Chaney, Deformable M-Reps for 3D Medical Image Segmentation. Internal report 2001 at website ftp://ftp.cs.unc.edu/pub/users/MIDAG/defmrep3d.final.pdf
8. Staib, LH, JS Duncan (1996). Model-based Deformable Surface Finding for Medical Images. *IEEE Trans. Med. Imaging* **15**(5): 1-12.
9. Styner, M, G Gerig, Medical Models Incorporating Object Variability for 3D Shape Analysis. *Information Processing in Medical Imaging* (IPMI 2001), MF Insana, RM Leahy, eds., Springer LNCS **2082**: 502-516.
10. Fletcher, PT, SM. Pizer, A Thall, P Yushkevich with S Joshi. Medial Geometry and Interpolation through Medial Correspondence. In preparation (2001).
11. Willis, L, A Geometric Description of Lung Shape During Respiration via M-reps and Normalized Mutual Information. MS thesis 2001, Dept. of Biomedical Engineering, UNC in preparation
12. Yushkevich, P, SM Pizer, S Joshi, JS Marron, Intuitive, Localized Analysis of Shape Variability. *Information Processing in Medical Imaging* (IPMI 2001), MF Insana, RM Leahy, eds., Springer LNCS **2082**: 402-408.

Half Fourier Acquisition Applied to Time Series Analysis of Contrast Agent Uptake

Andreas Degenhard[1], Christine Tanner[2], Carmel Hayes[1], David J. Hawkes[2], and Martin O. Leach[1]

[1] CRC Clinical MR Research Group
The Institute of Cancer Research and the Royal Marsden NHS Trust
Sutton, Surrey SM2 5PT, UK
andreasd@icr.ac.uk
[2] Division of Radiological Sciences and Medical Engineering
The Guy's, King's and St. Thomas' School of Medicine and Dentistry
Thomas Guy House, Guy's Hospital, London SE1 9RT, UK

Abstract Magnetic Resonance Imaging (MRI) has emerged as a powerful tool in medical diagnosis and research. Dynamic Contrast Enhanced MRI (DCE-MRI), which involves the administration of a paramagnetic contrast medium, has been shown to provide additional sensitivity in detecting abnormality. In particular, in imaging of the breast and axilla the ability to differentiate between benign and malignant lesions depends, in part, on the enhancement profile. Evaluation of this requires a sufficient temporal resolution in the time series acquisition. Faster imaging in general requires that images are acquired with a lower spatial resolution or signal to noise ratio. In this paper we investigate a novel approach for increasing the temporal resolution in DCE-MRI without decreasing the accuracy of the measurement. The results clearly indicate a superior image quality compared to standard half Fourier techniques and the algorithm correctly recovers the time series characteristics of T_1 and T_2^*-weighted time series data.

1 Introduction

Magnetic Resonance Imaging (MRI) is a valuable imaging modality because of its high contrast sensitivity to many characteristics of tissues and body fluids, including proton density, T_1 and T_2 relaxation times. Dynamic Contrast Enhanced MRI (DCE-MRI) using a paramagnetic contrast medium with a non-selective extracellular distribution, such as gadolinium diethylene triamine pentaacetic acid (Gd-DTPA), is currently essential in the detection and evaluation of breast cancer with MRI [1,2]. Observation of contrast enhancement is typically achieved using dynamic imaging techniques where the contrast agent is injected during acquisition of a dynamic series of images. Following contrast agent administration, malignant breast lesions tend to enhance more rapidly than benign lesions, a phenomenon also seen in imaging involving lymph nodes [4].

W. Niessen and M. Viergever (Eds.): MICCAI 2001, LNCS 2208, pp. 872–880, 2001.
© Springer-Verlag Berlin Heidelberg 2001

In this work we apply dynamic acquisition techniques to T_1 and T_2^*-weighted MR imaging. Both imaging methods have been investigated for differentiating between benign and malignant breast [3] and brain lesions [7]. For an insufficient temporal resolution time-feature characteristics such as peak-enhancement or first pass perfusion drop are not accurately characterized. Furthermore, successful pharmacokinetic modeling of time series data depends on the numerical stability in the fitting procedure and this in turn depends on the number of available data points describing the enhancement profile [6].

Partial Fourier acquisition techniques improve the temporal resolution, although the reconstructed images suffer from a reduced signal to noise ratio, inferior spatial resolution or reconstruction artifacts affecting the accuracy of the time series data. In this work we present an image reconstruction algorithm based on the concepts of image recovery theory [9] which approximately doubles the temporal resolution. The proposed algorithm requires a full Fourier Space (FS) acquisition of a pre-contrast image, that is, prior to contrast agent administration. To test our algorithm, half Fourier data have been generated from a full post-contrast FS acquisition for two reasons: Firstly the fully acquired FS data provides the original or true post-contrast image which is then used as a reference image to evaluate the image quality of the reconstructed images in the time series. Secondly the full post-contrast phase data are used in the comparison of reconstruction methods. Phase retrieval algorithms applied to half Fourier data can introduce phase errors which interfere with the performance of the different constrained amplitude reconstruction algorithms [9].

2 Methods and Material

MR data are acquired in Fourier space (FS) and the corresponding real space (RS) image is calculated by a linear map, i.e. the Inverse Fourier Transform (IFT) [8]. According to the Hermitian symmetry of FS, the bulk of the signal intensities (SI) are distributed symmetrically within the centre or low frequency regime of FS, whereas most of the information about the shape and the structure of the RS image is included in the outer high frequency part [8].

In a MR image acquisition, the pixel intensity in the RS image is also a complex value, since motion and magnetic field inhomogeneities introduce a nonzero or nontrivial phase to the RS image data. The nontrivial phase structure in the RS image leads to a deviation from the perfect symmetry in FS. Nevertheless images may be reconstructed from a half sampled FS data set using Fourier reconstruction methods [5]. Half Fourier acquisition techniques sample approximately half of the complete FS data as shown in Figure 1(a), thus decreasing the image acquisition time. However, an IFT applied to the undersampled FS results in poor quality RS images and constrained methods are the mathematical tools developed to provide additional information required to restore unsampled FS data. In this paper we compare two standard phase constrained reconstruction methods, the Margosian method [5] and a so-called projection on convex sets technique (POCS) [9], with two new variations on the latter summarized as

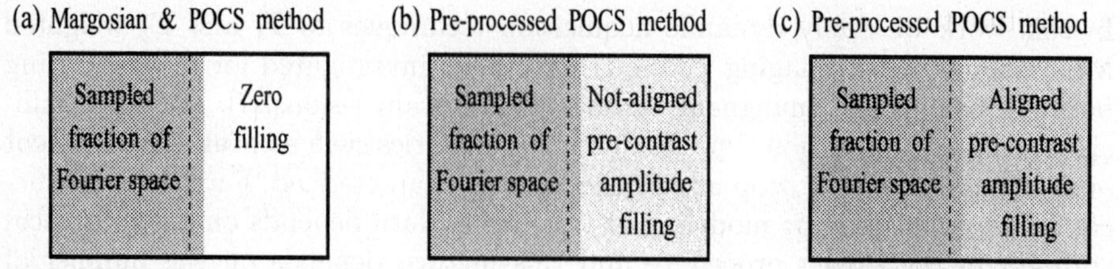

(a) Margosian & POCS method   (b) Pre-processed POCS method   (c) Pre-processed POCS method

Sampled fraction of Fourier space	Zero filling

Sampled fraction of Fourier space	Not-aligned pre-contrast amplitude filling

Sampled fraction of Fourier space	Aligned pre-contrast amplitude filling

Fig. 1. In the Margosian and the POCS method the unsampled fraction of FS is filled with zeros. For the pre-processed POCS method two possible filling procedures are shown. One half of FS and eight additional lines from the centre of FS are sampled.

pre-processed POCS methods. Both the Margosian and the POCS method are based on initial zero-filling of the unsampled half of FS and use the post-contrast phase to force or align the amplitude RS image according to the desired phase structure [5]. Unlike the Margosian approach, in the POCS method the post-contrast phase information is used iteratively to accomplish a sequence of phase constrained symmetrization steps. Each of the symmetrization steps starts with inserting the desired post-contrast phase information followed by a Fourier transform in RS or an inverse Fourier transform in FS to align the amplitude data to the post-contrast phase. Both methods require the acquisition of additional low frequency FS data for Hamming filtering to provide a smooth transition to the zero-filled part [5]. In the pre-processed POCS method, the unsampled half of FS is filled with pre-contrast amplitude data acquired prior to the dynamic series as schematically shown in Figure 1(b) and no Hamming filtering needs to be applied. The pre-contrast data can be aligned to the post-contrast phase using one or more symmetrization steps as in the conventional POCS method (c). After the unsampled half has been filled with unaligned or aligned pre-contrast data the conventional POCS method is applied.

In order to quantify the image quality of the different reconstruction methods the root-mean-square error (RMSE) is calculated by [6]

$$\text{RMSE}(S^*) = \sqrt{\frac{1}{N} \cdot \left[\sum_{i=1}^{N}(S_i^* - S_i)^2 - \frac{1}{N} \left(\sum_{i=1}^{N} S_i^* - S_i \right)^2 \right]} \quad . \quad (1)$$

In equation (1), N denotes the total number of pixels in the image and S_i and S_i^* denote the SI of a pixel in the true image S and the reconstructed image S^* respectively.

Images were acquired on a 1.5 Tesla Siemens Vision MR System. For the T_1-weighted dynamic imaging of the breast, a 3D fast gradient echo sequence was used with TR $= 12ms$, TE $= 5ms$, flip angle $= 35°$, FOV $= 340mm$ and spatial resolution of $1.33mm \times 1.33mm \times 2.5mm$ ($256 \times 128 \times 64$ voxels). T_2^*-weighted MR images of the brain with a matrix size of 256×256 pixels were acquired with TR $= 26.5ms$, TE $= 20ms$, flip angle $= 15°$ and FOV $= 250mm$. The acquisition time of an image is $90secs$ for the 3D and $11secs$ for the 2D dynamic sequence.

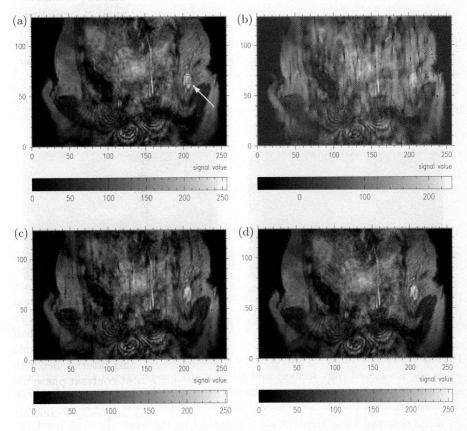

Fig. 2. A true post-contrast breast MR image showing the anatomy behind the breast wall including the axilla (a). The arrow is pointing to a malignant lymph node in the true image including a selected region of interest (ROI). Half Fourier reconstructed MR images are shown generated by the Margosian method (b) and the POCS method (c) using eight additional lines in the centre of FS. The image reconstructed using the pre-processed POCS method with aligned pre-contrast amplitude filling and eight additional lines in the centre of FS (d) shows no visible differences by comparing with the true image (a). The images for the conventional and the pre-processed POCS method are reconstructed using five final POCS iterations.

3   Results

Figure 2(a) shows a coronal slice of a T_1-weighted 3D breast MR image after contrast agent injection. A malignant lymph node (white arrow) has enhanced within the left breast and a ROI (63 pixels) was chosen from the true image Figure 2(a) for further time series analysis. Figure 2(b) and (c) show images reconstructed by the Margosian and the POCS method for the same slice using approximately half of the acquired full FS. For both reconstruction methods the eight additional lines in the centre of FS were used for asymmetric Hamming filtering providing a smooth transition to the zero-filled part [5]. Although it is clear from visual inspection that the POCS method has resulted in a considerable improvement in image quality, both images suffer from different types of artifacts not visible in the true image Figure 2(a). Increasing the number of iterations in the POCS method does not correct for the large reconstruction errors.

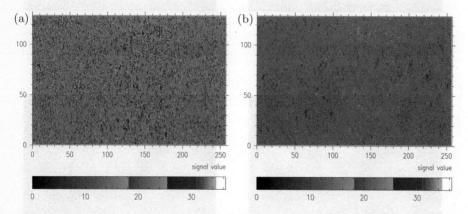

Fig. 3. Difference images generated by subtracting the reconstructed images using the unaligned (not shown) and the aligned pre-processed POCS method shown in Figure 2(d) from the true image Figure 2(a). Since differences between the reconstructed images were barely visible, the difference images are plotted on a discrete and logarithmic scale. Compared to the aligned counterpart (b) the difference image generated by the unaligned pre-processed POCS method (a) displays broad artifacts and also spurious high signal intensity changes.

Figure 3 compares difference images of the pre-processed POCS method using not-aligned (a) and aligned (b) pre-contrast amplitude filling by subtracting the reconstructed images from the true T_1-weighted post-contrast image shown in Figure 2(a). In Figure 4, signal intensity-time curves for the whole dynamic T_1-weighted imaging acquisition including two pre-contrast and five post-contrast volumes are displayed. The relative percentage signal increase during the first 90 secs after contrast injection compared to the pre-contrast volume was 245% which is a typical value for malignant tumors. In all cases the maximum signal enhancement is recovered within the calculated error. However, the characteristic washout behaviour (signal decrease immediately after early peak enhancement) can not be recovered by the Margosian or by the POCS method. In Figure 5, time series data for a T_2^*-weighted dynamic contrast enhanced single slice sequence

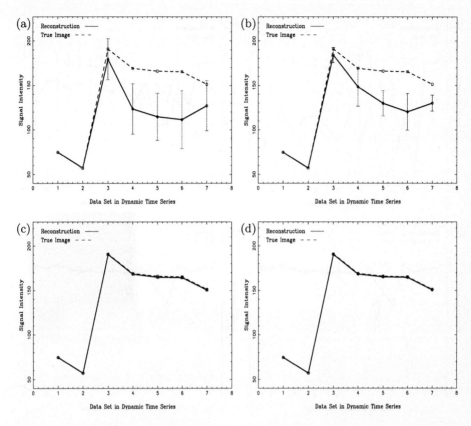

Fig. 4. T_1-weighted time series data for the 2D ROI shown in Figure 2(a). The Margosian method (a) and the POCS method (b) can not recover the correct temporal enhancement profile, although both reconstruction methods display the rapid enhancement for the first post-contrast volume. The results for the pre-processed POCS method are shown using unaligned (c) and aligned (d) pre-contrast amplitude data.

of the brain are displayed. The characteristic signal intensity loss for malignant tissue in the true signal-versus-time curve during the first 10 secs after contrast injection was 12% compared to the averaged baseline value. In Table 1 we summarize the results of all methods applied to brain and breast data calculating the time-averaged RMSE (1).

4   Discussion and Conclusions

We have applied a pre-processed half Fourier reconstruction method to different types of MRI time series data acquired dynamically following contrast agent administration. The method was evaluated on breast T_1-weighted image series' and brain T_2^*-weighted brain image series'. Unlike standard phase-constrained

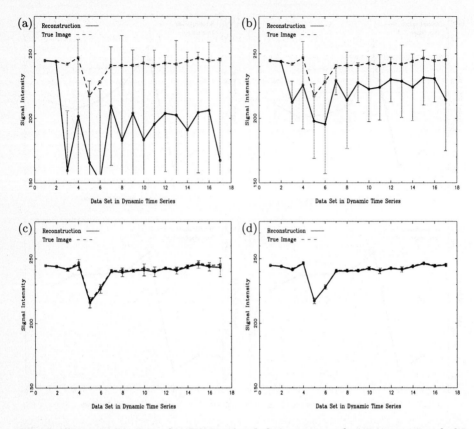

Fig. 5. Time series data for T_2^*-weighted first pass perfusion imaging of the brain. The perfusion drop after contrast agent injection has not been recovered using the Margosian method (a) and the POCS method (b). Both pre-processed POCS methods (c), (d) recover the perfusion drop.

reconstruction methods, the new algorithm, which is a variation of the POCS method, uses pre-contrast data to fill the unsampled part of Fourier space. Thus, Hamming filtering is not necessary to ensure a smooth transition in the centre of Fourier space. It was found that images reconstructed using the pre-processed POCS method have a far superior quality to those obtained using the standard methods. Furthermore, it was found that aligning the pre-contrast data with the post-contrast phase, yields images with an even better quality than those reconstructed without alignment. The image quality, as measured using the 'RMSE, improved by a factor of up to 90% on using the pre-contrast aligned data compared with that obtained using zero filling (see Table 1). In addition, it was found that a typical ROI in both breast and brain MR reconstructed images shows the same signal intensity-time curve profile as the original full Fourier images, with negligible error. This demonstrates that the algorithm has considerable potential in many MR imaging studies involving time series data. Future

Table 1. The RMSE averaged over all data sets in the time series, for the whole image and a selected ROI. The percentages given in brackets below the absolute RMSE values measure the improvement on the RMSE using an aligned pre-contrast amplitude.

Type of image data	Magosian method	POCS method	POCS method using pre-contrast amplitude not aligned	aligned
$256 \times 128 \times 64$ T_1 weighted breast image	25.33 (81.52%)	15.49 (69.79%)	2.73 (52.75%)	1.29
Selected ROI	27.77 (97.98%)	14.85 (96.23%)	1.12 (50.0%)	0.56
256×128 T_2^* weighted brain image	38.95 (95.96%)	16.78 (91.6%)	4.96 (71.57%)	1.41
Selected ROI	58.71 (98.25%)	25.47 (95.96%)	2.98 (65.44%)	1.03

work will consider the impact of the location, size and type of the tumor on the numerical evaluation. Combined with half Fourier acquisition techniques and phase estimation algorithms, the method can result in an improvement in the temporal resolution by a factor of approximately two. This is certain to be beneficial in any fast imaging acquisition, particularly when the spatial resolution and/or coverage should not be compromised.

Acknowledgments

The authors are greatful to EPSRC GR/M52762 for their financial support of this work. The support of the Medical Research Council [MRC] and the Cancer Research Campaign [CRC] is grateful acknowledged.

References

1. Heywang, S.H., Hahn, D., Schmidt, H., Krischke, I., Eiermann, W., Bassermann, R., Lissner, J.: MR imaging of the breast using Gadolinium-DTPA. J. Comp. Ass. Tomography **10** (1986) 199-204
2. Kaiser, W.A., Zeitler, E.: MR imaging of the breast: fast imaging sequences with and without Gd-DTPA. Radiology **170** (1989) 681-686
3. Kvistad, K.A., Lundgren, S., Fjosne, H.E., Smenes, E., Smethurst, H.B., Haraldseth, O.:: Differentiating Benign And Malignant Breast Lesions with T_2^*-Weighted First Pass Perfusion Imaging. Acta Radiologica **40** (1999) 45-51
4. Lernevall, A.: Imaging of Axillary Lymph Nodes. Acta Oncologica **39** (2000) 277-281

5. Liang, Z., Boada, F.E., Constable, R.T., Haacke, E.M., Lauterbur, P.C., Smith, M.R.: Constrained reconstruction methods in MR Imaging. Reviews of Magnetic Resonance in Medicine **4** (1992) 67-185
6. Press, W.H., Flannery, B.P., Teukolsky, S.A., Vetterling, W.T.: Numerical Recipes in C *The Art of Scientific Computing*. Cambridge University Press, Cambridge (1988)
7. Roberts, T.P.L., Chuang, N., Roberts, H.C.: Neuroimaging: do we really need new contrast agents for MRI? European Journal of Radiology **34** (2000) 166-178
8. Russ, J.C.: The Image Processing Handbook. CRC Press, Springer, Heidelberg (1998).
9. Stark, H.: Image Recovery: *Theory and Application*. Academic Press, New York (1987)

Analysis of Brain Functional MRI Time Series Based on Continuous Wavelet Transform and Stimulation-Response Coupling Distance

Laurent Thoraval[1], Jean-Paul Armspach[2], and Izzie Namer[2]

[1] Laboratoire des Sciences de l'Image, de l'Informatique et de la Télédétection,
LSIIT/GRI - UPRES-A CNRS 7005,
ENSPS, Bd. Sébastien Brandt, F-67400 Illkirch, France
Laurent.Thoraval@ensps.u-strasbg.fr
http://lsiit.u-strasbg.fr
[2] Institut de Physique Biologique,
Faculté de Médecine - UPRES-A CNRS 7004,
4, Rue Kirschleger, F-67085 Strasbourg Cedex, France
{armspach,namer}@ipb.u-strasbg.fr
http://ipb.u-strasbg.fr

Abstract. Analytical techniques applied to functional magnetic resonance imaging (fMRI) data require restrictive assumptions about the shape of the blood oxygenation level dependent (BOLD) time series observed at each voxel in response to a stimulation paradigm. In this paper, a radically different and fundamentally pattern recognition-oriented fMRI brain activation mapping approach is proposed. Neural activity is assessed at each voxel on a coupling distance principle between the deterministic alternation sequence of the stimulation paradigm and the sequence of BOLD response nonstationarities detected and characterized by a continuous wavelet transform (CWT). The voxel's stimulation-response coupling distance is measured using an adapted version of the string edit distance algorithm. fMRI studies conducted on synthetic and real data demonstrated the superiority of the "coupling distance" brain activation mapping approach over against the Student's t-test.

1 Introduction

Through the BOLD effect that links neural activity to blood oxygenation levels in the vessels near active neurons, fMRI enables to image and study functional activity of the human brain. A typical fMRI experiment consists in alternating the acquisition of blocks of N_a images ($N_a \sim 10$) of the brain while the subject is in an active state, that is, performing a specific task, with the acquisition of blocks of N_c images ($N_c \sim 10$) while the subject is in a control state. This active-control or ON-OFF cycle, when repeated M times ($M \sim 10$), constitutes the so-called stimulation paradigm.

Brain activation mapping consists in detecting regions of the brain activated by the stimulation paradigm. In standard practice, activation mapping is performed by means of the Student's t-test (TT), the cross-correlation (CC) or the

W. Niessen and M. Viergever (Eds.): MICCAI 2001, LNCS 2208, pp. 881–888, 2001.

statistical parametric mapping (SPM) approach. All three techniques are voxelwise: each BOLD response is analyzed independently. Neural activity is then declared at the voxel level if the corresponding BOLD response is determined by the stimulation paradigm somehow.

In essence, the TT measures a distance between two sample sets, one corresponding to the active fMRI samples, the other to the samples observed in the control state. The main drawback of the TT is that the time dimension of the BOLD fMRI signal is lost as the only information taken into account is the binary variable "stimulated" or "not stimulated". CC techniques are computationally efficient but rely on a priori knowledge about the reference waveform to be used. It can be either a boxcar function, a sine wave, or some mathematical model representative of the expected BOLD response [1]. The selected waveform can have a profound effect on the activation mapping results. Moreover, CC techniques consider the BOLD response as uniform across the brain. In the SPM approach [2], the BOLD response is fitted to a set of basis functions using a linear regression analysis. The basis functions are predefined according to the experimental protocol. They model either effects of interest that are sought or low frequency nuisance effects. A contrast map can then be obtained for any combination of the basis functions of interest with respect to the ones of no interest. SPM is a more powerful and versatile data processing approach than CC. But like CC, SPM requires morphological assumptions about the BOLD response which is unknown and may vary not only with the stimulation paradigm but also spatially within the brain.

In this paper, a new voxelwise brain activation mapping approach is developed that keeps the time dimension of the analysis while relaxing as much as possible traditional morphological assumptions about the ideal BOLD response expected at each voxel. Rather than considering the shape of the local BOLD response in its whole, the proposed approach focuses on its dynamics changes. In the presence of a regional neural activity, these are assumed to be time-locked to some extent onto the successive transitions of the stimulation paradigm.

2   Methods

A continuous wavelet transform (CWT) is first applied to each voxel's fMRI signal under test to detect and characterize dynamics changes of interest. The derived sequence of events, R, is then compared to the deterministic event sequence, S, that models the successive transitions of the stimulation paradigm. A "coupling distance", $dist(R \rightarrow S)$, between the response R and the stimulation S is finally worked out using a dynamic event matching procedure.

2.1   Detection / Characterization of fMRI Signal Changes by CWT

Wavelet multiresolution analysis has been widely used in multiscale representation and analysis of signals and images [3]. The wavelet-based brain activation mapping approach presented here differs significantly from the pioneering work of Ruttimann et al. [4]. Rather than detecting neural activity based on a discrete wavelet transform of the average difference image from the input fMRI sequence as proposed by Ruttimann et al., neural activity is detected here based on the discrete space-time field of signal sharp variations underlying the raw 3-D fMRI sequence. The ability of the CWT to detect and characterize such nonstationarities in the time-scale domain is here of great interest. For any finite energy signal $f(t)$, the CWT is defined by [3]:

$$(W_\psi f)(a, b) = \frac{1}{\sqrt{a}} \int_{-\infty}^{+\infty} f(t)\psi^* \left(\frac{t - b}{a} \right) dt \qquad (1)$$

The parameters a and b denote the scale and the translation parameter respectively of the complex conjugate of the mother wavelet $\psi(t)$ where:

$$\psi(t) = \begin{cases} C.(1 + \cos 2\pi f_0 t).e^{2i\pi k f_0 t} & \text{for } |t| \leq \frac{1}{2f_0} \\ 0 & \text{elsewhere} \end{cases} \qquad (2)$$

k is set to 2 to satisfy with the required admissibility conditions while f_0 denotes the normalized frequency $(0 < f_0 < 1/2)$ and C a normalizing constant. $\psi(t)$ is chosen complex valued to benefit from the phase information of the fMRI signal CWT. Indeed, it has been demonstrated in [3] that symmetry singularities of a signal $f(t)$ are associated with particular values of the phase of its CWT. Specifically, a positive inflexion point at time t_0 $(f''(t_0^-) > 0, f''(t_0) = 0, f''(t_0^+) < 0, f'(t_0) > 0)$ is associated at high resolution (i.e., small values of the scale parameter "a") with phase value $+\pi/2$. Similarly, a negative inflexion point at time t_0 $(f''(t_0^-) < 0, f''(t_0) = 0, f''(t_0^+) > 0, f'(t_0) < 0)$ corresponds at high resolution to phase value $-\pi/2$. Then, assuming that the fMRI dynamics changes of interest exhibit a local positive or negative inflection point, detecting the occurrence times of these changes can be performed at a sufficient high scale of resolution by detecting the $\pm\pi/2$ crossings of the phase of the fMRI signal CWT. Moreover, while moving towards finest scales of analysis, $\pm\pi/2$ crossing points are increasing while describing curves known as fingerprints in pattern recognition. The length of a fingerprint, expressed in terms of the number of scales crossed from the finest scale of detection, is characteristic of the importance of the fMRI dynamics change associated with. Finally, as stated in [3], $\pm\pi/2$ crossing points correspond to maxima of the square modulus of the fMRI signal CWT.

As an example, the phase of the CWTs of an activated and a non-activated fMRI signal are plotted in figure 1. The horizontal time axis is indexed by the scan number in the fMRI sequence while the scale index i is reported on the vertical axis of figures 1c-d. The frequency $f_0 = 0.04$ and the scale parameters are $a_i = f_0/(f_0 - |i - 1|.\Delta)$, with $\Delta = 0.002$, $1 \leq |i| \leq 15$. Color jumps from white to black correspond to $+\pi/2$ crossings for $i \leq -1$ and $-\pi/2$ crossings for $i \geq 1$ so that the color jumps at the virtual scale $i = 0$ correspond to the occurrence times of the detected dynamics changes of interest.

In practice, a feature vector $\mathbf{v} = (v_1, \cdots, v_K)$ is derived for each dynamics change detection point. Two features are retained, namely, v_1, the length of the

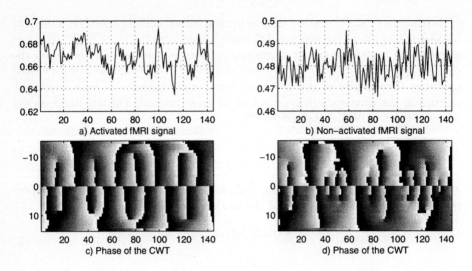

Fig. 1. Phase information of real fMRI data CWT.

corresponding fingerprint, starting at scale $i = \pm 1$ and corresponding to the integer number of associated levels of decomposition, and v_2, the sum of the square modulus along the fingerprint. Then, the event $r = (t, p, \mathbf{v})$ is formed by appending $\mathbf{v}$ to the pair (t, p) of integers where t and p denote the occurrence time and the "polarity" of the change, respectively. That is, p takes the value ± 1 according to the $\pm \pi/2$ value of the phase crossing at t. Finally, an ordered event sequence $R = r_1, r_2, \cdots, r_I$ of length $|R| = I$ is produced for every fMRI signal.

2.2   Modeling of the Stimulation Paradigm Dynamics

Dynamics modeling of a two states-based stimulation paradigm is straightforward. Every transition is modeled by an event $s = (t', p')$ where t' and p' represent the occurrence time and the "polarity" of the transition in the stimulation paradigm, respectively. As p, p' takes the arbitrary +1 or -1 value according to the OFF-ON or ON-OFF nature of the transition, respectively. Thus, the stimulation paradigm dynamics is modeled by the deterministic event sequence $S = s_1, s_2, \cdots, s_J$ of fixed length $|S| = J$, where $s_j = (t'_j, p'_j)$ models the j-th transition of the paradigm. By contrast to the multiple response sequences, it can be noticed that the stimulation sequence S is unique.

2.3   Matching of Event Sequences

The coupling distance between the stimulation sequence S and a response sequence R has been developed based on the string edit distance used in text processing [5,6]. First, "matching" operations are introduced in place of the well-known "edit" operations. A matching operation m is a pair $(x \rightarrow y) \neq (\emptyset \rightarrow \emptyset)$

where x (y) denotes either an event r_i of R (an event s_j of S) or the NULL event $\emptyset$, in place of the NULL string. Three matching operations can then be defined, namely, the insertion (ins), the deletion (del) and the valid matching (vm) which take the general forms $(\emptyset \to s_j)$, $(r_i \to \emptyset)$, $(r_i \to s_j)$, respectively.

As in the string edit distance, a specific cost $c(m)$ is assigned to each matching operation $m \in \{ins, del, vm\}$. An insertion can be considered as a misdetection of a fMRI dynamics change of interest in response to the paradigm transition s_j. Similarly, a deletion can be viewed as a false alarm. Defining the cost of a valid matching operation is less straightforward for many reasons. First, matching a fMRI dynamics change with a paradigm transition of opposite polarity is clearly unnatural and must be unvalidated as such. Second, one will assign a cost all the more low as the dynamics change to be matched is important in terms of feature magnitudes. Third, an activation delay d at a particular voxel has to be modeled. Based on these remarks, the costs of an insertion, a deletion and a valid matching operation are respectively defined by $c(ins) = w_{md}$, $c(del) = w_{fa}$, and $c(vm|d) = \alpha_0.c_0(d, t_i, t'_j) + \sum_{k=1}^{K} \alpha_k.c_k(v_k)$ where the misdetection weight w_{md} and the false alarm weight w_{fa} are preset constants. $\{\alpha_k\}$ are weighting coefficients verifying $\sum_{k=0}^{K} \alpha_k = 1$ while $\{c_k(.)\}$ are positive cost functions selected ad hoc and upper bounded (sup $(c_k(.)) = w_{max}, \forall k$). For any valid matching vm, w_{max} must verify $w_{max} \leq w_{md} + w_{fa}$. Indeed, depending on the feature magnitudes, if $w_{max} > w_{md} + w_{fa}$, it could be never useful to match two events, one can always delete and insert an event, instead. The cost functions used in our approach are simple and are plotted in figure 2. W models the detected change occurrence time

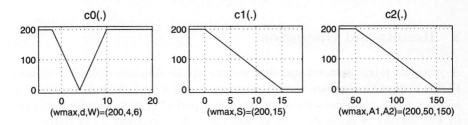

Fig. 2. Cost functions used for a valid event matching.

jitter allowed around the given delay d. S denotes the highest scale index of the CWT. $A1$ and $A2$ are real parameters arbitrarily set to the $\mu - \sigma$ and $\mu + \sigma$ values respectively where μ and σ represent the mean and the standard deviation of the feature v_2 estimated from the input voxel's sequence R.

Now, to measure the coupling distance between the stimulation sequence S and a response sequence R, one will typically need to successively apply different event matching operations. Let $M = m_1, \cdots, m_l, \cdots, m_L$ be a matching sequence of length L where $m_l \in \{ins, del, vm\}$. Then, the cost of M, $c(M)$, is defined as the sum of the costs of the elementary matching operations m_l making up the sequence, that is, $c(M) = \sum_{l=1}^{L} c(m_l)$. Given R and S, there may be more than one matching sequence M that couples R to S. If $M_{R \to S}$ denotes the set of all such sequences, then the coupling distance $dist(R \to S)$ is given by the matching sequence with the minimum cost, that is, $dist(R \to S) = min[c(M)|M \in M_{R \to S}]$. In practice, $dist(R \to S)$ is computed based on dynamic programming [5,6]. Given the activation delay $d \in D = [d_{min}, d_{max}]$, let $\delta(i, j, d)$ denote the partial minimum cost needed to match the first i events of R with the first j events of S. $\delta(i, j, d)$ is computed as follows:

> **for** i=1 **to** I **do**
> **for** j=1 **to** J **do**
> **for** d=d_{min} **to** d_{max} **do**
>   **if** $((t_i > t'_j + d - W)$ **and** $(t_i < t'_j + d + W)$ **and** $(p_i = p'_j))$ **then**
> $w(i, j, d) = c(r_i \to s_j|d);$
>   **else**
> $w(i, j, d) = w_{md} + w_{fa};$
>   **endif**
> $\delta(i, j, d) = min(\delta(i-1, j, d) + w_{fa}, \delta(i, j-1, d) + w_{md},$
> $\delta(i-1, j-1, d) + w(i, j, d))$
> **endfor**
> **endfor**
> **endfor**

The initialisations are $i)\delta(0, 0, d) = 0, \forall d$, $ii)\delta(i, 0, d) = i.w_{fa}, \forall i$, $iii)\delta(0, j, d) = j.w_{md}, \forall j$. Then, the coupling distance $dist(R \to S)$ is obtained by $dist(R \to S) = min_{d \in D} \delta(I, J, d)$, where $I = |R|$ and $J = |S|$ as stated previously.

3   Results and Discussion

A synthetic fMRI data set was first generated. To simulate distinct activated BOLD responses, a square wave, a sinus wave and a periodic Poisson signal in additive white gaussian noise were used. The period of each waveform was set to $T = 16$ ($N_a = N_c = M = 8$) so that $|S| = J = 16$ given a 145 fMRI samples time-series. The fluctuation of the synthetic BOLD response with respect to the constant baseline of magnitude 0.5 was set to $\pm 10\%$. The noise variance was set so that the SNR=20dB in the overall experiment. To simulate activation delay, the phase had a spatial random fluctuation uniformly distributed over $T/3$, along with a constant phase shift for any given activated voxel's time-series. The lag parameter of the Poisson waveform was arbitrarily set to $\lambda = 5$. The parameters used for the CWT were those mentionned in section 2.1. As a preliminary evaluation, the parameters of the coupling distance algorithm were set to $(w_{md}, w_{fa}, w_{max})$=(100,100,200) and (W, d_{min}, d_{max})=(4,-2,13) in accordance with the period T. Synthetic neural activity detection results obtained by the proposed method have been compared to those obtained by the Student's t-test. The corresponding ROC curves are plotted in figure 3. In all cases, the coupling distance method outperforms the t-test. However, the characterization

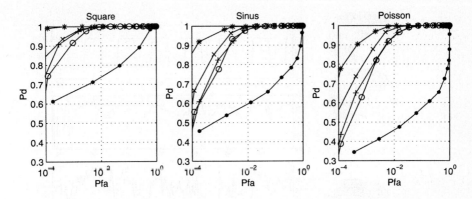

Fig. 3. Neural activity detection ROC curves obtained from synthetic fMRI data by the t-test (.) and the coupling distance method with $(\alpha_0, \alpha_1, \alpha_2) = (1, 0, 0)(*)$, $(.5, .5, 0)(+)$, $(.5, 0, .5)(x)$, $(.34, .33, .33)(o)$.

of the detected dynamics changes appears inadequate since the ROC curves for $(\alpha_0, \alpha_1, \alpha_2) = (1, 0, 0)$ remain all maximum compared with other triplets of values.

Language fMRI studies have also been conducted. Images were acquired with a 2T whole body S200 Bruker MRI system with a head volume coil. fMRI images were obtained with echo-planar imaging (EPI) using an axial slice orientation (32 slices,64x64 pixels,voxel size=4x4x4mm,TE=10ms,TR=5s). All fMRI images were registered to the first image in the series. Three testing procedures were designed to determine the cortical areas involved in word finding, auditory and visual lexical processing. Activation maps obtained for the verb generation task are compared in figure 4. Coupling distance activation maps demonstrated all together the ability of the method to detect additional activated regions with respect to the standard t-test. From a signal processing point of view, true-activated fMRI signals declared non-activated by the t-test where essentially corrupted by impulsive noise or baseline drift, or exhibited activation delays along with low SNRs.

4   Conclusion and Future Work

A new method for detecting activated voxels in fMRI brain activation studies has been presented. Unlike other methods, no a priori knowledge is required about the shape of the BOLD response expected at each voxel. In the presence of neural activity, BOLD response dynamics changes are assumed to be time-locked to some extent onto the active-control transitions of the stimulation paradigm. Time-locking is expressed in terms of a coupling distance between the sequence of dynamics changes of interest detected and characterized by a CWT and the deterministic transition sequence of the stimulation paradigm. The coupling distance is computed based on a modified version of the string edit

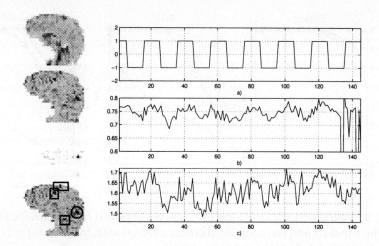

Fig. 4. Results on real fMRI data. Left side, from top to bottom: fMRI slice, coupling distance activation map, t-test activation map, copy of the coupling distance activation map with one common (circle) and three additional (rectangles) activated regions detected. Right side: a) paradigm transitions, b-c) two activated fMRI signals picked up from the rectangles of the coupling distance activation map.

distance algorithm used in text processing. The method has been compared to the standard Student's t-test on synthetic and real fMRI data. Results obtained in both cases demonstrated the superiority of the "coupling distance" approach.

The proposed method has now to be compared further. In addition, we plan to introduce spatial information in the measure of the coupling distance by reformulating the approach in terms of multiple dynamics change sequence alignment.

References

1. Bandettini, P.A., Jesmanowicz, A., Wong, E.C., Hyde, J.S.: Processing strategies for time-course data sets in functional MRI of human brain. Magn. Reson. Med., **30** (1993) 161–173
2. Friston, K.J., Jezzard, P., Turner, R.: Analysis of functional MRI time-series. Human Brain Mapping, **1** (1994) 153–171
3. Aldroubi, A., Unser M.: Wavelets in Medicine and Biology. CRC Press (1996)
4. Ruttimann, U.E., Unser, M., Rawlings, R.R., Rio, D., Ramsey, N.F., Mattay, V.S., Hommer, D.W., Frank, J.A., Weinberger, D.R.: Statistical Analysis of Functional MRI Data in the Wavelet Domain. IEEE Trans. Med. Imaging, **17** (1998) 142–154
5. Wagner, R.A., Fischer, M.J.: The string-to-string correction problem. J. Assoc. Comput. Machinery, **21** (1974) 168–173
6. Marzal, A., Vidal, E.: Computation of normalized edit distances and applications. IEEE Trans. Pat. Ana. Mach. Int., **15** (1993) 926–932

Cardiac Motion Analysis from Ultrasound Sequences Using Non-rigid Registration

María J. Ledesma-Carbayo[1], Jan Kybic[2], Manuel Desco[3], Andrés Santos[1], and Michael Unser[2]

[1] ETSI Telecomunicación,
Universidad Politécnica de Madrid,
Ciudad Universitaria s/n 28040 Madrid, Spain
mledesma@die.upm.es
[2] Department of Microengineering,
Swiss Federal Institute of Technology Lausanne,
CH-1015 Ecublens, Switzerland
Jan.Kybic@epfl.ch
[3] Unidad de Medicina y Cirugía Experimental,
Hospital General Universitario Gregorio Marañón,
Dr. Esquerdo 46, E-28007 Madrid, Spain
desco@mce.hggm.es

Abstract. In this article we propose a cardiac motion estimation technique that uses non-rigid registration to compute the dense cardiac displacement field from 2D ultrasound sequences. Our method employs a semi-local deformation model which provides controlled smoothness. We apply a multiresolution optimization strategy for better speed and robustness. To further improve the accuracy, the sequence is registered in both forward and backward directions. We calculate additional parameters from the displacement field, such as total displacement and strain.

We create an artificial ultrasound sequence of one heart cycle using a motion model and use it to validate the accuracy of the algorithm. Finally, we present results on real data from normal and pathological subjects that show the clinical applicability of our method.

1 Introduction

Cardiac motion estimation constitutes an important aid for the quantification of the elastic and contractility properties of the myocardium. Localized regions with movement abnormalities are related to the existence of ischemic segments, damaged by insufficient tissue microcirculation.

MR imaging and especially tagged MR are currently the reference modalities to estimate dense cardiac displacement fields with high spatial resolution. The deformation fields, as well as derived parameters such as myocardial strain, can be found with good accuracy [1, 2, 3].

Nuclear modalities, such as SPECT and PET were used [4] despite their low spatial and temporal resolutions, high cost and the requirement for specialized

W. Niessen and M. Viergever (Eds.): MICCAI 2001, LNCS 2208, pp. 889–896, 2001.
© Springer-Verlag Berlin Heidelberg 2001

equipment [5, 6]. Computed tomography has also been considered [7, 8] but has the drawback of high patient radiation dose.

Echocardiography is currently the imaging method most widely used to assess cardiac function. It offers significant advantages over the rest of the imaging techniques: availability, portability, low cost, and no adverse secondary effects. While new ultrasound techniques provide high image quality, increasing attention is being paid to the automatic processing of ultrasound image sequences [8, 9, 10, 11].

Many of the aforementioned approaches to cardiac motion analysis start by the segmentation of the myocardial wall, followed by geometrical and mechanical modelling using active contours or surfaces to extract the displacement field and to perform the motion analysis [8, 9, 3]. Some authors introduce temporal modelling of the cardiac motion to provide temporal smoothness and better motion tracking [1, 2]. Alternative methods use energy-based warping and optical flow techniques to compute the displacement of the myocardium [5, 6, 7].

For echocardiography, deformable and mechanical model-based techniques are the most popular. They require a presegmentation step which is particularly difficult in the case of cardiac ultrasound images due to the noise and the complexity of cardiac structure [8, 9, 10]. Speckle tracking techniques have also been proposed to estimate heart motion [11].

Here we propose to compute the dense cardiac displacement field from ultrasound sequences using a non-rigid registration algorithm based on a global pixel-based matching criterion. To the best of our knowledge, this kind of approach has not been pursued before, except for the simpler case of M-mode data where dynamic programming-based unidimensional registration has been used [12]. We present a fully automatic method that does not require segmentation. We use a semi-local deformation model that provides controlled smoothness of the motion field. Multiresolution strategy yields speed and robustness with respect to the speckle changes in time. While we deploy the methodology for bidimensional ultrasound sequences, it is also applicable to 3D data.

The accuracy of the algorithm was validated using an artificial heart motion model. Real data from normal and pathological subjects were also analysed to show the clinical applicability of the method.

2   Methodology

2.1   Non-rigid Registration Method

The workhorse of our approach is an elastic registration algorithm. Given a reference image f_r and a test image f_t, it finds a correspondence function $\mathbf{g}$, which relates coordinates in f_t and f_r. More specifically, we consider registration as a minimization problem. We search a correspondence function $\mathbf{g} : \mathbb{R}^2 \to \mathbb{R}^2$, such that the warped test image $f_w(\mathbf{x}) = f_t(\mathbf{g}(\mathbf{x}))$ is as close as possible to the reference image f_r. We measure the quality of the fit using a sum of squared differences (SSD) criterion

$$E = \sum_{i \in I} e_i^2 = \sum_{i \in I} \left(f_w(i) - f_r(i) \right)^2 \tag{1}$$

where the summation is taken over all the pixels in the reference image. We generate a continuous version f_t^c of the discrete image f_t by spline interpolation.

$$f_t^c(\mathbf{x}) = \sum_{i \in I} b_i \beta_q(\mathbf{x} - i) \tag{2}$$

where $\beta_q(\mathbf{x})$ is a tensor product of centered B-splines of degree q. It has the advantage of good accuracy and the possibility of evaluating spatial derivatives analytically. We represent the correspondence function $\mathbf{g}$ using splines as well.

$$\mathbf{g}(\mathbf{x}) = \mathbf{x} + \sum_{j \in \mathbb{Z}^N} \mathbf{c}_j \beta_r \left(\mathbf{x}/h - \mathbf{j} \right) \tag{3}$$

Therefore $\mathbf{g}$ is a linear combination of basis functions $\beta_r(\mathbf{x})$ placed on a rectangular grid. The scale parameter h governs the node spacing, the total number of parameters $\mathbf{c}_j$, and the smoothness of the solution. The advantages of this model are good approximation properties, fast evaluation of the deformation, local influence of the parameters, and automatically imposed smoothness.

The resulting problem of optimising (1) with respect to the coefficients $\mathbf{c}_j$ is solved using a standard multidimensional optimisation algorithm. We found that a Marquardt-Levenberg-like algorithm was fastest with respect to the number of iterations, while simple gradient descent-like optimizer converged in the least amount of time.

The original idea of the algorithm was described in [13] and its extensions to multiple dimensions in [14]. For the present application, the algorithm was completely redesigned, resulting in a major speed-up. It now registers 256×256 images pixels in less than 10 s with subpixel precision on a standard PC. The time required is essentially proportional to the number of pixels.

For the echocardiographic sequences we typically use a control grid of 8×8 points, represent the deformation using quadratic or cubic splines, and the image using cubic or linear splines.

2.2   Extraction of the Displacement Field

The input to our algorithm is an ultrasound sequence of a cardiac cycle composed of N images (frames). We apply the registration algorithm to consecutive pairs of frames within the sequence. The correspondence function $\mathbf{g}$ from (3) provides the displacement field between images i and $i + 1$ which we denote $\mathbf{r}_{i,i+1}^f$. That is, a point at position $\mathbf{x}$ in image i moves to position $\mathbf{x} + \mathbf{r}_{i,i+1}^f(\mathbf{x})$ in image $i+1$. The cumulative displacement field along the sequence for a given frame $i + 1$ is then computed as

$$\mathbf{r}_{0,i+1}^f = \mathbf{r}_{0,i}^f + \mathbf{r}_{i,i+1}^f \quad \text{with} \quad \mathbf{r}_{0,0}^f = 0 \tag{4}$$

where for brevity we have omitted the spatial coordinates $\mathbf{x} = (x, y)$. As our sequence is cyclic, $\mathbf{r}^f_{0,N} \equiv \mathbf{r}^f_{0,0}$ should be equal to zero. In practice, we find this error to be small, typically about one pixel. For even better precision, we carry on the registration backward, yielding $\mathbf{r}^b_{i,i-1}$ and a cumulative field

$$\mathbf{r}^b_{0,i} \equiv \mathbf{r}^b_{N,i} = \mathbf{r}^b_{N,i+1} + \mathbf{r}^b_{i+1,i} \tag{5}$$

If we consider the error distribution of the registration as independent, identically distributed and normal, then the maximum likelihood (ML) estimate of the cumulative displacement is

$$\mathbf{r}_{0,i} = \omega_i \mathbf{r}^f_{0,i} + (1 - \omega_i)\mathbf{r}^b_{0,i} \quad \text{with} \quad \omega_i = \frac{N - i}{N} \tag{6}$$

2.3   Spatio-temporal Derived Parameters

Once the displacement field is obtained, other parameters of clinical interest are computed. We calculate the velocity and acceleration fields

$$\mathbf{v}_i = \frac{\partial \mathbf{r}_i}{\partial t} \qquad \mathbf{a}_i = \frac{\partial^2 \mathbf{r}_i}{\partial t^2} \tag{7}$$

We compute also the Lagrangian strain, which provides information about my-ocardial contractility [15, 5]. Strain is defined as the spatial gradient $\boldsymbol{\varepsilon} = \nabla_\mathbf{x} \mathbf{r}$ where $\boldsymbol{\varepsilon}$ is the strain tensor, with diagonal terms $\partial r_x/\partial x$ and $\partial r_y/\partial y$ corresponding to normal directional strains, and antidiagonal terms corresponding to shear strains. The spline representation (3) allows for an analytical computation of the strain.

2.4   Simulated Sequence Model

An artificial ultrasound sequence has been generated to validate the algorithm. The sequence is generated by warping an end-diastole apical view image using cubic spline interpolation (2). We used the following motion model

$$\mathbf{r}_{0,i}(\mathbf{x}) = \begin{bmatrix} \sin^2(i\pi/T)a_x \sin \frac{\pi(x_0 - x)}{2|x_{\max} - x_0|} \\ \sin^2(i\pi/T)a_y \end{bmatrix}^T \tag{8}$$

where i is the frame index and x_0 is the coordinate of the left ventricular long axis, which is oriented vertically; i.e., parallel to axis y. We corrupted the deformed images by a multiplicative Rayleigh noise η_m representing speckle changes, and an additive Gaussian noise η_a to simulate acoustic attenuation [16, 17].

$$n(\mathbf{x}) = \eta_m \sqrt{f(\mathbf{x})} + \eta_a \quad \text{where} \quad \eta_a \sim \mathcal{N}(0, \sigma), \ \eta_m \sim \mathcal{R}(\alpha) = \frac{z}{\alpha^2}e^{-z^2/2\alpha^2}$$

and $f(\mathbf{x})$ is the original image. For our images in the $0 \sim 255$ range, we used $\sigma = 20$ and $\alpha \approx 0.8$, which corresponds to $\mathrm{E}[\eta_m] = 1$.

2.5 Real Sequences

Real data from normal volunteers and ischemic patients were acquired with a Siemens-ACUSON Sequoia© scanner (Mountain View, CA, USA). Two and four chamber view sequences of the left ventricle were analysed.

3 Experiments and Results

3.1 Simulated Sequence

This section presents the results with the artificial sequence described in Section 2.4. First, a series of experiments was conducted to choose the most suitable parameters for the registration algorithm. Figure 1 shows the accumulated displacement and velocity fields as small arrows superimposed on the ultrasound images.

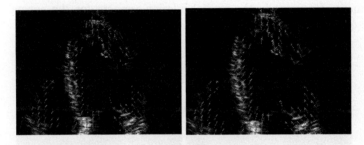

Fig. 1. Simulated sequence results. *Left*: Accumulated displacement field at the time of maximum contraction ($t = 320$ ms). *Right*: Velocity field during contraction ($t = 120$ ms).

Figure 2 shows the axial and longitudinal accumulated displacements for a middle septum point (a point in the middle of the vertical wall on the left in the images). Even in this noisy case we found good agreement between the true movement and the movement found by the algorithm. The mean square error over the whole sequence for 25 selected points within the myocardium was 1.3 mm.

3.2 Real Sequences

In this section, we describe experiments on real sequences from normal volunteers and ischemic patients. Figure 3 shows the computed displacement field vectors of two chamber view sequences from a normal volunteer and an ischemic patient. The ischemic patient presents an infarct in the inferior wall with severe hypokinesis and a normokinetic basal aneterior segment. For the healthy volunteer the accumulated displacement observed corresponds to normal left ventricular contraction. On the other hand the analysis of the ischemic patient

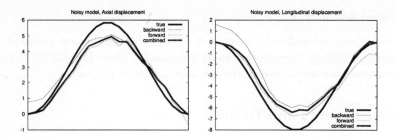

Fig. 2. Simulated sequence results. Axial *(left)* and longitudinal *(right)* displacements in mm for a middle septum point. Real displacements, results of the forward and backward registration, and the combined result.

confirms the pathological function of the inferior wall, having very small movement, and quasi normal motion of the basal anterior segment. These results are also shown quantitatively in Figure 4 that represents the axial and longitudinal displacement of a point in the medial inferior segment for the normal and the ischemic cases.

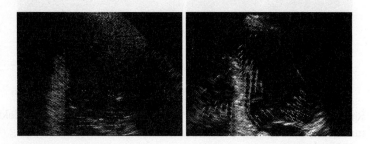

Fig. 3. Accumulated displacement field at the mechanical systole for a normal subject *(right)* and an ischemic patient with inferior infarct *(left)*.

Figure 5 shows the results of the analysis of a four chamber sequence from an ischemic patient with hypokinetic function of the lateral wall and basal and distal septum segments. The displacement field correlates well with the diagnosis. Strain analysis shows constantly low lagrangian longitudinal strain and normal axial strain for the medial and distal septum segments.

4   Conclusions

We have presented a fully automatic method to compute myocardial displacement and deformations from ultrasound sequences. The method has been validated on simulated and real sequences. Results show that the proposed method is able to estimate heart motion and to provide plausible displacement and velocity fields. The results of applying the method to data from normal and ischemic

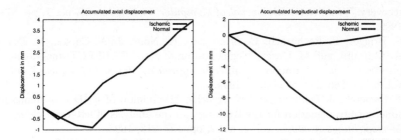

Fig. 4. Axial and longitudinal systolic displacements of a medial inferior segment point for a normal volunteer and an ischemic patient with inferior infart.

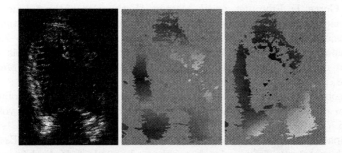

Fig. 5. Accumulated displacement for a four chamber sequence of an ischemic patient *(left)*. Axial *(middle)* and longitudinal *(right)* strain images for mid-systole ($t = 120$ ms).

patients is promising and encourages clinical applicability. Further clinical validation is planned for the immediate future.

Acknowledgements

This work was supported in part by grant No 3200-059517.99/1 from the Swiss Science Foundation, and the Spanish projects TIC99-1085 and III-PRICYT.

References

[1] P. Clarysse, C. Basset, L. Khouas, P. Croisille, D. Friboulet, C. Odet, and I. Magnin, "Two-dimensional spatial and temporal displacement and deformation field fitting from cardiac magnetic resonance tagging," *Medical Image Analysis*, vol. 4, no. 4, pp. 253–268, 2000.

[2] J. C. McEachen, A. Nehorai, and J. S. Duncan, "Multiframe temporal estimation of cardiac nonrigid motion," *IEEE Trans. Med. Imag.*, vol. 9, pp. 651–664, April 2000.

[3] P. Shi, A. J. Sinusas, R. T. Constable, and J. S. Duncan, "Volumetric deformation analysis using mechanics-based data fusion: applications in cardiac motion

recovery.," *International Journal of Computer Vision*, vol. 35, no. 1, pp. 87–107, 1999.

[4] P. Brigger, S. Bacharach, G. Srinivasan, K. Nour, J. A. Carson, V. Dilsizian, A. Aldroubi, and M. Unser, "Segmentation of gated Tl-SPECT images and computation of ejection fraction: A different approach," *Journal of Nuclear Cardiology*, vol. 6, pp. 286–297, May-June 1999.

[5] J. Declerck, J. Feldmar, and N. Ayache, "Defininion of a 4D continuous planispheric transformation for the tracking and the analysis of left-ventricle motion," *Medical Image Analysis*, vol. 2, no. 2, pp. 197–213, 1998.

[6] J.-P. Thirion and S. Benayoun, "Myotrack: A 3D deformation field method to measure cardiac motion from gated SPECT," in *Proc. MICCAI 2000, Lecture Notes in Computer Science, vol. 1935* (B. J. Scott L. Delp, Anthony M.DiGioia, ed.), pp. 697–706, Springer Verlag, Berlin, Oct. 2000.

[7] J.-M. Gorce, D. Fibroulet, and I. Magnin, "Estimation of three dimensional cardiac velocity fields: assessment of a diferential method and application to three-dimensional CT data," *Medical Image Analysis*, vol. 1, no. 3, pp. 245–261, 1996/7.

[8] C. Nastar and N. Ayache, "Frequency-based nonrigid motion analysis application to four dimensional medical images," *IEEE Trans. Pattern Anal. Mach. Intell.*, vol. 18, pp. 1067–1079, November 1996.

[9] G. Jacob, A. Noble, M. Mulet-Parada, and A. Blake, "Evaluating a robust contour tracker on echocardiographic sequences," *Medical Image Analysis*, vol. 3, no. 1, pp. 63–75, 1999.

[10] X. Papademetris, A. J. Sinusas, D. P. Donald, and J. S. Duncan, "Estimation of 3D left ventricular deformation from echocardiography," *Medical Image Analysis*, vol. 5, pp. 17–28, March 2001.

[11] F. Yeung, F. Levinson, D. Fu, and K. J. Parker, "Feature-adaptive motion tracking of ultrasound image sequences using a deformable mesh," *IEEE Trans. Med. Imag.*, vol. 17, pp. 945–956, Dec. 1998.

[12] M. Unser, G. Pelle, P. Brun, and M. Eden, "Computer analysis of M-mode echocardiograms: estimation of spatial deformation with time," in *Cardiovascular Dynamics and Models*, pp. 304–310, Paris: Institut National de la Santé et de la Recherche Médicale, 1988.

[13] J. Kybic, P. Thévenaz, A. Nirkko, and M. Unser, "Unwarping of unidirectionally distorted EPI images," *IEEE Trans. Med. Imag.*, vol. 19, pp. 80–93, Feb. 2000.

[14] J. Kybic and M. Unser, "Multidimensional elastic registration of images using splines," in *Proceedings of ICIP*, (Vancouver, Canada), 2000.

[15] J. D'hooge, A. Heimdal, F. Jamal, T. Kukuslki, R. F. Bijnens, B. and, L. Hatle, P. Suetens, and G. Sutherland, "Regional strain and strain rate measurements by cardiac ultrasound: Principles, implemantation and limitations.," *Eur J. Echocardiography*, vol. 1, pp. 154–170, 2000.

[16] X. Zong, A. Laine, and E. Geiser, "Speckle reduction and contrast enhancement of echocardiograms via multiscale nonlinear processing," *IEEE Trans. Med. Imag.*, vol. 17, no. 4, pp. 532–540, 1998.

[17] T. Loupas, W. McDicken, and P. Allan, "An adaptive weighted median filter for speckle suppression in medical ultrasonic images," *IEEE Trans. Circ. Syst.*, vol. 36, pp. 129–135, Jan. 1989.

A Mean Curvature Based Primal Sketch to Study the Cortical Folding Process from Antenatal to Adult Brain

A. Cachia[1,4,5], J.-F. Mangin[1,5], D. Rivière[1,5], N. Boddaert[2,5], A. Andrade[1,5], F. Kherif[1,5], P. Sonigo[2,5], D. Papadopoulos-Orfanos[1,5], M. Zilbovicius[1,5], J.-B. Poline[1,5], I. Bloch[4,5], F. Brunelle[2,5], and J. Régis[3]

[1] Service Hospitalier Frédéric Joliot, CEA, 91401 Orsay, France
mangin@shfj.cea.fr, http://www-dsv.cea.fr/
[2] Service de Radiologie Pédiatrique, Hopital Necker, Paris
[3] Service de Neurochirurgie Fonctionnelle et Stéréotaxique, La Timone, Marseille
[4] Département Traitement du Signal et des Images, CNRS URA 820, ENST, Paris
[5] Institut Fédératif de Recherche 49

Abstract. In this paper, we propose a new representation of the cortical surface that may be used to study the cortex folding process and to recover foetus sulcal roots usually burried in the depth of adult brains. This representation is a primal sketch derived from a scale space computed for the mean curvature of the cortical surface. This scale-space stems from a geodesic diffusion equation conditionaly to the cortical surface. The primal sketch is made up of objects defined from mean curvature minima and saddle points. The resulting sketch aims first at highlighting significant elementary folds, second at representing the fold merging process during brain growth. The relevance of the framework is illustrated by the study of central sulcus sulcal roots in antenatal, baby and adult images.

1 Introduction

The most striking, interesting, yet poorly understood gross morphological features of the human cerebral cortex are the diverse and complex arrangements of gyri and sulci [22]. Cortical folding patterns exhibit various forms in different individuals [13]. This prevents the brain mapping community from using them as a straightforward and accurate referential to localize functional activations. Recent works claim that the solution should stem from a better understanding of the brain growth process [14, 18]. The primary cortical folds that appear on the foetus cortex, indeed, seem to be especially stable across individuals. During ulterior stages of brain growth, these sulcal roots merge with each other and form different patterns depending on the subjects. Deformations of the depth of adult cortical sulci corresponding to burried gyri, however, may be some clues to the sulcal root fusions (see Fig. 1) [14, 10]. Therefore, a map of these sulcal roots

W. Niessen and M. Viergever (Eds.): MICCAI 2001, LNCS 2208, pp. 897–904, 2001.

may turn out to be the adequate generic model required to match different adult folding patterns. Moreover, a map including statistics on sulcal roots chronology and dates of appearance may become a precious tool for early detection of development problems suspected from antenatal MR images.

In this paper, we propose a new representation of the cortical surface that may be used to study the cortex folding process and to recover sulcal roots usually buried in the depth of adult brains. This representation is a primal sketch [12, 1] derived from a scale space [23, 7] computed for the mean curvature of the cortical surface. This scale-space stems from a diffusion equation geodesic to the cortical surface. The primal sketch is made up of objects defined from mean curvature extrema and saddle points, like in previous approaches [8, 9]. The resulting sketch aims first at highlighting significant elementary folds, second at representing the fold merging process during brain growth. The method has been tested with antenatal, baby and adult MR images. Antenatal and children images have been acquired for clinical purposes.

2   Spherical Mesh of the Cortical Surface

The first stage of the method consists in extracting a smooth mesh representing the cortical surface. This mesh is endowed with the actual spherical topology of this surface, which allows the implementation of geodesic diffusion or inflation operations. In the case of children and adult brains, T1-weighted MR images obtained from an inversion recovery sequence are used. In the case of antenatal or small baby brains, the axon myelinisation is still in progress, which means that T1-weighted images show no contrast between gray and white matters. Hence T2-weighted images, which provide a better contrast (see Fig. 1) but a larger slice thickness, are acquired.

An automatic robust method for detecting a white matter interface of spherical topology from T1-weighted images has been previously described [11]. This method has been adapted to T2-weighted images in order to yield a semi-automatic toolbox dedicated to fetus and baby brains. Designing a fully automatic method was beyond the scope of this adaptation because of the frequent artefacts induced by fetus motions. The interface currently detected to represent the cortical surface is located between the cerebro spinal fluid and the brain tissues. While this choice is sufficient to detect dimples bound to become a fold, further work should be done to detect the gray/white matter interface.

The method mentioned above provides a binary mask endowed with a spherical topology interface. A standard facet tracking algorithm is used first to compute a spherical graph made up of facets [5]. Then, the center of each facet is connected to the center of the neighboring facets in order to yield a smooth spherical mesh of triangles. This algorithm which preserves the initial topology relies on a look-up table of configurations like in the marching cube algorithm. Finally, a decimation including smoothing is performed to discard stair artefacts related to the underlying discretization. The decimation algorithm is inspired by the algorithm used in the Vtk package [20]. The embedded smoothing operation slightly moves nodes towards their neighborhood gravity center, which may be related to some usual surface evolution processes [15].

3   Mean Curvature

Different approaches can be used to study fine details of the cortical surface folding patterns. Depth maxima have been used to detect a concept similar to sulcal roots in [10]. In this paper, mean curvature (H) is proposed as a richer descriptor (than the depth) of the various features that can be observed along sulcus bottoms and walls, which is illustrated in figure 2: fold bottoms appear as local minima of H while gyrus crown appear as maxima. Hence, buried gyri appear as areas of positive curvature along the sulcus walls. Other curvature related features, such as Koenderink's curvature metric C (the L2 norm of the principal curvatures, or the logarithm thereof) or the maximum principal curvature, may be interesting for our purpose and will be investigated in the future. In this paper, mean curvature is directly estimated from the mesh thanks to its relative smoothness. We used an approximation proposed in [19] that takes into account some local properties of the mesh, as triangle angles and areas, dihedral angles between normals and edge lengths (see Fig. 2). This method is considered to be as accurate and robust as quadratic patch based approaches.

4   Scale Space and Geodesic Diffusion

The curvature map of the cortical surface contains much geometrical information that may be related to the anatomical elements that have to be detected (sulcal roots, sulci, etc). These elements, however, correspond to different levels of scale (see Fig. 3). Moreover, a scale based point of view is required to distinguish anatomical elements from noise features bound to appear in curvature approximations (see Fig. 2). The scale-space paradigm has been developed to deal with such problems where all the scales can be of interest. Among the many possible scale-space approaches that could be used to study cortex shapes, we have chosen in this paper a standard heat equation [7] applied to mean curvature. One intriguing feature of our method that will be discussed later is the fact that heat equation has been implemented geodesically to the surface from which the mean curvature map stems.

The fact that the 2D lattice is embedded in a volume raises a problem concerning the parameterization upon which to base the estimation of the local partial derivatives. The parameterization adopted was a simple local transformation that maps each surface element (a node and its first neighbours) into a plane, while keeping unchanged both edge distances and angular proportions between the edges [21, 2]. An individual parameterization is defined for each node. Locally mapping each surface element into the plane avoids the severe areal distortion that would result from a global flattening.

Implementation of partial differential equations on irregular lattices can lead to complex problems. The causality property usually required by the scale-space framework may be lost because of discrete phenomena. This point is beyond the scope of this paper and would require further study. Our implementation is carried out as an iterative process of the form:

$$H(M, t + \delta t) = H(M, t) + \delta t \widehat{\Delta} H(M, t) \qquad (1)$$

for each point M and each temporal iteration step δt, where $\widehat{\Delta}$ is an estimate of a Laplacian. Using the 2D parameterization, the Laplacian can be estimated using the approach proposed in [6], based on Taylor series expansion of a function around a point. For each neighbor (u_i, v_i) of a given point $M = (u_0, v_0)$, this expansion has the form:

$$H_i = H_0 + h_i \frac{\partial H_0}{\partial u} + k_i \frac{\partial H_0}{\partial v} + \frac{h_i^2}{2} \frac{\partial^2 H_0}{\partial u^2} + \frac{k_i^2}{2} \frac{\partial^2 H_0}{\partial v^2} + k_i h_i \frac{\partial^2 H_0}{\partial u \partial v} + O(\delta^3) \quad (2)$$

$H_i = H(u_i, v_i)$, $\frac{\partial H_0}{\partial u} = \frac{\partial H}{\partial u}(u_0, v_0)$, $h_i = u_i - u_0$, $k_i = v_i - v_0$, and $\delta = \sqrt{h_i^2 + k_i^2}$. Writing Equation 2 for all neighbors $i = 1, 2, ...m$, we obtain for each point M the set of equations

$$[A][DH] - [H] = [0]$$

$$[A] = \begin{bmatrix} h_1 & k_1 & \frac{h_1^2}{2} & \frac{k_1^2}{2} & h_1 k_1 \\ h_2 & \cdots & \cdots & \cdots & \cdots \\ \vdots & & & & \\ \vdots & & & & \\ h_m & & & & \end{bmatrix}$$

$$[H] = [H_1 - H_0, ..., H_m - H_0]^T, [DH] = \left[\frac{\partial H_0}{\partial u}, \frac{\partial H_0}{\partial v}, \frac{\partial^2 H_0}{\partial u^2}, \frac{\partial^2 H_0}{\partial v^2}, \frac{\partial H_0^2}{\partial u \partial v} \right]^T.$$

This system of equations is solved once at the beginning of the diffusion process.

The initial mesh construction includes some smoothing operations that may remove some interesting anatomical information. This smoothing process appears important to get initial acceptable mean curvature maps, but other diffusion processes could be less restrictive. Surface evolution according to a function of mean curvature could be an interesting alternative to our geodesic smoothing process [15]. This evolution, however, can not be implemented according to the powerful level set framework, because of the implicit definition of the surface. This framework, indeed, allows topological modification of the tracked isosurface, and provides no constant parameterization that may be used to track objects across scales. A mesh based implementation, in return, may be used for the evolution process. While a similar implementation is used to inflate our cortical surfaces [4], this last algorithm includes additional constraints minimizing local distortions. Therefore, no such attempt has been done for the moment. It should be understood, however, that mean curvature should be recomputed during each iteration, which could be incompatible with the causality constraint of the scale-space framework. Finally, anisotropic diffusion scheme could lead to other interesting improvements of our framework [16].

5   The Primal Sketch of the Mean Curvature

A primal sketch is constructed from the mean curvature scale-space using the algorithm proposed by Lindeberg applied to the opposite of the mean curvature [9]. Grey level (GL) blobs are extracted first from each level of scale. One GL blob is defined from each local minimum of the smoothed mean curvature. The blob extent is defined from a water rise like algorithm which is stopped by saddle points or background. Hence, each GL blob is defined by two extremal points,maximum and *stop* point, whose behavior in the scale-space is well known from a theoretical point of view. These extremal points appear or disappear according to events called anihilation, merge or split. GL blobs are linked across scales in order to create scale-space blobs supposed to correspond to the objects embedded in the initial curvature map. A scale-space blob is made up of a chain of GL blobs beginning and ending by one of the events mentionned above.

6   Results and Discussion

Figure 4 provides a glimpse on the primal sketch focused on the central sulcus of an adult brain. The structure of this sub-sketch is consistent with our initial aims. First, the three highest scale-space blobs are linked by an event which seems to correspond to the merge of the central sulcus sulcal roots described by neuroanatomists [14]. Second, the two sulcal roots have a longer life time throughout scales than noise related blobs. A fine analysis of the lower part of the sketch, however, shows that some instabilities may stem from spurious *split* events induced by the elongated shape of the sulcus related blobs. This will lead us to add some pruning operation into the standard approach.

The new representation of the sulcal folding patterns presented in this paper will be used to infer a finer grained than usual generic model of the human corti-cal surface. While such results would greatly improve our current understanding of the cortex inter-individual matching issues, a lot of anatomical work remains to be done to find the link between foetal patterns of sulcal roots, and their pri-mal sketch analogue. While a first manual exploration is required to match the new representations with our current sulcal root maps, an automatic strategy should be devised to get a more reliable generic model. Few approaches have been proposed for such inference of high level models of brain anatomy. Some ideas could stem from similar work done from skull crest lines [17]. Another attractive direction consists of Markovian models for the comparison of primal sketches developed to match activation maps across individuals [3].

References

[1] H. Asada and M. Brady. The curvature primal sketch. *IEEE PAMI*, 8:2–14, 1986.
[2] A. Andrade, F. Kherif, J.-F. Mangin, K. Worsley, A.L. Paradis, O. Simon, S. Dehaene, D. Le Bihan and J.-B. Poline Detection of fMRI activation using cortical surface mapping *Human Brain Mapping*, 12(2):79-93, 2001.

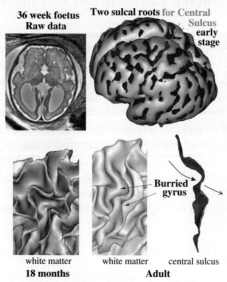

36 week foetus Raw data

Two sulcal roots for Central Sulcus early stage

Burried gyrus

white matter
18 months

white matter   central sulcus
Adult

Fig. 1. *Evolution of the central sulcus shape during brain growth.* **Up:** *Antenatal images allow the reconstruction of the foetus cortex surface on which shallow dimples corresponding to negative mean curvature areas are highligted in blue. At that stage, the central sulcus is made up of two sulcal roots.* **Down left:** *18 months after birth, the gyrus separating the two sulcal roots is still visible on white matter surface.* **Down right:** *At adult stage, only slight deformations of the central sulcus walls give clues on the presence of a burried gyrus.*

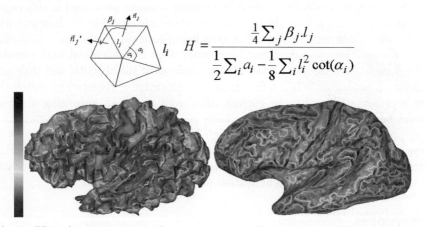

$$H = \frac{\frac{1}{4}\sum_j \beta_j . l_j}{\frac{1}{2}\sum_i a_i - \frac{1}{8}\sum_i l_i^2 \cot(\alpha_i)}$$

Fig. 2. **Up:** *Approximation of mean curvature from an irregular mesh.* **Down:** *Mean curvature of the white matter surface (adult brain), mapped on itself (left) and on an inflated version [4] (right). Red (negative) areas correspond to sulci, while blue (positive) areas correspond to gyri.*

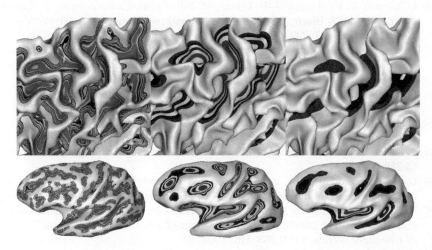

Fig. 3. *Some isophotes of mean curvature at different scales. Central sulcus includes two curvature minima at middle scale, and finally only one minima at highest scale. The middle scale minima will correspond to two blobs in the final primal sketch. The saddle point which separates these two blobs is located at the level of the burried gyrus related clues. Hence, these blobs may correspond to central sulcus sulcal roots.*

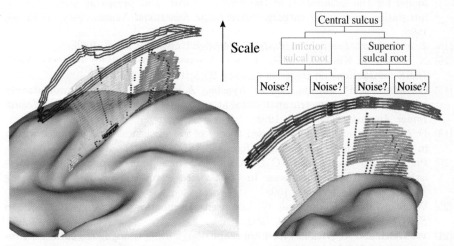

Fig. 4. *Primal sketch of the mean curvature of the central sulcus. Each scale-space blob has its own color. Red points correspond to the curvature minima from which the grey level blob growth begins. Purple points between two blobs and green points between one blob and the background, correspond to points stopping blob growth.*

[3] O. Coulon, J.-F. Mangin, J.-B. Poline, M. Zilbovicius, D. Roumenov, Y. Samson, V. Frouin, and I. Bloch. Structural group analysis of functional activation maps. *NeuroImage*, 11:767–782, 2000.

[4] H.A. Drury, D.C. Van Essen, C. H. Anderson et al. Computerized mappings of the cerebral cortex : a multiresolution flattening method and a surface based coordinate system. *Journal of cognitive neuroscience*, 8(1):1–28, 1996.

[5] D. Gordon and J. Udupa. Fast surface tracking in three-dimensional binary images. *Computer Vision, Graphics, and Image Processing*, 45(6):196–214, 1989.

[6] G. Huiskamp. Different formulas for the surface Laplacian on a triangulated surface. *Journal of computational physics*, 95:477–496, 1991.

[7] J. Koenderink and A. van Doorn. The structure of images. *Biological Cybernetics*, 53:383–396, 1984.

[8] L. Lifshitz and S. Pizer. A multiresolution hierarchical approach to image segmentation based on intensity extrema. *IEEE Trans. PAMI*, 12(6):529–540, 1990.

[9] T. Lindeberg. Detecting salient blob-like image structures and their scales with a scale-space primal sketch: a method for focus-of-attention. *International Journal of Computer Vision*, 11(3):283–318, 1993.

[10] G. Lohmann and D. Y. von Cramon. Automatic labelling of the human cortical surface using sulcal basins. *Medical Image analysis*, 4(3):179–188, 2000.

[11] J.-F. Mangin, V. Frouin, I. Bloch, J. Regis, and J. López-Krahe. From 3D MR images to structural representations of the cortex topography using topology preserving deformations. *J. Mathematical Imaging and Vision*, 5(4):297–318, 1995.

[12] D. Marr. *Vision*. W. H. Freeman, NewYork, 1982.

[13] M. Ono, S. Kubik, and C. D. Abernethey. *Atlas of the Cerebral Sulci*. Georg Thieme Verlag, 1990.

[14] J. Régis, J.-F. Mangin, V. Frouin, F. Sastre, J. C. Peragut, and Y. Samson. Generic model for the localization of the cerebral cortex and preoperative multimodal integration in epilepsy surgery. *Stereotactic Functional Neurosurgery*, 65:72–80, 1995.

[15] J. A. Sethian. *Level set methods*. Cambridge University Press, 1996.

[16] N. Sochen, R. Kimmel, and R. Malladi. A general framework for low level vision. *IEEE transactions on image processing*, 20(5):100–107, 1999.

[17] G. Subsol, J.-P. Thirion, and N. Ayache. A general scheme for automatically building 3D morphometric anatomical atlases: application to a skull atlas. *Medical Image Analysis*, 2(1):37–60, 1998.

[18] D. C. Van Essen. A tension-based theory of morphogenesis and compact wiring in the central nervous system. *Nature*, 385:313–318, 1997.

[19] Ph. Veron, D. Lesage, and J-C. Leon. Outils de base pour l'extraction de caracteristiques de surfaces numerisees. In *7eme assises europeene du prototypage rapide - Ecole Centrale de Paris*, 1998.

[20] W. Schroeder,J. Zarge, and W. Lorensen Decimation of triangle meshes. In *SIGGRAPH'92*, pages 65–70, 1992.

[21] W. Welch and A. Witkin. Free-form shape design using triangulated surfaces. *Proceedings of SIGGRAPH '94, Computer Graphics Proceedings, Annual Conference Series (July 1994, Orlando, Florida)*, pages 247–256, 1994.

[22] W. Welker. Why does the cerebral cortex fissure and fold. *Cerebral Cortex*, 8B:3–135, 1989.

[23] A. Witkin. Scale-space filtering. In *Int. Joint. Conf. on Artificial Intelligence*, pages 1019–1023, 1983.

Adaptive Entropy Rates for *f*MRI Time-Series Analysis*

John W. Fisher III[1], Eric R. Cosman, Jr.[1], Cindy Wible[2], and
William M. Wells III[1,2]

[1] Massachusetts Institute of Technology,
Artificial Intelligence Laboratory,
Cambridge, MA, USA
{fisher, ercosman, sw,}@ai.mit.edu
[2] Harvard Medical School,
Brigham and Women's Hospital,
Department of Radiology,
Boston, MA, USA
cindy@bwh.harvard.edu

Abstract. In previous work [Tsai *et al* , 1999] we introduced an information theoretic approach for analysis of *f*MRI time-series data. Subsequently, [Kim *et al* , 2000] we established a relationship between our information theoretic approach and a simple non-parametric hypothesis test. In this work, we describe an adaptive approach for incorporating the temporal structure that relates the *f*MRI time-series to both the current *and* past values of the experimental protocol. This is achieved via an extension of our previous approach using the information-theoretic concept of entropy rate. It can be shown that, despite a differing implementation, our prior method is a special case of the new approach. The entropy rate of a random process quantifies future uncertainty conditioned on the past and side-information (e.g. the experimental protocol, confounding signals, etc.) without making strong assumptions about the nature of that uncertainty (e.g. Gaussianity). Furthermore, we allow the form of the dependency to vary from voxel to voxel in an adaptive fashion. The combination of the information theoretic principles and adaptive estimation of the temporal dependency allows for a more powerful and flexible approach to *f*MRI analysis. Empirical results are presented on three *f*MRI datasets measuring motor, auditory, and visual cortex activation comparing the new approach to the previous one as well as a variation on the general linear model. Particular attention is paid to the differences in the type of phenomenology detected by the respective approaches.

* J. Fisher was supported in part by an NSF ERC grant, Johns Hopkins Agreement #8810274. E. Cosman was supported under the NSF award #IIS-9610249. C. Wible was supported in part under NIMH grants MH40799 and MH52807. W. Wells was supported by the same ERC grant, and by NIH 1P41RR13218.

W. Niessen and M. Viergever (Eds.): MICCAI 2001, LNCS 2208, pp. 905–912, 2001.

1   Introduction

Previously, we have discussed the application of an information theoretic formalism to the analysis of fMRI time series. In [8] we presented a novel information theoretic approach for calculating fMRI activation maps by estimating the mutual information between an encoding of the experimental protocol and fMRI voxel time-series. Subsequently in [5] we demonstrated the equivalence of the method to a statistical hypothesis test when the underlying densities are unknown. As a consequence, the computation of the activation map can be formulated as a binary MAP detection problem using the Ising model as a spatial prior and solved *exactly* in polynomial time using the Ford and Fulkerson method [4]. The information-theoretic framework is appealing in that it is a principled methodology requiring few assumptions about the structure of the fMRI signal. It is capable of detecting unknown nonlinear and higher-order statistical dependencies. Furthermore, it is relatively straightforward to implement. An implicit assumption of [8] and [5] is that samples of the time-series are statistically independent. That is, time structure was neither assumed nor exploited. This is in contrast to approaches based upon the general linear model (GLM) in which strong assumptions about the time structure are made through the choice of a set of basis vectors or equivalently a signal subspace [3].

In this work, we consider a natural extension to the information theoretic method in which we learn and then exploit the time structure of the fMRI voxel time-series and its dependence on the time structure of the protocol. Whereas when we assumed sample independence, mutual information was a natural way to relate the protocol to the fMRI time series, the information theoretic notion of *entropy rate* is the natural quantity when we consider time structure. As a consequence of the adaptive learning approach, we do not make strong assumptions about the exact nature of the time structure á *priori*, merely that it exists and can be estimated. In fact, time dependence of the fMRI time-series is allowed to vary from voxel to voxel. In doing so, the determination of whether or not a voxel is declared active relies upon the methodology described in [2]. That work discusses a general approach for random process analysis. The assumption is that the dependency is distributed across many samples in the past, but may be approximated using low-dimensional functions of the past. In this work we examine a special case for which the methodology of [2] is appropriate.

We compare the new method to an approach based on the general linear model (GLM) popularized by Friston *et al* [3] using data from three fMRI data sets testing motor, auditory, and visual cortex activation.

2   Entropy Rates

We model the fMRI time series as a random process, denoted $\{Y\} \equiv \{y\}_0^\infty \equiv \{y_0, y_1, \cdots\}$ in which a sample y_k statistically depends on the past values $\{y\}_0^{k-1} \equiv \{y_0, \cdots, y_{k-1}\}$, and perhaps on the present and past values of the protocol time-series, $\{u\}_0^k$. This dependence is quantified by the information theoretic notion of *entropy rate*, defined as [1]

$$H\left(Y\right) \equiv \lim_{N \to \infty} \frac{1}{N+1} h\left(\{y\}_0^N\right) = \lim_{N \to \infty} h\left(y_N|\{y\}_0^{N-1}\right) \tag{1}$$

where $h(\ )$ is differential entropy. Note that equality assumes the process is stationary, however, the second form is also valid for a wide class of nonstationary processes and is the form we use in practice. The entropy rate quantifies the average uncertainty about future values conditioned on the past. We can also condition on side information (e.g. the protocol) by

$$H\left(Y|\{u\}_0^N\right) = \lim_{N \to \infty} h\left(y_N|\{y\}_0^{N-1}, \{u\}_0^N\right) \tag{2}$$

It can be shown that, in general, conditioning reduces entropy, that is

$$H\left(Y|\{u\}_0^N\right) \leq H\left(Y\right) \tag{3}$$

with equality only when $\{y\}_0^N$ and $\{u\}_0^N$ are statistically independent [1]. Equations 1 and 2 imply that we must consider the joint densities over all samples of the process which is generally intractable. However, we make two assumptions that reduce the complexity. First, we assume the process depends on the finite past, that is

$$h\left(y_k|\{y\}_0^{k-1}\right) = h\left(y_k|\{y\}_{k-M_y}^{k-1}\right) \tag{4}$$

$$h\left(y_k|\{y\}_0^{k-1}, \{u\}_0^k\right) = h\left(y_k|\{y\}_{k-M_y}^{k-1}, \{u\}_{k-M_u}^k\right) \tag{5}$$

limiting the dimensionality to $M_y + M_u + 1$. Furthermore, we assume the information about y_k in the samples $\{y\}_{k-1}^{k-M_y}$ and $\{u\}_k^{k-M_u}$ can be summarized by lower dimensional functions,

$$h\left(y_k|\{y\}_{k-M_y}^{k-1}\right) \approx h\left(y_k|f_a\left(\{y\}_{k-M_y}^{k-1}\right)\right) \tag{6}$$

$$h\left(y_k|\{y\}_{k-M_y}^{k-1}, \{u\}_{k-M_u}^k\right) \approx h\left(y_k|f_a\left(\{y\}_{k-M_y}^{k-1}\right), f_b\left(\{u\}_{k-M_u}^k\right)\right) \tag{7}$$

where $f_a(\ )$ and $f_b(\ )$ are parameterized. Fisher *et al* [2] describe a generalized approach for both learning the parameterized functions and then using them to compute entropy rates. Note that when using the methodology of [2] the approximation of equations 6 and 7 are close in the Kullback-Leibler sense and thus consistent with a hypothesis testing framework [6]. For reasons of brevity we shall only consider the class of linear predictive models.

2.1   Hypothesis Testing and Entropy Rates

For the moment we put aside the question of estimating the functional parameters to examine the relationship between hypothesis testing and entropy rates. Consider the following hypothesis test.

$$H_0 : y_k \sim p_Y(Y_k|\{y\}_0^{N-1})$$
$$H_1 : y_k \sim p_{Y|U}(Y_k|\{y\}_0^{N-1}, \{u\}_0^N)$$

Hypothesis H_0 states that the random process Y depends only on the past of Y, while H_1 states that the random process depends on the past of both Y and U. We compute the log of the likelihood ratio

$$T_n = \sum_{k=1}^{n} \log \left(p_{Y|U}(y_k | \{y\}_0^{N-1}, \{u\}_0^N) \right) - \log \left(p_Y(y_k | \{y\}_0^{N-1}) \right) . \qquad (8)$$

It can be shown that [1]

$$\lim_{n \to \infty} T_n = n \left(H(Y) - H\left(Y | \{u\}_0^N \right) \right) = \mathrm{E}\{T_n\} , \qquad (9)$$

consequently, the difference in entropy rates used as the activation statistic is equivalent to the aforementioned hypothesis test. In practice we substitute the Parzen density estimate and, as in equations 6 and 7, substitute functions $f_a(\ )$ and $f_b(\ )$ to summarize the dependency on the past.

The preceding analysis is similar to that presented in [5] which shows the equivalence between a simpler hypothesis test and mutual information as the test statistic. We note here that when the process is independent from sample to sample and is dependent on the coincident (or a delayed) sample of the protocol then the hypothesis test is equivalent to that described in [5]. In [8], the test was performed for a range of delays modeling a type of hemodynamic response. Here, since we consider past samples jointly this is not necessary and consequently more general forms of the hemodynamic response are modeled. This will be further elaborated in the experimental results section.

3   Modeling the Temporal Structure of fMRI Time-Series

We now discuss a method for estimating the time dependence of the fMRI time-series y_k on past samples of both y_k and the protocol u_k. We restrict ourselves to linear functionals of past samples, a special case of the more general approach described in [2]. Note the information theoretic principles play a role both in quantifying the dependence of the voxel time-series on the protocol and in estimating the parameters of the functions. Letting y_k represent the time-series at some voxel, we consider two signal components.

$$y_k^a = - \sum_{i=1}^{M_y} a_i y_{k-i}^a + n_k \qquad y_k^b = \sum_{i=0}^{M_u} b_i u_{k-i} \qquad (10)$$

where n_k is an i.i.d. noise sequence and u_k is the protocol signal. We assume that n_k is independent of u_k. The estimates of $\{a_i\}$ and $\{b_i\}$ should reflect this assumption. This condition partially distinguishes our approach from standard ARMA (auto-regressive moving-average) models. Consequently, y_k^a is an AR (auto-regressive) process with a random noise source while y_k^b is a MA (moving-average) process with the protocol as the input. The fMRI time-series is modeled as the sum of these two signals.

$$y_k = y_k^a + y_k^b = y_k^a + \sum_{i=0}^{M_u} b_i u_{k-i} = \sum_{i=1}^{M_y} a_i y_{k-i}^a + n_k + \sum_{i=0}^{M_u} b_i u_{k-i} \qquad (11)$$

Ordinarily, solving for ARMA parameters is a nonlinear optimzation problem. However, since u_k is known, the parameters can be obtained using linear least squares estimation [7] with the additional constraint that n_k is statistically independent of u_k. Furthermore, it can be shown for linear predictive models (such as in equation 10) that the solution obtained by minimizing the squared error in the prediction has the same expected value as that obtained by minimizing the entropy rate (equations 6 and 7).

Standard least squares methods do not ensure the independence of n_k and u_k, in general. If an active voxel obeys the model (even approximately) past samples will contain some dependence on the protocol which will be transmitted through the $\{a_i\}$ coefficients. That dependence must be removed so that we can isolate contributions from u_k and pass them only through the $\{b_i\}$ coefficients. A straigtforward approximation is to solve for the coefficients sequentially.

$$\{b_i\} = \arg\min_{\{b_i'\}} \sum_k \left(y_k - \sum_{i=0}^{M_u} b_i' u_{k-i} \right)^2 \qquad (12)$$

$$\{a_i\} = \arg\min_{\{a_i'\}} \sum_k \left(y_k - y_k^b - \sum_{i=1}^{M_y} a_i' y_{k-i}^a \right)^2 \qquad (13)$$

To the degree that the model order is correct, predictions of y_k from y_k^a will be independent of y_k^b. Furthermore, the entropy rates of the processes are equivalent to the entropy of the error residuals (with and without the protocol contribution). That is, under the model,

$$H(Y) = h(y_k - y_k^a) \quad \text{and} \quad H(Y \mid \{u\}_0^k) = h(y_k - y_k^a - y_k^b), \qquad (14)$$

where $(y_k - y_k^a)$ and $(y_k - y_k^a - y_k^b)$ are our estimates of n_k under the two hypotheses. As follows from equation 8, the difference of these entropies form our ARMA-based entropy rate statistic (ER).

Note that the MA model y_k^b is the same model implicit in a GLM approach when the basis is $M_u + 1$ shifted versions of the protocol signal. This is only the case when we restrict ourselves to *linear* functions of the past, and represents a principled way to choose a GLM design matrix and to include noise modeling. In Section 4, we contrast the ER-test to a classical F-test that approximates incorporating our modified ARMA model into a GLM design matrix.

4   Empirical Results and Discussion

We present results on three fMRI datasets, whose respective protocols were designed to activate the motor cortex (dominant hand movement protocol), auditory cortex (verb generation protocol), and visual cortex (visual stimulation with alternating checkerboard pattern). Each data set contains 60 whole brain acquisitions taken three seconds apart, each consisting of 21 coronal slices. Each protocol consists of a 30 second rest phase followed by a 30 second task phase repeated three times. In all cases, the MA and AR systems are sixth-order.

We compare the two versions of the new method to a baseline GLM (the protocol signal is the basis) and MI [8]. The first estimates the entropy rates nonparametrically (ER) while the second assumes Gaussian statistics, whereby the difference in entropy rates is equivalent to a variance ratio (an F-test, and in effect, a GLM with our ARMA model in the design matrix). For each protocol the GLM threshold was set so that the number and location of activations was consistent with the protocol. In the comparison methods, the thresholds were set such that all of the GLM activations were detected. This resulted in additional detections, some spurious and some not. Results for the visual cortex are shown in Figure 1. Visual inspection of the signals of the new activations in the ER maps (contrast Figure 1 (a) and (c)) suggested a relationship to the protocol. Figures 2 and 3 present four such activations, from visual, auditory, and motor protocols, which the GLM only detects when its threshold is siginificantly lowered. The lowered GLM threshold produced many additional detections as well. This is illustrated in Figure 4, which contrasts the detections in slice 6 before and after the threshold change. In this particular case, all activations detected with the lower threshold (Figure 4(d)) had very small MI and ER values and were judged to be spurious by inspection. One such false positive is shown in Figure 5.

We found that the ARMA-based F-statistic and the GLM statistic are both small for the active voxels plotted in Figure 2 (a) and (e). This is likely due to their inherent assumption of Gaussianity. Figure 2 (c) and (g) suggests a bi-modal error density for these cases. The ER statistic does not make this assumption and can more robustly detect these depedencies on the protocol.

The hemodynamic response is modeled implicitly by the MA term in the model. When calculating MI and GLM statistics, this delay is found by searching a range of delays. Figure 2(b) shows the MA signal estimate as a solid line overlying the dotted line representing the protocol period (and the fMRI signal, dashed) and is slightly delayed. Note that this delay corresponds roughly to the centroid or peak of the MA weights shown in Figure 2(d), which is between 2 and 3 delays. The active voxel shown in Figure 3 is one whose MI value erroneously indicates a vanishing dependency on the protocol, but which ER accurately detects. We have observed that MI and GLM poorly detect signals like this one, which are characterized by high-amplitude, high-frequency variation (relative to the protocol period).

While these results are not exhaustive, we feel that they are indicative of the potential of the method, particularly in the cases where it is difficult to model phenomenon á priori.

References

[1] T. M. Cover and J. A. Thomas. *Elements of Information Theory*. John Wiley & Sons, Inc., New York, 1991.

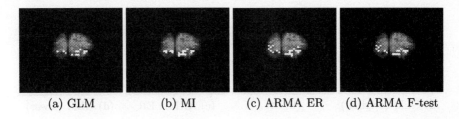

(a) GLM   (b) MI   (c) ARMA ER   (d) ARMA F-test

Fig. 1. Comparison of *f*MRI analysis results from visual experiments (2nd slice)

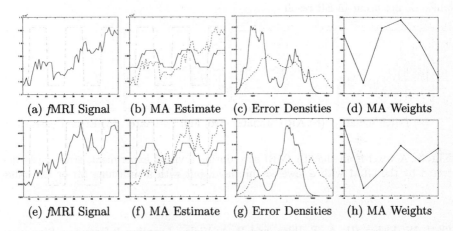

(a) *f*MRI Signal   (b) MA Estimate   (c) Error Densities   (d) MA Weights

(e) *f*MRI Signal   (f) MA Estimate   (g) Error Densities   (h) MA Weights

Fig. 2. The "partial-responders" (a,e) appear to be cases in which the subject did not respond during all task phases (visual - top, auditory - bottom). Consequently, the error residuals exhibit a bimodal density (solid lines in (c,g)). The residual error density using only past signal values (dotted lines) has lower entropy, but similar variance, so ER detects the lower entropy rate, while ARMA F-test and baseline GLM do not.

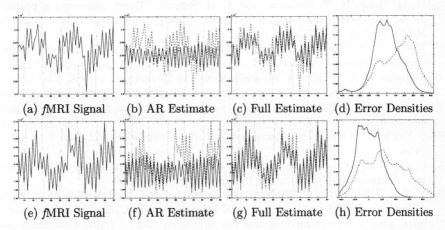

(a) *f*MRI Signal   (b) AR Estimate   (c) Full Estimate   (d) Error Densities

(e) *f*MRI Signal   (f) AR Estimate   (g) Full Estimate   (h) Error Densities

Fig. 3. The ER statistic finds dependencies on the protocol that was apparently hidden from both MI and GLM by the low SNR in both these signals. (a)-(d): A voxel in the visual protocol   (e)-(h): A voxel in the motor protocol

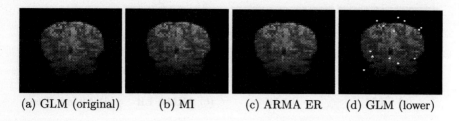

| (a) GLM (original) | (b) MI | (c) ARMA ER | (d) GLM (lower) |

Fig. 4. Visual experiment, slice 6: spurious GLM detections due to lowered threshold which do not occur in ER result.

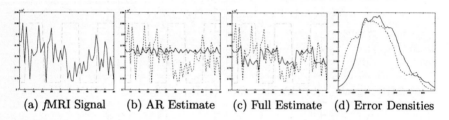

| (a) fMRI Signal | (b) AR Estimate | (c) Full Estimate | (d) Error Densities |

Fig. 5. A voxel from the 6th fMRI slice during a visual experiment, erroneously detected by the GLM with a lowered threshold, but with a vanishing MI or ER value

[2] J. W. Fisher III, A. T. Ihler, and P. A. Viola. Learning Informative Statistics: A Nonparametric Approach. In S. A. Solla, T. K. Leen, and K. R. Müller, editors, *Proceedings of 1999 Conference on Advances in Neural Information Processing Systems 12*, 1999.

[3] K. J. Friston, P. Jezzard, and R. Turner. The Analysis of Functional MRI Timeseries. *Human Brain Mapping*, 1:153–171, 1994.

[4] D. M. Greig, B. T. Porteous, and A. H. Seheult. Exact maximum a posteriori estimation for binary images. *Journal of the Royal Statistical Society. Series B(Methodological)*, 51(2):271–279, 1989.

[5] J. Kim, J. W. Fisher III, A. Tsai, C. Wible, A. Willsky, and W. M. Wells III. Incorporating Spatial Priors into an Information Theoretic Approach for fMRI Data Analysis. In S. L. Delp, A. M. DiGioia, and B. L. Jaramaz, editors, *Third International Conference on Medical Image Computing and Computer-Assisted Intervention*, volume 1935 of *Lecture Notes in Computer Science*, pages 62–71 Springer, Oct 2000.

[6] S. Kullback. *Information Theory and Statistics*. John Wiley and Sons, New York, 1959.

[7] L. L. Scharf. *Statistical signal process: detection, estimation, and time series analysis*. Addison-Wesley Publishing Company, New York, 1990.

[8] A. Tsai, J. Fisher III, C. Wible, W. M. Wells III, J. Kim, and A. Willsky. Analysis of Functional MRI Data using Mutual Information. In C. Taylor and A. Colchester, editors, *Second International Conference on Medical Image Computing and Computer-Assisted Intervention*, volume 1679 of *Lecture Notes in Computer Science*, pages 473–480. Springer, Sept 1999.

Automatic Non-linear MRI-Ultrasound Registration for the Correction of Intra-operative Brain Deformations

Tal Arbel[1], Xavier Morandi[1], Roch M. Comeau[2], and D. Louis Collins[1]

[1] Montreal Neurological Institute, McGill University, Montréal, Québec, Canada
{taly,morandi,louis}@bic.mni.mcgill.ca, http://www.bic.mni.mcgill.ca
[2] Rogue Research Inc., 4398 St-Laurent, Suite 206, Montréal, Québec, Canada
roch@rogue-research.com, www.rogue-research.com

Abstract. Movements of brain tissue during neurosurgical procedures reduce the effectiveness of using pre-operative images for intra-operative surgical guidance. In this paper, we explore the use of acquiring intra-operative ultrasound (US) images for the quantification of and correction for *non-linear* brain deformations. We will present a multi-modal, automatic registration strategy that matches pre-operative images (e.g. MRI) to intra-operative ultrasound to correct for the non-linear brain deformations. The strategy involves using the predicted appearance of neuroanatomical structures in ultrasound images to build "pseudo ultrasound" images based on pre-operative segmented MRI. These images can then be registered to intra-operative US in a strategy based on cross-correlation measurements generated from the ANIMAL [1] registration package. The feasibility of the theory is demonstrated through its application to clinical patient data acquired during 12 neurosurgical procedures. Qualitative examination of the results indicate that the system is able to correct for non-linear brain deformations.

Key words: Image-guided Neurosurgery, ultrasound, magnetic resonance, brain shift, multi-modal registration, non-linear registration

1 Introduction

The precise localization of anatomical structures and pathological features within the complex three-dimensional architecture of the brain is one of the major challenges of neurosurgery. Image-guided neurosurgical (IGNS) systems that embed neuronavigation are becoming widely used for intra-cranial procedures [2, 3]. There are numerous benefits reported from the increased usage of IGNS. These include (i) minimally invasive cranial openings, (ii) accurate localization of sub-cortical lesions, (iii) reduction in blood loss, (iv) reduction in surgical time, and (v) a decrease in the complication rate and thus on intensive care unit and hospital stays [4, 5]. However, the requirements for a precise, reliable and accurate surgical guidance system include: low system error and a high degree

W. Niessen and M. Viergever (Eds.): MICCAI 2001, LNCS 2208, pp. 913–922, 2001.

of correspondence between the pre-operative images and the surgical anatomy. Errors in IGNS caused by geometrical distortions in the pre-operative images, patient-to-image registration errors and errors in tracking the surgical instruments are well-defined for various systems in existence [3, 6]. However, another important source of error is the deformation of the brain tissue from the time of pre-operative image acquisition to the time of the surgical procedure and, more importantly, during the surgery. Brain deformation is a complex, spatiotemporal phenomenon with a wide variety of causes, including both chemical and physical factors [3, 4, 7]. IGNS systems based on pre-operative data alone cannot properly account for this type of deformation, which is estimated to range from $5mm$ to $20mm$ [4, 7].

In order to quantify and correct for spatial errors resulting from intra-operative brain deformations, registration strategies based on intra-operative MRI have been proposed and implemented [8, 9]. This approach has several strengths and weaknesses. Among the advantages are safer tumor resections, a better assessment of the resections, the quantification and visualization of brain deformations, and detection of intra-operative complications such as hemorrhage. Nevertheless, a number of technical and logistical problems still require solutions. These include restricted surgical access to the patient due to the confining layout of the MR system, the shortage of MR compatible auxiliary equipment and surgical instruments, and inconsistent image quality. Finally, the significant expense of the solution, both in terms of acquisition equipment and MRI-friendly surgical tools, leads to questions regarding the cost-effectiveness of the solution [9].

Another recently proposed approach for the correction of deformations consists of using pre-operative MR images to generate a 3D patient-specific model of the brain resulting from simulated surgical procedures [10, 11]. Since the causes of brain deformations are complex, predicting the physical and chemical processes that can be encountered in each case would be difficult. Moreover, the presence of pathologies increases the complexity of the processes, particularly cases that lead to tissue removal and water displacement (e.g. cerebrospinal fluid, edema, etc).

Ultrasound (US) has a long established track record for intra-operative use in neurosurgical practice. Intra-operative US systems cost less than 10% of a typical MRI system, are portable (enabling them to be shared), have few special logistical requirements and are compatible with existing operating room equipment [12]. Nevertheless, owing to limited image quality and limited experience in interpreting such images, the first period of enthusiasm in the 1980s was followed by disappointment. Since the mid-1990s, Trobaugh et al. [13], followed by other researchers [14, 15, 16, 12, 17] have developed the concept of correlating intra-operative US with pre-operative MRI using 2D and 3D images. Some techniques have been developed to match pre-operative MR images to intra-operative US to correct for linear deformations [19]. However, to the best of our knowledge, this paper presents the first report of an automatic[1] non-linear registration technique that successfully corrects for non-linear brain deformations. It should be noted that other groups have also developed non-linear correction methods, but they depend on manually identified landmarks to drive the warp [18]. In our approach, we propose using a surgical guidance system that incorporates an automatic non-linear MRI-US registration method for the correction of intra-operative brain deformations. The feasibility of the theory has been demonstrated in a clinical context on a series of 12 patients.

2 Methods

The goal of this work is to update the patient's pre-operative MR images based on US images acquired intra-operatively, given the presence of non-linear brain deformations. Our strategy is to first acquire pre-operative patient MRI and store the result as a 3D volume. During the surgical procedure, a series of US images are acquired. The specific aims of this work are: (i) to compute an initial linear transformation that maps the position and orientation of the US images into the coordinate space defined by the pre-operative MR volume, (ii) to construct a full 3D composite US volume from the images acquired and (iii) to compute the non-linear deformation field from the US volume to the corresponding MR volume in order to correct for non-linear brain deformations as well as errors in the linear registration stage. The resulting deformation field will be used to provide the surgeon with an update of the patient's MR images during the procedure. In this section, we will describe the various processing steps required to meet these goals.

2.1 Linear Registration

Pre-operative patient MRI are acquired and stored as a 3D volume in MINC format, a publicly available medical image file format developed at the Montreal Neurological Institute that was designed as a multi-modal, N-dimensional, cross-platform format [20]. The file format is self-describing, portable and simplifies inter-process communication through transform files that allow one data set to be mapped to another.

In order to perform comparisons between the two data sets, US images acquired intra-operatively must then be mapped to the same space as the corresponding pre-operative MRI. Three rigid body or affine transformations are required to perform the mapping, as described in [16], by making use of a Polaris tracking system (Northern Digital Inc.). At the start of the surgical procedure, MR image space is mapped to the Polaris reference space by identifying homologous anatomical landmarks on the patient head using a tracked pointer, and on the MR images using a mouse, and employing a least squares (SVD) minimization fit. Normally, five to nine points are used to define the transformation.

---

[1] The registration strategy is fully automatic, however pathologies must be manually processed pre-operatively.

During the surgical procedure, the tracker monitors the orientation and position of the US transducer through a tracked rigid body, or "US tracker", permanently mounted on the US transducer. US images are implicitly acquired in Polaris reference space as the US image-to-US tracker transformation is determined prior to surgery, using a calibration tool designed for this purpose, and the tracker itself provides the transformation from US tracker to the Polaris reference space. Thus, as US images are acquired during surgery, the resulting transformation can be used to extract a corresponding oblique slice from the MRI volume, permitting the simultaneous display and comparison of the pre-operative MRI and intra-operative US. The system stores the coordinates of the acquired US image in the appropriate coordinate space within the MINC format.

2.2   3D Composite US Volume

Once the sequence of acquired US images[2] are stored in the appropriate coordinate space, a composite 3D US is created by superimposing and averaging the slices into a full 3D volume (originally zero-valued) in the same coordinate frame as the MR volume acquired earlier. The methodology chosen uses a nearest neighbour approach to place each intensity pixel into the nearest voxel in the volume image, in a strategy similar to that in [21]. Because the images are stored in MINC format, tools are available to average the slices in the areas where they intersect. A blurring operator is applied to the volume to remove the effects of acoustic artifacts such as speckle noise. An example of an US volume superimposed onto a patient's MRI can be seen in Figure 1.

2.3   Non-linear Registration

In previous work, we have developed a versatile 3D volume registration and segmentation package, termed ANIMAL (Automatic Non-linear Image Matching and Anatomical Labeling) [22, 1]. In this project, ANIMAL is primarily used to compute the non-linear spatial transformation required to map intra-operative US to pre-operative MRI. The procedure for estimating this transformation is to compute dense field of 3D deformation vectors, mapping each voxel of one image volume to match those in a target image volume. The algorithm builds up a 3D non-linear deformation field in a piecewise linear fashion, recursively fitting local spherical neighborhoods. Each local neighborhood from one volume is translated to achieve an optimal match within the other volume using cross-correlation similarity metrics to estimate the local transformation. The local neighborhoods are arranged on a 3D grid to fill the volume and each grid node moves within a range defined by the grid spacing. This procedure is applied in a hierarchical fashion, first using blurred data to estimate the largest and most global deformations, and then refining the transformation by using less blurred data and finer grid sampling to account for more local deformations. The process stops when reaching a $2mm$ grid size.

---

[2] A minimum of $20 - 30$ images per sweep is required.

ANIMAL requires similar features in the source and target volumes in order to perform either cross-correlation or optical flow computations between the two data sets. Since US and MRI have very different characteristics, we have decided to generate *pseudo US* images - images whose appearance closely matches the predicted appearance of real US images that will be acquired during surgery - from data derived from the pre-operative MRI[3]. In this manner, the ANIMAL routine can be used to correlate the pseudo US to the real, intra-operative US images acquired. To compute the pseudo US volumes, the ANIMAL segmentation package is used to segment major brain structures from the MRI volume. The segmentation is then further refined to create a volume that includes only those structures that are clearly visible in US. The resulting volume of anatomical structures is then submitted to a radial gradient operator in order to generate gradient magnitude data that reflects the appearance (in terms of intensity values) of acoustic boundaries visible in the US image. In future work, other structures prevalent in the US image (such as the cerebral falx) will be added to the pseudo US images, and more realistic physical simulations will be developed. However, the current technique allows for a proof-of-principal to be demonstrated here. For the time being, pre-operative segmentation of pathologies is performed manually[4]. Figure 2 shows an example of each of the steps involved in creating a pseudo US image ($0.5mm^2$ pixel size).

ANIMAL then estimates the non-linear spatial transformation required to match a pseudo US image volume to real US images acquired during surgery. This same transformation can be used to update the patient's MRI during surgery, thus permitting the neurosurgeon to make use of the pre-operative images during the intervention, even in the presence of a brain deformation (and errors in the linear registration from the patient to the pre-operative images).

3 Clinical Applications

The method was applied to 12 surgical cases, including those with brain tumors ($n = 8$) and selective amygdalo-hippocampectomies ($n = 4$). Pre-operative MRI were acquired using a Philips 1.5T Gyroscan (The Netherlands) machine. Intra-operative images were acquired using an Ultramark 9, Advanced Technologies Laboratories Inc. (Bothwell, WA) machine with an ATL P7-4 multi-frequency probe, and a Capsure^{TM} frame grabber on a Macintosh computer (Apple Computer, Cupertino, CA). Tracking was achieved with the use of a Polaris tracking system with a passive probe.

The feasibility of the approach is demonstrated through examination of the qualitative results from two clinical cases. Figure 4 shows the case of an amygdalo-hippocampectomy for intractable epilepsy. US images were acquired at two different stages of the operation: before and after the opening of the dura. The figure illustrates how the system is able to correct for brain deformations at these two stages of surgery. The extent of the correction can be seen in

---

[3] The current strategy does not take acoustic properties or physics into account.

[4] The automatic segmentation of pathologies is currently an open research topic.

Figure 3^5. Figure 5 illustrates the case of a tumor resection. Here, US images were acquired after the dura opening, when significant brain deformation (on the order of $8mm$) had occurred. The strategy was able to correct for the deformations of both pathological and anatomical structures. In all cases, it took approximately 30 seconds of processing time to provide a corrected MRI volume on average.

4   Discussion and Conclusions

In the context of image-guided craniotomies for brain lesions, there are three important issues to address: (i) finding the lesions, (ii) avoiding the eloquent, functional brain tissue, and (iii) determining the borders between pathological and normal brain tissues. Over the past decade, advances in IGNS systems have permitted neurosurgeons to reach these objectives in a large number of situations [2]. However, because of the frequent occurrence of brain deformations during craniotomies, the accuracy of the neuronavigation system is often compromised. In this paper, we have demonstrated preliminary clinical results for the automatic correction of brain deformations during craniotomies by using a non-linear registration strategy that automatically matches pre-operative MRI to intra-operative US. The strategy is based on cross-correlation computations within ANIMAL that register pseudo US images, derived from segmented pre-operative MRI, to intra-operative US images. Current work involves building more sophisticated US simulations, based on the identification of a larger number of neuro-anatomical structures in clinical US data, and better physical modeling of the acoustic phenomenon.

One important advantage of the intra-operative system described in this paper is its relative speed. Pre-operative processing time for the creation of the pseudo US image, including the segmentation and gradient computations, is less than 10 minutes. The linear registration is a one-step process that lasts less than 5 minutes. Intra-operative computations include: performing the US acquisition ($2-3$ minutes), computing the composite US volume (2 minutes) and finally, computing the deformations and updating the MRI takes 30 seconds. Optimization of the US composition should take that step down to several seconds.

The standard criticism associated with the use of US during neurosurgical procedures are its poor spatial and contrast resolutions. Our approach minimizes these concerns by providing the neurosurgeon with high resolution MR, warped to reflect the surgical reality, based on US images acquired intra-operatively. The technique has been applied to the images of 12 patients to demonstrate the feasibility and the reliability of the method. Further work is required to quantitatively validate the method, as well as to assess the added clinical value to the patient outcomes. Future work will also include a *quantification* of the registration error, and an interface to provide the neurosurgeon with the means to participate in the error control process.

---

[5] Figure references are not in sequence to ensure that all color figures appear on the same page.

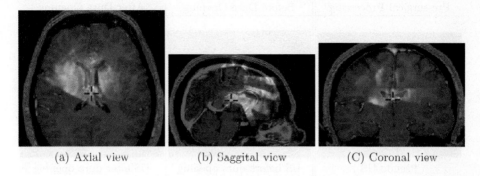

(a) Axial view   (b) Saggital view   (C) Coronal view

Fig. 1. 3D Composite US Volume: MRI in grey with US overlayed in a hot-metal color scale.

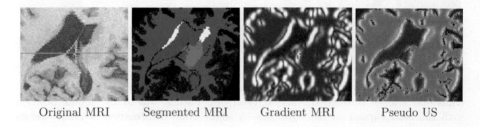

Original MRI   Segmented MRI   Gradient MRI   Pseudo US

Fig. 2. Generating Pseudo US. The original MRI is segmented using ANIMAL, a radial gradient is then applied, and these are merged to create a pseudo US image (see text for details).

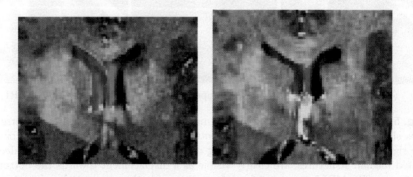

Fig. 3. Case from Figure 4 illustrating US (in green) after dura opening over original MRI (left) and over corrected MRI (right). Notice the distinct collapse of the left lateral ventricle.

920   T. Arbel et al.

| Pre-surgical Processing | Before Dura Opening | After Dura Opening |

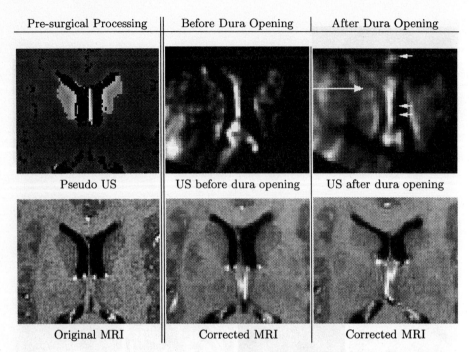

| Pseudo US | US before dura opening | US after dura opening |
| Original MRI | Corrected MRI | Corrected MRI |

Fig. 4. Left selective amygdalo-hippocampectomy for intractable epilepsy: zoom of transverse images through the lateral ventricles. Patient was in the supine position with the head turned on the right side. A slight brain deformation is visible before the dura opening (column 2). A larger gravitational displacement (towards the right of the image) of the median structures is observed after dura opening (column 3). The deformation mainly involves the anterior horn of the left lateral ventricle (white arrow), whereas the falx (arrowhead) and septum pellucidum (double arrowhead) do not move. Correction of the deformation is demonstrated during these two surgical steps.

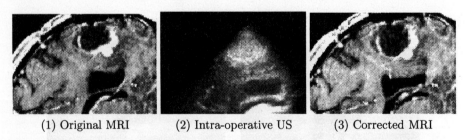

(1) Original MRI   (2) Intra-operative US   (3) Corrected MRI

Fig. 5. Case with right frontal recurrent malignant tumor. These near-transverse images show the tumor (top), ventricles (bottom), with the front of the head towards the right. After dura opening, the sinking of the entire tumor, as well as the deeply-seated median structures, are clearly visible as a displacement towards the bottom of the image. The MRI is corrected for deformations of both pathological and anatomical structures (e.g. The ventricle is displaced and slightly compressed. The tumor is displaced as well.) The posterior part of the septum drops, but the anterior part does not as the registration system confuses it with the choroid plexus. This will be fixed with proper representation of the septum and choroid plexus in the simulations. Note that the falx does not move.

References

[1] D. L. Collins and A. C. Evans, "Animal: validation and applications of non-linear registration-based segmentation," *International Journal and Pattern Recognition and Artificial Intelligence*, vol. 11, pp. 1271–1294, Dec 1997.

[2] N. Dorward, "Neuronavigation – the surgeon's sextant," *British Journal of Neurosurgery*, vol. 11, pp. 101–103, 1997.

[3] J. Golfinos, B. Fitzpatrick, L. Smith and R. Spetzler, "Clinical use of a frameless stereotactic arm: result of 325 cases," *Neurosurgery*, vol. 83, pp. 197–205, 1995.

[4] D. Hill, C. Maurer, R. Maciunas et al., "Measurement of intraoperative brain surface deformation under a craniotomy," *Neurosurgery*, vol. 43, pp. 514–528, 1998.

[5] T. Paleologos, J. Wadley, N. Kitchen, and D. Thomas, "Clinical utility and cost-effectiveness of interactive image-guided craniotomy: clinical comparison between conventional and image-guided meningioma surgery," *Neurosurgery*, vol. 47, pp. 40–48, 2000.

[6] C. Maurer, G. Aboutanos, B. Dawant et al., "Effect of geometrical distortion correction in MR on image registration accuracy," *Journal of Computer Assisted Tomography*, vol. 20, pp. 666–679, 1996.

[7] D. Roberts, A. Hartov, F. Kennedy et al., "Intraoperative brain shift and deformation: a quantatative analysis of cortical displacement in 28 cases," *Neurosurgery*, vol. 43, pp. 749–760, 1998.

[8] P. Black, E. Alexander, C. Martin et al., "Craniotomy for tumor treatment in an intraoperative magnetic resonance unit," *Neurosurgery*, vol. 45, pp. 423–433, 1999.

[9] M. Bernstein, A. Al-Anazi, W. Kurcharczyk et al., "Brain tumor surgery with the Toronto open magnetic resonance imaging system: preliminary results for 36 patients and analysis of advantages, disadvantages, and future prospects," *Neurosurgery*, pp. 900–907, 2000.

[10] D. Roberts, M. Miga, A. Hartov et al., "Intraoperatively updated neuroimaging using brain modeling and sparse data," *Neurosurgery*, vol. 45, pp. 1199–1207, 1999.

[11] D. Roberts, M. Miga, A. Hartov et al., "Model-updated image guidance: Initial clinical experiences with gravity-induced brain deformation," *IEEE Transactions on Medical Imaging*, vol. 18, pp. 866–874, Oct 1999.

[12] R. Comeau, A. Sadikot, A. Fenster, and T. Peters, "Intraoperative ultrasound for guidance and tissue shift correction in image-guided neurosurgery," *Medical Physics*, vol. 27, pp. 787–800, 2000.

[13] J. Trobaugh, W. Richard, K. Smith, and R. Bucholz, "Frameless stereotactic ultrasonography: Methods and applications," *Computerized Medical Imaging and Graphics*, vol. 18, no. 4, pp. 235–246, 1994.

[14] R. Bucholz, C. Sturm, and J. Henderson, "Detection of brain shift with an image guided ultrasound device," *Acta Neurochirurgica*, vol. 138, p. 627, 1996.

[15] R. Bucholz, D. Yeh, J. Trobaugh et al., "The correction of stereotactic inaccuracy caused by brain shift using an intraoperative ultrasound device," *CVRMed-MRCAS*, pp. 459–466, 1997.

[16] R. M. Comeau, A. Fenster, and T. Peters, "Intraoperative US in interactive image-guided neurosurgery," *Radiographics*, vol. 19, no. 4, pp. 1019–1027, 1998.

[17] D. Gobbi, R. Comeau, and T. Peters, "Ultrasound/MRI overlay with image warping for neurosurgery," in *MICCAI 2000*, (Pittsburgh, PA, USA), pp. 106–114, Oct. 2000.

[18] D. Gobbi, B. K. H. Lee, and T. M. Peters, "Correlation of preoperative MRI and intraoperative 3D ultrasound to measure brain tissue shift," in *Medical Imaging 2001: Visualization, Display, and Image-Guided Procedures, Proceedings of SPIE 2001*, (San Diego, CA, USA), Seong Ki Mun (ed.), Vol. 4319, pp. 264–271, Feb. 2001.

[19] A. Roche, X. Pennec, M. Rudolph et al., "Generalized correlation ratio for registration of 3D ultrasound with MR images," in *MICCAI 2000*, (Pittsburgh, PA, USA), pp. 567–577, Oct. 2000.

[20] P. Neelin, D. MacDonald, D. Collins, and A. Evans, "The MINC file format: from bytes to brains," *NeuroImage*, vol. 7, no. 4, p. 786, 1998.

[21] A. King, J. Blackall, G. Penney et al., "An estimation of intra-operative deformation for image-guided surgery using 3-D ultrasound," in *MICCAI 2000* (Pittsburgh, PA, USA), pp. 588–597, Oct. 2000.

[22] D. L. Collins, P. Neelin, T. M. Peters, and A. C. Evans, "Automatic 3D intersubject registration of MR volumetric data in standardized Talairach space," *Journal of Computer Assisted Tomography*, vol. 18, pp. 192–205, 1994.

A Novel Nonrigid Registration Algorithm and Applications

J. Rexilius[1], S.K. Warfield[1], C.R.G. Guttmann[1], X. Wei[1], R. Benson[2], L. Wolfson[2],
M. Shenton[1], H. Handels[3], and R. Kikinis[1]

[1] Surgical Planning Laboratory, Harvard Medical School & Brigham and Women's Hospital,
75 Francis St., Boston, MA 02115, USA.
rexilius@bwh.harvard.edu
[2] Department of Neurology, University of Connecticut Health Center, USA.
[3] Institute for Medical Informatics, Medical University of Luebeck, Germany.

Abstract. In this paper we describe a new algorithm for nonrigid registration of brain images based on an elastically deformable model. The use of registration methods has become an important tool for computer-assisted diagnosis and surgery. Our goal was to improve analysis in various applications of neurology and neurosurgery by improving nonrigid registration.

A local gray level similarity measure is used to make an initial sparse displacement field estimate. The field is initially estimated at locations determined by local features, and then a linear elastic model is used to infer the volumetric deformation across the image. The associated partial differential equation is solved by a finite element approach. A model of empirically observed variability of the brain was created from a dataset of 154 young adults. Both homogeneous and inhomogeneous elasticity models were compared. The algorithm has been applied to medical applications including intraoperative images of neurosurgery showing brain shift and a study of gait and balance disorder.

1 Introduction

Developed about twenty years ago, nonrigid registration has meanwhile become a fundamental method for brain analysis in computer-assisted neurology and neurosurgery. An important issue thereby is the generation of deformation fields that reflect the transformation of an image in a realistic way with respect to the given anatomy. Due to lack of image structure, noise, intensity artifacts, computational complexity and a restricted time frame e.g. during surgery, it is not suitable to measure the deformation for each voxel. This leads to estimates of the deformation field only at sparse locations which have to be interpolated throughout the image.

In the last few years physically based elastic and viscous fluid models for nonrigid registration have become more and more popular [3] because they can constrain the underlying deformation in a plausible manner. However viscous fluid models [10],[11] have to be chosen carefully, since they allow large deformations which is not always suitable for medical applications concerning the brain. Furthermore, viscous fluid models driven by alignment of similar gray values may allow anatomically incorrect matches

W. Niessen and M. Viergever (Eds.): MICCAI 2001, LNCS 2208, pp. 923–931, 2001.

of different but adjacent structures through the same mechanism that allows large deformation matches. For example, one gyri may flow from the source brain to match two or more different gyri in a target brain, in a manner that may or may not be desirable.

In terms of physically based elastic models various algorithms have been described. Recent work (e.g. [7],[8]) proposed an active surface algorithm computed at the boundary of a regarded structure for an initial estimate of the deformation field. A drawback of this method is, that although it has been shown to be accurate close to the object's boundary, away from the boundaries the solution could potentially be less accurate. In [11] this idea was improved using statistical shape informations based on a set of images with hand-labeled points on the boundary of a structure which was included as an additional matching criterion. Even though such methods are promising for specific structures of the brain a robust 3D shape representation of the whole brain still remains difficult to achieve.

A different approach was proposed by Collins et.al. (see [6]). Their nonrigid registration algorithm was based on an iterative refinement of a local similarity measure using a simplex optimization. As this approach is constrained only by smoothing after correspondence estimation, the derived deformation field can only be accurate for specific regions of the brain. To achieve better results the method was improved by introducing various gyri and sulci of the brain as geometrical landmarks [5].

The aim of this paper is to present a new algorithm for computer-assisted neurology and neurosurgery. In order to get realistic deformations we propose an physically based elastic model, without requiring a segmentation or having the drawback that initial estimates of the deformation are only generated for the boundary of a considered structure. Therefore we used an enhanced approach based on the local similarity measure proposed by Collins et.al.. Furthermore we incorporated a model for inhomogeneous elasticities into our algorithm. The discretization of the underlying equation was done by a finite element technique, which has become a popular method for medical imaging applications (e.g. see [4] and [8]).

2   Method

The process of registration can be described as an optimization problem that minimizes both the difference between a template and a reference image and the deformation energy. We present a registration method, which basically runs in two steps. Based on a set of points extracted out of an image as described in (2.1), an initial sparse estimate of the deformation field is found by a local normalized cross-correlation (2.2). In a second step nonrigid registration is performed using an elastic model (2.3) which is constrained at the sparse estimates computed before.

2.1   Feature Point Extraction

Let Ω denote the domain of a volume $S : \Omega \to \mathbb{R}$ with voxel positions $\mathbf{x} = (x, y, z)^\top$, $\mathbf{x} \in \Omega$. In order to obtain suitable feature points for an initial sparse estimate of the deformation field, first the gradient magnitude is calculated out of blurred image intensities where only voxel higher than two standard deviations above the mean of the magnitude of the gradient are used for the correspondence detection (2.2). Figure 1 shows this process for one slice of a Magnetic Resonance (MR) scan of the brain.

To overcome the poor edge preserving properties of linear low-pass filters, we use a nonlinear diffusion filter which can be described as a solution of the partial differential equation (PDE)

$$\partial_t S = \operatorname{div}\left(g(|\nabla S_\sigma|^2)\,\nabla S\right) \tag{1}$$

with Neumann boundary conditions [15]. In order to reduce the noise sensitivity, the diffusion function $g : \mathbb{R} \to \mathbb{R}$ depends on the magnitude of the gradient of smoothed image intensities, computed by convolving S with a Gaussian kernel of standard deviation σ. In our method, we use a diffusion function proposed by Weickert in [15]:

$$g(x) = \begin{cases} 1 & \text{for } x \le 0 \\ 1 - \exp(\frac{-C}{(x/\lambda)^4}) & \text{for } x > 0 \end{cases} . \tag{2}$$

The parameter λ separates regions of low contrast from those of high contrast. For the constant C Weickert proposes $C = 3.31448$ which gives visually good results and sets the flux $f(x) = x \cdot g(x)$ to an expected behavior, i.e. f is increasing for values smaller or equal λ and decreasing for values greater than λ. In our approach λ was set interactively according to the considered volume. Furthermore for computational efficiency we use a parallel additive operator splitting (AOS) scheme which is stable for arbitrary large time steps and can be solved in linear time in terms of the image size. See [14] for details.

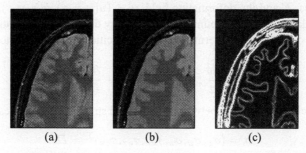

(a)   (b)   (c)

Fig. 1. Illustration of feature point extraction. For a better visual impression we only show a detail of the image. (a) Slice of MR scan; (b) Blurred image using a nonlinear diffusion filter; (c) Magnitude of the gradient of the blurred image after thresholding.

2.2 Correspondence Detection

After extracting feature points, the correspondence between the reference R and template volume T is computed for these points. We use the local normalized cross-correlation (NCC) as a similarity measure [6]

$$\text{NCC}(R, T, d) = \frac{\sum_{k \in \mathcal{N}(\mathbf{x})} f(R, k) \cdot f(T, d(k))}{\sqrt{\sum_{k \in \mathcal{N}(\mathbf{x})} f^2(R, k) \cdot \sum_{k \in \mathcal{N}(\mathbf{x})} f^2(T, d(k))}} , \forall \mathbf{x} \in \Omega , \tag{3}$$

which is maximized in terms of the deformation function d by a brute force search. The search space in our method is restricted to translations because other transformations like rotations or scaling would be of higher computational complexity. Assuming a window of size $(w \times w \times w)$, the local neighborhood of a voxel $\mathbf{x}$ is described by $\mathcal{N}(\mathbf{x}) \in \{(x - w, y - w, z - w)^\top, \ldots, (x + w, y + w, z + w)^\top\}$. The spatial points used for the NCC are computed by $f : (\mathbb{R}, \Omega) \to \mathbb{R}$, whose output $f(S, \mathbf{x})$ is given for voxels with high gradient magnitudes calculated out of blurred image intensities, as described in section (2.1).

2.3 Interpolation from Sparse Displacement Estimates

The sparse deformation estimates obtained for the feature points computed by a local NCC, are now introduced as external forces into an elastic model described in Equation (4). The underlying idea is to restrict the the registration process so that the resulting deformation field is a priori fixed by the estimates at these points.

For a three dimensional elastic body Ω the total potential energy is defined as the work of the internal strains minus the potential of the external forces and can be expressed as [18]:

$$E(\mathbf{u}) = \frac{1}{2} \int_\Omega \sigma^\top \epsilon \, d\Omega - \int_\Omega F^\top \mathbf{u} \, d\Omega , \qquad (4)$$

where the variables are given in terms of the strain vector, σ, the stress vector, ϵ, the external forces, F and the deformation field, $\mathbf{u} = (u(x, y, z), v(x, y, z), w(x, y, z))^\top$. We seek the deformation that minimizes the energy described in Equation (4). As we assume small deformations in terms of linear elasticities, the strain vector ϵ is given by

$$\epsilon = \left(\frac{\partial u}{\partial x}, \frac{\partial v}{\partial y}, \frac{\partial w}{\partial z}, \frac{\partial u}{\partial y} + \frac{\partial v}{\partial x}, \frac{\partial v}{\partial z} + \frac{\partial w}{\partial y}, \frac{\partial w}{\partial x} + \frac{\partial u}{\partial z} \right)^\top . \qquad (5)$$

The elastomechanical relation between stresses and strains can be expressed as

$$\sigma = (\sigma_x, \sigma_y, \sigma_z, \tau_{xy}, \tau_{yz}, \tau_{zx})^\top = D\epsilon \qquad (6)$$

with the elasticity matrix D. See [18] for the full details.

For the discretization we choose the finite element method (FEM), i.e. the domain Ω is approximated by a sum of elements. In our approach we use a regular mesh of tetrahedra. For every element the deformation $\mathbf{u}^e$ can now be described as a linear combination of so-called shape functions $N_i^e(x, y, z) = \frac{1}{6V}(a_i + b_i x + c_i y + d_i z)$. A detailed computation for the volume V of a tetrahedron and the coefficients is given in [18]. We assume a uniformly continuous transition between two elements, which leads to

$$u^e(x, y, z) = \sum_{i=1}^{4} u_i^e(x, y, z) N_i^e(x, y, z) \quad , \forall e \in \Omega_a , \qquad (7)$$

where Ω_a represents an approximation of the continuous domain Ω.

A large system of equations can be computationally expensive to solve. To work against this, the resulting system of equations is solved in parallel with the Portable Extensible Toolkit for Scientific Computation (PETSc) package [2] in less than five minutes for a $256 \times 256 \times 124$ volume. Usually the NCC search is much more expensive than solving this system.

Typically elasticity parameters have been set arbitrarily and homogeneously [3]. Recently Lester et.al. [10] applied an inhomogeneous viscous fluid model to brain and neck registration using the manually segmented bone of the reference image as a region of high stiffness. Davatzikos et.al. [7] applied inhomogeneities to brain warping setting the elasticity parameters of the brain four times higher than their value in the ventricles.

Our approach differs in that the inhomogeneous elasticity parameters are derived from an empirical estimate of anatomical variability. We used a set of 154 MR scans of the brain, first segmented into white matter, grey matter, cerebro-spinal fluid (CSF) and background using an EM-based statistical classification algorithm [16]. Then the head of each scan was aligned to an arbitrarily selected scan out of this database, using global affine transformations [13] and our nonrigid registration. In order to generate a model for inhomogeneous elasticities, we use a maximum-likelihood classification, where for each voxel the most likely structure and its frequency of occurrence at the voxel on all cases was stored. According to these results, the elasticity parameters are computed for every voxel. We choose a linear mapping for the computed frequency of occurrence of the identified brain tissues where the Poisson ratio ν was scaled in a range of $\nu \in [0.1, 0.4]$ while Young's elasticity modulus E has a range of $E \in [2000kPa, 10000kPa]$. The background was set to a low stiffness $E = 1000kPa$ and incompressibility parameter $\nu = 0.05$, respectively. Figure 2 shows a slice of the computed model and the associated intensities for ν.

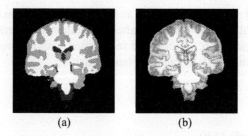

(a)   (b)

Fig. 2. Computed model of empirically observed variability. (a) Slice of the model after maximum-likelihood classification; (b) Computed incompressibility parameter (Poisson ratio ν) for each voxel of the same slice. Dark regions imply a low value for ν.

3 Experimental Results

To evaluate the two different methods presented in this paper, we show some results obtained for varying medical applications. In case of homogeneous elasticities we use $E = 3000kPa$ for the Young elasticity modulus, and $\nu = 0.4$ for the Poisson ratio, as used by Ferrant et. al. [8].

3.1 Illustration of Nonrigid Registration with Homogeneous and Inhomogeneous Elasticities

In order to show the behavior of a deformation model with homogeneous and inhomogeneous elasticities, the algorithm was applied to register 159 MR scans of the brain of young adults. Therefore each scan was first globally registered to an arbitrarily chosen dataset by an affine transformation [13]. The nonrigid registration with homogeneous and inhomogeneous elasticities was then applied to the aligned data (Figure 3).

An analysis of the summed squared differences showed an improvement of 2% using inhomogeneous elasticities. This rather small effect is due to the setting of feature points in our experiments. As it can be seen in Figure 2 large regions of white matter only have a small range of anatomical variability, i.e. large number of fixed deformation estimates constrain the interpolation done by the elastic model. Further research will investigate new approximation schemes to address this.

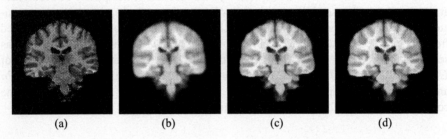

(a)	(b)	(c)	(d)

Fig. 3.   Results of study applying rigid and nonrigid registration to 159 subjects. (a) Slice of reference volume; (b)-(d) Result after registration and averaging over all scans using: (b) affine registration; (c) nonrigid registration with homogeneous elasticities; (d) nonrigid registration with inhomogeneous elasticities.

3.2 Capturing Brain Shift

During neurosurgery the shape of the brain changes which can be considered as nonrigid deformation. Recently a fast biomechanical simulation of this brain shift was proposed in [12]. This algorithm used segmentation to identify key structures and to remove noise and intensity artifacts. In our new method we can derive sparse estimates without a segmentation so long as noise and intensity artifacts are minimal. This allows estimates to be obtained in a larger region of the brain. Figure 4 shows images of the brain before (Fig. 4 (a)) and after craniotomy (Fig. 4 (b)) as well as the reference image after craniotomy with overlayed initial (Fig. 4 (c)) and deformed image (Fig. 4 (d)). It can be observed, that the brain shift was successfully captured. Even though the results show some artifacts in the area of the brain surface. This is due to a massive change in the patients brain structure during craniotomy resulting in a large cavity which cannot be computed with an elastic model out of the initial image. As this area only contains

cerebro-spinal fluid we haven't addressed this issue in our current studies. More validation experiments will be required to appropriately assess the potential for this method.
These are currently under way.

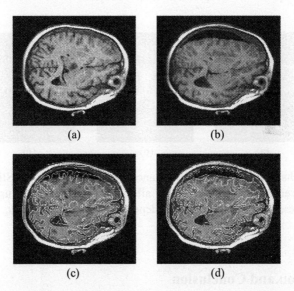

Fig. 4.   Elastic matching applied to MR scan of the brain obtained during neurosurgery. (a) Image at the beginning of the surgery; (b) Image after craniotomy; (c) Slice
of reference volume with overlayed contours of initial scan; (d) Slice of reference volume with overlayed contours of deformed volume;

3.3   Analysis of Balance and Gait Disorders

Impaired mobility caused by gait and balance disorders is common in older adults. Central nervous system disease, as revealed by white matter signal abnormalities (WMSAs)
observed by MRI, is believed to play a significant role in gait disorder while still being
common in asymptomatic elderly subjects [9]. Therefore it is interesting to understand
the spatial distribution of WMSAs in impaired and asymptomatic subjects. The alignment of impaired mobility subjects and controls in a common coordinate system can
help to determine the spatial distribution of such WMSAs. A commonly applied but
relatively low order nonrigid registration algorithm is that provided by SPM [17],[1].
We wished to investigate the use of our high dimensional nonrigid registration to determine spatial distribution of WMSAs associated with gait disorder by comparing the
spatial distribution of WMSAs between two groups - 16 subjects with impaired mobility, and 12 age matched control subjects without impaired mobility.

Figure 5 (a) shows the slice of one subject used as reference image. The results of the
nonrigid registration after averaging over all scans are presented in Figure 5 (b). Figure
5 (c) illustrates the results of a Chi-square test, with values significant at the $\alpha = 0.01$

level shown as bright pixels, and with lower values scaled linearly in intensity to zero (black). The results show clearly that people with balance and gait disorders have a statistically significant increase in lesions in two specific regions of the white matter of the brain, as compared to asymptomatic elderly subjects.

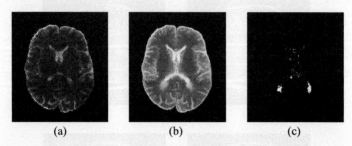

(a)   (b)   (c)

Fig. 5.   Results of a study analyzing balance and gait disorders. (a) Slice of reference volume; (b) Averaged cases of the study after nonrigid registration using inhomogeneous elasticities; (c) Result of a voxel independent chi-square statistic.

4   Discussion and Conclusion

We have presented a method for nonrigid registration which was used for various applications in neurology and neurosurgery including simulation of brain shift and a study of balance and gait disorders. The applied elastic model provides us thereby with the ability to simulate realistic deformation applying inhomogeneous elasticities derived by a model of empirically observed variability. A local similarity measure was used to constrain the model which was discretized by the finite element method.

Further work will investigate alternative similarity measures and features extractions, e.g. local structure features. We also plan to enhance this approach incorporating the anisotropy of certain brain tissue structures.

Acknowledgements: This investigation was supported by NIH P41 RR13218, NIH P01 CA67165 and NIH R01 RR11747.

References

1. J. Ashburner and K.J. Friston: Spatial Normalization. In Brain Warping. Ed. Arthur W. Toga, (Academic Press) Ch.2:27-44, 1999.
2. S. Balay, W.D. Gropp, L.C. McInnes and B.F. Smith: PETSc 2.0 users manual. Tech. Rep. ANL-95/11 - Revision 2.0.28, Argonne National Laboratory, 2000
3. R. Bajcsy and S. Kovacic: Multiresolution Elastic Matching. Computer Vison, Graphics and Image Processing, 46:1-21, 1989.
4. M. Bro-Nielsen: Finite element modeling in medical VR. Journal of the IEEE, 86(3):490-503, 1998.

5. D.L. Collins, G. Le Goualher and A.C. Evans: Non-linear Cerebral Registration with Sulcal Constrains. In MICCAI 1998, Cambridge, MA, USA, 1998 pages 974-984.
6. D.L. Collins: 3D Model-based segmentation of individual brain structures for magnetic resonance imaging data. PhD thesis, 1994.
7. C. Davatzikos: Spatial Transformation and Registration of Brain Images Using Elastically Deformable Models. Comp. Vis. and Image Understanding, Special Issue on Medical Imaging, 66(2):207-222, May 1997
8. M. Ferrant, S.K. Warfield, A. Nabavi, F.A. Jolesz and R. Kikinis: Registration of 3D Intraoperative MR Images of the Brain Using a Finite Element Biomechanical Model. In MICCAI 2000, Pittsburgh, Pennsylvania, USA, 2000, pages 19-28.
9. C.R.G. Guttmann, R. Benson, S.K. Warfield, X. Wei, M.C. Anderson, C. Hall, K. Abu-Hasaballah, J.P. Mugler and L. Wolfson: White matter abnormalities in mobility-impaired older persons. Neurology, 54:1277-1283, 2000
10. H. Lester, S.R. Arridge, K.M. Jansons, L. Lemieux, J.V. Hajnal and A. Oatridge: Non-linear Registration with the Variable Viscosity fluid Algorithm. In IPMI 1999, pages 238-251, 1999.
11. Y. Wang, L.H. Staib: Physical model-based non-rigid registration incorporating statistical shape information. Medical Image Analysis, 4(2000) pages 7-20, 2000.
12. S.K. Warfield, M. Ferrant, X. Gallez, A. Nabavi, F.A. Jolesz and R. Kikinis: Real-Time biomechanical Simulation of Volumetric Brain Deformation for Image Guided Neurosurgery. High Performance Networking and Computing Conference, Dallas, USA, 230:1-16, 2000.
13. S.K. Warfield, F.A. Jolesz and R. Kikinis: A High Performance Computing Approach to the Registration of Medical Imaging Data. Parallel Computing 24:1345-1368, 1998.
14. J. Weickert, B. ter Haar Romeny, M.A. Viergever: Efficient and reliable schemes for nonlinear diffusion filtering. IEEE Trans. Image Processing, Vol. 7, pages 398-410, March 1998.
15. J. Weickert: Anisotropic diffusion in image processing. Teubner Verlag, Stuttgart, 1997.
16. W.M. Wells, R. Kikinis, W.E.L. Grimson, F. Jolesz: Adaptive segmentation of MRI data. IEEE Transactions on Medical Imaging, 15:429-442, 1996
17. K.J. Worsley, S. Marrett, P. Neelin, A.C. Vandal, J.J. Friston and A.C. Evans: A unified Statistical Approach for Determining Significant Signals in Images of Cerebral Activation In Human Brain Mapping, pages 58-73, 1996
18. O.C. Zienkewickz, R.L. Taylor: The Finite Element Method. McGraw Hill Book Co., 1987.

Analysis of the Parameter Space of a Metric for Registering 3D Vascular Images

Stephen R. Aylward, Sue Weeks, and Elizabeth Bullitt

Department of Radiology
Computer-Aided Diagnosis and Display Lab
The University of North Carolina at Chapel Hill

Abstract. We present a new metric for registering 3D images of vasculature, and we analyze the rigid-body transformation parameter space of that metric and its derivatives. To quantify and direct a source image's alignment with a target image, this new vascular-image registration system models the vessels in the source image and makes measurements in the target image at a sparse set of transformed points from the centerlines of those models. The system is fast and effective because the measures made at the transformed centerline points incorporate the general geometric properties of tubes and specific model-quality information calculated during the vessel model generation process. Additionally, by adjusting the sample density or scaling the centerline point measures, coarse-to-fine registration strategies are directly enabled. We present visualizations of the metric and its derivatives over a range of mis-registrations given different sample densities and different measure scalings using magnetic resonance angiograms, x-ray computed tomography images, and 3D ultrasound images.

1 Introduction and Background

The registration of 3D medical images is critical to many clinical tasks. Most computer-based registration research focuses on registering tissue images. Many clinical applications, however, are driven by the patient's vasculature. Vascular imaging modalities include x-ray computed tomography after contrast injection (CTA), magnetic resonance angiography (MRA), and 3D ultrasound (3D-US). Applications that benefit from the registration of vascular images include: quantifying treatment effectiveness for arterio-venous malformations (AVM) as captured by MRA and planning adult-to-adult partial liver transplants using registered CTA to generate digital-subtraction CTA of liver vasculature.

We know of no other vessel-specific 3D image registration metric. If image intensities or vessel centerline features are used to register vascular images, the sparseness and local similarity of these features produce a multitude of local maxima in the transformation parameter space. Others have developed methods for model-based segmentation of coronary arteries (e.g., [1]), but such work assumes one model fits every patient and does not fully exploit ridge criteria

W. Niessen and M. Viergever (Eds.): MICCAI 2001, LNCS 2208, pp. 932–939, 2001.

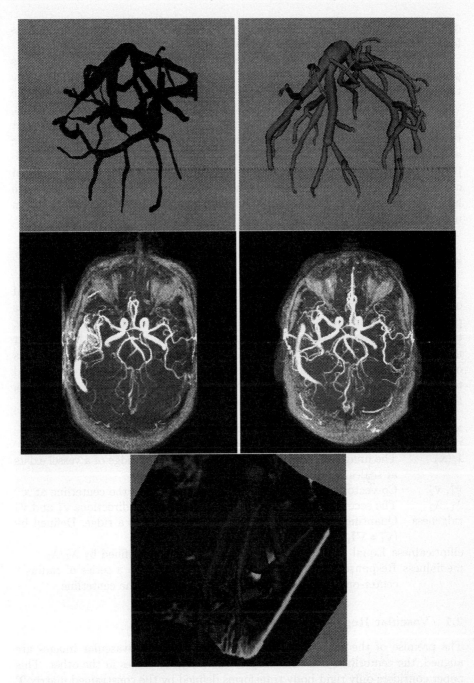

Fig. 1. (*Top row*) Vessel models from two liver CTA datasets: (*left*) from data collected during the arterial-phase of contrast and (*right*) from the venous-phase of contrast. (*Middle row*) Maximum intensity projections of two MRA datasets (an AVM is visible on the left side of each image): (*left*) pre-treatment data and (*right*) three months after radiation therapy treatment. (*Bottom row*) Vessel models from 3D-US data.

during registration. We [2] and others [1,3] have previously presented methods for registration of 3D vascular models with their 2D projections.

In this paper, we present our 3D vascular registration metric and illustrate its parameter space using clinical MRA, CTA, and 3D-US data (Fig 1). We show that the metric is maximal when two vascular images are aligned; the metric varies smoothly about that maximum; and for a broad range of transformations, the metric's derivatives point towards the maximum. Additionally, we show that the parameters of this metric control the extent and smoothness of the metric and its parameters about the maximum, thereby enabling coarse-to-fine registration strategies. Furthermore, the metric and its derivatives require minimal computation - even at high sample density, these calculations usually require less than one-half second, so complete 3D registration can be accomplished in under one minute.

2   Method and Results

The registration metric builds on our vessel modeling work [2, 4]. A summary of other vessel modeling methods is given in [5], but none of these other methods provides the information that we have found useful for registration. Specifically, the registration metric requires models of the vessels in the "source image." Our model extraction method produces sub-voxel representations of the centerlines of vessels via a multi-scale ridge traversal process. The centerlines are then used to stabilize a vessel-width estimation process. At each centerline point, therefore, the following information is defined in our vessel models:

$\mathbf{x}$ The position of the centerline point in the source image, $\mathbf{x} \in \Re^3$

r The radius of the vessel at $\mathbf{x}$

$\mathbf{I}_r(\mathbf{x})$ The image intensity at $\mathbf{x}$ at scale r (the height ridge of a vessel exists at scales related to the width of the vessel)

$\vec{\mathbf{v_1}}, \vec{\mathbf{v_2}}$ Co-vectors that define the directions normal to the centerline at $\mathbf{x}$

λ_1, λ_2 The second derivative of the image intensity in directions $\vec{\mathbf{v_1}}$ and $\vec{\mathbf{v_2}}$

ridgeness   Quantifies how well a centerline point localizes a ridge. Defined by $\left(\vec{\mathbf{v_1}} \bullet \nabla \mathbf{I}_r(\mathbf{x})\right)^2 + \left(\vec{\mathbf{v_2}} \bullet \nabla \mathbf{I}_r(\mathbf{x})\right)^2$

ellipticalness Equal to 1 if cross-section at $\mathbf{x}$ is circular. Defined by λ_2/λ_1

medialness Response from convolving the image at $\mathbf{x}$ with a series of radius r center-on, surround-off kernels oriented along the centerline.

2.1   Vascular Registration Metric

The premise of the registration metric is that when two vascular images are aligned, the centerlines from one map to the intensity ridges in the other. This paper considers only rigid-body transforms defined by the constrained matrix $\mathbf{T}$ which we parameterize by its offset vector $\mathbf{o}$ and the Euler rotation parameters α, β, and γ. The registration metric, $f(\mathbf{T})$, is a weighted, w_i, sum of scaled, κr_i, intensities in the target image, $\mathbf{I}$, at a sub-sampling, n, of the transformed centerline points, $\mathbf{x}_i \mathbf{T}$.

$$f(\mathbf{T}) = \frac{1}{\sum_{i=1}^{n} w_i} \sum_{i=1}^{n} w_i \mathbf{I}_{\kappa r_i}(\mathbf{x}_i \mathbf{T}) \tag{1}$$

The centerlines are sub-sampled to reduce the number of points at which a volume must be evaluated to quantify the quality of an alignment. This greatly reduces the computation requirements of the metric. Furthermore, we reject any sub-sample point if its ridgeness or its medialness (see Section 2) is less than 0.2 (to eliminate points which are poorly localized). This actually increases the accuracy of the metric when few points are used. The effect of sub-sampling on the shape of metric surface about the metric maximum is illustrated in Fig. 2. On a 500 Mhz Pentium III, for the CT data, to calculate the metric and its gradients requires 0.06 seconds when 46 points (~1 of every 100 centerline points in the vessel models) are used, 0.39 seconds when 279 points (~1 of 20) are used, and 1.97 seconds when 1360 points (~1 of 5 = ~1 point per voxel a centerline passes through) are used. For the MRA data, instead of evaluating the 10,485,760 voxels in the data, to calculate the metric and its gradients requires 0.02 seconds for 76 points, 0.09 seconds for 513 points, and 0.49 seconds for 2559 points. The MRA data requires less time per evaluation since the typical centerline point exists at a smaller scale in the MRA data compared to the CTA data. A coarse-to-fine registration strategy can by implemented by changing the density of the sub-sampling during transformation parameter optimization.

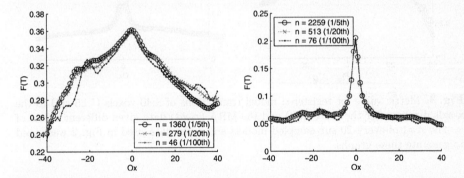

Fig. 2. Metric value for model translations of ±40 voxels (~±5 cm) in the x-axis direction for the CTA (*left*) and the MRA (*right*) data given different sub-samplings. For CTA, vessel models from arterial-phase data were registered with venous-phase data. For MRA, vessel models from pre-treatment data were registered with post-radiation treatment data. For MRA and CTA, the registered models defined the 0-offset transformations (the location of the metric maximum). These datasets contained non-rigid deformations including missing and extra vessels, but the metric is insensitive.

Since the spatial extent of small vessels is limited, they are more drastically affected by image noise, and they are less informative given large-scale mis-registrations. We therefore weight vessels based on their radius (Equ. 2). This weighting could be balanced during transformation optimization to impliment a coarse-to-fine registration strategy.

$$w_i = \frac{2}{1 + e^{-2r_i}} \tag{2}$$

Via the scalings κr_i in Equ. 1, the measurements made in the target image are made using aperatures proportional to the radius of the vessel expected at that point in the target image. This local blurring creates an intensity ridge, if the point is transformed to a vessel's centerline in the target image. This scaling can be controlled using the metric parameter κ. If κ is increased beyond 1.0, the capture radius of the metric increases, the effect of noise is decreased, and larger vessels are given additional emphasis in determining the qualify of the registration. By starting with κ large, and decreasing κ to 1.0 as a registration process iterates, a coarse-to-fine registration strategy is effected (Fig. 3). Note the multiple local maxima at $\kappa = 0.0$.

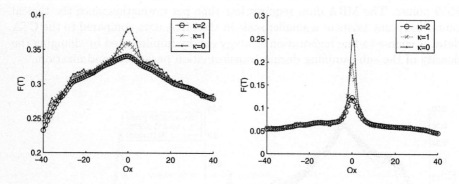

Fig. 3. Metric value for registered model translations of ±40 voxels ($\tilde{}\pm5$ cm) in the x-axis direction for the CTA (*left*) and the MRA (*right*) data given different values of κ. The n=1-of-every-20 sub-sampled models and same data used in Fig. 2 were used to generate these graphs.

2.2   Gradients of the Vascular Registration Metric

The strength of the vascular registration system comes from the incorporation of ridge criterion into the calculation of the metric's gradient. First, to reduce the number of local maxima in the gradient space, we limit each transformed point's influence to the directions normal to its centerline. When aligned, this prevents points from traveling along a centerline and when mis-aligned, this limits, for example, horizontal vessels to inducing vertical changes in the transformation parameters. The normal plane at a point $\mathbf{x}_i$ is the matrix (where * indicates co-vector transform by $\mathbf{T}$ and $\times$ indicates cross-product)

$$\mathbf{N}_i = (\mathbf{v}_{1i} * \mathbf{T}) \times (\mathbf{v}_{1i} * \mathbf{T}) + (\mathbf{v}_{2i} * \mathbf{T}) \times (\mathbf{v}_{2i} * \mathbf{T}) \tag{3}$$

Therefore, the weighted, normal-plane component of the gradient is

$$\nabla \mathbf{I}(\mathbf{x}_i \mathbf{T})_{\mathbf{v}} = w_i \nabla \mathbf{I}_{\kappa r_i}(\mathbf{x}_i \mathbf{T}) \mathbf{N}_i \tag{4}$$

Second, we normalize the gradient by the distribution (weighted sum) of the normal-planes' orientations. This prevents the metric gradient from being biased when the vessels models have a favored orientation. The bias matrix is

$$\mathbf{B} = \sum_{i=1}^{n} w_i \mathbf{N}_i \tag{5}$$

Therefore, the normal-plane, unbiased gradient of the metric is defined as (where $J(\mathbf{T})$ denotes the jacobian of $\mathbf{T}$)

$$f(\mathbf{T})d\mathbf{T} = \frac{1}{\sum_{i=1}^{n} w_i} \sum_{i=1}^{n} J(\mathbf{T}) \nabla \mathbf{I}(\mathbf{x}_i \mathbf{T})_{\mathbf{v}} \mathbf{B}^{-1} \tag{6}$$

The utility of the proposed modifications is illustrated in Fig. 4. It depicts the components of $f(\mathbf{T})d\mathbf{T}$ for vessels extracted from and registered with the 3D-US data. This illustrates the situation in which the vessel models match the image data exactly. There are no non-rigid effects in the data, and the ideal transformation parameter values (the identity matrix) are known. Note that the translation components are valid for a broad range of rotations, but the rotation components require the resolution of the translation components. These and similar observations are driving our research into defining a fast optimization strategy.

Using our existing gradient ascent optimization strategy, the arterial and venous phase CTA data were registered as well as the pre and post-treatment MRA data (Fig. 5). For the CTA datasets, very few vessels exist in both datasets, but the registration method is still effective. For the MRA datasets, the vessels are well registered away from the AVM but at the AVM, significant non-rigid deformations have occured since the vessels have shifted and several are missing.

In a final evaluation of the vascular registration metric, we attempted to register the arterial and venous-phase CTA data using a mutual information metric. The mutual information metric with rigid-body transform required significant intensity windowing and fine-tuning to focus its alignment on the liver. It instead favored the alignment of the bones or lungs. Even when mutual information was finally tuned to focused on the liver, surrounding organs interfered with the quality of the registration. The method presented in this paper is better for the registration of specific vascular organs.

3   Conclusions

The proposed vascular registration metric and its gradients are fast to calculate (require less than one-half second per evaluation), are maximal at the optimal

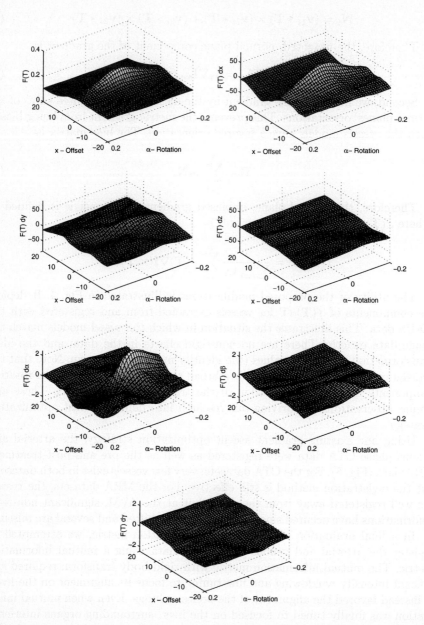

Fig. 4. Using the modified metric gradient (Equ. 6) and the 3D-US data (vessels were extracted from and registered with the same data), these graphs depict (in order from top left to bottom right) the metric and its gradient with respect to the transformation offset components o_x, o_y, o_z and rotation components α, β, and γ for a range of x-offsets (± 20 voxels - y-axis on graphs) and α rotations (± 0.2 radians - x-axis on graphs). The metric is maximal at the ideal transformation (i.e., no transformation), the metric and its gradients vary smoothly from the ideal, gradients point towards the ideal for a large extent for the effected tranformation parameters, and gradients of un-effected transofrmation parameters remain near zero.

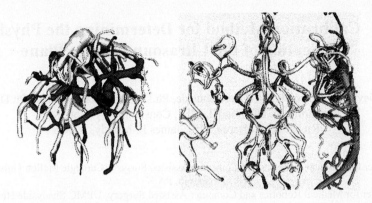

Fig. 5. (*left*) Gradient ascent was used to register the arterial-phase vessel models with the venous-phase CTA data. Shown are models from both sets of data (arterial-phase in dark gray and venous-phase in light gray). (*right*) Vessel models from the registered pre and post-treatment MRA data are shown (pre-treatment in wireframe and post-treatment as surfaces).

parameter settings, and smoothly vary about that maximum. These are the features that a metric should have to be effective for image registration.

A WWW site containing additional illustrations of this and related work is at http://caddlab.rad.unc.edu. Portions of this work were implemented using the NLM's Visible Human Segmentation and Registration Toolkit ("Insight Toolkit"). This work was supported in-part by the NIH/NCI R01-CA67812, the NIH/NCI P01-A47982, and an equipment and software grant from the Microsoft Corporation. Aspects of this work have been licensed (patent pending) to Medtronic Inc. (Minn., Minn.) and R2 Technologies (Los Altos, CA).

References

1. K Harris, SN Efstraatiadis, N Maglaveras, C Pappas, J Gourassas, and G Louridas, "Model-based morphological segmentation and labeling of coronary angiograms." IEEE Transactions on Medical Imaging, 18(10):1003-1015, October 1999
2. E Bullitt, A Liu, S Aylward, C Coffey, J Stone S Mukherji, and S Pizer, "Registration of 3D Cerebral Vessels with 2D Digital Angiograms: Clinical Evaluation," Academic Radiology, 6:539-546 1999
3. N Alperin, DN Levin, and CA Pelizzari, "Retrospective registration of x-ray angiograms with MR images by using vessels as intrinsic landmarks," Journal of Magnetic Resonance Imaging, 4:139-144 1994
4. SR Aylward, E Bullitt, SM Pizer, and D Eberly, "Intensity Ridges and Widths for Tubular Object Segmentation and Registration," in *IEEE Workshop on Mathematical Methods in Biomedical Image Analysis*, 131-138 1996
5. PJ Yim, PL Choyke, and RM Summers, "Gray-scale skeletonization of small vessels in magnetic resonance angiography," IEEE Transactions on Medical Imaging, 19(6); 568-576, June 2000.

Calibration Method for Determining the Physical Location of the Ultrasound Image Plane

Devin V. Amin, Ph.D.[1], Takeo Kanade, Ph.D[1]., Branislav Jaramaz, Ph.D.[2],
Anthony M. DiGioia III, MD[2], Constantinos Nikou, MS[2],
Richard S. LaBarca, MS[1], James E. Moody, Jr, MS[2]

[1]Center for Medical Robotics and Computer Assisted Surgery, Carnegie Mellon University,
Pittsburgh, PA
[2]Center for Medical Robotics and Computer Assisted Surgery, UPMC Shadyside Hospital,
Pittsburgh, PA
{Devin V. Amin}da2q@andrew.cmu.edu

Abstract. This paper describes a calibration method for determining the physical location of the ultrasound (US) image plane relative to a rigidly attached 3D position sensor. A calibrated US probe can measure the 3D spatial location of anatomic structures relative to a global coordinate system. The calibration is performed by aiming the US probe at a calibration target containing a known point (1 mm diameter sphere) in physical space. This point is repeatedly collected at various locations in the US image plane to produce the calibration dataset. An idealized model of the collection process is used to eliminate outliers from the calibration dataset and also to examine the theoretical accuracy limits of this method. The results demonstrate accurate and robust calibration of the 3D spatial relationship between the US image plane and the 3D position sensor.

1   Introduction

Intraoperative ultrasound images allow non-invasive measurement of the bone surface location. This information can be used to perform intraoperative registration to enable computer assisted surgery for minimally invasive procedures that involve limited direct access to the bone surface [1,4,5,7]. In order to determine the precise location of the ultrasound (US) image plane, a 3D position sensor (tracker) must be attached to the US probe and the spatial relationship between the tracker and the ultrasound imaging plane must be defined with a calibration routine [1,2,3,8,9]. In this study an optical tracker was attached to a removable shell that fit uniquely over the US probe. The calibration data was collected in order to evaluate two hypotheses. The first hypothesis was that the idealized model based outlier elimination process would allow the accuracy of the calibration method to approach the theoretical accuracy limit imposed by the experimental setup. The second hypothesis was that removal and re-attachment of the molded shell would not affect the spatial relationship between the ultrasound image plane and the 3D position sensor attached to the molded shell.

W. Niessen and M. Viergever (Eds.): MICCAI 2001, LNCS 2208, pp. 940-947, 2001.

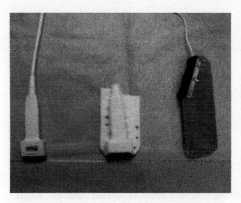 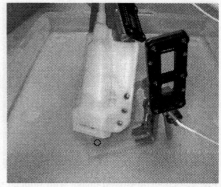

Fig. 1. Left - Ultrasound probe, molded shell and optical position sensor attached to aluminum plate. Right - US probe aimed at fiducial (1 mm diameter sphere; located at the center of the circle) on the calibration target.

2   Methods

The calibration routine that defines the spatial relationship between the optically tracked molded shell and the US image data is performed once for a given US probe (with fixed imaging parameters such as the depth) and then the removable shell can simply be reattached to the US probe prior to each use in the OR. To attach a 3D position sensor (optical tracker) to the ultrasound probe in a reproducible manner, a two-piece removable molded shell was constructed that fit precisely over the US probe. The first piece was molded to the shape of the US probe using a thermally sensitive plastic (Aquaplast™, Smith Nephew, 2.4 mm thickness). The optical tracker was then permanently attached to a rectangular aluminum plate which served as the second piece of the removable shell.

The first step of the calibration process is to determine the physical location of a 1 mm sphere, termed the US fiducial, using the Optotrak™ device (Northern Digital Inc., Waterloo, Ontario, Canada). An optically tracked US fiducial tool was calibrated to measure the center of the spherical US fiducial and data was collected to assess the accuracy with which the physical location of the US fiducial could be measured. The physical location was collected 100 times with the US fiducial tool pivoting about the center of the US fiducial; the maximum difference from the mean of the collected locations was less than 0.3 mm. A graphical user interface was used to manually determine the location of the fiducial in each US image (see Fig. 2).

2.1   Calibration Target

A calibration target was constructed from by mounting a spherical US fiducial (1 mm diameter steel ball bearing; Applied Industrial, Pittsburgh, PA) to the surface of a rectangular piece of plexiglass. An optical tracker was attached to the calibration target to allow continuous measurement of the physical location of the US fiducial

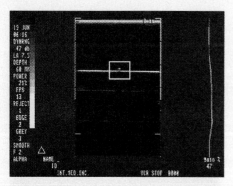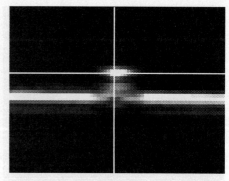

Fig. 2. Left - Ultrasound image with fiducial profile near mid-point of surface contour. Right - Close-up with crosshairs indicating the center of the US fiducial in the Image.

(see Fig. 1). The calibration target was submerged in a water medium and images of the US fiducial were obtained.

The ultrasound probe was aimed at the fiducial and images were acquired showing the location of the fiducial within the image (see Fig. 2). The US images were obtained from the video output of the US machine, the position of the fiducial was then specified manually using a graphical user interface, enabling the user to select the x and y coordinate of the center of the fiducial marker, as viewed in the US image. The z coordinate (i.e out of plane direction) was taken to be zero since there was no information available in this direction (i.e. in each calibration image, the US image plane was assumed to intersect the physical center of the US fiducial).

$$^{US}P_{Fiducial} = {}^{US}T_{CB} \text{ x } {}^{CB}P_{Fiducial} \qquad (1)$$

The physical location of the fiducial, originally collected in the calibration target coordinate frame ($^{CB}P_{Fiducial}$) was transformed to the coordinate frame of the US probe ($^{US}P_{Fiducial}$) for each US image using the transform ($^{US}T_{CB}$) collected by the Optotrack™ device. The calibration transform ($^{US}T_{IM}$) was then computed using the two sets of corresponding 3D points (in the image and US coordinate system) with a closed form least squares solution for the absolute orientation [6].

In addition to the six parameters that define the rotation and translation of the calibration transform we must also solve for the scale or ratio of pixels to mm in the US image. Beginning with an approximate initial value (estimated from the screen) the scale was varied over the range +/- 0.1 pixel/mm in 0.001 pixel/mm increments and the scale producing the minimum residual error was used as the scale for the remainder of the calibration studies.

2.2   Idealized Model Based Outlier Elimination Method

An idealized model of the calibration process was used to eliminate outlier points from the calibration dataset. The idealized model assumes that the US image plane is infinitely thin (the real US image plane has a thickness in the out of plane direction

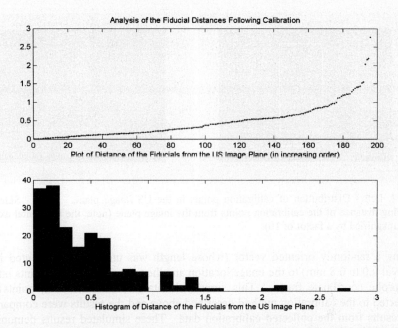

Fig. 3. Analysis of residual distances from the calibrated location of the US image plane.

that varies as a function of distance from the US probe). The physical location of the fiducial can be measured by the US fiducial tool within 0.3 mm (see section 2). The radius of the US fiducial is 0.5 mm. Therefore, according to the idealized model the maximum distance that a calibration point could be from its closest point on the computed location of the US image plane is 0.8 mm (0.5 mm for the radius of the fiducial and 0.3 mm for the measurement error). Points further than 0.8 mm must have some additional source of error contributing to the residual error.

Thus, outliers were defined as points further than 0.8 mm from the computed location of the US image plane. However, removing one of these outliers from the dataset affects the computation of the US image plane location. Hence, the outliers were eliminated one at a time and after the elimination of each outlier point from the dataset, the calibration transform was recalculated to update all of the residual errors. In this manner, outliers were eliminated until all of the remaining points of the calibration dataset were within 0.8 mm of the computed location of the US image plane (typically, less than 25 % of the points were eliminated).

2.3 Theoretical Accuracy

The idealized model can also be used to evaluate the theoretical accuracy of the calibration method. A simulated calibration dataset was produced using the diameter of the fiducial and the measurement error of the Optotrak device. The image locations ($z = 0$ for each point) were used as the true locations of the US fiducial, the corresponding location in the US probe coordinate frame was then produced by

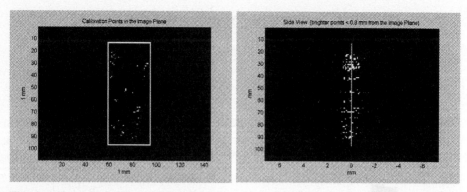

Fig. 4. Left - Distribution of calibration points in the US image plane. Right - Side view showing distance of the calibration points from the image plane (note: the horizontal axis has been magnified by a factor of 10).

adding a randomly oriented vector (whose length was uniformly distributed in the interval 0.0 to 0.8 mm) to the image location and then transforming the points into the US probe coordinate frame. This simulated dataset (100 calibration points) was subjected to the calibration method described above and the results were compared to the results from the collected calibration data. These simulated results demonstrate the limitations on the achievable accuracy imposed by the experimental setup of the calibration protocol.

2.4   Consistency of the Calibration Following Reattachment of the Molded Shell

To evaluate whether the spatial relationship between the optical tracker and the US image plane was identical when the molded shell was reattached, two sets of 100 US images were collected. Between the collection of the first and second set of 100 images the molded shell was removed completely from the US probe and then reattached. The first dataset collected, dataset A, was randomly partitioned into two mutually exclusively sets of 50 points to produce dataset A_1 and A_2. In a similar manner, the second dataset collected, dataset B, was partitioned to produce dataset B_1 and B_2.

By comparing the calibration transform obtained from dataset A_1 (or A_2) to either B_1 or B_2 we can test the hypothesis that the molded shell attaches in a unique and repeatable manner each time. This comparison is called Inter, since we are comparing calibration transforms obtained before and after removal and reattachment of the molded shell. The other comparison, between dataset A_1 and A_2 (or B_1 and B_2) is called Intra. In both cases (the Intra or the Inter comparison) the outlier removal procedure described above was performed on both datasets prior to the computation of the calibration transforms. Since some variation in the calibration transform would be expected simply from partitioning the dataset, the Intra dataset comparison serves as a control for the variance from partitioning the dataset. If the molded shell did not reattach with an identical spatial relationship between the US probe and the optically tracked molded shell, this difference would be observable as an increased difference in the Inter results as compared to the Intra results.

3   Results

Prior to performing the calibration studies, the scale was optimized with respect to the residual error and determined to be 4.415 pixels per mm (for the particular fixed settings on the US machine used to collect the US images).   Six parameters (3 rotations and 3 translations) define the calibration transform that specifies the relationship between the optical tracker and the US image plane.   The rotational parameters, Rx, Ry, and Rz are reported in degrees and the translational parameters Tx, Ty, and Tz are reported in millimeters. The results are presented as the absolute differences in the six parameters that define the two calibration transforms being compared.

3.1   Theoretical Accuracy

The first results reported are for the theoretical accuracy study. Tables 1 and 2 display the results using the simulated dataset as compared to the real collected calibration data. The differences between the six calibration parameters using the simulated data indicate the accuracy limitations of this particular experimental setup, and thus are referred to as the theoretical accuracy.

	Rx	Ry	Rz	Tx	Ty	Tz
Real	0.5394	0.1248	0.5147	0.1422	0.3335	0.0378
Simulated	0.1680	0.1252	0.2089	0.1104	0.1210	0.0525

Table 1. Theoretical Accuracy Study: Average Differences

	Rx	Ry	Rz	Tx	Ty	Tz
Real	1.0849	0.3329	1.4918	0.3392	0.8126	0.1178
Simulated	0.2946	0.3119	0.5345	0.2292	0.2356	0.1015

Table 2. Theoretical Accuracy Study: Maximum Differences

3.2   Consistency of Calibration Following Removal and Reattachment

The second set of results evaluate the consistency of reattachment of the molded shell to the US probe. Table 3 lists the average differences and table 4 lists the maximum differences between the six calibration parameters over the set of ten trials of random partitioning of the data. Again, the resulting transforms were compared with the absolute differences between the six parameters that define the calibration transforms. The Inter label indicates that one calibration transform was computed from data collected before and the other after removal of the molded shell. The Intra label indicated that both calibration transforms were obtained withouth removing the molded shell. The results demonstrated that the calibration transforms obtained using data collected without removing the shell were not significantly different than those obtained using data collected after removal and reattachment of the molded shell.

	Rx	Ry	Rz	Tx	Ty	Tz
Inter	0.6096	0.2772	0.6052	0.1804	0.2506	0.3263
Intra	0.5394	0.1248	0.5147	0.1422	0.3335	0.0378

Table 3. Consistency of Calibration Study: Average Differences

	Rx	Ry	Rz	Tx	Ty	Tz
Inter	1.2498	0.4675	1.2468	0.4108	0.7310	0.4072
Intra	1.0849	0.3329	1.4918	0.3392	0.8126	0.1178

Table 4. Consistency of Calibration Study: Maximum Differences

4   Discussion

The results using the real data were nearly as accurate (within a factor of two on average) as the results using the simulated data indicating that the calibration results are approaching the limit of accuracy attainable given the experimental setup. However, even after application of the outlier elimination method based on the idealized model, the differences using the collected data were still larger than the differences with the simulated data. This may suggest that modeling the residual errors with a uniform distribution underestimates the typical distribution of the residual errors.

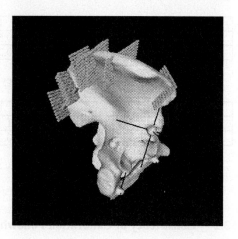

Comparisons between the Intra and Inter results for the collected data indicated that the molded shell did in fact reattach in a unique and reproducible manner as there was not any significant difference between the calibration transforms obtained before and after removal and reattachment of the molded shell.

Fig. 5. Set of 2D ultrasound image planes shown relative to pelvic surface model.

5   Conclusion

The calibration method presented here has several advantages in terms of the accurate and robust determination of the calibration transform. The outlier elimination routine provides a principled method for removing points that are not consistent with the rest of the calibration dataset. Using a large number of calibration points (e.g. 100 or more) allows averaging of the distribution of calibration points to reduce the error associated with the out of plane thickness of the US imaging region. Having the calibration points well distributed throughout the image plane also increases the accuracy by providing a longer baseline to confine the rotational degrees of freedom.

We gratefully acknowlege support for this work from the Medical Robotics and Computer Assisted Surgery Fellowship of the Shadyside Hospital Foundation.

References

[1] Amin D.V., Ultrasound Registration for Surgical Navigation. PhD Thesis, Carnegie Mellon University, 2001.

[2] Barbe C., Troccaz J., Mazier B., Lavallee S., Using 2.5D Echography in Computer Assisted Spine Surgery. IEEE Engineering in Medicine and Biology Society Proceedings, 1993; 160-161.

[3] Blackall J.M., Rueckert D, Mauer C.R., Penney G.P., Hill D.L.G.,Hawkes D.J. An Image Registration Approach to Automated Calibration for Freehand 3D Ultrasound. MICCAI 2000 Proceedings, pp. 462-471, 2000

[4] Carrat L., Tonetti J., Lavallee S. et al, Treatment of pelvic ring fractures: percutaneous computer assisted iliosacral screwing, MICCAI '98 Proceedings, pp. 84-91, 1998

[5] DiGioia A.M., Jaramaz B., Blackwell M., et al. Image Guided Navigation System to Measure Intraoperatively Acetabular Implant Alignment. Clinical Orthopedics and Related Research 355 (1998): 8-23.

[6] Horn B.K.P. Closed form Solution of Absolute Orientation Using Unit Quaternions. Journal of the Optical Society of America A. 4(4):629-642, April, 1987

[7] Ionescu G., Lavallee S., Demongeot J., et al, Automated Registration of ultrasound with CT images: Application to computer assisted prostate radiotherapy and orthopedics, MICCAI '99 Proceedings, 1999

[8] Leotta D.F., Three-dimensional spatial compounding of ultrasound images acquired by freehand scanning: Volume reconstruction of the rotator cuff, PhD Thesis, University of Washington, 1998

[9] Prager, R., Rohling R., Gee A., Berman L., Rapid calibration for 3D freehand ultrasound. Ultrasound in Medicine and Biology, 24(6):855-869, 1998.

Non-linear Local Registration of Functional Data

Isabelle Corouge[1], Christian Barillot[1], Pierre Hellier[1], Pierre Toulouse[2], and
Bernard Gibaud[2]

[1] IRISA, INRIA-CNRS, Campus de Beaulieu, 35042 Rennes Cx, France
{icorouge, cbarillo, phellier}@irisa.fr
http://www.irisa.fr/vista
[2] IDM laboratory, Faculty of Medicine, University of Rennes I, 35043 Rennes Cx,
France
{Pierre.Toulouse, Bernard.Gibaud}@univ-rennes1.fr

Abstract. Within the scope of three-dimensional brain imaging we propose an inter-individual fusion scheme to register functional activations
relatively to anatomical cortical structures, the sulci. This approach is
local and non-linear. It relies on a statistical sulci shape model accounting for the inter-individual variability of a population of subjects, and
providing deformation modes relatively to a reference shape (a mean
sulcus). The deformation field obtained between a given sulcus and the
reference sulcus is extended to a neighborhood of the given sulcus by
using the thin-plate spline interpolation. It is then applied to the functional activations associated with this sulcus. This approach is compared
with other classical matching methods.

1 Introduction

In the context of inter-individual normalization, we address in this paper the
registration of 3D anatomical and functional data, *i.e.* data from various subjects and/or acquired according to various modalities (e.g. magnetic resonance
imaging (MRI) for anatomical data, magnetoencephalography (MEG) or functional magnetic resonance imaging (fMRI) for functional data). We intend to
grasp the high inter-individual variability implied by such data with a shape
model. Deformable models are a powerful tool to image analysis [1]. Some of
them use modal analysis techniques lying on a physical approach [2], [3] or on a
statistical approach [4], [5]. In this kind of model, adequation between model and
data is improved by introducing *prior* knowledge thanks to a training set. These
models are able not only to represent the shape of an object but also the way it
can vary. They are generally used for segmentation purpose. Within the framework of anatomo-functional normalization, it is interesting to use the modeling
of deformations to register scattered data associated with modeled structures
of interest. Thus to register functional activations we rely on the modeling of
anatomical structures, the sulci, which are relevant landmarks for such purpose;
the registration being finally achieved thanks to a technique based on the thin-
plate spline interpolation [6], [7].

W. Niessen and M. Viergever (Eds.): MICCAI 2001, LNCS 2208, pp. 948–956, 2001.
© Springer-Verlag Berlin Heidelberg 2001

In Sect. 2 we describe the construction of the statistical model of cortical sulci by learning a set of shapes. The training stage is first detailed, then we present the statistical analysis we use, *i.e* the principal component analysis (PCA). In Sect. 3 we present the thin-plate spline method and its use combined to the model exploitation in the local and non-linear registration of functional activations, MEG dipoles. We compare this approach with a local rigid approach and with global methods (rigid and non-rigid).

2   Statistical Model of Cortical Sulci

2.1   Training

Cortical sulci are anatomical structures whose shape is complex. We dispose of a parametric representation of these shapes of interest [8] describing them by their median surface. This one is extracted from MRI volumes by the "active ribbon" method and is eventually modeled by a cubic B-spline surface, which is well adapted to model free form objects. The spline, parameterized by u and v, is described by nbp knots and $nbc = nbc\_u * nbc\_v$ control points where nbc_u (resp. nbc_v) is the number of control points in the direction associated with parameter u (resp. v). In the case of sulci, the parametric direction u represents the length of the sulcus and the direction v its depth. Giving nbc control points completely defines the sulcal surface. Consequently, we can represent a sulcus by the vector of its knots or its control points. The ratio nbc/nbp defines the smoothing factor: the smaller this ratio, the smoother the surface (we have chosen $nbc/nbp = 1/24$). The main advantages to use control points are their lower number and their complete representation of each surface.

The statistical technique used here needs to establish the point to point correspondences between all shapes of the training set. This implies a resampling stage so that the sulci have the same number of points and a registration stage in order to express them in the same system of reference. Each sulcus is initially expressed in its image reference system which is different from one patient to another. The idea is to associate its own system of reference with each sulcus, built so that it is common to all sulci. We call it "local system of reference". It is then just needed to determine the rigid transformation (rotation+translation) aligning all local systems of axes and to apply it to the associated shapes.

Let $\mathcal{R}_s(O_s, \mathbf{u_s}, \mathbf{v_s}, \mathbf{w_s})$ be the system of reference local to the sulcus. The axes $\mathbf{u_s}$, $\mathbf{v_s}$ and $\mathbf{w_s}$ are defined as the axes of inertia of the sulcal surface, and are decided to be so that $\mathbf{u_s}$ follows the length of the sulcus, $\mathbf{v_s}$ its depth and $\mathbf{w_s}$ its normal. This discrimination between the 3 axes is first carried out by considering that $\mathbf{u_s}$ (resp. $\mathbf{v_s}$) is the axis of inertia the "most collinear" with the nbc_u (resp. nbc_v) pseudo-parallel directions; each of them being defined by the two extremities of a sulcus' line in direction u (resp. v). Then $\mathbf{w_s}$ is obtained by vector product: $\mathbf{w_s} = (\mathbf{u_s} \wedge \mathbf{v_s})$. At last the origin O_s is the center of mass of the sulcus.

The sulci have now to be expressed in their local systems of reference. It amounts to determining, for each sulcus, the matrix $\mathbf{M}$ defining the change of basis from the local system of reference $\mathcal{R}_s$ towards the image system of reference, let it be $\mathcal{R}(O, \mathbf{u}, \mathbf{v}, \mathbf{w})$. Let $\mathbf{R}$ and $\mathbf{t}$ be the rotation matrix and the translation vector of the inverse change of basis $\mathbf{M}^{-1}$ (*i.e.* from $\mathcal{R}$ towards $\mathcal{R}_s$). Then in homogeneous coordinates:

$$\mathbf{R} = (\,\mathbf{u_s}\ \mathbf{v_s}\ \mathbf{w_s}\,),\ \mathbf{t} = \overrightarrow{OO_s}\ \text{ and }\ \mathbf{M}^{-1} = \begin{pmatrix} \mathbf{R} & \mathbf{t} \\ 0\,0\,0 & 1 \end{pmatrix}$$

Since $\mathbf{R}$ is orthogonal: $\mathbf{M} = \begin{pmatrix} \mathbf{R}^T & -\mathbf{R}^T\mathbf{t} \\ 0\,0\,0 & 1 \end{pmatrix}$.

Applying this rigid transformation to all the points of each sulcus aligns the training set as illustrated on Fig. 1a. Since the image data are acquired to the same scale, we decided not to perform any homothety. First, it enables to avoid one more transformation, then the inter-individual size variation will thus be grasped by the shape model.

The next stage consists in resampling the sulci of the training set. We resample the elements of the training population on the one which has the most sample points, spline properties ensuring that the original shapes are preserved. Once the sulci are resampled and aligned, the matching is performed by just assigning control point to control point according to their curvilinear abscissa.

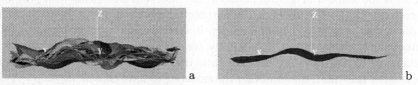

a   b

Fig. 1. a) A side view of a database of 18 left central sulci aligned in the local system of reference. b) A side view of the mean left central sulcus of this database.

2.2 Statistical Analysis of Deformations

The statistical analysis of the training set leads to a modeling of cortical sulci and of their variations. The model captures the shape variability observed within the training set. Indeed, the statistical analysis reveals the main modes of variation relative to a prototype shape, representative of the considered class. We use a principal component analysis which enables to represent data in a new basis, orthogonal, and which suppresses the redundancy of information. Moreover, this analysis enables a modal approximation.

Principal Component Analysis. Let $\mathcal{P}$ be the training population made up of N elements, $\mathbf{x}_i \in \mathcal{P}$ a shape, $\bar{\mathbf{x}}$ the mean shape on $\mathcal{P}$, $\mathbf{C}$ the covariance matrix. A shape $\mathbf{x}_i$ is represented by the vector of control points of the spline which models the median surface of the sulcus:

$$\mathbf{x}_i = (x_{i_1}, y_{i_1}, z_{i_1}, \ldots, x_{i_n}, y_{i_n}, z_{i_n})^T \ \text{ with } n = nbc \ .$$

The mean shape, representative of the studied class, and the covariance matrix are given by:

$$\bar{\mathbf{x}} = \frac{1}{N}\sum_{i=1}^{N}\mathbf{x}_i \text{ and } \mathbf{C} = \frac{1}{N}\sum_{i=1}^{N} d\mathbf{x}_i d\mathbf{x}_i^T \text{ with } d\mathbf{x}_i = \mathbf{x}_i - \bar{\mathbf{x}} \ .$$

Diagonalizing the covariance matrix $\mathbf{C}$ provides the new modal basis $\boldsymbol{\Phi}$:

$$\mathbf{C} = \boldsymbol{\Phi}\boldsymbol{\Lambda}\boldsymbol{\Phi}^T \ , \ \Lambda = diag(\lambda_1, \ldots, \lambda_{3n}) \text{ with } \lambda_1 \geq \lambda_2 \geq \ldots \geq \lambda_{3n} \ .$$

Then any shape $\mathbf{x}$ can be written: $\mathbf{x} = \bar{\mathbf{x}} + \boldsymbol{\Phi}\mathbf{b}$ where $\mathbf{b} = (b_1, \ldots, b_{3n})^T$ is the vector of modal amplitudes of deformation and $(-\boldsymbol{\Phi}\mathbf{b})$ corresponds to the deformation vectors in each point of $\mathbf{x}$ towards the mean shape. Since the eigenvalue λ_i is the variance explained by the ith mode, a large part of the variability can be explained by retaining only the first m modes. The value m is chosen so that $\sum_{i=1}^{m} \lambda_i$, the variance explained by the first m modes, represents a proportion, sufficiently important of the whole variance: $\lambda_T = \sum_{i=1}^{3n} \lambda_i$. Retaining only m modes enables us to achieve a modal approximation:

$$\begin{cases} \mathbf{x} = \bar{\mathbf{x}} + \boldsymbol{\Phi}_\mathbf{m}\mathbf{b}_\mathbf{m} \\ \mathbf{b}_\mathbf{m} = \boldsymbol{\Phi}_\mathbf{m}^T(\mathbf{x} - \bar{\mathbf{x}}) \end{cases}$$

where $\boldsymbol{\Phi}_\mathbf{m}$ is a submatrix of $\boldsymbol{\Phi}$ containing the first m eigenvectors of $\mathbf{C}$, thus defining the modal approximation basis. The vector $\mathbf{b}_\mathbf{m} = (b_1, \ldots, b_m)^T$ represents a shape in the m-dimensional space defined by the principal components. This space is interesting since it is of lower dimension (dim m). However, $\mathbf{b}_\mathbf{m}$ must be constrained in order to represent an "allowable" shape (*i.e.* a shape consistent with the learnt shapes). Given the assumption that the distribution of vectors $\mathbf{x}_i$ is normally distributed (*i.e.* gaussian distribution), the range of variability of each b_i is typically such as: $-3\sqrt{\lambda_i} \leq b_i \leq +3\sqrt{\lambda_i}$.

Results. Several tests have been carried out by making the cardinal of the training population vary (up to 85 sulci) and also by changing the type of sulci (central right and left sulcus, lateral sulcus, superior frontal sulcus, ...). We present the results obtained on a training set made up of the 18 left central sulci registered in the previous stage. Figure 2 shows the predominance of the first modes. Indeed, the first 5 modes explain a large part of the total variation (about 70%). The first mode explains on its own almost 30% of the total variation (whereas a sulcus is described by 104 control points, that is to say 312

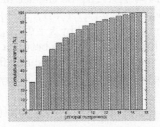

Fig. 2. Cumulative variance according to the number of principal components retained.

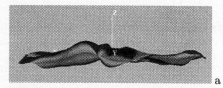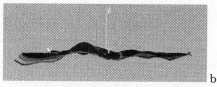

a   b

Fig. 3. a) Variations of the first mode around the mean sulcus, $-3\sqrt{\lambda_1} \leq b_1 \leq +3\sqrt{\lambda_1}$. b) Variations of the 15th mode around the mean sulcus, $-3\sqrt{\lambda_{15}} \leq b_{15} \leq +3\sqrt{\lambda_{15}}$.

variables, and by more than 8000 variables if knots are considered). The statistical modeling seems to be appropriate to express the shapes and the variations in a compact way. Figure 3a shows the variations due to the first mode. They are mainly relative to the length and to the torsion of the sulcus. On the contrary, Fig. 3b illustrates the minor influence of the 15th mode: the deformations are hardly distinct, all the sulci are almost superimposed to the mean shape.

3 Deformation Fields and Non-linear Registration

The deformation field $(-\Phi_{\mathbf{m}}\mathbf{b_m})$ obtained between a given sulcus and the reference sulcus (the mean sulcus in our case) can be extended to a local neighborhood of the considered sulcus by using the thin-plate spline interpolation [6]. It can then be applied to any object associated with this sulcus. We take advantage of this extension of the deformation field $(-\Phi_{\mathbf{m}}\mathbf{b_m})$ to register scattered data located in the left central sulcus area towards a mean space.

3.1 The Thin-Plate Spline Method

The use of thin-plate spline interpolation for registration purpose in medical imaging was first proposed by Bookstein. In [6], he proposes an algebraic approach to describe deformations specified by two sets of corresponding points. This method provides an interpolation function f which maps one of the two sets of corresponding points, the source set, onto the other one, the target set. Moreover, the function f is defined in some neighborhood of the set of source points so that it can be applied to a point in the source space to find its homologous in the target space.

Let $\mathcal{P} = \{P_i(x_i, y_i, z_i), i = 1, \ldots, n\}$ be the set of source points in the Euclidean space, and $\mathcal{V} = \{V_i = (x'_i, y'_i, z'_i), i = 1, \ldots, n\}$ the set of target points. The set $\mathcal{P}$ describes a shape $\mathbf{x}$, expressed by $\bar{\mathbf{x}} + \Phi_{\mathbf{m}}\mathbf{b_m}$ according to our model. Let $r_{ij} = |P_i - P_j|$ be the Euclidean distance between two source points P_i and P_j. Then the function f is the sum of two terms: an affine part which represents its behavior at infinity, and a second part which is asymptotically flat:

$$f(x, y, z) = a_1 + a_x x + a_y y + a_z z + \sum_{j=1}^{n} w_j U(|P_j - (x, y, z)|) \qquad (1)$$

where

- the basis function U is the fundamental solution of the biharmonic equation $\Delta^2 U = \delta(0,0)$, δ being the Kronecker's function. It can be shown [7] that the equation of a thin uniform metal plate originally flat and now bent by vertical displacements is directly related to the biharmonic equation. In 3D the function U is $U(r) = |r|$;
- the coefficients $\mathbf{a} = (a_1, a_x, a_y, a_z)^T$ and $\mathbf{w} = (w_1, w_2, \ldots, w_n)^T$ are obtained by solving the linear system:

$$\begin{cases} \mathbf{Kw} + \mathbf{Pa} = \mathbf{v} \\ \mathbf{P}^T\mathbf{w} = 0 \end{cases} \quad \text{where} \quad \mathbf{P} = \begin{pmatrix} 1 & x_1 & y_1 & z_1 \\ \vdots & \vdots & \vdots & \vdots \\ 1 & x_n & y_n & z_n \end{pmatrix},$$

$\mathbf{K}$ is a $n \times n$ matrix having the general term $(U(r_{ij}))$, and $\mathbf{v}$ is the vector of one coordinate of the target set (e.g. $\mathbf{v} = (x_1', \ldots, x_n')$, what implies that (1) must be declined for $f_x(x,y,z)$, $f_y(x,y,z)$, $f_z(x,y,z)$).

Regarding the target set as the mean shape $\bar{\mathbf{x}}$, the deformation field $(-\mathbf{\Phi_m b_m})$ is then represented by the elements of $(\mathbf{w} \mid \mathbf{a})$, and it is extended outside the source shape $\mathbf{x}$ thanks to the function f.

3.2 Results

The statistical modeling of anatomical structures such as cortical sulci can now be used to register functional activations in a non-linear and local way by using the method described above. We first detail the results obtained through this method (NLL), and second we compare this approach with the following methods:

- a global rigid method (GR): the registration by maximization of mutual information [9], [10];
- a global piecewise affine registration (PS): the Talairach Proportional Squaring [11];
- a non-linear global registration (NLG): a method based on optical flow and a robust optimization scheme [12];
- a local rigid method (LR): the local registration realized through the transformation described by the matrix $\mathbf{M}$ (see Sect. 2.1). This method will be evoked over all this part since it is a constant in all methods.

For all methods, the functional data to register are MEG dipoles corresponding to a somatosensory activation of right hand fingers (thumb, index, little finger) performed for 15 subjects of the 18 subjects of our database (see Sect. 2). MEG current dipoles have been reconstructed using a spatiotemporal algorithm [13] and selected by choosing the most significant one in the 45+/-15 ms window. These functional activations are located in the central sulcus area.

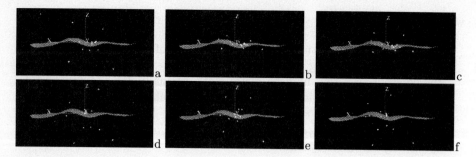

Fig. 4. Registration of MEG dipoles (somatosensory activation of the thumb): the sulcus is the mean left central sulcus. a) Method LR: the dipoles are rigidly registered. b), c) Method NLL: the dipoles are registered via the deformation field , b) $m = 17$, c) $m = 5$. d) Method GR. e) Method PS. f) Method NLG.

Method NLL. We apply the thin-plate spline method to merge anatomical and functional information in the central sulcus mean space. First, we rigidly register each dipole towards the local space by applying the transformation described by the corresponding matrix $\mathbf{M}$ (see Sect. 2), *i.e.* by using the LR method. Then, for each subject, we compute the "field" $(\mathbf{w} \mid \mathbf{a})$ between the left central sulcus of this subject and the mean sulcus. We apply it to the 3 dipoles of this subject, the field $(-\mathbf{\Phi_m b_m})$ being computed with all the modes ($m = 17$). Figure 4b shows that dipoles gather around the plane of the mean sulcus. Moreover, the covariance along x, y and particularly z is considerably reduced (see Table 1, first row). We present a second test in which we consider only 5 modes in the construction of $(-\mathbf{\Phi_m b_m})$. This approximation smoothes the sulcus and discards minor modes possibly resulting from potential segmentation errors of initial data. Results are presented Fig. 4c and Table 1. The gathering towards the mean plane and the decrease of the covariance are less than the ones of the previous test, but still significant.

Table 1. The covariance along x, y and z of MEG dipoles for somatosensory activations (thumb, index, little finger) after local rigid registration (LR), thin-plate splines interpolation based registration (NLL) for $m = 17$ and $m = 5$, and global registration (methods GR, PS, NLG).

	LR	NLL ($m = 17$)	NLL ($m = 5$)
thumb	90.8 25.41 69.99	77.33 21.98 7.3	80.88 20.39 16.67
index finger	90.89 31.58 71.85	85.46 26.25 5.96	82.39 26.99 11.81
little finger	97.79 33.36 81.94	90.18 34.26 8.05	88.29 32.99 21.91
	GR	PS	NLG
thumb	92.01 22.93 111.18	76.67 16.98 69.21	81.56 25.37 98.11
index finger	94.13 27.75 97.98	83.31 25.26 69.41	86.52 38.51 90.01
little finger	99.39 28.68 111.31	89.36 22.93 62.83	91.69 39.31 102.99

Comparison. We apply each of the 3 global methods to MEG data; then, for comparison purpose, we place the resulting dipoles in the local space via the LR method. Figure 4 shows that method NLL gathers the dipoles around the reference mean sulcus more than the other ones. This visual result is confirmed by computing the dipole localization covariance along each axis (see Table 1). Global methods, linear or not, lead to quite similar dispersion. However method PS leads to inferior covariances than method GR and NLG. This may be explained since method PS is by construction relevant and precise in the central sulcus area. To light the significant difference observed between global methods and method NLL we may note that global methods GR, PS and NLG rely more on luminance information than on anatomical information, whereas the NLL method is fully based on anatomical constraints. That point may be a motivation to introduce local anatomical contraints in global registration process [14], [15].

4   Conclusion

We have presented a statistical model of cortical sulci built by performing a modal analysis (PCA) on a training population. This model accounts for the deformations of the sulci between individuals, and the achieved tests show the relevance of the obtained deformation modes. This modeling has the advantage to lie in a "mean space". The sulci thus modeled can be used as landmarks in the registration of MEG dipoles towards the mean space. This registration is carried out via the thin-plate spline method. Results show a significant difference between this local and non-linear method and the global methods we presented. Interpretation remains delicate all the more so as no ground truth is available. Finally, the registration framework presented here is general and not restricted to MEG activities.

References

1. McInerney, T., Terzopoulos, D.: Deformable Models in Medical Image Analysis: A Survey. Medical Image Analysis, 1(2):91–108 (1996).
2. Subsol, G., Thirion, J.P., Ayache, N.: A General Scheme for Automatically Building 3D Morphometric Anatomical Atlases: Application to a Skull Atlas. MedIA, 2(1):37–60 (1998).
3. Martin, J., Pentland, A., Sclaroff, S., Kikinis, R.: Characterization of Neuropathological Shape Deformations. IEEE Trans. on PAMI, 20(2):97–112 (1998).
4. Kervrann, C., Heitz, F.: A Hierarchical Statistical Framework for the Segmentation of Deformable Objects in Image Sequences. IEEE CVPR, 724–728 (1994).
5. Cootes, T.F., Taylor, C.J., Cooper, D.H., Graham, J.: Active Shape Models - their training and application. CVIU, 61(1):38–59 (1995).
6. Bookstein, F.: Principal Warps: Thin-plate splines and the decomposition of deformations. IEEE Trans. on PAMI, 11(6):567–585 (1989).
7. Bookstein, F.L., Green, D.K.: A Feature Space for Derivatives of Deformations. IPMI, LNCS, 687:1–16 (1993).

8. Le Goualher, G., Barillot, C.,Bizais, Y.: Modeling Cortical Sulci with Active Ribbons. IJPRAI, 8(11):1295–1315 (1997).
9. Collignon, A., Vandermeulen, D., Suetens, P., Marchal, G.: 3D Multi-Modality Medical Image Registration using Feature Space Clustering. CVRMed, 195–204 (1995).
10. Viola, P., Wells, W.: Alignment by Maximization of Mutual Information. Proc. Int. Conf. Computer Vision, 15–23 (1995).
11. Talairach, J., Tournoux, P.: Co-planar Stereotaxic Atlas of the Human Brain. Georg Thieme Verlag, Stuttgart (1988).
12. Hellier, P., Barillot, C., Mémin, E., Pérez, P.: An energy-based framework for dense 3D registration of volumetric brain image. IEEE CVPR, 2:270–275 (2000).
13. Schwartz, D., Badier, J.M., Bihoué, P., Bouliou, A.: Evaluation with realistic sources of a new MEG-EEG spatio-temporal localization approach. Brain Topography, 11(4):279–289 (1999).
14. Collins, L., Le Goualher, G., Venugopal, R., Caramanos, A., Evans, A., Barillot, C.: Cortical Constraints for Non-linear Cortical Registration. VBC, LNCS, 1131:307–316 (1996).
15. Hellier, P., Barillot, C.: Cooperation Between Local and Global Approaches to Register Brain Images. IPMI, LNCS, 2082:315–328 (2001).

Registration of Reconstructed Post Mortem Optical Data with MR Scans of the Same Patient

E. Bardinet[1], A.C.F. Colchester[2], A. Roche[1], Y. Zhu[2], Y. He[2], S. Ourselin[1],
B. Nailon[3], S.A. Hojjat[2], J. Ironside[3], S. Al-Sarraj[4], N. Ayache[1], and
J. Wardlaw[3]

[1] INRIA, Epidaure Project, Sophia Antipolis, France
[2] KIMHS, University of Kent at Canterbury, UK
[3] National Creutzfeldt-Jakob Disease Surveillance Unit, WGH, Edinburgh, UK
[4] Institute of Psychiatry, London, UK
ebard@sophia.inria.fr

Abstract. We present a method for registration of macroscopic optical images with MR images of the same patient. This forms a key part of a series of procedures to allow *post mortem* findings to be accurately registered with MR images, and more generally provides a method for 3D mapping of the distribution of pathological changes throughout the brain. The first stage of the method involves a 3D reconstruction of 2D brain slices and was presented in a previous paper [2]. In the current paper, we focus on the registration of the reconstructed volume with corresponding MR images.

1 Introduction

The correlation of pathological findings with abnormalities on MR images is important in many neurological conditions. In Creutzfeldt-Jakob disease (CJD), MR signal changes have been observed in certain locations, for example (in variant CJD) in the posterior thalamus (pulvinar) [10], but pathological changes are known to be more widespread, and it is likely that grey matter signal abnormality occur in a much wider distribution. Accurate 3-D registration of MR and large field-of-view pathology images could help to clarify the distribution and mechanism of MR signal changes.

In a previous publication [2], we described work on the 3D reconstruction of macroscopic optical images of brain slices into a a 3D coordinate frame. During routine clinical neuropathology, such slices are cut by hand, the slice thickness being controlled by a simple guide on which a knife is rested while cutting. 3D reconstruction of the macroscopic optical data would be easier to accomplish if thin sections could be obtained from a macrocryotome [8]. However cryosections have to be cut from fresh frozen ("unfixed") brain which is highly infectious in CJD. The apparatus would thus have to be retained for use on CJD brains only, and the subsequent specialised processing of large thin sections would also

W. Niessen and M. Viergever (Eds.): MICCAI 2001, LNCS 2208, pp. 957–965, 2001.

require dedicated equipment which could not be used for any other types of patients. The precaution needed would be complex, very expensive, and probably prohibitive. Furthermore, the large cryosections could not be proceed in the way needed for routine diagnostic neuropathology. Therefore, we have devoted considerable effort into developing methodology for reconstruction of macroscopical optical brain slice images which can be incorporated into a routine clinical environment [2].

In the present paper, we take such 3D reconstructions of optical brain slice data and show that these can be successfully registered with MR scans of the same patient. This is a further major step towards our goal of relating microscopic pathology data to the exactly corresponding locations in MR scans.

2   Methods

The left hemisphere of a formalin-fixed *post mortem* brain was examined for this preliminary study. First, several MR images were acquired (Proton-Density, T1, T2, FLAIR) with the brain suspended in a water-filled container which reduced brain distortion due to gravity and dampened oscillations transmitted from the scanner. The brain was aligned in the scanner following the normal clinical procedure as far as possible, but it was not expected that the MR slice planes would correspond exactly to the physical brain slices which were to be cut later. Fig. 1 shows three orthogonal views of the Proton-Density image. After brain fixation, the pathologist cut 14 coronal slices 12 mm thick through the brain. The anterior (A) and posterior (P) faces of each slice were photographed. A perspex jig was constructed to hold each slice during photography [2]. Accurate circular fiducial marks were machined at each corner. Slices were numbered from front to back (Fig. 2 shows the images from slices 2, 3 and 4).   Section 2.1

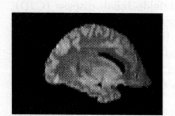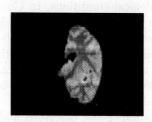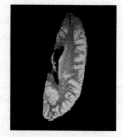

Fig. 1. *Post mortem MR Proton-Density image. From left to right: sagittal, coronal and axial views.*

briefly summarizes the method used to realign the optical sections, allowing the reconstruction of a 3D block. Details are found in [2]. In the present paper, we restricted ourselves to *rigid* slice realignment when reconstructing 3-D optical data sets. Although more complex 2-D transformations between adjacent slices

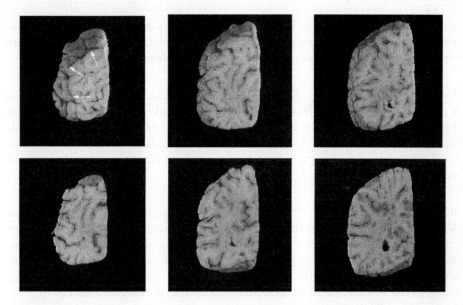

Fig. 2. *Macroscopic optical images of three brain slices. Top row: anterior images (A2, A3, A4); bottom row: corresponding posterior images of the same slice (P2, P3, P4). In image A2, arrows show the boundary between the cut surface of the slice and the oblique (non-cut) surface forming the side of the slice.*

can be estimated from the optical data alone [2], the lack of 3D prior information makes it hard to evaluate accuracy and deformations in the z direction cannot be retrieved. The geometric distortions in the optical data compared to the MR data can in theory be fully recovered during 3D/3D registration between the reconstructed block and an MR image of the same patient. Schormann *et al.* [7] previously proposed a method based on a series of slice-by-slice block-matching strategies to estimate a global 3-D affine transformation, but they assumed that out-of-plane motion could be neglected, which is not valid for our application. We thus propose another 3D multimodal affine registration method in section 2.2.

2.1   3D Reconstruction of Macroscopic Optical Brain Slice Images

To reconstruct the original 3D relationships, two different types of registration had to be computed. The first was to register the anterior and posterior sides of each slice, i.e. within-slice registration. The second was to register the images of surfaces on either side of the cut which separates two adjacent slices, i.e. between-slice registration. Finally by propagating the 2D registrations through the volume and using the known slice thickness, the 3D volume was reconstructed.

Within-Slice Co-registration Using Artificial Landmarks The cut surfaces on each side of a slice are separated in the direction perpendicular to the faces by several millimetres. We therefore cannot rely on sufficient similarity between image features to match them correctly. Instead, fiducials on the jig were detected automatically and point-based rigid registration computed.

Between-Slice Intensity-Based Registration The surfaces on either side of a single cut were derived from the cleavage of a single tissue plane and natural features on the two cut surfaces should correspond exactly to each other. Although, distortions occur during cutting and during later movement of a slice, rigid co-registration using a robust block matching algorithm provided a good match [4].

3D Reconstruction by Propagation of 2D Registrations through the Volume The known slice thickness was used to calculate the antero-posterior coordinate (z value) of each image. The alternating within-slice and between-slice rigid registrations were propagated from slice 7 (approximately the largest slice) near the middle of the volume, forwards and backwards through smaller slices in the volume, to allow each image to be transformed in x and y.

2.2 Registration between Reconstructed Optical Data and MR Images of the Same Patient

3D Rigid Registration: Surface-Based Method We first perform a rigid Iterative Closest Point (ICP) registration [1,11] between the brain surfaces extracted from both the MR and optical volumes. Notice that the MR surface has a much higher resolution along the z-axis than the reconstructed optical block surface (3 mm vs 12 mm thickness).

In the optical images, the surface extracted automatically was in fact the outer silhouette rather than the boundary of the cut surface (see Fig. 2, slice A2). This causes the ICP algorithm to match surface points from the MR image with some non-corresponding points from the optical block. Therefore, one sees that the accuracy of a surface-based registration is intrinsically limited by the amount of visible non-cut surfaces. Nevertheless, it provides a fair starting estimate for the subsequent intensity-based registration, a method generally quite dependent on good initialisation.

3D Affine Registration: Intensity-Based Method In order to improve the ICP result and to achieve affine registration, we use an intensity-based approach which enables us to match homologous regions rather than contours. Starting from the rigid estimate provided by the ICP, we search for the affine transformation that maximises a similarity measure between the MR image and the reconstructed optical block.

A robust variant of the correlation ratio based on the Geman-McClure scale estimator was used as the similarity measure, as in our previous work [6]. The assumption underlying the correlation ratio is that there exists an unknown mapping from the MR intensities to the reconstructed optical block intensities. This assumption actually does not hold in the whole image overlap whenever regions with small intensity variance in the MR image are expected to match regions with high intensity variance in the optical block. This will typically occur here because MR background voxels are expected to match non-cut surfaces voxels. The use of a robust correlation measure prevents the registration from being biased by such outliers. Other similarity measures such as mutual information [3,9,?] could also be used. However, we found the correlation ratio measures to be generally easier to optimise as they yield fewer local maxima [5].

3   Results and Discussion

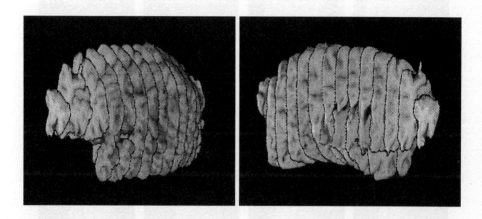

Fig. 3. *3D reconstruction of macroscopic optical brain slice images from a left hemisphere (only images of the anterior faces are shown). Left: antero-lateral view. Right: antero-medial view.*

We present in Fig. 3 the 3D reconstructed block obtained after rigid re-alignment of the macroscopic optical brain slices. The result of the 3D affine registration between the reconstructed block and the MR Proton-Density image is shown in two different ways in Figures 4 and 5. Fig. 4 presents four different optical slices overlaid with brain contours extracted from the MR image, respectively: before registration, after ICP rigid registration, and after correlation ratio-based affine registration. In order to better assess the effect of registration in 3D, we show in Fig. 5 three different perspective views of the MR and optical volumes, respectively before and after registration.

Our results show that the methods we have developed do indeed allow successful registration between images of physically-cut post-mortem slices and MR data from the same post-mortem brain acquired before cutting. In the present paper, evaluation of the success of registration has been based on visual inspection of 2D slices through the volume data. It is relatively easy to judge the

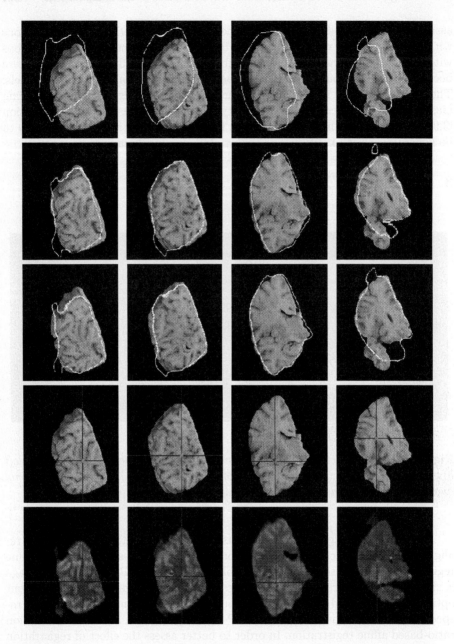

Fig. 4. *Rows 1, 2, 3: contours of post mortem MR image (outer surface of brain hemisphere) superimposed on optical slices; row 1: before matching; row 2: after contour-based rigid matching; row 3: after intensity-based affine matching. Rows 4, 5: optical and MR slices after intensity-based affine registration, with cursor superimposed to help visual inspection of the correspondence between visible features in the two modalities. Columns correspond to different slices in the volumes.*

correspondence of outlines of 2D sections through the registered 3D data. However, the optical data are digital photographs of a physically sliced brain; in addition to the *cut surface*, the *non-cut surface* may be visible adjacent to the *cut surface* in the same photograph, if the *non-cut surface* is at an appropriate angle to the camera viewpoint so that it is not occluded. Therefore, evaluation by visual inspection of the quality of the matching after registration needs to take account of the fact that the boundary of a thin MR section should correspond to the boundary of the *cut surface* in the optical data set, which is not necessarily the same as the outer silhouette of the optical image. Inspection of the registered outlines in Fig. 4 confirms that a good result has been achieved. Judicious use of outlier rejection in the final stage of 3D intensity-based affine registration has ensured that the match has been successful. Inspection of the correspondence between visible features in the two modalities in Figures 4 and 5 confirms the good matching even in the presence of a substantial amount of non-cut surface in some optical images.

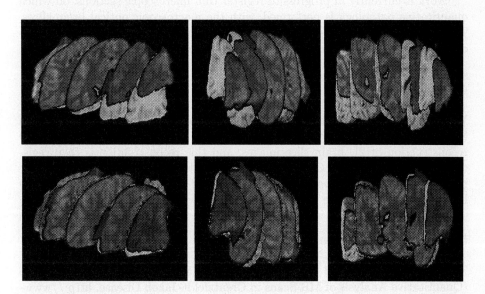

Fig. 5. *Perspective views of five selected corresponding slices of the post mortem MR image and the reconstructed macroscopical volume. First row: before registration. Second row: after 3D affine registration. Left column: antero-superior view. Middle column: antero-lateral view. Right column: antero-medial view.*

When brain slices are cut by the pathologist, new distortions are inevitably introduced. Apart from smooth distortions, which may be visualised as those occurring when a loaf of bread is cut, there are additional problems when separated fragments of brain can move independently of each other. Thus, if a coronal section is cut through the frontal lobe and also the temporal pole, the temporal fragment may be completely disconnected from the remainder of the hemisphere, and it is impossible to avoid some degree of independent movement between the two fragments. In the current work, the aim was to register the majority of the slice correctly, leaving fragments which had moved independently as outliers (i.e. not registered at this stage). Future refinements will include methodology to allow free-form movement of discrete parts relative to each other. Within parts, affine deformation is likely to remain a good approximation to the real deformations in continuous blocks of fixed brain tissue.

Just as there are deformations between post-mortem MR of a fixed brain hemisphere and reconstructed 3D volumes from optical images of brain slices, so also there are deformations between in vivo MR and subsequent MR of post-mortem brains. However, if care is taken to suspend the brain during fixation in formalin, we believe that most of the latter deformations are less complex than those between post-mortem MR and post-mortem optical data, and we expect to be able to apply the same basic approach to direct registration between *in vivo* MR and *post mortem* optical data.

Work is currently in progress to register thin microscopic sections, on which quantitative pathology is performed, with the macroscopic optical brain slices. This will complete the sequence of transformations necessary for mapping microscopic data into in vivo MR scans of the same patient.

4   Conclusion

We have developed a method for registration of macroscopic optical images with MR images of the same patient. The first stage of the method involved a 3D reconstruction of 2D brain slice images, and this reconstruction is then registered with the MR data. Our preliminary evaluation indicates that an excellent registration can be achieved. This is a key part of a series of procedures to allow histological findings to be accurately registered with *in vivo* MR images.

5   Acknowledgements

This work was supported by the EU-funded QAMRIC project BMH 4-98-6048 (Quantitative Analysis of MR Scans in Creutzfeldt-Jakob Disease, http://www-sop.inria.fr/epidaure/qamric). The imaging was performed at the SHEFC Brain Imaging Research Centre for Scotland. We thank Hervé Delingette for the visualisation software.

References

1. P.J. Besl and N.D. McKay. A Method for Registration of 3-D Shapes. *IEEE Transactions on Pattern Analysis and Machine Intelligence*, 14(2):239–256, 1992.
2. A.C.F. Colchester, S. Ourselin, Y. Zhu, E. Bardinet, Y. He, A. Roche, S. Al-Sarraj, B. Nailon, J. Ironside, and N. Ayache. 3-D Reconstruction of Macroscopic Optical Brain Slice Images. In S.L. Delp, A.M. DiGioia, and B. Jaramaz, editors, *Proceedings of MICCAI'00*, volume 1935 of *LNCS*. Springer, 2000.

3. F. Maes, A. Collignon, D. Vandermeulen, G. Marchal, and P. Suetens. Multimodality Image Registration by Maximization of Mutual Information. *IEEE Transactions on Medical Imaging*, 16(2):187–198, 1997.
4. S. Ourselin, A. Roche, G. Subsol, X. Pennec, and N. Ayache. Reconstructing a 3D Structure from Serial Histological Sections. *Image and Vision Computing*, 19(1-2):25–31, January 2001.
5. A. Roche, G. Malandain, and N. Ayache. Unifying Maximum Likelihood Approaches in Medical Image Registration. *International Journal of Imaging Systems and Technology*, 11:71–80, 2000.
6. A. Roche, X. Pennec, M. Rudolph, D. P. Auer, G. Malandain, S. Ourselin, L. M. Auer, and N. Ayache. Generalized Correlation Ratio for Rigid Registration of 3D Ultrasound with MR Images. In S.L. Delp, A.M. DiGioia, and B. Jaramaz, editors, *Proceedings of Medical Imaging Computing And Computer-Assisted Intervention (MICCAI'00)*, volume 1935 of *LNCS*, pages 567–577. Springer, 2000.
7. T. Schormann, M. Von Matthey, A. Dabringhaus, and K. Zilles. Alignment of 3-D Brain Data Sets Originating From MR and Histology. *Bioimaging*, 1:119–128, 1993.
8. V. Spitzer, M.J. Ackerman, A.L. Scherzinger, and D. Whitlock. The visible human male: a technical report. *Journal of American Medical Informatics Association*, 3(2):118–130, 1996.
9. P. Viola. Alignment by Maximisation of Mutual Information. *International Journal of Computer Vision*, 24(2):137–154, 1997.
10. M. Zeidler, R.J. Sellar, D.A. Collie, R. Knight, G. Stewart, M.A. Macleod, J.W. Ironside, S. Cousens, A.C.F. Colchester, D.M. Hadley, and R.G. Will. The pulvinar sign on magnetic resonance imaging in variant Creutzfeldt-Jakob disease. *Lancet*, 355(9213):1412–1418, April 2000.
11. Z. Zhang. Iterative Point Matching for Registration of Free-Form Curves and Surfaces. *International Journal of Computer Vision*, 13(2):119–152, 1994.

A Model for Relations between Needle Deflection, Force, and Thickness on Needle Penetration

Hiroyuki Kataoka[1], Toshikatsu Washio[2], Michel Audette[2], and
Kazuyuki Mizuhara[3]

[1] NEDO Industrial Technology Researcher, Surgical Assist Technology Group,
National Institute of Advanced Industrial Science and Technology(AIST)
[2] Surgical Assist Technology Group,
National Institute of Advanced Industrial Science and Technology(AIST)
[3] Dept. of Mechanical Engineering, Tokyo Denki University

Abstract. A force-deflection model of needle penetration is proposed and evaluated experimentally. The force at the fixed end of the needle and the needle deflection were measured using a force sensor and a bi-plane X-ray imaging system, and the model was evaluated with the data. We define a physical quantity ω, which we call infinitesimal force per length, analogous to traction (force per surface area). The model predicts ω to be constant over the length of the inserted portion of the needle. However the results indicate that this assumption does not fully account for the real deflection. It is strongly suggested that there is an additional degree of freedom: a moment or a rotational force acting on the needle.

1 Introduction

Needle penetration is one of the least invasive treatments and some surgical robots are designed for this treatment [1]. However, it is known that it is not easy for surgeons to precisely reach the planned target inside soft tissue with a needle because a thin needle can be deflected in the tissue and the tissue itself also can be deformed by the needle, even if surgeons attempt to lead the needle in a straight direction. This problem makes the needle path planning difficult, and finally surgeons have to repeat the penetration by trial-and-error. Therefore clarifying the dynamics of both needle deflection and soft tissue deformation is expected to contribute to more efficient treatment through the precise planning of needle penetration with the help of preoperative simulation.

In order to model the tissue deformation and needle deflection, the relation between the locally applied force and motion of both the tissue and the needle have to be measured. However, there is no way to measure the local force directly since force sensors can only detect the force at their attached point, and it is also difficult to measure the local motion with enough temporal resolution. CT and MRI provide excellent 3D images, but these images are insufficient in both space and time resolution. Therefore we propose a new method of estimating the local force and

W. Niessen and M. Viergever (Eds.): MICCAI 2001, LNCS 2208, pp. 966–974, 2001.
© Springer-Verlag Berlin Heidelberg 2001

motion of the needle based on the mechanical analysis of both the needle deflection and the force.

In order to achieve this estimation, a force-deflection model of a needle is required. There are some reports about needle force and deflection in the field of anesthesia [2-3]. Dentists have also reported significant needle deflection in dental anesthesia [4]. Though these reports measured the deflection of commercial needles corresponding to their length in the tissue in different gauges, tip types and target materials, they didn't investigate the relation between the force and the deflection of the needle. In addition, since the diameter of commercial needles is non-linear in gauge representation and the wall thickness of needles is different for product companies, the results in the reports cannot be compared quantitatively. Brett [5] measured the axial component of the needle force to detect the epidural puncture. However, he didn't investigate the transverse force, which has a strong effect on the needle deflection.

For these reasons we simultaneously measured the needle deflection and the transverse force at the fixed end of the needle on penetration in regularized conditions. In order to observe the needle deflection, we introduced a bi-plane X-ray imaging system for its ability to observe the needle deflection in three-dimensions and for its superior resolution in space and time, in comparison with MRI and CT.

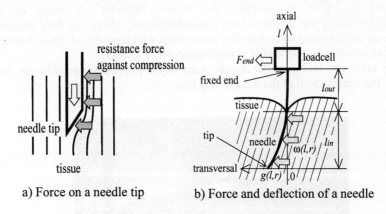

a) Force on a needle tip   b) Force and deflection of a needle

Fig. 1. A force-deflection model of a needle on penetration. $\omega(l,d)$ is the infinitesimal force per length on the needle side.

In this report we propose a novel force-deflection model: a needle with a bevelled tip goes forward while compressing the tissue around the tip, as shown in Fig.1a, and the needle is deflected by the resistance force against the compression. We introduce an assumption that the resistance force appears at the needle in a simple distribution (ie: with a constant direction everywhere along the length of inserted needle.) as shown in Fig.1b. The physical quantity used in the stress studies is the traction defined for a surface element as the limit of the surface force per area $\lim_{\Delta s \to 0} \Delta F_s / \Delta s$ [6]. However this quantity is less useful for a long thin shapes such as a needle, so we adopt the infinitesimal force per length $\omega = \lim_{\Delta l \to 0} \Delta F_l / \Delta l$, whereby ΔF_l is the force acting the segment of a curve, Δl is the length of short segment. From the transverse force at the fixed end F_{end}, measured by a three-axis loadcell, we can predict the deflection $g(l,d)$ and the resistance force per length $\omega(l,d)$, as a function of axial position l and neelde diameter d. We evaluated the model by comparing the predicted deflection $g(l,d)$ and the measured deflection $\hat{g}(l,d)$. Since ω is supposed to be related to the volume of the inserted potion of the needle, which is the same as the volume of tissue displaced by the needle, the correlation between ω and the needle diameter is also investigated.

The study shows that the constant direction of ω assumed in the model does not fully account for the real deflection, and strongly suggest that there is an additional degree of freedom: a moment or rotational force acting on the needle.

2 Materials and Methods

2.1 Measurement of the Force to a Needle

We selected swine's hip muscle as a soft tissue penetration target. The skin was removed in order to simplify the needle behavior. A mass of muscle (200x200x70mm) was prepared from a slaughterhouse, whose size fully encompassed the tissue deformation caused by the penetration with a needle of 1mm diameter, the extent of which was determined in preliminary experiments.

The mass was laid on a flat styrene foam in the penetration machine as shown in Fig.2. The outside wall of the muscle was free.

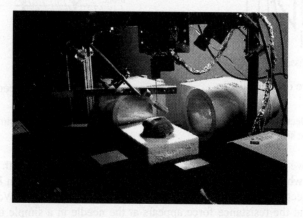

Fig. 2. A picture of the bi-plane X-ray imaging system. A sample muscle is on the penetration stage at the center.

A needle was located vertically above the center of the muscle, and both a three-axis loadcell (Nissho Co., 400N in axial and 100N in transverse direction is maximum) and a linear guide to drive the needle in its axial direction were attached at the fixed end of the needle. Some needles of different diameters (0.65mm, 1.00mm, 1.35mm, 1.55mm) were prepared. They were made from a solid cylindrical shaft to simplify the influence of the tip shape. The needle tips were bevelled at an angle of 14 degrees to emphasize the deflection. Each needle was driven forward into the muscle at a constant speed of 5mm/sec, and stopped before the tip reached the tissue bottom. The output of the loadcell was recorded by a PC at the rate of 10Hz, 50Hz sampling followed by 5 sample averaging. The penetration was carried out twice for each needle, and the penetration point on the muscle was changed each time to prevent the needle from being inserted into the incision created by the previous penetration.

2.2 3D Reconstruction of the Needle Deflection from Stereo Images

Two sets of X-ray generators and detectors (EXM-60P, Toshiba IT & Control Systems Co.), whose maximum power is 60kv/1.2mA, were located diagonally around the muscle. The FOV of each X-ray is 40x30mm at the center of the penetration machine. Its imaging rate is 30 frames per second. To measure the three-dimensional needle deflection, the shape of the needle has to be reconstructed from the stereo images of the bi-plane X-ray system.

At first, the needle area in each image was extracted and skeletonized. Then the correspondences of the image coordinates of this skeletonized needle were checked with the following equation relating the stereo images [7]:

$$m_a F m_b = 0 \qquad (1)$$

where m_a and m_b are the image coordinates of the needle represented by the homogeneous coordinate system, and F is the fundamental matrix which is uniquely determined according to camera positions. In our system F can be determined as a unique matrix from preliminary X-ray calibration as X-ray generators and detectors are fixed. Once the correspondences were found, the 3D coordinates of the points comprising the needle were estimated by solving the following equations of a perspective camera model:

$$\lambda_a m_a = P_a x_{3D} \qquad (2)$$

$$\lambda_b m_b = P_b x_{3D} \qquad (3)$$

where x_{3D} represents the 3D coordinate of the needle in the homogeneous coordinate system, P_a and P_b are the perspective camera matrices which map the 3D coordinate system to the respective image coordinate systems. These matrices are also determined uniquely by X-ray calibration. Lastly λ_a and λ_b are arbitrary variables.

After the 3D coordinates of the needle were obtained, the deflection plane on which the needle mainly deflects was calculated to consider the deflection two-dimensionally. This plane is defined as being spanned by z and by the vector in the x-y plane, coinciding with the line regression of projections of the needle points on x-y plane as shown in Fig.3. Then the needle was projected on the deflection plane.

Finally, we consider the horizontal component of the loadcell output $F_{load-xy}$ and project it onto the deflection plane. We call this projection F_{end}, the transverse force at the fixed end of the needle.

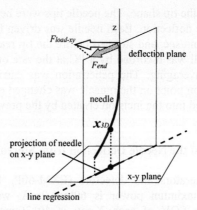

Fig. 3. The deflection plane on which the needle deflects. The plane is defined as being spanned by z and by the vector in the x-y plane, coinciding with the line regression of projections of the needle points on the x-y plane.

2.3 The Force-Deflection Model of a Needle

Following Fig.1 and [8], the needle deflection $g(l,d)$ caused by $\omega(l,d)$ can be described by solving the following equation:

$$\frac{d^2 g(l,d)}{dl^2} = -\frac{1}{EI} \int \omega(l,d) \, l \, dl \qquad (4)$$

where l is the axial position of the needle whose origin is at the needle tip without deflection, E is Young's Modulus and I is the moment of inertia of the needle, d is the diameter of the needle. The transverse force at the fixed end of the needle F_{end} can be described as follows:

$$F_{end} = \int_0^{l_{in}} \omega(l,d) \, dl \qquad (5)$$

where l_{in} is the insertion depth (refer to Fig.1b). By differentiating Eq.5 over l_{in}, ω can be represented as follows:

$$\frac{dF_{end}}{dl_{in}} = \omega(l,d) \qquad (6)$$

We obtained w from F_{end} by Eq.6, and calculated the needle deflection by Eq.4 to compare with the real deflection.

To investigate the relation between ω and the needle diameter d, ω was plotted against d^2 as suggested by the dependence of the displaced tissue volume on the cross-sectional area.

3 Results

3.1 Measurement of the Force on the Needle

The transverse force at the fixed end of the needle is shown in Fig.4. The needles were penetrating the muscle during $t=3$ to $t=10$ seconds. Note that all curves show linear correspondence between the insertion depth and the force, as the penetration speed is constant therefore the time is linearly related with insertion depth in this time period. Also, note that the force remained constant after stopping the needle motion ($t>10$).

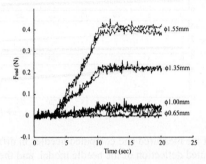

Fig. 4. The transverse force at the fixed end of the needle vs time for needles of different diameters. All needles stopped the penetration at $t=10$sec

3.2 3D Reconstruction of the Needle Deflection from Stereo X-ray Images

Figure 5 shows stereo images of a needle observed by the bi-plane X-ray imaging system. The gray area is the X-ray projection of the muscle, and the black line in the middle is the needle. The needle is deflected away from the vertical direction. The black dots in the muscle are the shadows of lead balls, which are used in tissue motion tracking research currently under way.

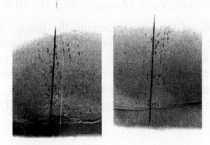

Fig. 5. Stereo X-ray images of a needle inside a mass of muscle. The gray area is the X-ray projection of the muscle, and the black line in the middle is the needle.

Figure 6 is the reconstructed deflection of the needles of different diameters on the deflection plane. The predicted and measured deflections as a function of *l* are linear and have comparable slopes, but differ by an offset (~2mm). This offset is explained by the model underestimating the deflection outside the tissue.

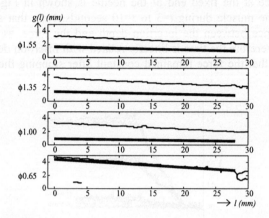

Fig. 6. The deflection of the measured and computed needles in different needle diameters. The thick lines are the computed deflection of the needle model, and the thin lines are the measured deflection of the real needle. The needle tip coincides with l=0mm, and the muscle surface is at l=28mm.

3.3 The Force-Deflection Model of the Needle

Figure 4 shows that the transverse force at the fixed end is proportional to the insertion depth. Hence, according to Eq.6, $\alpha(l,d)$ can be defined as a constant value along the axial position of the needle. By defining this value as $W(d)$, the needle deflection can be now described as follows [8]:

$$g(l,d) = \frac{W(d)}{24EI}(l^4 - 4l_{in}(l_{in}^2 + 3l_{in}l_{out} + 3l_{out}^2) l \qquad (7)$$
$$+ l_{in}(3l_{in}^3 + 12l_{in}^2l_{out} + 18l_{in}l_{out}^2 + 8l_{out}^3)) \quad (0 \leq l \leq l_{in})$$

where l_{out} is the length of the needle outside the tissue. The needle deflections calculated by Eq.7 are shown as thick lines in Fig.5, where $E = 2.0\times10^2$GPa for stainless material, $l_{in} = 28$mm, $l_{out} = 77$mm. $W(d)$ is the value estimated from Fig.3 for each needle. The deflections of the reconstructed needles from X-ray images at the time the needles stopped are also shown in Fig.5 as thin lines.

The force per length $W(d)$ is plotted against the square of the needle diameter in Fig.7.

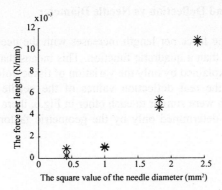

Fig. 7. The distribution forces to the square of the needle diameters (marked as *) and a regression line of the plots.

4. Discussion

4.1 Deflection Force

The transverse force at the fixed end in Fig.4 remained constant after the needle motion was stopped. This means that the origin of this force is not dynamic such as cutting force at the tip of the needle.

The transverse force Fend appeared proportional to the incremental insertion depth. This would imply that as insertion length increased the resistance force per length ω was constant, i.e., the incremental force from the tissue was constant regardless of the progress of needle deflection. However, an additional offset was caused by deflection outside the tissue ($g{\neq}0$ at $l{=}28$), which the model underestimated as one can observe in Fig.6 at the muscle surface ($l{=}28$mm). This added deflection should cause ω to increase. Therefore, we need to consider other models of force distribution, resulting in ω varying with the insertion depth.

4.2 Model-Experiment Agreement

As shown in Fig.6 the predicted and measured deflections as a function of l are linear and have comparable slopes, but differ by an offset (~2mm). This offset is explained by the model underestimating the deflection outside the tissue.

In order to keep the same transverse force at the fixed end of the needle, the deflection offset $\left| \hat{g}(l,d) - g(l,d) \right|$ should be supplied by either an additional moment at the needle tip or a force per length, featuring a rotational component, whose integration is equal to the transverse force at the fixed end of the needle. We will try to apply the force-deflection model with this new ω in the next model.

4.3 Force per Length and Deflection vs Needle Diameter

Figure 7 suggests that the force per length increases with the needle diameter as the function of higher order than a quadratic function. This means that the variation of ω with needle size is not explained by only the variation of tissue volume displacement.

Finally, considering the real deflection values of the needle at 1.55, 1.35 and 1.00mm diameters which were similar to each other in Fig.6, there is a possibility that the needle deflection is determined only by the geometric factor such as the bevel angle of the needle tip.

5 Conclusions

The relation between the force on a needle and its deflection during needle puncture into biological tissue was investigated. A simple infinitesimal force per length relation was assumed as the force-deflection model and the predicted deflection was compared to the measured deflection. These showed a good agreement in the slope of the displacement vs length at different needle diameters. However, the predicted deflection was smaller than the measured deflection.

The transverse force at the fixed end was proportional to the needle length inside tissue, which would imply the constant force per length along the needle. However, the observed needle deflection exhibited a large component outside the tissue, which is incompatible with a constant force per length. Therefore, it is strongly suggested that an additional moment or rotational component is required.

References

1. Stoianovici, D., et.al., "An efficient needle injection technique and radiological guidance method for percutaneous procedures," In proc. of CRVMed-MRCAS '97, pp.295-298, 1997.
2. Sitzman, B.T.,et.al., "The effects of needle type, gauge, and tip bend on spinal needle deflection ," Anesth Analg, 82(2), pp. 297-301, 1996
3. Drummond, G.B., et.al., "Deflection of spinal needles by the bevel," Anaesthesia, 35(9), pp. 854-7, 1980
4. Robinson, S.F., et.al., "Comparative study of deflection characteristics and fragility of 25-, 27-, and 30-gauge short dental needles," JADA, 109, pp.920-924, 1984
5. Brett, P.N., et.al., "Schemes for the Identification of Tissue Types and Boundaries at the Tool Point for Surgical Needles," IEEE trans on Inf Technol Biomed, Vol.4, No.1, pp.30-36, 2000
6. Malvern, L.E., "Introduction to the Mechanics of a Continuous Medium," Prentice-Hall, Inc., New Jersey, 1969
7. Jun Sato, "Computer Vision - Geometry of Vision -," Corona Publishing Co. Ltd., Tokyo, 1999
8. JSME ed., "JSME Mechanical Engineers' Handbook," JSME, Tokyo, 1987

In Vivo Data Acquisition Instrument for Solid Organ Mechanical Property Measurement

Mark P. Ottensmeyer[1] and J. Kenneth Salisbury, Jr.[2]

[1] Simulation Group, CIMIT, HGX-2, Massachusetts General Hospital
55 Fruit St., Boston, MA 02114, USA,
mpo@alum.mit.edu

[2] Intuitive Surgical, Inc., 1340 W. Middlefield Rd., Mountain View, CA, 94043, USA

Abstract. Surgical simulation systems need not only models that capture the behaviors of living tissue, but also parameters measured from real tissues to make such models meaningful. A portable system called the TeMPeST 1-D (Tissue Material Property Sampling Tool) that can acquire force-displacement responses *in vivo* has been developed. By fitting these data to the form of a chosen model, the tissue parameters can be obtained.

The data acquisition tool is suitable for minimally invasive or open surgical use. It measures normal indentation force-displacement response over a frequency range from DC to approximately 100Hz. This permits the investigation of the visco-elastic properties of living solid organ tissue. It can exert forces up to 300 mN, and has a range of motion of $\pm 500\mu m$. The TeMPeST 1-D was used to measure the frequency-dependent stiffness of porcine liver *in vivo* in a proof-of-concept demonstration, and is being used in a more comprehensive series of tests. Based on simple tissue models, preliminary estimates for tissue stiffness are presented and the frequency-dependent and non-linear characteristics are discussed.

1 Introduction

Our work has focused on providing support for the development of a simulator for laparoscopic surgery. Some of the structures of interest include solid organs such as liver, spleen and kidney. This paper will describe a surgical instrument that permits the measurement of the mechanical response of tissue *in vivo*. By substituting the response data into a suitable tissue model, the parameters characterizing the tissue can be determined.

Generally speaking, surgical simulations that generate accurate force feedback and deformations depend on knowledge of the mechanical properties of biological tissues. While many groups are developing such simulators ([8], [5], [11]), most must rely on estimated values or measurements typically made *in vitro*. Various reviews of tissue properties include [3], [21] and [4], but these and most other sources of data, use cadaver or animal tissues. The properties of non-living tissues are known to be significantly different from those of living organisms, due to temperature and strain state differences, and the absence of

W. Niessen and M. Viergever (Eds.): MICCAI 2001, LNCS 2208, pp. 975–982, 2001.
© Springer-Verlag Berlin Heidelberg 2001

blood perfusion, among other factors ([21], [4]). To provide the necessary data, tools must be developed to measure properties in the living state.

Some of the groups pursuing these data are using MRI, ultrasound and other imaging methods that scan broad regions of the tissue to measure properties such as elastic (Young's) or shear moduli ([18], [20], [19]). By making a static or oscillatory deformations and simultaneously scanning, the strain field in the tissue and tissue moduli can be calculated. However, for the static techniques, only relative values are available and no technique covers the range of frequencies relevant to haptic feedback (i.e. DC to 100s of Hz). The relationship between elasticity and sonic velocity in a material has been investigated with limited success [9].

Other groups are developing tools to measure organ properties by imposing deformations in a variety of ways. The Dundee Single Point Compliance Probe (DSPCP), a hand-held tool [2], records indentation depth and force while the user presses a rigid indenter against tissue. Frequency dependence cannot be determined, but the DSPCP has a range of motion sufficient to investigate non-linearity in stiffness. Stiffness could also be measured with a piezoelectric tube device [16]. Anisotropy in stiffness is related to the variation in the cantilevered tube's resonant frequency with direction of vibration tangential to the tissue surface. A number of groups have modified laparoscopy tools [17], [15] to measure the force-displacement characteristics of tissue, but typically with the intention of augmenting the sensations perceived by the surgeon rather than determining material properties. Recent results on porcine liver and spleen are beginning to be presented [1], as well as data and models for porcine brain [10].

Due to the limited data and lack of standard instruments, we developed the TeMPeST 1-D (Tissue Material Property Sampling Tool) to precisely deform tissues and record the force-displacement response ([12], [13], [14]). This device will be described in the next section.

2   TeMPeST 1-D: Tissue Material Property Sampling Tool

The TeMPeST 1-D is a minimally invasive tool that passes through standard 12mm cannulas and can be fixed to the operating table with a modified laparoscope holder. It is designed to have a range of motion of $\pm 500 \mu$m and an open-loop bandwidth of approximately 100Hz[1]. The small range of motion was intended to cover the linear regime of tissue response, thus enabling determination of the linear elastic modulus, and also to investigate whether the limits of linearity lay within this range.

The TeMPeST 1-D makes use of a voice-coil linear actuator to drive a right cylindrical indenter. The maximum force that can be exerted is 0.3N, with a resolution of approximately 70μN. The device can impose sinusoidal, chirp[2],

---

[1] varies slightly depending on stiffness of material being tested
[2] sinusoidal signal with time-varying frequency

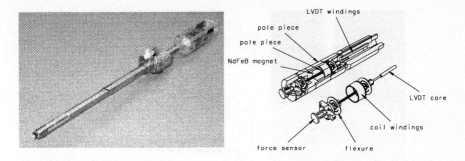

Fig. 1. TeMPeST 1-D in 12mm cannula (left) and details of indenter, actuator, force sensor and LVDT (right) showing cut-away sensor/actuator package and details of moving core.

step, and other force profiles on the tissue, while independently recording the force exerted with a force sensor at the tip, and the deformations imposed with an LVDT position sensor (see Figure 1). Force and position measurement resolutions are $\pm 70 \mu$N and $\pm 0.2 \mu$m.[3]

As an ideal case, tissue can be modeled as a linear elastic, isotropic, homogeneous and incompressible ([18], [20]) medium. In this instance, only Young's modulus is required to describe the material. If force and deformation are known, and if the tissue geometry can be approximated by a semi-infinite body undergoing normal indentation by a right circular punch, the parameters are related by equation (1) [6], as illustrated in Figure 2.

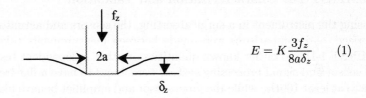

$$E = K \frac{3f_z}{8a\delta_z} \qquad (1)$$

Fig. 2. Indentation of semi-infinite elastic body with rigid, right circular punch.

δ_z and f_z are the displacement and force normal to the surface, a is the cylindrical indenter radius, and E is Young's modulus. For a semi-infinite body, K is unity [7], but if the elastic material is a layer of thickness h bonded to a flat, rigid surface, K increases with increasing a/h and δ_z/h.

Since living tissue is known to have viscous and other dissipative mechanisms, it may exhibit a frequency-dependent sinusoidal response. In the case of normal indentation, the static expression of equation (1) can be extended to the dynamic case through the correspondence principle [4], so that $E(\omega)$ is determined from

---

[3] A 12-bit motion controller card was used for control and data input.

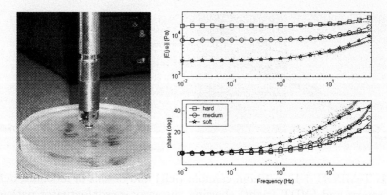

Fig. 3. TeMPeST 1-D testing silicone gel sample (left). Comparison of results from TeMPeST 1-D (dots) and parallel plate rheometer (symbols). Note close match between two data sets over wide frequency range (right).

$\delta_z(\omega)$ and $f_z(\omega)$. These results can provide data on damping coefficients and time constants of the material.

A preliminary survey of inhomogeneity could be made by taking data from numerous locations on the same organ, but anisotropy cannot be measured with the TeMPeST 1-D. However, until simulation systems become sufficiently powerful, providing $E(\omega)$ will be a significant first step, especially since these data will be based on living tissue.

2.1   TeMPeST 1-D Characterization and Validation

Before using the instrument in a surgical setting, the sensors and actuators were characterized, and comparisons were made between measurements taken with the TeMPeST 1-D and either known quantities or other independent tests. The position sensor and signal processing system were found to have a flat frequency response to at least 100Hz, while the force sensor and amplifier behave like a first order filter with a break frequency of approximately 380Hz. This behavior reflects the small output signal of the force sensor and the gain-bandwidth product limits of the instrumentation amplifier. The break frequency can be increased with better amplifiers, but the inverse of the force sensor transfer function can be applied to frequency-dependent measurements to compensate for the filtering effect. Finally, the actuator has both a flat frequency response and a constant current/force proportionality over its range of motion.

Tests were performed on lumped elements including a series of mechanical springs and standard laboratory masses. The measured spring frequency responses were flat, with magnitudes agreeing with static load cell tests. Impedance measurements on five and ten gram masses showed slopes of -40dB/decade and calculated masses within 10% of the correct values.

Figure 3 shows a comparison between swept-sine wave-based measurements made with a parallel plate rheometer on three silicone gel samples, each with a

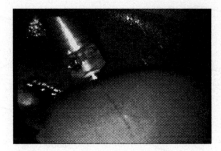

Fig. 4. Typical laparoscope view of TeMPeST 1-D approaching porcine liver.

different stiffness, with those made with the TeMPeST 1-D using chirp signals. The rheometer applies torsional loading to a thin sample of the gel, recording torque and angular displacement, from which elastic moduli can be directly calculated. The force-displacement response of the TeMPeST 1-D was converted to elastic modulus values using equation (1). Good agreement is shown between the two methods, despite completely different deformation modes. The low frequency measurements, especially for the softest materials, are subject to numerical errors, which can be reduced by increasing the sampling duration and indenter radius.[4] This shows that the TeMPeST 1-D, together with the results from solid mechanics, can be used to determine acceptable values of material properties.

2.2 *In Vivo* Liver Tests

The TeMPeST 1-D has been used under both laparoscopic and open surgical conditions to measure the elastic modulus of porcine liver *in vivo*.[5] A typical view from the laparoscope is shown in Figure 4.

The initial phase of testing included tests using fixed frequency sinusoids and chirp signals. Using the semi-infinite approximation described above (equation (1)), the Young's modulus for liver, over 0.1 to 60Hz is shown in Figure 5. The lowest measured value was approximately 2.2kPa. Simple preliminary analysis, including a least-squares fit using the less noisy sinusoidal data shows that a plane of the form of equation (3) captures the dominant characteristics of the data.

$$\log_{10} E = c_0 + c_f \log_{10} f + c_\sigma \sigma^*_{med} \tag{2}$$
$$\log_{10} E = 3.31 + 0.161 \log_{10} f + 2.152 \times 10^{-4} \sigma^*_{med} \tag{3}$$

---

[4] to increase low frequency content and applied force.

[5] Approval for the animal use protocols were obtained from the Dartmouth College IACUC for tests at the Dartmouth Medical School Animal Resource Center, and the Harvard University Standing Committee on Animals for tests at the Harvard Center for Minimally Invasive Surgery, as well as by the MIT Committee on Animal Care and the USAMRMC to permit the participation of the first author in the testing.

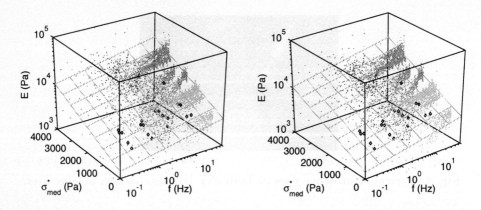

Fig. 5. Elastic modulus based on semi-infinite elastic body approximation, showing variation with both frequency and median nominal applied stress. Fixed frequency sinusoidal tests labeled by ◇, chirp transform data by shaded clouds of points. Shading corresponds with median nominal stress (y-axis) value. This image can be viewed as a stereogram by crossing one's eyes.

E is the elastic modulus, f the frequency in Hertz, and σ^*_{med} is the median nominal stress, which is the median applied force (considered over the full testing interval) divided by the cross sectional area of the indenter tip.

3   Discussion and Conclusions

The TeMPeST 1-D has been designed to measure mechanical properties of solid organ tissue in the living state. The instrument was tested on a series of standard materials, demonstrating that its measurements corresponded with independent tests. It has further been used to measure the elastic modulus of porcine liver *in vivo*. The results obtained are more complex than pure linear elastic or standard linear visco-elastic tissue models, but the measured range of elasticities falls within that expected from limited available *in vitro* data.

The preliminary expression used to fit the data has a number of characteristics which bear comment. First, there is an increase in modulus with frequency, likely due to viscous behavior of the tissue. While this is expected, the available data do not indicate what the minimum, steady-state value is. Additional tests at lower frequencies are required to address this issue. Second, there is a non-linear, exponential relationship between the nominal applied stress and elasticity. Because linear elasticity was expected, absolute depth of indentation was not measured, only the relative motion from the depth established by the preload was measured. In future tests, the controller and sampling sequence will be altered so that the absolute depth can be recorded. From the fit of the available data, however, and by recognizing that $E = \frac{d\sigma}{d\varepsilon}$, equation (3) can be solved for stress as a function of strain (equation (5)).

$$\ln \frac{d\sigma}{d\varepsilon} = \frac{c_0}{\log e} + c_f \ln f + c_\sigma \tag{4}$$

$$\Rightarrow \sigma = \frac{-\log e}{c_\sigma} \ln(1 - \frac{c_\sigma}{\log e} e^{\frac{c_0}{\log e} + c_f \ln f} \varepsilon) \tag{5}$$

These results will be validated as ongoing testing continues, and will be extended with tests at higher and lower frequencies, as well as over a wider range of applied loads. Further, due to the high uncertainties produced from the chirp measurements, fixed frequency sinusoidal measurements will be made, especially at lower frequencies. In addition, other solid organ tissues will be tested, including spleen.

While highly realistic surgical simulation is still some way off, collection of better tissue property data is a crucial step along the path.

Acknowledgements

This work was supported in part by the Department of the Army, under contract number DAMD17-99-2-9001. The views and opinions expressed do not necessary reflect the position or the policy of the government, and no official endorsement should be inferred.

References

1. Brower, I., Ustin, J., Bentley, L., Sherman, A., Dhruv, N., Tendick, F.: Measuring In Vivo Animal Soft Tissue Properties for Haptic Modeling in Surgical Simulation, Medicine Meets Virtual Reality 2001, Studies in Health Technology and Informatics, **81**, Newport Beach, CA (24-27 Jan 2001) 69–74
2. Carter, F.J.: University of Dundee Surgical Technology Group, 2/3/2000, last modified, 4/19/1999, http://surgtim.medschool.dundee.ac.uk/compprobe/main.html
3. Duck, F.A.: Physical Properties of Tissue, a comprehensive reference book. ISBN: 0-12-222800-6 Academy Press, Harcourt Brace Jovanovich, London (1990)
4. Fung, Y.C.: Biomechanics: Mechanical Properties of Living Tissues. ISBN: 0-387-97947-6, Springer-Verlag, New York (1993)
5. Gibson, S., Samosky, J., Mor, A., Fyock, C., Grimson, E., Kanade, T., Kikinis, R., Lauer, H., McKenzie, N., Nakajima, S., Ohkami, H., Osborne, R., Sawada, A.: Simulating arthroscopic knee surgery using volumetric object representations, real-time volume rendering and haptic feedback. Proceedings of First Joint Conference, Computer Vision, Virtual Reality and Robotics in Medicine and Medical Robotics and Computer-Assisted Surgery, Grenoble, France (19-22 Mar. 1997) 369–78
6. Hayes, W.C., Keer, L.M., Herrmann, G., Mockros, L.G.: A Mathematical Analysis of Indentation Tests of Articular Cartilage, Journal of Biomechanics, **5** (1972) 541–51
7. Johnson, K.L.,: Contact Mechanics. ISBN: 05-2125576-7, Cambridge University Press, Cambridge (1985)
8. Kühnapfel, U.G., Kuhn, Ch., Hübner, M., Krumm, H.-G., Maaß, H., Neisius, B.: The Karlsruhe Endoscopic Surgery Trainer as an example for virtual reality in medical education. Minimally Invasive Therapy and Allied Technologies, **6** (1997) 122–5

9. Maaß, H., Kühnapfel, U.G.: Noninvasive measurement of elastic properties of living tissue, Computer Assisted Radiology and Surgery (CARS '99): proceedings of the 13th international congress and exhibition (1999) 23–6

10. Miller, K., Chinzei, K., Orssengo, G., Bednarz, P.: Mechanical properties of brain tissue in-vivo: experiment and computer simulation. Journal of Biomechanics **33** (2000) 1369–76

11. O'Toole, O., Playter, R., Krummel, T., Blank, W., Cornelius, N., Roberts, W., Bell, W., Raibert, M.: Assessing skill and learning in surgeons and medical students using a force feedback surgical simulator, Proceedings of Medical Image Computing and Computer-Assisted Intervention – MICCAI'98. First International Conference, Cambridge, MA (11-13 Oct. 1998) 899–909

12. Ottensmeyer, M.P.: Minimally Invasive Instrument for In Vivo Measurement of Solid Organ Mechanical Impedance, Doctoral Thesis, Department of Mechanical Engineering, MIT (2001)

13. Ottensmeyer, M.P., Ben-Ur, E., Salisbury, J.K.: Input and Output for Surgical Simulation: Devices to Measure Tissue Properties in vivo and a Haptic Interface for Laparoscopy Simulators, Proceedings of Medicine Meets Virtual Reality 2000, Studies in Health Technology and Informatics, **70**, Newport Beach, CA (27-30 Jan 2000) 236–242

14. Ottensmeyer, M.P., Salisbury, J.K.: In vivo mechanical tissue property measurement for improved simulations, Proceedings of Digitization of the Battlespace V and Battlefield Biomedical Technologies II, R. Suresh and H.H. Pien, Eds., Proc. SPIE 4037, Orlando, FL (24-28 Apr 2000) 286–293

15. Rosen, J., Hannaford, B., MacFarlane, M.P., Sinanan, M.N.: Force Controlled and Teleoperated Endoscopic Grasper for Minimally Invasive Surgery-Experimental Performance Evaluation, IEEE Transactions on Biomedical Engineering, **46**(10) (1999) 1212–1221

16. Sarvazyan, A., Schafer, M.E., Ponomarev, V.: Method and device for measuring anisotropic mechanical properties of tissue, United States Patent 5,706,815 (13 Jan 1998)

17. Scilingo, E.P., DeRossi, D., Bicchi, A., Iacconi, P.: Haptic display for replication of rheological behavior of surgical tissues: modelling, control, and experiments, Proceedings of the ASME Dynamics, Systems and Control Division, Dallas, TX (16-21 Nov 1997) 173–176

18. Skovoroda, A.R., Lubinski, M.A., Emelianov, S.Y., O'Donnell, M.: Reconstructive elasticity imaging for large deformations, IEEE Transactions on Ultrasonics Ferroelectrics & Frequency Control, **46**(3) (1999) 523–35

19. Suga, M., Matsuda T., Okamoto, J., Takizawa, 0., Oshiro, O., Minato, K., Tsutsumi, S., Nagata, I., Sakai, N., Takahashi, T.: Sensible Human Projects: Haptic Modeling and Surgical Simulation Based on Measurements of Practical Patients with MR Elastography–Measurement of Elastic Modulus, Medicine Meets Virtual Reality 2000, Studies in Health Technology and Informatics, **70**, Newport Beach, CA (27-30 Jan 2000) 334–40

20. Sumi, C., Suzuki, A., Nakayama, K.: Estimation of shear modulus distribution in soft tissue from strain distribution, IEEE Transactions on Biomedical Engineering, **42**(2) (1995) 193–202

21. Yamada, H.: Strength of Biological Materials. SBN: 683-09323-1, Williams & Wilkins Company, Baltimore (1970)

Patient-Specific Simulation of Internal Defibrillation

Daniel Mocanu[1], Joachim Kettenbach[2], Michael O. Sweeney[3],
Bruce H. KenKnight[4], Ron Kikinis[2], and Solomon R. Eisenberg[1]

[1] Department of Biomedical Engineering, Boston University,
Boston, MA, U.S.A.
{mocanu,sre}@bu.edu
http://bme.bu.edu/Fieldsandtissues
[2] Surgical Planning Laboratory, Brigham and Women's Hospital,
Boston, MA, U.S.A.
{kettjo,kikinis}@bwh.harvard.edu
[3] Cardiac Pacing and Implantable Device Therapies, Brigham and Women's Hospital,
Boston, MA, U.S.A.
mosweeney@partners.org
[4] Department of Therapy Research, Guidant/CPI,
St.Paul, MN, U.S.A.
bruce.kenknight@guidant.com

Abstract. The objective of this study is to investigate the predictive capacity of computational models of electrical defibrillation by comparing the results of patient-specific simulations to clinically determined defibrillation metrics. Finite volume models of the thoracic conductive anatomy and *in situ* electrodes were constructed for seven patients who received implantable defibrillators. These models were based on segmented X-ray CT images taken shortly after implant. The models were solved for electric field (current density) distributions corresponding to a defibrillation shock. The defibrillation parameters were calculated from these distributions based on critical mass and inexcitability criteria for successful defibrillation. Preliminary results show good agreement between clinical and simulated thresholds for four of the seven patients modeled to date. The defibrillation parameters for the remaining three patients are underestimated. The correspondence between the predicted and measured defibrillation metrics observed in four of the seven patients is encouraging and provides preliminary support to the potential utility of the modeling approach. This approach may allow for patient specific presurgical planning, as well as provide a convenient computational testbed for evaluating new electrode configurations. Although these results are promising additional subjects are needed to further validate the modeling method.

1 Introduction

Ventricular fibrillation (VF) is a severe heart condition that can lead to sudden cardiac death (SCD) if not treated promptly. VF often starts with a premature

W. Niessen and M. Viergever (Eds.): MICCAI 2001, LNCS 2208, pp. 983–990, 2001.

excitatory stimulus during the vulnerable period (rising phase of the T wave) when the cardiac myocytes are in various states of recovery. The only effective clinical intervention to extinguish VF is electrical defibrillation. With the advent of smaller generators, catheter electrodes and active can technologies, implantable cardioverter defibrillators (ICD) have been shown to be very effective in protecting against SCD and have become the treatment of choice for patients with drug-resistant heart arrhythmias.

Determining the energy that the defibrillator must deliver in order to extinguish fibrillation and return the heart to a normal sinus rhythm continues to be primarily an empirical process. ICD implantation requires induction of VF to set the delivered energy and to confirm that the device can defibrillate at an energy 10 J below the maximum device output to assure an adequate safety margin. Typically, at least two, and often three, VF inductions are performed. Since each VF induction has some element of risk, including the possibility of non-conversion and death, ICD implantation might be improved by providing an estimate of the patient's defibrillation energy requirement prior to implant.

Previous computer modeling studies [1], [2], [3] have shown a good correlation with the overall mean of reported clinical defibrillation metrics. These findings suggest a possible use for computational models in the presurgical planning of ICD implantation. The goal of our current research is to assess the predictive capacity of patient-specific computer models of internal defibrillation by comparing patient-specific simulated and clinical[1] defibrillation metrics (the current threshold I_{th}, the voltage threshold V_{th} and the energy threshold DFT). To date, solutions for seven patient-specific models have been completed. These models were created from segmented cross-sectional CT images obtained post-implant from Brigham and Women's Hospital[1]. This paper presents the modeling results, and compares the predicted and clinical defibrillation parameters for the recruited patients.

2   Methods

2.1   Clinical DFT Determination

The defibrillation threshold (DFT) is defined as the smallest amount of energy that can be delivered to extinguish VF and return the heart to normal sinus rhythm. ICD implantation and DFT testing procedures follow a standardized clinical protocol. In all but one of the patients, the Endotak catheter lead system (Guidant/CPI) was implanted. A similar lead system (Medtronic) was used in the remaining patient. ICDs were implanted in the left pectoral region with venous access via the subclavian vein (Fig. 1). In all cases, the catheter electrode surface in the right ventricle (RV) adjacent to the apex was the cathode. The catheter electrode surface in the superior vena cava (SVC), and the surface of the implanted pulse generator (can) were the anodes. Fluoroscopic imaging

---

[1] The study was carried out in accordance with the guidelines established by the Human Research Committee at the Brigham and Women's Hospital, Boston MA.

was used to verify the correct lead placement. Clinical DFT testing was performed following a step-down procedure. VF was induced by applying a pulse of alternating current and the defibrillation shock was delivered 10 seconds later. The defibrillation waveform had a biphasic shape (Fig. 2a), with 60% tilt in the positive phase and 50% tilt in the negative phase. The pulse width of the first phase (PW1) and the second phase (PW2) were 60% and 40% respectively, of the total waveform duration (typically 10-15 msec). Typical trials started at 20 J and decremented until VF was no longer terminated (an example is shown in Fig. 2b).

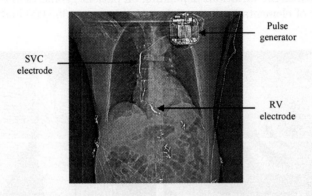

Fig. 1. X-ray image showing the implanted pulse generator and the catheter electrodes in the superior vena cava (SVC) and right ventricle (RV)

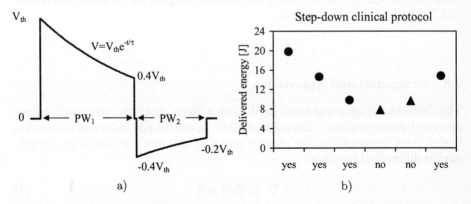

Fig. 2. a) CPI/Guidant biphasic waveform; b) Step-down clinical protocol for DFT testing. Solid circles represent successful shocks. Unsuccessful trials are shown with solid triangles

2.2 Model Construction

All patients were scanned on a spiral CT scanning system (Somatom Plus 4, Siemens Medical Systems, NJ) post-implant with the transvenous catheter electrodes in place. For each patient, nine tissue labels were segmented to generate the following objects: skin, subcutaneous fat, ribs and spine, thoracic wall muscles, lung, mediastinum, heart muscle, aorta and pulmonary vessels, catheter electrodes and ICD can [4]. Each of the 3-D computer models was constructed with a structured meshing algorithm, using low resolution images (128x128) in which each voxel in the segmented image data set was defined as a volume element in the computational model (Fig. 3). The size of a volume element is 3x3x6mm, with slight variations depending on patient geometrical features. The total number of elements in the models varied between 350,000 and 450,000.

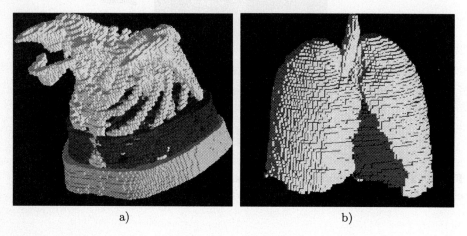

a)   b)

Fig. 3. Voxel based finite volume mesh. For clarity, only indicated parts of the model are shown: a) bone structure and bottom layers of the thoracic wall muscle and fat; b) heart muscle and lungs

2.3 Computational Approach

The thoracic anatomy was considered to be a linear, isotropic, piece-wise homogeneous volume conductor having negligible capacitive and inductive properties. Under these assumptions, the electric potential ϕ is the solution of the elliptic partial differential equation:

$$\nabla \cdot (\sigma \nabla \phi) = 0 \tag{1}$$

subject to boundary conditions:

$$\phi = \Phi_i \tag{2}$$

on the electrodes (RV, SVC, can), and

$$\frac{\partial \phi}{\partial n} = 0 \tag{3}$$

on the thorax surface, where σ is the electric conductivity, Φ_i is the constant potential on the i_{th} electrode surface and n is the surface normal. The electrical conductivity values for the six tissues were selected from literature reported estimates [5], [6]: $\sigma_{blood} = 8$ mS/cm, $\sigma_{myocardium} = 2.5$ mS/cm, $\sigma_{muscle} = 2.5$ mS/cm, $\sigma_{lung} = 0.7$ mS/cm, $\sigma_{bone} = 0.1$ mS/cm, $\sigma_{fat} = 0.5$ mS/cm. Equation (1) was solved using the I-DEAS/TMG software package (Structural Dynamics Research Corporation, Milford, OH, USA) which uses a finite volume approach to find the electric potential distribution. Current density distributions were computed from the potential distribution.

2.4   Defibrillation Metrics Calculation

Four defibrillation metrics (impedance Z; the current threshold I_{th}, the voltage threshold V_{th} and the energy threshold DFT) were calculated for each simulation to aid in the interpretation and evaluation of the solutions. The critical mass hypothesis of defibrillation states that in order to extinguish fibrillation wavefronts, a critical mass of the ventricular myocardium has to be exposed to electric fields equal to or greater than the inexcitability threshold (E_{th}) required to render a fibrillating myocyte inexcitable. Thus, in this study, each simulation was assumed to defibrillate with the minimum delivered energy that exposed 95% of the ventricular myocardium to electric fields greater than or equal to $E_{th} = 3.5$ V/cm [7], [8].

In the simulation, a unit voltage was applied between the RV cathode, and the SVC and can anodes. The resulting electric field magnitudes in the heart muscle were then scaled such that 95% of the ventricular myocardium was exposed to an electric field equal to or greater than $E_{th} = 3.5$ V/cm. Thus, the voltage threshold V_{th} and the current threshold I_{th} are scaled versions of the voltage applied in the simulation and the resulting delivered current. The DFT was calculated from the threshold voltage V_{th} and threshold current I_{th} based on the Guidant/CPI biphasic waveform features (Fig. 2a) using equation (4):

$$DFT = \int_0^{1.61\tau} V_{th} I_{th} e^{-2t/\tau} dt = 0.48 C V_{th}^2. \tag{4}$$

where $\tau = ZC$ is the time constant and $C = 150\mu F$ is the capacitance of the pulse generator.

3   Results

Simulated electric current pathways during a defibrillation shock are shown in Fig. 4. Patient-specific clinical and model-predicted defibrillation metrics (DFT, I_{th}, V_{th} and Z) are compared in Figs. 5a-d. Individual patients are encoded

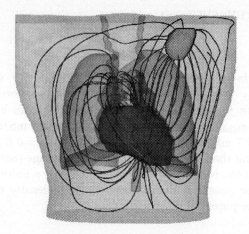

Fig. 4. Flux lines representing the electric current pathways during a defibrillation shock (simulation)

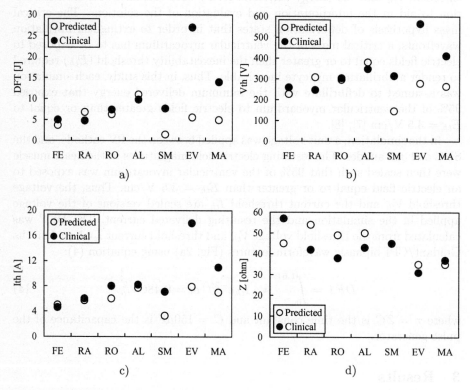

Fig. 5. Model predicted and clinical defibrillation metrics: a) Energy threshold (DFT); b) Voltage threshold, V_{th}; c) Current threshold, I_{th}; d) Interelectrode impedance, Z

using the following identifiers: AL, FE, RA, RO, SM, MA, EV. Clinical values correspond to the lowest energy shock that defibrillated.

4   Discussion

This paper presents comparisons between model-predicted and clinical defibrillation metrics determined for individual patients. The model-predicted defibrillation metrics were determined from patient-specific computational models using methods similar to those developed previously to simulate electric field (current density) distributions produced by a defibrillation shock and to extract defibrillation metrics corresponding to a successful defibrillation episode [1].

Model-predicted defibrillation metrics yielded good estimates of the clinically determined metrics in four of the seven patients examined (FE, RA, RO, AL). It is significant to note that the respective clinical defibrillation metrics DFT, V_{th}, I_{th} for these patients spanned an approximately 2-fold range, suggesting that the goodness of the achieved match was not due to the similarity of the patients examined. The model-predicted impedances all correlate well with the clinical measurements (Fig. 5d). The prediction is closest for the three patients that were not well matched by the respective threshold predictions of the model.

Each of the three patients whose clinical metrics were not well matched by the model-predicted values exhibited clinical anomalies. In one case (EV), the patient's left ventricle contained a large infarct region and exhibited a substantially compromised ejection fraction. The poor correspondence between the predicted and clinical metrics for this patient might well be due to the fact that the critical mass criterion used to extract the predicted defibrillation metrics needs to be modified to account for the substantial volume of the infarct region. In another (MA), the patient had substantial pleural effusion, which would impact the effective conductivity of the lungs and pleural space.

Although the preliminary results show that the simulated defibrillation metrics obtained using the critical mass criterion for defibrillation are generally in good agreement with clinical metrics for four of the seven patients examined, there are a number of limitations of this study. The modeling approach used can only capture geometry-based differences in defibrillation thresholds reflected in the patient population. Factors related to the underlying cellular electrophysiology enter the model only through the ad-hoc inexcitability threshold E_{th} and critical mass criterion. Hence, the model will not be able to predict defibrillation parameters for patients with cellular electrophysiology that differs substantially from the norm.

Numerical methods can also introduce errors. One source of error in the finite volume computational approach is associated with the approximation of the continuum domain with discrete, brick shaped elements. Finer meshes not only render the surfaces more smoothly, but provide more numerically accurate results. Another source of computational error is due to the values used for tissue conductivities, which may not adequately characterize the true electrical conductivity values found in the patient population.

The correspondence between the predicted and measured defibrillation metrics observed in four of the seven patients is encouraging and provides preliminary support of the potential utility of the modeling approach. This approach may allow for patient specific presurgical planning, and may also provide a convenient computational testbed for evaluating new electrode configurations. Although these results are promising, additional subjects are needed to further validate the modeling method.

Acknowledgment. This study was supported in part by a grant from Cardiac Pacemakers, Inc., St. Paul, MN, and the Trustees of Boston University. The authors would like to thank to Dr. Michael Benser from Cardiac Rhythm Management Laboratory, Guidant, for his valuable suggestions. The excellent support provided by the Scientific Computing and Visualization Group, Boston University, is also acknowledged.

References

1. Kinst, T.F., Sweeney, M.O., Lehr, J.L., et al.: Simulated Internal Defibrillation in Humans Using an Anatomically Realistic Three-Dimensional Finite Element Model of the Thorax. J. Cardiovasc. Electrophysiol., vol.8, 537-547, 1997.
2. Min, X., Mehra, R.: Finite Element Analysis of Defibrillation fields in a Human Torso Model for Ventricular Defibrillation. Prog. Biophys. & Mol. Biol., vol. 69, 353-386, 1998.
3. De Jongh, A.L., Entcheva, E.G., Replogle, J.A., et al.: Defibrillation Efficacy of Different Electrode Placements in a Human Thorax Model. Pace, vol. 22, 152-157, 1999.
4. Kettenbach, J., Schreyer, A.G., Okuda, et al.: 3-D Modeling of the Chest in Patients with Implanted Cardiac Defibrillator for Further Bioelectrical Simulation. In: Vannier, M.W., Inumra, K. (eds): Proc. C.A.R., Elsevier Science, 194-198, 1998.
5. Geddes, L.A., Baker, L.E.: The Specific Resistance of Biological Material: A Compendium of Data for the Biomedical Engineer and Physiologist. Med. Biol. Eng. Comput., 5:271-293, 1967.
6. Tacker, W.A. Jr., Mercer, J., Foley, P., et al.: Resistivity of Skeletal Muscle, Skin, and Lung to Defibrillation Shocks. Proc. AAMI 19th Annual Meeting, p. 81, 1984.
7. Zhou, X., Daubert, J.P., Wolf, P.D., et al.: Size of the Critical Mass for Defibrillation (abstract), Circ., vol. 80:II-531, 1989.
8. Zhou, X., Wolf P.D., Rollins P.D., et al.: Potential Gradient Needed for Defibrillation with Monophasic and Biphasic Shocks (abstract), Pace, vol. 12-651, 1989.

Registration of 3D Photographs with Spiral CT Images for Soft Tissue Simulation in Maxillofacial Surgery

Pieter De Groeve[1], Filip Schutyser[1], Johan Van Cleynenbreugel[1], and
Paul Suetens[1]

Medical Image Computing (Radiology - ESAT/PSI), Faculties of Medicine and
Engineering, University Hospital Gasthuisberg, Herestraat 49, B-3000 Leuven,
Belgium
Pieter.DeGroeve@uz.kuleuven.ac.be

Abstract. Prediction of the facial outcome after maxillofacial surgery is
not only of major interest for surgeons but also for patients. A mirror-like
image of the expected surgical outcome gives important information for
the patient and provides the surgeon with a good communication tool.
This paper presents a method for registration of 3D photographs with
3D CT images, to provide the patient with a realistic view of the natural
complexion of the simulated postoperative outcome of his/her face. A
rigid ICP-based registration algorithm, followed by a non-rigid transformation produces a close match between the two surfaces.

Keywords Surface registration, soft tissue modeling, image guided therapy,
maxillofacial surgery simulation

1 Introduction

Prediction of the facial outcome after maxillofacial surgery is not only of major
interest for surgeons but also for patients. A mirror-like image of the expected
surgical outcome is the goal for soft tissue simulators in maxillofacial planning
environments.

Besides realistic modeling of the facial soft tissues, a natural visualization of
the results is very important. Currently, CT-imaging is needed as input for maxillofacial planning environments [1]. Bone structures, skin surfaces, geometric
descriptions of the facial soft tissues can be extracted from these data. However,
when inspecting skin surfaces from CT, is it hard to recognize the patient. This
is due to the lack of color information. In fact, we need a skin surface extracted
from CT together with the natural complexion of the face. This paper presents
a method to generate 'colored CT skin surfaces'.

3D photography acquires both shape and texture. Combining this information together with CT-data provides 'colored CT skin surfaces'. Laser scanners
are well-known 3D photography systems. They generate accurate surfaces. However, these systems are very expensive and the acquisition time is long. Other

W. Niessen and M. Viergever (Eds.): MICCAI 2001, LNCS 2208, pp. 991–996, 2001.
© Springer-Verlag Berlin Heidelberg 2001

systems generate 3D photographs from some 2D photos with a pattern projected. These systems are less expensive, have short acquisition times, but are less accurate.

This paper focuses on an algorithm for registration of 3D photographs acquired by the latter type of systems, and CT surfaces resulting in 'colored CT skin surfaces'. Special attention has to be paid to the robustness of the system because of the different acquisition conditions: lying in a CT-scanner with a rather serious facial expression, and sitting on chair with a smile for the photograph. These elements turn registration into a nontrivial task.

Section 2 describes the registration algorithm. Results are presented in section 3. Concluding remarks finish the paper.

2   Methods

For the acquisition of 3D photographs an "active" 3D system is used. Figure 2 shows a face under structured ligth conditions. Surface information is recovered from the deformation of the pattern on the 2D picture.

On the other hand, the skin surface of the patient is extracted from CT image data by thresholding. The 3D photograph is then registered with the skin surface from using a 3D surface matching algorithm. Our algorithm is based on the *Iterated Closest Point* (ICP) algorithm, see [2]. Some fine-tuning was needed to meet the constraints of this application.

A first adaptation is needed when the CT skin-surface does not completely covers the surface of the 3D photograph. Then some points of the 3D photograph won't have a corresponding point on the CT surface. For each these points no corresponding points are found. These sets of correspondences must be rejected,to avoid bad convergence. Therefore a constraint is added : two points can only be two corresponding points, if the distance between them is less or equal than some threshold. This treshold is arbitrary chosen with respect to the accuracy of the acquired 3D photorgaph. An other method, using a generalized Mahalanobis distance, is mentioned in [3].

To improve accuracy in finding corresponding points, not only Euclidean distance, but also difference in normal orientation and difference in principal curvatures can be taken in account, see [3]. In our case, only coordinates and normals are used. We define a new distance between a point $P(x, y, z)$ with normal (n_x, n_y, n_z) and point $Q(x', y', z')$ with normal (n'_x, n'_y, n'_z) as :

$$D(P,Q) = [(x - x')^2 + (y - y')^2 + (z - z')^2] + \\ \alpha * [(n_x - n'_x)^2 + (n_y - n'_y)^2 + (n_z - n'_z)^2] \tag{1}$$

where α is a weight factor, controlling the importance of difference in normal orientation.

A 3D search data-structure is applied to find corresponding points in a fast way. The 3D-space is equally divided in cubes, all of the same dimensions. Every point of the 3D CT-data belongs to one cube. For each point of the 3D photograph corresponding points are searched for only in the cubes surrounding the point. An other technique using k-D trees is proposed in [4]. For further speed improvement, the data can be downsampled. To increase accuracy, the data is downsampled only the first few iterations. In this way the initial rough alignment converges rapidly to a better match in the first iterations. Then, without downsampling, the next iterations proceed a more accurately registration between the two surfaces. The rigid registration is stopped if the change between two succeeding transformations is less than some tolerance, or if a maximum number of iterations has been exceeded.

Due to inaccuracies in the 3D photograph, mostly in regions around the eyes, nose and mouth, rigid registration is insufficient, especially when used in surgery simulation, where an almost perfect match with CT-data is required. Therefore a non-rigid transformation is needed for a better and closer match between the two surfaces. Once the best rigid displacement is found, a projection-like transformation is applied by non-rigidly and individually translating every point of the 3D photograph toward the CT surface. The direction for translating a point is found by defining a local normal, given by the average of the normals of the two corresponding points. The distance between the point and the surface is approximated by projecting the Euclidean distance between the point and its corresponding point onto this local normal, see figure 1. After non-rigid transformation the two surfaces match very closely, and texture of the 3D photograph can be added to the CT skin-surface.

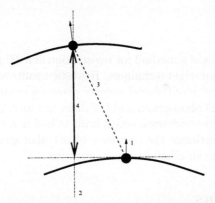

Fig. 1. Non-rigid transformation. From the corresponding points, each with its normal(1), a local normal is calculated(2). The Euclidean distance between the two points(3) is projected on this local normal, resulting in the approximate distance between the point and the surface(4).

3   Results

In this section, we present results of the registration algorithm. In figure 3 the top image represents the two unregistered surfaces. These surfaces must be roughly aligned before the algorithm can start. This is done by interactive manual matching of the two surfaces.

Once initialized, the rigid registration is applied and the images in the second row are obtained. Both surfaces have about 20.000 points. The maximum distance between two corresponding points is chosen to be 5mm. This should take in account the inaccuracies of the 3D photograph. For speeding up the searching of correspondences, cube dimensions of the search-structure are also 5mm in each dimension. This leads to an average of 5 points in each cube. The rigid transformation is found after 50 iterations with downsamplefactor 5 within five seconds CPU time on a SGI Octane R10000 175MHz, followed by another 50 iterations without downsampling in about 1 minute CPU time. The results are shown on the second row of figure 3.

We can see, however that the surfaces do not match exactly. For more tightly matching the surfaces, non-rigid transformation is applied (in less then two seconds CPU time), resulting in the images on the third row. This result is used to add the texture of the registrated photograph to the CT-data, shown in the bottom row images. This example illustrates that after rigid registration, the non-rigid displacement is needed for an almost perfect match.

4   Conclusion

In this paper we proposed a method for registration of a 3D photograph with CT-data using rigid and non-rigid techniques. Realistic results are obtained which are useful in the domain of maxillofacial surgery planning environments. Only when differences between 3D photograph and CT differ to much, problems might occur in finding correct correspondences, which leads to bad non-rigid transformations. However, efforts to optimize the accuracy of 3D photography and to improve non-rigid registration can alleviate these problems.

Acknowledgments

The work discussed here belongs, partly to the EU-funded Brite Euram III PISA project (nr. BRPR CT97 0378), a collaboration between Materialise NV, Belgium; Philips Medical Systems BV, the Netherlands: ICS-AD; DePuy International Ltd, UK; Ceka NV, Belgium; K.U. Leuven, Belgium: ESAT/Radiology Div. Biomechanics; University of Leeds, UK: Research School of Medicine, partly to the grant GOA/99/05 (VHS+ Variability in Human Shape and Speech) of the K.U.Leuven Research Council, and to a grant for research specialization from the Flemish Institute for stimulation of the scientific-technological research in the industry (IWT) to Filip Schutyser.

References

1. F. Schutyser, J. Van Cleynenbreugel, M. Ferrant, J. Schoenaers, P. Suetens: Image-based 3D planning of maxillofacial distraction procedures including soft tissue implications. Proceedings 3rd international conference on medical image computing and computer-assisted intervention - MICCAI2000, lecture notes in computer science, vol. 1935, pp. 999-1007, October 11-14, 2000, Pittsburgh, Pennsylvania, USA
2. P.J. Besl, N.D. McKay: A method for registration of 3-D shapes. IEEE Trans. PAMI 14 (2), p. 239-256, 1992.
3. J. Feldmar, N. Ayache: Rigid, affine and locally affine registration of smooth surfaces. INRIA Technical Report No. 2220, 1994.
4. Iterative point matching for registration of free-from curves and surfaces. Int. J. Comp. Vision 13 (2), 119-152.

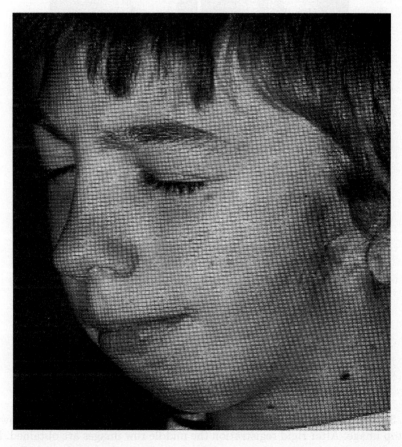

Fig. 2. For the acquisition of 3D photographs structured ligth is used, projecting a pattern onto the face. 3D structure can be extracted from the deformation of this pattern.

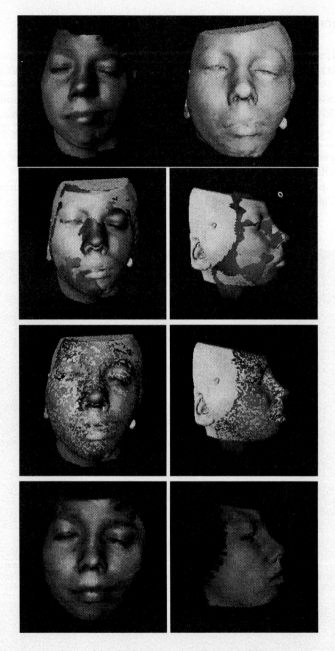

Fig. 3. The skin surfaces from 3D photography and CT imaging are shown on the top image. After rigid registration the middle row images are obtained. Non-rigid registration matches the two surfaces more closely (third row). Based on this result, the texture of the 3D photograph is added to the CT derived data resulting in the bottom row images.

TBNA-protocols

Guiding *TransBronchial Needle Aspirations* Without a Computer in the Operating Room

M. Kukuk, B. Geiger, and H. Müller

[1] SIEMENS Corporate Research, Imaging & Visualization, Princeton, NJ, USA
[2] University of Dortmund, Computer science VII, Germany
kukuk@scr.siemens.com

Abstract We attempt to maximize the success probability for "blind" biopsies by preoperatively estimating four parameters. These parameters well-define the procedure, given that the bronchoscope resides "somewhere" inside the target branch of the tracheobronchial tree. The calculations are based on a patient specific lung model (CT scan) and a digital model of a flexible bronchoscope. Using both models, we simulate the biopsy and derive frequency distributions for each parameter. Based on these distributions, we choose several parameter sets that together maximize the success probability. The parameters are provided to the surgeon in form of detailed step-by-step instructions (protocol) of how to handle the bronchoscope. To control the parameters in the operating room (OR) we use passive controls. First lung phantom experiments show that we could hit in worst-case 12 mm targets (average-case: 5 mm) with three aspirations.

1 Introduction

1.1 Motivation

Transbronchial needle aspiration (TBNA) is a valuable minimally invasive procedure in the bronchoscopic diagnosis and staging of patients with lung cancer [1]. The procedure allows nonsurgical access to lymph nodes from the inside of the tracheobronchial tree. Traditionally this biopsy is performed by maneuvering a bronchoscope to a suitable site within the tracheobronchial tree. Then the surgeon inserts a needle through the bronchoscope and punctures the bronchial wall in order to hit the target behind. This is literally a "blind" puncture since the target object is at no time visible by the bronchoscope. In order to increase the chance of hitting the tumor, the surgeon takes more than one tissue sample for every biopsy. Studies have shown that up to *eight* needle aspirations in the same site can be safely performed, although the optimal number of aspirations is yet to be clarified [2]. However, there is no strategy of how to place the up to eight aspirations beside a simple *trial-and-error* approach.

Despite the fact that the surgeon performs more than one needle aspiration in a single biopsy, this procedure has a failure rate of 60 to 80%, if the bronchial

W. Niessen and M. Viergever (Eds.): MICCAI 2001, LNCS 2208, pp. 997–1006, 2001.

998   M. Kukuk, B. Geiger, and H. Müller

wall is not yet affected [3]. The relatively "blind" nature of the procedure and the physician's lack of confidence about where to position the needle are obstacles to the widespread use and positive diagnostic yield of TBNA. Performing a TBNA requires 3D imagination (coordination of the learned three dimensional anatomy with a fish-eye distorted 2D video image) together with the handling of the endoscope (hand-eye-coordination).

1.2   Related Work

Techniques used to guide TBNA can be classified into three different groups: usage of standard imaging technology, on-line visualization of the target and tracking of the bronchoscope.

In the first group we have imaging techniques like fluoroscopy, CT and CT fluoroscopy. These techniques show the endoscope, the advanced needle and the target lesion. Fluoroscopy produces a real-time two-dimensional projection image with poor contrast. The target lesion is usually not visible [4]. Conventional CT produces images of adequate quality but the procedure is cumbersome and time-consuming since real-time imaging is not possible and each sequence must be prescribed in advance. CT fluoroscopy is a term for continuous-imaging CT that allows the visualization of dynamic processes in real-time, like the insertion of a needle into the target lesion. However, this technique is limited to axial images and requires significant CT-scanner time and relatively high radiation dosage.

In the second group we have a technique that tries to visualize the target lesion by inserting a ultrasound transducer through the working channel of the bronchoscope [2]. The study shows no significant difference in sensitivity compared to unguided TBNA.

In the third group we find techniques that try to track in real-time the tip of the bronchoscope to guide the TBNA. One subgroup tries to track the bronchoscope's tip solely by processing the endoscope images [5], [6], [7]. The Biosense intrabody navigation system [8] uses electromagnetic fields to track a sensor that can be attached to the bronchoscope's tip. In an in vivo study [9], 10 to 20 markers were secured on the animals' chest and the respiratory motion was monitored using a second sensor to compensate for breathing motion. The study showed an accuracy of 4.2 mm +-2.6 mm (+- SD).

1.3   Our Approach

We found that the following four parameters non-ambiguously describe how to handle a bronchoscope to perform a successful TBNA (compare to Fig. 1, left):

1. Bronchoscope insertion depth l
2. Shaft rotation about the principal axis α
3. Angle of tip deflection β controlled by the bronchoscope's angling wheel
4. Needle length d

We denote these parameters as *endoscope configuration* $C = (l, \alpha, \beta, d)$.

Our goal is to maximize the success probability for a TBNA by providing these parameters and detailed step-by-step instructions (protocol) to the surgeon. The four parameters are calculated prior to the intervention, based on a patient specific model of the tracheobronchial tree (derived from a CT scan) and a digital endoscope model. By using both models, we simulate the biopsy by calculating all possible endoscope configurations that reach to the target site. From all configurations, we derive frequency distributions for each parameter. To exploit the fact that it is common practice to perform several (up to eight) aspirations for one biopsy, we select several sets of the most frequent parameters from these distributions. During the intervention, we use *passive controls* (non electronic) to monitor all four parameters. This approach allows us to systematically perform several aspirations, instead of the currently used trial-and-error method. Registration of the calculated parameters to the patient's reference frame is done by using an anatomical landmark based method.

Our digital model of a flexible bronchoscope takes the physical characteristics like flexibility, *bending section*, diameter and length of our real bronchoscope into account. The bending section of a bronchoscope is its highly flexible distal end. It can be controlled using the *angling wheel* located at the bronchoscope's control head, to "look around" and guide the needle to the target.

2 System Overview

2.1 Basic Steps

Fig. 1 center shows an example scenario that gives an overview of the basic components of a TBNA. It shows the tracheobronchial tree and the target mass (tumor) outside the airways. The planned biopsy site B is shown in form of the endoscope's tip together with two possible shaft shapes. Note, that B is the position and orientation of the tip before the alignment and therefore doesn't necessarily have to point towards the target. The calculation of the protocol parameters l, α, β, d is based on our digital model $\mathcal{M}$ of a bronchoscope (see chapter 4) and includes four principal steps:

1. Physician preoperatively plans biopsy site B.
2. Calculation of bronchoscope length l to reach B: $l = \mathcal{M}(B)$
3. Calc. of the *endoscope-space* E to reach B with length l: $E = \mathcal{M}(l, B)$.
4. For all $e \in E$: Calculation of $\alpha(e), \beta = \mathcal{M}(e), d = \mathcal{M}(e)$

Firstly, the physician preoperatively plans the ideal biopsy site. The biopsy site B represents roughly the position and orientation of the bronchoscope's tip within the tracheobronchial tree from where to perform the biopsy.

Secondly, we regard the whole procedure of performing a TBNA as a two-step process: (1) inserting the bronchoscope into the branch that contains the biopsy-site and (2) aligning it with the target lesion. This allows us *to fix the inserted length l* and to calculate the *alignment parameters* α, β, d based on the fixed

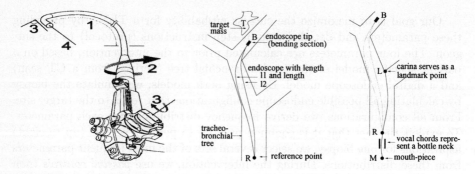

Figure 1. Left: Protocol parameters. Center: TBNA scenario. Right: Referencing

inserted length. Thirdly, we use our model $\mathcal{M}$ to calculate a set of endoscope shapes where each element represents an endoscope of length l that reaches into the branch containig the biopsy site B. We refer to this set as the endoscope-space E, since it describes all possibilities of a real bronchoscope to reach the biopsy site.

Finally, given the endoscope-space E we calculate for each endoscope shape the alignment parameters α, β, d. For β and d this is done on the basis of our digital bending section model.

2.2   Registration Between the Virtual and Real Bronchoscope

To register the calculated insertion depth l and shaft rotation α to the patient's reference frame, we use a landmark based approach. We have chosen the *carina*, a keel-shaped part of the tracheobronchial tree that marks the bifurcation of the trachea into the left and right lung as our anatomical landmark.

The situation is shown in Fig. 1, right. It shows the "ideal" biopsy-site B and two possible endoscope length (dotted) from B to the point of reference R. The point of reference is chosen to lie in a bottleneck (vocal chords) in terms of all possible paths an endoscope can take. To calculate the bronchoscope length to B measured from M, we first let the physician touch the landmark L with the bronchoscope (ML) and then have him insert (or withdraw for lesions proximal to the carina) the bronchoscope by the difference between RB and RL.

As the mutual zero-point for the shaft-rotation we choose the rotation of the bronchoscope that shows the carina to appear vertically. In the planning phase the physician rotates a virtual endoscopic camera and during the intervention he rotates the bronchoscope until their views shows the carina to appear vertically.

2.3   Controling the Protocol Execution

In order to set the bronchoscope to the configuration given by the protocol parameters, we need control over the inserted length l, the shaft rotation α, the tip

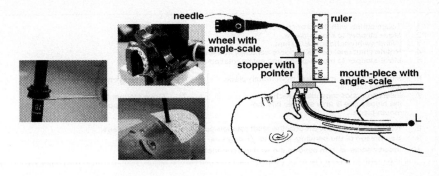

Figure 2. Passive controls for monitoring the protocol parameters.

deflection β and needle length d. Since we perform the needle aspirations based on a fixed bronchoscope length, we use a stopper to prevent the bronchoscope from penetrating the body deeper than desired, see Fig. 2. To control shaft rotation, we attach a goniometer (angle-scale) to the base plate of the mouth-piece and a pointer to the stopper (see detail figures). When the base plate stops the insertion of the bronchoscope, any shaft rotation moves the pointer along the angle-scale. We control the tip bending with an angle-scale that we attach to the angling wheel located at the bronchoscope's control head (top detail figure). During the planning phase, we use a look-up table to map the angle of tip deflection to the wheel angle. We control the needle length by marks on its proximal end and using the opening of the biopsy port as a reference point.

3   The TBNA-protocol

The following box shows the universal TBNA-protocol. It can be divided in three parts: Lines 1-5 contain the registration instructions and lines 6-7 describe the insertion / withdrawal of the bronchoscope to the biopsy-site. Lines 8-10 describe the alignment of the bending section with the target lesion. Only the protocol parameters l, α, β, d represent the patient specific part of the protocol. The instructions themselves remain unchanged for different patients.

Depending on the location of B relative to the current endoscope position we either execute the left or right column of lines 6-7. After execution of line 7, the bronchoscope reached the biopsy-site and the following instructions 8-10 use parameters α, β, d to align the bronchoscope with the target lesion. The arrow indicates that it is then possible to systematically perform a series of biopsies.

4   Endoscope Model

Our model $\mathcal{M}$ describes a flexible endoscope as a chain of rigid cylinders interconnected by discrete ball-and-socket joints. The chain interacts with the patient

1.	Touch carina with the bronchoscope tip.	
2.	Move stopper to mouth-piece.	
3.	Withdraw bronchoscope 30 mm.	
4.	Rotate shaft until carina appears vertically in the bronchoscope's view.	
5.	Move stopper to mouth-piece and set its rotation-pointer to 0 degrees.	

6.	Move stopper *l* mm away from mouth-piece and lock stopper.	6.	Withdraw bronchoscope *l* mm.
7.	Insert bronchoscope into branch of the biopsy-site B until stopper hits the mouth-piece.	7.	Move stopper back to mouth-piece and lock stopper.

8.	Rotate endoscope shaft until the shaft rotation-pointer points to α degrees.
9.	Set rotation of the bending-wheel to β degrees.
10.	Insert needle *d* mm beyond the working channel outlet.

specific anatomical model via our collision detection method [10]. Each cylinder of the chain is approximated by a cloud of sample points on its surface. Checking for collision of all sample points with the organ model allows us to verify if a chain configuration represents a valid endoscope shape. The flexibility of the chain is modeled by the choice of link length s (span) and joint range θ and is based on the notion *minimal radius* [11].

The overall idea is to exhaustively enumerate all possible chain configurations, given a start cylinder and the following four constraints: organ geometry, gravity, medial-axis and stopping-criteria. Using a recursive backtracking algorithm we create a tree data structure where the nodes represent the joints of the chain. The bending section (95 mm long) is modeled accurately to reflect the properties of our real bronchoscope.

A link is represented by a reference frame (4×4 homogeneous transform matrix) L, where the centerline of the cylinder is the z-axis of the frame and the cylinder bases lie in the $z = 0$ and $z = s$ plane. Given a link L_i of level i, the 9 connected links of the next level are given by:

$$L_{i+1}^j = R(r_j, \theta) \, L_i \, T(\hat{z}s) \,, \text{ for } j = 1, \ldots, 9 \,,$$

where T is a translation and R a rotation matrix, $\hat{x}, \hat{y}, \hat{z}$ denote the three 4×1 unit vectors, r_j is the jth rotation vector of the set $\left\{ (x \ y \ 0)^T \mid x, y \in \{-1, 0, 1\} \right\}$ and θ is the rotation angle.

For calculating the endoscope length to a given target link (biopsy-site) the stopping criteria is fulfilled when a link L docks to the target link. For calculating the endoscope-space E the stopping criteria is the recursion depth, see Fig. 3.

For each path from the root to a leaf, we calculate the alignment parameters. The shaft rotation α is only dependant on the orientation of the bronchoscope's bending plane. The bending plane of an endoscope is the plane in which the tip moves under the rotation of the bending wheel at the endoscope's control head. Let tip link L and target vector t be known with respect to the same global reference frame and let L's $y = 0$-plane be the bending plane. The desired shaft rotation is the rotation angle about $\hat{z}$ that rotates the $y = 0$-plane into target t:

$$\alpha = \cos^{-1} \left(\frac{t' \cdot \hat{x}}{|t'||\hat{x}|} \right) \text{ with } t' = (L^{-1}t)(1 \ 1 \ 0 \ 1).$$

The left-hand-side of the formula calculates the angle between unit vector $\hat{x}$ and t'. Vector t' equals t known with respect to L and orthogonally projected into the z=0-plane.

After shaft rotation, target t lies in the $y = 0$ bending plane and we need to calculate the angle of bending wheel rotation needed to align the tip with t. We found that not the current tip position, but the transition point q from the shaft to the bending section determines the angle of wheel rotation. This is probably because of the used pull-wire mechanism. We also found that the bending movement of the straight tip to the left and right can be approximated by a semi-circle with its center $c - 49$ mm away from the endoscopes end. We determine link Q of the chain that contains q and move it along its $\hat{z}$-axis by $a = 95 - 49 = 46$ mm. We regard the new origin of Q as the center of the semi-circle. The desired angle of wheel rotation is then given by the angle between $\hat{z}$ and target t:

$$\beta = \cos^{-1}\left(\frac{Q'^{-1}t \cdot \hat{z}}{|Q'^{-1}t||\hat{z}|}\right) \quad \text{with } Q' = Q\,T(\hat{z}a). \quad \text{Needle length } d = |Q'^{-1}\,t| - c.$$

5   Lung Phantom Experiments

5.1   Material

We have implemented this approach on a SGI PC540, 550Mhz (single), 0.5 GB RAM, running Windows 2000 and OpenGL. We have built a lung phantom (Fig. 3, left) using transparent (for visual verification) PVC tubes. We randomly placed 37 marker sticks (4 mm diameter, cardboard) in the model, so that they are aligned with the inner surface of the tubes. The phantom was then scanned (512x512x382, 1 mm slice distance, 1.2 thickness). After the scan, we identified manually these surface points as our target points. The lung phantom is 1.5 times the size (trachea diameter: 30 mm) of an adult lung, to compensate for the fact that no bronchoscope (average shaft diameter: 6.0 mm) but a "Gastrointestinal Videoscope" (Olympus GIF 100, shaft diameter: 9.5 mm) was available for non sterile experiments.

5.2   Objective and Design

We are interested in two questions: (1) What is the repeatability of the *real* configurations $C_r = (l_r, \alpha_r, \beta_r, d_r)$ needed to hit a target incision point? In other words, we need to know the variation of each parameter. (2) How accurate match our *predicted* configurations C_p the configurations C_r?

The experimental setup is shown in Fig. 3. Out of all 37 markers we choose five (arrows in Fig. 3) as target points, three of them close to the carina. For each target, we execute the protocol 20 times and record the configuration parameters needed to touch the marker stick with the biopsy needle. Note, that the markers can be seen by the endoscopic video camera as a white 4 mm disk.

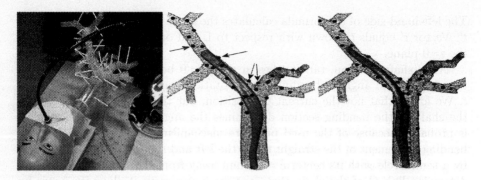

Figure 3. Left: experimental setup. Center: calculated endoscope-space E and five selected targets (arrow). Right: docking to the biopsy-site with a slightly stiffer endoscope.

To estimate the parameters for each target, our software generates for each parameter a dataset of at least 100 (and up to 25,000) measures. We then read each dataset with a data-analyzing package (IDL, Research System, Inc.) and create frequency distributions to draw histograms and calculate the mean and standard deviations.

5.3   Results

(1) Repeatability: To calculate the variation of the experimentally obtained parameters, we rejected the smallest and largest outlier of all 15 datasets (20 measures each) and calculated the range of each dataset. We found the largest range of α, β and d to be 7°, 6° and 7 mm and the average range to be 6°, 4° and 4 mm respectively.

(2) Accuracy of the prediction: The real error of a configuration $C = (\alpha, \beta, d)$ is given by the distance between the target point and the needle tip after setting the endoscope to configuration C. Since it is not possible to measure distances inside the plastic model we use a theoretical error model to obtain an upper bound error estimation for our parameter prediction. Our results show, that shaft rotation α is by far the most sensitive parameter with an average error of 12°, whereas β (3°) and d (1 mm) can be predicted more accurately. To exploit this fact, we performed a test where we took the configuration $(\bar{\alpha}, \bar{\beta}, \bar{d})$ for the first aspiration, $(\bar{\alpha} + \sigma, \bar{\beta}, \bar{d})$ for the second and $(\bar{\alpha} - \sigma, \bar{\beta}, \bar{d})$ for the third, where the dashed parameter denotes the mean and σ the standard deviation of the respective distribution. The test shows that we could hit in worst-case targets of 24 mm diameter with one aspiration and 12 mm targets with three aspirations. In average we could hit 13 mm targets with one aspiration and 5 mm targets with three aspirations.

6 Conclusion

In this paper, we have presented a method to guide "blind" biopsies by preoperatively calculating parameter sets that describe how to handle the bronchoscope to maximize the success probability. During the intervention, the surgeon follows step-by-step instructions (protocol) which are based on these parameter sets, to perform a series of systematic needle aspirations.

The most important feature of this approach is its simplicity. We don't need any additional devices or computer that need to be calibrated or operated in the OR. All our controls are passive, intuitive to operate and remain outside the body. After the intervention they can be easily removed and the bronchoscope can be sterilized as usual. Our approach is inherently "real-time" during the intervention, in contrast to some image based approaches. The surgeon operates at his/her own speed. We can use any off-the-shelf bronchoscopes (fiberoptic or video). This makes our system very cost efficient, since hospitals and doctors can use their existing equipment. Registration is not based on external markers, which move considerably during respiration, but on an anatomical landmark that only moves marginally relative to the target.

First results with a lung phantom show that the repeatability is high enough to expect a maximum accuracy of 5 mm. Our tests show that we are able to hit in worst-case targets of ≥ 12 mm diameter (average-case: 5 mm) with three aspirations.

Acknowledgments

This work was partly supported by a DAAD-Doktorandenstipendium (Ph.D. scholarship) HSP III financed by the German Federal Ministry of Science and Research. We would like to thank Timothy Scanlin for his support in building and Lisa Reid for her support in scanning the phantom.

References

1. Ko Pen Wang et al. Flexible Transbronchial Needle Aspiration for Staging of Bronchogenic Carcinoma. In *CHEST*, volume 84,5, pages 571 – 576, 1983.
2. John J. Shannon et al. Endobronchial Ultrasound-Guided Needle Aspiration of Mediastinal Adenopathy. In *Am J Respir Crit Care Med*, volume 153, 1996.
3. Udaya B. S. Prakash, editor. *Bronchoscopy*. Raven Press - New York, 1993.
4. C. S. White et al. CT-Assisted Needle Aspiration. In *Am J Roentgenol 169*, 1997.
5. I. Bricault, G. Ferretti, and P. Cinquin. Multi-level Strategy for Computer-Assisted Transbronchial Biopsy. In *MICCAI '98*, LNCS 1496. Springer.
6. Kensaku MORI et al. A method for tracking camera motion of real endoscope by using virtual endoscopy system. In *Proc. of SPIE Medical Imaging*, volume 3978, 2000.
7. Anthony J. Sherbondy et al. Virtual Bronchoscopic Approach for Combining 3D CT and Endoscopic Video. In *Proc. of SPIE Medical Imaging*, volume 3978, 2000.
8. Biosense Webster. EP Navigation, www.biosensewebster.com.

1006   M. Kukuk, B. Geiger, and H. Müller

9. Stephen B. Solomon et al. Real-time Bronchoscope Tip Localization Enables Three-dimensional CT Image Guidance for Transbronchial Needle Aspiration in Swine. In *CHEST '98*, volume 114/5, pages 1405–1410.
10. B. Geiger. Real–Time Collision Detection and Response for Complex Environments. *Proceedings Computer Graphics International 2000.*
11. Markus Kukuk and Bernhard Geiger. Registration of Real and Virtual Endoscopy - A Model and Image Based Approach. In *MMVR2000*, pages 168–174. IOS Press.

3D Reconstruction of the Human Jaw: A New Approach and Improvements

Moumen T. Ahmed, Ahmed H. Eid, and Aly A. Farag

Computer Vision and Image Processing Laboratory
University of Louisville, KY 40292
moumen,ahmdhamd,farag@cvip.uofl.edu
http://www.cvip.uofl.edu

Abstract. This paper presents a new, practical approach for 3D reconstruction of the human jaw from a sequence of intra-oral images. This research has an immense value in various dental practices including implants, tooth alignment, and craniofacial surgery. Our approach is based on the recently-proposed space carving algorithm for shape recovery. This algorithm provides more flexibility to the reconstruction process and eliminates several constrains imposed by other traditional approaches such as stereo and shape from shading. Our experimental results have shown that the approach is able to reconstruct 3D models of the human jaw with sub-millimeter accuracy.

1 Introduction

Orthodontic treatment involves the application of force systems to teeth over time to correct malocclusion. In order to evaluate tooth movement progress, the orthodontist monitors this movement by means of visual inspection, intra-oral measurements, fabrication of plastic models (casts), photographs and radiographs, a process which is both costly and time consuming. Obtaining a cast of the jaw is a complex operation for the orthodontist, an unpleasant experience for the patient and may not provide all the details of the jaw. Current technology in dental radiography can provide the orthodontist with 3D information of the jaw. While dental radiology is now widely accepted as a routine technique for dental examinations, the equipment is rather expensive and the resolution, being adequate for maxillofacial imaging, is still too low for 3D dental visualization. Furthermore, the dose required to enhance the resolution is unacceptably high. Some efforts have been devoted to computerized diagnosis in orthodontics, e.g., [2,7]. Usually, most of these 3D systems for dental applications found in the literature rely on obtaining an intermediate solid model of the jaw (cast or teeth imprints) and then capturing the 3D information from that model. User interaction is needed in such systems to determine the 3D coordinates of fiducial reference points on a dental cast. Other systems that can measure the 3D coordinates have been developed using either mechanical contact [8] or a traveling light principle [9].

Our research lab has been involved for the last five years in a project, the *jaw project*, to develop a system for dentistry to go beyond traditional approaches

W. Niessen and M. Viergever (Eds.): MICCAI 2001, LNCS 2208, pp. 1007–1014, 2001.

in diagnosis, treatment planning, surgical simulation, and prosthetic replacements ([1,4,5,6]). Our ultimate goal is to transform a number of orthodontic protocols and maxillofacial practices from art into science. The jaw project builds a 3D model of the jaw, not from a cast, but from the actual human jaw. The system can obtain sequences of calibrated images of the upper/lower jaw using small intra-oral cameras, provide accurate 3D reconstruction from the acquired images and register robustly the 3D models built from multiple views. This research has an immense value in various dental practices including implants, tooth alignment, and craniofacial surgery. The research has also wide applications in teledentistry, dental education and training.

Our focus in this paper is on developing accurate, practical techniques to build 3D models of the human jaw. Several different approaches have been examined. The stereo approach has been by far the most widely used for shape recovery. However, one of the main problems of stereo is the correspondence problem. Due to the difficult nature of the correspondence problem, several constraints have been imposed on stereo. A large number of stereo techniques rely heavily on assumptions such as the existence of specific features in the images to produce satisfactory results. For example, featureless scenes are hard to reconstruct in stereo because corresponding points between the different images cannot be accurately found. Also, stereo is difficult to apply to images taken from arbitrary viewpoints. This is because corresponding image points become very hard to find if the images are taken from viewpoints far apart. As a consequence, stereo is inefficient approach for reconstruction of objects like human teeth, which, in addition to having many occlusion edges, have no specific geometric features. On the other hand, area-based stereo methods (also known as correlation-based methods) perform poorly due to the common homogeneous, textureless regions of the teeth. Figure 1 depicts a typical situation in which, feature-based stereo fails to deliver a sufficient number of correct matches (despite the use of a highly-robust method [10]). In addition, the constraints on the viewpoints make the stereo hard to apply for the jaw reconstruction since they are difficult to satisfy with the hand-held arm and CCD camera.

In our previous approach [1,5], we have successfully reconstructed the human jaw using the shape from shading (SFS) algorithm. However, since the SFS does not provide metric information, the reconstruction result from the SFS was fused with several range measurements to enhance its performance. These measurements help also in removing the ambiguity of the 3D visible surface discontinuities produced by the SFS. The depth measurements were obtained with the help of the digitizer arm and small laser projector mounted on the arm. The laser was employed to highlight the point in the captured image for which a depth measurement is acquired by the arm. The main drawback of this approach is its dependence on laser which, although being eye-safe, is unfavorable when human subjects are involved (actually it was a discouraging factor for some of our test patients). Moreover, the SFS algorithm would have problems with any tooth fillings due to the difference in albedo between tooth surfaces.

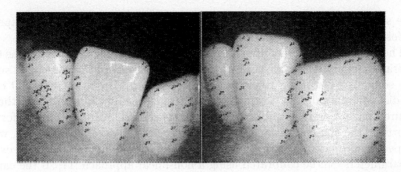

Fig. 1. *Few correct and incorrect matches are obtained by a robust feature-based stereo [10] applied to a pair of jaw sequence: the labeled corresponding points, shown in crosses, were produced by Zhang's "image-matching" program after extraction of points of interest, doing correlation and rejection of some false matches using relaxation.*

In this paper, we present an alternative 3D reconstruction method that does not require using the laser projector, any additional sensors or hardware. Yet this method recovers a complete, accurate 3D model of the jaw teeth from multiple views. Moreover, it alleviates the shortcomings of the stereo-based methods. On selecting this method, we depart from the traditional shape recovery approaches, e.g., stereo and SFS, which start off with images to find 3D surfaces, by employing a technique recently proposed by Kutulakos and Seitz called space carving [3]. Our choice for the space carving technique is guided by several concerns. Reconstruction using space carving does not rely on assumptions of the presence of specific image features, or on the positioning of the cameras, or the object geometry or texture. This technique allows us to reconstruct accurately 3D models that agree with the input images without the need to solve the difficult correspondence problem. In addition, since space carving is an "object-centered" reconstruction method, it becomes easy and straightforward to make use of any available *a priori* information on the shape of the object (which is true in our case), a key advantage of this method over the classical approaches. As such, this approach is more suitable and practical for our application.

This paper is organized as follows: Section II describes the overall system setup. Sections III presents our approach to tooth reconstruction using the space carving algorithm. Our experimental results are shown in Section IV followed by the concluding remarks in Section V.

2   System Setup and Overview

The experimental setup that we use consists of a MicroScribe 3D digitizer, an Ultra-Mirco CCD camera with a 5.5mm lens, a regulated white light source, and an SGI Indigo2 machine that hosts the software required for data processing. For more details about the system hardware, please refer to [5], which uses the same setup except for the laser projector that we do not use in this paper on purpose.

The CCD camera is mounted on the stylus of the 3D digitizer and it has to be calibrated before its use. Because of the small focal lens of the camera, it suffers from some lens distortion (mainly radial distortion). The first coefficient of radial distortion is calibrated using a straight line-based technique [12] so that all acquired images can be undistorted before processing. After correcting for lens distortion, the camera can be safely modeled as an ideal pinhole camera, whose perspective projection matrix that encompasses the camera intrinsic and extrinsic parameters can be calibrated using a non-linear approach [11]. If the camera is stationary, we do not have to re-calibrate again. Yet in the proposed system, the camera will be moving; This implies the recalculation of the perspective projection matrix. Being mounted on the digitizer arm, the camera location in the 3D space can be measured. Moreover, the arm provides the transformation that relates the new position and orientation of the camera to the world coordinate system. This transformation is used to update the camera extrinsic parameters and thus the camera perspective projection matrix. As such, the camera is maintained calibrated in all positions. In addition, the arm provides the position of the initial volume enclosing the tooth or any part of the jaw, which is to be carved by the space carving algorithm until the shape is reconstructed.

The five degrees of freedom provided by the arm enable the acquisition of a sequence of intra-oral images covering different parts of the jaw. Using the space carving algorithm, sets of voxels that represent the different parts of the jaw are computed. A fast registration technique [13] is employed to merge the resulting 3D models to obtain a complete 3D description of the jaw parts. The final stage transforms this model into patches of free form surfaces using a triangulation technique. This step enables the development of a 3D solid model for visualization. A cast can be fabricated from this model via rapid prototyping. Further processing that can be carried out on the digital model includes tooth separation, force analysis, implant planning, and surgical simulation.

3   Space Carving

In 3D object reconstruction, we attempt to achieve the reverse process of image formation by regenerating a 3D shape from various 2D projections. Space carving [3] attempts to produce the maximal 3D shape that is consistent with all the images. Space carving starts with an initial volume, V, that includes the object(s) to be reconstructed. This 3D space is then discretized into a finite set of voxels $v_1, v_2, ..., v_n$. The idea is to successively carve (remove) some voxels until the final 3D shape, V^*, agrees with all the input images. An outline of the algorithm is given below.

Space carving Algorithm:

Step 1: Initialize V based on arm position and discretize it.

Step 2:
- Determine the set of voxels $Vis(V)$ on the surface of V.
- Project each voxel v on $Vis(V)$ to the different images where v is visible.
- Determine the photo-consistency of each voxel v on $Vis(V)$.

Step 3: If no non-photoconsistent voxel is found, set $V^* = V$ and terminate. Otherwise, set $V = V$ - {non-photoconsistent v's} and return to Step 2.

Each voxel on the surface of the volume, i.e., in $Vis(V)$, is projected back to the different images using their respective projection matrices. To decide whether a voxel should be carved or not, the idea of color-consistency is used. The Lambertian model for the surface of the object is assumed. Under this model, light reflected from a single point on the surface of the object has the same intensity in all directions. Therefore, for a voxel to belong to the surface of the object, it must have the same color intensity, within some tolerance to allow for some light variations and some calibration inaccuracy, for all its projections to the different images provided. Voxels that are inconsistent with a single color, are viewed as free space in which different light rays intersect. By removing all color-inconsistent voxels, we are able to approximate a maximal photo-consistent shape that is defined by all the input images. The basic idea of space carving is illustrated in Figure 2. Three input images are used to generate the 3D model of the shape shown in the images. Voxels that project on the input images to pixels of similar color are kept and assigned that color. Voxels that project on the input images to pixels of different colors are removed.

Although the general idea in space carving is straightforward, modeling an algorithm to provide the desired results is not an easy task as the problem of occlusion must be treated. This is carefully taken care of in a multi-sweep fashion [3]. One important requirement by the algorithm is segmenting the objects from the background. This does not represent a problem with objects like teeth, since teeth are brighter than the interior of the mouth and have distinctive color from the gum. Therefore teeth can be easily segmented from the background in the image sequences.

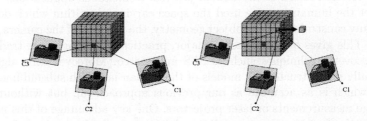

Fig. 2. *Basic idea of space carving. Voxels are projected to the input images using their respective projection matrices. C1, C2 and C3 represent the optical centers of the three cameras. (a) Consistent voxels are assigned the color of their projections. (b) Inconsistent voxels are removed from the volume.*

4   Experimental Results and Validation

After calibrating the camera, sequences of images are captured for overlapping segments of the jaw. Each segment consists of about 3-5 images. The process of taking the images was relatively fast, taking less than a minute for each segment and a total of 10-12 minutes to cover the upper/lower jaw. The patient's jaw should not move during the acquisition time of each segment (less than a minute). However, movements between segments are permitted because the registration technique can align the individual segments. Figure 3 shows some images taken of a patient's jaw segment. We applied the space carving algorithm to the acquired images of each segment. The initial volume was selected as a cube and discretized into 70x70x70 voxels for a total of 343,000 voxels. Each segment is reconstructed after 4-5 passes of the space carving algorithm, which took about 16 seconds on an SGI Indigo2 machine. On average, the final volume contained 4,500 voxels. We used a 15% standard deviation threshold of the grayscale values to determine whether or not the voxels should be declared photo-inconsistent and consequently carved. This relatively high threshold was chosen in order to compensate for calibration errors, possible light changes from one image to another and any deviation from the Lamertian assumption (e.g., presence of specularities in some images). Figure 3 shows also the reconstructed result of one segment of the lower jaw from two different views. Once each segment of the jaw is reconstructed, they are registered [13] to compose the whole jaw, of which a part is shown in Figure 4 from two different views. The part shown in the figure took about 84 seconds of processing time for reconstruction and registration. Quantitative assessment and validation of the reconstruction is obtained by comparing some tooth measurements (e.g., height and width) from the reconstructed model to those of the real tooth as shown in Figure 5. The comparison showed accuracy within 0.47 mm, which shows that the system can achieve sub-millimeter accuracy, similar to our previous approach but without the need for any range measurements.

5   Conclusions and Future Extensions

The 3D reconstruction of the human jaw has tremendous applications. To reconstruct the human jaw, we used the space carving algorithm which does not impose any constraints on the object geometry, the position of the camera, or the texture. This gives our approach a major, practical advantage over traditional shape recovery techniques such as SFS and stereo. Moreover, this algorithm successfully reconstructed 3D models of the human jaw with sub-millimeter accuracy, which is as accurate as our previous approach [5], but without using any range measurements or laser projectors. One key advantage of this new approach is the fact that it can easily exploit any available a prior information about the shape of the tooth. The algorithm can thus start with an initial volume whose shape is closer to the target object. This is expected to enhance and speed up the results of our approach. Our current research direction is directed to investigating this possibility.

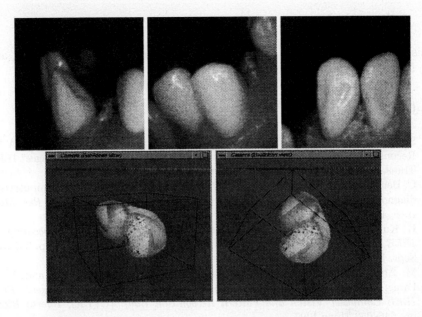

Fig. 3. *Reconstruction results of a jaw segment consisting mainly of two teeth: (a)-(c) images of the two teeth acquired by the CCD camera. (d) and (e) The reconstructed teeth shown from two different views.*

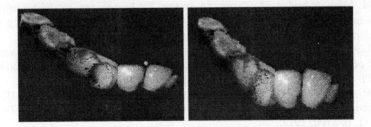

Fig. 4. *Reconstructed part of the lower jaw shown from two views.*

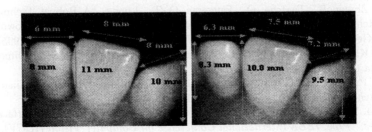

Fig. 5. *Validation of the reconstructed model: (a) measurements from the real jaw, (b) measurements from the reconstructed model.*

6   Acknowledgment

This work was supported in part by grants from the Whitaker Foundation, and the NSF (ECS-9505674) institutions.

References

1. Sameh M. Yamany, Aly A. Farag, David Tasman and Allan G. Farman " A 3D Reconstruction System for Human Jaw Using a Sequence of Optical Images" IEEE Trans. on Medical Imaging,vol. 19(5), pp. 538-547, May 2000.
2. C. Bernard, A. Fournier, J. M. Brodeur, H. Naccache, and R. Guay, "Computerized diagnosis in orthodontics," *Proc. 66th Gen. Session Int. Assoc. Dental Res. Montreal*, 1988.
3. K. Kutulakos and S. Seitz. "Theory of Shape by Space Carving." *Proceedings of IEEE International Conference On Computer Vision*, Corfu, Greece, pp. 307-314, Sept. 1999.
4. M. Ahmed, S. M. Yamany, E. E. Hemayed, S. Roberts, S. Ahmed, and A. A. Farag, "3d reconstruction of the human jaw from a sequence of images," *Proc. IEEE Computer Vision and Pattern Recognition Conf. (CVPR), Puerto Rico* , pp. 646–653, June 1997.
5. S. M. Yamany, A. A. Farag, D. Tasman, and A. G. Farman, "A robust 3D reconstruction system for human jaw modeling," *2nd International Conference on Medical Image Computing and Computer-Assisted Intervention (MICCAI'99), Cambridge, England*, pp. 778–787, Sept. 1999.
6. S. M. Yamany and A. A. Farag, "A system for human jaw modeling using intraoral images," *Proc. IEEE Engineering in Medicine and Biology Society (EMBS) conference, Hong Kong* 20, pp. 563–566, Oct. 1998.
7. D. Laurendeau and D. Possart, "A computer-vision technique for the acquisition and processing of 3D profiles of dental imprints: An application in orthodontics," *IEEE Transactions on Medical Imaging* 10, pp. 453–461, Sept 1991.
8. F. P. van der Linden, H. Boersma, T. Zelders, K. A. Peters, and J. H. Raben, "Three-dimensional analysis of dental casts by means of optocom," *J. Dent. Res.* 51(4), p. 1100, 1972.
9. A. A. Goshtasby, S. Nambala, W. G. deRijk, and S. D. Campbell, "A system for digital reconstruction of gypsum dental casts," *IEEE Transactions on Medical Imaging* 16, pp. 664–674, Oct. 1997.
10. Z. Zhang, R. Deriche, O. Faugeras, Q.-T. Luong, "A Robust Technique for Matching Two Uncalibrated Images Through the Recovery of the Unknown Epipolar Geometry," *Artificial Intelligence Journal*, 78, pages 87-119, Oct. 1995.
11. R. Klette, K. Schluns and A. Koschan, "Computer Vision: Three-Dimensional Data from Images," *Springer*, 1998.
12. B. Prescott and G. McLean, 'Line-based correction of radial lens distortion," *Graph. Models and Img. Process.*, 59(1), Jan. 1997.
13. S. M. Yamany and A. A. Farag, "Free-form surface registration using surface signatures," *Proc. IEEE International Conference on Computer Vision (ICCV), Greece* 2, pp. 1098–1104, Sept 1999.

Real-Time Surgical Simulation with Haptic Sensation as Collaborated Works between Japan and Germany

Naoki Suzuki[1], Asaki Hattori[1], Shigeyuki Suzuki[2], Max P. Baur[3],
Andreas Hirner[3], Susumu Kobayashi[4], Yoji Yamazaki[4], Yoshitaka Adachi[5]

1 Institute for High Dimensional Medical Imaging, Jikei Univ. School of Med.
4-11-1 Izumi-honcho, Komae, Tokyo 201-8601 JAPAN
nsuzuki@jikei.ac.jp
2 School of Science and Engineering, Waseda Univ., 3 Bonn Univ.,
4 Dept. of Surgery, Jikei Univ. School of Med., 5 Suzuki Motor Corp, R&D Center

Abstract. As part of an application of tele-virtual surgery and a force feedback device, surgeons in Japan and Germany examined a hepatectomy simulation system. Surgeons in each country could be performed various surgical maneuvers upon the same patient by using our system. Surgeons palpated abdominal skin, made electrical scalpel incisions and widened the incision line by using surgical tools in virtual space. The user can convey tactile sensations by the force feedback device while surgeons performed a virtual operation. Two graphic workstations of equal capability and force feedback devices were engaged in each location. As each workstation communicated only event signals through an ISDN (64Kb) line, it made possible to obtain real time tele-virtual surgery without a large capacity communication infrastructure.

1 Preface

Up to the present, three dimensional images reconstructed from MRI or CT images used in various applications. In our future medical treatments, the application of virtual reality (VR) techniques to 3D images has a large potential through tele-diagnosis and tele-medicine.

We report the results of a tele-virtual surgery experiment between Japan and Germany in this paper. Apparatus at both sites were connected by an ISDN line and equipped with a VR surgery system with a force feedback function. Having this system, surgeons in each plane shared identical tactile sensations.

2 Surgical Simulation System

A surgical simulation system has the useful application in the medical field. The system allows a user to repeatedly perform virtual surgery until a suitable procedure is established. This is especially useful for educational medical training.

We have been developing a virtual surgical simulation system upon the following requirements:

W. Niessen and M. Viergever (Eds.): MICCAI 2001, LNCS 2208, pp. 1015-1021, 2001.
© Springer-Verlag Berlin Heidelberg 2001

1). The system should provide a design for the user and determine surgical procedures based on 3D model reconstructed from the patient's data.
2). The system must transmit authentic tactile sensations to the user during organ manipulations by using force feedback device.
In our system, the surgeon (user) is able to perform various surgical maneuvers with

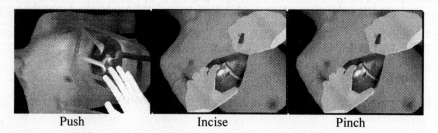

Push   Incise   Pinch

Fig. 1. Application of surgical simulation used in this experiment

suitable surgical tools as interactive actions in a virtual space. This system allows the surgeon to make a scalpel incision, widen the incision line and secure it with forceps (Fig.1). All surgical procedures on a 3D object in a virtual space are proceeded in real-time. Also 3D human structures are reconstructed from 3D patient data that gives such anatomical characteristics as vascularity. Numerical parameters such as location, depth, direction to the targeted organ and excised tissue volumes are measurable with quantitative accuracy.

Various viewpoints such as scale and angles can be displayed the basic system function. It can also alter the transparency of an organ's multiple layers. Rendering by wire frames is also possible. In addition, each organ model is shaded by light sources set in the system's space and separated by easily distinguishable colors. In order to determine possible incision points, these models are texture mapped by using images of the patient's skin and extracted organ texture.

3 Force Feedback Device

A haptic device, which giving authentic tactile sensations for the operator, was confirmed very recently. We also have been developing a force feedback device which possesses 16 degrees-of-freedom (DOF) for manual interactions with virtual environments. Followings are summarization of the features of the device manufactured for our virtual surgery system.

1) The force feedback system is composed of two types of manipulators: a force control manipulator and a motion control manipulator.
2) Three force control manipulators are attached to the end of the motion control manipulator.
3) Both ends of each force control manipulator are attached to the thumb, forefinger, and middle finger of the operator.
4) The force control manipulator has a joint structure with minimal inertia and less friction.
5) The motion control manipulator has mechanical stiffness.

Fig.2 shows the device for the right hand. The three force control manipulators are mounted at the pointed end of this device. These manipulators are attached to user's thumb, forefinger, and middle finger respectively. Fig.3 illustrates the user's fingers are attached to the manipulators. A user and the device attached to both hands were shown in Fig.4. These left and right force feedback devices have the same internal structure. The force feedback device for the right hand is a mirror image of the left one. These devices communicate data (finger location etc.) with the surgical simulation system through a LAN. As soon as an interaction occurs between the user's fingers and a 3D object in a virtual space, a force parameter of tactile sensations calculated by the surgical simulation system, is transferred to these devices. This allows the user to experience tactile sensations in each finger.

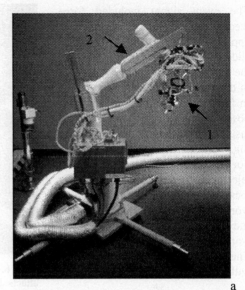

a

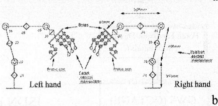

Left hand   Right hand

b

Fig. 2. A view of the force feedback device and the block diagram

4 Tele-Surgical Simulation System

Since we intended to examine tele-virtual surgery without a large capacity communication infrastructure, we used a 1ch ISDN line (64Kb/s), in this experiment. However, it was difficult to transfer images of simulation results to each location in real-time. Therefore, we installed a simulation program and the patient's 3D modeling into each system. The MRI images produced 3D data of the skin surface, liver, liver vessels, liver tumor and colon. The system transmitted and received only event signals related to the simulation.

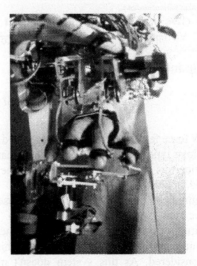

Fig. 4. Force feedback device attached to fingers of the right hand

The event signal included force feedback device location data, the application's GUI event (buttons, sliders etc.) and calculated force of the force feedback device. The size of data per event is about 200 bytes. In this way, both sites were able to observe an identical simulation result in real-time.

Fig.5 shows the system's outline. For the surgical simulation and teleconference, participants at each location employed two graphic workstations (Japan site: Octane, Indy, German site: Octane, O2. All workstations are SGI inc. products). These workstations were connected with an ISDN line via an ISDN

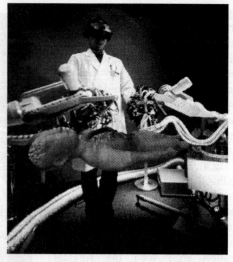

Fig. 6. User with force feedback device attached to both hands

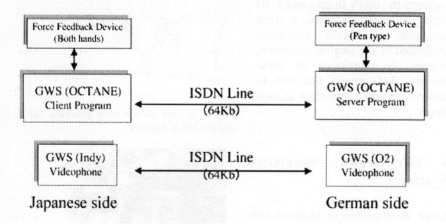

Fig. 5. System outline of tele-virtual surgery

router. A force feedback device was prepared at each workstation. The force feedback was a glove type device attached to both hands in Japan. On the other hand, a pen type device was used in Germany. During the virtual surgical operation, these devices conveyed tactile sensations to the surgeons.

For communicating between each site, we used a teleconference application InPerson (SGI inc.) and video image and audio functioning at 300x200 pixels. This application's video frame was about 0.5 frame/sec.

When using network communication as in this experiment, the data transfer delay has to be considered. As this system doesn't manage event time, the delay causes a different result between two sites. The delay between Japan and Germany was measured by using UNIX command ping. Ping command result was 300ms (round-trip time). At this speed, it is no necessary for the user to wait for the processing completion. However, if both users in each site interact with a 3D object simultaneously, each site's simulation result will be different. Therefore, each user conducts their procedures in turns.

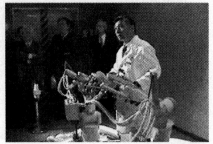

a. Japanese site

5 Results

For the experiment, a simulated hepatectomy was chosen. Fig.6 shows a scene of the experiment at the both sites. Surgeons in each location palpated the patient's abdominal skin (Fig.7a) and discussed an incision position while observing location of the tumor and vascularity of the liver by changing skin and liver surface transparency. While a Japanese surgeon widened the incision line using a surgical tool, surgeons in Germany

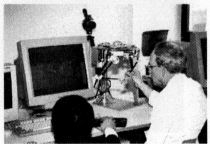

b. German site

Fig. 7. Scene of the experiment at both sites

made an incision on the skin surface (Fig.7b). After widening, they palpated the exposed liver and deliberated upon an incision to the liver (Fig.7c). Finally, a German surgeon made an incision to the liver to complete the hepatectomy (Fig.7d).

In this system, the display's frame rate was 6-7 frame/sec. However, considering the surgeons action in surgical simulation, the frame rate was acceptable for the simulation. The two surgeons in Japan and Germany also had no comment on the frame rate.

Both surgeons evaluated this system and the experiment. The Japanese surgeon commented that he felt in close proximity the German surgeon and didn't sense any delay in the operation. On the other hand, the German surgeon observed that he could discuss surgery procedures in detail with the Japanese surgeon in order to find a solution to the surgical problem.

6 Discussion

We have demonstrated the virtual surgery with two surgeons while sharing identical tactile sensations over a long distance. It was possible to obtain real-time tele-virtual surgery without a large capacity communication infrastructure.

However, this system has a limitation. Both sites operated on a 3D object in turn, due to time delays when communicating event signals. Different results were caused by the delay between two sites. Therefore, evaluating the effects of time delay on the

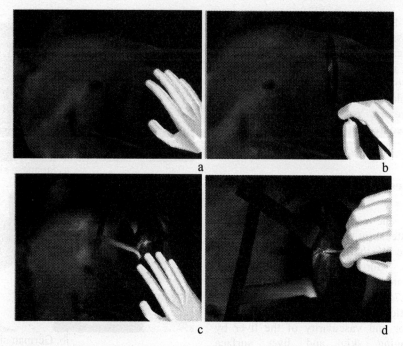

a b

c d

Fig. 8. Images of hepatectomy simulation. a) palpating the abdominal skin, b) making an incision to the abdominal skin, c) palpating the exposed liver, d) making an incision to the liver

surgical simulation and develop a system which enable users to manipulate a 3D object simultaneously was needed. The revised system will be the basis of the tele-surgery system.

A 3D model structure caused the drawbacks of the force feedback function. Elasticity of this model's is configured only on the surface, and it doesn't depend on an organ's internal structure. Now, we are developing another 3D model "Sphere filled model". This model is reconstructed as a surface model filled with small element spheres with which a force acting on the internal structure can be calculated. We can improve tactile sensations by applying this model.

References

1. Suzuki. N, Takatsu. A, Kita. K, Tanaka. T, Inaba. R, Fukui. K: Development of a 3D image simulation system for organ and soft tissue operations.: Abstract of the World Congress on Medical Physics and Biomedical Engineering 1994; 39a: 609.
2. Robb RA, Hanson DP: The ANALYZE software system for visualization and analysis in surgery simulation. In: Computer Integrated Surgery, Eds. Steve Lavalle, Russ Taylor, Greg Burdea and Ralph Mosges, MIT Press, 1995, pp.175-190.
3. Robb RA, Cameron B: Virtual Reality Assisted Surgery Program. In: Interactive Technology and the New Paradigm for Healthcare, Eds., R. Satava, et al., Vol. 18, 1995, pp.309-321

4. Kikinis R, Langham Gleason P, Jolesz FA: Surgical planning using computer-assisted three-dimensional reconstructions. In: Computer Integrated Surgery, Eds. Russel Taylor, Stephane Lavallee, Grigore Burdea, and Ralph Mosges. MIT Press, 1995, pp.147-154.
5. N. Suzuki, A. Hattori, A. Takatsu: "Medical virtual reality system for surgical planning and surgical support", J. comput. Aided Surg., 54-59, 1(2), 1995.
6. N. Suzuki, A. Hattori, S. Kai, T. Ezumi, A. Takatsu: "Surgical planning system for soft tissues using virtual reality", MMVR5, Eds: K.S. Morgan et al., pp.159-163, IOS Press, 1997.
7. D. Terzopoulos and K. Fleischer: "Modeling inelastic deformation: Viscoelasticity, plasticity, fracture", Computer Graphics, vol.22, NO.4, pp.269-278, 1988.
8. A. Norton, G. Turk, B. Bacon, J. Gerth, and P. Sweeney: "Animation of fracture by physical modeling", The Visual Computer, vol.7, pp.210-219, 1991.
9. H. Delingette: "Simplex Meshes: a General Representation for 3D Shape Reconstruction", Technical Report 2214, INRIA, Sophia-Antipolis, France, 1994.

Phase-Based User-Steered Image Segmentation

Lauren O'Donnell[1], Carl-Fredrik Westin[1,2], W. Eric L. Grimson[1],
Juan Ruiz-Alzola[3], Martha E. Shenton[2], and Ron Kikinis[2]

[1] MIT AI Laboratory, Cambridge MA 02139, USA
`odonnell, welg@ai.mit.edu`
[2] Brigham and Women's Hospital, Harvard Medical School, Boston MA, USA
`westin, kikinis@bwh.harvard.edu`
[3] Dept. of Signals and Communications, University of Las Palmas de Gran Canaria,
Spain
`jruiz@dsc.ulpgc.es`

Abstract. This paper presents a user-steered segmentation algorithm
based on the livewire paradigm. Livewire is an image-feature driven
method that finds the optimal path between user-selected image locations, thus reducing the need to manually define the complete boundary.
We introduce an image feature based on local phase, which describes local edge symmetry independent of absolute gray value. Because phase is
amplitude invariant, the measurements are robust with respect to smooth
variations, such as bias field inhomogeneities present in all MR images. In
order to enable validation of our segmentation method, we have created
a system that continuously records user interaction and automatically
generates a database containing the number of user interactions, such as
mouse events, and time stamps from various editing modules. We have
conducted validation trials of the system and obtained expert opinions
regarding its functionality.

1 Introduction

Medical image segmentation is the process of assigning labels to voxels in order
to indicate tissue type or anatomical structure. This labeled data has a variety of
applications, for example the quantification of anatomical volume and shape, or
the construction of detailed three-dimensional models of the anatomy of interest.

Existing segmentation methods range from manual, to semi-automatic, to
fully automatic. Automatic algorithms include intensity-based methods, such as
EM segmentation [14] and level-sets [4], as well as knowledge-based methods such
as segmentation by warping to an anatomical atlas. Semi-automatic algorithms,
which require user interaction during the process, include snakes [11] and livewire
[1,7]. Current practice in many cases, however, is computer-enhanced manual
segmentation. This involves hand-tracing around the structures of interest and
perhaps employing morphological or thresholding operations to the data.

Although manual segmentation methods allow the highest degree of user
control and enable decisions to be made on the basis of extensive anatomical
knowledge, they require excessive amounts of user interaction time and may

W. Niessen and M. Viergever (Eds.): MICCAI 2001, LNCS 2208, pp. 1022–1030, 2001.
© Springer-Verlag Berlin Heidelberg 2001

introduce high levels of variability. On the other hand, fully automatic algorithms may not produce the correct outcome every time, hence there exists a need for hybrid methods.

2   Existing Software Platform

The phase-based livewire segmentation method has been integrated into the 3D Slicer, the Surgical Planning Lab's platform for image visualization, image segmentation, and surgical guidance [9]. The Slicer is the laboratory's program of choice for manual segmentation, as well as being modular and extensible, and consequently it is the logical place to incorporate new algorithms for our user base. At any time during an average day, one would expect to find ten people doing segmentations using the 3D Slicer in the laboratory, which shows that any improvement on manual methods will be of great utility. Our system has been added into the Slicer as a new module, Phasewire, in the Image Editor.

3   The Livewire Algorithm

The motivation behind the livewire algorithm is to provide the user with full control over the segmentation while having the computer do most of the detail work [1]. In this way, user interaction complements the ability of the computer to find boundaries of structures in an image.

Initially when using this method, the user clicks to indicate a starting point on the desired contour, and then as the mouse is moved it pulls a "live wire" behind it along the contour. When the user clicks again, the old wire freezes on the contour, and a new live one starts from the clicked point. This intuitive method is driven only by image information, with little geometric constraint, so extracting knowledge from the image is of primary importance.

The livewire method poses this problem as a search for shortest paths on a weighted graph. Thus the livewire algorithm has two main parts, first the conversion of image information into a weighted graph, and then the calculation of shortest paths in the graph [6,12].

In the first part of the livewire algorithm, weights are calculated for each edge in the weighted graph, creating the image forces that attract the livewire. To produce the weights, various image features are computed in a neighborhood around each graph edge, transformed to give low edge costs to more desirable feature values, and then combined in some user-adjustable fashion. The general purpose of the combination is edge localization, but individual features are generally chosen for their contributions in three main areas, which we will call "edge detection," "directionality," and "training." Features such as the gradient and the Laplacian zero-crossing [13] have been used for edge detection; these features are the main attractors for the livewire. Second, directionality, or the direction the path should take locally, can be influenced by gradients computed with oriented kernels [7], or the "gradient direction" feature [13]. Third, training is the process by which the user indicates a preference for a certain type of boundary, and the image features are transformed accordingly. Image gradients and intensity values [7], as well as gradient magnitudes [13], are useful in training.

In the second part of the livewire algorithm, Dijkstra's algorithm [5] is used to find all shortest paths extending outward from the starting point in the weighted graph. The livewire is defined as the shortest path that connects two user-selected points (the last clicked point and the current mouse location). This second step is done interactively so the user may view and judge potential paths, and control the segmentation as finely as desired. The implementation for this paper is similar to that in [6], where the shortest paths are computed for only as much of the image as necessary, making for very quick user interaction.

4   Phase-Based Livewire

4.1   Background on Local Phase

The local phase as discussed in this paper is a multidimensional generalization of the concept of instantaneous phase, which is formally defined as the argument of the analytic function

$$f_A = f - if_{Hi} \tag{1}$$

where f_{Hi} denotes the Hilbert transform of f [2,3].

The instantaneous phase of a simple one-dimensional signal is shown in Figure 1. This simple signal can be thought of as the intensity along a row of pixels in an image. Note that in this "image" there are two edges, or regions where the signal shape is locally odd, and the phase curve reacts to each, giving phase values of $\pi/2$ and $-\pi/2$.

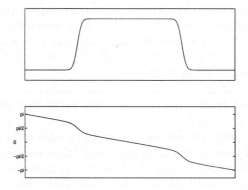

Fig. 1. A simple signal (top), and its instantaneous phase (bottom).

The output from a local phase filter, i.e. a Gabor filter, is an analytic function that can be represented as an even real part and an odd imaginary part, or an amplitude and an argument. Consequently, this type of filter can be used to estimate both the amplitude (energy) and the local phase of a signal. As local phase is invariant to signal energy, edges can be detected from small or large signal variations. This is advantageous for segmentation along weak as well as strong edges. Another advantage is that local phase is in general a smoothly varying function of the image, and provides subpixel information about edge position.

4.2   Implementation

To estimate the phase we are using quadrature filters which have a radial frequency function that is Gaussian on a *logarithmic* scale:

$$\nu(\rho) = e^{-\frac{4}{\log 2}B^{-2}\log^2(\frac{\rho}{\rho_i})} \tag{2}$$

where ρ_i is the center frequency and B is the 6 dB sensitivity bandwidth in octaves. In contrast to Gabor filters, these filters have zero response for negative frequencies, ensuring that the odd and even parts constitute a Hilbert transform pair and making the filters ideal for estimation of local phase [10]. We multiply the filters with a cos^2 radial function window in the frequency domain to reduce ringing artifacts arising from the discontinuity at π when using filters with high center frequencies and/or large bandwidth.

The local phase is our primary feature, serving to localize edges in the image: the livewire essentially follows along low-cost curves in the phase image. The phase feature is scaled to provide bounded input to the shortest-paths search. Figure 2 shows a phase image derived from the original image shown in Figure 4.

Since the argument of the phase is not sensitive to the amount of energy in the signal, it is useful to also quantify the certainty of the phase estimate. In image regions where the phase magnitude is large, the energy of the signal is high, which implies that the the phase estimate in that region has high reliability and thus high certainty.

We define the certainty using the magnitude from the quadrature filters, mapped through a gating function. By inverting this certainty measure, it can be used as a second feature in the livewire cost function. The weighted combination of the phase and certainty images produces an output image that describes the edge costs in the weighted graph, as in Figure 2.

5   Applications

In this section, we describe the behavior of our phase-based segmentation technique through a series of experiments with medical images.

In the first set of experiments, we show the stability of phase information across different scales [8]. The input to the quadrature filters was blurred using a Gaussian kernel of variance 4 pixels. Figure 3 demonstrates the robustness

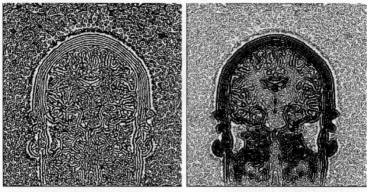

Local Phase Image   Combined Image

Fig. 2. Local phase images. The left-hand image shows the local phase corresponding to the grayscale image in Figure 4. This is the primary feature employed in our phase-based livewire method. The right-hand image displays the weighted combination of the phase and certainty features, which emphasizes boundaries in the image. Darker pixels correspond to lower edge costs on the weighted graph.

of phase information to changes in scale, as the two segmentations are quite similar. The leftmost image is the original grayscale and its segmentation, while the center image shows the result of Gaussian blurring. The rightmost image displays the segmentation curve from the blurred image over the original image for comparison.

The second experiments contrast the new livewire feature, phase, with our original intensity-based livewire implementation. Phase is more intuitive to use, produces smoother output, and is generally more user-friendly than the intensity-based method as illustrated in Figure 4. In contrast to the intensity-based method, no training step is required to bias the phase-based method towards the desired edge type, as the phase information can be used to follow weak or strong edges.

6   Discussion and Validation Framework

We have presented a user-steered segmentation algorithm which is based on the livewire paradigm. Our preliminary results using local phase as the main driving force are promising and support the concept that phase is a fairly stable feature in scale space [8]. The method is intuitive to use, and requires no training despite having fewer input image features than other livewire implementations.

In order to enable validation of phase-based livewire, we have created a system that continuously records user interaction and can generate a database containing the number of user interactions and time stamps from various editing modules. A selection of the items which are recorded is listed in Table 1. An

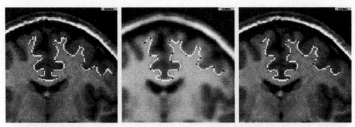

Original Image   Gaussian Blurring Overlay of Segmentation

Fig. 3. Illustration of insensitivity to changes in scale: initial image, result of Gaussian blurring, and overlay of second segmentation (done on the blurred image) on initial image. Note the similarity between the segmentation contours, despite blurring the image with a Gaussian kernel of four pixel variance.

ongoing study using this system will enable evaluation of the performance and utility of different image features for guiding the livewire.

Analysis of the logged information has shown that great variability exists in segmentation times, partially due to users' segmentation style, learning curve, and type of image data, and also due to factors we cannot measure, such as time spent using other programs with the Slicer Editor window open. A complete comparison of the phasewire and manual segmentations systems, consequently, is difficult, and perhaps the most reliable indication of the system performance can be found in the opinions of doctors who have used it.

Table 2 demonstrates the utility of the segmentation method using information from the logging system, and Table 3 gives doctors' opinions regarding ease of use and quality of output segmentations. For example, Figure 5 shows a liver segmentation done with phasewire, in which the doctor remarked that the three-dimensional model was more anatomically accurate than the one produced with the manual method, where both segmentations were performed in approximately the same amount of time. This is likely due to the smoothness of the contour obtained with phasewire, in comparison with the contour obtained with the manual method.

Item Logged	Details
mouse clicks	recorded per slice, per label value, per volume, and per editor module
elapsed time	recorded per slice, per label value, per volume, and per editor module
description	includes volumes viewed and location of scene description file
username	will allow investigation of learning curve

Table 1. Selected items logged by the 3D Slicer for validation and comparison purposes.

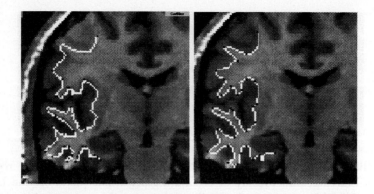

Fig. 4. Comparison of phase-based and intensity-based implementations of livewire. On the left is our original implementation of livewire, which uses image-intensity based features. It does a poorer job of segmenting gray and white matter. Training was performed on the region in the upper left of the image. The segmentation was more difficult to perform than the phase-based segmentation because more coercing was necessary to force the livewire to take an acceptable path. The right image shows segmentation of the same boundary using the phase-based livewire. Contrary to the intensity-based method, no training was necessary before beginning to segment. The conclusion is that the phase-based implementation is more intuitive to use than the intensity-based version, since the phase image gives continuous contours for the livewire to follow. Rather than being distracted by unwanted pixels locally, the phase livewire is generally only distracted by other paths, and a small movement of the mouse can set it back on the desired path. It can be quite fluid to use, with clicks mainly necessary when the curve bends in order to keep the wire following the correct contour.

7   Acknowledgements

The work was funded in part by CIMIT and NIH P41-RR13218 (RK,CFW), by a National Science Foundation Graduate Research Fellowship (LJO), by NIH R01 RR11747 (RK), by Department of Veterans Affairs Merit Awards, NIH grants K02 MH 01110 and R01 MH 50747 (MS), and by European Commission and Spanish Gov. joint research grant 1FD97-0881-C02-01 (JR). Thanks to the Radiation Oncology, Medical Physics, Neurosurgery, Urology, and Gastroenterology Departments of Hospital Doctor Negrin in Las Palmas de Gran Canaria, Spain, for their participation in evaluation of the system. Also thanks to Aleksandra Ciszewski for her valuable feedback regarding the Slicer system.

References

1. W. A. Barrett and E. N. Mortensen. Interactive live-wire boundary extraction. *Medical Image Analysis*, 1(4):331–341, 1997.

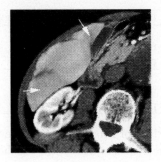

Fig. 5. A surface model of the liver, created from a phasewire segmentation, shows well-defined surfaces between the liver and the kidney and gallbladder.

study	method	total clicks	clicks/slice	time/slice (sec)	volume (mL)
CT brain tumor	manual	234	26.0	39.3	68.5
	phasewire	97	10.8	28.7	67.3
	phasewire	109	12.1	25.5	69.2
CT bladder	manual	1488	28.1	31.7	715.6
	phasewire	359	6.8	21.5	710.8

Table 2. Example segmentations performed with Phasewire. Clicks and time per slice are averages over the dataset.

2. Boualem Boashash. Estimating and interpreting the instantaneous frequency of a signal - part 1: Fundamentals. *Proceedings of the IEEE*, 80(4), 1992.

3. Boualem Boashash. Estimating and interpreting the instantaneous frequency of a signal - part 2: Algorithms and applications. *Proceedings of the IEEE*, 80(4), 1992.

4. V. Caselles, R. Kimmel, G. Sapiro, C. Sbert. Minimal Surfaces: A Three Dimensional Segmentation Approach. Technion EE Pub 973, 1995.

5. E. W. Dijkstra A Note On Two Problems in Connexion With Graphs *Numerische Mathematik*, 269–271, 1959.

6. A. X. Falcao, J. K. Udupa, and F. K. Miyazawa. An Ultra-Fast User-Steered Image Segmentation Paradigm: Live Wire on the Fly. *IEEE Transactions on Medical Imaging*, 19(1):55–61, 2000.

7. A. X. Falcao, J. K. Udupa, S. Samarasekera, and S. Sharma. User-Steered Image Segmentation Paradigms: Live Wire and Live Lane. *Graphical Models and Image Processing*, 60:233–260, 1998.

8. D. J. Fleet and A. D. Jepson. Stability of Phase Information *IEEE Trans. PAMI*, 15(12):1253–1268, 1993.

9. D. T. Gering, A. Nabavi, R. Kikinis, W. E. L. Grimson, N. Hata, P. Everett, and F. Jolesz and W. Wells. An Integrated Visualization System for Surgical Planning and Guidance Using Image Fusion and Interventional Imaging. *Medical Image Computing and Computer-Assisted Intervention - MICCAI'99*, 809–819, 1999.

study	method	ease of use	segmentation quality
CT brain tumor	manual	3	3
	phasewire	4	4
CT bladder	manual	2.7	3
	phasewire	4	4

Table 3. Doctors' comparison of Phasewire and Manual segmentation methods on the datasets from Table 2. The scale is from 1 to 5, with 5 being the highest.

10. H. Knutsson and C.-F. Westin and G. H. Granlund. Local Multiscale Frequency and Bandwidth Estimation *Proceedings of IEEE International Conference on Image Processing*, 36–40, 1994.
11. T. McInerney, D. Terzopoulos. Deformable Models in Medical Image Analysis: A Survey. Medical Image Analysis, 1(2):91–108, 1996.
12. E. N. Mortensen and W. A. Barrett. Interactive Segmentation with Intelligent Scissors. *Graphical Models and Image Processing*, 60(5):349–384, 1998.
13. E. N. Mortensen and W. A. Barrett. Intelligent Scissors for Image Composition. *Computer Graphics (SIGGRAPH '95)*, 191–198, 1995.
14. W. M. Wells, R. Kikinis, W.E.L. Grimson, F. Jolesz. Adaptive segmentation of MRI data. *IEEE Transactions on Medical Imaging*, 15:429–442, 1996.

Comparison of Two Restoration Techniques in the Context of 3D Medical Imaging*

Miguel A. Rodriguez-Florido[1], Karl Krissian[2], Juan Ruiz-Alzola[1], and
Carl-Fredrik Westin[3]

[1] Departamento de Señales y Comunicaciones
[2] Departamento de Informática y Sistemas
Universidad de Las Palmas de Gran Canaria - Las Palmas, Spain
{marf,jruiz}@dsc.ulpgc.es ; krissian@dis.ulpgc.es
[3] Surgical Planning Lab. - BWH - Harvard Medical School - Boston(MA) - USA
westin@bwh.harvard.edu

Abstract. In this paper, we compare two restoration techniques applied
to 3D angiographies and to femoral CT scans. The first technique uses a
Partial Derivative Equation and the second one is based on an extension
of adaptive Wiener filters. We first present each method. Then, we discuss and compare the estimation of the local orientations in 3D images
obtained either by the smoothed gradient and the principal curvature
directions or by the eigenvectors of the structure tensor. A good estimation of the orientations is essential because it directs the restoration
process. Finally, we compare the restored images on both synthetic and
real images for the two studied applications.

1   Introduction

Image enhancement is especially important in medical imaging because it allows
physicians to obtain a better visual interpretation, especially when viewing weak
structures (i.e. thin vessels), differentianting false joint regions (i.e. space between
femoral head and hip) and in other numerous clinical applications. Moreover,
enhancement is a preprocessing step for subsequent automated medical analysis,
such as segmentation of different tissues or registration of images from different
modalities. In this sense, this paper presents a qualitative comparison between
anisotropic diffusion [5, 9, 11] and anisotropic adaptive frequency filtering [4, 13],
that will permit future algorithmic improvements or a feedback process between
both. We also compare the local structure estimation that each technique uses,
analyzing which one is the best in different cases. The paper is structured as
follows: first, we present a brief description of both restoration methods, second
we compare two orientation extraction techniques, and finally we present our
results.

---

* This work was partially funded by the European project ERB-4061-PL-97-0777, by
European Comission and Spanish Gov. joint research grant 1FD97-0881-C02-01, and
by CIMIT and NIH P41-RR13218. The first author is funded by a FPU grant at the
University of Las Palmas de Gran Canaria.

W. Niessen and M. Viergever (Eds.): MICCAI 2001, LNCS 2208, pp. 1031–1039, 2001.

2   Presentation of the Two Methods

In this section, we present two 3D anisotropic filtering techniques. The first is based on anisotropic diffusion and uses the gradient and the principal curvature directions. The second technique is designed in the Fourier domain and uses the eigenvectors of the structure tensor to drive the filtering.

2.1   Flux-Based Anisotropic Diffusion

In [5, 6], a multi-directional flux-based diffusion scheme is proposed. The general expression of the diffusion equation is:

$$\begin{cases} u(x,0) = u_0 \\ \frac{\partial u}{\partial t} = div(\mathbf{F}) + \beta(u_0 - u). \end{cases} \tag{1}$$

where $\mathbf{F}$ is the diffusion flux that drives the diffusion and β is a data attachment term which allows a convergence of the diffusion scheme to an image u that remains close to the initial data u_0. The expression of the differential equation as the divergence of a vector field ensures conservation of image intensity. Particular cases of this equation with $\beta = 0$ are:
• the heat diffusion equation $\mathbf{F} = \nabla u$ which is equivalent to a Gaussian convolution that reduces noise, but does not preserve the contours of the image, smoothing the information in an isotropic way.
• the Perona and Malik equation [9] with $\mathbf{F} = g(\parallel \nabla u \parallel)\nabla u$ where g is a diffusion function that reduces the diffusion for "high" gradients. To achieve this goal, a *threshold* δ on the norm of the gradient is introduced. g is chosen in such a way that it diffuses a little when $\parallel \nabla u \parallel$ is higher than δ ; it tends to a positive constant when $\parallel \nabla u \parallel$ is close to zero, acting like heat diffusion. However, the flux is always oriented in the gradient direction.
• the matrix diffusion, developed by Weickert [11], uses a matrix diffusion D with a flux $\mathbf{F} = D\nabla u$. Then the flux can be expressed as $\mathbf{F} = D\nabla u = \sum_{i=0}^{2} \lambda_i u_{\mathbf{v}_i} \mathbf{v}_i$ with λ_i and $\mathbf{v}_i$ the eigenvalues and eigenvectors of D and $u_{\mathbf{v}_i} = \nabla u.\mathbf{v}_i$ is the first order derivative of the intensity in the direction of $\mathbf{v}_i$.
Let $(\mathbf{e}_0, \mathbf{e}_1, \mathbf{e}_2)$ denote any orthogonal unit basis of $\mathbb{R}^3$ that generally depends on the local structures of the image. Then, the diffusion flux proposed in [5, 6] for this basis is written as:

$$\mathbf{F} = \sum_{i=0}^{2} \phi_i(u_{\mathbf{e}_i})\mathbf{e}_i. \tag{2}$$

It is equivalent to tensor diffusion where the eigenvectors of the diffusion matrix are $(\mathbf{e}_i)_{i \in \{0,1,2\}}$ and the eigenvalues are functions of the first order derivative of the intensity in the direction of the associated eigenvector: $\lambda_i = \lambda_i(u_{\mathbf{e}_i})$ leading to diffusion functions $\phi_i(u_{\mathbf{e}_i}) = \lambda_i(u_{\mathbf{e}_i})u_{\mathbf{e}_i}$. This choice allows the separation of diffusion in different directions so that the diffusion in a given direction does not depend on the intensity variations in the other directions. Some interpretation of this diffusion scheme is given in [5, 6, 7].

For the local orientations, we use the gradient and principal curvature directions computed on the smoothed image u^*, where the smoothing is obtained by convolution with a Gaussian of standard deviation σ. This basis corresponds respectively to unit vectors in the directions of the gradient ($\mathbf{e}_0 = \frac{\nabla u^*}{\|\nabla u^*\|}$), and of the maximal and minimal curvature of the smoothed image. The principal curvature directions can be computed as two of the eigenvalues (eigenvectors respectively) of the matrix PHP, where H is the Hessian matrix of the image and P is the projection matrix orthogonal to the gradient direction, that is $H' = PH_\sigma P$ with $P = I - \mathbf{e}_0\mathbf{e}_0^t$, where H_σ is the Hessian matrix of the smoothed image previously computed and I is the identity matrix. One of the eigenvectors of this matrix is the gradient of the smoothed image with a zero associated eigenvalue, and the two others are the directions of principal curvature.

The diffusion functions Φ_i of eq. (2) are chosen as $\Phi_0(x) = x\,e^{-(\frac{x}{\delta})^2}$ with a threshold δ on the intensity derivative in the gradient direction, $\Phi_1(x) = 0$ and $\Phi_2(x) = x\,\alpha$, where α is a positive constant allowing a diffusion only in the minimal curvature direction.

2.2   Anisotropic Adaptive Filtering

Here we describe a method based on an adaptive extension of the well-known Wiener filter. The adaptive filter is steered by means of a local estimation of structure as provided by an auxiliary bank of filters which enhances the local orientation and the degree of anisotropy [3, 4].
Consider the Wiener filter $H = \frac{S_{ff}}{S_{ff}+\sigma_n^2}$, where σ_n is the noise standard deviation and S_{ff} is the power density spectrum. Based on the conventional unsharp masking technique used by photographers [10], Abramatic and Silvermann [1] proposed to use the filter $H_\alpha = H + (1 - \alpha)(1 - H)$ in order to isotropically trade-off a low-pass and a high-pass component weighting them with a visibility function $0 \le \alpha \le 1$. Knutsson et al.[4] introduced an anisotropy component to this filter:

$$H_{\alpha,\gamma} = H + (1 - \alpha)(\gamma + (1 - \gamma)cos^2(\phi - \theta))(1 - H) \tag{3}$$

where γ weights the degree of anisotropy of the filter and θ is the main orientation of the image local structure. The $cos^2(\phi - \theta)$ term is a polar function which shapes the high pass component of the filter preventing any smoothing along θ. In order to generalize this idea to N-dimensions, it is convenient to describe the local structure by means of a second order symmetric positive semidefinite tensor $\mathbf{T}$, which principal eigenvector is aligned along the main direction of the local structure. This can be visualized as a local ellipsoid elongated along such direction. Different approaches can be used to estimate the local structure tensor [2, 4, 12]. Here we combine the output from a bank of spherically separable quadrature filters; details can be found in [3, 12].
An extension to the 2-D filter for the N-dimensional case is [13]:

$$H_\gamma = H + (1 - H) < \mathbf{C}, \mathbf{U} > \tag{4}$$

where $\mathbf{C} = \sum_{k=1}^{N} \gamma_k \hat{\mathbf{e}}_k \hat{\mathbf{e}}_k^T$ is a control tensor, $\mathbf{u}$ is a vector of spatial frequencies, $\mathbf{U} = \hat{\mathbf{u}}\hat{\mathbf{u}}^T$ is the outer product of the unit frequencies and $<\mathbf{C}, \mathbf{U}>$ is an inner product. The eigenvalues of the control tensor indicate the degree of smoothing along the associated directions and hence the control tensor must be related to the tensor structure.

In our implementation, the control tensor is obtained from $\mathbf{C} = m(\lambda_1)\mathbf{T}'$, where m is the mapping function

$$m(\lambda_1) = \gamma(1 - \lambda_1) + \frac{\lambda_1^{\beta}}{\lambda_1^{(\alpha+\beta)} + \sigma^{\beta}}, \qquad (5)$$

$\mathbf{T}'$ is the local structure tensor normalized by the globally largest eigenvalue over the whole dataset, and λ_1 is the maximum eigenvalue of $\mathbf{T}'$ for every voxel. Details can be found in [13].

3   Orientation Extraction

In this section we compare on 3D synthetic images the orientations obtained by the gradient of the smoothed image $\mathbf{e}_g$ and the maximal and minimal curvature directions $\mathbf{e}_M$ and $\mathbf{e}_m$, with the orientations obtained by the eigenvectors of the structure tensor, denoted by $\mathbf{e}_{\lambda_1}, \mathbf{e}_{\lambda_2}, \mathbf{e}_{\lambda_3}$, and ordered decreasingly according to associated eigenvalues.

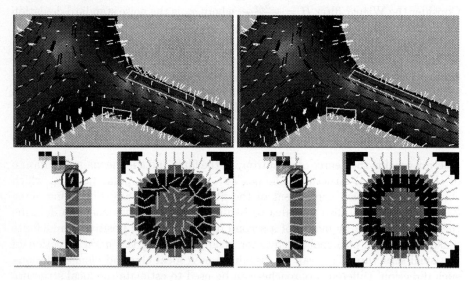

Fig. 1. Top row, comparison of the estimated orientations on a synthetic 3D junction. Bottom row, comparison of the estimated orientations on a synthetic 3D joint, where each image on the left represents a YZ slice, and on the right, an XY slice. The left column shows orientation obtained by the gradient and the minimal curvature, and the right column shows the first and the last eigenvectors of the structure tensor.

We use two synthetic 3D images to test these orientations. The first one is a synthetic 3D junction of vessels and the second one is a synthetic 3D hip joint (fig. 3). The intensity of the synthetic junction is 100 while the background is 0, and the vessel radii are 4, 3 and 2 voxels. The image has been convolved with a Gaussian kernel of standard deviation 1 and a white Gaussian noise of standard deviation 30 has been added (top left of fig. 3). Top row of fig. 1 shows results of $\mathbf{e}_g$ in white and $\mathbf{e}_m$ in black on the left, computed with $\sigma = 2$, and $\mathbf{e}_{\lambda_1}$ in white and $\mathbf{e}_{\lambda_3}$ in black on the right, computed with $\rho_0 = \pi/2$ and $B = 2$. For both direction estimations, the results on the two widest vessels are very similar. However, the orientations are different near the junction and on the smallest vessel. On the one hand, the top white square on the two images shows points of the surface where $\mathbf{e}_g$ gives much better results than $\mathbf{e}_{\lambda_1}$. In this case, while the vectors $\mathbf{e}_g$ are well oriented, the vectors $\mathbf{e}_{\lambda_1}$ are parallel to the point of view of the projection and seem very small. This can be explained by a global deviation of $\mathbf{e}_{\lambda_1}$ in the direction orthogonal to the 3D plane that contains the junction, which is globally the direction of maximal intensity variation. On the other hand, the bottom small white square shows that the black vectors $\mathbf{e}_{\lambda_3}$ are better oriented than $\mathbf{e}_m$, due to the Gaussian smoothing that displaces the contour position. Globally, the basis of the gradient direction and the principal curvature directions give a better orientation estimation than the basis of the structure tensor eigenvectors.

In the second case, we present a synthetic hip joint (see bottom row of fig. 3) with a sphere and a semi-cylinder that simulate femoral head and hip. This 3D image has a size of $40 \times 40 \times 23$ and a $1 \times 1 \times 3.04$ voxel size. It has been generated with a binary image using the same parameter values as the synthetic junction and a noise standard deviation of 10. We observe (fig. 1 bottom row) a better orientation of $\mathbf{e}_{\lambda_1}$, computed with $\rho_0 = \pi/4$ and $B = 2$, (see XY slice and circle in the YZ slice) than $\mathbf{e}_g$, computed with $\sigma = 1$. This better definition of the local structure is due to the fact that the gradient is very weak between the sphere and the semi-cylinder, so the normalized gradient orientation is not accurate. However, the tensor structure responds well in this case and points in the right direction, because it averages the orientations without taking into account opposite directions.

4   Restoration

An intuitive analogy can be made between the two filtering techniques. First, the low pass filter used by the first method is a heat diffusion equation with a data attachment, while the second method uses a Wiener filter, which also has low-pass characteristics. Second, anisotropic diffusion uses a diffusion function based on a threshold parameter δ on the first derivative of the intensity in the gradient direction to decide whether a region should be enhanced or smoothed. The proposed adaptive filtering uses a mapping function based on the first eigenvalue of the structure tensor to decide whether high frequencies should be increased or decreased. However, the PDE scheme progressively cools the solution while the

adaptive filter obtains it in a single step. In this section, we compare restoration
of noisy synthetic and real images using both methods.

4.1 Synthetic Images

Three synthetic images were created. The first synthetic image is a 3D image of
size $15 \times 15 \times 60$ containing two bar-like structures of width 3 voxels separated
by 2 voxels. This image varies only along z axis and we represented an intensity profile at the center of XY plane and along Z axis in figure 2. The image

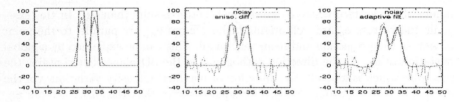

Fig. 2. Intensity profiles on a synthetic image.

was first convolved with a Gaussian of standard deviation 1 and then Gaussian
white noise of standard deviation 15 was added. The solid line in the left graph
in figure 2 shows the intensity profile of the binary image that we created, and
the dashed line shows the convolved image. The middle graph in Figure 2 shows
the restored image after anisotropic diffusion ($\sigma = 1, \delta = 7, \beta = 0.05, \alpha = 1$)
superimposed on the noisy image. Then, the right-hand graph in figure 2 shows
the noisy image in slashed line and the restored image after adaptive filtering ($\rho_0 = \pi/3, B = 2, \alpha = \gamma = 0, \beta = 10, \sigma = 0.9$) in plain line. We remark that the adaptive filtering tends to give a result that is closer to the
convolved image, and the anisotropic diffusion attempts to converge to a segmented image with constant areas. The second synthetic image (top row of

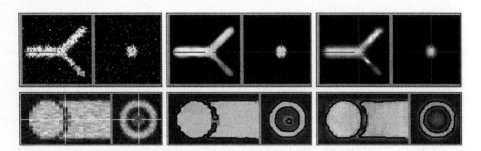

Fig. 3. Top row, comparison of the filtering on a synthetic 3D junction. Bottom
row, comparison of the filtering on a synthetic 3D joint. Left, initial image with
noise; middle, restoration using anisotropic diffusion; right, restoration using
adaptive filtering.

fig. 3) represents a 3D synthetic junction between vessels. This image was described in section 3. We use the following definition of the Signal to Noise Ratio (SNR): $SNR(I) = 10 \ log_{10} \frac{\sigma^2(I)}{\sigma^2(I_b - I)}$ where I_r is the image to evaluate, I_b is the initial binary image, and σ denotes the standard deviation. Its value is 0.4 for the noisy image, 5.7 for the image restored by anisotropic diffusion ($\sigma = 1, \delta = 10, \beta = 0.1, \alpha = 1$) and 2.0 for the image restored by adaptive filtering ($\rho_0 = \pi/2, B = 2, \alpha = \gamma = 0, \beta = 10, \sigma = 0.9$). This means that we can obtain a better restoration using the anisotropic diffusion which corresponds to the visual impression in fig. 3, and which can be explained by the better estimation of the directions using the gradient and the principal curvature directions. The third synthetic image (bottom row of fig. 3), described in section 3, represents a 3D synthetic joint. The parameters used for the anisotropic diffusion are $\sigma = 1, \delta = 10, \beta = 0.05, \alpha = 1$ and for the adaptive filtering are $\rho_0 = \pi/4, B = 2, \alpha = \gamma = 0, \beta = 2, \sigma = 0.9$. An iso-intensity contour of threshold 60 was superimposed in black on the restored images to show that the adaptive filtering allows a better contrast enhancement. This is coherent with the better estimation of the orientations obtained by the structure tensor.

4.2   Real Images

Figure 4 presents results on two real images. The top row is a XY slice representation of a $94 \times 52 \times 26$ sub-volume from a 3D Magnetic Resonance Angiography. The voxel size is $0.93 \times 0.93 \times 1.5mm$. We remark that the anisotropic diffusion ($\sigma = 1, \delta = 5, \beta = 0.2, \alpha = 0.3$) provides a more homogeneous background than the adaptive filtering ($\rho_0 = \pi/2, B = 2, \alpha = \gamma = 0.5, \beta = 1.5, \sigma = 0.5$), while the conservation of the small vessels is similar. This conservation depends on the parameters of each method. The bottom row presents a $85 \times 83 \times 20$ sub-volume of a hip joint CT scan of voxel size $0.82 \times 0.82 \times 3mm$. We display on the top left of each image a zoom on the joint region that confirms that better enhancement is obtained by adaptive filtering ($\rho_0 = \pi/4, B = 2, \alpha = \gamma = 0.5, \beta = 1.5, \sigma = 0.1$) compared to anisotropic diffusion ($\sigma = 1, \delta = 30, \beta = 0.1, \alpha = 1$) as in the synthetic case.

5   Discussion and Future Work

We presented a comparison between two different types of anisotropic filtering. The first one uses the gradient and the principal curvature directions to steer the diffusion and the second one uses the eigenvectors of the structure tensor to weight the frequencies. We first compared the orientations used by each method and showed on synthetic 3D images that the gradient and principal curvature directions are better oriented in the case of vascular structures while the eigenvectors of the structure tensor respond better in regions of closed structures. We also made a qualitative comparison between the filtering results on both synthetic and real images applied to vessels and hip joint. As far as we know,

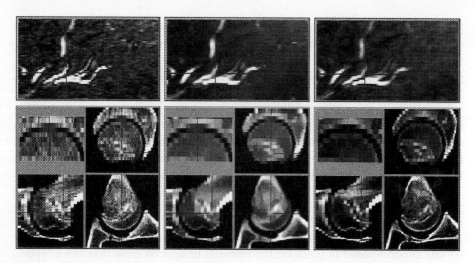

Fig. 4. Top row, 3D Magnetic Resonance Angiography. Bottom row, hip joint CT scan. Left, initial real image; middle, restoration using anisotropic diffusion; right, restoration using adaptive filtering.

this work is the first comparison that has been done between these two distinct filtering methods. An extended version of this work, including quantitative evaluation on synthetic images, is presented in [8]. In future work we also plan to use the same best estimation of orientation in boths methods, according to the application, and quantify the restoration of real images based on a specific segmentation algorithm and manually segmented images from physicians.

Acknowledgements

Thanks to L. Alvarez for supporting the second author as a post-doctoral grant, and to Miguel Aleman and Lauren O'Donnell for their help editing this paper.

References

[1] Abramatic J.F. and Silverman M. Nonlinear restoration of noisy images. *IEEE Trans. of Pattern Analysis and Machine Intelligence*, 4(2):141–149, 1982.

[2] Bigün J. and Granlund G. H. and Wiklund J. Multidimensional orientation: texture analysis and optical flow. *IEEE Transactions on Pattern Analysis and Machine Intelligence*, PAMI–13(8), August 1991.

[3] Knutsson H., Haglund L., Bårman H. and Granlund G. H. A framework for anisotropic adaptive filtering and analysis of image sequences and volumes. In *Proceedings ICASSP-92*, San Fransisco, CA, USA, March 1992. IEEE.

[4] Knutsson H., Wilson R. and Granlund G. H. Anisotropic non-stationary image estimation and its applications-part i: Restoration of noisy images. *IEEE Trans. on Communications. COM-31*, 3:388–397, 1983.

[5] Krissian, K. Flux-based anisotropic diffusion: application to enhancement of 3d angiographies. Technical Report 0011, Instituto Universitario de Ciencias y Tecnologías Cibernéticas, Las Palmas, Spain, Dec. 2000.

[6] Krissian, K. *Traitement multi-échelle: applications à l'imagerie médicale et à la détection tridimensionnelle de vaisseaux.* PhD thesis, Univ. de Nice-Sophia Antipolis, Av. Joseph Vallot, 06108 Nice cedex 2, 2000.

[7] Krissian, K. and Malandain, G. and Ayache, N. Directional anisotropic diffusion applied to segmentation of vessels in 3d images. In *Scale-Space Theory in Computer Vision (Scale-Space)*, volume 1252 of *Lecture Notes in Computer Science*, pages 345–348, Utrecht, The Netherlands, July 1997. Springer Verlag.

[8] Krissian K., Rodriguez-Florido M.A., Ruiz-Alzola J., Westin C.-F. Comparison between two multidimensional anisotropic filtering techniques. Technical Report 18, Instituto Universitario de Ciencias y Tecnologías Cibernéticas, Las Palmas, Spain, 2001.

[9] Perona, P. and Malik, J. Scale-Space and edge detection using anisotropic diffusion. *IEEE Trans. on Pattern Analysis and Machine Intel.*, 12(7):629–639, July 1990.

[10] Schriber W.F. Wirephoto quality improvement by unsharp masking. *J.Pattern Recognition*, 2:117–121, 1970.

[11] Weickert, J. *Anisotropic Diffusion in image processing.* Teubner-Verlag, Stuttgart, 1998.

[12] Westin C.-F. and Bhalerao A. and Knutsson H. and Kikinis R. Using Local 3D Structure for Segmentation of Bone from Computer Tomography Images. In *CVPR*, pages 794–800, Puerto Rico, June 1997.

[13] Westin C.F., Richolt J., Moharir V., Kikinis R. Affine adaptive filtering of CT data. *Medical Image Analysis*, 4:161–177, 2000.

Robust Segmentation of Medical Images Using Geometric Deformable Models and a Dynamic Speed Function

Benoit M. Dawant[1], Shiyan Pan[1], and Rui Li[1]

[1] Vanderbilt University, Department of Electrical Engineering and Computer Science, Box 1662 Station B, Nashville, TN 37235
{Benoit.Dawant, Shiyan.Pan, Rui.Li}@vanderbilt.edu

Abstract. A number of methods based on geometric deformable models have been proposed recently to segment medical images. These methods require the definition of a speed function that governs model deformation. In this paper we propose a new speed function that is modified dynamically as the front progresses. This new speed function is particularly well adapted to situations where edges are ill-defined, adjacent structures have comparable intensity values, and images are noisy. We illustrate qualitatively the performance of our approach on a variety of MR, CT, and ultrasound images. The examples show the generality of our approach and its insensitivity to parameters. We also evaluate it quantitatively on several CT scans of the liver.

1. Introduction

In recent years, geometric deformable models have been proposed as an alternative to parametric deformable models such as snakes originally proposed by Kass et al. [1]. In the geometric deformable model framework, the evolution of an initial contour toward the true object boundary is considered as a front propagation problem. This permits the use of the level set and fast marching methods introduced by Sethian [2] to model propagating fronts with curvature-dependent speeds. Following the level set formulation, the boundary of a 3D object is embedded as the zero-level set of a time-dependent function Φ. As time progresses, the value of the function Φ evolves and the boundary is given by its zero-level set. In practice, the function Φ is computed iteratively as follows:

$$\Phi_{i,j,k}^{n+1} = \Phi_{i,j,k}^{n} - \Delta t \cdot F \mid \nabla_{i,j,k} \Phi_{i,j,k}^{n} \mid, \tag{1}$$

in which F is the speed function, i.e., the function that specifies the speed at which the contour evolves along its normal direction. The main challenge when using front propagation methods is to produce an adequate speed function for a specific application. Malladi et al. [3] have proposed a general model for image segmentation defined as

$$F = g_I(F_0 - \varepsilon \kappa), \tag{2}$$

W. Niessen and M. Viergever (Eds.): MICCAI 2001, LNCS 2208, pp. 1040-1047, 2001.
© Springer-Verlag Berlin Heidelberg 2001

in which g_I is a multiplicative term derived from the image itself. It is used to stop the propagation of the contour near desired points such as points with high gradient or pre-specified intensity values, κ represents the curvature of the front and acts as a regularization term; F_0 is a constant; and ε is a weighting parameter. But except if hard thresholds are set on the value of g_I (i.e. if g_I is set to zero when the gradient exceeds a certain value or when intensity values fall outside a predefined range), contours never stop completely at weak edges. Given enough time these will eventually "leak" outside the desired regions. This problem has been recognized and a solution has been proposed by Casselles *et al.* [4] who introduced an additional term in the speed function designed to attract contours toward boundaries. Although this term offers a partial solution to the leakage problem it is still not very well adapted to situations with weak edges in noisy and non-uniform images [5]. To address this problem speed functions that take into account probability density functions of regions inside and outside the structures of interest have been proposed [5,6]. This class of solution is well adapted to situations where adjacent structures have different intensity distributions but are challenged by applications that require the segmentation of structures surrounded by other structures with similar intensity values and separated by weak edges.

In this paper, we propose a new expression for the speed function that greatly increases the robustness of geometric deformable models for the segmentation of 2D and 3D noisy images with weak edges. The major difference between the approach we propose and previous approaches is the dynamic adaptation of the speed function. We call this new dynamic speed functions the accumulative speed function because its value depends on the path of the front. The next sections describe our approach and present qualitative and quantitative results we have obtained on a variety of medical images.

2. Method

2.1   The Accumulative Speed Function

In traditional speed functions, the terms related to the underlying image are static, i.e., they do change spatially but for a fixed location, they do not change as time progresses or as a function of the path followed by the front. To stop the front propagation at weak boundaries, speed functions have to be designed to decelerate the fronts very rapidly. This necessitates the choice of large values for the weights assigned to the gradient or intensity terms with the possible drawback of stopping the front at spurious edges. The novel approach we propose is to progressively slow the front down as it passes over the boundary points. In essence, we build memory into the process. If the front passes over one boundary point it slows down some. If it passes over two boundary points in sequence, it slows down more, etc., until it comes to a complete halt. This speed function allows the front to step over noisy points (for instance speckle noise in ultrasound images) while stopping at the object boundary even if it is not clearly defined.

2.2   Computation of the Accumulative Speed Function

The algorithm we propose to implement our dynamic speed function is as follows:

1. Define a standard image-dependent static multiplicative term as described earlier and call it g_{bas} .

2. Define g_0 as the actual multiplicative term to be used in the speed function and let $g_0 = g_{bas}$.

3. At each iteration, compute $\{(x, y, z) \mid \Phi(x, y, z) = 0\}$, the zero level set of the embedding function. For every point in this set, retrieve $g_{bas}(x, y, z)$ and extend it to a narrow band around the zero level set (the notion of extension is defined later). This creates an additional multiplicative term which we call g_{ext}

4. Let $g_0 = g_0 \cdot g_{ext}$

5. Use g_0 as the multiplicative term in the speed function that governs the propagation of the front. For example, to include curvature in the final speed function, define it as $F = g_0 (1 - \varepsilon \kappa)$

6. Compute Φ^{n+1}, the value of the embedding function, using equation (1)

7. After a predefined number of iterations or if the zero level set does not move, stop. Otherwise, go to step 3

Step 3 in the algorithm requires the computation of an extended multiplicative term. Here, the notion of extension is the same as the one proposed by Adalsteinsson and Sethian [7] for velocities defined on zero level sets only. Loosely speaking, for voxels close to the zero level set, we set $g_{ext}(x, y, z) = g_{bas}(c(x, y, z))$ in which $c(x, y, z)$ is the closest point in the zero level set. Following Adalsteinsson's approach, this can be achieved by computing an extended multiplicative term that satisfies the following equation:

$$\nabla g_{ext} \cdot \nabla \varphi = 0, \tag{3}$$

in which φ is the standard signed distance function computed from the zero level set. This equation is solved using the Fast Marching Method as proposed by Sethian.

The key step in our algorithm is step 4. If a section of the front is over a region where the underlying static multiplicative term is small albeit non-zero, the actual multiplicative term decreases exponentially toward zero and the front stops within a few iterations. When this happens, the front is stopped permanently. Because of this, we do not need to design speed functions that are exactly zero to stop the front at the desired boundaries. We have the much easier task to design speed functions that have small values over the object boundaries. Examples will show that it lets us define generic speed functions that require tuning of very few parameters.

2.3   The Static Multiplicative Term g_{bas}

Our approach still requires the definition of an underlying static multiplicative term. The underlying multiplicative term we have used in all the experiments presented herein is simple and it is shown in Figure 1 (the left panel of the figure shows its analytical expression; the function is plotted on the right panel). In this equation, I_{min} and I_{max} are two parameters used to specify the minimum and maximum intensity values expected in the structure of interest, σ is the standard deviation of these intensity values, and γ is used to control the rate at which g decreases; the smaller the value of γ, the faster the reduction in speed at weak boundaries.

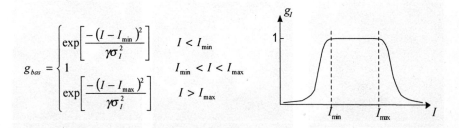

Fig. 1. Function used to define the static multiplicative term

3. Results

3.1 Qualitative Results

We have experimented with this multiplicative term combined with the new dynamic update scheme we have developed on a series of segmentation tasks ranging from the segmentation of structures and substructures in MR images of the brain, the ventricles in MR and ultrasound images of the heart, to the liver in MR images of mice. In every case the same underlying multiplicative term was used and the only parameters that were adjusted were I_{min}, I_{max}, and ε, the parameter used to weigh the contribution of the curvature term; γ and σ were kept constant. The overall speed function we have used for these experiments is as in (2) with $F_0 = 1$. Note that the formulation we propose does not include any term related to the intensity gradient which has little meaning in noisy images or in images with weak edges.

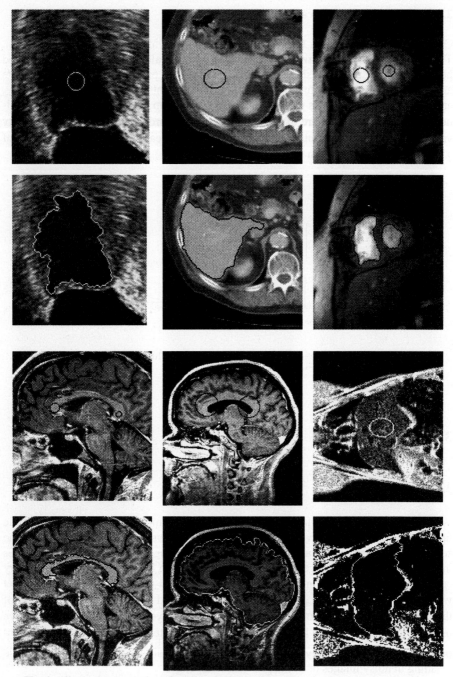

Fig. 2. Illustrative examples of results obtained with our method. For each pair of images, the top one shows the original contour; the bottom one shows the final contour.

	Imin	Imax	Epsilon	Gamma
Heart US	10	60	3.0	100
Liver CT	90	200	3.0	100
Heart MR	140	400	3.0	100
Corp. Call.	70	85	2.0	100
Brain MR	40	85	3.0	100
Mouse MR	25	50	3.0	100

Table 1. Parameters used to generate the resutls shown in Figure 2.

A number of movies showing results we have obtained can be seen at http://www.vuse.vanderbilt.edu/~dawant/levelset_examples. In each of these movies, the contours have been initialized with small circles shown on the first frames of the movies and the end of the movies shows the final contours. Figure 2 presents a static view of some of these results obtained on a variety of images. From left to right and top to bottom, this figure shows results obtained on an ultrasound image of the heart, a CT image of the liver, an MR image of the heart, an MR image of the head focused on the corpus callosum, an MR image of the head showing the entire brain, and an MR image of a mouse focused on the liver. In every instance, a pair of image is presented. The top one shows the original contour, the bottom one shows the final contour. For the final mouse image, the contrast and intensity values have been adjusted to highlight the final contour because the amount of noise present in the image prevents the simultaneous display of the tissues and the contour on a gray level image. Table 1 lists the parameters that were used in each case. This figure clearly shows that the results are largely insensitive to the choice of parameters. The value of ε had to be reduced for the corpus callosum image because the structure is narrow and a larger value for the curvature term did prevent the propagation of the front. Further experiments have also revealed that the results are insensitive to the precise values of I_{min} and I_{max}. The human liver and corpus callosum images illustrate the performance of our algorithm for the segmentation of structures with similar intensity values that are separated by weak edges. In the liver image, the liver and the kidney have similar intensity values and are separated by a blurred edge. Observe how the front stopped at the correct position and also that it did not penetrate the vena cava. The corpus callosum image shows the posterior part of this structure as a region of white matter surrounded by a thin layer of gray matter and then white matter again. Here, the contour stopped correctly at the narrow white/gray matter interface. The mouse image has been chosen to show the behavior of the algorithm on images with very poor signal-to-noise ratio.

3.2 Quantitative Results

To validate the proposed method quantitatively, we tested it on five abdominal CT scans, three of which are from normal subjects and two others contain abnormal livers with tumors for a total of 280 slices. Scans were selected to include livers with different size, shape, and position in the abdomen. Experiments were conducted in 2D and 3D in all five scans. The voxel size for all scans is 0.625mm x 0.625mm x 3mm. In 2D, the algorithm was initialized by drawing a small circle within the liver in each slice. In slices where the liver consists of several disconnected structure, one small circle was placed within each structure. The 3D algorithm was initialized by placing a sphere somewhere inside the liver. For each of these volumes, we kept the same parameters except for I_{min} and I_{max} which were adjusted to compensate for slight contrast differences between volumes due to the injection of a contrast agent.

Even though the speed function and update scheme we propose are able to stop contours when edges are ill defined, we found it to be insufficient for this particular application. Indeed, between the ribs, the edge at the liver/muscle is virtually non-existent and both tissues are iso-intense. The approach we have taken to address this problem is to constrain the propagation using a priori anatomic information. We locate the skin/air interface and the position of the ribs. We compute an average distance between the ribs and the skin and we constrain the propagation of the front using this distance.

All segmentation results were compared with manual delineations inspected and approved by an experienced surgeon. For each point in the plots shown in Figure 3, the X and Y coordinates correspond to the area of manual and automatic segmentations in the same slice, respectively. The majority of points cluster near the straight line with slope of 1 and passing through the origin, which indicates a good match between the two sets of segmentations. Some scattered points are found above the line in the 3D plot and below the line in both the 3D and 2D plots. Points above the line repre-

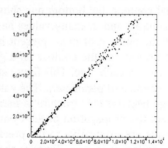 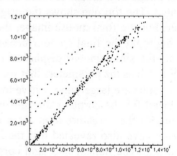

Fig. 3. Areas of automatic contours versus areas of manual contours for every slice; left 2D, right 3D.

sent slices in which leakage did occur. Points below the line represent slices in which the automatic segmentation was unable to capture the entire liver.

This figure shows that the results we have obtained with both the 2D and 3D versions of our algorithm are in close agreement with manual delineation, it also indicates a rate of failure that is slightly higher for the 3D version than for the 2D version. Closer investigation of this phenomenon has shown that this is due to one image volume in which leakage occurred across slices. It is caused by the anisotropic nature of the image volumes we have used (the slice thickness of the images is 5 times larger than the in-plane resolution). In this volume, the boundary between the heart and the liver is not resolved between two slices. The 3D algorithm leaked from the liver into the heart between these two slices and then expanded into the heart in 3D. This, in turn, caused large segmentation errors on a number of slices. For the other volumes, 2D and 3D results are identical. Movies that illustrate the behavior of the algorithm we propose for liver segmentation can be viewed at the aforementioned URL (files liver2d.mpg and liver3d.mpg).

4. Discussion

The dynamic update scheme we propose for image segmentation using geometric deformable models permits the 2D and 3D segmentation of vastly different images and structures with only few parameter adjustments. Examples presented show that the algorithm we propose is able to cope with ultrasound images that are notoriously difficult to segment because of speckle noise as well as with images with low signal-to-noise ratio and poorly defined edges. The key feature of our algorithm is its ability to stop the propagation of the front even if the underlying multiplicative term in non-zero. If the front encounters one voxel with a low value for the multiplicative term, it slows down but does not stop. But if it passes several voxels in a row all with a low value it slows down exponentially until it comes to a complete halt. This property led us to call the speed function we propose the accumulative speed function because the likelihood of being at a real boundary point increases if several possible boundary points are encountered in sequence.

References

1.   M. Kass, A. Witkin, and D. Terzopoulos, "Snakes: active contour models." *Int'l J. Comp. Vis.*, **1**(4):321-331, 1987
2.   J.A. Sethian, "Numerical algorithms for propagating interfaces: Hamilton-Jacobi equations and conservation laws", *J. of Differential Geometry*, vol. **31**, pp. 131-161, 1990
3.   R. Malladi, J.A. Sethian, and B.C. Vemuri, "Shape modeling with front propagation: A level set approach", *IEEE Trans. PAMI*, **17**(2):158-175, 1995
4.   V. Caselles, R. Kimmel, and G. Sapiro, "Geodesic active contours", *Proc. Int'l Conf. Comp. Vis.*, pp. 694-699, 1995
5.   C. Xu, A. Yezzi Jr., and J. Prince, "On the relationship between parametric and geometric active contours", Technical Report JHU/ECE 99-14, Dec. 1999
6.   C. Baillard and C. Barillot, "Robust 3D segmentation of anatomical structures with level sets", *Proceedings of MICCAI 2000*, pp. 237-245, 2000.
7.   D. Adalsteinsson and J.A. Sethian, "The fast construction of extension velocities in level set methods", *L. Comp. Phys.*, **138**, 1, pp. 193-223, 1997.

Hybrid Segmentation of Anatomical Data

Celina Imielinska[1], Dimitris Metaxas,[2] Jayaram Udupa[3], Yinpeng Jin[4], Ting Chen[2],

[1] College of Physicians and Surgeons, Office of Scholarly Resources,
Medical Informatics Dept. and Dept. of Computer Science, Columbia University
ci42@columbia.edu
[2] Dept. of Computer and Information Science, University of Pennsylvania
[3] Medical Image Processing Group, Dept. of Radiology, University of Pennsylvania
[4] Department of Biomedical Engineering, Columbia University

Abstract. We propose new hybrid methods for automated segmentation of radiological patient data and the Visible Human data. In this paper, we integrate boundary-based and region-based segmentation methods which amplifies the strength but reduces the weakness of both approaches. The novelty comes from combining a boundary-based method, the deformable model-based segmentation with region-based segmentation methods, the fuzzy connectedness and Voronoi Diagram-based segmentation, to develop hybrid methods that yield high precision, accuracy and efficiency. This work is a part of a NLM funded effort to provide a fully implemented and tested Visible Human Project Segmentation and Registration Toolkit (Insight).

1 Introduction

In this paper we develop and test new hybrid methods for segmenting radiological (patient) data (e.g. CT, MRI, PET) and the Visible Human data. The novelty stems from the integration of deformable model-based segmentation methods with a variety of region-based methods which aims toward the development of segmentation methods that yield high precision, accuracy and efficiency. This is a collaborative project between the University of Pennsylvania and Columbia University, a part of a larger effort, funded by NLM, to provide the Visible Human Project Segmentation and Registration Toolkit (Insight, http://visual.nlm.nih.gov/insight/).

We have developed powerful region and contour-based segmentation tools that we plan to further extend to meet the above goals [5],[7], [8], [9], [17], [18]. Radiological image data of internal organs are routinely used at the University of Pennsylvania, where the Interactive Virtual Environment for Modeling Anatomy and Physiology has been developed, in addition to 3DVIEWNIX, [18], a Unix-based software system for the visualization, manipulation, and analysis of multidimensional multi-parametric, multi-modality images. Highly detailed segmentations and 3D visualizations of the Visible Human dataset are used in interactive applications, such as the Vesalius™ Project at Columbia University, an interdisciplinary effort to create an environment for anatomy and other medical applications [6]. Integration of boundary-based and region-based segmentation methods amplifies the strengths but reduces the weaknesses of both approaches.

W. Niessen and M. Viergever (Eds.): MICCAI 2001, LNCS 2208, pp. 1048-1057, 2001.
© Springer-Verlag Berlin Heidelberg 2001

2 Approach and Methodology

Automatic internal organ segmentation from various imaging modalities is a very important yet open research problem. Over the past several years, a variety of segmentation methods have been developed. Boundary-based techniques such as snakes [11] start with a deformable boundary and attempt to align this boundary with the edges in the image. The solution to these systems generally involves minimizing an energy functional which quantifies the shape of the model and image information near the boundary of the model. To avoid becoming stuck in local minima, most model based techniques require that the model be initialized near the solution. User steered methods such as live wire that are used in day-to-day clinical research find a global optimum through dynamic programming. Region-based or statistical techniques such as region growing [3],[7] or MAP-based methods [2] assign membership to objects based on homogeneity statistics. The advantage here is that image information inside the object is considered as well as on the boundaries. However, in the region based framework, there is no provision for including the shape of the region in the decision making process, which can lead to noisy boundaries and holes in the interior of the object.

Like several other recent approaches [4],[20], our design integrates the boundary and region-based techniques into a hybrid framework. By combining these techniques, hybrid approaches offer greater robustness than either technique alone. However, most previous work still requires significant initialization to avoid local minima. Furthermore, most of the earlier approaches use prior models for their region-based statistics, which we would rather avoid to increase usefulness in situations where a comprehensive set of priors may not be available.

We have recently developed a new approach to internal organ segmentation that is based on the integration of region-based and physics-based boundary estimation methods [8],[9]. Starting from a single pixel within the interior of an object, we make an initial estimate of the object's boundary using the fuzzy connectedness method [17] and clustering. A deformable surface model is then fitted to the extracted boundary data to fill in the missing boundary data and to override the spurious boundary data due to image noise. This is achieved by generalizing the formulation of our deformable models [12] to incorporate simple domain-specific knowledge.

In this paper we will further develop this approach by integrating deformable models with fuzzy connectedness, and the region-based color segmentation method developed at Columbia [7]. In addition, we will present a method based on an integration of Markov Random Field (Gibbs prior) and deformable models. In particular we develop two types of automatic segmentation algorithms: 1) Hybrid Method I: Integration of fuzzy connectedness, Voronoi Diagram; 2) Hybrid Method II: Integration of Gibbs prior and deformable models.

3 Hybrid Method I: Integration of Fuzzy Connectedness and Voronoi Diagram

We present a hybrid segmentation method which requires minimal manual initialization, where we integrate the fuzzy connectedness, and Voronoi Diagram

(VD). We will start with fuzzy connectedness algorithm to generate a region with a sample of tissue which we plan to segment. From the sample region, we will generate automatically homogeneity statistics for the VD-based algorithm which will produce an estimation of the boundary in a number of iterations. We will give an overview of the component algorithms used in the hybrid segmentation algorithm below.

3.1 Fuzzy Connectedness Algorithm.

This method described in detail in [17], uses the fact that medical images are inherently fuzzy. We define *affinity* between two *elements* in an image (e.g. pixels, voxels, spels) via a degree of *adjacency* and the *similarity* of their intensity values. The closer the elements are and more similar their intensities are, the greater is the affinity between them. There are two important characteristics of a medical image. First, it has graded composition coming from material, blurring, noise and background variation. Second, the image elements that constitute an anatomical object hang together in a certain way. Both these properties, *graded composition and hanging togetherness* are fuzzy properties. The aim of fuzzy connectedness is to capture the global hanging togetherness using image-based local fuzzy affinity.

Let us define a scene over a digital space (Z^n, α) as a pair $\Omega=(C,f)$, where C is an n-dimensional array of spels (elements) and $f: C \to [0,1]$. Fuzzy affinity κ is any reflexive and symmetric fuzzy relation in C, that is:

$$\kappa = \{((c,d), \mu_\kappa(c,d)) \mid c,d \in C\}$$
$$\mu_\kappa: C \times C \to [0,1]$$
$$\mu_\kappa(c,c) = 1, \text{ for all } c \in C \qquad (1)$$
$$\mu_\kappa(c,d) = \mu_\kappa(d,c), \text{ for all } c,d \in C.$$

The general form of μ_κ can be written as follows. For all $c,d \in C$,

$$\mu_\kappa(c,d) = g(\mu_\alpha(c,d), \mu_\psi(c,d), \mu_\phi(c,d), c, d)$$

where: $\mu_\alpha(c,d)$ represents the degree of adjacency of c and d; $\mu_\psi(c,d)$ represents the degree of intensity homogeneity of c and d; $\mu_\phi(c,d)$ represents the degree of similarity of the intensity features of c and d to expected object features. Fuzzy κ-connectedness K is a fuzzy relation in C, where $\mu_K(c,d)$ is the strength of the strongest path between c and d, and the strength of a path is the smallest affinity along the path. To define the notion of a fuzzy connected component, we need the following hard binary relation K_θ based on the fuzzy relation K. Let $\Omega=(C,f)$ be a membership scene over a fuzzy digital space (Z^n, α), and let κ be a fuzzy spel affinity in Ω. We define a (hard) binary relation K_θ in C as

$$\mu_{K_\theta}(c,d) = \begin{cases} 1, & \text{iff } \mu_\kappa(c,d) \geq \theta \in [0,1] \\ 0, & \text{otherwise} \end{cases} \qquad (2)$$

Let O_θ be an equivalence class [14, Chap.10] of the relation K_θ in C. A *fuzzy κ-component* Γ_θ *of C of strength* θ is a fuzzy subset of C defined by the membership function

$$\mu_{\Gamma_\theta} = \begin{cases} f(c), & \text{iff } c \in O_\theta \\ 0, & \text{otherwise.} \end{cases} \qquad (3)$$

The equivalence class $O_\theta \subset C$, such that for any $c,d \in C$, $\mu_\kappa(c,d) \geq \theta$, $\theta \in [0,1]$, and for any $e \in C - O_\theta$, $\mu_\kappa(c,d) < \theta$. We use the notation $[o]_\theta$ to denote the equivalence class of K_θ that contains O for any $O \in C$. The *fuzzy κ-component of C that contains* O, denoted $\Gamma_\theta(O)$, is a fuzzy subset of C whose membership function is

$$\mu_{\Gamma_\theta(o)} = \begin{cases} f(c), & \textit{iff } c \in [o]_\theta \\ 0, & \textit{otherwise.} \end{cases} \tag{4}$$

A *fuzzy $\kappa\theta$-object of Ω* is a fuzzy κ-component of Ω of strength θ. For any spel $O \in C$, a fuzzy $\kappa\theta$-object of Ω that contains O is a fuzzy κ-component of Ω of strength θ that contains O. Given κ, O, θ, and Ω, a fuzzy $\kappa\theta$-object of Ω of strength $\theta \in [0,1]$ containing O, for any $O \in C$, can be computed via dynamic programming [17].

3.2 Voronoi Diagram(VD)-Based Algorithm

This algorithm, which is described in detail in [7], is based on repeatedly dividing an image into regions using VD and clasifying the Voronoi regions based on a selected homogeneity classifier for the segmented anatomical tissue. We will use the algorithm as a component in the hybrid method where the classifiers for different tissue type will be generated automatically from the region segmented by the fuzzy connectedness method. VD and Delaunay triangulation (DT) play a central role in the algorithm. In 2D, the VD for a set V of points is a partition of the Euclidean plane into Voronoi regions of points closer to one point of V than to any other seed point [14]. For any $p_i \in V$, $V = \{p_1,...,p_n\}$,

$$VD(p_i) = \{x \in R^2 \mid d(x,p_i) \leq d(x,p_j), \forall j \neq i, 1 \leq j \leq n\} \tag{5}$$

Similarly, we define the VD in 3D:

$$VD(p_i) = \{x \in R^3 \mid d(x,p_i) \leq d(x,p_j), \forall j \neq i, 1 \leq j \leq n\} \tag{6}$$

Two Voronoi regions are adjacent if they share a Voronoi edge. The DT, of V is a dual graph of the Voronoi diagram of V, obtained by joining two points whose Voronoi regions are adjacent.

3.3 The Hybrid Method I

The algorithm integrates two methods, the fuzzy connectedness and VD-based algorithm. We will outline the algorithm first, and explain the component steps later. The fuzzy connectedness algorithm is used to segment a fragment of the target tissue. From the sample, a set of statistics is generated automatically, in RGB and HVC color spaces, to define the homogeneity operator. The homogeneity operator will be used as a multi-channel classifier for the VD-based algorithm. As we mentioned, we will use, in the future, the deformable model, to determine the final (3D) smooth boundary of the segmented region. Below, we outline the hybrid method:

Step 1. We run the fuzzy connectedness algorithm to segment a sample of the target tissue, and generate statistics, average and variance, in three "strong" color channels, in two color spaces, RGB and HVC.

Step 2. Run the VD-based algorithm using multiple color channels, until it converges: (a) For each Voronoi region, classify it as interior/exterior/boundary region using multi-channel homogeneity operator; (b) Compute DT and display segments which connect boundary regions; (c) Add seeds to Voronoi edges of Voronoi boundary regions; (d) GoTo Step 2(a) until the algorithm converges to a stable state or until the user chooses to quit.

Step 3. (future) Use the deformable model to determine the final (3D) boundary and re-set the homogeneity operator.

Implementation of Step 1.   To initialize the fuzzy connectedness algorithm and establish the mean and standard deviation of spel values and their gradient magnitudes. The user collects the pixels within the region of interest, by clicking on the image and selecting at each time a square region with 7x7 pixels. Then an initial seed spel is selected to compute the fuzzy connectedness, using the dynamic programming approach [17]. We determine the strength of the fuzzy connectedness θ, $\theta \in [0,1]$, by letting the user to select interactively its threshold value, such that the initially segmented sample of the target tissue resembles the shape of the underlying image. For a binary image with a roughly segmented sample of a tissue, we generate the "strongest" three channels in two color spaces, RGB and HVC [15], for average and variance, respectively. First, we define for the binary image, the smallest enclosing rectangle, a region of interest (ROI), in which we identify the segmented image and its background. Within the ROI, we calculate the mean and variance in each of the six color channels (R,G,B,H,V,C) for the object and its background, respectively. Then three channels with the largest relative difference in mean value and in variance value between the object and its background are selected, respectively. The homogeneity operator for the VD-based algorithm uses the expected mean/variance values of the object together with tolerance values, computed for each selected channel, for classifying the internal and external region

Implementation of Step 2.   We build an initial VD by generating some number of random seed points (Voronoi points) and then run the QuickHull, [1], to calculate the VD. Once the initial VD has been generated, the program visits each region to accumulate classification statistics and makes a determination as to the identity of the region. For each Voronoi region, the mean/variance value for the preselected channels are computed, if they are similar, then it is marked as internal, otherwise external. Those external regions that have at least one internal neighbor are marked as boundary. Each boundary region is divided for next iterations until the total number of pixels within it is less than a chose number.

4 Hybrid Method II: Integration of Gibbs Prior and Deformable Models

Most medical images are Markov Random Field (MRF) images, that is, the statistics of a pixel is related to the statistics of pixels in its neighborhood. According to the Equivalent Theorem proved by Hammersley and Clifford, the MRF is equivalent to the Gibbs field under certain conditions. Thus for medical images which are MRF images, their joint distribution can be written in the Gibbsian form, which is shown as follows.

$$\Pi(x) = Z^{-1} \exp(-H(x)), Z = \sum_{z \in X} \exp(-H(z)) \tag{7}$$

where $H(x)$ represents the energy function of image x, X is the set of all possible configuration of the image, Z is the normalization factor or partition function in the terminology of statistical mechanics. The local and global properties of images will be incorporated into the model by designing an appropriate energy function. The lower the value of the energy function, the higher the value of the Gibbs distribution, the better the image is fit to the prior distribution. We began the establishment of the Gibbs model by designing the energy function as

$$H(X) = H_1(X) + H_2(X) + H_3(X) \tag{8}$$

$H_1(X)$ models the piecewise homogeneity statistics and $H_2(X)$ models the continuity of the boundary, $H_3(X)$ is the noise model term. For $H_2(X)$ we use the 3 by 3 clique. Local characteristics in the clique are given different weight. The local characteristics that more likely to appear in the image has lower weight. So when the energy function is minimized, such kind of local characteristics will increase. This will help to locate the boundary if the difference between object and background is not so big. A set of suitable parameters will enable the Gibbs prior model to: (a) Find the boundary according to the variance between objects and background. ($H_1(X)$); (b) If the variance is not large enough or the object gradually turns into the background, $H_2(X)$ is capable of finding a smooth and continuous boundary estimation; (c) Erase the noise using term $H_3(X)$.

We use the iterated conditional mode (ICM) method to minimize the energy function. This will give an estimation of the object boundary which can be used by the deformable model. Our deformable model is a superellipsoid with local deformations. The global parameter of the model is its natural shape, and the local deformations determine its displacement from the natural shape for discrete nodes on the surface of the model. Given the reference shape $\mathbf{s}$ and displacement $\mathbf{d}$, points on a model $\mathbf{p}$ are defined by:

$$\mathbf{p} = \mathbf{s} + \mathbf{d} \tag{9}$$

To keep the continuity of the model surface, we impose a C^0 continuous deformation strain energy on it.

$$\varepsilon_m(d) = \int \omega_{10} (\frac{\partial d}{\partial u})^2 + \omega_{01} (\frac{\partial d}{\partial v})^2 + \omega_{00} d^2 du, \tag{10}$$

where d is the node local deformation, ω_{00} controls the local magnitude and ω_{10}, ω_{01} control the local variation of the deformation. We can calculate the stiffness matrix $\mathbf{K}$ of the model based on the strain energy. The model nodes will move under the influence of internal and external forces. The internal forces constrain the deformation of a model according to the stiffness matrix to maintain its natural shape, while the external forces make the model expand until they meet a balance with the internal forces. The dynamics can be described by the first order Lagrangian method:

$$\overset{*}{d} + Kd = f, \tag{11}$$

where f is the summation of external forces and boundary forces. The nodes of the model are forced outward in the direction of their normal vector. So the model will expand like a balloon being filled with gas. When the model is reaching the estimated boundary, it will also move under the influence of boundary forces, which is in the opposite direction of the balloon force. Thus the model will fit to the estimated boundaries. When the shape of the object is complicated such as at sharp corners, new nodes will be added to the model. The Finite Element Analysis (FEA) method is used in our work to calculate the deformation on each node. The deformation is updated using Euler step:

$$d_{n+1} = d_n + t\overset{*}{d}, \tag{12}$$

where t is the time step. When most nodes (>90%) on the surface stop moving, the model stops. When the model is fitted to the estimated boundaries, we do statistics in the model region, updating the parameters for the Gibbs Prior model according to the result. The mean intensity, standard error of the object and the threshold of boundary existance will be recalculated. Weights of the local characteristics will be changed according to the global shape of the model.

The whole method can be summarized as follows: (Step 1) First create the Gibbs prior models using parameters calculated according to statistics result over a small region inside the object; (Step 2) Use the Gibbs prior models to estimate the boundaries of objects; (Step 3) Fit the deformable models to this data according to the combination of balloon and the boundary forces. (Step 4) Recalculate the parameters for the Gibbs prior model according to the results of Step3. Then go back to Step 2.

5 Hybrid Method I: Results

In this section we present the results from experiments using Hybrid Method I. We tested different tissue types: muscle tissue (VH data, Fig.1.) and brain tissue (VH, Fig.2, and MRI patient data, Fig.3. In Fig.1, we segment temporalis muscle, a structure in the head region. In Fig.2, we segment brain gray matter. We would like to note that we have used fuzzy connectedness extensively, in 3D, to segment gray and white matter in patient image data [19]. Gray matter and white matter are fuzzy connected entities in 3D. With a few seed points they can be, and they are, routinely segmented.

We show that the Hybrid I algorithm can generate automated statistical homogeneity classifiers for a variety of human tissue. We tested the method with the Visible Human data and as well with a sample of MRI patient data. The method will be formally validated, in the future using our rigorous validation methodology.

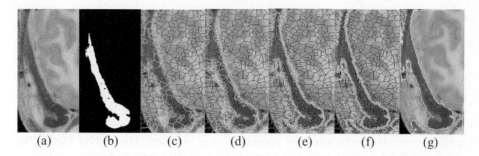

Fig.1. Hybrid Method I (segmentation of temporalis muscles): (a) Color VH male cryosection slice, (b) a fuzzy connected component, (c)-(f) iterations of the VD-based algorithm , (g) an outline of the boundary.

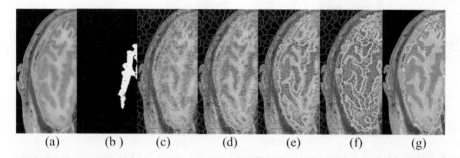

Fig.2. Hybrid Method I (segmentation of brain gray matter): (a) Color VH male cryosection slice, (b) a fuzzy connected component, (c)-(f) VD-based algorithm, (g) an outline of the boundary.

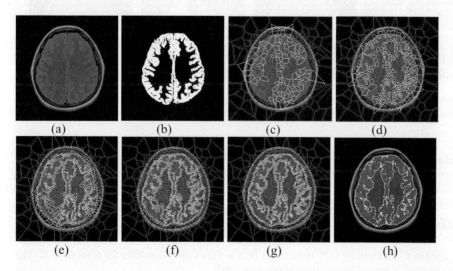

Fig.3. Hybrid Method I (segmentation of (MRI) gray matter): (a) MRI patient slice, (b) fuzzy connected component, (c)-(g) iterations of the VD-based algorithm, (h) an outline the boundary.

6 Hybrid Method II: Results

We segmented below, using Hybrid Method II, structures using the VH data (rectus muscle, Fig.4., and eyeball, Fig.5) and MRI patient data (white brain matter, Fig.6). In this method, by using the Gibbs prior, we generate a better estimation of the boundary and it is used as an initialization for the deformable model. We show that Gibbs prior method can estimate the boundary well in a variety of. The deformable model provides updated parameters to the Gibbs prior model, and the iterative algorithm is applied recursively until a refined segmentation is obtained. The Hybrid Method II, will be validated, in the future, using our rigorous validation methodology.

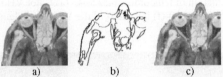

a)   b)   c)

Fig.4. Hybrid Method II (segmentation of rectus muscle): (a) VH slice, (b) Gibbs prior estimation (c) deformable model result.

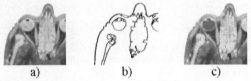

a)   b)   c)

Fig.5. Hybrid Method II (segmentation of eyeball (small scale)) : (a) VH slice, (b) Gibbs prior estimation (c) deformable model result.

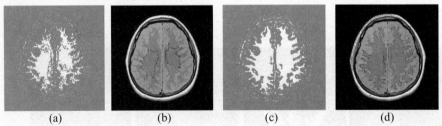

(a)   (b)   (c)   (d)

Fig.6. Hybrid Method II (segmentation of white matter from Fig. 3(a): (a)(c) Gibbs prior estimation, (b)(d) deformable model result.

Acknowledgements. This work was supported in part by NLM contract on the "VHP Segmentation and Registration Toolkit" - NLM99-103/DJH.

References

1. Barber, C.B.; Dobkin, D.P, Huhdanpaa H.:The Quickhull Algorithm for Convex Hull, The Geometry Center, University of Minnesota, 1995.
2. Blake, A., Zisserman, A.: Visual Reconstruction. MIT Press, 1987.

3. Bertin, E., Parazza, F.; Chassery, J.M., Segmentation and Measurement Based on 3D Voronoi Diagram: Application to Confocal Microscopy, *J. CMIG*, 1993, 17(3), p.175-182.
4. Chakraborty, A., Duncan, J.S.: Integration of Boundary Finding and Region-Based Segmentation Using Game Theory, In Y. Bizais et al., editor, Information Processing in Medical Imaging, Kluwer, 1995, p.189-201.
5. Falcao, A., Udupa, J.K., Samarasekera, S., Sharma, S., Hirsch, B.E.; Lotufo, R.: "User-Steered Image Segmentation Paradigm: Live wire and Live Lane", *Graphical Models and Image Processing*, vol.60, pp.233-260, 1998.
6. http://cpmcnet.columbia.edu/vesalius
7. Imielinska, C., Downes, M., Yuan, W.: Semi-Automated Color Segmentation of Anatomical Tissue, *J. of CMIG* ., 24(2000), 173-180, April, 2000.
8. Jones, T, Metaxas, D.: Automated 3D Segmentation Using Deformable Models and Fuzzy Affinity, *Proc. XVth Intern. Conf. on Image Processing in Medical Imaging*, June 1997.
9. Jones, T., Metaxas D,: Image Segmentation based on the Integration of Pixel Affinity and Deformable Models, *Proc. IEEE CVPe*, Santa Barbara, CA, June 1998.
10. Kaufmann, A.: *Introduction to the Theory of Fuzzy Subsets*, Vol. I, Academic Press, New York, 1975.
11. Kass, M., Witkin, A., Terzopoulos, D.: Snakes: Active Contour Models, *Intl. J. of Computer Vision*, 1998, 1(4), p.321-331.
12. Metaxas, D., Physics-Based Deformable Models: Applications to Computer Vision, Graphics and Medical Imaging, Kluwer-Academic Publishers, 1996.
13. Panel on ``Technical Challenges" at the Second User Conference of the National Library of Medicine's Visible Human Project, Oct. 1-2nd, 1998, Bethesda, MD.
14. Preparata, F.P.; Shamos, M.I.: *Computational Geometry*, New York, Springer, 1985.
15. Gong,Y., Sakauchi, M.: Detection of Regions Matching Specified Chromatic Features, *Computer Vision and Image Understanding*, 61(2), p.263-269, 1995.
16. Udupa, J., Odhner, D., Samarasekera, S., Goncalves, R., Iyer, K., Venugopal, K., Furuie, S.: 3D VIEWNIX: An Open, Transportable, Multidimensional, Multimodality, Multiparametric Imaging Software System", *SPIE Proceedings*, 2164:58-73, 1994.
17. Udupa, J.K., Samarasekera, S.: Fuzzy Connectedness and Object Definition, In *SPIE Proceedings*, vol.2431, pp. 2-11, 1995.
18. Udupa, J.K., Samarasekera, S.: Fuzzy Connectedness and Object Definition: Theory, Algorithms, and Applications in Image Segmentation, *Graphical Models and Image Processing*, 58(3), pp.246-261, 1996.
19. Udupa, J.K., Wei L., Samarasekera, S.: Miki, Y.; van Buchem, M.A.; Grossman, R.I.; Multiple sclerosis lesion quantification using fuzzy Connectedness principles, *IEEE Trans, Med Imaging*, vol. 16, pp. 598-609,1997.
20. Zhu, S.C, Lee, T.S., Yuille, A.L.: Region Competition: Unifying Snakes, Region Growing, and Bayes/mdl for Multi-Band Image Segmentation, *In Proc. Intl. Conf. on Computer Vision*, 1995, p.416-423.

Segmentation of Dynamic N-D Data Sets via Graph Cuts Using Markov Models

Yuri Boykov[1], Vivian S. Lee[2], Henry Rusinek[2], and Ravi Bansal[1]

[1] Siemens Corporate Research, Imaging & Visualization, Princeton NJ 08540, USA
yuri@scr.siemens.com, ravi@scr.siemens.com
[2] NYU School of Medicine, Radiology, 550 First Avenue, New York NY 10016, USA
lee@mri.med.nyu.edu, hr18@homemail.nyu.edu

Abstract. This paper describes a new segmentation technique for multi-dimensional dynamic data. One example of such data is a perfusion sequence where a number of 3D MRI volumes shows the dynamics of a contrast agent inside the kidney or heart at end-diastole. We assume that the volumes are registered. If not, we register consecutive volumes via mutual information maximization. The sequence of n registered volumes is regarded as a single volume where each voxel holds an n-dimensional vector of intensities, or *intensity curve*. Our approach is to segment this volume directly based on voxels intensity curves using a generalization of the graph cut techniques in [7, 2]. These techniques use a spatial Markov model to describe correlations between voxels. Our contribution is in introducing a temporal Markov model to describe the desired dynamic properties of segments. Graph cuts obtain a globally optimal segmentation with the best balance between boundary and regional properties among all segmentations satisfying user placed hard constraints. Flexibility, coherent theoretical formulation, and the possibility of a globally optimal solution are attractive features of our method that gracefully handles even low quality data. We demonstrate results for 3D kidney and 2D heart perfusion sequences.

1 Introduction

Dynamic data show how the intensity of different tissues changes with time. Typical examples of dynamic data are perfusion sequences of heart, brain, kidney, etc. The observed voxel intensity changes as a contrast agent propagates through an organ. Such dynamic contrast-enhanced data are commonly used in medicine to analyze blood circulation and to examine proper functioning of organs. Functional MR of brains is another example of dynamic data where intensity of certain groups of neurons change while a patient performs given tasks. Dynamic data reveal geometric structure of an organ in a fashion distinct from most other types of data in computer vision; intensity dynamics vary in different parts of the organ while no visible motion takes place.

In most applications segmentation is a necessary step to analyze dynamic data. Segmentation is a process in which image elements representing the same

W. Niessen and M. Viergever (Eds.): MICCAI 2001, LNCS 2208, pp. 1058–1066, 2001.

tissue class are grouped together and labeled. Such tissue classification is used for monitoring of volume changes (atrophy, tumor growth), 3D rendering and visualization, measurement of tracer concentration etc.

The list of most commonly used segmentation techniques includes thresholding, region growing, split-and-merge, segmentation by clustering, snakes, level set methods, and others. Multi-dimensional dynamic data presents significant challenges for segmentation techniques. Each volume of a dynamic sequence has to be quickly obtained over a short period of time. As a result, the data sets may have very low resolution with strong "partial voluming" effects. Certain perfusion applications [11, 13] use low doses of contrast-enhancing agent which may further reduce the contrast in each volume. Many segmentation techniques can easily fail by "leaking" through a large number of weak object boundaries.

In this paper we present a segmentation technique that addresses the difficulties of dynamic data. Our main idea is as follows. Note that a dynamic sequence of n volumes with grey-level data describes the same geometric structures. Normally, the sequence is either registered or can be registered. If necessary, we obtain such registration via mutual information maximization between pairs of consecutive volumes. The registered dynamic sequence is treated as a single volume where each voxel has an n-dimensional intensity vector, i.e. an *intensity curve*. Then we directly segment this single volume of intensity curves. We approach this potentially treacherous multi-dimensional segmentation problem via graph cut methods [7, 2] that offer a solid theoretical framework based on posterior energy minimization. These methods model correlation between voxels using spatial Markov models.

The graph cut method in [7] allows us to find a globally optimal binary segmentation in case of the Potts energy that combines certain regional and boundary properties of segments. Exact minimization of an appropriate energy solves many of the problems due to low resolution and weak contrast. The technique works on images or volumes. The method in [2] adds a possibility of intuitive user inputs to impose hard constraints for energy minimization. These hard constraints give an efficient way to correct any imperfections in the results. In practice, segmentation imperfections are almost guaranteed in case of low resolution/contrast dynamic data and any completely automatic technique is very likely to fail in such cases.

The graph based energy minimization techniques in [7, 2] use data gradients to describe boundary properties of segments. The desirable regional properties of segments are summarized by intensity distributions or histograms $\Pr(I|L)$ for all regions (labels L) of interest. There are certain difficulties in applying these methods to a volume of intensity curves that we get with dynamic data. In particular, each voxel has n-dimensional intensity vector rather than a simple gray-scale value. The histograms $\Pr(I|L)$ become very difficult to handle numerically when the dimension of I is larger than 4 or 5. Given that a typical perfusion sequence can easily have n greater than 15 or more, we introduced a temporal Markov model for intensity curves. In fact, this model effectively simplifies the

n-dimensional histograms $\Pr(I|L)$ into a product of n 2-dimensional transitional histograms.

Graph based energy minimization methods are quite flexible, easy to implement, work for N-dimensional volumes, and generate globally optimal segmentation that can have arbitrary topological properties. These methods are used in a large number of applications previously reported in computer vision literature, e.g. [12, 9, 1, 16, 14, 15]. In the context of dynamic medical data, [10] demonstrated that the graph based method in [7] can be used to segment functional MRI of brains. They implicitly assume that each intensity curve is a sequence of independent observations. The regional properties of segments are described by mutual information between intensity curves and the time-line of "tasks" given to a patient. In fact, their assumption of independence strips intensity curves of most of its useful "dynamic" content. Our Markov assumption is much more general and allows a wider scope of problems with dynamic data.

The rest of the paper is structured as follows. In Section 2 we provide background information on energy minimization and graph cut techniques that we use. Details of our segmentation method are described in Section 3. In particular, our temporal Markov model for intensity curves is explained in Section 3.2. In Section 4 we show experimental results for 2D heart and 3D kidney perfusion sequences.

2   Background on Potts Energy Minimization

Greig et. al. [7] was first to discover that powerful graph cut algorithms from combinatorial optimization [6, 4] can be used to minimize certain important energy functions in vision. The energies addressed by Greig et. al. and by later graph based methods (e.g. [9, 1, 2]) can be represented as a posterior energy in a standard MAP-MRF[1] framework that assumes a spatial Markov property for a volume labeling. The typical a posteriori energy function is

$$E(L) = \sum_{p \in \mathcal{P}} D_p(L_p) + \sum_{(p,q) \in \mathcal{N}} V_{p,q}(L_p, L_q), \tag{1}$$

where $L = \{L_p \,|p \in \mathcal{P}\}$ is a labeling (segmentation) of volume $\mathcal{P}$, $D_p(\cdot)$ is a data term, $V_{p,q}$ is an interaction potential, and $\mathcal{N}$ is a set of all pairs of neighboring pixels/voxels. The first and the second terms in (1) represent regional and boundary properties of segments, correspondingly.

Greig et.al. developed a technique based on graph cuts that gives a globally optimal binary segmentation L in case of the Potts model of interaction in (1):

$$V_{p,q}(L_p, L_q) = K_{(p,q)} \cdot T(L_p \neq L_q) \tag{2}$$

where $K_{(p,q)}$ is a discontinuity penalty and $T(\cdot)$ is 1 if condition inside the parenthesis is true and 0 otherwise. This method was generalized in [2] to include

---

[1] Maximum A Posteriori estimation of a Markov Random Field.

additional hard constraints (seeds) that may be placed by a user. The same seeds can also be used as sample points to summarize regional properties of desirable segments. In [2] such properties are represented by intensity histograms $\Pr(I|L)$ for each possible label value L. The underlying MAP-MRF formulation in [7, 2] suggests the data penalty function based on the likelihood $\Pr(I_p|L_p)$ of intensity I_p at pixel p :

$$D_p(L_p) = -\ln \Pr(I_p|L_p). \tag{3}$$

A fast implementation of graph based energy minimization methods in [7, 2] is possible via min-cut/max flow algorithm discussed in [3].

3   Our Technique for Dynamic Data

Here we provide details of our segmentation technique. In Section 3.1 we describe our registration method in case when original dynamic sequence can not be viewed as "perfectly" registered. After registration we treat dynamic sequence of n volumes as a single volume of intensity curves $I_p = \{I_p^t | 1 \le t \le n\}$. We use graph cut techniques in [7, 2] to find a globally optimal segmentation $L = \{L_p | p \in \mathcal{P}\}$ where each voxel label L_p is either "object" or "background". Our energy is given by equations (1), (2), and (3). The data term, D_p in (3), is set by assuming a Markov property for the distributions $\Pr(I_p|L_p)$ of intensity curves. This Markov model is explained in Section 3.2. Our choice of parameters for the Potts interaction penalty, $V_{p,q}$ in (2), is explained in Section 3.3.

3.1   Mutual Information Based Registration

Let $\mathcal{F} = \{F_1, F_2, \ldots, F_n\}$ denote the random field from which one of the volumes, called the *float* volume, is sampled. Similarly, let $\mathcal{R} = \{R_1, R_2, \ldots, R_m\}$ be the random field from which the other volume, called the *reference* volume, is sampled. Assuming that the random variables $\{F_1, F_2, \ldots, F_n\}$ are independently and identically distributed (i.i.d.), let F be the random variable which represents the voxel intensities in the *float* volume. Similarly, assuming that $\{R_1, R_2, \ldots, R_m\}$ are i.i.d, let R be the random variable representing the voxel intensities in the *reference* volume. Then the mutual information $I(F, R)$ between the two random variables F and R with marginal probability density functions $P_F(f)$, $P_R(r)$ and joint probability density function $P_{F,R}(f, r)$ is defined to be $I(F, R) = \sum_{f,r} P_{F,R}(f, r) \, \log_2 \left(\frac{P_{F,R}(f,r)}{P_F(f) \times P_R(r)} \right).$

Let α denote the set of rigid transformation parameters, three translations and three rotations, by which the *float* volume is being transformed. Then the probability density function of the transformed *float* volume, as a function of α is denoted as $P_{F,\alpha}(f)$. Similarly, the joint density function will be denoted by $P_{F,R,\alpha}(f, r)$. The probability density function, $P_{R,\alpha}(r)$, is a function of α because we are evaluating the mutual information on the overlapping region of the two volumes. The various joint and marginal probability density functions are estimated by using the Parzen window method [5]. Using these notations, the mutual information, $I_\alpha(F, R)$, is evaluated as a function of α as

$$I_\alpha(F, R) = \sum_{f,r} P_{F,R,\alpha}(f, r) \log_2 \left(\frac{P_{F,R,\alpha}(f, r)}{P_{F,\alpha}(f) \times P_{R,\alpha}(r)} \right). \tag{4}$$

The optimal set of transformation parameters α, which maximize $I_\alpha(F, R)$, are then found using the stochastic gradient descent approach [8, 17].

3.2   Temporal Markov Model for Intensity Curves

If we have dynamic sequence of n volumes then intensity I_p at voxel p becomes an n-dimensional vector $I_p = (I_p^1, \ldots, I_p^n)$, that we call an intensity curve. Remember that the general n-dimensional distribution $\Pr(I_p|L_p)$ in (3) cannot be handled in practice for n greater than 4 or 5 and additional assumptions should be made about intensity curves I_p.

Assuming independence of $\{I_p^t\}$ for $1 \leq t \leq n$ reduces $\Pr(I_p|L_p)$ to a product of n one dimensional distributions $\Pr(I_p^t|L_p)$ and may look as an attractive solution. In fact, this can significantly oversimplify dynamic information contained in intensity curves I_p. For example, information on "continuity" between I_p^t for consecutive values of t is completely lost if I_p^t are treated as independent. If an object of interest contains several types of tissue with different intensity dynamics then independence based probability model can assign high probability to a random curve that "jumps" between curves representing these different tissues. In such a case probability distribution is not very meaningful.

In our formulation we make a more general assumption that intensity curves I_p have a Markov property. This property means that for any time instance t the conditional distribution of intensity I_p^t given the whole history of intensities $I_p^1, \ldots, I_p^{t-1}$ at the previous time instances, in fact, depends only on the most recent observation I_p^{t-1}, i.e. $\Pr(I_p^t|I_p^1, \ldots, I_p^{t-1}) = \Pr(I_p^t|I_p^{t-1})$. This assumption is quite reasonable in the context of dynamic medical data like perfusion or functional MR. It is easy to show that the Markov property implies that the joint distribution $\Pr(I_p|L_p)$ can be written as a product of two-dimensional distributions

$$\Pr(I_p|L_p) = \Pr(I_p^1|L_p) \cdot \prod_{t=2}^{n} \Pr(I_p^t|I_p^{t-1}, L_p). \tag{5}$$

From computational point of view, two dimensional histograms $\Pr(I_p^t|I_p^{t-1}, L_p)$ are quite manageable. We use equation (5) to describe desirable "dynamical" properties of segments summarized in the data term (3) of energy (1).

3.3   Setting Up the Potts Interactions

It remains to explain our choice of parameters for the Potts interaction term (2) of energy (1). We can choose the discontinuity penalty $K_{(p,q)}$ to vary over different pairs of neighboring voxels. The goal is to encourage segmentation discontinuities where image gradient forces are large and to discourage discontinuities inside regions with low texture. One typical example of such discontinuity penalty is used in a number of graph based techniques in vision

$$K_{(p,q)} = \lambda \cdot \exp\left(-\frac{||I_p - I_q||^2}{\sigma^2}\right).$$

The fact that I_p is an n-dimensional vector makes one interpret $||\cdot||$ as a vector norm, e.g. Euclidean norm.

In general, we can have $K_{(p,q)} \neq K_{(q,p)}$. In the context of gray-scale volume segmentation, [2] showed that this can help to differentiate between the boundary from "bright" to "dark" and the boundary from "dark" to "bright". If the properties of the object-to-background boundary are known this may help to draw the boundary in the right place. For multi-dimensional intensity curves I_p we can use asymmetrical function

$$K_{(p,q)} = \beta \cdot (C(I_p) - C(I_q)) + \lambda \cdot \exp\left(-\frac{||I_p - I_q||^2}{\sigma^2}\right).$$

The scalar function $C(\cdot)$ can represent, for example, a "center of mass" of the corresponding curve, or its average intensity, or any other property of intensity curve that can characterize the desirable properties of the object-to-background segmentation boundary.

4   Experimental Results

We have two choices when estimating the histograms/distributions (5) for object and background intensity dynamics. We can use some historic histograms that were "learned" from intensity curves in the previous segmentation/classification experiments. In this case the initial segmentation can be computed automatically and additional user placed seeds (hard constraints) would be needed only to correct imperfections, if any. Such a version can be created for a specific application where the data does not vary too much.

Here we present results for a more flexible alternative approach that can be used to segment a variety of data sets. A user places seeds even for initial segmentation. These seeds indicate a few voxels that he is certain to be object (red seeds) or background (blue seeds). Similar to [2] we make a dual use of these seeds. First, they work as hard constraints for energy minimization. Second, they give an "expert" sample of intensity curves for object and background. These samples are used to set the histograms in equation (5). Then, an optimal segmentation can be computed. Any imperfections can be still efficiently removed by placing additional correcting seeds (hard constraints). Normally, the results are robust and do not depend on exact positioning of seeds. Below we show some of the results for 2D heart and 3D kidney perfusion data sequences.

In Figure 1(a-d) we show a 2D segmentation example for a single slice of perfusion data of heart at end-diastole. The sequence of 35 images was well

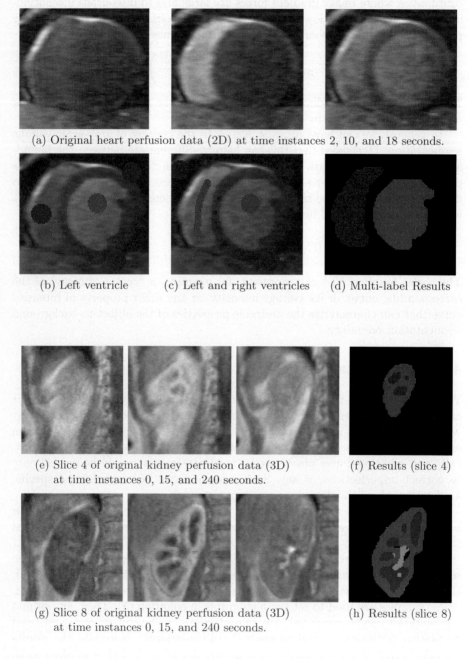

(a) Original heart perfusion data (2D) at time instances 2, 10, and 18 seconds.

(b) Left ventricle   (c) Left and right ventricles   (d) Multi-label Results

(e) Slice 4 of original kidney perfusion data (3D)   (f) Results (slice 4)
    at time instances 0, 15, and 240 seconds.

(g) Slice 8 of original kidney perfusion data (3D)   (h) Results (slice 8)
    at time instances 0, 15, and 240 seconds.

Fig. 1. 2D (heart) and 3D (kidney) examples of dynamic data segmentation.

registered and MI based registration (Section 3.1) was not necessary. In separate experiments we segment the left ventricle alone (b) and both the left and the right ventricles together (c). The segmentation results in (b) and (c) are shown by highlighting the object and background segments with, correspondingly, red and blue colors. Note that multi-label segmentation is possible if the method is used iteratively. An additional binary segmentation can separate the left and the right ventricles starting from the results in (c). The resulting multi-label (red, blue, black) segmentation is shown in (d). All results are obtain in under 10 seconds including time that it takes a user to place seeds (Pentium III, 333MHz).

In Figure 1(e-h) we show an example of kidney perfusion data (a sequence of 18 volumes of size $100 \times 100 \times 17$). The original sequence requires registration. The resolution in each volume is $1 \times 1 \times 3.6$ mm and there are severe defects due to partial voluming. The goal is to segment the cortex, the medulla, and the collecting system of the kidney. Given nontrivial topological properties of the tissues and extremely poor data quality (to date, the best possible) no automatic segmentation seems possible and the use of an interactive technique looks very appropriate.

Registration using MI maximization takes about 3-4 minutes. Then we obtain a multi-label segmentation in three iterations. First, the whole kidney is separated from the background. Then we separate the medulla versus the cortex and the collecting system. The last step is to cut the collecting system from the cortex. Each iteration takes around one minute (50% user input and 50% computation). The seeds were placed in two or three (out of 17) slices in the volume. In (f) and (h) of Figure 1 we show 3D segmentation results. We use "red" for cortex, "blue" for medulla, "green" for collecting system, and "black" for background.

References

[1] Y. Boykov, O. Veksler, and R. Zabih. Markov random fields with efficient approximations. In *IEEE Conference on Computer Vision and Pattern Recognition*, pages 648–655, 1998.

[2] Yuri Boykov and Marie-Pierre Jolly. *Interactive graph cuts* for optimal boundary & region segmentation of objects in N-D images. In *International Conference on Computer Vision*, July 2001.

[3] Yuri Boykov and Vladimir Kolmogorov. An experimental comparison of min-cut/max-flow algorithms for energy minimization in vision. In *3rd. Intnl. Workshop on Energy Minimization Methods in Computer Vision and Pattern Recognition (EMMCVPR)*. Springer-Verlag, September 2001.

[4] William J. Cook, William H. Cunningham, William R. Pulleyblank, and Alexander Schrijver. *Combinatorial Optimization*. John Wiley & Sons, 1998.

[5] R. O. Duda and P. E. Hart. *Pattern Classification and Scene Analysis*. John Wiley & Sons, 1973.

[6] L. Ford and D. Fulkerson. *Flows in Networks*. Princeton University Press, 1962.

[7] D. Greig, B. Porteous, and A. Seheult. Exact maximum a posteriori estimation for binary images. *Journal of the Royal Statistical Society, Series B*, 51(2):271–279, 1989.

[8] S. Haykin. *Neural Networks: A Comprehensive Foundation.* Macmillan College Publishing, 1994.

[9] H. Ishikawa and D. Geiger. Segmentation by grouping junctions. In *IEEE Conference on Computer Vision and Pattern Recognition*, pages 125–131, 1998.

[10] Junmo Kim, John W. Fisher III, Andy Tsai, Cindy Wible, Alan S. Willsky, and William M. Wells III. Incorporating spatial priors into an information theoretic approach for fMRI data analysis. In *Medical Image Computing and Computer-Assisted Intervention (MICCAI)*, pages 62–71, 2000.

[11] V.S. Lee, H. Rusinek, G. Johnson, N. Rofsky, G.A. Krinsky, and J.C. Weinreb. Ultra-low dose Gadolinium-DTPA MR renography for the diagnosis of renovascular disease. *Radiology*, 2001, in press.

[12] Sebastien Roy and Ingemar Cox. A maximum-flow formulation of the n-camera stereo correspondence problem. In *IEEE Proc. of Int. Conference on Computer Vision*, pages 492–499, 1998.

[13] H. Rusinek, V.S. Lee, and G. Johnson. Optimal dose of Gd-DTPA for dynamic MR studies. *Magnetic Resonance in Medicine*, 2001, in press.

[14] Dan Snow, Paul Viola, and Ramin Zabih. Exact voxel occupancy with graph cuts. In *IEEE Conference on Computer Vision and Pattern Recognition*, volume 1, pages 345–352, 2000.

[15] B. Thirion, B. Bascle, V. Ramesh, and N. Navab. Fusion of color, shading and boundary information for factory pipe segmentation. In *IEEE Conference on Computer Vision and Pattern Recognition*, volume 2, pages 349–356, 2000.

[16] Olga Veksler. Image segmentation by nested cuts. In *IEEE Conference on Computer Vision and Pattern Recognition*, volume 1, pages 339–344, 2000.

[17] P. Viola and W. M. Wells. Alignment by maximization of mutual information. In *International Conference on Computer Vision*, pages 16–23, 1995.

Unsupervised and Adaptive Segmentation of Multispectral 3D Magnetic Resonance Images of Human Brain: A Generic Approach

Chahin Pachai[1,3], Yue Min Zhu[1], Charles R.G. Guttmann[3], Ron Kikinis[3], Ferenc A. Jolesz[3], Gérard Gimenez[1], Jean-Claude Froment[2], Christian Confavreux[2], and Simon K. Warfield[3]

[1] CREATIS, CNRS Research Unit UMR 5515, INSA de Lyon, France
{pachai, zhu, gimenez}@creatis.insa-lyon.fr

[2] Departments of Neurology and Radiology-MRI, Hôpital Neurologique et Neurochirurgical, Pierre Wertheimer, Lyon, France
{christian.confavreux, jean-claude.froment}@chu-lyon.fr

[3] Surgical Planning Laboratory, Department of Radiology-MRI, Brigham and Women's Hospital, Harvard Medical School, Boston, MA, USA
{guttmann, kikinis, jolesz, warfield}bwh.harvard.edu

Abstract. A generic algorithm is presented for the segmentation of three-dimensional multispectral magnetic resonance images. The algorithm is unsupervised and adaptive, does not require initialization, classifies the data in any number of tissue classes and suggests an optimal number of classes. It uses a statistical model including Bayesian distributions for brain tissues intensities and Gibbs Random Fields (GRF)-based spatial contiguity constraints. The classification is unsupervised, that is to say the intensity-based signatures of brain tissues and the spatial hyperparameters of the underlying GRF are derived from the data. Adaptivity is achieved through the variation of the size of the neighborhoods used for the estimation of the intensity characteristics. This allows slow variations of signal intensity in space to account for MRI intensity nonuniformity. Segmentation results with proton density, T2 and T1-weighted data are provided. The algorithm can be used as an independent segmentation module within a brain MRI data processing pipeline.

1. Introduction

The aim of this paper is to describe a generic algorithm for unsupervised segmentation of brain MR images, from which one could derive practical solutions to a variety of applications such as quantification and visualization of white matter (WM), gray matter (GM), cerebrospinal fluid (CSF) and pathological structures such as multiple sclerosis (MS) lesions and tumors. The goal of the present work is to provide a unique framework for the processing of brain data, a context in which several parameters may change from one application to the other. These parameters are the number of MRI input channels, their spatial resolutions, the number of brain tissues to be segmented, and the size of the smallest features to be segmented. The

W. Niessen and M. Viergever (Eds.): MICCAI 2001, LNCS 2208, pp. 1067–1074, 2001.

proposed framework supports multichannel MRI input, adaptive and unsupervised 3D segmentation based on Gibbs-Markov random fields (GRF-MRF). It accounts for the piecewise contiguity of brain regions (WM, GM) and, in a certain amount, for intensity nonuniformity without being dependent upon any specific initialization.

Markov Random Field (MRF) models were used with brain MR images in an important number of works to add spatial smoothness into the process of image segmentation [1-9]. These works reported that adding an explicit, local and low-level tissue-contiguity model within the segmentation framework could consistently improve the quality of the segmentation, especially in regions with low signal to noise ratio or corrupted by a strong white (salt and pepper) noise. However, these works did not identically address all the important issues. These issues are parameter estimation, cluster validation, problem dimensionality (MRI input channels, 2D or 3D implementation), the use of mixture models for partial volume effect correction, and whether the model accounts for intensity nonuniformity. In this contribution, we particularly stress on the integration of an MRF model within a completely unsupervised segmentation scheme. We briefly describe the statistical model, the resulting segmentation algorithm, the implementation issues and give visual results.

2.   Segmentation Model

As described by Derin and Elliott in [10] and the related works [11-14] we defined a discrete 3D random field over a finite lattice of voxels and introduced a neighborhood system on it. A second order neighborhood system was used. The clique definition was similar to the one described by Derin *et al*. We did not consider single site cliques because we did not have prior information regarding the percentage of voxels in each region type (the missing prior information on the distribution of voxels in each tissue class could be obtained from a probabilistic atlas of human brain). This class of Gibbs distributions is used to characterize the spatial clustering of voxels into regions. It introduces prior spatial information regarding the size, the shape and the orientation of the regions to be segmented. The spatial smoothness constraint accounts for the natural contiguity of voxels belonging to the same tissue type, say WM, GM or CSF. If a voxel is of a certain tissue type, the neighboring voxels should also have a high probability of being of the same tissue type.

The segmentation vector or the scene was considered as a discrete random variable. This variable can be associated with a Gibbs Random Field defined on the lattice and with respect to the neighborhood system under conditions defined in [10]. The digital MRI data or the observation can be considered as a realization from a random field. At each voxel, the observation is a multidimensional vector, each component of which represents an MRI channel. The segmentation process consists of finding the scene realization (or segmentation), which produced the observation. We used a maximum a posteriori (MAP) criterion to estimate the realization, which maximized the a posteriori distribution. Using Bayes' theorem, the posterior probability was written as the sum of two contributions: the data term and the spatial term. The data term is the model providing a measurement given a scene realization (or segmentation) and the spatial term is the prior model of the spatial interaction between adjacent voxels. Both terms have intuitive meanings: the Gibbs term gives a prize for smoothness and the data term matches the fitted class means to the intensity.

At each voxel site, the observation vector can be modeled as the sum of the mean intensity of tissue class at that voxel and an additive, tissue (class) dependent, space variant, zero mean, Gaussian white noise. The diagonal elements of the associated covariance matrix (positive-definite symmetric) are the intensity variances and the off-diagonal elements are the correlation coefficients of the different input images. At each voxel site, the probability of observing an intensity given the tissue class label can be modeled with a multidimensional Gaussian function. To determine the data model (or the measurement model), tissue class parameters (means and covariances matrices) representing an intensity-based signature of the current segmentation were computed. The optimal segmentation was obtained by maximizing the posterior probability. Instead of finding the global minimum of this function, which is computationally prohibitive, we used Besag's Iterated Conditional Mode (ICM) to separate the segmentation process into two steps [15-16].

First, segmentation by maximization of the posterior probability: given the current estimates of the spatial and data models, a new segmentation is obtained at each voxel site, by minimizing the conditional density of equation 1. This new segmentation only depends on the intensity estimates and the values of the neighboring voxels.

$$F_s\left(x_s|y_s, x_{s'}, s' \in \eta_s\right)=$$
$$\sum_{c \in C} V_c\left(x_s|\eta_s\right) + \frac{1}{2}\left\{\ln\left(\det\left(\Sigma_{x_s}\right)\right) + \left(y_s - \mu_{x_s}\right)^T \Sigma_{x_s}^{-1}\left(y_s - \mu_{x_s}\right)\right\} \qquad (1)$$

where x_s is the segmentation, y_s the observation (multispectral MRI) at voxel site s, η_s the neighborhood system centered at s, c a clique belonging to clique ensemble C, V_c the potentiel associated with clique type c, $(\mu_{x_s}, \Sigma_{x_s})$ class dependent and spatially varying intensity functions (means and covariance matrices, respectively)

Second, estimation of the statistical model: given the current segmentation, new estimates of the spatial term and the data term are to be calculated. The data model is estimated by computing at each voxel site and for all tissue classes, means and covariance matrices are estimated locally using a neighborhood [17].

To estimate the hyperparameters of the prior model, Besag's Maximum Pseudo-Likelihood (MPL), the product of local conditional probabilities, was used [15-16], [6], [11]. The estimate of the current spatial model was obtained by maximizing the MPL product over all voxels. For a given segmentation, the pseudo-likelihood only depends on the current segmentation and the neighborhood system. An adaptive simulated annealing (SA) algorithm was used to minimize this function and find the hyperparameters. SA is a stochastic relaxation algorithm suitable to search the global minimum of a non convex function with many local minima.

The ICM algorithm is a partial optimal solution to the optimization problem and converges to a local minimum of the energy function. Therefore, the initialization issue has a major importance in the overall success of the segmentation. In order to initialize the algorithm, a one-class model was adopted. For a given tissue class number, all the clusters were split, one at a time, and the split which maximized the posterior probability was kept as the best segmentation. To increment the number of tissue classes, we split each tissue class in two, one at a time, to obtain different segmentations [6]. For splitting a given tissue class in two, we first split a given tissue class independently of the remaining voxels and then, using the resulting classification, we classified the data using a K-Means algorithm. This class-dependent initialization of the K-Means algorithm was repeated for all the current classes, so that each one initiated a different segmentation. The splitting algorithm is based on an initial division of a given cluster in two, following the principal component of the corresponding (multichannel) intensity distribution. The initial perturbation initiates a 2-Means algorithm (K-Means with 2 classes). The resulting classification initializes a global K-Means algorithm within the ICM cycle.

In order to find the optimal number of regions that gives the best fit (cluster validation issues), information criteria such as minimum description length [18], Akaike information criterion [19] or MAP criteria [6], [11] can be used. We considered a MAP criterion: the configuration that leads to the best segmentation is also the one which maximizes the MAP value over all the possibilities. Hence, cluster validation can be carried out along with the class splitting process.

3.   Implementation Issues

The signal intensity of a given brain structure may exhibit important variations due to normal and pathological intra-tissue variations or the MRI system. These variations are slowly varying in space. The statistical model should accordingly allow the tissue classes to have slowly varying intensity functions. For this purpose, local estimates of means and covariance matrices at all voxel sites were computed over a neighborhood around each voxel. The size of this neighborhood is an important parameter for a good appreciation of intensity variations within a tissue class. To account for slowly varying (low frequency) phenomena, large parts of brain should be used for computing the estimations while accurate segmentation at the interfaces of tissue classes requires local estimates of intensity functions [17].

Local measures of means and covariance matrices for all tissue classes make the segmentation algorithm adaptive. In order to reduce the computation time, estimates were only calculated on a grid of points and the remaining values were computed using interpolation. The initial size of the neighborhood should be approximately equivalent to the size of the head and be progressively reduced, until a minimum size is reached. Since MRI data sets may have different resolutions, the size of the neighborhood should take into account this anisotropy.

For a given tissue class, the robustness of the estimations of its intensity functions at a given voxel site increases as the number of voxels with the same label and available in the neighborhood around that voxel grows. Estimates for a given class are then supposed valid if there are more than a minimal number of voxels with the same label in the neighborhood.

The spatial prior model based on a homogeneous and isotropic GRF has a major importance in regularizing the interfaces between different tissue classes. Increasing the value of the hyperparameters favors the clustering of voxels and imposes a stronger smoothness constraint. The relative difference between the data term and the Gibbs term has an impact both at the voxel level, for the computation of a new segmentation within the ICM and at the global level, where the MAP values are used to split the existing classes. We used an adaptive simulated annealing algorithm (ASA) implemented by Lester Ingber [20] to minimize Besag's maximum pseudo-likelihood function. Even if estimating the hyperparameters by SA is time consuming, our experiments showed that changes in the values of hyperparameters might influence the outcome of the segmentation. Setting the hyperparameters to constant values may cause oversmoothing and undersmooting.

4. Result

Figure 1 shows the result of the segmentation of a double channel, PD and T2-weighted data set. WM, GM and CSF are segmented and we further processed the data set to remove features which did not belong to the intracranial cavity. Figure 2 shows 3D reconstructions of WM, GM and CSF from a segmented millimetric T1-weighted data set. Figure 3 shows the result of the segmentation of a millimetric T1-weighted data set (one axial slice among 150). Successive segmentations are obtained as intermediary results. They are shown for 2, 3, 4 and 5 tissue classes. We also provide the segmentation prior to the iterations of the ICM algorithm. The resulting segmented images confirm the necessity of introducing spatial smoothness constraints through Gibbs prior. We can also notice the improvement of the overall segmentation result as the number of tissue classes increases. The best visual result was obtained with 5 tissue classes. This number was also suggested by the MAP stop criterion (cluster validation).

5. Discussion and Conclusion

The class of Gibbs distributions, used as a spatial prior, was an effective way to account for the piecewise contiguity of brain tissues. Data resolution, the number of tissue classes and the number of iterations within the ICM algorithm influenced the hyperparameter values. Our experiments confirmed that using multispectral MRI was an efficient way for more robust tissue identification. The adaptivity of the segmentation algorithm through the variation of the neighborhood size in estimating intensity functions allows slow intra-tissue variations of class intensities. In a certain amount, this ability accounts for intensity nonuniformity and normal or pathological intra-tissue intensity variations. Since the segmentation algorithm does not need to be initialized, any set of registered (if necessary) MRI channels can be used as input. The MAP-based cluster validation criterion provides a good indication for the best choice of the number of tissue classes to be segmented. The regularization model consistently and automatically improves the quality of the underlying segmentation. Reproducible measures and high quality visualization can be carried out using different MRI input configurations.

The implementation of this approach was useful to investigate the advantages and the limits of a completely unsupervised segmentation to reach both accuracy and reproducibility. The segmentation algorithm can be improved by incorporating a global model accounting for intensity nonuniformity. The low-level Markovian regularization process may be insufficient to successfully reconstruct strongly biased data. Using additional spatial prior from a probabilistic brain atlas after an atlas-to-patient elastic matching step can also lead to more robust classification by assigning the GRF single site clique potentiels to relevant values derived from the atlas.

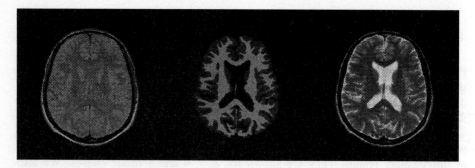

Fig. 1. Segmentation of double channel proton density (left) and T2-weighted (right) MRI. The intracranial cavity (WM, GM and CSF) is extracted from segmented data (middle).

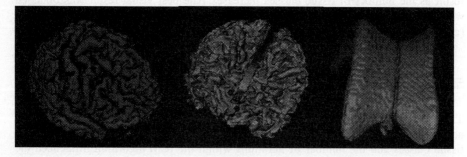

Fig. 2. 3D reconstruction of GM, WM and CSF from millimetric T1-weighted segmented data

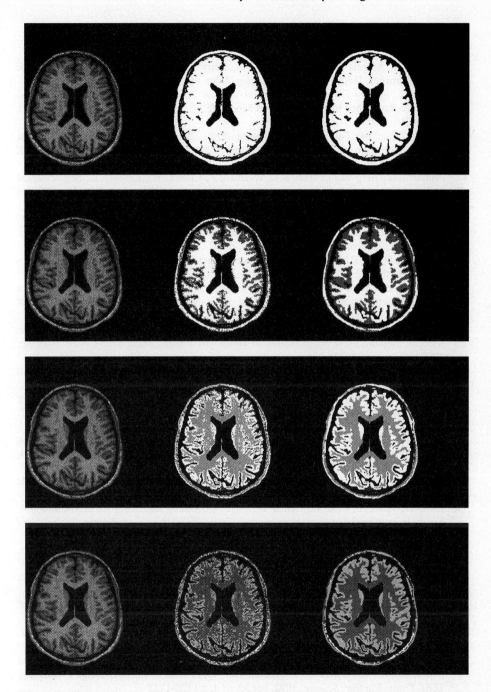

Fig. 3. Segmentation of single channel T1-weighted MRI in 2, 3, 4 and 5 tissue classes (top-down) : original image (left), segmentation without (middle column) and with (right column) MRF spatial regularization

References

1. Hurn M.A., Mardia K.V., Hainsworth T.J., Berry E., Bayesian Fused Classification of Medical Images, *IEEE Trans. Med. Imaging*, 1996, vol 15, n° 6, p 850-858
2. Choi H.S., Haynor D.R., Kim Y., Partial Volume Tissue Classification of Multichannel Magnetic Resonance Images – A Mixel Model, *IEEE Trans. Med. Imaging*, 1991, vol 10, n° 3, p 395-407
3. Liang Z.R., MacFall J.R., Harrington D.P., Parameter estimation and tissue segmentation from multispectral MR images, *IEEE Trans. Med. Imaging*, 1994, vol. 13, no. 3, p 441-449
4. Ashton E.A., Berg M.J., Parker K.J., Weisberg J., Chen C.W., Ketonen L., Segmentation and feature extraction techniques, with applications to MRI head studies, *Magn Reson Med*, 1995, vol 33, n° 5, p 670-677
5. Rajapakse J.C., DeCarli C., McLaughlin A., Giedd J.N., Krain A.L., Hamburger S.D., Rapoport J.L., Cerebral Magnetic Resonance Image Segmentation Using Data Fusion, *J. Comput. Assist. Tomogr.*, 1996, vol 20, n°2, p 207-218
6. Fwu J.K., Djuric P.M., Unsupervised Vector Image Segmentation by a Tree Structure - ICM Algorithm, *IEEE Trans. Med. Imaging*, 1996, vol 15, n° 6, p 871-880
7. Chang M.M., Sezan M.I., Tekalp A.M., Berg M.J, Bayesian segmentation of multislice brain magnetic resonance imaging using three-dimensional Gibbsian priors, *Optical Engineering*, 1996, vol 35, n° 11, p 97-106
8. Held K., Rota Kops E., Krause B. J., Wells W. M., Kikinis R., Müller-Gärtner H.-W., Markov Random Field Segmentation of Brain MR Images, *IEEE Trans. Med. Imaging*, 1997, vol 16, n° 6, p 878-886
9. Kapur T., Grimson W.E.L., Wells W.M., Kikinis R., Segmentation of Brain Tissue from Magnetic Resonance Images. *Medical Image Analysis.*, 1996, vol 1, p 109-127
10. Derin H., Elliott H., Modeling and Segmentation of Noisy and Textured Images Using Gibbs Random Fields, IEEE Trans. on Pattern Analysis and Machine Intelligence, 1987, vol 9, n° 1, p 39-55
11. Won C.-S, Derin H., Unsupervised Segmentation of Noisy and Textured Images Using Markov Random Fields, *Computer Vision Graphics and Image Processing*, 1992, vol 54, n° 4, p 308-328
12. Derin H., Cole W.S., Segmentation of textured images using Gibbs random fields *Computer Vision, Graphics, and Image Processing*, 1986, vol 35, p 72-98
13. Derin H., Elliot H., Cristi R., Geman D., Bayes smoothing algorithms for segmentation of binary images modeled by markov random fields, *IEEE Trans. on Pattern Analysis and Machine Intelligence*, 1984, vol 6, n° 6, p 707-720
14. Lakshmanan S., Derin H., Valid parameter space for 2-D Gaussian Markov random fields, *IEEE Trans. Information Theory*, 1993, vol 39, p 703-709
15. Besag J., Spatial interaction and the statistical analysis of lattice systems, *J. R. Statist. Soc. B.*, 1974, vol 2, p 192-236
16. Besag J., On the statistial analysis of dirty pictures, *J. R. Statist. Soc. B.*, 1986, vol 48, n° 3, p 259-302
17. Pappas T.N., An Adaptative Clustering Algorithm for Image Segmentation, *IEEE Trans. Sig. Processing*, 1992, vol 40, n° 4, p 901-913
18. Liang Z., Jaszczak R.J., Coleman R.E., Parameter Estimation of Finite Mixtures Using the EM Algorithm and Information Criteria with Application to Medical Image Processing, *IEEE Trans. Nuclear. Science*, 1992, vol 39, n° 4, p 1126-1133
19. Akaike H., A new look at the statistical model identification, *IEEE Trans. Automat. Contr.*, 1974, vol. 19, p 716-723
20. Ingber L., Adaptive simulated annealing (ASA): Lessons learned, *Control and Cybernetics*, 1996, vol 25, p 33-54, URL : http://www.ingber.com/

Image Guided Radiotherapy of the Prostate

David Jaffray[1], Marcel van Herk[2], Joos Lebesque[2], and Alvaro Martinez[1]

[1] William Beaumont Hospital, Royal Oak, MI USA
djaffray@beaumont.edu
[2] Radiotherapy Department, The Netherlands Cancer Institute, Amsterdam, The Netherlands
portal@nki.nl

Abstract. This paper describes the prototype of an integrated system for cone-beam CT guided radiotherapy of prostate cancer. The system works by acquiring a 3D image set just prior to treatment delivery. This image set is matched automatically with bones and prostate defined in the planning CT to determine the required couch translation and to determine a best fitting treatment plan which is subsequently delivered. Because of the improved localization of the prostate on the treatment machine, potentially smaller safety margins can be applied and a higher dose can be delivered leading to a higher cure rate without increasing damage to healthy tissues.

1 Introduction

External beam radiotherapy aims at killing a tumor with high-energy photons, while sparing as much as possible surrounding healthy tissues. In general, the treatment is planned on CT and/or MR images, and it is delivered in daily fractions over a period of several weeks. To focus the radiation on the required spot, individually shaped beams are delivered from multiple directions by a small linear accelerator mounted in a rotating gantry. A complicating factor is the limited precision of tumor localization on the treatment machine, due to tumor delineation inaccuracies, movement of the tumor within the body and variations in daily positioning of the patient. For this reason, a safety margin must be applied, i.e., a larger volume is treated than the actual tumor to compensate for geometric inaccuracies [e.g., 11]. As the precision increases, the safety margin can be reduced and a higher dose can be given to the target without unacceptable damage to surrounding healthy tissues.

Several methods have been investigated to improve the precision of prostate irradiation. Electronic portal imaging, imaging the patient with the treatment beam, has been shown successful in measuring and reducing the errors in repositioning of the bony anatomy [e.g., 1, 3]. More recently, ultrasound imaging has been applied to improve the localization of the prostate on the treatment machine [e.g., 8]. Another localization approach that has been explored is X-ray radiography of metal markers implanted into the prostate [7] (projected radiography has insufficient contrast to visualize the prostate directly). The aim of this project is to develop an integrated delivery system that performs three-dimensional localization of the prostate on the treatment machine just prior to treatment delivery. The system has the following re-

W. Niessen and M. Viergever (Eds.): MICCAI 2001, LNCS 2208, pp. 1075-1080, 2001.

1076   D. Jaffray et al.

quirements. The technique must not be invasive (no markers) and must not require physical contact with the patient to avoid deformation of soft tissues in the pelvis (this happens with ultrasound localization). Furthermore the localization, analysis and treatment process should be as fast as possible to maintain an acceptable patient throughput and in particular to reduce the probability of patient or tumor movement in the time interval between imaging and treatment.

2 Material and Methods

A cone beam CT scan will be acquired on the treatment machine for each treatment fraction (Fig. 1). This 3D CT data set is analyzed automatically to localize the prostate and the treatment prescription is adapted to match the actual position and orientation of the prostate. Finally, the treatment is delivered.

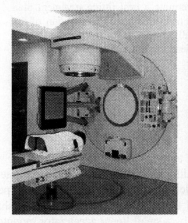 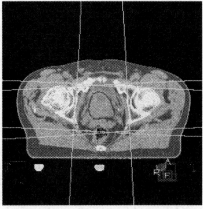

Figure 1. (a) Prototype cone beam CT scanner mounted on the gantry of a commercial medical linear accelerator. A diagnostic X-ray tube (right) and a flat panel imager (left) have been added. (b) Conventional treatment planning is based on delineation of the target in 3D. Multiple beams are planned that encompass the target with a safety margin for geometrical errors.

Image acquisition. The cornerstone of the system is a kilovoltage cone-beam CT system that is integrated on the gantry of an Elekta SL-20 linear accelerator [4]. The radiation source of the system is a diagnostic x-ray tube, with its beam axis perpendicular to the treatment beam. Opposite the tube is a 41 x 41 cm flat panel imaging device (consisting of a fluorescent screen coupled to an 1024x1024 pixel amorphous silicon photodiode array on a glass substrate), mounted at 160 cm from the isocenter. To obtain sufficient field of view to image the whole pelvis, the detector will be offset by 20 cm, and half field images are made over 360 degrees of rotation in a single gantry rotation.

A three-dimensional image of the patient is obtained by cone beam reconstruction using the Feldkamp algorithm for limited cone reconstruction [2]. Because of the retractable construction of the imaging system, there is a substantial flex of the components as function of gantry rotation. This flex is reproducible and has been taken into account in the reconstruction algorithm to obtain a high image quality [5].

Image analysis. CT-based treatment planning in a routine clinical setting typically takes several hours per patient (Fig. 1b). On-line application, i.e., while the patient is on the treatment table, requires considerable acceleration of this process. The model that will be applied is based on the observation that the movement of the prostate relative to the pelvis can be well described by a rotation and translation, where most rotation occurs around the left-right axis of the patient [10]. The proposed image analysis algorithm first registers the segmented bony anatomy of the on-line CT scan with a planning CT scan using a chamfer matching algorithm [9]. Then the displacement of the prostate relative to the pelvis is measured using a registration algorithm similar to the one developed by Woods et al [13]. For this purpose, prostate contours are manually defined in the planning CT, which is also part of planning for conventional radiotherapy. The planned prostate shape is then aligned to the on-line CT by minimization of the variance of the gray values of the on-line CT under the predefined prostate shape. The minimum corresponds with the rotation and translation of the prostate from its position in the initial treatment plan.

Treatment planning, delivery and verification. Existing treatment planning technology can be employed in a novel manner to minimize the on-line planning time by identifying the most probable degrees of prostate motion and preparing a set of plans to accommodate this motion. First, the patient couch is translated to account for translation of bone and prostate relative to the treatment room. Then a best fitting treatment plan is selected from the set of pre-defined treatment plans to account for prostate rotation.

The selected treatment plan will be delivered by means of a step-and-shoot intensity delivery technique using 5 beam angles and about 20 treatment segments. The beam shaping occurs by means of a standard multi-leaf collimator.

During treatment, regular verification such as electronic portal imaging and in-vivo dosimetry will be performed. In addition, cone beam acquisition is repeated after treatment delivery. Off-line re-planning based on the pre- and post-treatment CT images will be performed to determine the cumulative radiation dose delivered to prostate and critical structures. For this purpose, the prostate shape and position will be interpolated between the pre- and post-treatment scans. Because the off-line planning is performed under less time pressure, the progress of the treatment will be more carefully monitored compared to the on-line procedure. In addition, the safety is increased because possible deficiencies in each fraction can be rectified on later fractions.

3 Results

Image acquisition. Prototypes of the hardware and software of the system have been constructed. Cone-beam CT of anthropomorphic phantoms has been acquired on the treatment machine, with an acquisition time of 3 minutes (Fig. 2), but a reconstruction time of hours. The final system will acquire a scan in 1 minute and will use a hardware accelerated reconstruction system. With flex calibration, the image quality of the cone beam CT data is similar to a diagnostic CT scan.

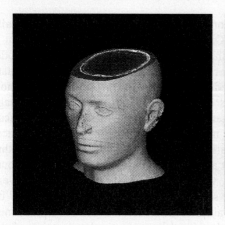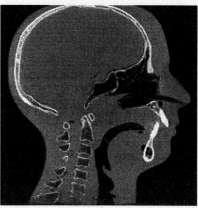

Figure 2. Cone-beam reconstruction of a head phantom acquired with the cone beam CT scanner of Fig. 1. The image was made with 320 projections at 120 kVp and 200 mAs in 180 s. (a) Surface rendering with axial slice. (b) Sagittal cut. The image quality is similar to a diagnostic CT scan.

Image analysis. The results of the proposed algorithm for on-line prostate localization are shown in Figs. 3a-d. In the baseline CT, the pelvic bone and the prostate are pre-defined. On-line matching of the planning CT with the proposed cone-beam CT (both with calibrated isocenter positions) on the pelvic bone determines the setup error (translation and rotation) of the bony anatomy. Figs. 3a and b represent on-line CTs and have been taken from an organ motion study, matched in this way to the planning CT. The motion of the prostate is apparent because the prostate contours (dotted white line), which were delineated in the planning CT, do not fit the prostate in these 'on-line' images. The motion of the prostate relative to the bony anatomy is quantified by translating and rotating the prostate contours until they cover a homogeneous area, i.e., an area with minimal standard deviation of gray values (Figs 3b and c). The flow chart in Fig. 3e illustrates the algorithm. The gray boxes correspond to a-priori available information. Because the bone matching can be performed accurately on fairly low resolution CT and the prostate matching only requires a small part of the cone-beam CT volume, the complete image analysis can be performed in less than 10 s on a 700 MHz PC.

For this particular problem, this procedure corresponds closely with that of manual delineation. It is important to note that in the case of CT, such algorithms do not necessarily localize the prostate, but rather the contrasting structure defined in the 3D template. Although this is the best result that can be obtained using CT data, any systematic deviations between the actual prostate location (defined best by MR) and the CT-defined prostate must be considered separately [6, 11].

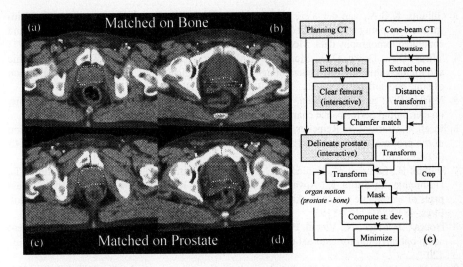

Figure 3. Automated localization of the prostate. (a,b) Reference prostate contour overlaid on the "on-line" CT based on registration to bony anatomy. This transformation is adjusted using Woods' algorithm to locate the prostate in the on-line set (c,d). Much improved coverage of the prostate is thus achieved. (e) Flow-chart summary of the algorithm (priors are gray).

4 Discussion and Conclusions

We implemented a system for cone beam CT on a clinical accelerator. The phantom tests show excellent spatial resolution and contrast to noise performance. The image quality is adequate to resolve tumors visible on diagnostic CT. A software system has been developed for image reconstruction and processing. The image analysis is very fast, but the cone beam CT reconstruction is at present prohibitively slow (hours). In the final system, a specialized hardware accelerator will be applied to reduce the reconstruction time to 1 minute. One problem that needs to be addressed in more detail is the mobility of the patient and his organs on the treatment machine in the time between image acquisition and delivery. We will perform repeat MRI studies on volunteers and patients to determine the time dependent statistics of prostate movement. The results will determine the amount of margin reduction that can safely be achieved with this approach.

References

1. Bel, A., van Herk, M., Bartelink, H., Lebesque, J.V.: A verification procedure to improve patient set-up accuracy using portal images. Radiother. Oncol. 29 (1993) 253-260
2. Feldkamp, L.A., Davis, L.C. and Kress, J.W.: Practical cone-beam algorithm. J. Opt. Soc. Am. A. 1 (1984) 612-619

3. Gilhuijs, K.G.A., van der Ven, P.J.H. and van Herk, M.: Automatic three-dimensional in-spection of patient setup in radiation therapy using portal images, simulator images, and computed tomography data. Med. Phys. 23 (1996) 389-399
4. Jaffray, D.A., Drake, D.G., Moreau, M., Martinez, A.A., and Wong, J.W.: A radiographic and tomographic imaging system integrated into a medical linear accelerator for localization of bone and soft-tissue targets. Int. J. Radiat. Oncol. Biol. Phys. 45 (1999) 773-789
5. Jaffray, D.A. and Siewerdsen, J.H.: Cone-beam computed tomography with a flat-panel imager: initial performance characterization. Med. Phys. 27 (2000) 1311-1323
6. Rasch, C., Barillot, I., Remeijer, P., Touw., A., van Herk, M. and Lebesque, J.V.: Definition of the prostate in CT and MRI: a multi-observer study. Int. J. Radiat. Oncol. Biol. Phys.43 (1999) 57-66
7. Shirato, H., Shimizu, S., Kunieda, T., Kitamura, K., van Herk, M., Kagei, K., Nishioka, T., Hashimoto, S., Fujita, K., Aoyama, H., Tsuchiya, K., Kudo, K., Miyasaka, K.: Physical as-pects of a real-time tumor-tracking system for gated radiotherapy. Int. J. Radiat. Oncol. Biol. Phys. 48 (2000) 1187-1195
8. Troccaz, J., Laieb, N., Vassal, P., Menguy, Y., Cinquin, P., Bolla, M., Giraud, J.Y.: Patient setup optimization for external conformal radiotherapy. J. Image. Guid. Surg. 2 (1995) 113-120
9. van Herk, M. and Kooy, H.M.: Automatic three-dimensional correlation of CT-CT, CT-MRI, and CT-SPECT using chamfer matching. Med. Phys. 21 (1994) 1163-1178
10. van Herk, M., Bruce, A., Kroes, A.P., Shouman, T., Touw, A., Lebesque, J.V.: Quantifica-tion of organ motion during conformal radiotherapy of the prostate by three dimensional im-age registration. Int. J. Radiat. Oncol. Biol. Phys. 33 (1995) 1311-1320
11. van Herk, M., de Munck, J.C., Lebesque, J.V., Muller, S., Rasch, C. and Touw, A.: Auto-matic registration of pelvic computed tomography data and magnetic resonance scans in-cluding a full circle method for quantitative accuracy evaluation. Med. Phys. 25 (1998) 2054-2067
12. van Herk, M. Remeijer, P. Rasch, C. Lebesque, J.V.: The probability of correct target dos-age: dose-population histograms for deriving treatment margins in radiotherapy. Int. J. Ra-diat. Oncol. Biol. Phys. 47 (2000) 1121-1135
13. Woods, R.P., Mazziotta, J.C. and Cherry, S.R.: MRI-PET registration with automated algorithm. J. Comput. Assist. Tomogr. 17 (1993) 536-546

A Quantitative Comparison of Edges in 3D Intraoperative Ultrasound and Preoperative MR Images of the Brain

Karen E. Lunn [1], Alex Hartov[1,2,3], Eric W. Hansen[1], Hai Sun[a],
David W. Roberts[2,3], and Keith D. Paulsen[1,2,3]

[1]Thayer School of Engineering, Dartmouth College, Hanover, NH 03755 USA
[2]Dartmouth Hitchcock Medical Center, Lebanon, NH 03766 USA
[3]Norris Cotton Cancer Center, Lebanon, NH 03766 USA

Abstract. The displacement of brain tissue during neurosurgery is a significant source of error for image-guidance systems. We are investigating the use of a computational model to predict brain shift and warp preoperative MR images accordingly. 3D ultrasound appears to be a valid means of acquiring intraoperative images to use as sparse data for guiding the model calculations. We present here a study of edge detection in MR and ultrasound images to investigate the accuracy of our ultrasound system and explore methods of extracting sparse data. Ultrasound images are acquired prior to deformation and compared to their corresponding oblique MR/CT images. Results from phantom images show misalignment by an average of 2.2 ± 1.67 degrees, 0.90 ± 0.82 mm in x, and 0.87 ± 0.87 mm in y. Patient images are misaligned by an average of 2.2 ± 1.4 degrees, 1.24 ± 0.89 mm in x, and 0.97 ± 0.87 mm in y.

1. Introduction

The introduction of image-guidance systems has been a significant advancement in the field of neurosurgery, giving surgeons a powerful navigational tool and an increased level of accuracy. MR images of the patient are acquired prior to surgery, and registered to the patient in the operating room. Surgical tools can then be tracked and related to the MR images through coordinate transformations obtained from the registration procedure. This system provides feedback to the surgeon to help more accurately place surgical tools and navigate through the brain.

The accuracy of an image-guidance system depends on the assumption that registration involves a rigid transformation of the patient's brain in the operating room (OR) to the preoperative image volume. A number of studies have shown, however, that the brain shifts with respect to the skull, thus making the assumption of a rigid transformation invalid [1-4]. Strategies for reducing this source of error are being explored, with intraoperative MR, brain deformation modeling, and intraoperative ultrasound, or some combination of the three, emerging as the most common solutions. [5-10]. While MR has the advantage of being high contrast with high signal to noise ratio, it also has the drawbacks of being expensive, time consuming, and bulky. Ultrasound images can also provide intraoperative updates of the brain during surgery, and has the advantages of being real-time, portable, and far less expensive. However, due to the low signal to noise ratio and speckle

W. Niessen and M. Viergever (Eds.): MICCAI 2001, LNCS 2208, pp. 1081-1090, 2001.

characteristic of ultrasound data, a full volume representation of brain deformation would be difficult to construct from ultrasound alone. In contrast, a computational model could retain the advantages of MR image quality by warping preoperative images based on computed displacements. In previous studies, we have demonstrated the feasibility of using a model based on consolidation physics to recover brain shift [11-13]. Nonetheless, it is likely critical to obtain sparse intraoperative data to help drive model calculations. The advantages of ultrasound make it well suited for providing this information.

This paper describes an initial study designed to validate the use of 3D ultrasound as sparse data. We outline our procedure for relating the ultrasound image to the MR stack and matching homologous features. As a measure of error, we present the degree of rotation and translation needed to align each pair of images. Finally, we explore the results of edge detection in MR and ultrasound in the context of extracting sparse displacement data. Specifically, we investigate the level of feature congruence that may be obtainable in the OR during clinical cases that lack high contrast structures (e.g. tumor margins) or well-demarked surfaces (e.g. ventricles) that may not be present or visible in many cases.

2. Method

The initial registration of ultrasound and MR data is performed using an optical tracking system, which records the location of the ultrasound scanhead in real time. In this stage of registration, each ultrasound image is registered to the MR image stack, making it possible to reconstruct an oblique MR slice in the same orientation as the ultrasound image plane. The registration is then refined locally by aligning the edges of corresponding features in ultrasound and MR data. This image-based re-registration is classical in nature, and still in preliminary stages of development. Others groups have shown success in using mutual information (MI) or correlation ratio (CR) to co-register ultrasound and MR images (or other multimodal data) [14-17]. These image-based methods seek to register ultrasound and MR without the aid of tracking systems, and therefore the registration is performed over a larger volume. Our goal is somewhat different; we seek to improve the initial tracking-based registration over a localized region of interest, by exploiting some operator input, in order to investigate the visibility of less obvious feature edges in both ultrasound and MR. As a result, we opted to use the relatively simple techniques described here, rather than more sophisticated image-based registration strategies despite the fact that future work may benefit from incorporation of MI or CR into this refinement process.

2.1 Materials

Our 3D ultrasound system consists of a 5MHZ intraoperative ultrasonography system (Aloka Model 633; Corometrix Medical Systems, Wallingford, CT), a computer equipped with a frame grabber (model DT3155; Data Translation, Marlboro, MA), and a 3D optical tracker (Polaris; Northern Digital, Waterloo, Ontario, CAN). Image processing was performed using intrinsic functions available in Matlab (Version 6.1, Mathworks), as well as custom-built software, also written in Matlab.

2.2 MR Reconstruction

Points in ultrasound coordinates are mapped to MR coordinates through a series of coordinate transformations. These successive mappings are summarized in Eq.1,

$$P_{mr} = {}^{mr}T_w \, {}^{w}T_{tr} \, {}^{tr}T_{us} P_{us} ,$$ (1)

where P_{mr} is a vector containing points in MR coordinates, P_{us} is the corresponding vector for points in ultrasound coordinates, and the remaining terms are the three transformation matrices: the transformation from ultrasound to tracker coordinates $({}^{tr}T_{us})$, which is obtained through a complex calibration procedure; the transformation from tracker coordinates to world coordinates $({}^{w}T_{tr})$, which is provided by the Polaris optical tracking system; and the transformation from world coordinates to MR coordinates $({}^{mr}T_w)$, which is obtained through patient registration. Previous analysis of our calibration procedure has shown that by mapping the ultrasound calibration points to world coordinates, we can recover the original world coordinates to within an average RMS of 1.5 mm. Furthermore, an independent test of our ability to map a point in ultrasound to its world coordinates showed that we could do so with an average error of 2.32 mm. [19]. Our Polaris optical tracker has been found to have an accuracy of approximately 0.33 mm, which is comparable to results reported by other groups [5, 20].

Reconstructing an oblique MR image begins by mapping each pixel in an ultrasound image to the MR coordinate system, using Eq.1. The corresponding MR pixel is then obtained by finding the nearest voxel. This is completed for every pixel in the ultrasound image, resulting in two images of the same resolution (480×640 pixels). With an accurate registration, this pair of images should depict the same features, though they may appear different in each modality. As a qualitative approach to assessing alignment, we also create a colored composite of the two images superimposed, with MR in the red channel, and ultrasound in the green channel. This helps to visually identify common features in the two images.

2.3 Image Processing

We assess the accuracy of the MR reconstruction by extracting homologous features from the two images using classical methods, which are mostly manual. Before running an edge detection algorithm, the images are preprocessed to reduce noise and enhance edge features. The ultrasound images are first are smoothed and enhanced using a mean (averaging filter), followed by a median filter. For an n × n kernel, the mean filter calculates the average of the pixels in the neighborhood, and reassigns the mean intensity to the center pixel. This has the effect of blurring the image, with a larger kernel creating greater blurring. The median filter calculates the median of its n × n neighborhood, and assigns that value to the center pixel. MR images are enhanced using an anisotropic diffusion algorithm [21]. This filter is designed to smooth homogenous regions, while retaining sharp edges. The level of smoothness imposed can be increased or decreased by changing the level of iterations, as well as the degree of diffusion. For more challenging images, sometimes a combination of median, mean and anisotropic diffusion filters were used on both ultrasound and MR images. A custom designed graphical user interface allows the user to interactively change the size of the median and mean filters, as well as the iterations and diffusion level, to enhance features that are recognizable in both ultrasound and MR.

Following preprocessing, the edges in the images are identified using classical edge detection algorithms. For ultrasound images, edges are defined as the zero crossings of the Laplacian of a Gaussian filter. For MR images, we search for the maximum of the gradient, employing the Sobel approximation calculate the magnitude of the gradient. The threshold of these operators can be interactively changed to produce fewer or more edges. These operations are prepackaged functions in the Matlab Image Processing Toolbox. Edge patterns that appear in both images are selected. Selected edges are dilated to assist the edge matching algorithm in searching for common edges.

To match edges, the user must initialize the alignment by identifying a matching feature in the ultrasound and MR images. The algorithm then automatically searches for the proper alignment of the edges, by searching ± 5 units in rotation and translation for the combination of these parameters that results in a minimum value in the absolute difference between the two binary images. This method was tested on a simple simulation, where a binary image of a triangle edge was rotated and translated by a known amount, and those parameters were recovered using the algorithm described above. For all trials of initialization, the automatic search proved to capture the rotation and translation better than a manual approach. The original transformation was recovered with exact matching in rotation, and to within 0.3 pixels in x and y translation.

3. Results

3.1 Phantom

This edge matching procedure was performed on both phantom images and clinical data. The phantom consisted of a Plexiglas water tank strung with wires. These features were displayed clearly and with bright contrast in both ultrasound and CT images. As a result, edge detection and edge matching was a simple process. Figure 1A. shows a sample image pair, with the walls and wires of the tank clearly visible in both modalities. Before processing, both images are cropped to the same size to limit the computation to the region of interest. The ultrasound image of the phantom was filtered using a 5x5 mean filter, followed by a 15x15 median filter. The CT image of the phantom was filtered using an anisotropic filter, with 15 iterations and a diffusion level of 10. The resulting edges, after deleting artifacts, are displayed in the last row. For the image shown in figure 1A, the CT image was rotated by 0 degrees, and translated approximately .34 mm (2.5 pixels) in x and 0.69 mm (5 pixels) in y to match with the ultrasound image. For the remaining 34 images, using four different ultrasound scale settings, images were rotated by an average of 2.2 degrees, and translated by 0.89 mm in x and 0.89 mm in y, to match the edges. Table 1 presents the results obtained for each scale.

Table 1. Phantom results. Shows rotation and translation necessary to align US and CT images.

depth scale	rotation (degrees)	x translation (mm)	y translation (mm)
6cm	1.91 ± 1.51	0.65 ± 0.39	0.59 ± 0.25
8cm	2.18 ± 2.09	0.83 ± 0.48	0.50 ± 0.34
12cm	2.10 ± 1.37	1.02 ± 1.00	0.69 ± 0.57
16cm	2.77 ± 1.69	1.07 ± 1.12	1.57 ± 1.29

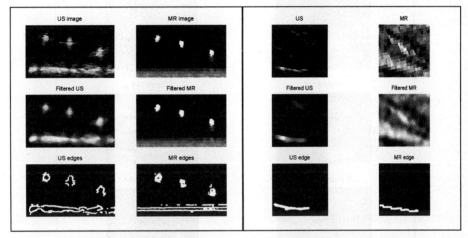

Figure 1. A. Images on left show ultrasound (far left) and CT (middle left) images of phantom tank, filtered images, and detected edges used to align images. B. Images on right show ultrasound (middle right) and MR (far right) of section of patient's brain. Below original image, filtered images and detected edges are displayed.

3.2 Patient

This combination of preprocessing, selection of edges, and semi-automatic alignment was also performed for 18 images of one patient. All of these images were obtained after the craniotomy, before the dura was removed. Therefore, we can assume that little or no deformation has occurred. Figure 1b illustrates a typical example from this case, where the white to gray matter boundary displayed in MR corresponds to a bright line in ultrasound. For this image set, the ultrasound image was preprocessed with a 5x5 mean filter, followed by a 15x15 median filter. The MR image was smoothed using an anisotropic diffusion filter, with 30 iterations and diffusion level 30. These images were matched with approximately 2 degrees rotation, 0.8 mm (6 pixels) in x, and 1.4 mm (10.2 pixels) in y. A more difficult case is displayed in figure 2. The images show similar, but less exact patterns. In this case, the both pairs of images were first filtered with mean and median filters to blur the edges and reduce noise. Next, they were filtered using the anisotropic diffusion algorithm to further blend homogenous regions while retaining sharp edges. The smoothed images are displayed in the middle row of figure 2. The last row depicts the resulting edges from these filtered images, overlaid on the original images. This particular image set was determined to be misaligned by -3 degrees, 1.3 mm (9.5 pixels) in x, and 1.6 mm (11.7 pixels) in y. The results of all of the images show that they are properly aligned by rotating by an average of 2.2 ± 1.4 degrees and translating by an average of 1.24 ± 0.89 mm in x and 0.97 ± 0.87 mm in y.

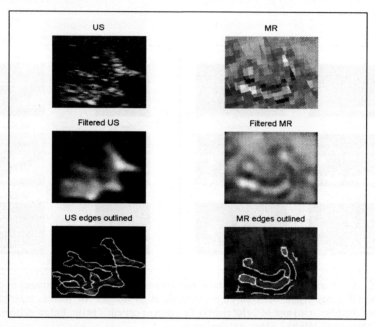

Figure 2. Ultrasound (left) and MR images of patient brain, with filtered and edge detected results. Images represent a region of approximately 1.5 by 2.0 cm.

4. Discussion and Conclusions

The results of these studies validate the accuracy of our 3D ultrasound system and provide some insight into possible methods of extracting quantitative sparse data from intraoperative ultrasound images. The level of accuracy achieved in matching the phantom images represent a significant achievement in our goal of using intraoperative ultrasound in conjunction with a brain deformation model. The phantom provided an excellent set of test images, as its features produced clear, high contrast images of its walls and wires. The clarity of edge contours in both ultrasound and CT left little ambiguity in choosing the correct features to match. Therefore, we have confidence in our conclusion that for a given ultrasound image, we can properly reconstruct the corresponding oblique MR image to within approximately 1 mm.

It would be convenient if MR and ultrasound edges were always as apparent as they are in the phantom; unfortunately, this is not usually the case. Images of brain features such as the falx, tumors, and ventricles, which can be high contrast and easy to recognize, have been used in other studies to register images or characterize deformation [6,16,22]. However, these features are not always present in the region of interest. With the patient data from this study, we show that it is possible to match more subtle brain features, such as the interface between white and gray matter, as well as sulcal patterns. Furthermore, we propose that when similar patterns emerge in both images, these could be used for matching, even if the exact nature of the feature is unclear.

The results of the phantom study lead us to conclude that edges which appear to line up in the MR and ultrasound image do, in fact, represent the same features. For example, the distinction between white and gray matter is readily apparent in MR images. By superimposing the ultrasound images on their oblique MR counterparts, it was clear that strong ultrasonic reflections were produced at the white/gray matter interface. Figure 2 shows a typical example of this echogenicity. Note that the bright line in the ultrasound image is located in the same region as the gray/white matter boundary displayed in the MR image.

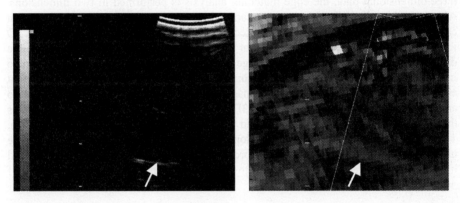

Figure 3. Cropped ultrasound image (left) and its corresponding oblique MR reconstruction (right). Arrow points to white/gray matter interface in both images. For reference, the ultrasound scale and wedge shape are overlayed on the MR image

By searching within a region of interest in the two images, we were also able to match edges of more complex features with correlating patterns. For example, the images shown in Figure 3 show similar patterns of parallel horizontal edges in the lower left corner, and diagonal edges in the center. In this case, the features appear to be sulcal patterns. It is important to note, however, that the features do not need to be correctly categorized in order to recognize patterns in edges and find the translation and rotation necessary to align the two sets of edges. Furthermore, while these features were already closely aligned, it seems feasible to use this method of pattern searching in ultrasound images depicting deformed brains, where features have moved from their preoperative location. The region of interest would have to be greater in order to find patterns in the displaced tissue that match patterns in the MR.

After identifying similar features, the rotation and translation could be calculated using a similar edge matching technique. Finally, the results of this displacement calculation would be used as inputs to the computational model. Obviously, this strategy needs to be explored further to validate its usefulness in the deformed case. It may be that more sophisticated, automatic, image-based registration methods, such as MI or CR, will need to be employed in order to realize a robust global edge-matching technique.

The results of the patient case should be interpreted with some caution. The images analyzed represent the best ultrasound/MR pairs, in the sense that the features present in one image are clearly related to those in the second image. Nonetheless, the results are valuable in that they demonstrate the level of accuracy that can be achieved. Furthermore, this selective process is a practical strategy for using sparse ultrasound data in conjunction with the brain model. That is, it seems reasonable to use only the best ultrasound/MR pairs to calculate local displacement as input to the model. Since our motivation for using intraoperative ultrasound is to gain sparse displacement data, rather than a full volume description, this limited selection is compatible with our strategy.

Another possible drawback of the method described here is that while we have three-dimensional data, the edge matching analysis is performed in two dimensions. Although this simplification is acceptable for an initial study, the displacement calculated would represent only the projection of the actual displacement onto the 2D image plane. It has been pointed out that if the 2D image lines up with the principle direction of displacement, the 2D image may be adequate [6]. We have begun to investigate the use of 3D data, with some encouraging initial results. Our current approach still uses the 2D ultrasound image plane, but searches for a better match to an oblique MR plane by integrating the 3D MR image volume. Figure 4 demonstrates the results from matching one ultrasound image with an improved oblique MR slice. This 3D method warrants further development; it does not yet incorporate multiple ultrasound images in 3D, which may prove to be more robust. More sophisticated image processing techniques also need to be developed in order to attain our goal of predicting shift in real time.

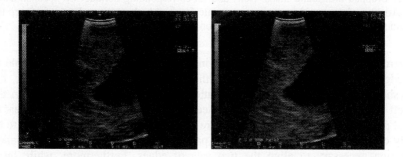

Figure 4. Results from 3D edge matching on one set of ultrasound and MR images. Left figure displays overlap of images before re-registration. Right figure displays images after 3D edge matching isperformed.

Finally, we have proposed that less obvious features, such as gray/white matter interfaces and sulcal patterns are potentially useful for extracting sparse intraoperative data on brain tissue motion. While we present some initial findings on the relative appearance of these structures in ultrasound and MR, a more extensive comparison of the characteristics of brain features in various modalities would be quite helpful. Such a study could provide a priori knowledge concerning feature boundaries, which would be useful in automating the steps of segmentation and edge matching.

The underlying assumption in the work presented here is that the features occurring in both image sets do in fact correspond to the same physical structures Given this premise questions also arise as to whether the simple image processing and feature extraction techniques we used apply appropriately across the differing image scales of the two modalities. Certainly, the results from the phantom study (Fig. 1) and high contrast in vivo data (Fig. 4) which exploited the same techniques suggest they do. However, further study is required to thoroughly substantiate the approach in more subtle low contrast cases (e.g. Fig. 2,3). Our intent was not to definitively validate the methodology described herein, or even to necessarily endorse the approach above other possibilities, but rather to indicate that opportunities exist for localized low-contrast feature matching between intraoperative US and preoperative MR that could constitute sparse data for full-volume MR updates achieved through computational modeling.

References

1. D.W. Roberts, A. Hartov, F.E. Kennedy, M.I. Miga, K.D. Paulsen: Intraoperative Brain Shift and Deformation: A Quantitative Analysis of Cortical Displacement in 28 Cases. *Neurosurgery*, vol.43: 49-760, 1998.
2. N. Hata, A. Nabavi, W.M. Wells, S.K. Warfield, R. Kikinis, P.M. Black, F.A. Jolesz: Three-dimensional optical flow method for measurement of volumetric brain deformation from intraoperative MR images. *Journal of Computer Assisted Tomography*, vol.24(4): 531-8, 2000.
3. C.R. Maurer, D.L. Hill, A.J. Martin, H. Liu, M. McCue, D. Rueckert, D. Lloret, W.A. Hall, R.E. Maxwell, D.J. Hawkes, C.L. Truwit: Investigation of intraoperative brain deformation using a 1.5-T interventional MR system: preliminary results. *IEEE Transactions on Medical Imaging*, vol.17(5): 817-25, 1998.
4. D.L. Hill, C.R. Maurer, R.J. Maciunas, J.A. Barwise, J.M. Fitzpatrick, M.Y. Wang: Measurement of intraoperative brain surface deformation under a craniotomy. *Neurosurgery*, vol.43(3): 514-26, 1998.
5. D.G. Gobbi, R.M. Comeau, and T.M. Peters: Ultrasound Probe Tracking for Real-Time Ultrasound/MRI Overlay and Visualization of Brain Shift. *Medical image computing and computer-assisted intervention--MICCAI '99 : second international conference :* 920-927, 1999.
6. R.M. Comeau, A. Fenster, T.M. Peters: Intraoperative US in Interactive Image-guided Neurosurgery. *RadioGraphics*, vol. 18(4): 1019-1027, 1998.
7. A. Jödicke, W. Deinsberger, H. Erbe, A. Kriete, D.K. Böker: Intraoperative Three-Dimensional Ultrasonography: An Approach to Register Brain Shift using Multidimensional Image Processing. *Minim. Invas. Neurosurg* 41: 13-19, 1998.
8. D.G. Gobbi, R.M. Comeau, T.M. Peters: Ultrasound/MRI Overlay with Image Warping For Neurosurgery. *Medical image computing and computer-assisted intervention--MICCAI 2000*: 106-114, 2000.

1090   K.E. Lunn et al.

9. D.W. Roberts, M.I. Miga, A. Hartov, S. Eisner, J.M. Lemery, F.E. Kennedy, K.D. Paulsen: Intraoperatively Updated Neuroimaging Using Brain Modeling and Sparse Data. *Neurosurgery,* vol.45(5): 1199-1207, 1999.
10. C. Nimsky, O. Ganslandt, S. Cerny, P. Hastreiter, G. Greiner, R. Fahlbusch: Quantification of, Visualization of, and Compensation for Brain Shift Using Intraoperative Magnetic Resonance Imaging. *Neurosurgery,* vol.47(5): 1070-1080, 2000.
11. M.I. Miga, K.D. Paulsen, P.J. Hoopes, F.E. Kennedy, A. Hartov, D.W. Roberts: In Vivo Quantification of a Homogeneous Brain Deformation Model for Updating Preoperative Images During Surgery. *IEEE Transactions on Biomedical Engineering.* vol. 47(2): 266 – 273, 2000.
12. K.P. Paulsen, M.I. Miga, F.E. Kennedy, P.J. Hoopes, A. Hartov, D.W. Roberts: A Computational Model for Tracking Subseruface Tissue Deformation During Stereotactic Neurosurgery. *IEEE Transactions on Biomedical Engineering,* vol.46(2): 213-225, 1999.
13. L. Platenik: Investigation of Retraction Deformation Modeling for Model-Updated Image-Guided Stereotactic Neurosurgery. M.S. Thesis, Thayer School of Engineering, Dartmouth College, January 2001.
14. J.M. Blackall, D. Ruechert, C.R. Maurer, G.P. Penney, G.L.G. Hill, and D.J. Hawkes. An Image Registration Approach to Automated Calibration for Freehand 3D Ultrasound. *Medical image computing and computer-assisted intervention--MICCAI 2000*: 462-471, 2000.
15. A. Roche, G. Malandain, and N. Ayache. Unifying Maximum Likelihood Approaches in Medical Image Registration. *International Journal of Imaging Systems and Technology,* vol.11, (2000) 71-80
16. A. Roche, X. Pennec, M. Rudolf, D.P. Auer, G. Malandain, S. Ourselin, L.M. Auer, and N. Ayache. Generalized Correlation Ratio for Rigid Registration of 3D Ultrasound with MR Images. *Medical image computing and computer-assisted intervention--MICCAI 2000*: (2000) 567-577
17. J.P.W. Pluim, J.B.A. Maintz, and M.A. Viergever. Image Registration by Maximization of Combined Mutual Information and Gradient Information. *Medical image computing and computer-assisted intervention--MICCAI 2000:* (2000) 452-461
18. A. Hartov, S.D. Eisner, D.W. Roberts, K.D. Paulsen, L.A. Platenik, M.I. Miga: Error analysis for a free-hand three-dimensional ultrasound system for neuronavigation. *Neurosurgical Focus,* vol.6(3), 1999. <http://www.neurosurgery.org/focus/mar99/6-3-5.html>
19. K.E. Lunn, A. Hartov, F.E. Kennedy, M.I. Miga, D.W. Roberts, L.A. Platenik, K.P. Paulsen: 3D Ultrasound as Sparse Data for Intraoperative Brain Deformation Model. In *Proceedings of SPIE--The International Society for Optical Engineering. Medical Imaging 2001: Ultrasonic Imaging and Signal Processing.*
20. Northern Digital, Inc. Products: POLARIS, <http://www.ndigital.com/polaris.html>, 12/01/00
21. P. Perona, J. Malik: Scale-Space and Edge Detection Using Anisotropic Diffusion. *IEEE Transactions on Pattern Analysis and Machine Intelligence.* vol.12(7): 629-639, 1990.
22. H. Erbe, A. Kriete, A. Jödicke, W. Deinsberger, D.K. Böker: 3D-Ultrasonography and Imaging Matching for Detection of Brain Shift During Intracranial Surgery. *Computer Assisted Radiology: Proceedings of the International Symposium on Computer and Communication Systems for Image Guided Diagnosis and Therapy:* 225-230, 1996.

Constructing Patient Specific Models for Correcting Intraoperative Brain Deformation

A.D. Castellano-Smith[1], T. Hartkens[1], J. Schnabel[1], D.R. Hose[2], H. Liu[3], W.A. Hall[3], C.L. Truwit[3], D.J. Hawkes[1], and D.L.G. Hill[1]

[1] Computational Imaging Sciences Group, Radiological Sciences, Guy's Hospital, King's College London, London SE1 9RT, UK
Andrew.Castellano Smith@kcl.ac.uk
[2] Medical Physics Department, Clinical Sciences Division, University of Sheffield, UK.
[3] Depts. of Radiology and Neurosurgery, University of Minnesota, Minneapolis, MN, USA.

Abstract. In this work we present a Mesh Warping technique for the construction of patient-specific Finite Element Method models from patient MRI images, and demonstrate how simulated surgical loading can be applied to these models. We compare the results of this simulation with observed deformation during surgery, and show that our model matches well with the observed degree of deformation.

1 Introduction

Brain deformation during neurosurgery can substantially degrade the utility of pre-operative imaging as a surgical guidance tool. Structures on or below the surface of the brain have been found to move by 10mm or more [1].

Biomechanical models have the potential to predict brain deformation and may in future, be incorporated into image guided surgery systems to improve accuracy [2]. For these models to be successful, they are likely to need to treat different parts of the brain in different ways. The generation of patient-specific brain models is extremely time-consuming, as it requires segmentation of relevant structures within the patient, generation of a 3D mesh with appropriate properties allocated to each element, and finally solving the model using suitable conditions.

We propose a technique for building a finite element model of an individual patient by non-rigid registration of a carefully meshed atlas image to the pre-operative image of a specific subject. We demonstrate this meshing approach on 4 patients. Once the data mesh has been generated, each element in the mesh can be assigned appropriate mechanical properties (including any expected volume change), and then the finite element model is solved after applying appropriate forces.

2 Methods

2.1 Patient Selection and Imaging

To assess the effectiveness of the techniques used in this paper, we selected patients who were undergoing surgery at the interventional MR facility at the University of

W. Niessen and M. Viergever (Eds.): MICCAI 2001, LNCS 2208, pp. 1091–1098, 2001.
© Springer-Verlag Berlin Heidelberg 2001

Minnesota. Typical scanning protocol consisted of acquiring multi-slice spin echo and MP-RAGE volume datasets prior to commencement of surgery, similar acquisitions immediately after surgery was completed while the patient is still in the operating position. Additional single-slice images were acquired intra-operatively.

From this set of patients (13 resection, 5 biopsy, 4 functional procedures), we selected four patients (2 resection cases, 2 functional surgery cases) to demonstrate our mesh warping algorithm. We then simulate deformation on one of these subjects (a functional surgery patient), comparing the modelled deformation with the deformation imaged at the end of surgery.

2.2 Quantification of CSF Volume Change During Surgery

For the 21 patients listed above, we estimated CSF volume loss during the procedure by manually segmenting the lateral ventricles from the pre- and post-surgery images.

2.3 FEM Model Generation - Mesh Warping

The use of Finite Element Methods (FEMs) for modelling brain deformation during surgery has been the subject of some study [2,3,4]. In order to simulate surgical loads on a patient dataset, it is necessary to construct a patient-specific FEM model incorporating salient features of that particular patient geometry. However, the construction of FEM meshes fitting to the features in an MR image of a head is very difficult and time-consuming. To model each patient head and brain in a realistic fashion, we have devised a technique for constructing FEM meshes based on an atlas mesh and a non-rigid registration technique, which we refer to as *Mesh-Warping*.

In this technique, the construction of patient-specific FEM meshes relies on the construction of a mesh fitting to an atlas brain. This mesh is then deformed according to the non-rigid registration solution found by registering the patient image to the atlas brain image. This technique is similar to the Mesh-Matching technique discussed in [5] but in our case, the whole image is used during the registration procedure as opposed to the surface-based registration in [5], providing a better fitting patient mesh.

Atlas Model The Brainweb brain atlas[1] was used as our brain model. In order to construct a FEM model from the segmented images in the atlas, surface models were constructed of the outer brain surface (grey-matter/CSF boundary) and the ventricular surfaces. These surface models were extracted from the images using a modified marching cubes technique [6] before being smoothed and decimated to remove small edges and small triangular facets using the "evolver" software package[2]. This smoothing and decimation process has been shown [7] to preserve salient features of surface shape, whilst providing a reduction in the number of facets making up the model surface.

The resulting surface models (brain surface and ventricles) were then loaded into ANSYS[3], a commercial FEM package we have used in previous work, the interior volumes of the surfaces constructed, and a combined volume produced. The techniques

---

[1] from http://www.bic.mni.mcgill.ca/brainweb/
[2] from http://www.susqu.edu/facstaff/b/brakke/evolver/evolver.html
[3] ANSYS Inc. http://www.ansys.com

presented in this paper do not rely on the use of a specific FEM package. This multi-component volume was then meshed with tetrahedral elements. The effect of meshing in this way is to preserve the internal boundaries within the object - in this case the ventricular surfaces, whilst producing a continuous mesh across that surface. The smoothed surface of the grey matter and ventricles is preserved within the mesh.

Segmenting white matter separately and constructing a surface model as for the grey matter and ventricular surfaces was not practicable, because the brainweb white matter is non-connected. In order to allow for the different biomechanical properties of grey matter, white matter and CSF we therefore chose to label the mesh with tissue-type labels after meshing. This labelling assigns to each tetrahedral element in the mesh a tissue type - grey matter, white matter or fluid. The result of such a labelling can be seen in Figure 1.

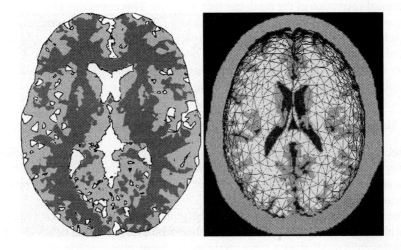

Fig. 1. The atlas mesh, labelled (Left) with fluid (white), white matter (dark grey) and grey matter (light grey). The ventricular surface was segmented and constructed separately, and is preserved in the mesh, whereas white matter regions are labelled within the mesh after construction. The atlas mesh (right) is displayed as a wireframe overlaid on an atlas slice.

Non-rigid Registration for Mesh Warping In order to construct a subject-specific mesh for each patient in the study, it would of course be possible to follow the process described for the construction of the atlas mesh, but for each patient. However, this process is slow and labour intensive - manual segmentation of ventricular surfaces, grey and white matter is required. Decimation and smoothing of the surface models requires user interaction, and meshing is computationally expensive, requiring several hours. The construction of the atlas mesh used in this work required several tens of hours from start to finish. Clearly this time-scale is clinically unacceptable, and for this reason, we propose a method for patient-specific mesh construction which avoids these problems.

The fully automated non-rigid registration in use in our centre [8,9] can accurately align the ventricular surfaces, the cortical surface and other salient features. This registration procedure produces a deformation field relating all points in the target image (in this case the atlas) to a position in the source image (the patient). In this way, the atlas mesh can be warped to fit the patient geometry. We believe that the use of a non-rigid intensity-based registration scheme to warp meshes to fit patient data has not been used before and has great potential for allowing patient-specific FEM models to be constructed in a clinically relevant timescale.

The warped, patient-specific mesh is only suitable for use if the elements produced meet quality criteria. Any folding during the registration procedure can produce elements which are also folded, and hence do not usefully model the patient geometry. Other "badly shaped" elements, such as tetrahedra with very extreme angles, must also be avoided. ANSYS provides mesh checking capabilities to identify such elements, and manual correction of the mesh can then be made. This correction process could be automated, if required, based on an examination of the mesh element surface normals.

Each of the four patients in the study was registered to the atlas image, and the pre-labelled atlas mesh then warped following the deformation field produced. The mesh quality was checked, in each case, for folding and badly shaped elements. These were manually corrected before further processing.

2.4   Simulation Scenarios

To simulate the surgical situation, we firstly fixed the position of all external points on the grey matter surface, simulating the connection of the brain to the inside of the skull by the arachnoid strands. The patient selected for modelling had a functional procedure involving no resection.

The Young's Modulus of the tissues, following [10] were set to $4 \times 10^3 NM^{-2}$ for white matter, and $8 \times 10^3 NM^{-2}$ for grey matter, with Poisson's ratio of 0.495 for near incompressibility. All tissues were modelled as linear elastic solids using 10-noded tetrahedral elements (the "solid187" element in ANSYS). The measurements of ventricular volume suggested that we should simulate CSF loss by shrinking the lateral ventricles by 10% during the procedure. The region of brain surface apendent to the electrode entry point was allowed to move freely on the side ipsi-lateral to the insertion. We then applied gravity to the model (a uniform vertical force on each element) and the ventricles were reduced in volume by 10% by applying a thermal load to the FEM mesh elements making up the ventricular system such that they uniformly shrink in volume by 10%.

Comparison of Real and Simulated Deformations   The FEM solution was used to produce a warped version of the pre-operative image, simulating an MR image of the post-operative brain. We visually compared this simulated image with the real intra-operatively recorded image data.

3   Results

3.1   Quantification of Deformation

Volume Vhange of Ventricles The ventricle ipsi-lateral to the craniotomy exhibites larger volume changes than the contra-lateral ventricle in cases where a substantial difference in volume change occurs between the ventricles. Larger volume changes occur in the resection cases than in the biopsy or functional cases. The variability in volume change measure assessed by repeated segmentation of a pre/post-operative ventricle image pair was 5.4%. This variability is similar to the variability in segmentation of cerebral hemispheres in earlier work [7].

Finite Element Meshes The patient-specific meshes for the four patients in this study are shown in Figure 2. Near some gyri the mesh is not aligned perfectly with the cortical surface, due to shrinkage of the mesh surface during the decimation used in the atlas construction. This should not cause large errors in the solutions, and will be addressed by the construction of a finer model.

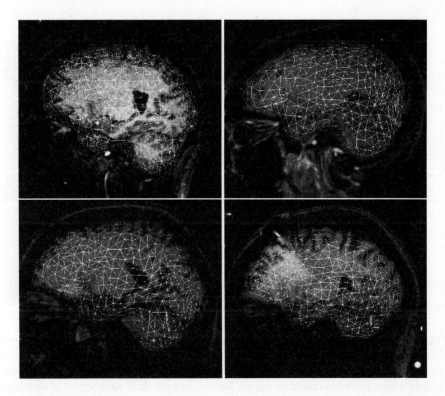

Fig. 2. FEM meshes of the four patients in the study. Top left - functional2; Top right - resection7; Bottom left - resection11; Bottom right - functional6. There is some shrinkage of the mesh away from the cortical surface due to the decimation and smoothing applied to the atlas model.

The meshes each contain 56747 nodes and 40310 tetrahedral elements - the same number as the atlas mesh. The mesh quality can be quantified by the number of folded and badly shaped elements in the mesh due to the registration and Mesh Warping procedure. In all cases, fewer than 20 elements were badly shaped. Only resection7 had a substantial number of folded elements (6276), caused by the abnormal structure of the brain making registration to the atlas difficult.

3.2   Comparison of FEM Solutions with Quantification of Brain Deformation

In Figure 3 the top two images show the FEM model after deformation, with the displacement of brain surface colour coded, lightest colour corresponds to 4.5mm displacement. The middle image pair shows the subtraction of the post-surgery image from the pre-operative image. The lower images show subtraction of the simulated post-surgery image from the pre-operative image. Note that the deformation of the frontal lobes is greater ipsi-lateral to the electrode insertion in both cases, and that the ventricular volume change appears visually similar in both the real and simulated images. The simulated data lacks the noise and RF inhomogeneity artefacts of the real data.

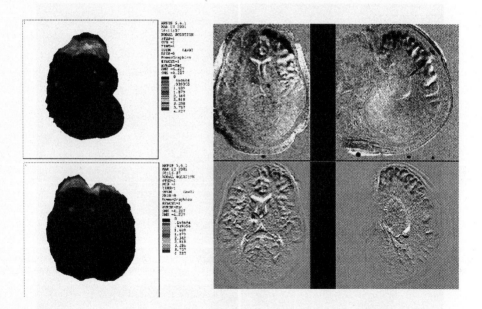

Fig. 3. Comparison of modelled deformation to true deformation. Top panels show the deformed FEM model (colour animated version of this at http://www-ipg.umds.ac.uk/a.d.smith/miccai2001/). Middle images show subtraction of post-surgery image from pre-operative image. Bottom images show subtraction of simulated post-operative image from pre-operative image.

4   Conclusions and Discussion

In this paper we have described a technique to generate a patient-specific finite element model for predicting intraoperative brain deformation. This technique, which we refer to as *Mesh Warping*, involves 3D registration of an atlas image that has been carefully meshed to a pre-operative MR image of the subject being studied. This assigns properties to grey matter, white matter and CSF in the model. We have applied this meshing technique to four neurosurgical subjects imaged in the interventional MR facility at the University of Minnesota. For one of these patients who had a functional surgical procedure, we then ran an example deformation scenario in which CSF volume was reduced by 10%, the attachment of the brain to the dura was broken appendant to the point of insertion of the electrode. We show that the model generates visually plausible deformation. The run time of the algorithm was 4 hours on a 300MHz Sun Ultra 10 using the commercial ANSYS finite element modelling software. Running the algorithm on a state-of-the art CPU may in the near future give a run-time that is compatible with the timescale of neurosurgical procedures.

Meshing with no user interaction saves a lot of time. The registration may in some cases be slow, but is fully automated. Our Mesh-Warping technique is not limited to the non-rigid registration technique in use in our centre, but may be applied using any suitable non-rigid registration algorithm.

Further work will involve the construction of a higher resolution atlas model, incorporating more detail of brain folds. The fidelity of the model's deformation predictions will be assessed in future work involving more intra-operative data collection during neurosurgical procedures to provide better localization of deformation. This work will also allow the testing of these techniques on a much larger set of patients. The interaction between sulcal walls will become important in this model, as deformations within the FEM model will need to take account of the unrealistic nature of deformations involving tissue moving through other tissue. All the FEM solutions presented here are equilibrium state solutions. We will explore the possibility of finding temporally varying solutions to allow a time-varying deformation to be predicted. More use of the intraoperative image data will allow a verification of the predictions made by this model.

We assume that the brain surface gravitationally lower than or contralateral to the craniotomy remains firmly tethered to the inner table of the skull. The degree to which this assumption is true in practice needs investigation, but displacements of these areas of brain surface, observationally at least, appear small compared to the displacements of other structures.

The simulation of actual resections by removing sections of brain from the mesh, remains a challenge to the current model which we are addressing in on-going work.

The measurement of mechanical properties of biological tissues is difficult, and more especially where they relate to abnormal tissues. In this work we have used literature values. Future work will assess the sensitivity of the model's solutions to differences in material properties over the ranges found in the literature.

Acknowledgements

We are grateful to the UK Engineering and Physical Sciences Research Council for funding ADCS and TH, Justin Penrose of Sheffield University for assistance with ANSYS and colleagues in CISG.

References

1. D. L. G. Hill, C. R. Maurer, Jr., R. J. Maciunas, J. A. Barwise, J. M. Fitzpatrick, and M. Y. Wang. Measurement of intraoperative brain surface deformation under a craniotomy. *Neurosurgery*, 43:514–528, 1998.
2. M. I. Miga, K. D. Paulsen, J. M. Lemery, S. D. Eisner, A. Hartov, F. E. Kennedy, and D. W. Roberts. Model-updated image guidance: initial clinical experiences with gravity-induced brain deformation. *IEEE Trans. Med. Imaging*, 18:866–874, 1999.
3. M. Bro-Neilsen. Finite element modelling in surgery simulation. *Proceedings of the IEEE*, 86:490–503, 1998.
4. M. I. Miga, K. D. Paulsen, P. J. Hoopes, F. E. Kennedy, A. Hartov, and D. W. Roberts. In vivo quantification of a homogeneous brain deformation model for updating preoperative images during surgery. *IEEE Trans. Biomed. Eng.*, 47:266–273, 2000.
5. B. Couteau, Y. Payan, and S. Lavallee. The mesh-matching algorithm: an automatic 3d mesh generator for finite element structures. *Journal of Biomechanics*, 33:1005–1009, 2000.
6. W.E Lorensen and H.E. Cline. Marching cubes: a high resolution 3d surface construction algorithm. *Computer Graphics*, 21(4):163–169, 1987.
7. A.D. Castellano Smith. *The Folding of the Human Brain: From Shape to Function*. PhD thesis, King's College London, September 1999.
8. D. Rueckert, L.I. Sonoda, C. Hayes, D.L.G. Hill, M.O. Leach, and D.J. Hawkes. Non-rigid registration using free-form deformations: Application to breast MR images. *IEEE Trans. Med. Imaging*, 18:712–721, 1999.
9. J. A. Schnabel, D. Rueckert, M. Quist, J. M. Blackall, A. D. Castellano Smith, T. Hartkens, G. P. Penney, W. A. Hall, H. Liu, C. L. Truwit, F. A. Gerritsen, D. L. G. Hill, and D. J. Hawkes. A generic framework for non-rigid registration based on non-uniform multi-level free-form deformations. *Proc. MICCAI 2001*, Springer LNCS:(in press), 2001.
10. H. Takizawa, K. Sugiura, M. baba, and J. D. Miller. Analysis of intracerebral hematoma shapes by numerical computer simulation using the finite element method. *Neurol Med Chir (Tokyo)*, 34:65–69, 1994.

Interface Design and Evaluation for CAS Systems

Cristiano Paggetti[1], Sandra Martelli[2], Laura Nofrini[2], Paolo Vendruscolo[2]

[1]MEDEA - MEDical and Engineering Applications, Firenze, Italy
c.paggetti@medea-italia.it
[2]Biomechanics Lab, Istituti Ortopedici Rizzoli, Bologna, Italy
{S.Martelli, L.Nofrini, P.Vendruscolo}@biomec.ior.it
http://www.ior.it/biomec/

Abstract. The use of Computer Assisted Surgery (CAS) systems is becoming very common in the clinical practice, therefore the evaluation of such systems in terms of clinical outcomes and ergonomic features is more and more relevant. This paper goals has been to define some domain specific guidelines for the design of Human Computer Interfaces (HCI) for surgical application and to provide an evaluation protocol of existing CAS systems. The demonstration application has been a planning system developed for the Total Knee Replacement (TKR), a high skill demanding procedure, where the planning phase is crucial for the success of the intervention. The results we have obtained can be extended also to surgical training systems and surgical navigation platforms.

1 Introduction

The use of Computer Assisted Surgery (CAS) systems is becoming very common in the clinical practice, therefore the evaluation of such systems in terms of clinical outcomes and ergonomic features is more and more relevant. This paper addresses the definition of some domain specific guidelines for the design of Human Computer Interfaces (HCI) for surgical application. Currently the literature does not provide much indications related to the HCI in such a framework [7] [8]. Starting from the application problem analysis and the user requirements, this paper explains how the system specifications have been implemented and which criteria have been applied for the evaluation of the HCI. The paper's goal is therefore to provide a consistent approach for the HCI design and an evaluation protocol of existing CAS systems. The domain addressed is related to the planning systems and it is suitable also for training and surgical navigation ones.

In this paper the demonstration application is the Total Knee Replacement (TKR), a high skill demanding procedure, where the planning phase is crucial for the success of the intervention. The aim of TKR is to restore the correct alignment of the mechanical axis of the limb and the correct function of the knee joint. In particular the HCI discussed in this paper assists the surgeon in the planning of correct size, orientation and position of the prosthesis components for TKR interventions.

W. Niessen and M. Viergever (Eds.): MICCAI 2001, LNCS 2208, pp. 1099-1106, 2001.
© Springer-Verlag Berlin Heidelberg 2001

2 Material and Methods

2.1 HCI Design

We recall that the main objectives of most Computer Assisted Systems (CAS) are[1][2]:

i. enhance surgeon's 3D perception of the surgical scenario;
ii. enhance surgeon's dexterity in performing high skill demanding actions;
iii. enhance the accuracy and repeatability of surgeon's action;
iv. reduce the invasiveness of the surgical intervention;
v. reduce the intraoperative decision time.

The universal access to a HCI to use CAS systems implies to address general requirements during its design, with a systematic approach related to the functionality implementation as well as the features of the specific application domain.
We suggest the following methodological approach:

1. identification of the users and of the working conditions
2. definition of the system's output (i.e. goals and specific outcomes)
3. definition of the system's input
4. definition of the system functionalities to treat input data to obtain required output
5. identification of the logical phases to subdivide and organize the overall procedure
6. definition of the user's interaction modality

We underline that the HCI design, although usually proposed by a scientist, needs a constant involvement of the users' in the selection of data, display layout and also testing

2.2 Evaluation Protocol for CAS HCI

The evaluation of CAS HCI was performed during repeated tests of the planning procedure. Trials were conducted on 10 patients by four surgeons (two expert surgeons and two junior surgeons), who planned the intervention on all patients; one of them repeated planning four times in different days.

In particular, it has been worked out an evaluation based on the analysis of the user's reactions as respect to the HCI implementation. Comments and reactions have been divided in two groups, those related to *features correctly implemented in the CAS system* and those *features that can be suggested in order to improve the usability and the user's satisfaction*.

Furthermore the outcomes of the questionnaire, based on the Guidelines for designing user interface software[9] from the MITRE Corporation, are discussed directly with the programmer and the HCI expert. It is worthwhile to carry out the evaluation without analysing the results of the surgeons involved in the HCI design.

The CAS HCI evaluation was based on three different aspects, originally defined by the authors:

1. evaluation of the user's satisfaction in using HCI, through interviews to the users and a specific questionnaire
2. evaluation of the user's ability and fatigue in using the HCI, through objective observation of the system's behavior by an independent scientist
3. evaluation of the planning repeatability as an index of the HCI efficacy.

The first item concerns the subjective feeling of the surgeons in using the system's tools: friendliness, ease of use, lack of tools that could be useful to successfully reach the system's aims.

The second item concerns the evaluation of objective aspects of the system: time necessary to complete a particular action, the implemented data control, errors' management, workspace layout.

The third item concerns quantitative evaluations of the system performances.

3 Results

3.1 Implementation of HCI Design

The six methodological criteria reported in §2.1 were applied to the TKR planning HCI design, with the following results:

1. users are orthopaedic surgeons working in a pre-operative framework;
2. the system's output is the prosthesis components location with respect to the patient anatomy;
3. the system's input are patient CT data and CAD drawings of different prosthesis,
4. system functionality include patient selection, anatomical marker selection, virtual prosthesis positioning,
5. the TKR planning can be divided in two phases: the Alignment phase and the Positioning phase
6. the user's interaction modality is mouse based; in particular the selection criteria is based on a "one click" approach, simple menus to deal with input data, data elaboration and on-line help.

In practice the TKR planner consists of two successive steps and corresponding screen: the *Alignment phase* and the *Positioning phase*.

In the first, the frontal and the lateral scouts of the limb are shown together with a well distiguished command menu with sorted buttons corresponding to the expected user's actions (Fig.1). The surgeon identifies the 'ideal' limb mechanical axis in the two scout views (the line connecting the hip center and the ankle center passing through the knee center), adjusting three geometrical frame-markers (a circle for the ankle center a cross for the knee center and a rectangle for the ankle center) to the patient's anatomy by drag and drop with the mouse. Two buttons, called UNDO and REDO, allow the surgeon to move across the ten latest performed actions. Moreover there is a DATA button that provides the surgeon with the information about the realignment angle: this is computed on the frontal scout view of the patient limb and is the 2D angle between the line joining the hip center and the center of the distal part of the femur and the line between the proximal tibia center and the ankle center.

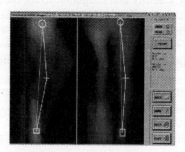

Fig. 1. Alignment phase

In the second planning step, the positioning phase (Fig.2), the surgeon defines the orientation, placement and size of the two prosthetic components. In this phase, the user interface includes four data windows: the frontal and the lateral projection of the joint (X-rays like image computed from CT data), a window displaying sections of the bone computed in any user's desired position and orientation and a windows with the 3D reconstruction of the joint.

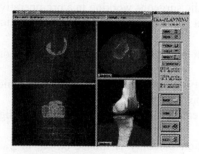

Fig. 2. Positioning phase

During the positioning phase, the arrangement of the components can be verified and interactively adjusted by the surgeon using the system tools: he can drag the prosthesis with the mouse onto a frontal projection, lateral and arbitrary oriented section planes of the knee joint. All the images can be zoomed and the system provides the surgeon with some 3D measures, such as current correction angle, that help the surgeon to verify if the current one is the desired result.

Moreover a command menu is present on the screen, with a position, layout and organization similar to that of the previous phase. It includes buttons similar to the previous ones and specific command buttons: UNDO and REDO, whose task is the same as for the alignment phase, RESET, that allows the system to restore the initial state, FEMUR and TIBIA that are the two buttons to enter the two prosthesis databases. These databases includes the prosthesis templates of different sizes both for the femur and for the tibia.

3.2 Evaluation of the Implemented CAS HCI

The evaluation was performed recording users' comments and suggestions and by means of a questionnaire based interview. The main outcomes have been summarized in three groups, one for each aspect described in §2.2.

As concerns the user's satisfaction about the system, the surgeons expressed positive judgements on data issuing methods: patients' data are loaded only one time at the beginning of the planning session, choosing the patient directly from a list. During all the planning session the system shows both patient's CT images and information (name, leg on which is planned to intervene) derived directly from patient's CT slice header; this way the surgeon is guaranteed that the patient is the right one, without any effort.
About issuing methods during the interaction with the system, the most appreciated aspect is that data are issued according only through the mouse, avoiding the shifting from the board to the mouse and back.
Other aspects that have been appreciated are that the visualisation of the areas used to issue data are sufficiently clear, even because the surgeon can easily zoom the images' areas he is interested in, and the fact that the data issuing rhythm is defined by the user and not imposed by the system: the surgeon can take as much time as he needs to fulfil any task.
Moreover the user's actions and the system's reactions are similar as concerns similar and always predictable actions and the set of words used to control the operations' sequence is always coherent.
Finally the transactions' sequence is logic from the user's point of view, reflecting the steps of the surgical technique.

In order to increase the software usability, users have suggested to introduce the visualization of the scale according which values are represented and what they refers to (for instance, angular values are visualized, but is not clear what they are referring to). Moreover, it could also be useful to visualize within a defined area of the screen an hint concerning data to be issued in order to fulfill the planning phase.
The prosthesis and the tools in general should be represented with the least number of particulars, so that the references on the underneath CT image remains as much as possible visible.
Finally the surgeons would be pleased to have a results' preview, to be sure of his work be correct.

Among the valuations done by an independent scientist in order to assess user's fatigue in using HCI, noteworthy is the fact that windows are never superimposed and the working area is very well organized, with all the information and buttons on the left of the screen and the patient's images on the other side. Buttons are labeled with self explanatory commands and correspondent buttons remains the same in all the phases (for instance, the EXIT button appears in all the phases, always in the same position)
Moreover has been appreciated the fact that there is always an immediate feedback between what appears on the screen and the issued or the given command: the system does not suffer delays in detecting the position of the cursor, the cursor itself is

always stable and visible, and when time needed at the end of the reckoning it is correctly shown through an indicator.

The lines tracking avails itself of the elastic effect, which allows to see immediately how the traced line will come out.

Further aspects positively valued have been that data can be cancelled or modified only by the user(only in one particular situation the user can delete data without being informed; we will describe this situation among the features that have to be included in the system in order to improve the usability), and that data processing starts always explicitly: the computer does never take the control automatically and in case of error's messages the program's execution is not interrupted.

Finally there is no chance of messing the system's messages and helps although the system never overload the user with too much information.

In order to improve the system's usability and to reduce the user's fatigue, some features have been suggested to be introduced, like a messages asking if data are required to be cancelled whenever destructive actions are carried (RESET) or asking if it is really required to exit and save the configuration currently on at the exit from the operative phase. Moreover it should be possible to save the intermediate data and eventually to go back automatically to the saved configuration.

Another feature that should be introduced is to unable buttons and tools when these are not usable.

Finally the cursor should vary the shape according to the area which is in. The use of the arrow cursor is not the best one in a graphic work area (a cross should probably be better).

Testing results concerning the planning repeatability are shown in Table 1.

TKA Computer Planning	
Accuracy of measures done on scout images (± 1 pixel)	0.6 mm
Accuracy of measures done on images derived from slices (± 1 pixel)	0.3 mm
Repeatability of interactive anatomical choices (anatomical points identification)	3.8 mm
Repeatability of interactive anatomical choices (long mechanical axis identification)	1 °
System's reliability (anatomical points identification)	6.2 mm
System's reliability (mechanical axis identification)	1.2 °

Table 1- Testing results

4 Discussion

It is difficult to evaluate if the proposed approach is "optimal", but we just observe that the general user's feeling is easy of use and confidence in the outcome (22 over 27.75, about 80%), that the use of the HCI is consistent and focused on the most important parameters. In fact the planner outcomes are very repeatable especially in the significant final variables, i.e. the mechanical axis (variability of 1° for the same surgeon and 1.2° for different surgeons).These data are the most important in Table 1, because determine the automatic prosthesis initial placement; the results show that the indication for the limb realignment guarantees quantitative reliable results.

Another important and original aspect of this paper is the proposed evaluation method. It is a new method, only partially inspired to standard techniques [3] [4] [5] [6] and absent in the previous descriptions of CAS system and also TKR planning[10] [11][13] [14].

We have proposed a detailed description of the main issues in the evaluation procedure (§2.2) and verified that in our TKR planning software they were able to provide useful indications of the HCI efficacy and also on further developments of its design and functionality. In particular the user's indications and the objective observation have allowed to correct mainly the user's interaction modality, increase the number of information that the user can easily handle, and this result confirm the impression that even a careful and systematic method to HCI design should be always followed by a similar careful and systematic testing phase, able to optimize the specific software outcome.

We remark that the methodological guidelines and most of the specific observations can be useful to other groups developing or testing surgical planners(especially in orthopaedics).

Moreover we underline that also surgical training systems and surgical navigation platforms share a similar data treatment and HCI layout, because the final goal is still an image guided definition of the optimal surgical strategy(preoperatively in our case, in simulation modality in training systems, intraoperatively in navigation platforms).

Therefore these kind of applications can benefit directly from the proposed approach to HCI design and evaluation. However this approach cannot yet be extended simply to registration or execution HCI for robotic or automatic systems, but just represent a first step toward a standardized procedure to design efficient and safe HCI in CAS systems.

References

1 "Computer Assisted Orthopedic Surgery (CAOS)", by L.P. Nolte and R. Ganz (eds.), Hogrefe Huber Publishers, Seattle-Toronto-Bern, 1999, ISBN 0-88937-168-7.

2. Taylor, R.H. , S. Lavalée. Computer Integrated Surgery. Cambridge: MIT Press, 1996.
   Clinical Orthopaedics and Related Research, Number 354 September 1998 (Special issue).
   Patkin M., Isabel L., "Ergonomics, engineering & surgery of endo_dissection" J. R. Coll. Surg. Edinb., 40 –April 1995.

3. Sater-Black K., Iversen N. "How to conduct a design review" Mechanical Eng., 89-92, March 1994

4. Picard F., Tourne Y., Saragaglia D. "Computer Assisted Knee Replacement/Ergonomic Evaluation" Proceedings of the Millennium Symposium on Computer Assisted Orthopaedics Surgery(CAOS 2000), Davos (Switzerland), February 17-19, 2000.

5. Zimolong a., Radermacher K., Mengel M., Friedrichs D., Rau G. "User-Interface and Input-Devices for the CRIGOS Surgical Robot" Proceedings of the Millennium Symposium on

Computer Assisted Orthopaedics Surgery(CAOS 2000), Davos (Switzerland), February 17-19, 2000.

6. Vendruscolo P., Martelli s., "Interfaces for computer and robot assisted surgical systems", Information and Software Technology, Vol. 43, N. 2 , pp. 87 - 96 , 2001 (Feb)

7. Ollson E., Boralv E., Goransson B., Sandblad B., "Domain specific style guides – design and implementation" Proceedings of the Motif and COSE International User Conference, Washington DC, 133 – 139 (1993).

8. Ameritech Standard for information systems, Ameritech services, 1993, 1994, 1995, 1996.

9. Smith S.L., Mosier J.N., "Guidelines for designing user interface software", the MITRE Corporation, 1986.

10. Fadda M., Bertelli D., Martelli S., Marcacci M., Dario P., Paggetti C., Caramella D., Trippi D.: "Computer assisted planning for total knee arthroplasty". In "Lecture Notes in Computer Science: CVRMed - MRCAS'97", Vol. 1205, Troccaz, Grimson and Mösges Eds., Springer (ISBN 3-540-62734), 619-28 , 1997.

11. Delp S.L., Stulberg S.D., Davies B., Picard F., Leiter F. "Computer Assisted Knee Replacement". Clin Ort. 354:51-56, 1998.

12. Martelli S., Marcacci M. et al. "Computer and robot assisted total knee replacement: analysis of a new surgical procedure". Annals of biomedical engineering Vol. 28 1-8, 2000

13. Muller W., Bockholt U., Voss G., Lahmer A., Borner M., "Planning System for Computer Assisted Total Knee Replacement" In Medicine Meets Virtual Reality- J.D. Westwood et al. (eds) IOS Press 214-219, 2000.

14. Wolsiffer K., Kalender W.A. "A feasibility study on computer assisted planning of total knee replacement surgery" Proceedings of the Millennium Symposium on Computer Assisted Orthopaedics Surgery(CAOS 2000), Davos (Switzerland), February 17-19, 2000.

Independent Registration and Virtual Controlled Reduction of Pelvic Ring Fractures

T. Hüfner[1], M. Citak[1], S. Tarte[2], J. Geerling[1], T. Pohlemann[4], H. Rosenthal[3], L.P. Nolte[2] and C. Krettek, M.D.[1]

[1] Trauma Department, Hannover Medical School, 30625 Hannover, Germany
Hüfner.Tobias@mh-hannover.de
[2] Department for Orthopedic Biomechanics, M. E. Müller Institute, Bern, Switzerland
[3] Radiology Dept., Hannover Medical School, Hannover, Germany
[4] Trauma Department, University of Saarland, 66421 Homburg, Germany

Abstract: This study presents a new developed software module for Computer Assisted Surgery (Surgigate, Medivision, Oberdorf, Switzerland), allowing independent registration of two fragments and real time virtual representation while reduction occurs.
Three fracture models were used to evaluate the accuracy: geometric foam blocks, a pelvic ring injury with symphysis and disruption of SI-joint and a pelvic ring fracture with symphysis disruption and transforaminal sacral fracture. One examiner performed both visual and virtual controlled reduction. To measure the residual displacement a magnetic motion tracking device was used. The results revealed significantly increased residual displacement with virtual compared with visual control. The differences were low, averaging 1 mm residual translation and 0.7° angulation respectively. This residual displacement may not be clinically relevant. Further development of the software prototype as integration of surface registration may lead to improved handling and facilitated multifragment tracking. Use in the clinical setting seems possible within a short time.

1 Introduction

Computer assisted surgery was introduced to increase the accuracy of selected procedures in orthopaedic and trauma surgery. Current clinically available software modules for CT based optoelectronic navigation systems are restricted to navigate a limited number of instruments or implants (pointer, chisels, pedicle probe, drill) within one solid bony structure. A real time visualization of fragment manipulation is not available for clinical applications, yet.
However, reduction is one of the key procedures in fracture surgery and can influence the immediate course of an operation, but the quality of reduction also directly affects the long-term outcome in the many cases. fractures This has been reported in several series especially for pelvic ring and acetabular fractures.
Within the current study we evaluated a new developed software for accuracy allowing independent registration and tracking of fragments.

W. Niessen and M. Viergever (Eds.): MICCAI 2001, LNCS 2208, pp. 1107-1113, 2001.
© Springer-Verlag Berlin Heidelberg 2001

2 Material and Methods

For the experiments a commercially Navigation system was used (Surgigate® Medivision, Oberdorf, Switzerland). The system included an Ultra 10 workstation (SUN Microsystems, Palo Alto, CA,) and an Optotrak 3020 optoelectronic localizer (Northern Digital Inc., Waterloo, Canada).

An alpha-version software for virtual controlled reduction based on standard software (Surgigate® Medivision, Oberdorf, Switzerland) was developed in cooperation with the Maurice Müller Institute of Biomechanics in Berne, Switzerland. The reduction software was developed within two major software platforms (imaging Application Platform -Cedara, Missassuga, Canada and Open Inventor, SGI, Mountain View, CA). The combination of this software allows the system to work with volumetric datasets (Voxel graphic) extracted from conventional CT datasets and surface models (vector graphics). The automatic generation of surface models from voxel data enables real time tracking of bone fragment motion. Currently registration is limited to paired-point matching and tracking is limited to two fragments.

2.1 Fracture Models

Commercially available plastic models (n=2) of the whole bony pelvic ring and osteoligamentous anatomic specimens (n=2) were used for similar experiments. Two different injury types were created:
combined symphysis and SI-joint disruption AO/OTA61 C 1.2 [1] and combined symphysis disruption and transforaminal sacral fracture AO/OTA 61 C 1.3 [1]
From each single object CT data were acquired (Somatom +4, Siemens, Erlangen, Germany) (140 kV, 171 mA, slice thickness 2mm, reconstruction index 2 mm, pitch 1 mm). After preoperative segmentation and surface model generation a dynamic reference base was attached to each fragment. Registration was done paired point with four titanium fiducials close to the fracture lines.

2.2 Measurement Devices

The fragments were fixed to 3D-arms allowing three-dimensional manipulation and easy fixation within a certain position (Figure 1). For measurement of the accuracy of reduction an electromagnetic three-dimensional tracking system was attached to the fragments and calibrated in a secure distance to metal bodies (Polhemus, Colchester, VT). The accuracy of the system was specified and tested by calibration with 0.1 mm in the translational planes (x, y and z planes), and 0.1° angulation deviation within the angles α, β and γ. The data processing was done with a new developed software.

For the reduction set-up the Pohlemus motion sensor was attached to each of the fragments (Figures 1, 2). The sensors were attached to the fragments by 105 mm plastic rods to avoid metallic artifacts affecting the electromagnetic motion tracker. The motion tracker unit was calibrated to an error less than 0.1 mm and 0.1° angulation. A data acquisition rate of 1 Hz was used.

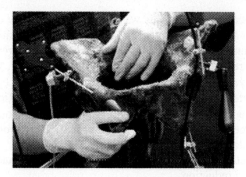

Fig. 1: For definition of the zero position the examiner reduces the fracture with full apposition without a step-off. Then, the motion tracker is calibrated to the zero position. In the same fashion visual controlled reduction takes place.

2.3 Reduction Protocol

First, the reduction under direct visualization and using tactile information was performed (Figure 2). Reduction was defined as complete fragment apposition without any step-off. This position was used to calibrate the motion tracker system to the start-up position with all axes and angles reset to zero.

One examiner did the reduction without limitation of time using two different methods: visual controlled reduction with full direct sight and tactile information for definition of the ideal results (n = 20) and solely virtual controlled reduction with the examiner completely blinded to the object only with monitor sight and manipulating only the 3D-arms (n = 20) (Fig. 2).

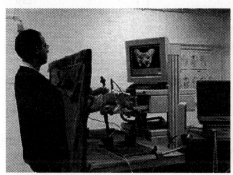
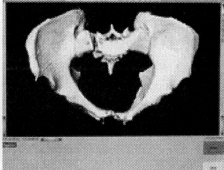

Fig. 2a: With virtual controlled reduction the examiner is blinded to the fracture model itself.

Fig. 2b: The virtual display allows all views, as an inlet view displayed here in this C 1.3 fracture.

The experiment was started after registration when the calculated system error within the navigation system was less than 1 mm, otherwise the registration was repeated. The endpoint of the experiment was defined as the position judged by the examiner as position of anatomical reduction. This was done using the view on the monitor. The 3D-arms were then fixed rigidly preserving the end-point position. Data recording was continued for another 10 seconds in the end position to create stable end point measurements. The residual displacement was measured in the x, y and z planes (mm) and in the α, β and γ angles (degrees). The ASCII data provided by the motion tracker system were imported to an Excel spreadsheet (Microsoft, Richmond, WA.) The resulting reduction accuracy was calculated using Euclidean geometry $d = \sqrt{x^2 + y^2 + z^2}$. The Euclid distance (translation) and the residual angulations were calculated compared with the start-up (zero) position.

A comparison of outcomes was done using systematic error analysis between direct and virtual controlled reduction.

Statistical analysis was done using the Levene test and a nonpaired t test. Significance level was set at $p < 0.05$. All analyses were performed using commercially available statistical software (SPSS, SPSS Inc, Chicago, IL).

3 Results

Pelvic Models and Specimen

C 1.2 injury. The residual translation is shown in Figures 3. Virtual controlled reduction led to increased residual translation compared with visual controlled reduction for foam models and specimen ($p < 0.01$), the average maximum deviation was 0.7 mm for the virtual-group.

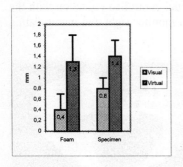
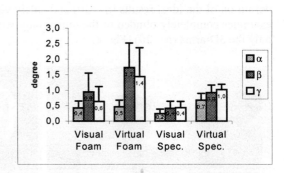

Fig. 3a: The residual translation (Euclid distance) was small after both, visual and virtual controlled reduction. With visual controlled reduction a significant lower residual translation was achieved compared to virtual control (p<0,01). No significant difference was appreciated between foam models and specimen (p>0,05).

Fig. 3b: Foam models: the residual angulation was lower only for the □-angle (p<0,01). Specimen: visual lead to lower residual angulation for all angles compared to virtual controlled reduction (p<0,05). The residual angulation of the specimen pelvis was lower compared to the foam pelvis models (p<0,05).

After visual controlled reduction of the foam pelvis the residual angulation was less only for the and γ angle (Figure 8). The differences averaged 0.3° for the α angle, and 0.7° for the β and γ angles respectively.

Compared with virtual controlled reduction visual controlled reduction with the pelvis specimen led to significantly lower residual angulation (p < 0.05).

The residual angulation of the pelvis specimen was lower than the foam models for visual and virtual controlled reduction (p < 0.05).

C 1.3 injury. With virtual controlled reduction residual translation was increased compared with visual control. The difference averaged 0.7 mm. With virtual controlled reduction residual angulation for foam models was increased for the γ angle only (p < 0.05), whereas with the pelvis specimen virtual controlled reduction led to increased β and γ angles (p < 0.05) compared with visual reduction. Generally the specimen models had lower residual angulation compared with the foam models (p < 0.05).

4 Discussion

The value of currently available navigation systems has been reported in several studies. Several standard procedures, e.g. pedicle screw insertion, pelvic osteotomies and cup and shaft implantation of hip prostheses require high intraoperative precision have been included in the available software [2-7]. However, these applications are limited to one bone or one fragment. In trauma surgery CT based optoelectronic systems have been used for pelvic fracture surgery, including internal fixation of pelvic ring fractures or pelvic nonunion [8, 9]. But these were situations with no further fracture movement.

Langlotz et al. introduced a new software for CAS controlled periacetabular osteotomies that allows the independent tracking of a second fragment [2]. Here the primary registration is limited to the intact pelvis and the second fragment can be generated only virtually. This software has been used successfully for osteotomies and reduction control in late reconstructions of malhealed pelvic ring fractures [10].

The software version introduced in this study overcomes these limitations by the option of independent and repetitive registration of each fragment and real time movement tracking of both. Although only paired-point registration is available, yet, it was sufficient for accurate virtual reduction control in this set-up. Furthermore the segmentation algorithm and generation of the surface models seemed reliable for foam models and specimens.

In some studies, accuracy analyses of CAS systems are related to the examination of the imaging technique [11], the camera unit [12, 13], the registration algorithms [14, 15] or to overall clinical applications. [2, 7, 16-19].

However, for the surgeon the overall clinically relevant error, as defined by Maciunas et al. [13] is a more relevant factor. This comprises the errors associated with imaging, registration and the technical accuracy of the CAS system. A standard acceptable error cannot be provided, because this is dependent on the application and the primary diagnosis.

The current set-up focused on the clinically relevant issue of residual displacement after the process of pelvic ring reduction being monitored and controlled either by the sight and tactile information or visual control. The use of an high precision three-dimensional magnetic based motion tracking device, the set-up, and the repetition of the experiments was facilitated and three-dimensional datasets were available.

The results showed differences between visual and virtual control of reduction, however, both groups are within a range which is accepted as an anatomic result when applied clinically to the evaluation of pelvic reduction.

The missing soft tissue envelope which influences the quality of a closed reduction is a disadvantage of the model used in the current study. Additional experiments are planned with a more realistic set-up. The lower residual angulations seen in the specimen compared with foam models seem to be attributable to a better fit of the fragments after reduction was done.

This new developed software module allows simultaneous, independent registration of two fragments and real time representation of both fragments. This led to reproducible high precision when used for virtually controlled reduction in this experimental set-up. Integration of surface registration and enhanced surface model generation as further developments may lead to improved handling and multifragment tracking. Use in the clinic seems possible within a short time.

References

1.   Orthopedic Trauma Association Committee for coding and classification, *Fracture and dislocation compendium*. J Orthop Trauma, 1996. **10**(Suppl 1): p. V-IX.

2.   Langlotz F, et al., *The first twelve cases of computer assisted periacetabular osteotomy*. Comput Aided Surg, 1997. **2**: p. 317-326.

3.   Langlotz F, et al., *Computer Assistance for Pelvic Osteotomies*. Clin Orthop, 1998. **354**: p. 92-102.

4.   Langlotz U, et al. *A novel system for complete THR planning and intraoperative free-hand navigation*. in *CAOS Computer Assisted Orthopaedic Surgery*. 2000. Davos, Switzerland.

5.   Lavallee, S., et al., *Computer-assisted spine surgery: a technique for accurate transpedicular screw fixation using CT data and a 3-D optical localizer*. J Image Guid Surg, 1995. **1**(1): p. 65-73.

6.   Lavallée S, et al., *Computer-assisted Spine Surgery Using Anatomy-based Registration.*, in *Computer-Integrated Surgery*, Taylor R, et al., Editors. 1996, MIT Press: Cambridge.

7.   Laine T, et al. *Accuracy of pedicle srew insertion with and without computer assistance - A randomized controlled clinical study in 100 consecutive patients*. in *CAOS Computer Assisted Orthopaedic Surgery*. 2000. Davos, Switzerland.

8.   Kahler DM, Zura RD, and Mallik K. *Computer guided placement of iliosacral screws compared to standard fluoroscopic technique*. in *5th Symposium on CAOS Computer Assisted Orthopaedic Surgery*. 2000. Davos.

9.   Zura, R.D. and D.M. Kahler, *A transverse acetabular nonunion treated with computer-assisted percutaneous internal fixation. A case report*. J Bone Joint Surg Am, 2000. **82**(2): p. 219-24.

10.   Hüfner T, et al. *Computer assisted surgery for correction of a malhealed pelvic ring fracture in a young female patient*. in *4th CAOS Computer Assisted Orthopedic Surgery*. 1999. Davos.

11.   Schneider, J., *Risikomanagement in der Medizintechnik. Methodik zur Überprüfung der geometrischen genauigkeit CT-basierter Verfahren in der computer-unterstützten Therapie.*, in *Medizinische Fakultät.* 2000, Friedrich-Alexander-Universität: Erlangen-Nürnberg. p. 87.

12.   Chassat F and Lavallee S. *Experimental protocol of accuracy evaluation of 6-D localizers for computer-integrated surgery: application to four optical localizers.* in *Proceedings of the First International Conference on Medical image computing and computer-assisted intervention - MICCAI '98.* 1998. Berlin Heidelberg: Springer.

13.   Maciunas, R.J., R.L. Galloway, Jr., and J.W. Latimer, *The application accuracy of stereotactic frames.* Neurosurgery, 1994. **35**(4): p. 682-94; discussion 694-5.

14.   Bächler R, *Oberflächenbasierte Registrierung für orthopädische und HNO-Anwendungen.*, in *Philosophisch-naturwissenschaftliche Fakultät.* 2000, Universität Bern: Bern, Switzerland. p. 114.

15.   Hüfner T, et al. *Registration using a modified external fixateur system for the pelvis.* in *5th International Symposium on CAOS.* 2000. Davos.

16.   Laine, T., et al., *Accuracy of pedicle screw insertion: a prospective CT study in 30 low back patients.* Eur Spine J, 1997. **6**(6): p. 402-5.

17.   Nolte LP, et al., *Image-guided insertion of transpedicular screws.* Spine, 1995. **20**(4): p. 497 - 500.

18.   Merloz, P., et al., *Pedicle screw placement using image guided techniques.* Clin Orthop, 1998(354): p. 39-48.

19.   Vandervelde D, Mahieu G, and Nuyts R. *Reduction in the variability of acetabular cup positioning using computer assisted surgery.* in *CAOS Computer Assisted Orthopaedic Surgery.* 2000. Davos.

Optimization in Prostate Cancer Detection

Ariela Sofer[1], Jianchao Zeng[2], and Seong K. Mun[2]

[1] Department of Systems Engineering and Operations Research
George Mason University, Fairfax, VA 22030
asofer@gmu.edu
http://www.gmu.edu/departments/ore/sofer.html
[2] Imaging Science and Information Systems Center (ISIS)
Department of Radiology, Georgetown University Medical Center
zeng@isis.imac.georgetown.edu (J. Zeng)
http://www.simulation.georgetown.edu

Abstract. Clinical diagnosis of prostate cancer is most often done by transrectal ultrasound-guided needle biopsy. Because of the low resolution of ultrasound, however, the urologist cannot usually distinguish between cancerous and healthy tissue. Therefore, most biopsies follow standard protocols based on long-term physician experience. Recent studies indicate that these protocols may have a significant rate of false negative diagnoses. This research develops optimized biopsy protocols. We use real prostate specimens removed by prostatectomy to develop a 3D distribution map of cancer in the prostate. We develop also a probability model of the needle insertion procedure. Using this model, the tumor map, and the geometry of the biopsy needle, we obtain estimates for the probability of obtaining a positive biopsy in various zones of prostates with cancer. We develop a nonlinear optimization problem that determines the protocols that maximize the probability of cancer detection for a given number of needles, and present new optimized protocols.

1 Introduction

Prostate cancer is the most prevalent male malignancy and the second leading cause of death by cancer in American men. The American Cancer Society estimates that there will be about 198,100 new cases of prostate cancer in the United States in 2001, and about 32,000 men will die of the disease. Current screening for the cancer includes the prostate specific antigen (PSA) test and the digital rectal exam. However the cancer can only be correctly diagnosed by needle biopsy of the prostate and histopathology of the sampled tissues. The most common technique for detection of prostate cancer is transrectal ultrasound-guided (TRUS) needle core biopsy.

Since normal prostate tissue cannot usually be differentiated from cancerous tissue during the biopsy, a number of standard protocols have been developed to assist the urologist in performing the biopsy. The protocol most commonly used is the systematic sextant biopsy [4]. Recent studies [1], [7] have shown, however, that this strategy has an unacceptable level of false negative diagnoses, and that

W. Niessen and M. Viergever (Eds.): MICCAI 2001, LNCS 2208, pp. 1114–1121, 2001.

many patients who have a negative initial biopsy are found to have cancer in repeat biopsies.

As a result, recent clinical studies have investigated new protocols that have higher detection rates [2], [3]. The improvement in detection is obtained by using additional needles (up to seven more) in the biopsy.

Our approach is different: our goal is to develop optimized biopsy protocols. For a specified number of needles, an optimal protocol is one that maximizes the probability of detection of cancer in a patient. The hope is that with optimized protocols one could achieve improved detection rates with fewer needles.

A major component of our effort is the development of a statistical distribution map of cancer in the prostate. The map is constructed from cancerous prostates that were removed via prostatectomy. Each of the prostates is first reconstructed into a 3D computerized model that accurately represent the anatomy of the prostate, and the distribution of cancer within it. Next, each model is divided into zones based on clinical conventions, and the presence of cancer in each zone is calculated. From this the 3D distribution map of tumor location is developed. Thus far, 301 prostates have been reconstructed and analyzed.

We have previously established a statistical distribution map and optimal biopsy protocols for a 48-zone division of the prostate [8], [10]. The rationale for the division is that it is likely the upper limit on the number of zones that can still be accessible by the physician. A drawback of the model, however, is that it assumes that a biopsy taken in a cancerous zone is bound to be positive. In practice, it is possible that a biopsy in a cancerous zone will be negative.

In this paper we address this issue. Although we still maintain a coarse grid (i.e., the 48-zone division) for the purpose of biopsy guidance for the physician, we use a much finer grid for the development of a cancer distribution map. Each of the 48 zones is thus further divided to a larger number of subzones, with each subzone smaller in volume (and sometimes much smaller) than the needle core size. The presence of cancer is evaluated in each subzone to create a fine-grid cancer distribution map. This information is then used to estimate, for each patient, the probability that a biopsy in a given zone will be positive, and in turn, the probability that a given biopsy protocol will detect cancer. This leads to more accurate estimates of detection rates, and improved biopsy protocols.

2   Reconstruction of the Prostate Models and Statistical Distribution Map

The reconstruction of the prostates involved several steps [9]. Each prostate was sectioned in 4μm sections at 2.25mm intervals, and each slice was digitized with a scanning resolution of 1500 dots per inch. Each digitized image was segmented by a pathologist to identify the key pathological structures, including surgical margins, capsule, urethra, seminal vesicle, and the tumor. The contours of each structure were identified on each slice, and then stacked up. Interpolation between pairs of contours was performed using a 3D elastic contour model. The 3D model of each structure in the prostate was finalized by tiling triangular patches onto the interpolated contours, using a deformable surface-spine model.

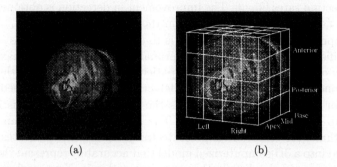

(a)   (b)

Fig. 1. Figure 1: 3D reconstruction of prostate models: (a) Final 3D reconstructed prostate model. (b) 48-zone grid superimposed over prostate.

Next we determine the statistical distribution map. The coarse grid 48-zone coarse grid used for biopsy guidance is illustrated in Figure 1. The grid has three transverse layers, base, mid, and apex. Each such layer is further divided into four coronal layers, which, following clinical conventions, are labeled from the posterior to the anterior as posterior 1, posterior 2, anterior 1, and anterior 2 respectively. Finally, the layers are divided from left to right into four sagittal layers, denoted as left lateral, left mid, right mid, and right lateral, respectively. It is noted that the size of the zones will vary with the size of a prostate model. A larger prostate model ends up with having a larger size for each of its 48 zones. This variation of zone sizes is the natural and consistent reflection of the original prostate, and it should not affect the accuracy of cancer distributions.

For determination of the statistical distribution map, each of the course-grid compartments is further divided to smaller subzones. We have used a total of 5^3 subzones per zone, so that the final grid superimposed over the prostate has 6000 subzones. The occurrence of cancer is calculated in each of the subzones for each of the patients; a subzone is considered positive for a given patient if it contains any part of a cancer. Subzones that contain no prostate tissue are marked accordingly.

Next, we estimate for each patient and for each of the coarse-grid zones, the probability that a needle biopsy in the zone will detect cancer. To ensure accuracy we will model the variability in the physician's placement of the needle. Specifically for each of the 48 zones we model (i) the depth of the needle insertion point (from apex to base); (ii) the longitudinal position of the needle insertion point (from posterior to anterior) and (iii) the firing angle of the needle. (Note that the physician controls the firing angle by rotating the ultrasound probe around its axis; there is only one degree of freedom, since the needle has a fixed angle with respect to the axis of the ultrasound probe.) We now assume that for each zone the three corresponding random variables controlling the needle trajectory are statistically independent Gaussian variables. (The parameters of these distributions will vary from zone to zone.) We then use a discretization of these distributions, to estimate for each patient, the probability that a needle probe in the zone will be positive. The analysis is based on the fine-grid cancer distribution map, the volume of each subzone, the geometry of the needle and the volume of the needle core.

3   The Optimization Problem

3.1   Problem Formulation

We now develop a mathematical model that determines the optimal locations for the biopsy needles based on the 3D cancer distribution model. The objective is to determine, for a specified number of needles, the protocol that maximizes the probability of detecting cancer. We note that while the detection rate increases with the number of needles, using optimized strategies could permit using fewer needles, thus avoiding patient discomfort and saving costs.

To formulate the problem, let n denote the number of zones in the coarse grid (here $n = 48$), and let m denote the number of patients in our sample ($m = 301$). Define variables x_j, $j = 1, \ldots, n$, by

$$x_j = \begin{cases} 1 \text{ if a biopsy is taken in zone } j, \\ 0 \text{ otherwise.} \end{cases}$$

Let p_{ij} be the estimated probability that a needle in zone j will detect cancer in patient i ($i = 1, \ldots, m$, $j = 1, \ldots, n$), and let $q_{ij} = 1 - p_{ij}$. We have that

$$(q_{ij})^{x_j} = \begin{cases} 1 & \text{if } x_j = 0 \\ q_{ij} & \text{if } x_j = 1. \end{cases}$$

Now in general, the occurrence of cancer in adjacent prostate zones is correlated. But for a given patient i in our sample the location of cancer is known, hence the occurrence of cancer is no longer a random variable (but its realization). In contrast, the outcome of a needle biopsy in a given zone for this patient is a random variable. The randomness is due only to the uncertainty in how the physician places the needle; if the placement of the needle were totally deterministic, the outcome of the needle biopsy would also be deterministic. Since the physician's positioning of different needles can be assumed to be statistically independent, the outcomes of needle biopsies in different zones can be assumed to be statistically independent. Thus the probability that a set of needle biopsies diagnoses cancer in patient i of our sample is

$$1 - \prod_{j=1}^{n} (q_{ij})^{x_j}.$$

It follows that the k-needle biopsy protocol that maximizes the probability of detection for a randomly selected patient in our sample solves

$$
\begin{aligned}
\text{maximize} \quad & \frac{1}{m} \sum_{i=1}^{m} (1 - \prod_{j=1}^{n} (q_{ij})^{x_j}) \\
\text{subject to} \quad & \sum_{j=1}^{n} x_j = k \\
& x_j \in \{0,1\}
\end{aligned}
\tag{1}
$$

Note that when scaled by m, the objective function is the expected number of patients in the sample to be diagnosed with cancer. Problem (1) can be written equivalently as

$$
\begin{aligned}
\text{minimize} \quad & \sum_{i=1}^{m} \prod_{j=1}^{n} (q_{ij})^{x_j} \\
\text{subject to} \quad & \sum_{j=1}^{n} x_j = k \\
& x_j \in \{0,1\}
\end{aligned}
\tag{2}
$$

Additional constraints reflecting physician preferences can also be added. For example, left-right symmetry of the protocols is obtained by the constraints $x_l = x_r$ for every pair of zones l and r that are left-right symmetric. One may also restrict biopsies to zones in the posterior area (since the anterior is more difficult to probe), by imposing the constraint $x_a = 0$ for all zones a in the anterior. For simplicity we will let X denote the feasible set—the set of vectors $x \in \{0,1\}$ that satisfy $\sum_{j=1}^{n} x_j = k$ and any additional desired constraint.

The optimization problem (2) is a nonlinear integer problem. In its current form the problem is difficult to solve, since its objective is a nonconvex function in the integer variables x_j. However we can transform it to a more tractable problem. Let ϵ be some (sufficiently) small positive tolerance (say, $\epsilon = 10^{-10}$), and define the $m \times n$ matrix U by $u_{ij} = -\log(\max\{q_{ij}, \epsilon\})$. Denoting $z_i = \sum_{j=1}^{n} u_{ij} x_j$, the optimization problem is equivalent to the problem

$$
\begin{aligned}
\text{minimize} \quad & \sum_{i=1}^{m} e^{-z_i} \\
\text{subject to} \quad & z - Ux = 0 \\
& x \in X
\end{aligned}
\tag{3}
$$

Although the resulting problem is still nonlinear and integer, the transformed form is more convenient, since the objective function is convex.

3.2 Solution of the Optimization Problem

To solve problem (3) we use a generalized decomposition algorithm [6] framework. The idea is to decompose the problem in a way that enables the creation of a sequence of easier subproblems that gradually provide tighter lower and upper bounds on the optimal objective. Here this is done as follows: We rewrite (3) as

$$\underbrace{\operatorname*{minimize}_{x \in X} \operatorname*{min}_{z} \quad g(z) = \sum e^{-z_i} \atop \text{subject to} \ z - Ux = 0}_{\text{primal problem}} \qquad (4)$$

Let $L(x, \lambda) = \sum_{i=1}^{m} e^{-z_i} - \lambda^T(z - Ux)$ be the Lagrangian for the primal problem. Now because the problem is convex, its objective is equal to that of its Lagrangian dual [6]. Hence (4) is equivalent to

$$\operatorname*{minimize}_{x \in X} \quad \operatorname*{max}_{\lambda} \operatorname*{min}_{z} \left(\sum e^{-z_i} - \lambda^T(z - Ux)\right). \qquad (5)$$

Problem (5) can be written in equivalent form

$$\operatorname*{minimize}_{x \in X, \delta} \quad \delta$$
$$\delta \geq \operatorname*{min}_{z}(\sum e^{-z_i} - \lambda^T(z - Ux)) \quad \forall \lambda$$

Suppose we start from an initial feasible integer point x^0. It is easy to show that for a given vector x^t, the solution to the primal problem in (4) is

$$z^t = Ux^t \quad \lambda_i^t = -e^{-z_i^t}.$$

This yields at iteration t an upper bound UB=min$\{UB, g(x^t\}$ on the optimal objective, where at iteration 0, UB=$g(z^0)$. Now given the iterates $x^0, \ldots, x^t$, the problem

$$\operatorname*{minimize}_{x \in X, \delta} \quad \delta$$
$$\delta \geq (\lambda^j)^T Ux + \sum e^{-z_i^j} - (\lambda^j)^T z^j, \quad j = 0, \ldots, t$$

is a "relaxation" of Problem 3.2, in the sense that it relaxes its constraints. Thus the solution provides a lower bound on the optimal objective LB=δ and a new starting x^{t+1} for the primal.

We can thus obtain a sequence of solutions to the primal problem and the dual problem, with the former yielding a nonincreasing sequence of upper bounds to the optimal objective value, and the latter yielding a nondecreasing sequence of lower bounds to this objective value. The algorithm terminates when the upper and lower bounds differ by less than a prescribed tolerance. The relaxed dual problems are linear programs with integer variables, and are easily solved by the software package ILOG CPlex 6.5 [5].

4   Optimized Protocols

We have obtained some preliminary results using the sample of 301 prostate analyzed so far. The resulting estimated detection rates for optimized 6-, 8-, and

10-needle biopsy protocols are shown in Table 1. As one can see, the estimated detection rate for our optimal 6-needle protocols is about 79%. In contrast, the estimated detection rate for the sextant method is about 67%. Thus it is possible to improve detection rates with 6 needles only, just by using optimized protocols. Additional needles will further improve the detection rates as indicated in the Table. The corresponding optimal biopsy protocols are shown in Table 2.

Table 1. Estimated detection rates with optimized symmetric protocols using 6, 8, and 10 needles. Estimated detection rate for sextant method is 67.3%

No. of Needles	Posterior Only	Entire Gland
6	78.8%	79.3%
8	81.6%	82.9%
10	84.2%	85.5%

5   Conclusions and Future Work

Preliminary results show that the optimal biopsy protocols have a substantial improvement over the protocols currently used clinically. Simulation using additional 100 prostate models is under way and initial results have also confirmed this improvement. A post-optimality sensitivity analysis will also be performed to assess the sensitivity of our solutions to the model's parameters.

A new generation of image-guided prostate biopsy system is now being developed. We are developing an image segmentation technique to acquire the boundary of a series of transverse ultrasound images of the prostate. These are used to construct a 3-D prostate surface model of the patient. The intersection of the ultrasound beam with the reconstructed 3-D model enables us to extract the corresponding cancer distribution information and optimized biopsy protocols and to superimpose the information onto the ultrasound image as highlighted grids. This information will significantly enhance the physicians' situation awareness and thus lead to a substantial improved performance of cancer detection.

Acknowledgements
Ariela Sofer is partially supported by National Science Foundation grant DMI-9800544. Jianchao Zeng is supported in part by The Whitaker Foundation Biomedical Engineering Program grant RG-99-0115. We wish to acknowledge the input of John J. Bauer (WRMC), Wei Zhang and Isabell A. Sesterhenn (AFIP), and Judd W. Moul (CPDR).

References

1. Bankhead C.: "Sextant biopsy helps in prognosis of Pca, but its not foolproof," Urology Times, Vol. 25, (1997) No. 8. (August).

Table 2. Optimal symmetric biopsy protocols for 6, 8, and 10 needles. x indicates a zone that is part of the biopsy; ll, lm, rm, and rl indicate left lateral, left mid, right mid, and right lateral respectively; p1, p2, a1, and a2 denote posterior 1 and 2, and anterior 1 and 2 respectively.

		Base				Mid				Apex			
		ll	lm	rm	rl	ll	lm	rm	rl	ll	lm	rm	rl
6 needles	a2												
	a1					x			x				
	p2										x	x	
	p1					x			x				
8 needles	a2												
	a1					x			x				
	p2	x			x						x	x	
	p1					x			x				
10 needles	a2												
	a1					x			x				
	p2	x			x						x	x	
	p1					x			x		x	x	

2. Chang J.J., Shinohara K., Bhargava V., Presti, J.C. Jr.: "Prospective evaluation of lateral biopsies of the peripheral zone for prostate cancer detection," J. Urology, Vol. 160, (1997), pp. 2111–2114.

3. Eskew, A.L., Bare,R.L., McCullough D.L.: "Systematic 5-region prostate biopsy is superior to sextant method for detecting carcinoma of the prostate." J. Urology, Vol. 157 (1997), pp. 199–202.

4. Hodge K.K, McNeal J.E., Terris M.K., and Stamey T.A.: "Random systematic versus directed ultrasound guided trans-rectal core biopsies of the prostate," J. Urology Vol. 142, (1989) pp. 71–74

5. ILOG CPLex 6.5 User Manual, ILOG, 1999.

6. Nash, S.G, and Sofer, A: Linear and Nonlinear Programming, McGraw Hill, 1996.

7. Rabbani F., Stroumbakis N., Kava B.R., Cookson M.S., and Fair W.R.: "Incidence and clinical significance of false-negtive sextant prostate biopsies," J. Urology Vol. 159 (1998), pp. 1247–1250.

8. Sofer, A., Zeng, J., Opell, B., Bauer, J., Mun, S.K., "Optimal Biopsy Protocols for Prostate Cancer," submitted for publication in Interfaces, October 2000.

9. Zeng, J., Bauer J.J., Yao X., Zhang W., Sesterhenn I.A., Connelly R.R., Moul J., and Mun S.K.: "Building an accurate 3D map of prostate cancer using computerized models of 280 whole-mounted radical prostatectomy specimens." Proc. of SPIE Medical Imaging Conference, Vol. 3976, 2000, pp. 466–477.

10. . Zeng, J., Bauer, J., Sofer, A., Yao, X., Opell, B., Zhang, W., Sestrehenn, I. A., Moul, J. W., Lynch, J., Mun, S. K.: Distribution of Prostate Cancer for Optimized Biopsy Protocols. In Proceedings of the Medical Image Computing and Computer Assisted Intervention Conference, 2000, pp. 287–296.

Automated Identification and B-spline Approximation of a Profiling Coil Centerline from Magnetic Resonance Images

S. Taivalkoski, L. Jyrkinen, and O. Silvén

Medical Imaging Research Group, University of Oulu, FINLAND
{staivalk, ljj}@ee.oulu.fi

Abstract. Incorporation of a radiofrequency coil extending over a length of the instrument body can be used in visualising long, flexible instruments such as catheters and guidewires in magnetic resonance. Acquiring images with this RF coil results in a profile of the coil. In this work, the algorithm for an automatic identification of the coil profile centerline is presented. The algorithm consists of image segmentation and consequent instrument profile approximation with B-spline curves. The performance of the algorithm was evaluated with two profiling coil designs.

1 Introduction

Magnetic resonance imaging (MRI) is a well established diagnostic method, the use of which is widening toward therapeutic procedures. Some minimally invasive operations in MR guidance have been done routinely for some time now. There are, however, many new challenges that the growing interest in using MRI in therapeutic procedures has raised. These need to be faced and met, if MRI is to settle its new role as an interventional modality. A crucial problem to solve is the real-time visualisation and guidance of interventional instruments.

The localisation of rigid instruments during an operation can be done quite easily and accurately by means of optical tracking [1]. However, the localisation of flexible instruments, like catheters and guidewires, is still problematic. Passive and active tracking and profiling have been proposed for monitoring the location of flexible instruments with an MR scanner [2]. Passive methods use signal voids and susceptibility artifacts for visualising instruments. Usually, no additional scanner hardware is needed. Sometimes contrast enhancing compounds or materials strengthening susceptibility artifacts are used to improve the visibility of the instrument. Active methods use either a miniature tracking RF coil embedded in the instrument or a longer profiling coil that detects signals along the length of the instrument. While tracking of the instrument tip provides information on the location of the tip position only, profiling shows the entire instrument body which is often desirable for flexible instruments.

The identification of instruments from MR images is required by both passive and active methods. Passive methods have proven more problematic in this respect [3]. It is difficult to attain a sufficient level of contrast necessary for clearly differentiating the instrument from the background. The reason for this is that thick slices are usually

W. Niessen and M. Viergever (Eds.): MICCAI 2001, LNCS 2208, pp. 1122–1129, 2001.

needed to ensure that the instrument is located within the imaging volume. In thick image slices, the instrument is easily lost in the ambient tissue because of partial volume effect. Furthermore, susceptibility artifacts used for gaining more contrast often distort the images.

Active profiling avoids the problems described above. In this method, signal is received only from the immediate vicinity of the profiling coil. This removes the partial volume distortion and gives a high contrast signal, which is not dependent on slice thickness. The slice selection gradient can be switched off, leading to a projection image of the profiling coil through the entire imaging volume like in x-ray fluoroscopy. Distortions may arise due to coil geometry, noise and possible signal voids in the coil surroundings. These distortions are, however, usually less severe than susceptibility artifacts in passive profiling.

So far the major effort has been devoted to making instruments visible in MR. Less attention has been paid to visualising the instruments and utilising location information of the instruments. A common visualisation method is to extract an outline of the instrument from the MR image and to overlay it on an anatomic road map image. As Ladd et al. [4] point out, precautions must be taken to ensure that the volume acquired for the road map contains the volume of anatomy where the instrument is to be manipulated, because the instrument may lie outside the road map volume. The use of instrument location information would remove this problem, since updates of the road map could be tied to the movements of the instrument. A 3-D model of the instrument contains complete information about the location, thus offering an ideal means of controlling image acquisition and of visualising the instrument from an appropriate direction.

We have demonstrated earlier that the three dimensional geometry and location of the instrument can be reconstructed from two to three projection images [5, 6]. The identification of profiling coil centerline from MR projection images is central to the 3-D reconstruction in our work. The centerline detection has been done semiautomatically in our former studies. Likewise, Bender et al. [7] have applied semiautomatic centerline detection for x-ray images as a part of their 3-D reconstruction algorithm. However, the need for a fully automated algorithm is evident. Semiautomatic centerline detection demands some user action to help the detection, typically selecting a starting point and a direction for the centerline. This is unacceptable if the goal is to use the algorithm in a real-time instrument guidance system.

The aim of this work has been to develop a fully automated centerline detection algorithm that is versatile and well-suited for the requirements of 3-D reconstruction. The centerline detection should be fast, and it should be able to handle images of various types of profiling coils. In addition, the algorithm should avoid any impractical restrictions of discontinuous instrument profiles and limited curvature of the centerline, which have been reported earlier [5].

2   Methods

2.1   Segmentation of the Centerline

The centerline detection algorithm can be divided into two main steps: centerline segmentation and spline fitting. The centerline detection begins with image segmentation.

The purpose of segmentation is to extract pixels belonging to a catheter from the background of MR images. The profiling coil excites spins and receives signals from only the immediate vicinity of the catheter. Thus the major part of the background in MR images is dark due to lack of signal. The surroundings of the profiling coil appear as a bright prolonged structure.

The background noise that complicates segmentation can be estimated to follow the Rician distribution [8]. In theory, although it would be possible to find the parameters of the noise distribution from images and then remove the noise with a suitable filter, the small number of signal pixels in an image, typically just a few per cent, makes this approach unpractical. We chose to filter the background applying several filters in cascade.

In background filtering, conditional dilation is applied first. This is a standard algorithm for noise reduction when the objects to be segmented are spatially simple and connected compared to the noise. Conditional dilation thresholds the grey scale MR image with high and low threshold values. For the upper threshold, we have used a value that selects 1 % of the brightest image pixels and for the lower threshold one that selects 4 % of the brightest pixels. Thresholding with the high value creates a binary image in which the pixels that are binary-1 belong almost certainly to the catheter. However, a number of pixels belonging to the catheter remain binary-0 labelled. Thresholding with the lower value creates another binary image in which almost all the pixels that belong to the catheter are labelled binary-1. There are, however, many binary-1 labelled noise pixels that are misdetected and not part of the catheter. Conditional dilation fills out the high thresholded image to the bounds allowed by the lower thresholded image without including spatially disconnected noise in the result image. This produces a binary image, in which binary-1 pixels are potential catheter pixels and binary-0 pixels belong to the background.

Small isolated groups of binary-1 pixels that still remain after conditional dilation are most probably caused by the noise. They are removed by applying erosion with a small kernel. Medial axis transformation is applied to the remaining binary-1 pixels. The purpose of this is to thin the centerline path so that only the pixels in the neighbourhood of the centerline are retained. The reduced number of pixels speeds up calculations during the following spline fitting procedure.

2.2   Spline Fitting

Prior to spline fitting, the segmented data points have to be ordered. The travelling salesman algorithm is used for this. The travelling salesman algorithm searches for the shortest path through the segmented data points without returning to the start point. The ordered data points form the input data set for spline fitting algorithm.

The segmented and ordered centerline data is represented in a compact mathematical form by fitting an approximating B-spline curve to the recognised data points. B-splines are a standard way of representing curves on computers. In this context, it is possible to give only a brief summary on the topic based on [9] to illustrate the calculation of B-splines.

The B-spline curve is defined by introducing the concepts of knots and basis functions. A nondecreasing sequence of real numbers $U = \{u_0, ..., u_m\}$, where $u_i \leq$

u_{i+1}, $i = 0, ..., m - 1$, is called the knot vector and the u_i are called knots. The ith B-spline basis function of p-degree, denoted by $N_{i,p}(u)$, is defined by a recurrence formula as

$$N_{i,0}(u) = \begin{cases} 1 & \text{if } u_i \leq u < u_{i+1} \\ 0 & \text{otherwise} \end{cases}$$

$$N_{i,p}(u) = \frac{u - u_i}{u_{i+p} - u_i} N_{i,p-1}(u) + \frac{u_{i+p+1} - u}{u_{i+p+1} - u_{i+1}} N_{i+1,p-1}(u) . \tag{1}$$

A pth degree B-spline curve is defined by

$$\mathbf{C}(u) = \sum_{i=0}^{n} N_{i,p}(u)\mathbf{P}_i \qquad 0 \leq u \leq 1 , \tag{2}$$

where the $\{\mathbf{P}_i\}$ are the control points, and the $\{N_{i,p}(u)\}$ are the pth degree B-spline basis functions (1) defined on the knot vector

$$U = \{\underbrace{0, ..., 0}_{p+1}, u_{p+1}, ..., u_{m-p-1}, \underbrace{1, ..., 1}_{p+1}\} \tag{3}$$

containing $m + 1$ knots. The polygon formed by the $\{\mathbf{P}_i\}$ is called the control polygon.

Catheter centerline is approximated to within a user-specified error bound, E. This error bound limits the maximum deviation between the data points and the B-spline curve to be less than E everywhere on the curve. For the approximating B-spline curve, it is not usually known in advance how many control points are required to obtain the desired accuracy E. Thus, the approximation is an iterative process. Iteration starts with a sufficient number of control points so that the first approximation satisfies E. Then the number of control points is reduced and another curve is fitted. If E is no longer satisfied with the new curve then the previous curve is used as the approximation curve. If E is satisfied the number of control points is reduced again and iteration is repeated.

The degree of the approximating curve is elevated in steps of one until the pth degree is reached. The first approximating curve is a 2nd degree curve, which is degree elevated to a 3rd degree curve. Then excess control points are discarded iteratively and the 3rd degree approximating curve is degree elevated to a 4th degree curve. This goes on until a pth degree approximating curve is reached. Working up to degree p in steps decreases wriggling in the final curve and settles the curve to follow the geometric characters of the data at a proper stage. The first degree is omitted and calculation starts directly with the second degree curve, i.e. quadratic interpolation. This is justified by the smoothness of the catheter centerlines.

Fitting of the B-spline curve requires solving a linear least squares problem for the unknown control points $\mathbf{P}_i$. Let n be the number of control points and let $\{\mathbf{Q}_k\}$, $k = 0, ..., m$ be a set of catheter points we want to approximate with a pth degree B-spline curve. We assume that $p \geq 1$, $n \geq p$ and $m > n$. To each point $\mathbf{Q}_k$ we assign a precomputed parameter value $\bar{u}_k$. These are chosen using the chord length d,

$$d = \sum_{k=1}^{m} |\mathbf{Q}_k - \mathbf{Q}_{k-1}| . \tag{4}$$

Then

$$\overline{u}_0 = 0, \qquad \overline{u}_m = 1 \qquad \text{and}$$

$$\overline{u}_k = \overline{u}_{k-1} + \frac{|\mathbf{Q}_k - \mathbf{Q}_{k-1}|}{d} \qquad k = 1, ..., m-1. \tag{5}$$

Knots are calculated using averaging

$$u_0 = \cdots u_p = 0, \qquad u_{m-p} = \cdots u_m = 1 \qquad \text{and}$$

$$u_{j+p} = \frac{1}{p} \sum_{i=j}^{j+p-1} \overline{u}_i \qquad j = 1, ..., m-2p-1. \tag{6}$$

We look for the pth degree B-spline curve

$$\mathbf{C}(u) = \sum_{i=0}^{n} N_{i,p}(u)\mathbf{P}_i \qquad u \in [0, 1] \tag{7}$$

satisfying $\sum_{k=0}^{m} |\mathbf{Q}_k - \mathbf{C}(\overline{u}_k)|^2$ is a minimum with respect to the $n+1$ variables, $\mathbf{P}_i$. This means that points $\mathbf{Q}_k$ are approximated in the least squares sense.

Let

$$f = \sum_{k=0}^{m} |\mathbf{Q}_k - \mathbf{C}(\overline{u}_k)|^2$$

$$= \sum_{k=0}^{m} \left[(\mathbf{Q}_k^2 - 2 \sum_{i=0}^{n} N_{i,p}(\overline{u}_k)(\mathbf{Q}_k \cdot \mathbf{P}_i) + (\sum_{i=0}^{n} N_{i,p}(\overline{u}_k)\mathbf{P}_i)^2 \right]. \tag{8}$$

To minimise f we set the partial derivatives of f with respect to the n variables, $\mathbf{P}_l$, equal to zero,

$$\frac{\partial f}{\partial \mathbf{P}_l} = \sum_{k=0}^{m} \left(-2N_{l,p}(\overline{u}_k)\mathbf{Q}_k + 2N_{l,p}(\overline{u}_k) \sum_{i=0}^{n} N_{i,p}(\overline{u}_k)\mathbf{P}_i \right) = 0. \tag{9}$$

Arranging terms in (9) it follows that

$$\sum_{i=0}^{n} \left(\sum_{k=0}^{m} N_{l,p}(\overline{u}_k)N_{i,p}(\overline{u}_k) \right) \mathbf{P}_i = \sum_{k=0}^{m} N_{l,p}(\overline{u}_k)\mathbf{Q}_k. \tag{10}$$

Equation (10) is a linear equation in the unknowns $\mathbf{P}_0, ..., \mathbf{P}_n$. Using (5) and (6) to compute the parameters $\{\overline{u}_k\}$ and the knot vector U leads to a positive definite and well-conditioned coefficient matrix which has a semibandwidth less than $p+1$. Thus the equation (10) can be solved by a standard LU decomposition technique, for instance.

The deviation checking against the user-specified limit, E, measures maximum distance between the catheter points $\mathbf{Q}_k$ and the B-spline curve,

$$\max_{0 \le k \le m} \left(\min_{0 \le u \le 1} |\mathbf{Q}_k - \mathbf{C}(u)| \right). \tag{11}$$

Generally

$$\min_{0 \le u \le 1} |\mathbf{Q}_k - \mathbf{C}(u)| \le |\mathbf{Q}_k - \mathbf{C}(\overline{u}_k)| \tag{12}$$

and thus $\{\overline{u}_k\}$ serves as a good start point for an iterative solution of (10).

3   Measurements

We tested our centerline detection algorithm with two prototype catheters equipped with different profiling coils. A twisted pair coil was constructed by coiling a 0.1 mm copper wire around the outer surface of a 4 French flush catheter. Secondly, a single loop coil was embedded inside a hollow catheter. The catheter contained three channels, two of which were used as a round trip path for a 0.1 mm copper wire and the third was filled with $MnCl_2$ solution. The length of both profiling coils was 40 cm.

The profiling coil designs were visualised in a 0.23 T open configuration magnet manufactured by Marconi Medical Systems. Both coils were used as transmit and receive coils. During the scanning, the catheters were immersed in 0.25 mmol $MnCl_2$ solution. The imaging sequences were FE-35/12 for the twisted pair coil and FE-21/8 for the single loop coil with a resolution of 128×256 without slice selection. Small 0.5 degree flip angle was used to reduce the RF transmit power to a practical level.

The profiling coils were imaged perpendicular to the main magnetic field, B_0, of the scanner. In this position, the signal to noise ratio and the apparent linewidth should be optimal for the twisted pair and suboptimal for the single loop coil [10]. We did not verify this. For the visualising purpose, we set catheters in different geometries during scanning and scanned them from axial, sagittal and coronal directions. The geometries tested were free form loop, helix and straight line.

4   Results and Discussion

Figures 1 and 2 show the results of the centerline detection using the projection images of catheters in different geometries as an input. It is marked on the left side of the images whether they have been taken with the twisted pair or with the single loop coil. In the series of three pictures the first one is the MR image of the profiling coil. The following two pictures show the results of segmentation and spline fitting.

The characteristic structures of the two profiling coils can be seen in these images. The twisted pair profiling coil produces a discontinuous beads-like profile of the catheter. The single loop coil has a more continuous profile, but shows a tendency to produce two parallel intense areas that are somewhat spaced from each other.

The algorithm has no difficulties in finding the centerline path of these profiles when the geometry is distinct. The algorithm is insensitive to segmentation errors in the neighbourhood of the signal intense area. A few misdetected catheter points do not disturb the correct centerline approximation. Likewise, moderate discontinuities of the segmented data are well tolerated and the spline approximation does not place restrictions on the curvature of the centerline.

On the other hand, with complex geometries like helix, the algorithm does not perform as well. In the worst cases, the centerline may not even resemble the real geometry of the coil, as it can be seen at the first three images of figure 1. The reason for this can be traced down to the travelling salesman algorithm used for arranging segmented centerline points before spline fitting. With complex geometries, the segmented data may be too complicated for travelling salesman to find the geometrically right order among the points. The shortest path is not always the correct one.

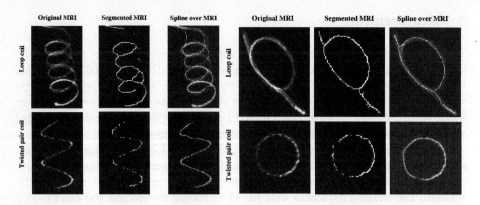

Fig. 1. Results of segmentation and spline fitting with helix and free from loop geometries

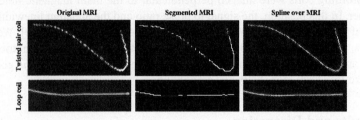

Fig. 2. Results of segmentation and spline fitting with geometries relevant to clinical applications

Failures in centerline detection may also be caused by some large intense signal areas outside the catheter profile that are missegmented to be a part of the profile. In this case, the approximating curve deviates far from the correct centerline. Fortunately, however, we found such intense noise to be relatively uncommon. If this becomes a problem, the solution is to improve the segmentation. It should be possible to find a criterion for isolated intense areas which are then excluded in the spline fitting phase.

The approximating B-spline curve is a continuous one. This causes back and forth loops in the centerline with some geometries. An example of this can be seen in the upper right corner of figure 1. Even though, it is not really a falsely detected centerline it is worth mentioning and considering, since such loops could potentially be problematic in some applications of the algorithm.

The diameter of the signal intense area is about 5 mm. The approximated centerline stays within this intense area and thus we have a rough estimate of the maximum deviation from the real centerline path. The time needed for the calculation of the centerline varied between 0.2 and 3.7 seconds on 700 MHz Athlon, the average time being 1.5 seconds. Compared with the image acquisition time, which was approx. 5 seconds, the image processing time is short, thus not limiting the overall performance of instrument localisation. All approximating B-spline curves are of 2nd degree. The parameter E that sets the maximum allowed deviation between segmented catheter points and B-spline curve had a value $E = 0.8$ in units of in-slice voxel size.

5 Conclusion

We have presented an automated algorithm for the identification of a profiling coil centerline from MR images and for representing the centerline by an approximating B-spline curve. The idea has been to develop a practical tool for further higher level image processing tasks, such as instrument visualisation, and to be employed in MRI guiding tools. The need for a fully automated algorithm became evident after a number of trials with some semiautomated centerline detection algorithms.

The algorithm has been tested with two different profiling coil designs. Catheters equipped with twisted pair and single loop coils were set up and imaged in different geometries. With both coil designs, the centerlines of distinct geometries were found without problems. The algorithm tolerates discontinuities in the imaged profile of the coil and does not set restrictions for the curvature of the centerline. Complicated geometries, like helix, tend to cause incorrectly detected centerlines. However, since the geometries in real applications are usually quite simple, this failure with complex geometries cannot be considered a serious drawback.

The speed of the algorithm is reasonable. As compared with the image processing time, the image acquisition time dominates. To improve the overall performance of image acquisition and processing, the imaging time and image transfer time between the scanner and the computer should be reduced. If this is possible, we will be able to hold a promise that the algorithm now presented could serve as a base for nearly real-time instrument visualisation and guiding tools for MRI.

References

[1] Robert B. Lufkin, editor. *Interventional MRI*, chapter Active tracking of interventional devices, pages 144–153. MOSBY, 1999.
[2] J.F. Debatin and G. Adam, editors. *Interventional Magnetic Resonance Imaging*, chapter Instrument Visualization in the MR Environment. Springer, 1998.
[3] Robert B. Lufkin, editor. *Interventional MRI*, chapter Vascular interventional MRI, pages 387–395. MOSBY, 1999.
[4] Mark E. Ladd, Gesine G. Zimmermann, Graeme C. McKinnon, Gustav K. von Schulthess, Charles L. Dumoulin, Robert D. Darrow, Eugen Hoffmann, and Jörg F. Debatin. Visualization of vascular guidewires using MR tracking. *Journal of Magnetic Resonance Imaging*, 8:251–253, 1998.
[5] T.J. Vaara, J.I. Tanttu, S. Taivalkoski, and L. Jyrkinen. Catheter RF-coil profile reconstruction from 2D-projections. In *Proc. of ISMRM'99*, page 1953, 1999.
[6] S. Taivalkoski, L. Jyrkinen, T. Vaara, J. Tanttu, O. Tervonen, and O. Silvén. Automated catheter 3-D profile reconstruction using spline approximation. In *3rd Interventional MRI Symposium, Leipzig*, May 2000.
[7] H.-J. Bender, R. Männer, C. Poliwoda, S. Roth, and M. Walz. Reconstruction of 3D catheter paths from 2D x-ray projections. In *Proc of the MICCAI'99 meeting*, pages 981–989, 1999.
[8] Hákon Gudbjartsson and Samuel Patz. The Rician distribution of noisy MRI data. *Magnetic Resonance in Medicine*, 34:910–914, 1995.
[9] Les Piegl and Wayne Tiller. *The NURBS Book*. Springer, 2nd edition, 1997.
[10] Mark E. Ladd, Peter Enhart, Jörg F. Debatin, Eugen Hofmann, Peter Boesiger, Gustav K. von Schulthess, and Graeme C. McKinnon. Guidewire antennas for MR fluoroscopy. *Magnetic Resonance in Medicine*, 37:891–897, 1997.

Performance and Robustness of Automatic Fluoroscopic Image Calibration in a New Computer Assisted Surgery System

Peter M. Tate, Vladimir Lachine, Liqun Fu, Haniel Croitoru, Marwan Sati

Surgical Navigation Specialists, 6509 Airport Rd, Mississauga ON, Canada L4V 1S7
ptate@surgnav.com

Abstract. In order to improve the clinical usefulness of computer-assisted fluoroscopic navigation, a new algorithm to automatically determine the calibration of fluoroscopic images has been developed. This is a challenging task since the intraoperative images acquired from fluoroscopic systems are often poor, making detection of the calibration grid difficult. Several feature-based methods have been implemented to perform bead detection for automatic detection of the calibration grids. The algorithms include support for multiple fields of view, a feature not supported on any computer assisted systems to date. In order to evaluate the performance of the algorithms, special phantoms were made and a cadaver study was performed to challenge the algorithms. One hundred images were acquired using three different C-Arms (OEC 9600, OEC 9800 and Philips BV-300+) using two different fields of view (nine and twelve inch). The chosen method successfully registered the images in ninety-six of the cases. The images that were not successfully registered were of limited clinical value anyway due to the very poor image quality.

1. Introduction

Computer-assisted fluoroscopic navigation has received strong interest as a new tool for spinal and orthopedic procedures[3][5][6][7]. Computer-assisted fluoroscopic navigation is a technique whereby a conventional C-Arm is equipped with an optically-tracked calibration device that consists of two fiducial grids and a collar that mounts to the image intensifier. When an image is acquired during surgery, the position of the C-Arm is captured and the image is transferred to the computer. After uploading the image onto the C-Arm, the computer detects the fiducial markers and calculates the calibration parameters (image distortions, image-patient transformation) and then superimposes instruments on multi-planar images for navigation. To improve image display, the grids are removed from the image, and the geometric image distortions are removed (the image is "unwarped"). The advantages over conventional fluoroscopy includes reduced radiation exposure, real-time guidance, no need to have the cumbersome image intensifier in the working area during the intervention, and navigation that is available in multiple planes.

Many current systems are challenged by the need to keep the C-Arm console settings constant throughout the surgical procedure (i.e. constant flip, rotation, and

W. Niessen and M. Viergever (Eds.): MICCAI 2001, LNCS 2208, pp. 1130-1136, 2001.
© Springer-Verlag Berlin Heidelberg 2001

field of view) before uploading the image. This can disturb the standard clinical workflow since image manipulation is often performed on the console to help the surgeon's orientation with the anatomy or to change the field of view for the area of interest. We have developed an asymmetric grid and an automatic grid detection technique that allows the user to use the C-Arm in a conventional fashion. This paper investigates the performance and robustness of this new technique.

Current systems miss fiducial markers in certain images and it is another objective of this work to improve fiducial detection rate through improved image processing algorithms. Fiducial beads with diameter larger than 3mm, used in some systems, are not desired since they noticeably obstruct the image, so another objective was to distinguish between 2 and 3mm beads arranged in an asymmetric grid for automatic detection of flip, rotate and field of view.

2. Materials and Methods

Three C-Arms (OEC 9600, OEC 9800 and Philips BV-300+) were used to acquire fluoroscopic images using the new fluoroscopic navigation system. The grids contained an asymmetric bead pattern that was used to identify flip, rotation and changes in the field of view in the image.

Spinal, hip, and femur phantoms, as well as images from three human cadaver trials were used in this study. The cadavers were specially ordered "large" specimens that provided worst-case quality images (due to the significant signal attenuation) and allowed us to test the robustness of the algorithm. Metallic surgical instruments and implants were placed in both the phantom images and the cadaver images to simulate worst-case obstruction of fiducial markers. One hundred images were analyzed in all.

Results were visually checked to determine accurate bead detection results, and were analyzed with respect to number of false positives, localization accuracy, number of beads detected per image. Ideally we would like to detect all the beads, however because of occlusions and image noise, this is not always possible.

The crucial step in automatic registration is robust bead detection. To perform bead detection, the beads were first segmented from the image by taking the difference between the original image and an image of the background intensity. The difference image was then thresholded using an adaptive method based on the intensity of the background image. This gave us a series of candidate bead positions, the orientation of the grid could then be determined using the Hough transform[4], parameterized using the normal representation of a line. Since the grids are laid out in rows and columns, inputting the candidate positions creates a pattern with strong responses when the rotation angle matches the orientation along the rows and columns, and along the diagonals of the grid. The proper orientation can be determined based on the spacing at that orientation since the spacing along the diagonal will be less than the spacing along the row/column direction. The translation and scale of the grid could be determined by taking projections along the rows and columns of the grids. Since the grid is symmetric, this determined the rotation to within integral intervals of 90 degrees. To resolve flip, the calibration grid was designed to have large beads placed along two rows and one column of the proximal plate (note the bead pattern in the first image of Figure 2).

After the initial grid orientation was determined, the rows and columns that may contain large beads were searched based on bead size to determine the final grid orientation. Searching is performed by calculating the average bead sizes of the possible rows and columns that may contain large beads and testing the candidates against each of the eight possible combinations by flipping and rotating the known bead pattern. The best fit is the pattern that yields the largest average size. The most challenging aspect of this process is to determine an appropriate size measure to differentiate the beads. We used the number of pixels in the segmented beads from the first step. Global thresholding provided inconsistent results, therefore an adaptive thresholding based on the background intensity was used which provided a more robust size metric, as well as better bead detection.

Two different algorithms were developed to find the background image, one is a grayscale morphological method based on Top Hat transformation[4], and the second is based on median filtering.

An example of bead detection can be seen in Figure 1. A special mode is shown where the system displays detected beads with crosses and large beads with circles. The standard mode does not show the bead location with crosses, but rather warns the system of a potential invalid registration.

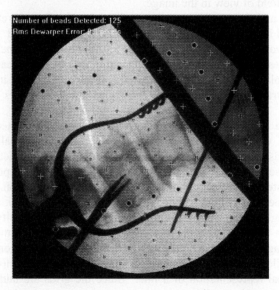

Number of beads Detected: 125
Rms Dewarper Error:

Fig. 1. Successful calibration. A special option allows the user to visualize the bead positions.

Validation of the bead detection was performed both automatically and visually. The automatic validation method was developed for intraoperative use to warn the surgeon of images that may not be properly registered. Automatic validation included checking for a minimum number of beads detected in each of the calibration grids, a check on the distribution of beads in the image, and a check on the magnitude of the distortion recovered from the image based on the unwarping function. The threshold for the minimum number of beads varied depending on the field of view of the image. We have found that the magnitude of the distortion in the image is bounded, so if the amount of distortion (measured as the difference between a bead's detected location, and its predicted "ideal" location after dewarping) for any bead is beyond the expected range, the calibration of that image was rejected. If the bead detection fails to meet these specified criteria (which varied depending on the field of view), the image calibration is rejected and a warning is displayed to the user.

After calibration, the beads are removed from the image to improve the surgeons view of the anatomy. Beads are removed by clipping the bead from the image, and performing surface fitting using a high order polynomial. The surgeon is also provided an option to not remove the beads.

3. Results

Results were evaluated in terms of the number of successful registrations, the average number of beads detected, the number of falsely detected beads, and the RMS dewarper error. The total number of beads that could be detected in the image varied with the field of view (241 for the twelve-inch field of view, and 137 for the nine-inch). The RMS dewarper error was found by calculating the difference between the detected location, and the predicted location found by the unwarping. In addition, each image was visually checked for false detections and to verify that the proper flip, shift, and rotation were determined.

Results from the study are shown in Table 1. The median method was successful on 96 out of 100 images compared with the morphological method's 92 out of 100. In each unsuccessful case the failed calibration was automatically found, thus ensuring that a failed image would not be navigated upon. On average the median method also found 3 more beads had a slightly improved RMS dewarper error.

Table 1. Results of automatic registrations.

Method	Number of Successful Calibrations	Number of falsely detected beads (Total)	Average number of beads detected	Average RMS dewarper error (mm)
Morphological	92	1	186	0.43
Median	96	1	189	0.41

A sample result from bead removal is shown in Figure 3. Bead removal generally performs very well, removing the grid from most parts of the image. Bead detection works well on edges, however bead removal on edges remains a challenge. The current bead removal may cause local blurring because the current surface matching interpolation method may be adversely affected by image content, showing smoothly varying "smudges" where the image contrast changes sharply.

1134   P.M. Tate et al.

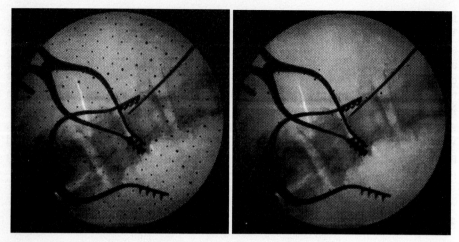

Fig. 2. Challenging image with beads removed. Note that some beads may be detected even if they are not removed.

4. Discussion

Of the two bead detection methods, results from median filtering are better than the morphological filtering, though marginally so (see results in Table 1). This is due to the morphological filtering increasing the average gray level of the image, hence the difference between the original and background images is reduced making thresholding more difficult.

Of the images that the bead detection failed, several were high-energy images and did not contain clinically interesting properties. In general, it is expected that some images cannot be automatically registered. This may be caused by a surgical tool in the field of view that obstructs one or more rows of large beads, making the final solution indeterminate, however this should be quite rare in practice. In these cases, users have the option to perform a manual calibration of the image, by setting the proper flip, rotation, and shift.

The system generally performed very well, and was able to find beads near edges and even through some metal instruments! (Figure 3) The performance of many other methods, especially signal-based methods such as cross-correlation, tend to suffer near edges.

A piece of electronics in a patient tracker that was obscuring a number of beads was falsely detected as a bead in one of the images, as is shown in Table 1. Because there were a sufficient number of beads detected elsewhere in the image, this did not affect the overall result.

The feature based technique proved extremely robust at determining the proper orientation of the grid, calculating the proper calibration in all cases where a sufficient number of beads were found. The feature-based method requires only that the beads in the image be aligned in a rectilinear grid, and that the center of the grid be close to the center of the image. The actual number of rows and columns in the grid is not important for determining the orientation or spacing.

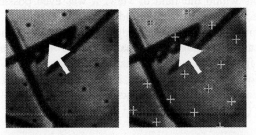

Fig. 3. Left hand image shows beads in the image, right hand image shows crosses representing the detected beads. Note the bead detected through the metal instrument.

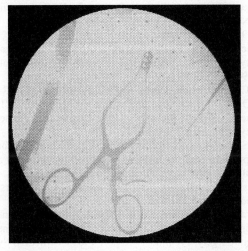

Fig. 4. Example of an unsuccessful calibration because of high-energy fluoroscopy. Note that there is no anatomy visible so the image would not be used clinically.

   The bead removal generally performed well, with beads removed near sharp edges causing some blurring. The current surface-fitting algorithm assumes smoothly varying intensity across the image. While this assumption is valid for most parts of the image, surgical tools and implants are characterized by sharp edges. By better modeling the intensity variation in the image, we anticipate that we can deliver better results. In order to minimize the visual artifacts caused by bead removal, the RMS error of the surface fitting is calculated, and if it is deemed too high, as often occurs near the edges of metal instruments, the bead is not removed from the field of view.

5.   Conclusions

This paper shows the performance and robustness of a new system for intra-operative fluoroscopic image registration.

- A very large percentage of fiducial beads were detected even under worst-case conditions of large human cadavers with simulated implants and surgical instruments within the field of view. It was even possible in some cases to detect beads that were normally hidden behind metal.
- The system was robust in distinguishing between 2 and 3mm beads and automatically detecting image manipulations at the C-arm console such as changing fields of view, image rotations and image flips.
- Bead removal is very satisfactory, however there is room for improvement for the grayscale interpolation to reduce blurring.

References

[1] Brack C, Burgkart R, Czopf A, Götte H, Roth M, Radig B, Schweikard A (1998) Accurate X-ray-based Navigation in Computer-Assisted Orthopaedic Surgery. Proc CAR Symposium 1998:716-722.
[2] Brack C, Götte H, Gossé F, Moctezuma J, Roth M, Schweikard A (1996) Towards Accurate X-Ray-Camera Calibration in Computer-Assisted Robotic Surgery. Proc CAR Symposium 1996:721-728.
[3] Foley, Kevin T., MD, Simon, David A, PhD, Rampersaud, Y. Raja MD (2000) Virtual Fluoroscopy. Operative Techniques in Orthopaedics 10(1) pp77-81
[4] Gonzalez, Rafael C., Woods, Richard E. (1992) Digital Image Processing – Third Edition. Addison-Wesley Publishing Company.
[5] Hofstetter R., Slomczykowski M., Sati M. and Nolte L.-P. "Fluoroscopy as an imaging means for computer assisted surgical navigation", 1999, Computer Aided Surgery 4:65-76.
[6] Hofstetter R., Slomczykowski M., Krettek C., Sati M. and Nolte L.-P. "Computer Assisted Fluoroscopy Based Reduction of Femoral Fractures and Anteversion Correction", 2000, Computer Aided Surgery 5:311-325
[7] Joskowicz L, Taylor RH, Williamson B, Kane R, Kalvin A, Guéziec A, Taubin G, Funda J, Gomory S, Brown L, McCarthy J, Turner R (1995) Computer Integrated Revision Total Hip Replacement Surgery: Preliminary Report. Proc 2nd MRCAS Symposium, 193-202.
[8] Viant WJ, Phillips R, Griffiths JG, Ozanian TO, Mohsen AMMA, Cain TJ, Karpinski MRK, Sherman KP (1997) A computer assisted orthopaedic surgical system for distal locking of intramedullary nails. Proc Instn Mech Engrs 211 (H):293-299.

An Architecture for Simulating Needle-Based Surgical Procedures

Alan Liu, Christoph Kaufmann, Daigo Tanaka
{aliu|ckaufmann|dtanaka@simcen.usuhs.mil}

National Capital Area Medical Simulation Center
Uniformed Services University of the Health Sciences
4301 Jones Bridge Road, Bethesda MD 20814, USA
http://simcen.usuhs.mil

Abstract. Many surgical procedures use cannulas, guidewires, and catheters in the treatment of life threatening conditions (e.g. cardiac tamponade and tension pneumothorax), or for diagnosis (e.g. diagnostic peritoneal lavage). Simulator development is costly in time and resources. Most computer-based trainers are procedure-specific. Each trainer uses a different hardware configuration. The cost of using multiple simulators for teaching is prohibitive. A result is decreased acceptance of simulation for teaching. A generalized software architecture has been developed that simplifies the process of constructing trainers for needle-based surgical procedures. Different procedures can use the same hardware platform. The architecture has been used to develop two trauma simulators. A third simulator is currently being developed using this architecture.

1 Introduction

Computer-based trainers have been developed for teaching many surgical procedures [1-4]. Simulator-based training has many advantages. Unlike cadavers or anesthetized animals, simulators require minimal setup and preparation. They are reusable, and provide a uniform training experience. Unlike animals, simulators present the student with the correct human anatomy. Simulators can also provide the appropriate physiological responses, unlike cadavers.

Despite these advantages, the acceptance of computer-based simulators for medical education has been weak. One reason is cost. Many simulators require a custom hardware configuration. The hardware may not be usable for a different procedure. Since each simulator is unique, their development and production cost is high. A course involving many different procedures will require several expensive systems. For many institutions, the expense cannot be justified.

This paper describes an architecture for developing trainers for needle-based procedures. Many procedures fall under this category. They include: Diagnostic peritoneal lavage (DPL), pericardiocentesis, needle thoracentesis, needle cricothyroidotomy, central line placement, intraosseous puncture, and needle biopsies of the thyroid and breast. An architecture using a common hardware platform and development approach for a class of procedures addresses the problems raised earlier.

W. Niessen and M. Viergever (Eds.): MICCAI 2001, LNCS 2208, pp. 1137-1144, 2001.

In this paper, section 2 describes the hardware and the architecture. Section 3 describes simulators constructed using this architecture. Section 4 describes the implications of this work.

2 Method

The architecture is based on the premise that a surgical procedure can be broken down into a series of discrete steps. The user is assumed to be familiar with the procedure's algorithm. A successful outcome requires the user to complete a sequence of steps correctly. Other outcomes with varying degrees of success are possible, depending on the user's actions and the number of errors made during the procedure.

Finite automata [5] provide a natural way of representing surgical algorithms. A finite automata consists of a set of states and transitions between states. Each state represents a specific action to be completed. The student's performance determines the transition between states. For example, when a cannula is incorrectly inserted, a transition back to the current state permits the student to try again. A correct insertion invokes a transition to a different state to perform the next step.

The architecture consists of several components: A state engine, a graphical user interface, a haptic interface, and a transition algorithm. Each is described in more detail.

2.1 State Engine

The state engine is the architecture's core. The engine incorporates a finite automata (FA), and a state transition algorithm. This algorithm is described in detail in section 2.4. The FA consists of a set of states, and a state transition table. Each state represents a step in a surgical procedure. The user interacts with state objects to perform the corresponding surgical action. A simulation consists of executing a series of steps. As the student performs each step, his performance together with the transition table will be used to determine the subsequent step.

Each state is defined by three functions. The *init()* function initializes the state. The *run()* function executes the surgical step. *get_result()* reports the result of that execution. Depending on the procedure, different states have different definitions for each function. A state may be distinguished as a start or an end state. The simulation will always begin on a start state. End states denote that the simulation has completed. An end state is characterized by having no other states to which that state can perform a transition. Depending on the student's actions, end states may denote a successful or unsuccessful completion. There is exactly one start state at least one end state.

2.2 Graphical User Interface

The GUI object consists of sequence window and an action window. Fig. 1 illustrates. The sequence window presents a randomized list of steps that must be performed in the procedure. The action window provides visual feedback on actions performed by the student during each step of the procedure. During a simulation, the user selects the current step using the sequence window. If the correct step is chosen, the action window becomes active and prompts the user to perform the chosen step (e.g., inserting a cannula). The user's actions are displayed in the action window. Successful completion of the current step re-activates the sequence window where the next step can be chosen.

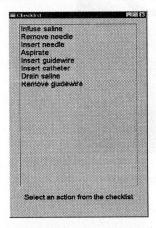 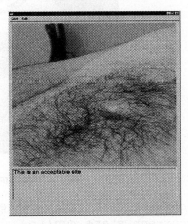

Fig. 1. GUI interface as configured for diagnostic peritoneal lavage.

2.3 Haptic Interface

The CathSim AccuTouch® device [6] by Immersion Medical (formerly HT Medical) is employed. The haptic interface consists of an enclosed needle carrier. Sensors on the needle carrier report pitch, yaw, and depth. The needle carrier accepts cannulas, catheters and guidewires. Encoders on the carrier can detect the depth to which a cannula or guidewire has been inserted. Up to two instruments (e.g., a cannula and a guidewire) can be simultaneously inserted and tracked. The needle carrier incorporates passive haptics in the depth direction. As the carrier is pushed or pulled, a variable amount of braking force can be applied. By dynamically controlling resistance, the sensation of a cannula penetrating various tissue layers can be accurately simulated. Fig. 2 illustrates.

2.4 Execution and Transition Algorithm

The sequence of states executed by the simulation is determined by this algorithm.

```
load_state_machine();
randomize_steps();
current_state = start_state;
current_result = initial_data;
while (current_state != NULL)
       {
       user_selected_state = get_user_input();
       while (user_selected_state != current_state)
              report("Incorrect next state chosen");
```

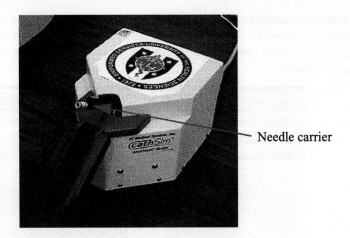

Needle carrier

Fig. 2. Haptic interface device.

```
    current_state.init(current_result);
    current_state.run();
    current_result = current_state.get_result();
    current_state = next_state(current_state,
                                    current_result);
    }

display_report();
```

The simulator begins by loading the state machine defining the procedure to be performed. The procedure's steps are randomized prior to display. The simulator is initialized with the start state and data from *initial_data*. The user is prompted to select the first step of the procedure. The function *get_user_input()* displays the sequence window and prompts the user to click on the correct step to perform. If an incorrect choice is made, an error message is displayed. When the correct state is chosen, that state is initialized (*current_state.init()*), then run (*current_state.run()*). The result of this execution is returned (*current_state.get_result()*) and stored in *current_result*. The next state executed is determined by the current state (*current_state*), and by the results in *current_result*. The results are also used to initialize the next state. This cycle is repeated until an end state is encountered. This is characterized by a state that does not select a new state (i.e., *next_state(current_state,current_result)* == NULL). Finally, the simulation displays a summary of the student's performance (*display_report()*).

3   Case Studies

This section highlights some of the simulators built using this architecture. At the time of writing, two simulations have been completed. A third simulator is currently being developed. We describe each in turn.

3.1 Pericardiocentesis

Pericardiocentesis is a surgical procedure performed to relieve fluid buildup between the heart and the pericardium. This condition (cardiac tamponade) interferes with the heart's ability to pump blood. Cardiac tamponade must be corrected rapidly, or the patient may die. Initial treatment involves inserting a cannula between the pericardium and heart, then aspirating the blood to relieve pressure buildup. An earlier version based on the Phantom haptic interface device was developed [4]. This simulation has been re-written using the architecture described in this paper. The CathSim device is used in place of the Phantom. Fig. 3 (left) is an image from the GUI.

3.2 Diagnostic Peritoneal Lavage

DPL is performed when intra-abdominal bleeding secondary to trauma is suspected. The procedure is performed when alternative diagnostic methods such as computerized tomography (CT) or ultrasound imaging are unavailable, or when the patient's condition does not allow them to be performed. The DPL procedure is complex, involving up to nine steps. Details of this procedure and the simulation have been previously described [3]. Fig. 3 (right) is an image from the GUI. The DPL simulation uses the architecture described in this paper. Fig. 4 illustrates the state machine.

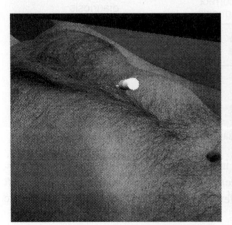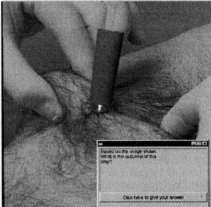

Fig. 3. (left) Pericardiocentesis. (right) Diagnostic peritoneal lavage.

3.3 Needle Thoracentesis of Tension Pneumothorax

Needle thoracentesis is used as an immediate treatment for life-threatening tension pneumothorax. This condition can result from chest trauma. Tension pneumothorax occurs when air leaks into the thoracic cavity and cannot escape. The increasing pressure compresses the heart and lungs, causing circulatory and respiratory problems. The procedure requires the insertion of a catheter in the second intercostal space, in the midclavicular line on the side of the tension pneumothorax. The catheter permits excess air pressure to escape. This simulation is currently being developed. The state

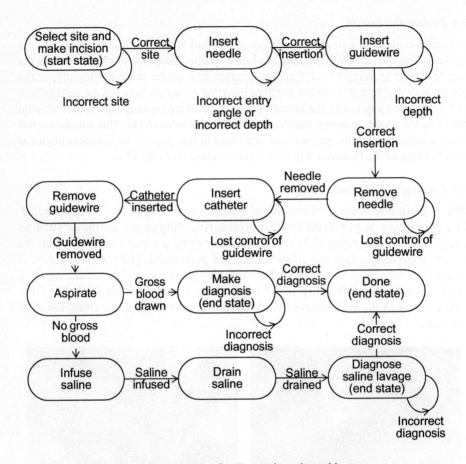

Fig. 4. State machine for diagnostic peritoneal lavage.

machine for this procedure is summarized in fig. 5. This simulation is more elaborate than the previous two in that the consequence of an incorrect action (e.g., incorrect needle insertion), is not apparent until a few steps later. The simulation permits the student to back up and correct the mistake.

4 Discussion

Surgical simulators can be an improvement over traditional methods of surgical education. Many simulators have been developed using unique and expensive hardware configurations. The hardware is procedure-specific. Multiple simulator platforms are required for different procedures. The cost of simulating multiple procedures is prohibitive.

Our approach uses a common platform to simulate a large class of procedures. These procedures are commonly taught or used. The chosen hardware platform is

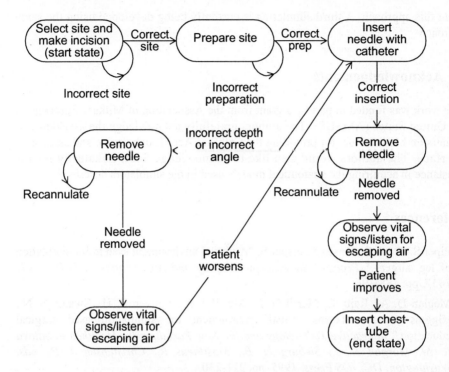

Fig. 5. State machine for needle thoracentesis.

commercially available and is relatively inexpensive. As all simulations built using our design run on the same hardware, no additional hardware investment is required.

Since needle-based procedures have many similarities, the architecture permits many needle-based procedures to be developed with minimal effort. Development effort is focused on defining the individual states, and the transition between states. User interface development, haptic device interface and other peripheral issues need not be considered. Our approach has limitations however. Since only basic hardware is assumed, the degree of realism may be limited. However, in many cases, a high level of realism is not required. Key aspects of learning a procedure include executing the surgical algorithm correctly, using the correct surgical instruments, and managing complications. Our simulation architecture permits these goals to be accomplished. In addition, haptic feedback is primarily limited to one DOF in needle-based procedures. Our choice of haptic interface is sufficient to provide the required feedback.

5   Conclusion

We described an architecture for developing needle-based procedures. Our approach is an improvement over conventional methods. Our method permits training simulators to be developed rapidly on a common, low-cost platform. We have validated our architecture by developing two simulations for different needle-based procedures using this approach. A third simulation is currently being developed using the same approach.

6 Acknowledgements

This work was funded in part by a grant from the Association of Military Surgeons of the United States (AMSUS). The authors gratefully acknowledge the assistance of Immersion Medical Inc. for providing the CathSim AccuTouch device and associated interface. The authors would also like to acknowledge Scott Zakaluzny for his assistance in acquiring the anatomical models used in the simulators described.

References

1. Piper S., Deph S., Rosen J., Fisher S. "A virtual environment system for simulation of leg surgery." *Proc. of Stereoscopic Display and Applications //. SPIE 1991; 1457.* pp. 188-196.
2. Meglan D. A., Raju R., Merril G. L., Merril J. R., Nguyen B. H., Swamy S. N., Higgins G. A. "Teleos virtual environment for simulation-based surgical education." *Interactive Technology and the New Paradigm for Healthcare, Satava R. M. Morgan K. s., Sieburg H. B., Masttheus R., Christensen J. P., eds. Washington, DC: IOS Press, 1995.* pp. 221-230.
3. Alan Liu, Kaufmann C., Ritchie T. "A computer-based simulator for diagnostic peritoneal lavage." *Medicine Meets Virtual Reality 2001. Westwood J. D., et al., eds. IOS press, 2001.* pp. 279-285.
4. Christoph Kaufmann, Zakaluzny S., Liu A. "First steps in eliminating the need for animals and cadavers in Advanced Trauma Life Support®." *Medical Image Computing and Computer-Assisted Intervention (MICCAI) 2000. Lecture Notes in Computer Science 1935, Springer.* pp. 618-623.
5. Hopcroft J. E., Ullman J. D. "Introduction to automata theory, languages, and computation." *Addision Wesley, 1979. ISBN 0-201-02988-X.*
6. Ursino, M.; Tasto, P.D.J.L.; Nguyen, B.H.; Cunningham, R.; Merril, G.L. "CathSimTM: an intravascular catheterization simulator on a PC." *Medicine Meets Virtual Reality. Convergence of Physical and Informational Technologies: Options for a New Era in Healthcare. MMVR 7, 1999, Netherlands.* pp. 360-366

Computer-Aided Hepatic Tumour Ablation

David Voirin[1,2], Yohan Payan[1], Miriam Amavizca[1], Antoine Leroy[1],
Christian Létoublon[2], Jocelyne Troccaz[1]

[1]Laboratoire TIMC - Faculté de Médecine - Domaine de la Merci
38706 La Tronche cedex - France
[2]Service de Chirurgie générale et digestive - CHU de Grenoble
BP 217 - 38043 Grenoble cedex 9 - France
Author for correspondence: Jocelyne Troccaz,
jocelyne.troccaz@imag.fr

Abstract. Surgical resection of hepatic tumours is not always possible. Alternative techniques consist in locally using chemical or physical agents to destroy the tumour and this may be performed percutaneously. It requires a precise localisation of the tumour placement during ablation. Computer-assisted surgery tools may be used in conjunction to these new ablation techniques to improve the therapeutic efficiency whilst benefiting from minimal invasiveness. This communication introduces the principles of a system for computer-assisted hepatic tumour ablation.

Introduction

Hepatic tumour destructions are traditionally performed under image control (intra-operative CT or intra-operative ultrasounds (US)). The operator introduces the surgical instrument whilst controlling its trajectory on the images. This significantly limits the range of possible trajectories. Our objective is to use a computer-assisted surgery (CAS) approach where pre-operative data are used for planning, intra-operative imaging is limited to registration and the execution of the planned trajectory is guaranteed by the use of a suitable assistance (navigation or robotic systems).

Over the last fifteen years, most of the CAS systems were developed in the context of specialities dealing with bony structures or with structures behaving with limited deformations and movements. Very little attention has been given to computer-assisted soft tissues surgery. Concerning hepatic surgery, the liver position depends both on the patient position and on the point in the respiration cycle. Moreover, hepatic tissues can get intrinsic deformations during surgery (for example, under the action of the surgical instruments). Some recent publications focused on motion evaluation and on registration for CAS liver surgery [1,2]. Meanwhile, registration experiments were performed on static phantoms. One purpose of this preliminary work was to quantitatively evaluate the feasibility of registration. The image modalities that were chosen for this evaluation were the ones that are traditionally selected for registration, namely pre-operative CT or MRI and intra-operative ultrasonic imaging.

W. Niessen and M. Viergever (Eds.): MICCAI 2001, LNCS 2208, pp. 1145-1146, 2001.
© Springer-Verlag Berlin Heidelberg 2001

Experiments

The main objective was to be able to quantitatively evaluate the algorithms that match *pre-operative data (CT or MRI) with 2.5D echography[1]* under rather realistic conditions. In the first stage of this study, it was assumed that the key steps of the protocol, namely image acquisitions and guidance, can be both executed at a same point in the respiration cycle, for instance after expiration. Because the experiments were conducted with a volunteer, MRI was preferred to CT. The acquisition was synchronized with the respiration cycle and occurred only during the expiration phase. In a second stage - that simulates intra-operative procedures - 2.5D echographic acquisitions were performed. Data were acquired during the apnoea that follows expiration. Based on these data, the registration algorithm - a surface rigid matching using a distance map recorded in an octree-spline data structure [3] - was quantitatively evaluated in terms of repeatability and accuracy.

Data registration was repeatable and the accuracy - even limited by data acquisition - allows envisioning the clinical applicability of the method. A detailed presentation and discussion of these results may be found in [4].

References

[1] Herline A.J., Stefansic J.D, Debelak J.P., Hartmann S.L., Wight Pinson C., Galloway R.L., Chapman W.C., Image-guided surgery: preliminary feasability studies of frameless stereotactic liver surgery, Arch. Surg., vol 134, (1999), 644-650.
[2] Herline A.J., Herring J.L., Stefansic J.D, Chapman W.C., Galloway R.L., Dawant B.M., Surface registration for use in interactive, image-guided liver surgery, Computer-Aided Surgery, 5, (2000), 11-17.
[3] Lavallée S., Szeliski R., Recovering the position and orientation of free-form objects from image contours using 3-D distance maps, IEEE PAMI (Pattern Analysis and Machine Intelligence), 17(4), (1995), 378-390
[4] Voirin D., Payan Y., Amavizca M., Létoublon C., Troccaz J., Computer-aided hepatic tumour ablation: requirements and preliminary results, Comptes-rendus de l'Académie des Sciences, in press, 2001.

Acknowledgements

This work has been supported by La Fondation de la Recherche Médicale. We thank Patrick Vassal, Pr Lebas, Pr Coulomb, Dr Sengel and Dr Teil for their assistance in the image acquisition processes.

---

[1] 2.5D echography is the process where the ultrasonic probe is localized in space thanks to a localizer (Optotrak in this experiment) allowing to get sparse 3D data.

Intra-operative Transfer of Planned Zygomatic Fixtures by Personalized Templates: A Cadaver Validation Study

Johan Van Cleynenbreugel[1], Filip Schutyser[1], Chantal Malevez[2], Ellen Dhoore[3], Charbel BouSerhal[4], Reinhilde Jacobs[4], Paul Suetens[1], Daniel van Steenberghe[4,5]

[1] Facultes of Medicine & Engineering
Medical Image Computing (Radiology - ESAT/PSI)
University Hospital Gasthuisberg, Herestraat 49, B-3000 Leuven, BELGIUM
Email: Johan.VanCleynenbreugel@uz.kuleuven.ac.be
[2] Department of Maxillo-facial Surgery, Université Libre de Bruxelles, BELGIUM,
[3] Materialise N.V., Technologielaan 15, B-3001 Leuven, and
[4] Department of Periodontology, Katholieke Universiteit Leuven, BELGIUM

1 Background

Our previously developed 3D CT-based oral implant planning system [1,2] has been extended recently towards zygoma fixtures [3]. Zygomatic implant surgery requires a meticulous pre-operative planning (Figure 1) due to factors such as the length of the implant's trajectory (> 40 mm), the complicated and curved anatomy of the sinus, the relative small size of the zygomatic target area, and a limited intra-operative visibility.

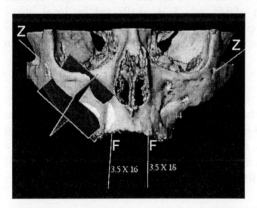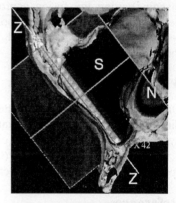

Fig. 1. *Left:* Two zygoma fixtures are shown at Z, and two frontal alveolar implants at F. *Right:* a CT reslice along a planned implant's axis is co-visualized with extracted bone structures. Note the nearby nasal cavity (N) and the course of the implant along the cortex of the sinus (S).

For conventional alveolar implants, personalized drilling templates have proven their efficiency and effectiveness, see [4]. However for zygomatic fixtures, where the problem of intra-operative transfer is even more important, it was up till now unknown whether personalized drilling templates could yield the necessary accuracy. Therefore a validation study was set-up with three cadavers (six zygoma fixtures).

---

[5] Daniel van Steenberghe holds the *P.-I.Brånemark Chair in Osseointegration* at K.U.Leuven, Belgium

W. Niessen and M. Viergever (Eds.): MICCAI 2001, LNCS 2208, pp. 1147-1148, 2001.

2 Materials and Methods

Based on pre-op CT images, fixture planning was done in the environment [3]. For each cadaver a personalized template was designed and manufactured in stereolithography, see Figure 2. Actual drilling did occur without opening the usual small 'window' in the outer cortex of the sinus. The latter procedure is typical for zygoma fixtures as it allows to adjust the drilling direction intra-operatively. In our study however, it was the intention to assess a complete dependency on the template. The template was only employed to guide drilling. Afterwards fixtures were inserted.

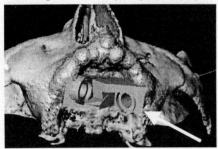 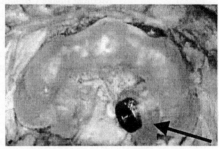

Fig. 2. *Left:* CAD design of the zygoma drill template visualized in the planning environment. *Right:* actual stereolithographic template generated from the design and applied intra-operatively. The template contains tubes, in which metal drill guides can be inserted (arrows).

Post-op CT images were acquired and matched to the pre-op CT images (and the planning) using the fusion approach of [5], which is unaffected by local image deformations. After resampling post-op over pre-op, the zygoma implants were easily segmented, which allowed to visualize and inspect them in in the pre-op space.

3 Results and Conclusions

One out of the six fixtures installed showed a deviation of 7° from the planned axis direction, of 6 mm. from the planned maxillar entry and of 8 mm. from the planned zygomatic exit. Considering the other five fixtures, the worst(best) case values were 3.1(0.6)°, 2.1(0.7) mm. and 2.7(0.8) mm. respectively. These results indicate that acceptable accuracy is to be expected from zygoma fixture drilling templates.

References

1. K. Verstreken, J. Van Cleynenbreugel, G. Marchal, I. Naert, P. Suetens, D. van Steenberghe, *Computer-assisted planning of oral implant surgery: a three-dimensional approach*, International Journal of Oral & Maxillofacial Implants, 11(6), 806-810, 1996
2. K. Verstreken, J. Van Cleynenbreugel, K. Martens, G. Marchal, D. van Steenberghe, P. Suetens, *An image-guided planning system for endosseous oral implants*, IEEE Transactions on Medical Imaging, 17(5), 842-852, 1998
3. J. Van Cleynenbreugel, F. Schutyser. P. Suetens, G. Marchal, D. van Steenberghe, C. Malevez, *A planning system for zygomatic fixtures based on 3D CT images*, First Prize Table Clinics Nobel Biocare International TeamDay, Göteborg, Sweden, July 2000
4. E.U. Brite-Euram project (BRPR CT970378) PISA 01-03-1997, 28-02-2001
5. F. Maes, A. Collignon, D. Vandermeulen, G. Marchal, P. Suetens (1997) Multimodality image registration by maximization of mutual information. *IEEE Transactions on Medical Imaging* 16(2), 187-98.

A PVA-C Brain Phantom Derived from a High Quality 3D MR Data Set

Kathleen J.M. Surry[1] and Terry M. Peters[1,2]

[1] Imaging Research Laboratories, Robarts Research Institute, London Canada
[2] Department of Medical Biophysics, University of Western Ontario, London Canada
kath@irus.rri.on.ca

Abstract. A brain mould was constructed by converting the digital surface of a high quality 3D magnetic resonance (MR) data set to a real model, using a stereo lithography apparatus (SLA). The tissue mimicking material (TMM) poly(vinyl alcohol) cryogel (PVA-C) was used to form a homogeneous phantom in the mould. 3D images of this phantom were then acquired in MR, CT and ultrasound. The surface contours of the phantom were compared between each modality and the source image. This phantom is employed in our laboratory as a model of a deformable brain.

1 Introduction

The neurosurgical image guidance tools that are being developed in our lab often make use of a high quality brain image [1] for testing and development. This reference brain image was created by averaging 27 magnetic resonance (MR) 3D images of the same brain to achieve a very high signal-to-noise ratio. To validate our research in ultrasound-MR integration to correct for brain shift, we required a deformable brain model which we based on this 3D MR image. We have developed a realistic, physical brain model, or phantom, from poly(vinyl alcohol) cryogel (PVA-C) [2], based on the surface of this human brain using a mould created from the reference brain data set.

2 Methods

Internal structures of the reference brain were masked and removed before a marching cubes algorithm extracted the surface. This surface was then cut at the cantho-meatal plane and appropriately formatted for input to a stereo lithography apparatus (SLA). The SLA built the mould by plastic deposition, with a layer resolution of 0.1 mm.

PVA-C liquid, 10% by weight in water, was poured into the mould and degassed. PVA-C is gelled by freezing to -20°C and thawing it back to room temperature in a standard chest freezer, with an internal fan to ensure air circulation.

MR, US and CT volumes were acquired of this phantom. These volumes were compared to the original reference brain volume using Register (3).

W. Niessen and M. Viergever (Eds.): MICCAI 2001, LNCS 2208, pp. 1149-1150, 2001.
© Springer-Verlag Berlin Heidelberg 2001

3   Results

A photograph of the mould can be seen in Figure 1. Registered slices of the reference brain and the phantom in MR and CT are shown in Figure 2. Registration of the phantom's MR scan with the original reference MRI demonstrated a fit accurate to ± 0.7 mm for homologous points on the cortical surface. The overall scaling factor for the fit was 1.044.

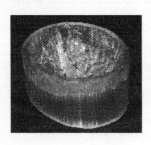   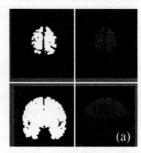   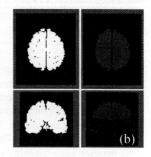

(a)   (b)

Fig. 1. Brain Mould   **Fig. 2.** Registered slices of the reference brain (white) and the phantom (grey) in (a) MR and in (b) CT.

4   Conclusions

We are satisfied with the external surface of this brain mould, and we are now adding internal structure to this phantom. While grey/white matter distinction is currently outside of our ability, we can produce water or PVA-C filled ventricles, or suspend fiducial markers (beads, wires etc) into the volume.

This "anatomically correct", deformable phantom can be manufactured with realistic tissue mechanical properties, and with imaging characteristics appropriate for MR, CT and US. It has application in the validation of stereotactic targeting procedures, multi-modality image registration studies and validation of 3D image warping algorithms.

5   References and Acknowledgements

We gratefully acknowledge Bill Wells and the NRC IMTI for building the SLA mould, and also David Gobbi, Sean Deoni, Chris Norley and Hua Qian for help in various stages of this project. This work was funded by the CIHR.

1   Holmes CJ, Hoge R, Collins L, Woods R, Toga AW and Evans AC 1998 Enhancement of MR images using registration for signal averaging *J Comput Assist Tomogr* **22** 324-333.
2   Nagura M, Nagura M and Ishikawa H 1984 State of water in highly elastic poly(vinyl alcohol) hydrogens prepared by repeated freezing and melting *Polym Comm* **25** 313-314.
3   Custom software from the McConnell Brain Institute, Montreal Neurological Institute, Montreal Canada.

3D Ultrasound Image Acquisition Using a Magneto-optic Hybrid Sensor for Laparoscopic Surgery

Yoshinobu Sato[1], Masaki Miyamoto[1], Masahiko Nakamoto[1],
Yoshikazu Nakajima[1], Mitsuo Shimada[2], Makoto Hashizume[3], and
Shinichi Tamura[1]

[1] Division of Interdisciplinary Image Analysis
Osaka University Graduate School of Medicine
[2] Department of Surgery II
[3] Department of Disaster and Emergency Medicine
Graduate School of Medical Science, Kyushu University
yoshi@image.med.osaka-u.ac.jp, http://www.image.med.osaka-u.ac.jp/yoshi

Abstract. A 3D ultrasound system suitable for laparoscopic surgery using a novel configuration of a magneto-optic hybrid 3D sensor is reported. A miniature magnetic sensor with five degrees of freedom (5D) is combined with an optical sensor outside the body to perform 6D sensing of the flexible probe in the abdominal cavity. The accuracy of the system is evaluated in comparison with a conventional 3D ultrasound system.

1 Introduction

In liver surgery, 3D ultrasound (3D-US) is a useful intraoperative imaging modality to assist the surgeon in recognizing spatial relationships between tumors and vessels. Although use of the laparoscope is becoming common as a minimally invasive procedure, using it in combination with 3D-US has not been reported. We have developed a 3D-US system that can be utilized in laparoscopic liver surgery. The tip of the ultrasound probe can be flexibly moved in the abdominal cavity. To measure six degrees of freedom (6D) for the position and orientation of the flexible probe tip, a novel magneto-optic hybridization configuration is employed. Conventional 6D magnetic sensors are too large to be inserted into the abdominal cavity without additional incision, while optical sensors suffer from the line of sight constraint. To circumvent these drawbacks, we combine a miniature magnetic sensor only 1 mm diameter which can be inserted into the abdomen without an additional incision but which measures only five degrees of freedom (5D), with an optical sensor outside the abdomen to localize the probe tip with 6D in the abdominal cavity.

2 Methods

The complete system is depicted diagramatically in Fig. 1(a). Registration of the coordinate systems of the magnetic and optical sensors is performed based on our

W. Niessen and M. Viergever (Eds.): MICCAI 2001, LNCS 2208, pp. 1151–1153, 2001.

previous framework of magneto-optic hybridization [1]. Figure 1(b) shows the ultrasound probe (Aloka, Tokyo) that we employ in laparoscopic surgery. The rigid body attached outside the abdomen defines the probe-centered coordinate system (PCS). The probe tip is flexible but its motion is restricted within a plane (Fig.1(c)). In the preoperative calibration stage, we determine the plane of the probe tip motion in PCS by gathering 5D measurements of the tip in various arrangements, thereby obtaining the fixed spatial relationship between the rigid body and the plane of the probe tip motion. In the intraoperative stage, the probe tip plane is estimated by combining the position and orientation of PCS measured using an optical sensor and the fixed relationship obtained in the calibration stage. The position and orientation within the probe tip plane are estimated using a miniature magnetic sensor (3D translation and 2D rotation). In this way, 6D parameters of the probe tip position and orientation are obtained, and the tip-centered coordinate system (TCS) is defined. Finally, the ultrasound image coordinate system (UICS) is determined by combining the relationship of TCS and UICS determined in the preoperative calibration stage [2].

3   Experimental Results

Experiments were performed to evaluate the accuracy of the system. Since our magnetic tracking system of choice, Aurora (Northern Digital Inc.), was not operational at the time we carried out the experiments, we provisionally substituted Fastrak (Polhemus Inc.) as the magnetic sensor and utilized only its 5D parameters so that it functioned in a similar manner to Aurora. Polaris (Northern Digital Inc.) was employed as the optical sensor. The 3D position of a phantom tip in a water bath (Fig.1(d)) was measured using the following three methods: (i) The Polaris pen-probe digitizer (Let $\mathbf{x}_p$ be its measurements). (ii) The proposed 3D-US system using a magneto-optic hybrid sensor ($\mathbf{x}_h$). (iii) A conventional 3D-US system with 6D magnetic sensor (Fastrak) directly attached to the probe tip ($\mathbf{x}_m$). The accuracies of the proposed and conventional 3D-US systems were evaluated by regarding the measurements of the Polaris pen-probe digitizer as the gold standard, that is, the errors were defined as follows: $\Delta\mathbf{x}_h = |\mathbf{x}_p - \mathbf{x}_h|$ and $\Delta\mathbf{x}_m = |\mathbf{x}_p - \mathbf{x}_m|$. Thirty measurements for the 3D position of the phantom tip were obtained with various probe tip arrangements. Table 1 shows the average (bias) and standard deviation (SD) of the errors. The accuracy of the proposed system, which is suitable for laparoscopic surgery, was comparable to that of the conventional one, which is difficult to use for that purpose.

4   Conclusion

We have described a 3D ultrasound system that employs a magneto-optic hybrid sensor and is suitable for use in laparoscopic surgery. The accuracy of the system was comparable to that of the conventional one, which is not suited to laparoscopic surgery. We will shortly replace the conventional magnetic sensor

Table 1. Accuracy evaluation. $(\delta_x, \delta_y, \delta_z)$ and $(\sigma_x, \sigma_y, \sigma_z)$ respectively denote bias and standard deviation (SD) with respect to each axis; $\sigma_D = (\sigma_x^2 + \sigma_y^2 + \sigma_z^2)^{0.5}$.

	Bias: $(\delta_x, \delta_y, \delta_z)$ (mm)	SD: $(\sigma_x, \sigma_y, \sigma_z)$, σ_D (mm)
Proposed 3D-US	(0.40, 0.31, 0.71)	(0.44, 0.84, 0.53), 1.08
Conventional 3D-US	(0.26, 1.38, 0.82)	(0.42, 0.99, 0.47), 1.18

(Fastrak) with a miniature one (Aurora) for 5D sensing in the abdominal cavity. We are planning to extend the system so as to realize augmented reality visualization, which superimposes 3D ultrasound images onto laparoscopic images [2].

Acknowledgement: This work was partly supported by JSPS Research for the Future Program JSPS-RFTF99I00903 and JSPS Grant-in-Aid for Scientific Research (B)(2) 12558033.

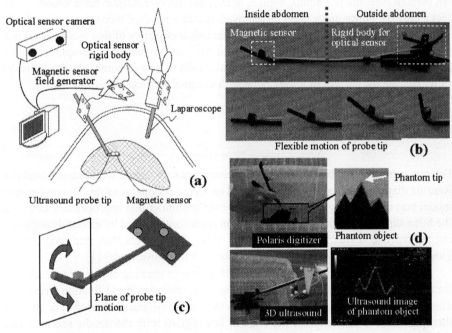

Fig. 1. 3D ultrasound system for laparoscopic surgery. (a) System diagram. (b) Ultrasound probe for laparoscopic surgery. (c) Plane of probe tip motion (probe tip plane). (d) Laboratory experiments for accuracy evaluation.

References

1. Nakamoto M et al., Magneto-optic hybrid 3-D sensor for surgical navigation, *LNCS*, **1935** (*Proc. MICCAI 2000*), 839–848 (2000).
2. Sato Y et al., Image guidance of breast cancer surgery using 3D ultrasound images and augmented reality visualization, *IEEE-TMI*, **17**(5), 681-693 (1998).

Minimally Invasive Excision of Deep Bone Tumors

R.E. Ellis, D. Kerr, J.F. Rudan, and L. Davidson

Computing and Information Science, Mechanical Engineering, and Surgery
Queen's University at Kingston, Canada
ellis@cs.queensu.ca

1 Rationale and Objectives

An osteoid osteoma is a small, benign, active, painful osteoblastic bone lesion. To effect a cure the entire nidus must be removed, because residual nidus is associated with recurrence of the osteoid osteoma [2]. The technical objective of this work was to perform minimally invasive excision of osteoid osteoma by means of computer-assisted guidance technology. The principal technical hurdle to be overcome was the difficulty of registering the surface of a long bone with minimal surgical exposure.

2 Materials and Methods

Patients were selected based on clinical presentations consistent with osteoid osteoma. Routine diagnostic CT scans were acquired on a conventional scanner. The registration model was extracted by determining a Hounsfield number that appropriately extracted the bone surface. An additional visualization model was formed by manually segmenting the reaction cortex that surrounded the nidus. The models were imported into the guidance system we have previously used for high tibial osteotomy [1].

Intraoperatively, a sterilized custom optoelectronic tracking object was attached to the affected bone through stab wounds, using conventional external-fixation screws. An 18ga hypodermic needle was attached to a tracked probe and calibrated. The surgeon then percutaneously contacted the bone in key regions with the needle and an initial registration was computed. Additional surface points were collected to refine the registration. The computer then tracked the drill and superimposed an image of the drill on the visualization model and on axial, sagittal, and coronal reformats of the CT scan.

Once the nidus was localized with image-guidance, a small hole (10mm) was drilled through the cortex. Unroofing of the nidus by gradual removal of the overlying reactive bone was undertaken prior to excision with curettes. The computer-related hardware was removed and the wounds were closed with SteriStrips. Patients were discharged within 24 hours of the procedure.

For each patient, the specimens were sent immediately for pathology analysis. Postoperative plain X-ray films were taken and the patient was permitted to bear weight as tolerated. Each patient was later examined in a followup clinic.

W. Niessen and M. Viergever (Eds.): MICCAI 2001, LNCS 2208, pp. 1154–1156, 2001.
© Springer-Verlag Berlin Heidelberg 2001

3   Results

We have operated on three cases of osteoid osteoma. The second patient, typical of the other two, presented with a sclerotic lesion in the posteromedial aspect of her tibia. Because of the difficulty of a direct surgical approach, a small incision was made in the anterior aspect of the leg. Images from the guidance phase of the procedure are shown in Figure 1.

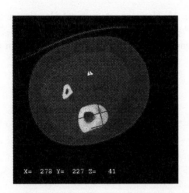 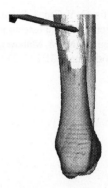

Fig. 1. Closeup images of from the use of a computer-tracked drill to localize an osteoma nidus. The cross-hairs in the left image, and the pointer in the right image, show the computed position and orientation of the drill bit. Note that the drill has approached from the anterior aspect, which would be challenging without some form of image guidance.

4   Discussion

The final pathology for all three cases reported specimen with the histologic features consistent with osteoid osteoma. All patients had immediate relief of their discomfort following the surgery and were permitted to bear weight as tolerated. There were no surgical complications.

This technique allows accurate localization of small lesions and is particularly useful for those that are deep within reactive bone. Accurate localization allows a small incision and a minimally invasive excision technique that does not destroy the integrity of the remaining bone. There is elimination of, or a lesser need for, postoperative immobilization, bone grafting, internal or external fixation and a shortened period of limited activity postoperatively. All of these factors make this technique particularly appealing to the young, active patient.

Osteoid osteoma is one of the most difficult tumors in the body to target. It is small, embedded deep in cortical bone, and the surrounding bone has few (if any) landmarks for registration to the CT scan. A system that can guide the excision of osteoid osteoma shows promise for use in removing, or biopsying, tissues located in or near any bone of the skeletal system.

1156   R.E. Ellis et al.

Acknowledgments

This research was supported in part by Communications and Information Technology Ontario, the Institute for Robotics and Intelligent Systems, and the Natural Sciences and Engineering Research Council of Canada.

References

[1] R. E. Ellis, C. Y. Tso, J. F. Rudan, and M. M. Harrison. A surgical planning and guidance system for high tibial osteotomy. *Journal of Computer Aided Surgery*, 4(5):264–274, 1999.

[2] D. H. Lee and M. M. Malawer. Staging and treatment of primary and persistent (recurrent) osteoid osteoma. 281:229–238, 1992.

A Multimodal Navigation System for Interventional MRI

K. Kansy[1], A. Schmitgen[1,2], M. Bublat[1,2], G. Grunst[1], M. Jungmann[1],
P. Wisskirchen[1], M. Moche[3], G. Strauss[3], C. Trantakis[3], and T. Kahn[3]

[1] GMD — German National Research Center for Information Technology,
D-53754 Sankt Augustin, Germany
kansy@gmd.de, http://fit.gmd.de/results/localite/
[2] LOCALITE GmbH, Graurheindorfer Str. 69, D-53111 Bonn, Germany
[3] Universitätsklinikum Leipzig, Liebigstrasse 20a, D-04103 Leipzig, Germany

Abstract. Medical imaging permits high precision minimally invasive
interventions even in very delicate situations but leads to complex medical procedures not easily applied in a hospital setting. The LOCALITE
Navigator is an interactive navigation system that comprises state-of-the
art registration and visualization of multimodal medical images for minimally invasive interventions with an interventional magnetic resonance
imaging (iMRI) system. The focus is on an intuitive and simple user interface that can be handled by the medical personnel themselves without
relying on computer experts. The system has got a CE certificate in 2001
and is used by all GE SIGNA SP installations in Germany.

1 Design of the LOCALITE Navigator

The LOCALITE Navigator was designed to improve the handling of interventional Magnetic Resonance Imaging systems, specifically the SIGNA SP (0.5 T)
of General Electric Medical Systems, Milwaukee, WI, USA. It tackles the following problems:

Image Quality. Due to the bad resolution (time and space) of real-time images, (some) experts regard them near to useless. LOCALITE complements them
with corresponding slices calculated from intra-operative 3D-data (a similar approach is used by 3D-slicer at Surgical Planning Lab at Brigham and Women's
Hospital [1]). The calculated slices are an excellent means for interpreting and
understanding the low quality real-time slices.

Interactivity. The SIGNA SP is equipped with a camera-based locator system
(Flashpoint, IGT, Boulder, CO, USA), which precisely measures position and
orientation of a hand piece at a rate of about 10 Hz. The real-time MR images
are scanned in any plane relative to the tip of device however with a delay of
several seconds. The calculated planes of LOCALITE can follow the speed of
the locator device.

Orientation. In real-time mode, the SIGNA SP only generates single 2D
slices. We have developed an abstract scene containing just the elements necessary for moving the device: markers for planned entry and target points and a

W. Niessen and M. Viergever (Eds.): MICCAI 2001, LNCS 2208, pp. 1157–1158, 2001.

virtual device showing the current position and orientation of the real device. This simple scene gives the surgeon sufficient orientation to perform positioning in seconds rather than minutes or even longer in delicate cases.

Multimodal Visualisation (Image Fusion). In addition to the interventional images, pre-operative data sets (CT, MR, fMR) may be required during the intervention. LOCALITE offers different presentation options for two data sets. Two data sets can be overlaid with transparency. Sliders allow a dynamic setting of the transparency levels. In this mode, the bright structures in both data sets will be shown. For typical mixes, predefined overlay modes can be selected by buttons, e.g., emphasizing a specific structure (bone) by colour or instantaneous switching to one data set.

Registration. Different data sets can only be displayed consistently within one scene after geometrical alignment of coordinate systems (registration). LO-CALITE includes a robust registration mechanism starting with a rough landmark-based registration followed by automatic registration based on mutual information which yields optimal precision for MR and CT. In the case of T2-weighted images of functional MR (fMR), this registration fails. Using a co-registered MR rather than the fMR data set (both scanned in one session with patient in a fixed position) solves the problem. The location of functional areas can now be related to the current position of the medical device.

2   Discussion

The LOCALITE Navigator is based on the LOCALITE system [2] and includes the functionality needed for a multimodal navigation system for iMRI and only this functionality. It has been developed in close cooperation with clinicians and is used inside and outside of a university setting by all SIGNA SP installations in Germany. Currently, we are working on a transfer of concepts to the imaging modality ultrasound, which is ubiquitously available and opens a wider market.

LOCALITE Navigator is programmed in Java on a standard PC with Windows NT 4.0 and graphics card supporting OpenGL.

References

1. David Gering (1999) *A System for Surgical Planning and Guidance using Image Fusion and Interventional MR.* MIT Master's Thesis.
2. Klaus Kansy et al. (1999) LOCALITE — a Frameless Neuronavigation System for Interventional Magnetic Resonance Imaging Systems. In: C. Taylor, A. Colchester (eds) *Medical Image Computing and Computer-Assisted Intervention — MIC-CAI'99.* Berlin: Springer (1999) 832-841

A Biomechanical Model of Muscle Contraction

J. Bestel, F. Clément, and M. Sorine

INRIA Rocquencourt, 78153 Le Chesnay Cedex, France

Models of the electro-mechanical activity of the cardiac muscle can be very useful in computing stress, strain and action potential fields from three-dimensional image processing. We designed a chemically-controlled constitutive law of cardiac myofibre mechanics, acting on the mesoscopic scale and devoted to be embedded into a macroscopic model. This law ensues from the modelling of the collective behaviour of actin-myosin molecular motors, acting on the nanoscopic scale to convert chemical into mechanical energy. The resulting dynamics of sarcomeres, acting on the microscopic scale, is shown to be consistent with the "sliding filament hypothesis", which was first introduced by A. F. Huxley [1].

Excitation-Contraction Model on the Myofibre Scale

The contractile elements (CE) of myofibres are able to produce stress while shortening in response to a chemical input $u(t)$, mainly depending on the calcium concentration. We propose, as a constitutive relation in the myofibre direction between stress σ and strain ε, the following set of controlled differential equations (modified from [2], [3]) of visco-elasto-plastic type:

$$\begin{cases} \dot{k}_c = -\left(|u| + |\dot{\varepsilon}|\right) k_c + k_0 |u|_+ & k_c(0) = \sigma_c(0) = 0 \\ \dot{\sigma}_c = -\left(|u| + |\dot{\varepsilon}|\right) \sigma_c + k_c \dot{\varepsilon} + \sigma_0 |u|_+ & \sigma = k_c \xi_0 + \sigma_c + \eta \dot{\varepsilon} \end{cases} \quad (1)$$

The system is able to account for : shortening from resting conditions ($\dot{\varepsilon} = 0$) in response to $u(t)$, passive behaviour of CE ($u = 0$) as described in [4], static relation between ε and σ, and isotonic contraction ($\dot{\sigma}_c = 0$ and $\dot{\varepsilon} < 0$) as in Hill's experimental model. For the purpose of ultrasonographic-image processing, the system is further being embedded into a partial differential equation model including reaction-diffusion equations to rule the propagation of action potential.

Excitation-Contraction Model on the Sarcomere Scale

On a microscopic scale, the sarcomere is made up of thin and thick parallel filaments. When ATP is available and the intracellular level of calcium reaches a threshold, myosin heads of the thick filament become likely to bind actin sites on the thin filament. The elastic free energy W of the actin-myosin interaction is responsible for muscle contraction: stress response to strain causes relative sliding of the actin over the myosin filament. Let $n(\xi, t)$ be the density of cross-bridges with strain ξ at time t and ε the strain (normalized by the ratio of rest to maximal length of cross-bridges). Then, Huxley's model is:

$$\partial_t n + \dot{\varepsilon} \, \partial_\xi n = f(1 - n) - gn, \quad \sigma(t) = -\int_{-\infty}^{+\infty} \partial_\xi W(\xi) n(\xi, t) d\xi + \eta \dot{\varepsilon} \quad (2)$$

W. Niessen and M. Viergever (Eds.): MICCAI 2001, LNCS 2208, pp. 1159–1161, 2001.

The following choice of $f(\xi,t)$ and $g(\xi,t)$, the positive rates at which cross-bridges respectively fasten and unfasten, is consistent with myofibre behaviour:

$$f(\xi,t)=|u(t)|_+ \text{ for } \xi \in [0,1] \;(=0 \text{ elsewhere}), \quad g(\xi,t)=|u(t)|+|\dot{\varepsilon}(t)|-f(\xi,t) \quad (3)$$

In the particular case $-\partial_\xi W(\xi) = k_0\xi_0 + \sigma_0\xi$, we notice, as in [5], that the total stiffness k_c and total elastic stress σ_c are respectively proportional to the zero and first-order moment of n:

$$k_c(t) = k_0 \int_{-\infty}^{+\infty} n(\xi,t)d\xi \quad \text{and} \quad \sigma_c(t) = \sigma_0 \int_{-\infty}^{+\infty} \xi n(\xi,t)d\xi \qquad (4)$$

where k_0 and σ_0 are constants related to physical parameters of crossbridges. The system (1) is a set of equations of moments derived from (2), (3) and (4).

Excitation-Contraction on the Molecular-Motor Scale

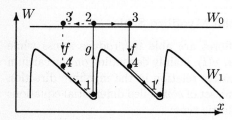

1 (1'). AM+ATP→M.ATP+A
g. Myosin unbinding
2. M.ATP→M.ADP.P
Myosin free motion
3 (3'). M.ADP.P+A→AM.ADP.P
f. Myosin binding controlled by Ca^{2+}
4 (4'). AM.ADP.P→AM+ADP+P
Myosin sliding on actin

Two-state model for a single motor[6] and Four-phase ATP-cycle

The motion of a myosin head is described by a Langevin equation with η, friction coefficient, b, thermal normalized gaussian white noise, and F_{ext}, external force:

$$\eta\dot{x} = -\partial_x W_i(x) + \sqrt{2\eta k_B T}b(t) + F_{ext}, \quad i = 0,\,1 \qquad (5)$$

The myosin is likely to move one way, as the thermal fluctuations are rectified by the periodic "sawtooth" potential W_1 (probable moves are 1→1 and 1→1'). *Collective behaviour of motors[6].* Applying the Fokker-Planck formalism to (5), $n(t,\xi)$ appears as the average density of myosin heads bound a distance ξ away from the nearest local minimum of W_1.

Conclusion and Perspectives

We have proposed a controlled contraction model on the myofibre scale consistent with models designed on the sarcomere and molecular scales. A more precise model accounting for detailed Ca^{2+} action is under development.

References

[1] A. F. Huxley. Muscle structure and theories of contraction. In *Progress in biophysics and biological chemistry*, volume 7. Pergamon Press, 1957.

[2] J. Bestel. PhD thesis, Université Paris 9, 2000.

[3] J. Bestel and M. Sorine. A differential model of muscle contraction and applications. In *Schloessmann Seminar on Mathematical Models in Biology, Chemistry and Physics*, Max Plank Society, Bad Lausick, Germany, May 19-23 2000.

[4] I. Mirsky and W. W. Parmley. *Cardiac Mechanics: Physiological, Clinical, and Mathematical Considerations*, chapter 4. J. Wiley, 1974.

[5] G. I. Zahalak. A distribution-moment approximation for kinetic theories of muscular contraction. *Mathematical Biosciences*, (114):55:89, 1981.

[6] F. Jülicher, A. Ajdari, and J. Prost. Modeling molecular motors. *Reviews of Modern Physics*, 69(4), October 1997.

A Framework for Patient-Specific Physics-Based Simulation and Interactive Visualization of Cardiac Dynamics

Wei-te Lin and Richard A. Robb

Mayo Foundation/Clinic, Rochester, Minnesota 55905

1. Introduction

Characterization of cardiac motion can be derived from a pre-operatively acquired image sequence of an entire cardiac cycle. However, changes in the patient's cardiac morphology and physiology during and after interventions will not be reflected in the pre-acquired data. What is needed is a faithful, patient-specific deformable model of the heart that can be used on-line with interventional cardiac procedures. Diffusion-encoded magnetic resonance imaging provides data for more precise modeling of a specific heart. A computer simulation which integrates fiber information with a physics-based mechanical model and a simulated electrical conduction model has been developed to realistically mimic cardiac dynamics. Such a model can ultimately be used to guide treatment interventions and to predict surgical outcomes.

2. Methods

Implementation of the simulation system includes four major components:

2.1 Reconstruction of Regional Fiber Orientation

Multiple MR images of an excised heart were acquired with diffusion encoded in six directions. The high resolution images were interpolated to produce 1 mm^3 voxels. Regional myocardial fiber orientation is defined for each voxel by the eigenvector corresponding to the largest eigenvalue of the diffusion tensor composed by the six MR images [1].

2.2 Cardiac Electrical Conduction Simulation

The conduction is simulated using a cellular automata model [2]. Each muscle voxel is modeled to have three conduction states: the resting state, the activation state, and the refractory state. Each muscle voxel performs shortening when activated by neighboring muscle voxels.

2.3 Cardiac Muscle Contraction Simulation

A contraction model is constructed for each muscle voxel. The muscle cell network is constructed by arranging muscle voxels in a 3-D grid with grid points connected by simulated springs (see Fig. 1). Muscle contraction is simulated by systematically performing shortening of individual muscle voxels. This leads to deformation of the entire heart.

2.4 Interactive Visualization

The surface model is deformed and displayed using a free-form deformation method. The surface model of the heart, reconstructed from the MR image, is embedded in the 3-D grid that is used to form the muscle cell network. Muscle voxel shortening results

W. Niessen and M. Viergever (Eds.): MICCAI 2001, LNCS 2208, pp. 1162-1163, 2001.

in displacements of the grid points, which deform the nearby space and cause the embedded surface model to deform.

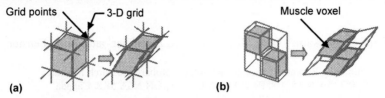

Fig. 1. Simulated muscle shortening. (a) Muscle voxel shortening results in deformation of the grid. (b) Muscle voxels are connected by a 3-D grid to form a muscle cell network.

3.   Results

Fig. 2 illustrates results of applying the model to a sheep heart. The images represent geometry changes of the left ventricle during systole.

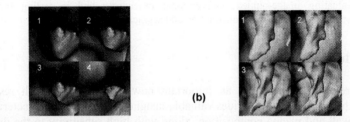

Fig. 2. Simulated heartbeat of the sheep heart. (a) Figure shows four time points during systole, viewing from inside the left ventricle toward the apex. (b) Deformation of the left ventricle.

4.   Discussion

Integrating regional fiber information with simulated electrical conduction and muscle contraction models provides realistic simulation of cardiac motion. With improving diffusion MR techniques, it will be possible to acquire high-resolution in vivo patient heart images for patient-specific muscle fiber mappings and models. For validation, images of an entire cardiac cycle acquired using high-speed CT scanners, 3-D ultrasound, and techniques such as MR tagging can be used for quantitative comparison. The extensible framework allows such factors as fluid dynamics of blood flow, reception of and response to signals from the central nervous system, and various genetic and acquired anomalies to be readily incorporated into the simulation.

References

1.   Hsu, E.W., Muzikant, A.L., Matulevicius, S.A., Penland, R.C. and Henriquez, C.S.: Magnetic resonance myocardial fiber-orientation mapping with direct histological correction. Am. J. Physiol. 274 (1998) H1627-H1634.
2.   Saxberg, B.E.H., and Cohen, R.J.: Cellular automata models of cardiac conduction. Theory of Heart: Biomechanics, Biophysics, and Nonlinear Dynamics of Cardiac Function. Edited by Glass, L., Hunter, P., and McCulloch, A., Springer Verlag, 1991.

A Pulsating Coronary Vessel Phantom for Two- and Three-Dimensional Intravascular Ultrasound Studies

Seemantini K. Nadkarni[1], Greg Mills[1], Derek R. Boughner[1] and Aaron Fenster[1]

[1]Imaging Research Laboratories, John P. Robarts Research Institute,
PO Box 5015, 100 Perth Drive, London, ON N6A 5K8, Canada.
Sknadkar@irus.rri.on.ca

Abstract. Intravascular ultrasound (IVUS) is an important new technique for high resolution imaging of coronary arteries. This paper describes a unique pulsating coronary vessel phantom to evaluate 2D and 3D IVUS studies. The elasticity and pulsatility of the vessel wall can be varied to mimic normal and diseased states of the human coronary artery. The phantom described is useful in evaluating image-guided interventional procedures and in testing the performance of 3D IVUS reconstruction and segmentation algorithms.

1. Introduction

IVUS has recently emerged as an important new technique for high resolution imaging of the coronaries. It provides valuable insight into the tissue characteristics of the arterial wall and plaque composition, along with high sensitivity to the detection of plaque calcification [1]. The purpose of this study was to develop an anthropomorphic pulsating coronary phantom for testing 2D and 3D IVUS techniques. This phantom is useful in evaluating the performance of image-guided interventional procedures of stent deployment, wall elasticity imaging studies, wall motion analysis, as well as 3D reconstruction and image segmentation algorithms.

2. Methods

The coronary phantom consists of an acrylic cylindrical casing with two discs attached at the ends of the casing (Fig.1a). A PVA vessel (r = 1.8mm; wall = 0.8mm) is inserted into the casing and attached to the two end discs. The acrylic casing is filled with water and sealed with a latex sheath attached over one of the end discs. The phantom is mounted on a platform in an acrylic tank filled with water (Fig.1b). The latex sheath, attached to a shaft connected to a servomotor, is stretched and relaxed causing pulsation in the PVA vessel wall. A servomotor controller is used to program motion waveforms into the servomotor, generating different vessel wall pulsation patterns. An UltraCross 3.2 IVUS catheter, driven by a motorized pull back unit at the constant speed of 1mm/s was used to image the phantom. The ClearView Ultra IVUS system was used to obtain 2D images of the phantom. Image digitization, at a frame rate of 30Hz and 3D IVUS reconstruction were controlled by a LIS L3D 3D ultrasound acquisition system (Life Imaging Systems Inc, London, Ontario).

W. Niessen and M. Viergever (Eds.): MICCAI 2001, LNCS 2208, pp. 1164-1165, 2001.
© Springer-Verlag Berlin Heidelberg 2001

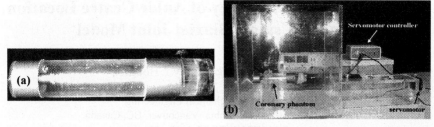

Fig 1. (a) Coronary phantom: the acrylic casing encloses the PVA vessel. (b) The coronary phantom setup: a servomotor drives the latex sheath to generate wall motion in the PVA vessel.

3. Results

Fig.2.a,b shows 3D images of the coronary vessel phantom with and without pulsation. The pulsation of the vessel wall is seen in Fig.2b. The wall pulsation was programmed using the cross-sectional area change waveform (solid line) shown in Fig.2c [2]. The resultant cross-sectional area change over one cardiac cycle, as measured from the 3D phantom image, is shown as the dotted line. The resultant phantom plot agreed with the input waveform to within 4.3%, with an r-value of 0.95.

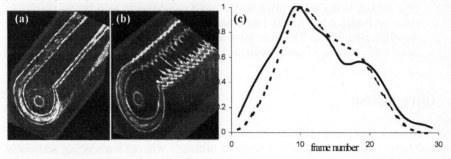

Fig.2 (a) and **(b)** 3D images of the coronary phantom: (a) no pulsation (b) with wall pulsation. **(c)** the programmed waveform (solid line) and the resultant phantom area change (dotted line) are plotted as a function of frame number. The frame interval was equal to 33ms.

4. Conclusions

We have described an *in vitro* experimental set up to test the development of new techniques in 2D and 3D IVUS imaging. The elasticity and pulsation of the phantom vessel wall can be accurately programmed to mimic normal and diseased coronaries.

References

1. Nissen, SE., Yock, P: Intravascular ultrasound: novel pathophysiological insights and current clinical applications. Circulation.(2001) 103:604-616.
2. Erbel, R., Roelandt JTC., Ge, J., Gorge G.: Intravascular ultrasound. Martin Dunitz (1998)

Repeatability and Accuracy of Ankle Centre Location Estimates Using a Biaxial Joint Model

Cameron A. Shute & Antony J. Hodgson

Department of Mechanical Engineering
University of British Columbia, Vancouver, BC, Canada
ahodgson@mech.ubc.ca

Abstract. In conventional total knee replacement (TKR) surgery, a significant fraction of implants have varus/valgus alignment errors large enough to reduce the lifespan of the implant, so we are developing a more accurate computer-assisted procedure aimed at reducing the standard deviation (SD) of the implant procedure. In this study we introduce a new method of locating the ankle joint centre (AJC) using a biaxial model (BM), and determine the accuracy and repeatability of this protocol compared to a digitization method and a sphere-fitting method used in a current computer-assisted procedure. Repeated *in vivo* measurements performed by a single operator were obtained from five normal subjects (450 measurements) using the three methods of AJC location. Based on these experiments we estimate the varus/valgus SD of defining the tibial mechanical axis in the frontal plane for the tested population to be 0.28° for the spherical model, 0.17° for the biaxial model, and 0.11° for the conventional digitizing point probe. The mean joint centre locations found by the motion-based models are significantly medial and anterior to the point probe centre.

1 Introduction

We are developing computer-assisted total knee replacement tooling that eliminates intramedullary rods and improves alignment accuracy without introducing additional imaging requirements (such as preoperative computed tomography scans) or invasive procedures (such as bone pins remote to the operating site). Currently there is no universally accepted method of defining the AJC, but there are two main approaches: anatomical determination (digitization) and biomechanical determination (motion-based). This work investigates the feasibility of using a biaxial model to define a biomechanically meaningful AJC by comparing the centre to those centres obtained with a spherical model and by direct digitization.

2 Methods

Digitization measurements were obtained using a 135 mm point probe, and calcaneal motion measurements were recorded with a optoelectronic three-emitter reference frame mounted to a calcaneal tracker (Flashpoint 5000 localizer). All measurements were relative to a three-emitter triangular local reference frame (120 mm on a side) mounted rigidly to a tibial tracker.

W. Niessen and M. Viergever (Eds.): MICCAI 2001, LNCS 2208, pp. 1166-1167, 2001.
© Springer-Verlag Berlin Heidelberg 2001

Study design: A simulated computer-assisted TKR setting was constructed, and a single operator performed 30 repeated trials on five live subjects (male, mean age 24, mean weight 80 kg), digitizing what was considered to be the extremes of both medial and lateral malleoli. Subjects then performed 30 trials of the following movements: dorsi/plantarflexion with the ankle in the neutral, inverted and everted positions, in/eversion with the ankle in the dorsiflexed, neutral and plantarflexed positions, and finally circumduction. The measured data was then used to fit a 12 parameter biaxial joint model developed previously [Bogert 1994]. The same motion data was also used to determine the AJC using a sphere-fitting method.

3 Results and Discussion

Table 1 summarizes the results of the experiment; the digitizing point probe method had significantly higher precision than either motion-based method in the frontal plane (P=0.002 Biaxial, P=0.0003 Spherical). The biaxial method was significantly less variable than the spherical method (0.17° SD vs 0.28° SD, P=0.004).

Table 1. Repeatability of joint centre location in the frontal plane

AJC Location Method	ML Direction SD (mm)	Varus/Valgus SD (°)	Bias relative to point probe centre (mm)	Range (mm)
Point Probe	0.69	0.11	N/A	2.75
Biaxial Method	1.14	0.17	7.24 (medial)	5.00
Sphere Method	1.84	0.28	10.80 (medial)	7.23

Varus/valgus alignment appears to have a strong effect on implant lifespan, so the repeatability of ankle centre identification is a key design parameter in computer-assisted TKR procedures. This is the first report on the precision of locating an AJC using a biaxial joint model.

Although the repeatability of locating the AJC with the point probe is significantly better than the motion-based methods, the anatomic centre so defined is only indirectly related to the loads carried by the implant. The kinematic centres defined by either the biaxial or spherical models are more relevant for load calculations.

Since only five subjects were tested in this preliminary study, we do not yet have enough data to say that the kinematically-determined centres are not colocated with the anatomical centres. However, the AJCs found using the motion-based methods were biased medially (7–11 mm) and slightly anteriorly (1–3 mm). A medial shift in the functional joint centre would imply that the knee is in greater varus than previously suspected and implants are known to tolerate varus alignments poorly.

References

1. van den Bogert AJ, Smith GD, Nigg BM: In Vivo Determination of the Anatomical Axes of the Ankle Joint Complex: an Optimization Approach. Journal of Biomechanics 27(12), 1994. pp 1477–1488.

A Whole Body Atlas Based Segmentation for Delineation of Organs in Radiation Therapy Planning

Sharif M. Qatarneh [1], Simo Hyödynmaa [2], Marilyn E. Noz[3],
Gerald Q. Maguire Jr.[4], Elissa L. Kramer[3], and Joakim Crafoord[5].

[1]Department of Medical Radiation Physics, Karolinska Institute and Stockholm University,
Box 260, S- 171 76 Stockholm, Sweden.
Sharif@radfys.ks.se
[2]Department of Oncology, Tampere University Hospital, Tampere, Finland.
[3]Department of Radiology, NewYork University, New York, USA.
[4]Department of Teleinformatics, Royal Institute of Technology, Stockholm, Sweden.
[5]Department of Radiology, Karolinska Hospital, Stockholm, Sweden.

Optimal radiation therapy (RT) can be achieved when accurate knowledge about the exact location of the target volume to be treated with respect to all organs at risk is available. A whole body atlas (WBA) can be utilized to convert the anatomy of a "standard man" into individual patients by applying warping on anatomical images and the anatomy of the atlas can be adjusted to an individual patient [2,3]. The purpose of this work is to propose a semi-automatic segmentation procedure that utilizes polynomial warping together with active contour models, which could be used with WBA to delineate different organs in RT planning [4].

Materials and Methods

The Visible Human Male Computed Tomography data set (VHMCT) was considered reference-man geometry. The body sections of interest were the hepatic region and the chest, while the liver, the spinal cord and the right lung were the organs of interest in this case. The organs were outlined manually in each of the VHMCT organ slices and a set of 7 landmarks for each particular VHMCT slice was selected [1]. Five organ CT slices from each of 12 patient studies were selected and matched with the closest slice from the VHMCT data set. After the corresponding 7 match points were selected on the patient's slice, the drawn outline of the organ was transformed from the VHMCT slice into the patient's slice. The initial warped contour was then refined by active contour model to find the true outline of the patient's organ (Figure 1).

Evaluation and Discussion

The snake-refined organs' outlines were compared to outlines manually drawn on the patient's slice by a radiologist. The area inside the snake-refined contour and the area inside the manually drawn contour agreed within –5 to +7% for the liver, while the values for the spinal cord were in the range of $\pm 28\%$ or ca. $\pm 1cm^2$. In the case of the lung study, that range was found to be -11 to -2%. The approximate volumes of liver

W. Niessen and M. Viergever (Eds.): MICCAI 2001, LNCS 2208, pp. 1168-1169, 2001.

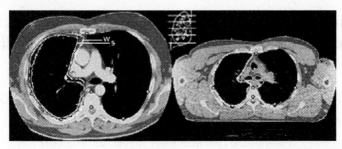

Fig. 1. The landmarks and the contour drawn on a VHMCT slice (right). The patient's match points, the warped contour (w) and the snake-refined outline (s) around the patient's lung (left).

for both segmentation methods agreed within ± 4%. The volumes of the abdominal spinal cord were found to agree within ± 21%, while lung volumes agreed within -8 to -5%. The average CT-number values inside the manually drawn liver and lung outlines were slightly lower and the standard deviation was found to be higher than in the case of active contour segmentation, which might be due to the partial volume effect. The center of gravity of the snake-refined liver contour was shifted to the left of the patient and posteriorly where structures of similar attenuation to liver are close. The active contour model has shown some limitations, particularly for the liver, where other structures of similar attenuation characteristics are close to the boundary [4]. The small size of the spinal cord provided limited control of the active contour but the high attenuation difference between the spinal cord and the spinal vertebrae has overcome that problem to a large extent. The large size of the lung and its high attenuation difference with surrounding tissue provided an ultimate environment of control and freedom for the active contour to find the lung boundaries.

The semi-automatic segmentation procedure can be applied to multiple organs at the same time for the purpose of radiation therapy. Active contour models can segment many organs, which have more attenuation difference when compared to surrounding organs and they have less shape complexity than the liver. The study addressed using 2D contours only, but 3D tools for warping and segmentation are needed, however, if a reliable whole body atlas is to be used with actual patients.

References

1. Crafoord J., Siddiqui F. M., Kramer E. L., Maguire Jr. G. Q., Noz M. E., and Zeleznik M. P., Comparison of Two Landmark Based Image Registration Methods for Use with a Body Atlas, Physica Medica XVI(2): (2000) 75-82.
2. Kimiaei S, Noz M. E., Jonsson E, Crafoord J. and Maguire Jr. G. Q. Evaluation of Polynomial image deformation using anatomical landmarks for matching of 3D-abdominal MR images and for atlas construction, IEEE Trans. Nucl. Sci. 46 (1999) 1110-1113.
3. Noz M. E., Maguire Jr. G. Q., Birnbaum B. A., Kaminer E. A., Sanger J. J., Kramer E. L. and Chapnick J. Graphics Interface for Medical Image Processing, J. Med. Systems 17 (1993) 1-16.
4. Qatarneh S. M., Crafoord J., Kramer E. L., Maguire Jr. G. Q., Brahme A., Noz M. E. and Hyödynmaa S. A Whole Body Atlas for Segmentation and Delineation of Organs for Radiation Therapy Planning. Nucl. Instr. and Meth. A (2001) (in press).

Automatic Modeling of Anatomical Structures for Biomechanical Analysis and Visualization in a Virtual Spine Workstation

Xuesong Chen[1], Chee-Kong Chui[1]*, Swee-Hin Teoh[2], Sim-Heng Ong[2], Wieslaw L. Nowinski[1]

1 Biomedical Lab, Kent Ridge Digital Lab, Singapore
* cheekong@krdl.org.sg
2 Laboratory for Biomedical Engineering & BIOMAT, National University of Singapore, Singapore

1 Introduction

With the advances in medical imaging, we can now extract quantitative information about human anatomical structures in three dimensions from images of various modalities. But visualization of anatomical structures and finite element analysis are two technical problems for representation of biomedical objects and simulation of physiological behavior. We describe the component of our workstation that contributes to the automatic generation of 3D physical-based meshes used in biomechanical engineering analysis and visualization of complex anatomical structures. This component extends the provision of visual information of the human spine to physical-based analysis for predicting the effects of treatment. These effects range from instrumentation in deformity correction, treatments on the courses of nerves and the resulting strains to the eventual interaction between bone and implants. One of the first applications of our approach was the used of the physical-based model to investigate the injury to human spine among airforce pilots in high G flying.

2 Automatic Modeling in the Virtual Spine Workstation

Figure 1 describes the processing pipeline of the virtual spine workstation. From medical images, after a preprocessing of identification and segmentation, we can start the automatic modeling of anatomical structures, which can generate physical-based meshes for biomechanical analysis and visualization. The automatic model generation process consists of several steps: Multiple Resolution 2D Meshing, 3D Meshing, Optimization and Validation.

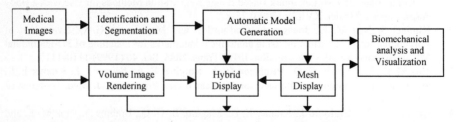

Figure 1. Processing pipeline of the virtual workstation

W. Niessen and M. Viergever (Eds.): MICCAI 2001, LNCS 2208, pp. 1170-1171, 2001.
© Springer-Verlag Berlin Heidelberg 2001

A grid plane approach for 2D meshing at each slice is proposed, which divides the area equally and generates regular elements. Firstly, the region on every slice is gridded at two orthogonal directions with a flexible resolution, which can be changed by the user to perform a better FEM analysis. Then, 2D meshes are generated using a two-dimensional marching cube algorithm. Regular elements of quadrilateral shape are constructed as interior core elements while triangular elements along the boundaries. Secondly, the nodes and elements are numbered to construct an FEM mesh system for engineering analysis.

The 3D meshing process joins 2D planar meshes at two adjacent slices to form volumetric meshes. A 3D grid frame structure establishes the topological relation of any two adjacent grid planes. The grid frame approach depicts the geometrical closeness of the contours at the adjacent slices, provides an accurate and convenient means to identify the topological connection of the anatomical contours. The 3D meshes are therefore built upon the grid frame by connecting corresponding nodes at adjacent grid planes.

Due to the complexity of the object's geometry, optimization and validation processes are performed to standardize the elements at the boundary to comply with the requirement for FEM analysis. In order to identify the related region accurately, the optimization process modifies the local coordinate system and performs adaptive meshing of the local region. After the process, the validation process checks each element by computing Jacobians, aspect ratios, volumes and areas of elements to meet the requirements of the FEM analysis software.

3 Results and Discussions

The generated 3D meshes of the anatomical structures allow for biomechanical analysis and visualization. Figure 2(a) shows the result of axial compression of L4 vertebrae after FEM analysis using ABAQUS packages. Figure 2(b) is a visualization of a human spine with the generated 3D meshes from VHD data [1]. Our modeling technique is applied to other anatomical structures. We are extending this workstation for clinicians to perform pre-operative planning for image guided spinal surgery.

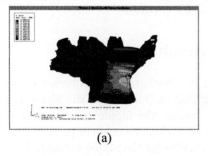
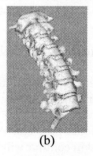

(a)   (b)

Figure 2. Biomechanical analysis and visualization with the 3D meshes

References

1. Spitzer VM, Whitelock DG (1998). *National Library of Medicine, Atlas of the Visible Human Male: Reverse Engineering of the Human Body*. Jones and Bartlett Publishers.

Matching Breast Lesions in Multiple Mammographic Views

Saskia van Engeland and Nico Karssemeijer

University Medical Center St Radboud, Department of Radiology, PO Box 9101,
6500 HB Nijmegen, The Netherlands

1 Introduction

By combining information from multiple mammographic views (temporal, medio-lateral oblique (MLO) and cranio-caudal (CC), or bilateral) it should be possible to improve the accuracy of computer-aided diagnosis (CAD) methods. In litera-ture various approaches have been described to establish correspondence between multiple views. Highnam et al. [1] used a model-based method to find a curve in the MLO view which corresponds to the potential positions of a point in the CC view. Kok-Wiles et al. [2] used a representation of the nested structure of 'salient' bright regions to match mammogram pairs. Karssemeijer et al. [3] and Lau et al. [4] both used a set of landmarks and applied a nonlinear interpolation to align the skin line of two breast images. Almost all matching approaches are based on acquiring a set of landmarks. In a mammogram the nipple is the most obvious landmark. Radiologists use the distance to the nipple to correlate a le-sion in MLO and CC view. It is generally believed that this distance remains fairly constant. The goal of this paper is twofold: first, to investigate to what extent this distance remains constant in multiple views, and second, to investi-gate if the accuracy of automated detection of the nipple is sufficient to use the distance to the nipple as a reliable measure for matching. For this purpose we used an annotated database which contained 327 corresponding mammogram pairs from the Dutch breast cancer screening program.

2 Method and Preliminary Results

After segmentation of the mammogram into background and breast tissue, the skin contour can be obtained. Assuming that the location of the nipple is some-where on this contour, the problem of locating the nipple can be reduced to a one-dimensional problem. When the nipple is clearly visible in profile the curva-ture of the skin contour will be a good indicator for the nipple position. However, when the nipple is not clearly visible, due to for instance suboptimal positioning or exposure, other features have to be used. Chandrasekhar et al. [5] used an intensity gradient in the direction normal to the skin contour and directed inside the breast for automatically locating the nipple. Previously, at our institute the nipple position was estimated by a relatively simple algorithm that was based on knowledge about the geometry of the breast. After automatically detecting the

W. Niessen and M. Viergever (Eds.): MICCAI 2001, LNCS 2208, pp. 1172–1173, 2001.

pectoral muscle using the Hough transform, this algorithm determined the point on the skin contour with the largest distance to the pectoral muscle (MLO) or the chest side of the mammogram (CC). Although this approach worked fairly well in 60 percent of the mammograms (error < 6 mm), it is not reliable enough to be used for matching lesions in a pair of mammograms.

This paper describes the on-going work on the development of a more accurate method for locating the nipple based on multiple features in combination with a neural network approach. The features that are used describe intensity gradients, shape of the skin contour, line patterns of the glandular tissue, and the geometry of the breast. The feature values are determined for every point on the contour and are fed into a three-layer backpropagation network. The network is trained using a set of 314 mammograms with known nipple position. Figure 1 gives some preliminary results. Although the network still relies very heavily on the distance algorithm, as described above, this new approach has improved the nipple detection accuracy. The variation in the distance to the nipple is approximately the same when using the indicated nipple positions and the nipple positions as determined by the network. To give an indication of the accuracy when using this measure for matching lesions: in 79 percent of the cases the distance to the nipple does not deviate more than 1.5 cm between both views.

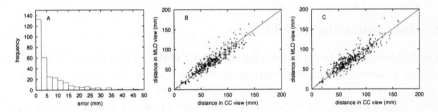

Fig. 1. Histogram of the distance from the actual to the estimated nipple position and scatter plots of the distance (mm) between a lesion and the nipple in MLO and CC view using the indicated nipple positions (B) and nipple positions as determined by the network (C).

References

[1] Highnam, R., Kita, Y., Brady, M., Shepstone, B., and English, R.: Determining correspondence between views. In Digital Mammography, Kluwer, Dordrecht (1998) 111–118
[2] Kok-Wiles, S., Brady, M., and Highnam, R.: Comparing mammogram pairs for the detection of lesions. In Digital Mammography, Kluwer, Dordrecht (1998) 103–110
[3] Karssemeijer, N., and te Brake, G.: Combining single view features and asymmetry for detection of mass lesions. In Digital Mammography, Kluwer, Dordrecht (1998) 95–102
[4] Lau, Y., and Bischof, W.: Automated detection of breast tumors using the asymmetry approach. Comp and Biomed Research **24** (1991) 273–295
[5] Chandrasekhar, R., and Attikiouzel, Y.: A Simple Method for Automatically Locating the Nipple on Mammograms. IEEE Trans Med Imag **16** (1997) 483–494

Automatic Detection of Large Misregistrations of Multimodality Medical Images

C.E. Rodríguez-Carranza[1,2] and M.H. Loew[1,2]

[1] Department of Electrical and Computer Engineering,
[2] Institute for Medical Imaging and Image Analysis,
The George Washington University,
Washington DC 20052, USA
claudia,loew@seas.gwu.edu

Abstract. Before a retrospective registration algorithm can be used routinely in the clinic, methods must be provided for distinguishing between registration solutions that are clinically satisfactory and those that are not [1]. One approach is to rely on a human observer. Here, we present an *algorithmic* procedure that discriminates between badly misregistered pairs and those that are close to correct alignment. We found that a new goodness measure based on brain contours appears to identify misregistrations on the order of 15 mm or more of RMS error.

1 Introduction and Design

The lack of ground truth in the clinical setting makes it essential to find methodologies to assess automated retrospective registration techniques (which sometimes converge at clinically unsatisfactory values). Visual assessment has been used [2,1] to distinguish registrations that were clinically useful from those that were not. We would like to find alternative automatic or semiautomatic assessment techniques that, at the very least, reduce the number of bad registrations reaching the clinician. Therefore, we propose and demonstrate an algorithmic assessment technique for 3D CT-MR brain registration based on contours.

The measure of the goodness of registration used in this research was R1 – the average fraction of MR contour voxels that were at a distance of zero or one (in the x-y plane) from a CT contour voxel. R1 lies in the range $[0, 1]$, and the larger R1 is, the closer the contours are. The aim is to use R1 to assign one of two possible labels to a registration result: "definitively bad" or "possibly good".

The measure was tested on CT, T1, and T2 images of three patients (practice set, patients 1 and 5) from the Vanderbilt study [3]. The registration error was defined as the RMS distance between the two sets of eight corner points of CT produced by its registration to MR using (1) the gold standard and (2) a given registration transformation.

To study the feasibility of R1 for assessing accuracy, we performed CT to T1 and CT to T2 registrations. A total of 800 misregistrations were generated per image pair per patient. The magnitudes of the resultant translational and rotational displacement vectors were confined to $0 - 8$ mm and $0 - 8°$, with corresponding RMS errors of $0 - 35$ mm.

W. Niessen and M. Viergever (Eds.): MICCAI 2001, LNCS 2208, pp. 1174–1175, 2001.

2   Results and Discussion

Figure 1 shows the results for the three patients ($801 \times 3 = 2403$ points per graph). Based on Wong et al. [2], we define registrations within both 3 mm and $4°$ from ground truth to be *good* registrations (diamonds), and outside that range to be *bad* registrations (dots). Observe that for R1 = 0.7 most of the bad points with RMS > 15mm could be identified. R1 is relatively insensitive to small rotations around the X or Y axes, so several bad points with RMS > 10mm have a large value of R1; this is something that clearly needs to be improved. Points with RMS < 10mm but R1 < 0.5 have large translational displacements, and therefore are real misregistrations.

How important to R1's usefulness is the accuracy of segmentation? The dependence is small because for registrations far from correct alignment the actual distance between contours will be much larger than the error induced by segmentation; work is underway on a general proof of this observation.

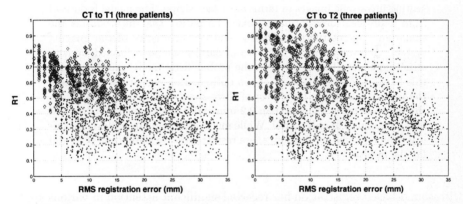

Fig. 1. Goodness of registration measure R1 against registration error.

3   Conclusions

We proposed a goodness measure based on brain contours as an aid to labeling registrations as either "definitively bad" or "possibly good". The results of the present study indicate that the use of R1 may be a good first step to reduce the number of badly registered images reaching the clinician.

References

1. Fitzpatrick, J.M., et al.: Visual assessment of the accuracy of retrospective registration of MR and CT images of the brain. IEEE TMI **17**(4) (1998) 571–585
2. Wong, J.C.H., et al.: Evaluation of the limits of visual detection of image misregistration in a brain F-18 FDG PET-MRI study. Eur. J. of Nuc. Med. **24**(6) (1997)
3. West, J., et al.: Comparison and evaluation of retrospective intermodality brain image registration techniques. JCAT **21**(4) (1997) 554–566

Registration of the Spine Using a Physically-Based Image Model for Ultrasound

Jason W. Trobaugh and R. Martin Arthur

Washington University, St. Louis, MO 63130, USA
jasont@ee.wustl.edu, http://www.ee.wustl.edu/pbuim/

Abstract. Despite significant efforts towards various applications of ultrasound-based tissue registration, ultrasound still plays a minor role in clinical computer-assisted intervention. Interpretation of the images is one major obstacle. Towards a robust and accurate approach to automated interpretation, we have developed a probabilistic model representing ultrasonic images in terms of surface shape. The model is derived from a physical description of image formation that incorporates the shape and microstructure of tissue and characteristics of the imaging system. A framework for inference of surface shape is formed by constructing a data likelihood from the probabilistic model. We have used this likelihood with a quasi-Newton optimization algorithm to estimate the pose of a vertebra from a set of three simulated images. In 20 trials, the estimate error was less than 0.2 mm and 0.4 degrees in 15 trials and over 1.0 degrees in only 1 trial. While much work remains to develop clinical utility in any application, these results indicate significant potential for the approach.

Ultrasound-based registration has received significant attention in various applications, e.g., assessment of intra-operative changes in the neuroanatomy, alignment of the prostate for radiotherapy, and registration of the spine for radiotherapy and for image-guided surgery [1]. Given a robust approach to image interpretation, the range of applications would be likely to increase rapidly. The accuracy and reliability requirements of these applications are significant, though, and success has been limited. These limitations have motivated our interest in a rigorous Bayesian approach to image analysis [2] that employs probabilistic models for the underlying structure and for observation via an imaging system. In addition to potential for improved registration, our work has provided a deeper understanding of the unique way in which shape is represented in ultrasound.

Our work has focused on the following ultrasonic image model for Bayesian image analysis. The image model is based on a physical description of image formation that incorporates surface shape, microstructure and the characteristics of the imaging system [3]. A probabilistic model is constructed from statistical images, mean, variance and SNR_0, that are computed directly from a mathematical representation of the physical description [4]. The computations are intensive, requiring several surface integrals for each pixel. The model assumes a complex Gaussian form for the intermediate RF image, from which amplitude statistics

W. Niessen and M. Viergever (Eds.): MICCAI 2001, LNCS 2208, pp. 1176–1177, 2001.

are computed numerically. From statistical images, Rayleigh and Gaussian density functions are assigned to individual pixels for the construction of a data likelihood representing the image conditioned on the underlying shape, in this case, the pose, i.e., rotation and translation, of the vertebra.

We have performed a preliminary investigation of our image model applied to registration of the spine. For this work, we isolated the surface shape from surrounding tissue by working with a phantom containing a cadaveric vertebra. Data from actual imaging systems included a volume of CT images and ultrasonic images acquired from a Tetrad imaging system using a 6 MHz linear array probe. A triangulated surface representing the vertebra was produced from a manual segmentation of the CT images using the Marching Cubes algorithm. The images and triangulated surface were co-registered using a StealthStation^{TM} Treatment Guidance Platform from Medtronic, Inc.

The data likelihood described previously was used as a cost function with a quasi-Newton optimization algorithm for estimating the pose of the vertebral surface. Performance was evaluated using the results of 20 trials, with each trial beginning from a random estimate 2 mm and 2 degrees from the known pose. Using a set of three simulated images, the resulting estimate error was less than 0.2 mm and 0.4 degrees in 15 trials, less than 0.2 mm and 1.0 degrees on 4 trials, and approximately 1 mm and 2 degrees in 1 trial.

These preliminary results are promising for such a small data set. We believe this early success is an indication of potentially significant value for our model and for this approach in computer-assisted intervention. In addition, the physical basis of the model provides a framework for understanding the problems as well as developing solutions.

The authors thank the following colleagues for their support and assistance in this work: Paul Kessman, Troy Holsing, Rob Teichman and Sarang Joshi at Medtronic, Surgical Navigation Technologies, and Jaimie Henderson, M.D. and Richard Bucholz, M.D. in the Department of Neurosurgery at the St. Louis University School of Medicine.

References

1. Trobaugh, J.W., Kessman, P.J., Dietz, D.R., Bucholz, R.D.: Ultrasound in Image Fusion: A Framework and Applications. Proc. IEEE Ultrason., Ferroelect., Freq. Contr. Symp. (1997) 1393–1396
2. Grenander, U., Miller, M.I.: Representation of Knowledge in Complex Systems. J. R. Statist. Soc.. **56** (1994) 549–603
3. Trobaugh, J.W., Arthur, R.M.: A Discrete-Scatterer Model for Ultrasonic Images of Rough Surfaces. IEEE Trans. Ultrason., Ferroelect., Freq. Contr. **47** (2000) 1520–1529
4. Trobaugh, J.W.: An Image Model for Ultrasound Incorporating Surface Shape and Microstructure and Characteristics of the Imaging System. Doctoral dissertation, Washington University in St. Louis, (May 2000)

Computing Match Functions for Curves in $\mathbb{R}^2$ and $\mathbb{R}^3$ by Refining Polyline Approximations

Brian Avants, Marcelo Siqueira, and James Gee

Departments of Computer and Information Science and Radiology,
University of Pennsylvania
Philadelphia, PA, USA 19104-6389
{avants,marcelos,gee}@grasp.cis.upenn.edu

1   Algorithm Summary

We believe geometry is particularly important in the medical domain because
shape descriptions can help quantify diagnosis. Our work follows the geometric
matching methods of [1] and [2] but is also related to [3] and [4].

Dynamic programming is used in [1] to find suboptimal matching with respect
to the following bending and stretching energy function:

$$E(g) = \int_0^L [\, |\cos(\psi) - \sin(\psi)| + R|\kappa_1 \cos(\psi) - \kappa_2 \sin(\psi)| \,]d\eta \ . \qquad (1)$$

Here, κ is curvature, L is the length of the match curve, and $\psi \in [0, \frac{\pi}{2}]$ is
the angle of its tangent vector with the x-axis (some details are omitted.) The
performance of the algorithm is very sensitive, in practice, to the value of R.
Also, no global knowledge of the curve is incorporated. Iteration over polygonal
curve approximations is used to restrict the problem in [2] while including global
geometric information.

Our solution builds on both approaches. We aim to minimize equation (1)
using polyline approximations to eliminate explicit choice of R. Therefore, our
goal is to find a function, g, such that, $g \colon C^1 \mapsto C^2$ and $g^{-1} \colon C^2 \mapsto C^1$. We
require that every point on C^1 maps optimally to a unique corresponding point
on C^2 (or is deleted). The algorithm is summarized here:

1. Re-parameterize each curve with constant arc length.
2. Initialize g_1 as a minimum stretching energy match.
3. Compute the $g_2, \ldots, g_n$ set of match functions, where each g_i corresponds
   to the match implied by pairing the vertices of the $i + 1$ sized best polygon
   fits with linear interpolation between vertices.
4. Evaluate the terms of the energy function for each g_i. Select the minimum.
5. Perform gradient descent to refine g_{min}.
6. Repeat the procedure between vertices of g_{min} until the distance between
   curves and approximations reaches a given tolerance $\epsilon \geq 0$.

W. Niessen and M. Viergever (Eds.): MICCAI 2001, LNCS 2208, pp. 1178–1179, 2001.

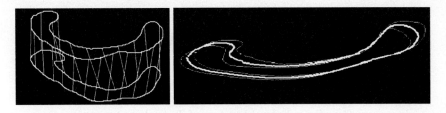

Fig. 1. A correspondence of corpora callosa with the associated match curves g and g^{-1} (left). Average human corpus callosum and one standard deviation of its shape (right).

2 Results

We used dynamic programming to implement a version of the algorithm that is fast (seconds) enough to be of use in clinical situations. Here, we give results of its use on an instance of real patient data as well as on a large dataset. The coronal direction of the corpus callosum was automatically segmented from MRI for each of 87 human controls matched roughly for age and handedness. No adjustments for scale were necessary.

3 Conclusions and Further Work

We summarized a novel solution to the curve correspondence problem. The statement of the solution is flexible and general enough that it may be adapted to find constrained minima of a large range of energy functions. In addition, it can be shown that dependence on explicit values of R in (1) can be eliminated. Automatic generation of the average callosa from a large dataset indicates the reliability of the method. Similar work is under way on open contours in $\mathbb{R}^3$. Future work will explore the effect of the polygon approximation, choice of refinement technique and incorporation of probability.

References

1. Sebastian T, Klein PN, Kimia BB, Crisco J: Constructing 2D Curve Atlases. MM-BIA. (2000) 70–77
2. Younes L. Computable Elastic Distance Between Shapes. SIAM J. Appl. Math, 1996. 58:565-586
3. Bakircioglu M, Grenander U, Khaneja N, Miller MI: Curve Matching on Brain Surfaces Using Induced Frenet Distance Metrics. Human Brain Mapping. (1998) 6(5):329–331
4. Xin Y, Truyen B, Pratikakis I, Cornelis J: Hierarchical contour matching in medical images. Image and Vision Computing. (1996) 417–433
5. Hobby J: Polygonal Approximations that Minimize the Number of Inflections ACM-SIAM Symposium on Discrete Algorithms. (1993)

A Multi-modal Approach to Segmentation of Tubular Structures

Matthias Harders and Gábor Székely

Swiss Federal Institute of Technology
Communication Technology Laboratory
ETH Zentrum, CH-8092 Zürich, Switzerland
{mharders,szekely}@vision.ee.ethz.ch

Abstract. In this paper we describe a new paradigm for interactive segmentation of medical 3D volume data. We are using a 3D haptic device to enhance the segmentation process with additional sensory feedback. The segmentation of tubular structures in the human body serves as an initial case study for our system. The haptic interaction allows the user to extract the centerline of a tubular structure, even if the image data quality is insufficient. The segmented path is then used to reorient cross-sections through the data volume, which helps to extract the boundary of the 3D object in a subsequent step.

1 Introduction

The segmentation of 3D medical datasets obtained from a variety of tomographic imaging modalities, such as CT or MRI, can be classified with regard to its degree of automation. In between the two extremes of manual and automatic segmentation lie semi-automated algorithms, which try to merge the advantages of both worlds. Rather than attempting to duplicate the complex and poorly understood human capability to recognize objects, they try to provide an interactive environment in which users control the segmentation process and exploit their expert knowledge. These algorithms can be further classified according to the underlying interaction paradigms in either two or three dimensions, but systems that exploit the possibilities of true interactive 3D segmentation are more seldom [2,4,3]. This is often justified by the problems that arise due to adding another dimension to the user interaction. Editing, controlling and interacting in three dimensions often overwhelms the perceptual powers of a human operator. Moreover, todays desktop metaphors are based on two-dimensional interaction and can not easily be extended to three dimensions. Finally, the visual channel of the human sensory system is not suitable for the perception of volumetric data. In the presented project these limitations are alleviated by enhancing the segmentation process with additional sensory feedback. We focus on providing perceptual information to the medical expert by using a haptic device, which provides 3 DOF translational feedback. We are currently concentrating on the semi-automatic detection and extraction of tubular structures in medical datasets. Usually this research area is subdivided with respect to the different medical fields the examined structures stem from. Nevertheless, several problems can be identified

W. Niessen and M. Viergever (Eds.): MICCAI 2001, LNCS 2208, pp. 1180–1182, 2001.
© Springer-Verlag Berlin Heidelberg 2001

which are common to segmentation tasks in all these subfields. Success or failure of reported algorithms is often largely dependent on the quality of the image data. For example, the variable intensity of an unevenly distributed contrast agent inside a vessel might cause artifacts during segmentation. Furthermore, the presence of pathological changes, which is often the case for the objects of interest, can cause problems for template or model based approaches that rely on the size or shape of the contour. Additionally, the handling of junctions in tubular structures often poses a difficulty, that has to be overcome. Also, two-dimensional approaches have limitations, because tubular structures often follow a tortuous and curved course through 3D space. This makes the accurate tracing of their geometry an extremely difficult task. Furthermore, tightly folded structures are often sliced at an oblique angle, resulting in extreme deterioration of image quality as tangential slicing direction is approached. These problems may make the slice-by-slice reconstruction of their 3D geometry a very complicated and error prone task.

2   Multi-modal Segmentation Tool

In order to overcome the described difficulties, we focus on using force-feedback as an additional channel to mediate information. The initial step of our multi-modal approach is the haptically assisted extraction of the centerline of a tubular structure. To do this we adopt an approach similar to the one used by Bartz for enhanced navigation [1]. First we create a binarization of our data volume by thresholding. From the resulting dataset S we compute an Euclidean distance: For each $(x, y, z) \in S$, we compute the distance map value

$$DM(x,y,z) = \min_{(x_i,y_i,z_i)\in S} d[(x,y,z),(x_i,y_i,z_i)],$$

where d denotes the Euclidean distance from a voxel that is part of the tubular structure to a voxel of the surrounding tissue. In the next step we negate the 3D distance map and approximate the gradients by central differences. Moreover, to ensure the smoothness of the computed forces, we apply a 5x5x5 binomial filter. This force map is precomputed before the actual interaction, to ensure a stable force-update. Because the force vectors are located at discrete voxel positions, we have to do a tri-linear interpolation to obtain the continuous gradient force map we need during interaction. The computed forces can now be utilized to guide a user on a path close to the centerline of the tubular structure. In the case of good data quality, the user "falls through" the dataset guided along the 3D ridge created by the forces. While moving along the path, the user can set control points which are used to approximate the path with a spline. The advantage of this approach becomes apparent in situations where the image data is not sufficient to discriminate the object boundaries. At regions with unclear image information, a user can exert forces on the haptic device to leave the precalculated path by pushing the 3D cursor into the direction, where the path continues. The segmentation of tubular structures can be optimally facilitated, if all cross-sections of the object would be orthogonal to the centerline. Therefore, we use the spline, that is generated interactively to determine the appropriate orientation of a free slice plane through the data volume. The next step is to use an active contour model to extract the 2D cross-sections of our structure of interest. The adaptive reorientation of the cutting slice allows us to make a rough assumption about the shape of the cross-section, which should be approximately circular. Furthermore, as we always update the slice orientation, we can use the segmentation of the previous step as a fairly good initialization for the next cross-section. This can be done, because the deviation between subsequent cross-sections in a tubular structure is usually small. To estimate the sensitivity of our approach and to understand its limitations, we performed a first case study as an initial proof of concept. As an area of high medical relevance, we selected virtual colonoscopy for the validation of our approach. The dataset used in our study, a 256 x 256 x 223 CT scan of the human abdomen, was acquired at the Institute of Diagnostic Radiology of the Zurich University Hospital.

3   First Results and Future Research

We used our interactive system to create the centerline through the tubular structure and obtained the reformatted cross-sections along the path. The cross-sections on each slice were extracted with an active contour model. Due to the reformatting of the cross-sections and the initialization propagating from slice to slice, this process could be done without any user interaction. Nevertheless, it has to be mentioned, that this processing step was eased by the good image quality of our dataset. Apart from the case study described in this paper, we also applied our system to the segmentation of the small intestines (A 256x256x147 CT-dataset of the abdomen, provided by the Department of Radiology, Semmelweis University Budapest). While in the former case conventional algorithms could also be used successfully, they failed on the latter one due to the problems described above. In contrast to this, our approach succeeded on this complex dataset, too. Nevertheless, we have to mention that a decrease of image data quality was accompanied by increased user interaction time and effort. Further evaluation, especially for more complex data has to be done in our on-going project. Especially, the suitability of this approach for clinical practice has to be studied.

References

1. Dirk Bartz and Özlem Gürvit. Haptic navigation in volumetric datasets. In *Proceedings of the Second PHANToM Users Research Symposium*. Swiss Federal Institute of Technology, 2000.
2. Ken Hinckley. *Haptic Issues for Virtual Manipulation*. PhD thesis, School of Engineering and Applied Science, University of Virginia, 1996.
3. Serra L., Ng H., Chua B.C., and T. Poston. Interactive vessel tracing in volume data. In *ACM 1997 Symposium on Interactive 3D Graphics*, pages 131-137, 1997.
4. Steven O. Senger. User-directed segmentation of the visible human data sets in an immersive environment. In Richard A. Banvard, Prof. Francesco Pinciroli, and Pietro Cerveri, editors, *The Second Visible Human Project Conference Proceedings*, 1998.

Segmentation of the Subthalamic Nucleus in MR Images Using Information Fusion - A Preliminary Study for a Computed-Aided Surgery of Parkinson's Disease

Vincent Barra[1], Jean-Jacques Lemaire[1,2], Franck Durif[3], Jean-Yves Boire[1]

[1] ERIM, [2] URN, [3] Department of Neurology, Faculty of Medicine, BP 38 63001
CLERMONT-FERRAND, France
{vincent.barra, j-yves.boire}@u-clermont1.fr

Abstract. Subthalamic nucleus (ST) stimulation is proved to have beneficial effects on the symptoms of Parkinson's disease. We propose a fully automated segmentation method of this structure on MR images based on an information fusion technique. Information is provided by both images and expert knowledge, and consists in morphological, topological and tissue constitution data. All this ambiguous, complementary and redundant information is managed using a three steps fusion scheme based on fuzzy logic. Information is first modeled into a common theoretical frame managing imprecision and uncertainty. Models are then fused and a segmentation is finally performed that reduce the imprecision and increase the certainty in the location of the structure. Computed locations are compared with those obtained during a stereotactic surgical procedure. Results on ten patients are very promising, and suggest that this method may be applied during the surgical procedure as an help for the location of the subthalamic nucleus.

Method

In order to segment the ST, we were first interested in locating the third ventricle (V3) and the two red nuclei (RN). V3 was defined as a "cerebrospinal fluid (CSF) area, roughly located in the inter hemispheric plane, at approximately 20mm under the lateral ventricles". RN as for them were defined as "ovoid-shape structures, almost symmetrical with respect to the inter hemispheric plane, approximately 7mm long in the left-right axis, and 9 mm long in the antero-posterior axis, with a white matter-like (WM) signal in T2-weighted images". Finally, the ST were defined by the neurosurgeon as "gray matter (GM) structure, almost symmetrical with respect to the inter hemispheric plane, 15 mm under or 10 mm under and anterior the RN, posterior and inferior to the V3 (at a distance of almost 8 mm)". We then defined the following scenario in order to precisely locate the ST:
- segmentation of the ventricular system and V3 using topological information ;
- segmentation of the RN from the V3 using topological and tissue information
- segmentation of the STN from the RN using topological, and tissue information

W. Niessen and M. Viergever (Eds.): MICCAI 2001, LNCS 2208, pp. 1183-1184, 2001.
© Springer-Verlag Berlin Heidelberg 2001

All the ambiguous information was modeled in a fuzzy logic frame, allowing the management of imprecision and incertitude inherent to the medical data. More precisely, each piece of information was theoretically modeled as a fuzzy map, where the gray level of a voxel represented its membership to the studied information (tissue constitution, distance, direction). All these fuzzy maps were then aggregated according to their redundancy and their complementarities, using concepts derived from data fusion. Finally a decision (*i.e.* a segmentation of ST) was processed following the aggregation step, and results of this segmentation were compared to those obtained during a stereotactic surgical procedure. All the interest of data fusion here was that decision was taken by managing all the available information. Moreover, further data (morphological aspect of the ST for example) might simply be added to the process.

Results and Conclusion

The following figure presents an overview of the process. Points of the ST were represented in black in the last image

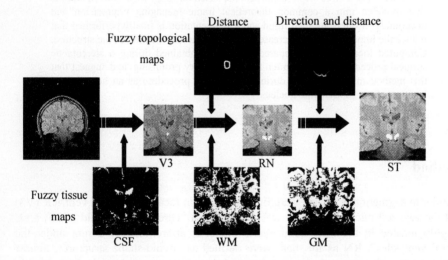

Ten patients were selected for electrical stimulation of ST. Three orthogonal MR images were acquired in stereotactic conditions (Leksell Model G frame and four unicortical fixations repositioning system, Elekta Instruments®) on a Magnetom 1T (Siemens). Stereotactic coordinates of the center of inertia of the computed ST were compared for the ten patients to stereotactic coordinates of the point considered as the most efficient for stimulation by neurosurgeons after the surgical procedure. Results of this preliminary study were quite encouraging, but still perfectible, and we now plan to improve the results by taking into account the real 3D shape of the ST using the three orthogonal MR sequences provided by the protocol.

Collaborative Multi-agent IVUS Image Segmentation

E.G.P. Bovenkamp, J. Dijkstra, J.G. Bosch, and J.H.C. Reiber

Leiden University Medical Center, Department of Radiology,
Building 1 C3-Q-50, Division of Image Processing, P.O. Box 9600,
2300 RC Leiden, The Netherlands
E.G.P.Bovenkamp@lumc.nl

Abstract. This paper describes a multi-agent segmentation approach in which asynchronous agents combine low-level image processing with high-level reasoning. Agents each have their own image processing specialty and communicate and collaborate with other agents to resolve conflicts with the mutual goal to come to a consistent overall interpretation of image runs. Agents locally adjust their behavior and control the image processing depending on image content.

1 Introduction

A typical problem encountered in efforts to automate the image interpretation process is that there is, generally speaking, no 'ultimate segmentation algorithm'. Therefore an approach is desired, which deals with combining results from different segmentation algorithms, selecting the best solution given the image evidence and possibly following multiple lines of reasoning. A more elaborate and explicit reasoning system may handle such problems and lead to a successful interpretation of these images.

2 System Design

A multi-agent approach was chosen to enable modularization of knowledge and allow for scalability and flexibility. Further a multi-agent approach almost naturally fits the requirements that the system should be able to deal with combinations of different segmentation algorithms and multiple lines of reasoning. We designed and implemented a multi-agent system which integrates our locally developed image processing platform with the Soar architecture where Soar is an architecture for constructing general intelligent systems.

Agents in the system can *interact* with other agents through communication, *act* on the world by performing image processing operations and *perceive* that same world by accessing images and image processing results.

We have designed and implemented an image processing agent knowledge model that currently contains over 300 rules. Most of these rules represent common knowledge for each agent in the architecture and describe how to do image

W. Niessen and M. Viergever (Eds.): MICCAI 2001, LNCS 2208, pp. 1185–1186, 2001.

processing (139 rules), how to communicate (33 rules), how to resolve conflicts (100 rules) and further general utilities and problem solving (26 rules).

On average only about 5 extra rules are necessary to determine an agent's specialization. These rules specify an agents capabilities and interests and specify how an agent is to build complex image processing tasks. Less that 2% of the agent's knowledge is thus agent specific. This makes the knowledge model of image processing agents highly modular resulting in easy construction and addition of new agents to the agent community.

3   Conflict Resolution

Agent conflict resolution is the process in which agents try to achieve consensus over their image interpretations in case there is a conflict. A conflict arises when two or more agents hold incompatible views on the segmentation of images or when an agent detects internal inconsistencies. The conflict resolution mechanism is designed as a separate category of problem solving expertise.

The conflict resolution mechanism causes local adaptation to image content, combines low-level image processing knowledge with high-level knowledge about relations between objects given the global interpretation context, and enforces global consistency of the image segmentation.

4   Results

Table 1 shows the qualitative interpretation results of the collaborative multi-agent image segmentation of 32 consecutive IntraVascular UltraSound (IVUS) images with 32 sidebranches and 13 shadows. The results compare the stand alone (sa) application of detection algorithms with their multi-agent application (ma). Optimal means a result matches segmentation by a human observer, suboptimal means acceptable but not perfect, and false means the result is not acceptable The table shows that no errors remain after conflict resolution (12 times) and algorithm adjustments (53 times) in the multi-agent approach, which illustrates its superior performance over stand alone application.

Table 1. Interpretation results of collaborative multi-agent IVUS image segmentation.

result	lumen		vessel		sidebranch		shadow	
	sa	ma	sa	ma	sa	ma	sa	ma
optimal	30	30	18	27	26	32	12	12
suboptimal	2	2	2	5	0	0	1	1
false	0	0	12	0	6	0	10	0

Acknowledgement

This work has been funded by the Dutch Innovative Research Program (IOP) under grant nr. IBV97008.

Segmentation of Chemical Shift Images
with Mixture Modeling

A.W. Simonetti, R. Wehrens, L.M.C. Buydens

Laboratory of Analytical Chemistry, Nijmegen University, Toernooiveld 1, 6525ED
Nijmegen, The Netherlands
A.Simonetti@sci.kun.nl

Introduction

Chemical shift imaging (CSI), a method which samples ^{1}H NMR-spectra from a grid of volume elements, produces an overwhelming amount of data. Each spectrum contains information about several metabolites in the sampled area. One approach for interpretation of this large amount of data is segmentation of the CSI grid in clusters which share the same features, followed by classification of each segment to a specific tissue type. We used mixture modeling to perform segmentation of CSI images for automatic identification of malignant areas in the human brain.

Mixture modeling is an approach to clustering in which the data are described as mixtures of distributions, usually Gaussians [Mc Lachlan, G.J., *Finite Mixture Models*, Wiley NY (2000)]. The parameters of the Gaussians are obtained through application of the EM algorithm [Dempster, A.P., J. Royal Statist. Soc. B 39(1) (1977) 1-38].

There are a number of advantages of mixture modeling over other more common forms of unsupervised clustering; it is possible to derive uncertainty estimates for individual classifications; with the Bayesian Information Criterion (BIC) [Schwarz, G., Ann. Statist. 6 (1978) 461-464] the optimal number of clusters as well as the clustering method can be chosen automatically -this is often a problem in other unsupervised approaches- and the visualization of the clusters is possible in the space of the original variables.

Results & Discussion

High resolution MRI images and CSI images were acquired from four patients with a histologically proven oligodendroglioma tumor on a 1.5 T Siemens whole body system. From each spectrum within the selection box 5 resonances were analyzed by numerical integration of 16 points under each resonance: myo-inositol (3.6 ppm); choline (3.2 ppm); creatine (3.0 ppm); N-aspartyl-aspartate (2.0 ppm) and lipids/lactate (1.3 ppm). These 5 quantitated resonances were used as input for the mixture modeling.

Segmentation was performed with the MCLUST software, which gives easy access to mixture modeling for clustering. The number of clusters were fixed between 3 and 5, which is a reasonable number from a medical point of view. From the BIC value

W. Niessen and M. Viergever (Eds.): MICCAI 2001, LNCS 2208, pp. 1187-1188, 2001.
© Springer-Verlag Berlin Heidelberg 2001

calculated by MCLUST the optimal number of clusters as well as the best model was automatically selected for each patient.

In Figure 1 the BIC values for patient G are presented. An ellipsoidal model with equal cluster volume and shape (EEE) gives the highest BIC value for 3 clusters, therefore this 3 cluster model is used.

In Figure 2 the segmentation (left) and uncertainty (right) values for each patient are depicted below a MRI image. Clearly the segmentation corresponds to areas suspected for malignancy for all patients. In all cases the segments can also be identified by visual inspection of the spectra. Also the agreement between clustering pixels in MRI images (not shown) and the segmentation presented is very good. In the case of patient M the 3 voxel segment at the top left of the tumor is suspected to be a bleeding. Segmentation for patient W is not convincing. This can be due to a low quality of the spectra.

The uncertainty values for all voxels are quit low. Uncertainties below 10% are common (white). The values can be used to expel voxels from a cluster. For example the isolated and right lower voxel belonging to the dark cluster in patient D may be removed from the cluster due to their high uncertainty value.

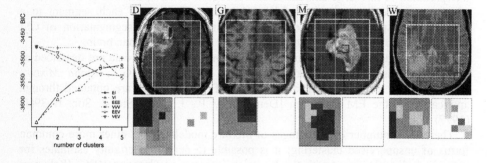

Fig. 1. BIC values for patient G. Clustering with 6 different models is tested.

Fig. 2. Segmentation (left) of CSI images from four patients. The number of clusters is automatically defined by MCLUST. For G and W 3 clusters are optimal, for D 5 and for M 4. The uncertainty values (right) for voxels are mostly below 10 % (white).

Conclusion

Mixture modeling can be used to identify malignant regions in the brain by segmenting CSI data. The characteristics of all spectra within one *segment* may be used instead of the spectrum in one *voxel*, which may lead to a more reliable identification of the tumor type by a (supervised) classification algorithm. If several clusters can be identified within the tumor, it may even be possible to take the heterogeneity of the tumor into account.

Voxels with a high uncertainty value can be identified and removed from a cluster, thus improving classification. CSI image segmentation may be performed automatically using the BIC criterion.

Analysis of 3D Deformation Fields for Appearance-Based Segmentation

Simon Duchesne and D. Louis Collins

Montréal Neurological Institute (MNI), McGill Univ., Montréal, Canada H3A 2B4
{duchesne,louis}@bic.mni.mcgill.ca

Segmentation methods for brain MR images typically employ manual and/or automatic knowledge-based models specific to the structure of interest (SOI). The technique presented here overcomes some of the limitations of current methods. It requires no manual intervention, is fast, fully 3D, and generic yet constrained by some form of prior structure information. The novelty of this work resides in its *a priori* Principal Components Analysis (PCA) of non-linear registration data of a volume of interest (VOI), represented by dense 3D deformation fields from ANIMAL [1]. The results are used in an Appearance Model, inspired by Cootes [2], able to segment any SOIs contained within the VOI, in the atlas-independent framework described by Collins [1]. This article presents the theoretical basis for and initial work towards hippocampus segmentation on subject images from the MNI International Consortium for Brain Mapping (ICBM) database.

Methods: In the appearance-based matching proposed by Cootes, a model of the grey-level variations is combined with an Active Shape model. For the former, PCA is used to reduce the dimensionality of the grey-level data and generate a linear grey variation model [2]:

$$\mathbf{g} = \bar{\mathbf{g}} + \mathbf{P_g}\mathbf{B_g} \tag{1}$$

where $\bar{\mathbf{g}}$ is the mean normalised grey-level vector, $\mathbf{P_g}$ is a set of orthogonal modes of variation and $\mathbf{B_g}$ is a set of grey-level parameters. In place of the 2D ASM we propose to use a 3D Warp Model, generated by statistical analysis of a large number of example deformation fields. To simplify computations, the 3D deformation vector fields are decomposed into volumes of orthogonal deformation components x, y, z. With PCA the linear warp variation model is expressed as:

$$\mathbf{x} = \bar{\mathbf{x}} + \mathbf{P_x}\mathbf{B_x}; \ \mathbf{y} = \bar{\mathbf{y}} + \mathbf{P_y}\mathbf{B_y}; \ \mathbf{z} = \bar{\mathbf{z}} + \mathbf{P_z}\mathbf{B_z} \tag{2}$$

Using the same notation as [2], this linear model allows any new warp instance $\mathbf{w}(\mathbf{x}, \mathbf{y}, \mathbf{z})$ to be approximated by $\bar{\mathbf{w}}$, the mean warp, $\mathbf{P_w}$, the set of orthogonal modes of warp variations, and $\mathbf{B_w}$, the set of warp parameters. The space of all possible elements expressed by eq. 2 is called the Allowable Warp Domain. Since there may be correlations between the grey-level and warp variations, grey-level and warp parameters are concatenated as follows

$$\mathbf{B} = [\mathbf{W'_g}\mathbf{B'_g} \ \mathbf{B'_x} \ \mathbf{B'_y} \ \mathbf{B'_z}] \tag{3}$$

W. Niessen and M. Viergever (Eds.): MICCAI 2001, LNCS 2208, pp. 1189–1190, 2001.

where $\mathbf{W_g}$ is a diagonal matrix of weights accounting for differences in dimensions between grey-level (intensity) and warp variations (distances). PCA of eq. 3 yields a super-set of parameters describing the complete appearance model

$$\mathbf{B} = \mathbf{QC} \tag{4}$$

where $\mathbf{Q}$ are appearance eigenvectors and $\mathbf{C}$ is a vector of parameters controlling both the warp and the grey-levels of the model. The core of the segmentation method consists then in matching a new grey-level image to one synthesized by the model using the appearance parameters. The iterative method described in [2] is used. After convergence, the solution explicitly contains warp variation parameters, which can be expressed back into x, y, z components of the warp field and concatenated into ANIMAL vector format. Segmentation of the VOI is then possible using any structure model defined on the ANIMAL reference volume. It is achieved by applying the inverse of the deformation field to structures defined in the standard volume and then mapping those onto the subject.

Results: The SOI for initial testing was the left hippocampus. Normal subjects ($n = 40$) were selected for the training set from the ICBM database. VOIs of $55 \times 79 \times 68$ voxels were defined on T1-weighted MR images, with isotropic resolution ($1mm^3$). This volume captured the hippocampus irrespective of normal inter- and intra-individual variability. VOIs were linearly registered into stereotaxic space to reduce positional variations which would propagate as unwanted noise in the morphometric PCA modelling. Segmentation of an additional 10 subjects from the same database was performed using ANIMAL [1] and the Appearance-based (AB) method. Overlap statistics between manual segmentation and ANIMAL ($\kappa = 0.69, \sigma_\kappa = 0.03$), and manual vs AB ($\kappa = 0.65, \sigma_\kappa = 0.05$) indicate that the two methods have similar accuracy. A 12-to-1 decrease in segmentation processing time (ANIMAL: 2 hr/side/subject; AB model: <10 min/side/subject) was observed.

Discussion and Conclusions: The principle and applicability of an Active Appearance model based on the analysis of 3D deformation fields for segmentation has been demonstrated. Accuracy and robustness remain to be thoroughly assessed but early results suggest that the AB method is as accurate as ANIMAL, while being significantly faster. Promising features of this novel approach include (1) its speed compared to locally available segmentation methods; (2) reliance on all grey-level voxels and deformation vectors as "landmarks" and hence maximum use of information; (3) fully 3D and automated; and (4) flexibility in the choice of SOI/VOI. The major constraint is the restriction to the domain of structure neighborhoods whose non-linear registration is achievable using ANIMAL for the training of the 3D Warp Model.

Acknowledgments: Fonds pour les Chercheurs et l'Aide à la Recherche (Government of Québec) and ICBM.

[1] D. L. Collins, *Human Brain Mapping*, vol. 3, pp. 190–208, 1995.
[2] T. F. Cootes, in *ECCV* (Springer), pp. 484-498, 1998.

3D Markov Random Fields and Region Growing for Interactive Segmentation of MR Data

Marc Liévin, Nils Hanssen, Peter Zerfass, and Erwin Keeve

Surgical Simulation and Navigation Group
Research center c a e s a r
Friedensplatz 16, 53111, Bonn, Germany
http://www.caesar.de/ssn

1 Introduction

Segmenting medical structures is mandatory in any computer assisted surgery system. This major field must be addressed in order to build realistic and accurate 3D models of patient individual anatomical structures. Magnetic Resonance Imaging (MRI) is becoming part of daily routine in clinical work. Whereas scanning speed and slice numbers increase each year, segmenting such data is still a challenging problem. Moreover, the segmentation stage remains time limiting in pre-operative planning and intra-operative guidance. Indeed, interactive tools, like live wire or intensity-based thresholding, requires a pre or post-filtering to homogenize areas. Common medical filters, such as median or morphology-based, are actually non adapted for MR noise removal. Their main side effect is to remove boundaries when applied on Gaussian corrupted data. Next, numerous steps spend efforts in reconstructing lost information and current approaches are therefore non interactive.

2 Methods

Our method mainly differs from the literature by grouping time-consuming steps in the first stage. In a multi-stage process, the framework uses statistical clustering as a pre-processing stage before region growing. To reduce the complexity of the filtering and to increase the interactivity with the user, the initial raw data is quantized in a sufficient but limited number of clusters (e.g. 16 quantization steps).

Next, a filtering based on Markov random fields (Mrfs) clustering is applied on the whole volume. The main purpose of the Mrfs is to link observations from data and relevant labels in a smart way. Considering our clustering as a non-linear filter, the observations are the raw data itself and our label set the corresponding values after quantization. The originality of our procedure is the definition of the metric neighborhood structure, which may contained from 6 to 26 neighbors in a 3D metric space, depending on how far accuracy is needed. The metric potential function is defined as the inverse of the Euclidian distance in millimeters between two neighbors. Next, less than 10 iterations on the field are enough to obtain homogeneous fields respecting boundaries and initial data value range.

W. Niessen and M. Viergever (Eds.): MICCAI 2001, LNCS 2208, pp. 1191–1192, 2001.

Region growing uses connectivity and homogeneity properties to link neighbors. The growth starts from one or several seed points located interactively by the user in the slice views. The homogeneity criterion is based on statistical distribution of the filtered values. The user interactively moves the threshold from low values to higher values until the result is acceptable.

3   Results and Discussion

Accuracy and relevance of our approach are validated on a high-resolution MR study of a male knee, with 512x512x120 images and a voxel size of 0.27x0.27x1.0 mm (50 Mbytes data set). Figure 1 presents the result of the 3D Mrfs filtering with 16 clusters of a whole slice. On RISC 400MHz architecture, the processing takes only between 0.5 and 1 sec. per slice, e.g. up to 5-10 min. for the whole volume. Next, the user may interact during the region growing process with an update rate under the second, 0.2 sec. for cartilage growth over 138000 voxels.

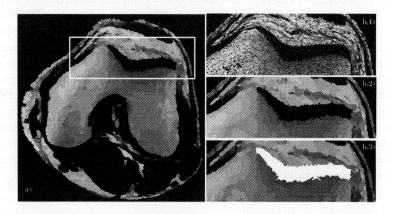

Fig. 1. Mrfs filtering and region growing results on the Femoral Cartilage area *(Transversal View; In white, the ROI)* a) MR slice filtered with 16 clusters; b) Zoomed Views of the ROI: 1) The raw data, 2) The Mrfs filtered data, 3) The Mrfs filtered data with superimposed in white region growing result of the cartilage.

The filtering algorithm only requires two tuning steps from the user: the neighborhood system (6 or 26 neighbors) and the quantization step. Integrated in a Vtk class (Kitware Inc.), this filter may be easily added to any medical pipeline. Extracting the 3D shape of challenging areas, such as cartilage in the knee, becomes easily and quickly feasible. We need now to extend this approach with new interactive tools like live wire or gradient methods. Integrating these procedures with volume rendering for advanced interactive segmentation is also under study.

Acknowledgment

We thank Ron Kikinis and the Surgical Planning Laboratory at Brigham and Women's Hospital Harvard Medical School, for making available the MR and manual segmented dataset of the knee.

Long Bone Panoramas from Fluoroscopic X-ray Images

Z. Yaniv and L. Joskowicz

School of Computer Science and Engineering
The Hebrew University of Jerusalem, Jerusalem 91904 Israel.
{zivy,josko}@cs.huji.ac.il

We have developed a new method for creating a single panoramic image of a long bone from a few individual fluoroscopic X-ray images [1]. Fluoroscopic X-ray panoramas can be useful in a variety of orthopaedic surgeries which require the presence in the same image of relevant anatomical features. In long bone surgery, they can be used for determining the mechanical axis of the bone, aligning bone fragments, measuring extremity length and anteversion, and assessing long implants positions. This data is difficult to obtain with existing methods and can help to improve diagnosis, shorten surgery time, and improve outcomes.

Our method uses a radiolucent ruler imaged alongside the long bone to establish the correlation between images. Before the surgery, an aluminum grid is imaged and a distortion correction map is computed [2]. Then, the radiolucent ruler is placed roughly parallel and at the same height of the long bone to be imaged. Several overlapping images (between 20% and 60% of their area) are taken by translating the fluoroscope parallel to the bone. The individual images are corrected for distortion, and the main thread and graduations of the ruler are extracted from the images using two-value histogram thresholding. The ruler graduations are matched using cross correlation as a similarity measure, and the rigid transformation that aligns them is computed. The undistorted images are then aligned according to the these transformations, and then composed into a single image by computing pixel values at locations where images overlap.

Our experiments show the method is robust and produces panoramas with an accuracy comparable to that of individual images, and are thus clinically acceptable. The advantages of our method are that it is fully automatic, uses readily available hardware, requires a simple image acquisition protocol and minimal user intervention, and works with most existing fluoroscopic units without modifications. [1]

1. Yaniv, Z. and Joskowicz, L., "Long bone panoramas from fluoroscopic X-ray images", *Proc. of the 15th Int. Congress on Computer-Assisted Radiology and Surgery*, CARS'2001, H.U. Lemke *et. al.* eds, Elsevier 2001.
2. Yaniv Z., Joskowicz L., Simkin A., Garza-Jinich M., Milgrom C. "Fluoroscopic Image Processing for Computer-Aided Orthopaedic Surgery", *1st Int.*

---

[1] This research was supported in part by a grant from the Israel Ministry of Industry and Trade for the IZMEL Consortium on Image-Guided Therapy.

Conf. on Medical Computing and Computer-Assisted Intervention, Lecture Notes in Computer Science 1496, Elsevier, Wells *et. al.* eds, 1998.

Long bone panorama construction

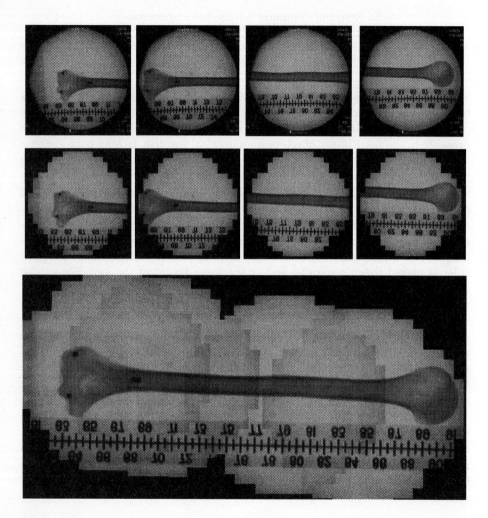

Fig. 1. Panorama construction of a dry humerus. The top row shows the original images with the ruler on the bottom, the middle row shows the images after distortion correction, and the bottom row shows the resulting panorama.

Augmented Reality in the Operating Theatre of the Future

Heinz Wörn and Harald Hoppe

Universität Karlsruhe (TH), Institute for Process Control and Robotics, Kaiserstraße 12,
76128 Karlsruhe, Germany
[woern,hoppe]@ira.uka.de

Abstract. While an increasing number of operation planning systems enable surgeons to preoperatively define and plan complex surgical interventions, providing these planning data intraoperatively in a reasonable way is still a challenging task. We have developed a new system using projector based augmented reality for the intraoperative visualization of preoperatively defined surgical planning data. Projector based augmented reality in medical applications represents a new field of research and yet shows results that are superior to techniques based on head mounted displays. The projector is not only used for visualization, but also for initial registration of the patient whose further movements are continuously tracked and taken into account for projection.

Introduction

Within the Sonderforschungsbereich SFB 414 "Information Technology in Medicine - Computer and Sensor Supported Surgery", the Institute for Process Control and Robotics/Universität Karlsruhe investigates new concepts for computer and robot based cranio-facial surgery in close collaboration with the Department of Oral and Maxillo-facial Surgery/University of Heidelberg. While operation planning systems enable surgeons to preoperatively define and plan complex surgical interventions, the most important step from the planning to the actual surgical intervention consists of providing the planning data intraoperatively in a reasonable way. Great efforts are being made to directly visualize the surgical planning data in the operation area where Head Mounted Displays enjoy great popularity [1] but also show some basic disadvantages.

Projector-Based Augmented Reality

We have developed a new system for the intraoperative visualization of surgical planning data consisting of an off-the-shelf video projector, two CCD-cameras and a state-of-the-art PC. The most important preoperative task consists of calibrating both the video projector and the CCD-cameras within the same coordinate system. Intraoperative registration of the patient normally makes use of artificial screw markers attached to the patient's bone before acquiring the diagnostic image data. In developing the presented system, our goal was to registrate the patient's position without attaching unpleasant screw markers to its bone in a precedent surgery. This is accomplished by projecting a sequence of stripe patterns (coded light) on top of the region of interest with the aid of the integrated video projector. The resulting point cloud can be matched to the preoperatively segmented surface of the diagnostic image data (CT,

W. Niessen and M. Viergever (Eds.): MICCAI 2001, LNCS 2208, pp. 1195-1196, 2001.
© Springer-Verlag Berlin Heidelberg 2001

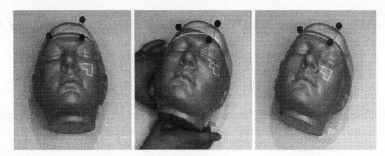

Fig. 1. Left: Phantom with projected planning data / Mid: Immediately after moving the phantom: planning data appear in wrong position / Right: After localizing the new marker positions, the projection is updated correctly.

MRI) on which the surgical plan was defined. This task is performed by a new algorithm which imitates the human strategy for the matching process of two corresponding surfaces by shifting one on top of the other where the surfaces remain in contact in at least three points. Afterwards, the fine tuning is realized by using the Iterative Closest Point algorithm described in [2]. The matching process provides an initial transformation from the coordinate system of the diagnostic image data to the initial position of the patient. Further movements are detected by observing artificial markers with the integrated cameras. The calculated transformations allow to continuously transfer the surgical planning data to the patient's coordinate system thus taking into account its actual position.

Results and Discussion

The described method enables the surgeon to visualize planning data on top of any preoperatively segmented and triangulated surface. The system allows to meet occlusion by simply moving around the video projector to an appropriate position since changes of position of the video projector are equivalent to those of the patient. Furthermore, the tracking system allows dynamic adjustment of the data to the patient's current position and therefore eliminates the need for rigid fixation with stereotactic frames or similar devices. While systems using HMDs generally require expensive navigation systems, the cost of the presented system is much lower than that of a corresponding system based on HMDs. Furthermore, it is currently superior to any HMD with regard to accuracy and resolution. The currently achieved accuracy of the projected surgical planning data is about +/- 1.5 mm using a resolution of 0.33 mm or less. Current efforts concentrate on improving the accuracy and on increasing the update frequency (currently 1.6 Hz). While the surgeon performs the intervention without any interference of his general practice, all surgically involved persons are able to share the same augmented reality view on the projected data.

References

1. S. Tang, C. Kwoh, M. Teo, N. W. Sing, and K. Ling, "Augmented Reality Systems for Medical Applications", IEEE Engineering in Medicine and Biology, pp. 49-58, June 1998.
2. K. S. Arun, T. S. Huang, and S. D. Blostein, "Least-Squares Fitting of Two 3-D Point Sets", IEEE Transactions on PAMI, vol. 9, no. 5, pp. 698-700, 1987.

Volume Visualization Using Gradient-Based Distance among Voxels

Shinobu Mizuta, Ken-ichi Kanda, and Tetsuya Matsuda

Graduate School of Informatics, Kyoto University, 606-8501 Kyoto, JAPAN
{smizuta,kkanda,tetsu}@i.kyoto-u.ac.jp

Abstract. The aim of this work is to visualize 3D objects in volume data with minimum numbers of user-defined models or parameters. In this report, we propose a novel method that utilizes the distances along the optimum paths between a seed voxel in a target object and other voxels. The distance here is defined using gradient between adjacent voxels along the path. The distance is also used as the criterion of path optimization. The visualization is carried out by rendering the volume where the initial voxel values are replaced with the distances. Experimental results for an image of human embryo obtained with MR microscopy have displayed the effectiveness of this method.

1 Introduction

Volume visualization is a key technology for the interpretation of 3D images and varieties of methods have been proposed [1]. In the conventional volume rendering techniques, it is quite difficult to observe the target object when the voxel values of an object of interest are similar to others. Meanwhile, most of the methods for the segmentation of target objects from 3D data are based on user-defined models or parameters, which influence the interpretations of resulting images. The aim of our research is to visualize 3D objects in volume data with minimum numbers of user-defined models or parameters to comprehend the meaning of images directly.

2 Methods

The procedure of volume visualization in the proposed method is as follows: (i) setting a seed voxel in a target object in input 3D volume data, (ii) calculating the distances between the seed voxel and all other voxels along the optimum paths based on Dijkstra algorithm [2], (iii) replacing the initial voxel values with the calculated distances, (iv) rendering the replaced volume. The optimization of paths between voxels is carried out by minimizing "roughness", which is defined by the largest value of absolute gradient between adjacent voxels along a path. The value is denoted by d (S, v, P) for a path P between the seed voxel S and another voxel v. The path P is regarded as "smooth" when d (S, v, P) is small. The minimum value of d (S, v, P) for various P is denoted by D (S, v), where the corresponding path is optimum. D (S, v) is used as the distance between the voxels S and v. The outline of the procedure is shown in Figure 1 (a).

W. Niessen and M. Viergever (Eds.): MICCAI 2001, LNCS 2208, pp. 1197-1198, 2001.

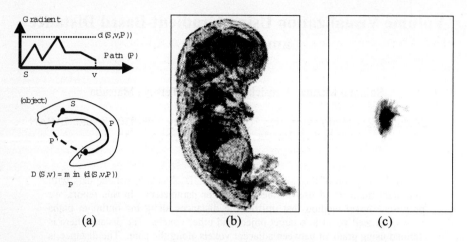

Fig. 1. (a) Outline of the proposed method. (b) Volume rendering result using conventional method (differences of voxel values from the seed voxel). (c) Volume rendering result using proposed method.

The procedure of finding optimum paths is similar as that of the region growing method for image segmentation [3] or "live-wire" method for interactive search of boundaries [4]. A unique point of our method is calculating the distances along the optimum paths for all voxels in order to utilize them to visualize volumes.

3 Results

A 3D image of a human embryo obtained with MR microscopy have visualized by the conventional and proposed methods. The target object is the lung area. The results are shown in Fig.1 (b)(c). By the proposed method, only the target object was visualized as the gradient-based distances from the seed point in the target object.

Acknowledgement

We would like to thank to K. Shiota and T. Nakatsu for the use of their specimens.

References

1. Sonka et al., "Handbook of Medical Imaging", SPIE Press, Bellingham, Washington (2000)
2. Cormen et al., "Introduction to Algorithms", McGraw-Hill, New York, NY (1990)
3. Zukker, Comput. Graph. Image Process., vol.5, no.3, pp.382-399 (1976)
4. Mortensen and Barrett, Proc. SIGGRAPH '95, pp.191-198 (1995)

The Evaluation of the Color Blending Function for the Texture Generation from Photographs

Daigo Tanaka, Alan Liu, Christoph Kaufmann
{dtanaka|aliu|ckaufmann}@simcen.usuhs.mil

National Capital Area Medical Simulation Center
Uniformed Services University of the Health Sciences
4301 Jones Bridge Road, Bethesda MD 20814, USA
http://simcen.usuhs.mil

Abstract. Mass-casualty triage simulation requires the realistic depiction of wounds and other signs of external injury on victims. Texture maps permit images of actual wounds to be rendered over computer models. Several images may be required to depict extensive injuries. Seamlessly combining these images requires an appropriate blending function. This paper compares two functions for their ability to create visually appealing integrations.

1 Introduction

Triage at a mass-casualty site includes a visual assessment of the patient's injuries. Traditionally, triage training required the use of healthy volunteers with moulage (i.e. special makeup). Computer simulations of mass-casualty situations have greater flexibility, require less planning and coordination, and can be performed more frequently. For realism, detailed images of actual wounds and other injuries can be acquired as texture maps, then applied over a generic human models. Texture maps of extensive injuries must be generated from two or more images. Blending these images seamlessly is necessary for realism. This paper evaluates two functions for this ability.

2 Method

The test object is a mannequin head. Images are taken of the head; one head-on (camera 1), the other from the mannequin's left side (camera 2) and perpendicular to the former. A 3D polygonal representation is also acquired. Let $\vec{c_1}$, $\vec{c_2}$ be the unit vector of the camera view directions, E_1, E_2 be camera center of projections, and I_1, I_2 be the camera image planes. Let p be a point on the head and $\vec{n_p}$ be the unit normal vector at p. Then $I_{k,p}$ is the point on image plane I_k intersected by line $E_k p$, where $k = 1, 2$. In addition, let $\alpha_{i,p}$ be the angle between $\vec{n_p}$ and $\vec{c_i}$ where $i = 1, 2$. A texture map of the head's front and left sides is generated using T_1, and T_2, where

W. Niessen and M. Viergever (Eds.): MICCAI 2001, LNCS 2208, pp. 1199-1200, 2001.

$$T_1(p) = \left(\sum_{i=1,2} (\vec{c_i} \cdot p)^2 I_{i,p} \right) \Big/ \left(\sum_{i=1,2} (\vec{c_i} \cdot p)^2 \right), \text{ and} \qquad (1)$$

$$T_2(p) = (\cos\alpha_{1,p} I_{1,p})^2 + (\sin\alpha_{1,p} I_{2,p})^2 . \qquad (2)$$

3   Results

Fig. 1 (left) is the head model with texture map generated by T_1. Fig. 1 (right) is the same model but with its texture map generated by T_2.

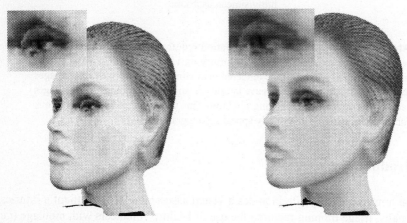

Fig. 1. (left) model of head using texture map generated by T_1. (right) same model but using texture map generated by T_2.

4   Conclusion and Discussion

T_1 produces noticeable artifacts, particularly around the eyes and in vertical bands across the left side of the face. T_1 uses an average of dot products, and is more sensitive to local variations of the surface normal. Regions where this changes rapidly (e.g., around the eye) are the most affected. T_2 produces smoother results with less objectionable artifacts around the eyes. T_2. This blending function produces more visually appealing results even across regions where the surface normal changes rapidly.

5   Acknowledgements

This work was funded by a grant from the Association of Military Surgeons of the United States (AMSUS), and by U.S. Army grant DAMD17-99-1-9022.

Anisotropic Volume Rendering Using Intensity Interpolation

Tae-Young Kim[1], Byeong-Seok Shin[2], Yeong Gil Shin[1]

[1] School of Computer Science and Engineering, Seoul National University
San 56-1, Shilim-Dong, Kwanak-Gu, Seoul 151-742, Korea
{tykim, yshin}@cglab.snu.ac.kr
[2] Dept. of Computer Science and Engineering, Inha University
253 YongHyeon-Dong Nam-Gu, Inchon, Korea
bsshin@inha.ac.kr

1 Introduction

In medical applications, anisotropic volume data sets are commonly used, of which the resolution in an axial plane is higher than that in the direction perpendicular to it. In this paper, we propose an efficient anisotropic volume rendering method based on intensity interpolation that obtains the intensity value at an interpolated position lying between voxels in two consecutive slices from the intensity values of the voxels. Unlike density interpolation method, it does not require long preprocessing time and extra memory for storing the interpolated slices. Experimental results show that this method improves rendering speed without significantly sacrificing image quality.

2 Anisotropic Volume Rendering Using Intensity Interpolation

In order to manipulate the anisotropic volume in rendering time, intensity calculation on missing voxels is required. Fig. 1 compares our method with a conventional density interpolation method to compute the intensity of an interpolated sample v_i divided internally as $m : (1-m)$ between the voxels in two adjacent slices, v_k and v_{k+1}. In the figure, $d(v_i)$, $N(v_i)$ and $I(v_i)$ is a density value, a normal vector and an intensity value of v_i, respectively. Since the conventional method computes $I(v_i)$ from

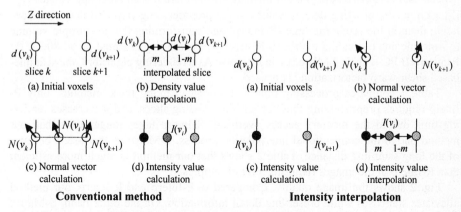

Fig. 1. Comparison of intensity calculation process.

W. Niessen and M. Viergever (Eds.): MICCAI 2001, LNCS 2208, pp. 1201-1203, 2001.

$N(v_i)$ obtained by interpolating density values of v_i and its neighbors, the normal calculation, with additional density interpolation is required for each interpolation position. On the other hand, intensity interpolation method computes $I(v_i)$ from $I(v_k)$ and $I(v_{k+1})$. It is not necessary to compute density values and normal vectors for intermittent samples. The normal calculation is only performed on the original voxels.

Consider the equation $I(v_k) = K_a I_a + K_d(L \bullet N(v_k))$ where K_a is an ambient-reflection coefficient, I_a is an ambient-light intensity, K_d is a diffuse-reflection coefficient, L is a light vector. Equation (1) proves that the intensity value $\tilde{I}(v_i)$, computed by intensity interpolation is equivalent to the intensity value calculated from the normal vector $\tilde{N}(v_i)$:

$$
\begin{aligned}
\tilde{I}(v_i) &= I(v_k)(1-m) + I(v_{k+1})m \\
&= (K_a I_a + K_d(L \bullet N(v_k)))(1-m) + (K_a I_a + K_d(L \bullet N(v_{k+1})))m \\
&= K_a I_a(1-m) + K_a I_a m + K_d L \bullet (N(v_k)(1-m) + N(v_{k+1})m) \\
&= K_a I_a + K_d L \bullet (N(v_k)(1-m) + N(v_{k+1})m) \\
&= K_a I_a + K_d(L \bullet \tilde{N}(v_i))
\end{aligned}
\tag{1}
$$

Compare the normal vectors along Z-axis of these methods. Following equations represent the normal vectors $N_Z(v_i)$ and $\tilde{N}_Z(v_i)$ (by equation (1)), which are for the conventional method and the intensity interpolation method, respectively.

$$
N_Z(v_i) = \frac{2(d(v_{k+1}) - d(v_k))}{\lambda}
\tag{2}
$$

$$
\begin{aligned}
\tilde{N}_Z(v_i) &= N_Z(v_k)(1-m) + N_Z(v_{k+1})m \\
&= \frac{(d(v_{k+1}) - d(v_{k-1}))(1-m) + (d(v_{k+2}) - d(v_k))m}{2\lambda}
\end{aligned}
\tag{3}
$$

In the equations, more samples are referenced for calculating $\tilde{N}_Z(v_i)$ compared to $N_Z(v_i)$. Thus the smoother images are obtained by the intensity interpolation.

3   Experimental Results

To evaluate the performance of our method, we compare it with other approaches [1]–[3] such as interpolating density values in the preprocessing step (P-Interp), interpolating them in the rendering time (R-Interp) and transforming the anisotropic volume to isotropic one by scaling matrix (S-Matrix). These are implemented on an 800 MHz Pentium III PC with 512 MB of main memory. As a rendering algorithm, the scanline-based shear-warp factorization [1] is used.

Table 1 compares processing time and storage. Among these methods, only P-Interp requires preprocessing time for creating missing slices, and it increases rendering time due to the memory access overhead. R-Interp takes longer time than our method due to the conventional interpolation process. S-Matrix is the fastest because of the long sampling distance. Table 2 shows that our method is much more efficient than R-Interp in the images requiring a lot of samples.

Fig. 2 shows the image quality. Compared to P-Interp and R-Interp, our method alleviates staircases while preserving detail information. On the other hand, S-Matrix produces excessive staircase artifacts, thus it is not practical in medical applications.

Table 1. Comparison of time and storage.

Data	Performance Test	Ours	P-Interp	R-Interp	S-Matrix
	Pre-interpolation Time (ms)	–	12684	–	–
Airway	Average Rendering Time (ms)	1108	1486	1513	673
	Storage (MB)	71.8	240.8	71.8	71.8

Table 2. Comparison of average rendering times between our method and R-Interp according to the number of contributed samples (colon data with $512 \times 512 \times 141$ resolution).

Structure	Samples	Ours (ms)	R-Interp (ms)	Speedup
Colon	0.6 M	1362	1992	1.46
Skin and Bone	8.1 M	5235	8802	1.68
Semitransparent Skin	13.3 M	8230	15047	1.83

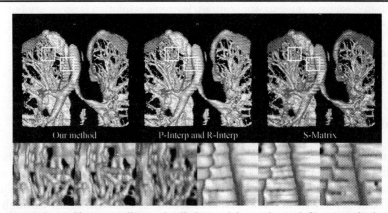

Fig. 2. Comparison of image quality on detailed parts (airway data): (left) our method; (middle) P-Interp and R-Interp; (right) S-Matrix.

4 Conclusion

We have presented an efficient way of calculating the intensity value on each sample in visualizing anisotropic volume data sets. We are currently extending our approach to avoid overblurring on high frequency area.

References

1. Lacroute P., Levoy, M.: Fast Volume Rendering Using a Shear-Warp Factorization of the Viewing Transformation. Computer Graphics (SIGGRAPH '94 Proceedings), Orlando, Florida, July (1994) 451–458
2. Mueller K., Shareef N., Huang J., Crawfis R.: High-quality splatting on rectilinear grids with efficient culling of occluded voxels. IEEE Transactions on Visualization and Computer Graphics, 5(2) (1999) 116–134
3. Pfister, H., Hardenbergh, J., Knittel, J., Lauer, H., Seiler, L.: The VolumePro Real-Time Ray-Casting System. Computer Graphics (SIGGRAPH '99 Proceedings), Los Angeles, CA, August (1999) 251–260

MRI Inter-slice Reconstruction Using Super-Resolution

Hayit Greenspan[1], Sharon Peled[2*], Gal Oz[1], and Nahum Kiryati[1]

[1] Faculty of Engineering, Tel Aviv University, Tel Aviv 69978, Israel
[2] Department of Radiology, Tel Aviv Sourasky Medical Center, Tel Aviv 64239, Israel

Abstract. MRI reconstruction using super-resolution is presented and shown to improve spatial resolution in cases when spatially-selective RF pulses are used for localization. In 2D multislice MRI, the resolution in the slice direction is often worse than the in-plane resolution. For certain diagnostic imaging applications, isotropic resolution is necessary but true 3D acquisition methods are not practical. In this case, if the imaging volume is acquired two or more times, with small spatial shifts between acquisitions, combination of the data sets using an iterative superresolution algorithm gives improved resolution and better edge definition in the slice-select direction.

1 Introduction

Conventional nuclear magnetic resonance imaging utilizes two main methods of encoding the spatial location of nuclear spins contributing to the NMR signal: (1) Spatially selective radio frequency (RF) pulses excite a certain frequency bandwidth. (2) Frequency and phase encoding of the MR signal through temporal variation of the magnetic field gradients before or during signal reception (after the RF excitation). Two-dimensional multislice MR imaging usually relies on selection of slices using the first method, and in-plane encoding using frequency encoding in one direction and phase encoding in the other in-plane direction. The thinner the slice that should be excited by the RF pulse (i.e. the narrower the frequency bandwidth), the longer the duration of the pulse, given the same magnetic field gradient strength. For reasons of RF power deposition, pulse sequence timing, and signal-to-noise ratio (SNR), there are disadvantages to thin-slice excitation.

Three dimensional MR imaging using true 3D data acquisition strategies would be the technique of choice when isotropic spatial resolution is required. Three-dimensional imaging techniques use an initial spatially selective RF pulse to define a "slab" which corresponds to a thick slice, within which thin slices are encoded using phase encoding, while the in-plane encoding is the same as the 2D method. 3D acquisition methods can be problematic, in terms of the time required for data acquisition, in terms of the achievable contrast, and in terms of image artifacts [1]. For T_1-weighted imaging, a 3D fast Fourier-encoding-based

---

* Currently with GE Medical Systems, Israel

W. Niessen and M. Viergever (Eds.): MICCAI 2001, LNCS 2208, pp. 1204–1206, 2001.
© Springer-Verlag Berlin Heidelberg 2001

gradient-echo sequence is in common use. On the other hand, T_2-weighting in a 3D acquisition can take too long for many clinical situations. Another prominent example in which 3D imaging fails is in echo-planar imaging (EPI) - the underlying technique of choice for functional MRI (fMRI) and diffusion tensor imaging (DTI).

2   MRI Reconstruction Using Super-Resolution

The method we present consists of: **1.** The acquisition of a small number of multislice data sets, each volume being shifted in the slice-select direction with respect to the other volumes. **2.** The use of super-resolution post-processing in the inter-slice (z) dimension. MRI fourier-encoded in-plane data has a sharp spatial frequency cut-off. This is due to the time limit of the acquisition mechanism and the fact that the information is gathered in the frequency domain (k-space). Thus the best we can do in the x and y dimensions is to interpolate the given data to the desired resolution, via zero-padding. The spatial frequencies in the inter-slice direction exhibit a less sharp cut-off thus providing the basis for using a super-resolution algorithm in enhancing the resolution. The iterative back-projection method of Irani-Peleg [2] is used as the super-resolution algorithm in our reconstruction of inter-slice data. This method is based on the minimization of differences between the original low-resolution images, and the low-resolution images that can be generated from down-sampling the current best guess of the high resolution image. The super-resolution algorithm terminates once the error difference between sequential iterations is below a predefined threshold.

3   Experimental Results

Experimental results using a "comb"-phantom object are shown in Figure 1. The phantom consists of long thin plastic partitions ("teeth"), lodged in a plastic block, placed 4mm apart, surrounded by Gd-DTPA-doped water. The imaging sequence consists of multislice fast spin-echo with 16 slices, 3mm thick, approximately parallel to the plastic partitions. Three sets of multislice data were acquired, with 1mm shifts in the slice-select direction. Figure 1 shows the results of zero-padding (left) and super-resolution (right). The visibility of the comb teeth has greatly improved by using super-resolution rather than zero-padding interpolation. Similar results for a pomegranate are shown in Figure 2. In both the comb and pomegranate examples, super-resolution brings out features that are inseparable in the source images.

4   Conclusions

We propose a novel framework of using super-resolution for MRI resolution augmentation. With inter-slice super-resolution we can effectively break limits on

slice thickness posed by the physical properties of existing MR imaging hardware. We are currently experimenting with human brain MRI data sets.

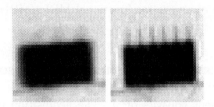

Fig. 1. Super-resolution applied to comb-phantom MRI data. The horizontal
axis is the slice-select direction. *Left:* Low-resolution data with zero-padding
interpolation. *Right:* Super-resolution output.

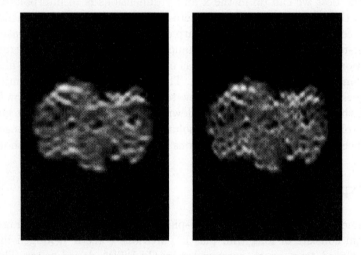

Fig. 2. Super-resolution applied to pomegranate data. The horizontal axis is the
slice-select direction. *Left:* Low-resolution data with zero-padding interpolation.
Right: Super-resolution output.

References

1. Mulkern, R.V., Wong, S.T.S., Winalski, C. and Jolesz, F.A. 1990. "Contrast
   manipulation and artifact assessment of 2D and 3D RARE sequences". Magn.
   Reson. Imag. 8:557-566.

2. Irani, M. and Peleg, S. 1993. "Motion analysis for image enhancement: resolution,
   occlusion and transparency" J. Vis. Comm. Image Rep. 4(4):324-335.

Assessment of Center of Rotation of the Glenohumeral Joint

Marjolein van der Glas, Frans Vos, and Albert Vossepoel

Pattern Recognition Group, Delft University of Technology,
Lorentzweg 1, 2628 CJ Delft, The Netherlands,
{marjolein, frans, albert}@ph.tn.tudelft.nl,
http://www.ph.tn.tudelft.nl/

1 Introduction

During a total shoulder replacement the glenohumeral joint is substituted by a prosthesis. The joint is a loose ball-and-socket joint, in which the humeral head is the ball and the glenoid is the socket. Most important for successful surgery is that the center of rotation of the glenohumeral joint is maintained [1]. During motion, the two geometric centers of both spherical surfaces coincide in the center of rotation of the glenohumeral joint [1]. In this paper we present a new technique to automatically determine the 3D center of a sphere in 3D images, using the direction and strength of the gradient.

2 Methods

The Hough transform [2] is a well accepted method used for sphere detection in binary, i.e. segmented, images. The novelty in our approach is the use of unsegmented 3D images.

Consider a parameterization of a sphere by (x_0, y_0, z_0, r), where x_0, y_0, z_0 refer to the position of the center, and r refers to the sphere radius. For the center detection, a 3D parameter space is defined, containing a probability count for all possible sphere centers. The parameter space is filled by going through the following step for every voxel in the grey-value image:

1. Determine the orientation and magnitude of the gradient, using Gaussian derivatives.
2. Project the gradient vector in parameter space.
3. Increase the count of the corresponding voxels in parameter space by the gradient magnitude.

The maximum in the parameter space corresponds with the center of the sphere. From the sphere center, the radius is determined using the radial histogram of the gradient magnitude of the image with respect to the detected sphere center. The maxima in this histogram correspond with the radii of the spheres.

W. Niessen and M. Viergever (Eds.): MICCAI 2001, LNCS 2208, pp. 1207–1209, 2001.

1208   M. van der Glas, F. Vos, and A. Vossepoel

3 Results

Artificial images, of size 84x84x84 voxels, are created with solid or hollow spheres. The center of the sphere is determined, using different values for the sigma of the Gaussian derivatives (table 1).

Table 1. Distance between the determined and the real sphere center in voxels, for various radii (vertically) and signal to noise ratio of Gaussian noise (horizontally) determined with the optimal sigma (between brackets) for solid complete spheres

R	no noise	26 dB	20 dB	16 dB	14 dB	12 dB	10 dB
26.00	0.093 (1.0)	0.109 (1.0)	0.089 (1.5)	0.111 (1.5)	0.114 (2.0)	0.088 (2.0)	0.125 (2.5)
30.00	0.106 (1.0)	0.112 (1.5)	0.080 (1.5)	0.098 (1.5)	0.106 (2.0)	0.103 (2.0)	0.101 (2.5)
34.00	0.103 (1.0)	0.125 (1.5)	0.082 (1.5)	0.088 (2.0)	0.099 (2.5)	0.102 (2.5)	0.126 (2.5)
38.00	0.105 (1.5)	0.087 (1.5)	0.075 (1.5)	0.100 (2.0)	0.097 (2.0)	0.101 (3.0)	0.104 (3.0)

In clinical images of the glenohumeral joint, the position of the center and the radius of the approximate sphere are determined. In both CT and MRI scans the method automatically detects the sphere that fits onto the spherical humeral head (figure 1). If a fitting method had been used, the sphere would be fitted onto the entire top of the humerus, as shown in [3].

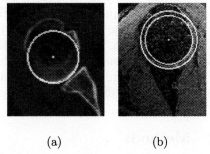

(a)   (b)

Fig. 1. Result sphere determination (a) in CT, (b) in MRI.

4 Conclusion

The method described in this paper is used to detect the center of solid and hollow spheres with high accuracy. The method is robust to noise and it does not need a complete sphere in order to detect the center. It can be used on isotropic as well as non-isotropic sampled images. As no segmentation is required, it can be directly applied to clinical images.

Detection of the center of rotation of the glenohumeral joint can be used for pre-operative planning for shoulder replacements. It will help the surgeon to optimally position the shoulder prosthesis. Furthermore the determined spheres can be used for fast visualization of bone surfaces during surgery.

Acknowledgements

This research is part of the DIPEX (Development of Improved endo-Prostheses for the upper EXtremities) program of the Delft Interfaculty Research Center on Medical Engineering (DIOC, http://www.wbmt.tudelft.nl/mms/dipex/).

References

1. O. de Leest, M.R. Rozing, and et al. Influence of Glenohumeral Prosthesis Geometry and Placement on Shoulder Muscle Forces. *Clin.Orthop.*, 330:p. 222–233, 1996.
2. V.F. Leavers. *Shape detection in computer vision using the Hough transform.* Springer Verlag, 1992.
3. J.J. Jacq and C. Roux. Automatic detection of articular surfaces in 3D image through minimal subset random sampling. In *CVRMedMRCAS'97 proceedings*, volume 1205, pages 73–82. Springer, 1997.

PET Studies of the Effects of ECT on Cerebral Physiology

M. Nobler, S. Yu, B. Mensh, S. Lisanby, L. Alkalay, R. Van Heertum, E. Heyer, H. Sackeim

Columbia University, New York, USA

Introduction

ECT is a remarkably effective treatment for major depressive disorder [MDD]. Neuroimaging studies of rCBF and rCMR are helpful in addressing mechanisms of therapeutic effects. We have reported that reductions in rCBF in prefrontal regions are associated with positive response to ECT[1], and that a course of bilateral ECT is associated with marked reduction in prefrontal rCMR[2]. We now report on a new study of patients receiving ECT for MDD. This study provides the first comparison of the relative acute effects of seizures on both rCBF and rCMR.

Methods

Fourteen inpatients met research diagnostic criteria for MDD. Each patient underwent positron emission tomography [PET]: (1) PreECT [following medication washout]: 1 rCBF [^{15}O-H$_2$O] and 1 rCMR [^{18}F-deoxyglucose; FDG] scan; (2) during ECT #3: rCBF scan just prior to ECT, rCBF scans at 20 and 40 min in the postictal state, rCMR scan at 50 min postictal; (3) 2-7 days post ECT course [medication free]: 1 rCBF and 1 rCMR scan. Prior to radioisotope injection [40 mCi O^{15} or 5 mCi FDG], a catheter was placed in the left radial artery for arterial sampling for full quantification. Scans were quantified using the autoradiographic method[3]. Scans were acquired with a Siemens ECAT HR+ scanner [63 slices, 4.2-5.4 mm FWHM] in 2D mode for rCBF and 3D mode for rCMR. Images were reconstructed using attenuation correction measured by a 15-min transmission scan.

We conducted two separate analyses: (1) After application of an anisotropic-diffusion filter, T1-weighted MRIs were segmented with a thresholding procedure and grossly parcellated into the following broad areas: CSF, cortical gray and white matter, subcortical gray matter, midbrain, pons, and cerebellum. The PET scans were registered to the MRIs. rCBF values for each of the 6 regions [excluding CSF] were determined using partial volume correction. (2) We also conducted a preliminary Statistical Parametric Mapping[4] [SPM-99] analysis of the changes in rCBF that occurred between the preECT baseline and the first ^{15}O measurement in the postictal state, using a corrected cluster size probability of P<0.001 [filter=12]. We conducted the same analysis on the FDG data collected at baseline and 50 min into the postictal state, using a cluster size probability of only P<0.01 [filter=12].

Results

Across a subgroup of the patients, ECT led to marked postictal reductions in fully quantified global cortical rCBF [P<0.001], with little impact in subcortical regions.

W. Niessen and M. Viergever (Eds.): MICCAI 2001, LNCS 2208, pp. 1210-1212, 2001.

The cortical effects were most pronounced 20-40 min post ECT, but persisted during the week post ECT. No consistent changes were seen within the broad categories of subcortical gray, midbrain, pons, cerebellum or white matter at either time point.

SPM data on 12 patients are available and revealed marked rCBF reductions in at the prefrontal pole and dorsolateral PFC, medial PFC, and parietal cortex [P's < .0001]. Clusters of significant rCBF reductions are represented in Figure 1. We conducted the same analysis on the FDG data collected at baseline and 50 min into the postictal state. This is represented in Figure 2. The pattern of significant rCMR reductions mirrored the rCBF changes, but the magnitude of rCMR reductions was much less marked [as indicated by the cluster size probability of only P<.01]. All increases in rCBF and rCMR occurred in posterior, occipital areas, suggesting a change in the anterior/posterior gradient and the increases reflecting the artifact that SPM does not account for absolute changes. Highly similar effects were observed when the resting rCBF scan conducted just prior to the treatment was compared to the first postictal scan, indicating that the postictal state was associated with marked topographic change. The divergence between rCBF and rCMR data indicates that ECT may result in uncoupling between cerebral perfusion and metabolic rate in the postictal state, with greater reductions in blood flow than metabolism.

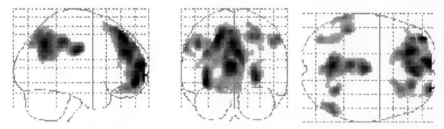

Figure 1. SPM Results for Acute Effects on rCBF Relative to preECT Baseline

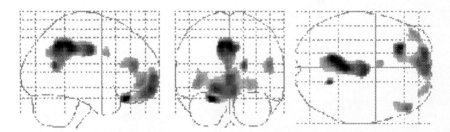

Figure 2. SPM Results for Acute Effects on rCMR Relative to preECT Baseline

Conclusions

The data thus far suggest that the rCBF and rCMR reductions in the immediate postictal state and following the ECT course are most marked in the neocortex, with inconsistent change when subcortical regions are treated as a single ROI. However, verification of these initial findings for views regarding the centrality of subcortical [eg, diencpehalic] structures for the efficacy of ECT, as well as the possibility of uncoupling of rCBF and rCMR in the immediate postictal period, must await fine grained ROI and voxel-based analyses, in particular implementing methods for full brain parcellation [ROI determination] and subsequent partial volume correction.

References

1. Nobler, M. S., Sackeim, H. A., Prohovnik, I., Moeller, J. R., Mukherjee, S., Schnur, D. B., Prudic, J., and Devanand, D. P.: Regional cerebral blood flow in mood disorders, III. Treatment and clinical response. Arch Gen Psychiatry **51** (1994) 884-97
2. Nobler, M. S., Oquendo, M. A., Kegeles, L. S., Malone, K. M., Campbell, C., Sackeim, H. A., and Mann, J. J.: Decreased regional brain metabolism following electroconvulsive therapy. Am J Psychiatry **158** (2001) 305-308
3. Raichle, M. E., Martin, W. R., Herscovitch, P., Mintun, M. A., and Markham, J.: Brain blood flow measured with intravenous H2(15)O. II. Implementation and validation. J Nucl Med **24** (1983) 790-798.
4. Friston, K. J., Holmes, A. P., Worsley, K. J., Poline, J. B., Frith, C. D., and Frackowiak, R. S. J.: Statistical parametric maps in functional imaging: A general approach. Hum Brain Mapping **2** (1995) 189-210

Fuzzy C-means Clustering Analysis to Monitor Tissue Perfusion with Near Infrared Imaging

Jeffrey Wallace[12], Homayoun Mozaffari N.[1], Li Pan[1], Nitish V. Thakor[12]

[1]Department of Biomedical Engineering,
[2]Engineering Research Center for Computer Integrated Surgical Systems and Technology
The Johns Hopkins School of Medicine, Baltimore, Maryland 21205 USA
nthakor@bme.jhu.edu

Abstract. During surgery, conventional or minimally invasive, a surgeon's ability to identify biological tissue properties is critical. Near Infrared (NIR) Imaging, a continuous, non-invasive imaging modality, offers a surgeon an augmented perception of the tissue characteristics (oxygenation, edema, etc.) In this paper, we present our NIR imaging setup and cluster analysis for localizing areas of similar NIR light absorbance, which relates directly to the tissue's Hb, HbO_2, and H_2O content. Through NIR imaging, a surgeon is equipped with auxiliary information to determine the extent and location of tissue injury.

1. Introduction

The ability of a surgeon to perceive the physiological state of biological tissue within the surgical field is paramount. Methods such as x-ray angiography and functional MRI give a surgeon vision into patient's physiology, but there are tradeoffs between functionality and hindrances, such as invasiveness and real-time functionality. Near Infrared (NIR) light has already been harnessed within the operating rooms as it is an 'optical window' [1] into the body. Several publications on NIR spectroscopy have been written detailing how NIR spectroscopy can be used to monitor physiological information [1, 2]. Spectrophotometry, however, is only a point measurement. NIR imaging, on the contrary, can give a surgeon both physiological and spatial information about the surgical field; it will give information that will aid the surgeon in localizing areas of injured tissue during surgery

In Mansfield's previous work [3] NIR imaging was used to monitor oxygenation and perfusion gradients on the reverse McFarlane skin flap model: a well-publicized model that creates an ischemia gradient across a section of tissue [4]. Fuzzy C-means clustering analysis was used on multi-spectral images to identify regions of adequately and poorly perfused tissue 1hr post surgery. Our work expands upon Mansfield's study by monitoring the tissue properties during perfusion changes.

2. Methods

A. Surgical procedures

The reverse McFarlane skin flap model [4] is ideal for establishing regions of tissue with a graded level of perfusion. For our experiments, we used anesthetized wistar rats (~400 g) with a maintained body temperature of 37°C. A 3x10 cm long skin flap was raised from the shaved dorsum of the rat and remained attached at the distal end, keeping only the sacral vessels intact for perfusion. Over time, the oxygenation gradient formed from limited perfusion.

W. Niessen and M. Viergever (Eds.): MICCAI 2001, LNCS 2208, pp. 1213-1214, 2001.
© Springer-Verlag Berlin Heidelberg 2001

B. Optical Setup and Image Processing

Monochromatic light was used for illumination at different wavelengths (750nm, 800nm, 830nm, 850nm, 925nm). The skin flap was illuminated while five spectral images were captured with a NIR enhanced camera (KPF2, Hitachi Denshi Corp.) in a dark room. All images were preprocessed with median filtering and a logarithmic residual correction method to calibrate the images [3]. Fuzzy C-Means cluster analysis (FCM)[3] was used to identify regions of tissue with similar spectral responses; responses that relate directly to tissue perfusion. The results of the FCM analysis are maps displaying each cluster and each cluster's NIR absorption spectrum.

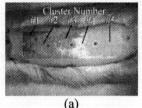

(a)

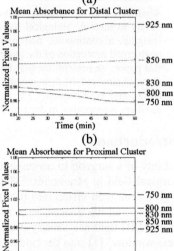

(b)

(c)

3. Results and Conclusion

Figure 1a shows an example of a skin flap image with the clustering map superimposed over the visual image (right side is the pedicle and the left side is distal to the pedicle). Figure 1b shows over time the absorption characteristics for the cluster farthest distal from the pedicle. There is an increase in absorbance for the 750 nm, which might reflect the presence of more Hb, while there is a decrease in the absorbance at 925 nm, which might be the absence of H_2O content. Figure 1c shows the absorption characteristics for the cluster most proximal to the pedicle, which shows very little absorption change over time. We believe this is due to the skin flap remaining adequately perfused. We conclude that NIR imaging has the ability to detect changes in tissue properties, both spatially and physiologically, which would be a great boon to a surgery.

Fig. 1: The clusters from FCM (a) were monitored over time. The most distal cluster (b) shows a decrease in 750 nm reflectance and an increase in 925 nm reflectance over time, while the proximal cluster (c) remains the same. We conclude that the distal cluster has an increase in Hb and a decrease in H_2O, while the proximal cluster remains adequately perfused.

References

1. Jobsis-vanderVilet, F.F., *Discovery of the Near-Infrared Window into the Body and the Development of Near-Infrared Spectroscopy.* J Biomed Optic, 1999. **4**(4): p. 392-396.
2. Thorniley, M.S., *et al.*, *The use of near-infrared spectroscopy for assessing flap viability during reconstructive surgery.* Br J Plast Surg, 1998. **51**(3): p. 218-26.
3. Mansfield, J.R., *et al.*, *Tissue viability by multispectral near infrared imaging: a fuzzy C-means clustering analysis.* IEEE Trans Med Imaging, 1998. **17**(6): p. 1011-8.
4. Mcfarlane, R. and D. G, *The design of a pedicle flap in the rat to study necrosis and its prevention.* Plast. Reconstr. Surg., 1965. **35**(2): p. 177-82.

A Method for μCT Based Assessment of Root Canal Instrumentation in Endodontics Research

Johan Van Cleynenbreugel[1], Lars Bergmans[2], Martine Wevers[3], Paul Lambrechts[2]

[1] Faculties of Medicine & Engineering,Medical Image Computing (Radiology - ESAT/PSI)
U.Z. Gasthuisberg, Herestraat 49
[2] BIOMAT, Department of Operative Dentistry and Dental Materials
[3] MTM, Department of Metallurgy and Materials Engineering
K.U.Leuven, B-3000 Leuven, BELGIUM
Johan.VanCleynenbreugel@uz.kuleuven.ac.be

The field of **endodontics** is devoted to the study and treatment of tissues inside (endo) the tooth (dontia). When a nerve within a tooth becomes necrotic and/or infected, so-called root canal therapy might be considered. In this case, a dental practitioner cleans and widens the inner root canal system by chemical irrigation and mechanical instrumentation with respect to the original canal morphology (see Figure 1). The success of this dental therapy largely depends on the safety and effectiveness - thorough cleaning and proper shaping - of the techniques employed for mechanical instrumentation (e.g. NiTi rotary files).

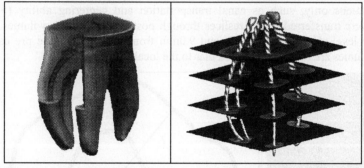

Fig. 1. *Left*: volume visualization of a μCT scanned extracted maxillary molar before instrumentation, partially showing its interior root canal system. *Right:* visualization by axial slices of the same tooth, now with the endodontic instruments (ProFile, Dentsply Maillefer, Ballaigues, Switzerland) in place (for illustrative purpose only).

Here we present a non-destructive approach, based on micro-focus CT (**μCT**) imaging [1], to study file-based preparation of root canals. A 3D methodology for quantitative evaluation of preparation effects is applied. The method was tested on ten in vitro phantoms (extracted mandibular molars). Each phantom was submitted to the five actions: 1) Acquisition of a 'pre' image volume. 2) Mechanical instrumentation of two mesial root canals by a LightSpeed file (Tulsa Dental Products, Tulsa, OK) in one canal, and by a GT Rotary file (Dentsply Maillefer, Ballaigues, Switzerland) in the other canal. 3) Acquisition of, a 'post' image volume after repositioning the phantom in the μCT device, using parameter values equal to 'pre'. 4) Post to pre registration: as only a small percentage of a phantom was affected by the instrumentation, a rigid geometric transformation could be assumed almost everywhere between the pre and post image volumes. The approach of [2], which is

W. Niessen and M. Viergever (Eds.): MICCAI 2001, LNCS 2208, pp. 1215-1217, 2001.
© Springer-Verlag Berlin Heidelberg 2001

unaffected by local image deformations, was applicable (see Figure 2). 5) Quantification of instrumentation influences.

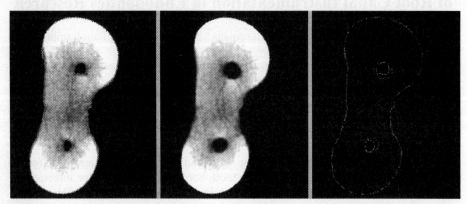

Fig. 2. *Left:* one slice from a pre image volume. *Middle:* corresponding slice from the post volume after image volume registration and resampling. Notice the effect of the endodontic instruments on both root canals. *Right:* overlay of the contours calculated on pre and post slice. Outer contours are aligned. Changes to the inner (canal) contours need to be quantified.

Instrumentation characteristics that were previously defined on 2D (destructive) cross-sections only, such as canal transportation and centering ability (Figure 3, right), were transferred to 2D reslices through post and pre image volumes. At five different levels (1.0, 3.0, 5.0, 7.0, and 9.0mm from the apex) of the pre canal axis these volumes are resliced perpendicular to the local tangent line.

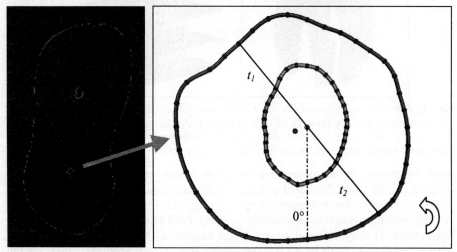

Fig. 3. Pre and post contours on a reslice plane (*left*), are represented in polar coordinates centered around the pre origin (*right*). 0° is taken at the buccal side of the root and each contour is sampled by a 10° increment counterclockwise. For each of the 18 directions thus obtained, **transportation** is defined by the distances t_1 and t_2, net transportation by $nt = |t_1 - t_2|$ and d is the distance between the opposite post boundary points, nt/d is the centering ratio. The **centering ability** of the instrument at this reslice is then defined as *max (nt/d)* over all directions.

Acknowledgements

Research support was obtained from the The European Society of Endodontology Research Grant 1999, the FWO, and Maillefer Instruments SA (Switzerland). The 3D quantification software was developed as part of the SuperVisie project (ITA-II 980302, IWT, Institute for the Promotion of Innovation by Science and Technology in Flanders).

References

1. SkyScan b.v.b.a., Aartselaar, Belgium, www.skyscan.be
2. F. Maes, A. Collignon, D. Vandermeulen, G. Marchal, P. Suetens (1997) Multimodality image registration by maximization of mutual information. *IEEE Transactions on Medical Imaging* **16(2)**, 187-98.

Reconstruction of Subcortical Brain Activity by Spatially Filtered MEG During Epileptic Seizures

H. Kober, O. Ganslandt, Ch. Nimsky, M. Buchfelder, and R. Fahlbusch

Neurocenter, Dept. of Neurosurgery, University Erlangen-Nuremberg, Germany
kober@nch.imed.uni-erlangen.de

Abstract. We analyzed the spontaneous brain activity of a brain tumor patient during an epileptic seizure. The current density reconstruction by spatial filtering (CLSF) revealed pathologic, neuronal activity originating from the hippocampus ipsilateral to the tumor which was confirmed by intraoperative electrocorticography. This study shows that subcortical brain activity can be localized noninvasively using MEG. Further MEG studies combined with depth electrode recordings will have to show the validity of our results and might help to improve our understanding of the pathophysiology of epileptogenesis.

Introduction Cortical interictal and subclinical ictal epileptic brain activity can be localized by Magnetoencephalography (MEG) [1]. Depth electrode recordings and lesion studies in epilepsy patients have shown that deep temporomesial structures like the hippocampus (HC) are important for the pathophysiology of epileptogenesis. However, depth electrode recordings show that with conventional dipole localization approaches activity originating from deep brain structures is likely to escape detection [2]. To non-invasively elucidate time course and location of these sources during epileptiform discharges we used a localization approach based on spatial filtering taking into account the spatio-temporal information of the measured MEG signal.

Methods We recorded bilateral spontaneous MEG activity in a 41 year old female patient with a brain tumor and focal epilepsy with a 2x37 channel biomagnetic system Magnes II (4-D Neuroimaging, San Diego, USA). Time course and location of ictal epileptiform discharges were investigated using a current density localization approach by spatial filtering (CLSF) [3]. The magnetic flux density B_i measured with a MEG sensor with lead field G_i which is generated by a current density distribution J can be calculated by $B_i = \int_\Omega \boldsymbol{J}(\boldsymbol{r}) \cdot \boldsymbol{G}(\boldsymbol{r}) dr^3$. The current density J_θ was reconstructed by a linear projection of the measured flux densities B_i at N sensor positions through a set of spatial filters w_i^θ:

$$J_\theta = \sum_{i=1}^{N} B_i w_i^\theta \ . \tag{1}$$

The N spatial filters for a target source at a specific location and current vector indicated by θ are constructed to minimize in a least-square sense the difference between the spatial response of the virtual sensor and an ideally selective delta function:

$$\chi^2 = \int_\Omega \left[\sum_{i=1}^{N} \boldsymbol{G}_i(\boldsymbol{r}) w_i^\theta(\boldsymbol{r}) - \boldsymbol{\delta}^\theta(\boldsymbol{r}) \right]^2 dr^3 \ . \tag{2}$$

W. Niessen and M. Viergever (Eds.): MICCAI 2001, LNCS 2208, pp. 1218–1219, 2001.

The filter coefficients minimizing this functional are given by $w = \Gamma^{-1} \cdot B$, where $\Gamma_{ij} = \int_\Omega G_i(r) \cdot G_j(r) dr^3$ is the Gram matrix and $B_i^\theta = \int_\Omega G_i(r) \cdot \delta^\theta(r) dr^3$ is the forward solution for the physical sensors due to a target dipole θ.

To improve the selectivity of the spatial filters for signal inherent sources the Gram matrix is substituted by the covariance matrix of the measured MEG data. Regularisation is achieved by a truncated singular value decomposition of the data covariance matrix including only the most significant singular values for the calculation of the spatial filter coefficients. Using equation (1) either a current density distribution of instantaneous source activity can be reconstructed using a set of equally spaced filters or the time course of a source at a specific voxel for successive measurement time instances.

Results During the seizure where the patient only perceived imaginary tones (no movement) two simultaneous sources could be localized ipsilateral to the low grade glioma, one source in the HC and the other one in the primary auditory cortex in the superior temporal gyrus (Heschl's gyrus) adjacent to the tumor which is perfectly consistent with the clinical symptoms. The reconstructed time course of the voxels with maximum CLSF current intensity in both foci revealed that the activity in the HC clearly preceded the activity in Heschl's Gyrus indicating a pacemaker function of the HC during the seizure (Fig. 1). Before the surgical removal of the tumor intraoperative electrocorticography confirmed the pathologic activity in the HC.

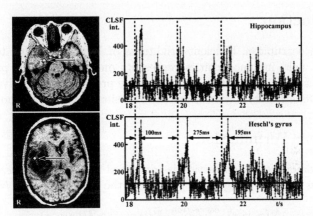

Fig. 1. Voxel with maximum CLSF intensity in axial MRI image (*left*) and the corresponding reconstructed time course (*right*) in the right hippocampus (*upper row*) and the right Heschl's gyrus (*lower row*) during an epileptic seizure with only auditory halluzinations (no movement).

References
[1] H. Stefan and C. Hummel. *Handbook of Clinical Neurology, The Epilepsies. Part I*, volume 72, chapter Magnetoencephalography, pages 319–336. Elsevier Science, 1999.
[2] C. Baumgartner, E. Pataraia, G. Lindinger, and L. Deecke. Neuromagnetic Recordings in Temporal Lobe Epilepsy. *J Clin Neurophysiol*, 17(2):177–189, 2000.
[3] S.E. Robinson and D.F. Rose. Current source image estimation by spatially filtered MEG. In M. Hooke, editor, *Biomagnetism: Clinical aspects*, pages 761–765. Elsevier Science, 1992.

Exploiting Voxel Correlation
for Automated MRI Bias Field Correction
by Conditional Entropy Minimization

Eduard Solanas and Jean-Philippe Thiran

Signal Processing Laboratory (LTS)
Swiss Federal Institute of Technology (EPFL)
CH-1015 Lausanne, Switzerland
{Eduardo.Solanas, JP.Thiran}@epfl.ch
http://ltswww.epfl.ch/~brain

Abstract. An unsupervised model-based strategy for bias field correction is proposed. We assume that information (in the sense of the information theory) in the corrupted image is greater than that in the uncorrupted one. The method exploits the fact that neighboring voxels are highly correlated to correct the bias field using a linear model.

1 Introduction

Besides noise corruption, deficient brightness of MR images due to radio frequency (RF) field inhomogeneities represents one of the major problems for image analysis. To correct this phenomenon we propose to take advantage from neighboring voxels' information using an extension of Likar's method [1].

2 Problem Formulation

Intensity inhomogeneities correction is concerned with finding $\widehat{U}(x, y, z)$, which best estimates the true image $U(x, y, z)$, from the acquired image $N(x, y, z)$

$$N(x, y, z) \xrightarrow{correction} \widehat{U}(x, y, z) \approx U(x, y, z) \tag{1}$$

$N(x, y, z)$ is usually described by a linear model of image formation (Beckers et al., 1994; Madisetti and Williams, 1998). Therefore, the corrected image can be calculated by inverting the image formation model (2).

$$N(x, y, z) = U(x, y, z)S_M(x, y, z) + S_A(x, y, z) \tag{2}$$

3 Neighborhood Information for Retrospective Bias Estimation (NIRBE)

Our method estimates the parameters for our correction model by optimizing a cost function that is a modified first order conditional entropy. Let X denote the

W. Niessen and M. Viergever (Eds.): MICCAI 2001, LNCS 2208, pp. 1220–1221, 2001.

entire set of symbols $x_1, x_2, ..., x_M$ where symbol x_i occurs with probability P_i and conveys the self-information I_i, and that satisfy $\sum_{i=1}^{M} P_i = 1$. If we suppose that a source has a *first order dependence*, so it is dependent on just their nearest symbols, then the conditional entropy, which represents the average information per symbol is defined as in eq. 3; where P_{ij} is the conditional probability that symbol x_i is chosen when its neighbor is symbol x_j. Averaging over all possible neighbor symbols we obtain the entropy of the source $H(X)$.

$$H(X|x_j) \triangleq -\sum_i P_{ij} log P_{ij} \Rightarrow H(X) = \sum_j H(X|x_j) \tag{3}$$

4   Experimental Results

For the evaluation of the proposed method we used a set of synthetic data without any pre-processing step. We used the *coefficient of variation (cv)* and *coefficient of joint variations (cjv)* to compare the performance between a model which assumes voxels' independence and ours. We assumed a linear model with polynomials of degree 2 for the correction, and the correlation between voxels is represented by the norm of the gradient though the method itself can use any neighborhood information taking into account hardware limitations.

Table 1. Correction of synthetic data using the Entropy (H) and the Conditional Entropy (CH) for information extraction

Mod	Bias	Correction	$cv(GM)$	$cv(WM)$	$cjv(GM, WM)$
T1	0%	-	0.17628	0.03668	0.58053
	40%	-	0.25057	0.16058	0.876
	40%	H	0.21089	0.15199	0.88807
	40%	CH	0.23469	0.10604	0.76078
T2	0%	-	0.20016	0.06213	0.95146
	40%	-	0.23691	0.22026	1.12067
	40%	H	0.23897	0.21384	1.24981
	40%	CH	0.19955	0.22807	0.94148
PD	0%	-	0.07473	0.01155	0.70667
	40%	-	0.12307	0.13825	1.9651
	40%	H	0.11985	0.13655	1.94841
	40%	CH	0.12151	0.13876	1.9972

References

1. Likar, B., Viergever, M. A., Pernus F.: Retrospective Correction of MR Intensity Inhomogeneity by Information Minimization. Medical Image Computing and Computer-Assisted Intervention (MICCAI 2000), 375-384.

Single Photon Emission Computed Tomography and 3 Dimensional Quantitative Evaluation in Renal Scintigraphy

M. Lyra[1], K. Skouroliakou[1], C. Georgosopoulos[2], C. Stefanides[3], J. Jordanou[1]

[1]Athens University, Radiology Department,
[2]Diagnostic Imaging Center,
[3]Pediatric Hospital "Aglaia Kyriakou" Athens, Greece (Hellas)

Abstract The evaluation of cortical damage to the kidneys, especially in children, is currently performed by means of Tc99m-DMSA renal scan. The routine involves the acquisition of planar images and their qualitative and quantitative evaluation. Many recent studies have dealt with the possible advantage that single photon emission tomography (SPECT) could possess on qualitative criteria. This study attempts to quantitatively deal with the issue by the calculation of an index, through the digitised slices' data. The results exhibit a clear advantage of tomographic and 3D reconstructed images over the conventional planar ones.

1 Introduction

Tc-99m DMSA renal scan is the method of choice for the detection and follow-up of any possible cortical damage to the kidneys. The test is widely performed in children in order to check for any possible signs of pyelonephritis, as well as for any suspected dysplasia of the kidneys. The usual procedure involves intravenous injection of Tc99m-DMSA and acquisition of four planar images (ANT, POST, RPO, LPO) 6 hours post injection. The evaluation of the results is qualitative by the physician as well as quantitative in the form of two indices denoting relative and absolute renal function for the two kidneys.

As single photon emission computed tomography (SPECT) become more popular, a number of studies dealt with the possible extra information that could be gained by the use of SPECT in renal studies. The comparison between the conventional planar technique and the tomographic acquisition was based on qualitative criteria. The tomographic procedure involves 32 posterior planar views over an 180^0 arc as it has been argued that a 360^0 arc does not offer any extra information. On the contrary it contributes to the presence of artifacts as the distance of the camera head from the kidneys is varying and the anterior projections involve an increased amount of soft tissue between the collimator and the kidneys.

In the present study the comparison between the planar and the tomographic imaging is attempted on quantitative basis by the computer extraction of two types of indices.

2 Material-Method

The patient sample consists of 50 children from 4 to 10 year old were admitted for a renal Tc-99m DMSA scan on the suspicion of pyelonephritis. The usual procedure,

W. Niessen and M. Viergever (Eds.): MICCAI 2001, LNCS 2208, pp. 1222-1223, 2001.

described above, was followed and an extra tomographic study was acquired.   It consisted of 32 planar views over a 180^0 arc (LLAT to RLAT). The tomographic study was reconstructed by typical parameters of filters (Hanning filter) and attenuation correction $(0.12cm^{-1})$. Three-dimensional reconstruction of the tomographic slices was obtained by a 25% threshold and a gradient factor of 15.

The typical procedure was followed by a tomographic reconstruction "by parts". That is, the images of kidneys were separated in three parts (upper, middle and lower), which were separately reconstructed for each kidney. A special program-routine was built to calculate the integrated number of counts over each reconstructed part, that is the number of counts Integrated Over the Volume of each part (IOV). This routine calculates the total number of counts over each "volume part" by integration of the transaxial slices corresponding parts. In order to avoid the background counts the routine was built so as to consider regions characterized by numbers of counts over a 20% threshold. This figure was extracted by measurements of the background to the kidney tissue ratio in a number of pathologic and normal images.

The result of this procedure was the calculation of three Integrated Over Volume (IOV) indices. These are the ratios of counts of upper to lower, upper to middle and lower to middle part. The corresponding count ratios were calculated from the posterior planar image.

3 Results

Indices were calculated from planar and tomographic (Integrated Over Volume [IOV] indices) images. Our Data concern 3 normal cases as well as pathologic cases (5 patients). In normal kidneys the results indicate a difference in the upper and lower kidney parts, the lower part is characterized by fewer counts than the upper one, a normal pattern that is not evident in the corresponding planar images. In pathologic cases the IOV concerning the kidney part where the focal defect is present is more representative than the corresponding planar index.   This fact is clearer if the corresponding images are viewed.

4 Discussion

It has been demonstrated by many studies that SPECT imaging of the kidneys, by Tc99m-DMSA, can provide the physician with extra qualitative information on the anatomy of the kidneys, especially when children are concerned. This conclusion has been drawn by studies based on qualitative criteria. The calculation of the indices in the present study offers a quantitative comparison of the planar, tomographic and 3D reconstructed images.

To conclude, where Tc99m-DMSA renal scan is concerned, the tomographic acquisition and reconstruction and the 3D display clearly offers additional valuable information to the physician, especially in the cases of children. This procedure does not require any extra quantity of radiopharmaceutical to be injected to the patient, therefore the radiation burden is the same. The extra time required is in the order of 15 minutes, therefore not presenting any inconvenience for the patient.

Automatic Analysis of the Left Ventricle in the Time Sequences of 3D Echo-Cardiographic Images

O. Gerard, M. Fradkin, A. Collet Billon, M. Jacob, J.-M. Rouet, and S.Makram-Ebeid

LEP - Philips Research
22 av. Descartes, F-94453 Limeil-Brevannes, France
{Olivier.Gerard|Maxim.Fradkin}@philips.com

1 Introduction

The 3D ultrasound imagery becomes more and more attractive for cardiac studies due to its simplicity, its improved reproducibility, and better precision, as compared to standard 2D echographic exams. However, automatic tools are needed to fully and efficiently analyze the large amounts of data obtained. In this paper, we present an automatic tool, aimed at the quantitative analysis of heart motion, based on the segmentation of the endo-cardium of the left ventricle. Using our method, quantitative measurements on volumes such as stroke and ejection-fraction (EF) are readily available (without needing any geometrical assumption), as well as regional wall motion parameters.

2 Method

The method is based on 3D model-based segmentation of time sequences images. Our 3D geometric model is described by a 2-simplex mesh. A 2-simplex mesh is a discrete non-parametric surface representation, defined by a set of 3-connected vertices. A great variability in possible cell shapes allows both very accurate and compact surface representation. The model deformation is expressed in displacement of mesh vertices, governed by two forces: *external*, attracting the model to the object boundaries, and *internal*, regularizing its surface (see [1]). Due to the limited scope of this paper, the reader may refer to [2] for details. The 3D+t segmentation procedure starts with the deformation of an initial model for the first image of the cardiac cycle. This initial model of the studied chamber is manually adjusted (with just 4 mouse clicks) to the data. Then the deformation procedure is repeated for the subsequent images, using the model derived from the previous image in the cardiac cycle as initial model. Another approach [3], in contrast with ours, uses a topological correspondence between the successive models. However, this topological correspondence does not necessarily imply the tracking of the same anatomical points of the heart, thus leading to an over-regularized final 4D model. Our approach, although quite simple, is very fast and completely automatic. Having the sequence of 3D models, one can easily calculate different heart parameters, such as the blood volume, stroke volume, and EF. Moreover, we can quantify the local wall motion of the heart.

W. Niessen and M. Viergever (Eds.): MICCAI 2001, LNCS 2208, pp. 1224–1225, 2001.

3   Results

For the validation of the proposed method, we have used 3D ultrasound data sets acquired using a rotating probe gated on the ECG (ATL, Seattle). The volume measurements have been validated using a dynamically pumped balloon-in-balloon phantom (D. J. Sahn, OSHU, Portland, OR), showing excellent accuracy (error less than the set-up precision) and a very good robustness with respect to initialization and parameter setting (with standard deviation < 1.2 ml).

The method is able to quantify the radial motion of the LV and to represent in color this information. It has been successfully tested on the LV for both trans-esophageal and trans-thoracic 3D acquisitions as well as on other cardiac chambers (RV, atrium). Fig. 1 shows the segmentation results for two phases of the cardiac cycle of a 3D trans-esophageal LV dataset of a patient suffering from a large mitral regurgitation. Complete volume calculation (and motion analysis) can be performed in less than 3 minutes on a standard PC. Clinical validations are under way to assess the accuracy of the whole process, so as to be ready when real-time 3D echocardiography becomes clinical routine procedure.

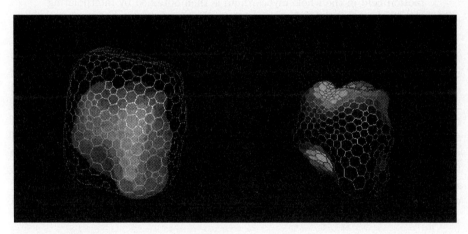

Fig. 1. Resulting model: superimposition of two active models, corresponding to end-systolic and end-diastolic phases (left); wall motion magnitude of systolic phase coding with gray levels (right)

References

1. Kass, M., Witkin, A., Terzopoulos, D.: Snakes: Active contour models. Int. J. Comp. Vision **4-1** (1988) 321–331
2. Delingette, H.: General Object Reconstruction Based on Simplex Meshes. Int. J. Comp. Vision **32-2** (1999) 111–146
3. Montagnat, J., Delingette, H.: Space and Time Shape constrained Deformable Surfaces for 4D Medical Image Segmentation. In: Delp, S., *et al.* (eds.): MICCAI-2000. Lecture Notes in Computer Science, Vol. 1935. Springer-Verlag, (2000) 196–205

Displacement Field Estimation from CSPAMM Images without Segmentation of the Myocardium

Sabine Dippel

Philips Research Laboratories, Division Technical Systems
Röntgenstrasse 24–26, D-22335 Hamburg, Germany
sabine.dippel@philips.com

Abstract. We present a method for the estimation of the displacement field in 2D CSPAMM tagged image time series for both ventricles which does not rely on a previous detailed segmentation of the myocardial contours. The automatic tag extraction is restricted to the myocardium by evaluating the motion characteristics of local maxima and minima. The motion field in the whole myocardium is then obtained by interpolating the displacement field of these points.

Introduction. In cardiac MR imaging, tagging techniques, where a spatial modulation of the magnetization is applied to the myocardium at end-diastole, permit a detailed imaging of the heart wall motion. CSPAMM (Complementary Spatial Modulation of Magnetization) tagging even allows slice following and produces relatively stable tags for a whole heart cycle [1]. However, since evaluation of such images is still quite cumbersome and usually involves a fair amount of user interaction, the method is not widely used yet. Besides, most studies so far have been restricted to the evaluation of the motion of the left ventricle. Here, we present a method which is related to that presented in [2]. However, our approach is applied to both ventricles, needs only the rough definition of a polygonal ROI, and does not make use of a functional fit to the motion field.

Material and Method. We use CSPAMM tagged images, where for the short axis slices a series with vertical and horizontal tags were acquired successively, but within one breath hold. In CSPAMM images, also the grey value maxima between the tag lines are quite pronounced. The tag extraction algorithm therefore first searches for local maxima and minima in the direction perpendicular to the tag direction. In the first frame, connected components are extracted and tags in all frames labeled according to their proximity to tags in the previous frame. To eliminate erroneously detected points (e.g. tags in the blood pool which disappear over time or tags in other tissue which do not move at all), the motion of tag points perpendicular to the tag line direction is evaluated. Tag points which do not exhibit a plausible motion characteristic, as well as tag points whose Laplacian changes too much over time, or is in general too small, are deleted. Only then, lines are fitted to the extracted tags in the first frame, and a previously defined polygonal ROI (see Fig. 1) is used to restrict this fitting

W. Niessen and M. Viergever (Eds.): MICCAI 2001, LNCS 2208, pp. 1226–1227, 2001.

to the myocardial region. This ROI is needed to eliminate points in other tissue outside of the heart which moves similarly to the heart and therefore could not be removed by evaluating the motion. On the basis of the calculated reference tag positions, a new evaluation of the motion of tag points is performed, and points moving inconsistently are again eliminated. Here, it is also taken into account that between two maxima there should be a minimum and vice versa. The resulting backward displacement [2] for the extracted tags (maxima and minima) is then used as a basis for interpolating the displacement for myocardial points not on a tag line. For each tagging direction, the displacement perpendicular to the tag direction is interpolated, and the results for both directions combined to give the 2D displacement field.

Results. Figure 1 shows a typical result from the procedure described above.

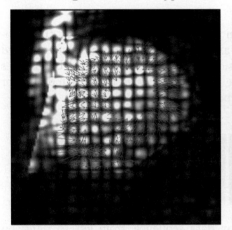 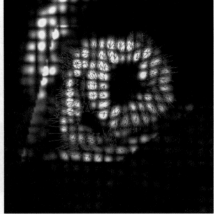

Fig. 1. Displacement from end-diastole to end-systole, superimposed on the corresponding end-diastolic (left) and end-systolic (right) image. The shaded polygonal ROI shown is only used in the evaluation of the displacement map. The arrows are derived from the displacement map obtained by interpolating the results for the tag lines for horizonal and vertical directions. The resulting image was created by multiplying the horizontally and vertically tagged images.

Acknowledgements. We thank Marcus Spiegel, ETH Zürich, for providing the image material, and our colleagues Peter Rösch and Rafael Wiemker of Philips Research Hamburg for helpful discussions.

References

1. M. Stuber, M. A. Spiegel, S. E. Fischer, M. B. Scheidegger, P. G. Danias, E. M. Pedersen, and P. Boesiger. Single breath-hold slice-following CSPAMM myocardial tagging. *MAGMA*, 9:85–91, 1999.
2. P. Clarysse, C. Basset, L. Khouas, P. Croisille, D. Friboulet, C. Odet, and I. E. Magnin. Two-dimensional spatial and temporal displacement and deformation field fitting from cardiac magnetic resonance tagging. *Med. Image Anal.*, 4:253–268, 2000.

Automatic Detection of Myocardial Boundaries in MR Cardio Perfusion Images

Luuk Spreeuwers[1] and Marcel Breeuwer[2]

[1] University Medical Centre Utrecht, Image Sciences Institute,
luuk@isi.uu.nl
[2] Philips Medical Systems,
Medical Imaging Information Technology - Advanced Development,
marcel.breeuwer@philips.com

1 Introduction

Cardiovascular diseases often result in reduced blood perfusion of the myocardium (MC). Recent advances in MR allow fast recording of contrast enhanced myocardial perfusion scans. For perfusion analysis the myocardial boundaries must be traced. Currently this is done manually. In this paper a method for automatic detection of the myocardial boundaries is proposed.

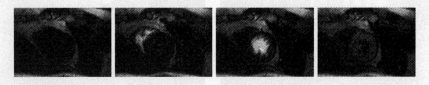

Fig. 1. Four images of a MRI perfusion data sequence; from left to right: no contrast, bolus passage in RV, bolus passage in LV, perfusion of the MC.

MR cardio perfusion scans are made by recording, during a period of 20-40 seconds, a number of short axis slices. The acquisition is controlled by the ECG so that each set of slices represents the same phase of the heart cycle. A few seconds after the beginning of the scan, contrast agent is injected. The contrast agent first enters the right ventricle (RV), then the left ventricle (LV) and finally the MC (see figure 1). The intensity as a function of time of a segment in the LV and RV and in the MC is sketched in figure 2a. The maximum upslope is most widely used [1,2] to characterise perfusion. To obtain the segments the boundaries of the MC have to be traced, see figure 2b.

2 Myocardial Boundary Detection

The most important consideration in the proposed approach is the use of both intensity-time and shape information to realise a robust segmentation. A block scheme of the myocardial boundary detection process is shown in figure 3.

W. Niessen and M. Viergever (Eds.): MICCAI 2001, LNCS 2208, pp. 1228–1231, 2001.

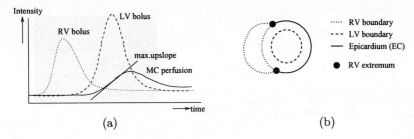

(a)   (b)

Fig. 2. a) Intensity-time profiles in the RV, LV and MC; b) boundaries to be traced.

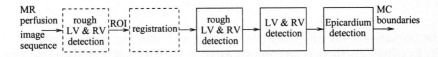

Fig. 3. Block scheme of the myocardial boundary detection process.

At bolus passage the LV and RV are very bright. Therefore, we search for very bright blobs in the image sequence. These blobs may be found by first smoothing in space and time to suppress smaller blobs caused by noise etc. and searching for the local maxima in space and time. Next feature images are constructed by correlating the time derivative of the intensity-time profiles of the RV and LV centres with those of all pixels in the image (figure 4a).

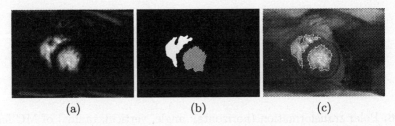

(a)   (b)   (c)

Fig. 4. LV and RV feature image (a), labelled regions (b) and boundaries (c).

The LV and RV are subsequently extracted by region growing from the RV and LV centres (figure 4b). The boundaries are extracted by tracing the outlines of the found regions. The extrema of the RV are detected by making a polar transform of the outline of the RV relative to the centre of gravity of the LV and searching for the extrema in the angles (figure 4c).

Detection of the EC is harder because the concentration of the contrast agent is much lower in the MC. Correlation of time-intensity curves did not result in usable features. To calculate a feature image for the MC, consider figure 5.

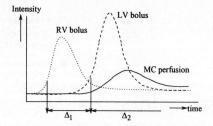
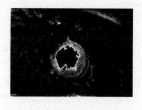

Fig. 5. MC feature image calculation. During Δ_1 the MC is dark, during Δ_2 the MC is bright. Subtracting MIPs of Δ_1 and Δ_2 gives an MC feature image (right).

The perfusion of the MC takes place during and after the bolus passage of the LV. In period Δ_1 there is no contrast agent in the MC and it is, therefore, dark. In period Δ_2 the contrast agent enters the MC and it becomes brighter, while the intensity elsewhere remains the same. By subtracting a maximum intensity projection (MIP) of period Δ_1 from a MIP of period Δ_2, the MC shows up bright, while the surrounding tissues are suppressed. The resulting feature is shown on the right in figure 5. The two RV extrema (figure 2) serve as starting points for the EC detection. Furthermore, it is assumed that the EC has a more or less circular shape. A polar transformation was generated from the MC feature image relative to the centre of gravity of the LV, see figure 6. Next a 5 node snake was fitted to the feature image, of which 2, the RV extrema, were fixed (arrows in figure 6). the nodes is linear (in polar domain). The spline maximises the contrast ratio. Finally the boundary is transformed back into spatial domain.

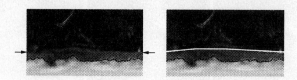

Fig. 6. Polar transformation (horizontal: angle, vertical: radius) of MC feature image (left). The RV-extrema are indicated by the arrows. Detected epicardium (right).

3   Results

The boundary detection procedure was tested on a total of 30 image sequences from 14 different scans. The scans varied in resolution (128*128 and 256*256 pixels) and number of slices (1-5). The detected boundaries were evaluated by visual inspection. From 26 out of 30 sequences the myocardial boundaries were

found correctly. The four remaining sequences contained severe motion artifacts. Segmentation of a 256*256*70 sequence took about 25 seconds on a Sun
UltraSPARC-IIi @440 MHz. Figure 7 shows some results.

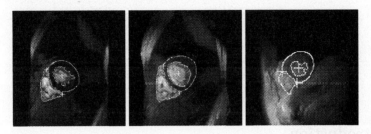

Fig. 7. Some results of the boundary detection method for different types of
images

References

1. N. Al-Saadi, E. Nagel, M. Gross, A. Bornstedt, B. Schnackenburg, C. Klein, H. Os-
   wald, and E. Fleck, "Non-invasive detection of myocardial ischemia from perfusion
   reserve based on cardiovascular magnetic resonance," in *Circulation*, No. 101, 2000.
   1st Virtual Congress of Cardiology, http://pcvc.sminter.com.ar/cvirtual.
2. M. Breeuwer, L. Spreeuwers, and M. Quist, "Automatic quantitative analysis of
   cardiac MR perfusion images," in *Proceedings of SPIE Medical Imaging*, (San Diego,
   USA), February 2001.

Using SPM to Detect Evolving MS Lesions

David Rey, Jonathan Stoeckel, Grégoire Malandain, and Nicholas Ayache

INRIA Sophia - Epidaure Project
2004 Route des Lucioles BP 93
06902 Sophia Antipolis Cedex, France
{David.Rey, Jonathan.Stoeckel, Gregoire.Malandain,
Nicholas.Ayache}@sophia.inria.fr
http://www-sop.inria.fr/epidaure/Epidaure-eng.html

1 Introduction

Clinicians need to study the effects of new treatments: it is sometimes possible to detect and quantify those effects by looking at evolutions in the medical images of a patient over time especially in the case of multiple sclerosis (MS) where lesions are related to clinical signs [1]. Some methods allow to compare two images to know where there are differences, typically between the last and the previous exam [2, 3]. However a retrospective analysis might be done on the whole set of images to find the moments when evolutions occur [4]. We propose to use the analogy between an activation in functional imaging (for instance PET, SPECT and fMRI) [5] and a signal change due to an evolving multiple sclerosis lesion. Voxels corresponding to evolving pathological areas are named ELV (Evolving Lesion Voxels) in this abstract.

2 Method

First of all we have to pre-process the image series: geometrical alignment [6] and temporal bias correction using the joint histogram of two images.

Considering the shape of ELV profiles over time (Fig. 1-a), we use a kind of asymmetric Gaussian (Fig. 1-b) with five parameters: amplitude, mean, rising time, decreasing time and vertical offset, $f(x) = p_1 \times \exp(-g(x - p_2)^2) + p_5$ with $g(x) = p_3 \times (x + \sqrt{1 + x^2}) + p_4 \times (x - \sqrt{1 + x^2})$. This model is fitted on a training set of ELV profiles and normalized to obtain an average model of evolving lesions (Fig. 1-c). The analysis is computed independently for each time point, thus resulting in as many analyses as the number of temporal images. Those separate analyses are due to the necessity to have enough data to preserve sensitivity. For each analysis, first the best linear combination of the average model and a constant value is estimated for each voxel (Fig. 2). Then we proceed to the statistical inference stage (using a t-test).

Thus our method takes into account both temporal and spatial cohesion of the evolving pathological areas: the temporal cohesion is due to the use of a temporal signal model of voxels in evolving lesions, and the spatial cohesion comes from the statistical analysis method that makes it possible to compute probabilities for clusters of voxels.

W. Niessen and M. Viergever (Eds.): MICCAI 2001, LNCS 2208, pp. 1232–1234, 2001.

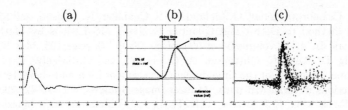

Fig. 1. *a) typical curves of evolving pathological voxel over time are composed of a rising part and a decreasing part. b) An instance of our model of evolving profile with five parameters. c) Normalized training set of profiles with the fitted. average model*

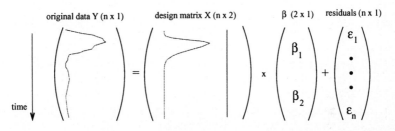

Fig. 2. *General linear model*

The described statistical analysis was applied on a time series of 24 T2-weighted MRI acquired over one year[1]. Each image has a size of $256 \times 256 \times 54$ with a voxel size of $0.9375 \times 0.9375 \times 3.0$ mm^3. We used the freely available SPM99 package[2] for the statistical analysis. We only kept the clusters which sizes have a probability smaller than 0.01.

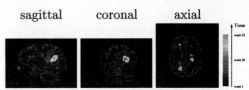

Fig. 3. *It is possible to superimpose evolving areas on an original image of the series.*

This new approach for detecting MS lesions combines temporal (model of ELV profiles) and spatial cohesion (SPM framework) providing promising results.

References

[1] C. R. G. Guttmann, S. S. Ahn, L. Hsu, R. Kikinis, and F. A. Jolesz. The Evolution of Multiple Sclerosis Lesions on Serial MR. *American Journal of NeuroRadiology*, 16:1481–1491, August 1995.

[2] D. Rey, G. Subsol, H. Delingette, and N. Ayache. Automatic Detection and Segmentation of Evolving Processes in 3D Medical Images: Application to Multiple Sclerosis. In *IPMI'99*, volume 1613 of *LNCS*, pages 154–167, June 1999.

---

[1] courtesy of Dr. Charles Guttmann and Dr. Ron Kikinis, Brigham and Women's Hospital, and Harvard Medical School

[2] http://www.fil.ion.ucl.ac.uk/spm

[3] D. Rey, C. Lebrun-Frénay, G. Malandain, S. Chanalet, N. Ayache, and M. Chatel. A New Method to Detect and Quantify Evolving MS Lesions by Mathematical Operators. In *AAN*, volume 54 of *Neurology (Supp. 3)*, page 123, May 2000.

[4] G. Gerig, D. Welti, C. Guttmann, A. Colchester, and G. Székely. Exploring the discrimination power of the time domain for segmentation and characterization of active lesions in serial MR data. *Medical Image Analysis*, 4(1):31–42, 2000.

[5] R.S.J. Frackowiak, K.J. Friston, C.D. Frith, R.J. Dolan, and J.C. Mazziotta. *Human Brain Function*. Academic Press, 1997.

[6] J. P. Thirion. New Feature Points Based on Geometric Invariants for 3D Image Registration. *International Journal of Computer Vision*, 18(2):121–137, May 1996.

Spherical Navigator Echoes for Full 3-D Rigid Body Motion Measurement in MRI

Edward Brian Welch[1], Armando Manduca[2], Roger C. Grimm[1],
Heidi A. Ward[1], Clifford R. Jack Jr.[1]

[1] MRI Research Lab, Dept. of Diagnostic Radiology, Mayo Clinic, Rochester, MN 55905
[2] Biomathematics Resource, Mayo Clinic, Rochester, MN 55905

Abstract. A 3-D spherical navigator (SNAV) echo technique for MRI that can measure rigid body motion in all six degrees of freedom simultaneously by sampling a spherical shell in k-space is under development. Rigid body 3-D rotations of an imaged object simply rotate the k-space data, while translations alter phase in a known way. A computer controlled motion phantom was used to execute known rotations and translations to evaluate the technique. Accurate detection was possible with a double SNAV echo acquisition following a 3-D helical spiral trajectory. Motion detection for retrospective or prospective correction in MRI with spherical navigator echoes is thus feasible and practical.

1 Introduction

Patient motion remains a significant problem in many MRI applications. Navigator echoes are commonly used to measure motion in one or more degrees of freedom and to compensate prospectively or retrospectively. An orbital navigator (ONAV) echo captures data in an origin-centered circle in some plane of k-space. This data can be used to detect rotational and translational motion in this plane (1). Multiple orthogonal ONAVs are required for general 3-D motion determination, and the accuracy of a given ONAV is adversely affected by motion out of its plane (2). The true 3-D spherical navigator (SNAV) echo can measure rigid body motion in all 6 degrees of freedom simultaneously by sampling an origin-centered sphere in k-space.

2 Theory

For all rigid body motions, if one ignores the effects of tissue entering or leaving the field of view, data never enters or leaves the k-space spherical shell. The relationship between a baseline position signal S measured at the original location (k_x, k_y, k_z) and a later signal S' measured at a new rotated location (k_x', k_y', k_z') or (k_ρ, θ', ϕ') plus a possible translation $(\Delta x, \Delta y, \Delta z)$ is expressed by the following equation.

$$S'(k_x',k_y',k_z') = S'(k_\rho,\theta',\phi') = S(k_\rho,\theta,\phi)e^{i2\pi k_\rho (\Delta x \cos\theta \sin\phi + \Delta y \sin\theta \sin\phi + \Delta z \cos\phi)} \qquad [1]$$

W. Niessen and M. Viergever (Eds.): MICCAI 2001, LNCS 2208, pp. 1235-1236, 2001.
© Springer-Verlag Berlin Heidelberg 2001

3 Methods

SNAV and ONAV data was acquired at several phantom positions. Magnitude registration to detect rotation was performed with a simplex minimization of sum of squared differences. Translation was detected by a weighted least squares fit to the phase differences. The 1008 sample SNAV helical spiral trajectory (3) begins at the equator and spirals toward the pole until the gradient slew rate limits are exceeded. Fig. 1 shows that less than 15% of the sphere's area is left unsampled at $k_\rho=0.39$ cm^{-1}. A second SNAV is acquired in the opposite hemisphere in order to make the total trajectory orthogonal to a possible motion-induced linear phase accrual term.

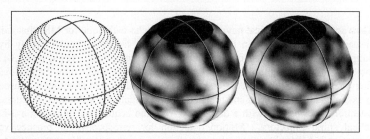

Fig. 1. The sampled SNAV trajectory (*right*) and two texture-mapped spheres (*middle and left*) showing the *k*-space magnitude ($k_\rho=0.39$ cm^{-1}) for the SNAV acquired at two phantom positions separated by 10°. The *k*-space features rotate in the expected manner. Great circles are drawn as a visual reference. The unsampled polar region of the sphere appears black.

4 Results

The motions detected by the SNAV agree well with ONAV results and are within the accuracy of the motion phantom, ±0.2 mm for translation and ±0.13° for rotation.

Table 1. SNAV Motion detection results compared to intended motion and ONAV results.

	Translation (mm)				Rotation (°)			
Intended Motion	-5.00	-3.00	+3.00	+5.00	-4.92	-3.16	+3.16	+4.92
SNAV Detection	-4.95	-2.93	+2.94	+4.89	-4.88	-3.18	+3.20	+4.90
ONAV Detection	-4.91	-2.88	+3.07	+4.97	-4.92	-3.16	+3.25	+5.27

References

1. Fu, Z.W., Wang, Y., Grimm, R.C., Rossman, P.J., Felmlee, J.P., Riederer, S.J., Ehman, R.L.: Orbital Navigator Echoes for Motion Measurements in Magnetic Resonance Imaging. Magnetic Resosnance in Medicine 34 (1995) 746-753
2. Ward, H.A., Riederer, S.J., Grimm, R.C., Ehman, R.L., Felmlee, J.P., Jack, C.R.: Prospective Multiaxial Motion Correction for fMRI. Magnetic Resosnance in Medicine 43 (2000) 459-469
3. Wong, S.T.S., Roos, M.S.: A Strategy for Sampling on a Sphere Applied to 3D Selective RF Pulse Design. Magnetic Resosnance in Medicine 32 (1994) 778-784

Phase Unwrapping for Magnetic Resonance Thermometry

Suprijanto[1], F.M. Vos[1], M.W. Vogel[2], A.M. Vossepoel[1], and H.M. Vrooman[2]

[1] Pattern Recognition Group, Department of Applied Physics
Delft University of Technology 2628 CJ Delft The Netherland
{supri, frans, albert}@ph.tn.tudelft.nl
[2] Department of Radiology, Erasmus University Medical Center
P.O. Box. 1738, 3000 DR Rotterdam, The Netherlands
vrooman@mi.fgg.eur.nl   mvogel@rdiag.fgg.eur.nl

1 Introduction

Magnetic resonance thermometry enables temperature measurement in a non-invasive way. A representation of the temperature is given by the phase shift of the MR signal[1]. Unfortunately, only "wrapped phase" is measured directly, yielding values between $-\pi$ and $+\pi$. However only the true phase("unwrapped phase") is proportional to temperature.

Phase unwrapping is essentially the process of recovering true phase from its wrapped representation. The unwrapping boils down to adding a multiple of 2π (the wrapped count) to each region enclosed by "fringe lines" marking a jump. In practical phase images, however, noise can cause such lines to merge, break them into parts, or create isolated segments. Locations where fringes merge or segments end are called *residues* or discontinuity sources. The problem of phase unwrapping is often solved by minimizing the number of discontinuities (phase jumps) over all choices of wrap count[2,3]. Unfortunately, the minimum discontinuity solution is not always appropriate for phase data that contains noise. To solve this problem "quality map" can be used to weight the discontinuities. Any further spurious discontinuities may be reduced by low pass filtering the complex image. In this paper we will investigate the effect of quality maps derived from MRI magnitude images. Additionally, we will look into noise filtering of the complex MRI images.

2 Method

The Minimum discontinuities algorithm proposed by Flynn [3] was used for phase unwrapping. The algorithm initially identifies fringes by a phase difference between adjacent pixels that exceeds π radians. A tree-growing approach is utilized to trace the paths of such discontinuities. The path formation proceeds until a loop is detected. Then, a multiple of 2π is added to the values of the enclosed image part. It performs this process iteratively until no more loops are detected.

W. Niessen and M. Viergever (Eds.): MICCAI 2001, LNCS 2208, pp. 1237–1239, 2001.

To weight the discontinuities in the presence of noise a *quality map* was introduced. The quality map was defined by the gradient magnitude of the MR signal. Additionally, filtering the wrapped phase data makes the phase unwrapping process considerably easier by reducing the number of residues. Unfortunately, direct filtering the wrapped phase data causes blurring of the fringe lines. Therefore, we propose to apply filtering to the complex data, using a Gaussian filter.

3 Results

The effect of our quality map and filtering on the unwrapped result was tested using two MRI images of the knee. The effect of preprocessing will be evaluated in two experiments: **(A)** unwrapping of the raw MRI wrapped phase without using a quality map and **(B)** unwrapping of the MRI wrapped phase after filtering, supported by the use of a quality map. To evaluate the outcome from experiments A and B, we will compare the number of remaining discontinuities(i.e. adjoining pixels whose values differ by more than π radians)on the solution.

Table 1. The number of discontinuities from Experiment-A and B for the axial and sagittal Knee MRI images.

MRI Images	Experiment-A	Experiment-B
Sagittal knee	6.3% of 65025 pixels	3.3% of 65025 pixels
Axial knee	11.4% of 65025 pixels	6.5% of 65025 pixels

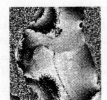  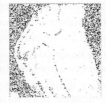 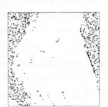

Wrapped phase   Unwrapped phase   Remaining discon-   Remaining discon-
                 from B   tinuities from A   tinuities from B

4 Conclusions and Further Research

We tested a quality representation derived from the magnitude component of MR images. To reduce the number of residues before unwrapping, filtering of the complex MR images was introduced. The experiments showed that both techniques are beneficiary to reduce the number of discontinuities that remain after unwrapping. Unfortunately, a drawback to be solved is that manual thresholding must be applied to mask out the low quality pixels. Currently, we work on techniques to determine a threshold based on the pulse sequence parameters that are applied during image acquisition.

References

1. J.R. MacFall, D.M. Prescott, H.C. Charles, T.V. Samulski. H^1 MRI phase thermometry in vivo canine brain, muscle, and tumor tissue, *Medical Physics*, Vol. 23, No. 10, pp. 1775-1782, October 1996,
2. Dennis C. Ghiglia. Mark D. Pritt. Two-Dimensional Phase Unwrapping, Theory, Algorithm and Software, John Willey and Sons, INC. 1998
3. Thomas J. Flynn. Two-dimensional phase unwrapping with minimum weighted discontinuity. *Journal of Optical Society of America A*,Vol. 14, No. 10, pp. 2692-2701,October 1977

A Simplified Field-of-View Calibration Technique for an Operating Microscope

A. Hartov, H. Sun, D.W. Roberts, K.D. Paulsen

Dartmouth College, Hanover, NH 03755

Abstract. We present a simplified camera calibration algorithm taking advantage of the geometry of our operating microscope, and requiring no special calibration target. Simulations showed that this algorithm is moderately sensitive to inaccuracies in S and f. For nominal values of S_n=6 pix/mm and fn=300 mm, we found that a 5% deviation in the value of S results in a mean error of 0.99 mm, while a 5% deviation in the actual value of f results in a 0.81 mm mean error.

1 Introduction

Our goal is to use the operating microscope's field of view (FOV) as a means to track shift between a preoperative MR and the operating field. This will provide data to update the preoperative study and compensate for the shift [1]. A necessary step consists of being able to predict where a point in world coordinates will appear in the FOV. Determining the required transformation matrices is usually referred to as the „camera calibration" problem. Camera calibration has been investigated by many and recent contributions include: Zhang [2], Devy et al. [3], Luong et al. [4], Stein [5], Hartley [6], Wei et al. [7], Faugeras [8], and Weng et al. [9], Caprile et al. [10]. It is also discussed in a textbook Gonzalez & Wintz [11] and Tsai [12]. We sought a much simpler approach allowing calibration on the fly during a procedure, and requiring no special calibration setup.

2 Materials and Methods

With a readily identifiable focal point, and the ability to physically make it coincide with any desired world feature we devised a method to express its location in world space using a suitable transformation matrix [13]. The result of this procedure is a vector V_f representing the location of the focal point in tracker coordinates. The series of transformations needed to map a point from world to image coordinates is:

$$^{I}P = {}^{I}T_{C} \cdot {}^{C}T_{T} \cdot {}^{T}T_{W} \cdot {}^{W}P$$

(1)

where the subscript and superscripts indicate image (I), camera (C), tracker (T) and world (W) coordinate systems. In equation 1, the location of the world-coordinates

W. Niessen and M. Viergever (Eds.): MICCAI 2001, LNCS 2208, pp. 1240-1242, 2001.

point, ^WP, is known; ^TT_W, the world to tracker transformation, is provided by the 3D positioning system; ^CT_T, the tracker to camera transformation, needs to be computed and the camera to image transformation, ^IT_C, is determined as explained here.

In the following discussion the desired point is known in tracker coordinates (i.e. the right-most multiplication in (1) has been performed). We expand here equation 1 in matrix form:

$$\begin{bmatrix} c \cdot x_I \\ c \cdot y_I \\ c \end{bmatrix} = \begin{bmatrix} S_x & 0 & 0 & 0 \\ 0 & S_y & 0 & 0 \\ 0 & 0 & 1/f & 0 \end{bmatrix} \cdot \begin{bmatrix} r_1 & r_2 & r_3 & t_x \\ r_4 & r_5 & r_6 & t_y \\ r_7 & r_8 & r_9 & t_z \\ 0 & 0 & 0 & 1 \end{bmatrix} \cdot \begin{bmatrix} x_T \\ y_T \\ z_T \\ 1 \end{bmatrix}$$

(2)

From (2), it can be seen that $c=z_C/f$, where z_C is the z coordinate of the point in camera coordinates. This coefficient is the nonlinear component of the overall transformation process, since it includes the z_C term and since the homogenous image coordinates must be normalized, (divided by c) to obtain x_I and y_I. Sx and Sy are the scaling factors translating distance (mm) to pixels in our system Sx=Sy (square pixels). The term f is the focal length of the optical system; when the focal point is aimed at the point of interest, z_C =f and c=1. Because of the nonlinear term in the camera to image transformation ^IT_C it is not possible to compute it directly. We chose to determine Sx and Sy directly from images and we also assume f to be the focal length specified by the microscope's manufacturer. The matrix containing the r1...r9 and tx...tz elements (^TT_C) relates tracker and camera spaces, and is the only term that needs computing. Having obtained estimates of the components of ^IT_C, we are able to solve for the remaining unknown terms using points whose coordinates are known in tracker and image frames.

3 Results

3.1 FOV Calibration: Simulations Results

Sx and Sy were fond from images of a ruler in the focal plane at each magnification setting. Evaluation of the FOV calibration is based on computer simulations at 4 different magnification settings with nominal values for Sn=6, 12, 24 and 48 pix/mm, (zoom factors of 1, 2, 4 and 8) and a fixed nominal value of 300 mm for the focal length fn. We used a 9x9 grid of test points forming a 20 mm square in camera space. From the test points defined in camera coordinates, homologous sets were produced in tracker, world and image coordinates. The image coordinates were computed using an actual focal length fa and an actual scaling factor Sa. These were varied by ±10% from their nominal values fn and Sn in 21 increments. Errors were computed from the Euclidean distances between the correct and calibrated points are summarized in table 1.

4. Tables

Table 1. Error in image point projection due to a disparity between the nominal (S_n, f_n) values for the scaling factor and focal distance and their actual values.

Conditions	10% error				5% error			
All units mm	S		f		S		f	
	mean	max	mean	max	mean	max	mean	max
Sn = 6, fn = 300	1.715	2.8808	1.8865	3.0641	0.9928	1.7552	0.8097	1.4142
Sn = 12, fn = 300	1.7175	2.8808	1.6824	2.7735	1.0373	1.7552	0.8244	1.3176
Sn = 24 fn = 300	0.9545	1.4404	0.8591	1.2964	0.5816	0.8776	0.4407	0.6482
Sn = 48 fn = 300	0.5464	0.7202	0.4918	0.6482	0.3329	0.4388	0.2459	0.3241

References

1. Roberts, D. W.; Miga, M. I.; Hartov, A.; Eisner, S.; Lemery, J. M.; Kennedy, F. E.; Paulsen, K. D. „Intraoperatively Updated Neuroimaging Using Brain Modeling and Sparse Data." Neurosurgery, Vol. 45, No. 5, Nov. 1999.
2. Zhang, Z. „A Flexible New Technique for Camera Calibration" Technical Report MSR-TR-90-71. Microsoft Research. http://research.microsoft.com/~zhang
3. Devy, M; Garric, V.; Orteu, J. „Camera Calibration from Multiple Views of a 2D Object, Using a Global Non Linear Minimization Method." Proc. IROS 97, pp 1583-1589.
4. Luong, Q.-T.; Faugeras, O.; „Self-Calibration of a Moving Camera from Point Correspondences and Fundamental Matrices. Int. J. of Computer Vision. 22(3):261-289, 1997.
5. Stein, G. „Accurate Internal Camera Calibration Using Rotation, with Analysis of Sources of Error." Proc. 5th Int. Conf. On Computer Vision. Pp 230-236, 1995.
6. Hartley, R. I. „An Algorithm for Self Calibration from Several Views." Proc. IEEE Conf. On Computer Vision & Pattern Recognition. Pp. 908-912, Seattle, WA, 1994.
7. Wei, G.; Ma, S. „Implicit and Explicit Camera Calibration: Theory and Experiments." IEEE Trans. On Pattern Analysis and Machine Intelligence. 16(5):469-480, 1994.
8. Faugeras, O.; „Three-Dimensional Computer Vision: a Geometric Viewpoint." MIT press, 1993
9. Weng, J.; Cohen, P.; Herniou, M. „Camera Calibration with Distortion Models and Accuracy Evaluation." IEEE Trans. On Pattern Analysis & Machine Intelligence, 14(10):965-980. 1992.
10. Caprile, B.; Torre, B. „Using Vanishing Points for Camera Calibration." Int. J. of Computer Vision, 4, pp. 127-140, 1990
11. Gonzalez, R. C.; Wintz, P.; „Digital Image Processing." 2nd edition. 1987.
12. Tsai, R. Y. „A versatile camera calibration technique for high-accuracy 3D machine vision metrology using off-the-shelf TV cameras and lenses." IEEE Journal of Robotics and Automation, Vol. RA-3, No. 4, Aug. 1987.
13. Hartov, A.; Eisner, S. D.; Roberts, D. W.; Paulsen, K. D.; Platenik, L. A.; Miga, M. I. „Error analysis for a free-hand three-dimensional ultrasound system for neuronavigation." Neurosurgical Focus Vol 6, No. 3, article 5, 1999. Online publication: http://www.neurosurgery.org/focus/mar99/6-3-5.html

Trans-urethral Ultrasound: A New Tool for Diagnostic and Therapeutic Imaging in Prostate Cancer

David R. Holmes III [1], Brian J. Davis [2], Richard A. Robb [1]

[1] Biomedical Imaging Resource and [2] Division of Radiation Oncology
Mayo Foundation, Rochester, MN 55902

We have developed a new imaging method for use in diagnosis and treatment of prostate cancer. Our laboratory is the first to publish[1,2] this method that involves inserting into the urethra a special small diameter catheter with a phased array ultrasound imaging module on the tip which images the surrounding prostate gland in real time and three dimensions, capturing both anatomy and physiology. It is well tolerated by patients, as the imaging catheters are only 2 to 3 mm in diamter. Since there are nearly 200,000 new cases of prostate cancer diagnosed each year, improved methods for real-time, high-resolution 3D visualizations of the prostate are ever more important for accurate differential diagnosis and for staging optimal therapy.

Screening for prostate disease involves a digital rectal exam and a prostate specific antigen (PSA) test. If a patient tests positive, a tissue biopsy is collected and analyzed to classify and stage treatment of the disease. Depending on the characterization of the disease as benign or malignant, one or more treatment methods may be pursued. These include "watchful waiting", hormonal therapy, prostatectomy, radiation therapy (external beam or local brachytherapy), microwave ablation or cryotherapy. Imaging is an essential tool in each of these forms of treatment. However, diagnostic and therapeutic imaging of the prostate is challenging. The prostate gland is surrounded by the heavy pelvic girdle and lies medially among adjacent tissues and organs. Currently no imaging modality can distinguish diseased tissue from normal tissue in the prostate. Experimental diagnostic imaging techniques, such as elastography and color Doppler imaging have potential but require sophisticated image processing. Therapy guidance imaging includes intraoperative transrectal ultrasound (TRUS), x-ray fluoroscopy and/or pre- and post-operative CT or MRI. Each of these modalities has advantages and disadvantages. Transurethral ultrasound (TUUS) imaging has potential to deliver many of the desired advantages with few disadvantages.

Imaging from the urethra has the obvious benefit of imaging from the center of the prostate. The reduced anatomic coverage (as compared to TRUS) allows higher frequency ultrasound to be used and consequently high-resolution images to be obtained. Therefore, TUUS images provide clear delineation of the prostate capsule, excellent tissue differentiation, improved contrast between tissue and radioactive seeds, and improved visualization of small structures, such as microvessels. In addition, TUUS imaging is inexpensive, real-time and both 2D and 3D.

We have performed a number of preliminary experiments with TUUS imaging of the prostate. Comparisons between TUUS, TRUS and CT illustrated several favorable advantages of TUUS images. These were quantitatively demonstrated with a prostate

W. Niessen and M. Viergever (Eds.): MICCAI 2001, LNCS 2208, pp. 1243-1244, 2001.
© Springer-Verlag Berlin Heidelberg 2001

1244   D.R. Holmes III, B.J. Davis, and R.A. Robb

phantom. TUUS provided much higher differentiation between the prostate and surrounding tissues, more accurate measurement of prostate volume, and more accurate measurement of seeds planted in the phantom, as noted in Table 1.

Initial animal studies (canines) demonstrated the viability and utility of TUUS as a unique real-time 3D imaging tool. Excellent differentiation between the prostate, rectum, bladder and neurovascular bundle was obtained. Color flow Doppler imaging with TUUS demonstrated potential for assessment of angiogenesis. Preliminary patient studies have demonstrated usefulness of TUUS for intraoperative imaging. The resolution of TUUS images in patients is superior to that of both CT and TRUS, providing clear differentiation between the prostate and surrounding tissue. Localization of implanted seeds in brachytherapy procedures was superior in TUUS compared to TRUS. TUUS was better than CT in determining total prostate volume. Figure 1 illustrates how TUUS images may be used in a brachytherapy application.

Table 1

Imaging Modality	Voxel size (mm)	Seed Size Measured (True: 0 .8 x 4.5 mm)
TRUS	.2 x .2 x 5	1.2 mm x 7.5 mm
CT	.35 x .35 x 3	2.1 mm x 8.4 mm
TUUS	.1 x .1 x .1	.63 mm x 4.4 mm

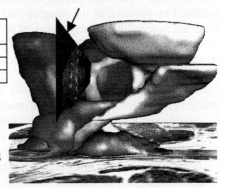

Figure 1: Real-time TUUS image (arrow) fused with 3D model segmented from MRI scan. Note clear delineation of radioactive seeds in TUUS image (2-D sector scan).

As a therapeutic tool, TUUS imaging has already been used in our institution during local brachytherapy procedures. Future TUUS devices will help to provide intraoperative feedback to the clinician during placement of radioactive seeds into the patient. Other treatments that might benefit from intraoperative TUUS include microwave therapy and cryoablation by monitoring the temperature of the prostate tissue during the procedure.

In conclusion, TUUS imaging has the potential to dramatically improve reliable detection and treatment of prostatic disease. It provides high-resolution, real-time 2D and 3D images for intra-operative applications, such as local brachytherapy. Utilizing ultrasound elastographic techniques with TUUS may provide a stiffness measure of the prostate. Doppler imaging with TUUS can help assess angiogenesis in the prostate. Further validation needs to be carried out, but preliminary results are very promising. Additional development will help provide systems and protocols for TUUS imaging in a variety of diagnostic and therapeutic scenarios.

1. Holmes DR and Robb RA. Trans-Urethral Ultrasound (TUUS) Imaging for Visualization and Analysis of the Prostate and Associated Tissues. Proc. Medicine Meets Virtual Reality. 70:126-132, 2000.

2. Holmes DR and Robb RA. 3-D Trans-urethral Ultrasound: a New View of the Prostate Gland. Computer Aided Radiology and Surgery, 2000.

Resection of Recurrent Carcinomas in the Pelvis - A New Field of Computer Aided Surgery

J. Geerling[1], T. Hüfner[1], R. Raab[3], M. Citak[1], T. Pohlemann[4], H. Rosenthal[2], C. Krettek[1]

[1] Trauma Dept., Hannover Medical School, Carl-Neuberg-Str. 1, D-30625 Hannover
jens.geerling@planet-interkom.de
[2] Radiology Dept., [3] Dept. of Surgery, Hannover Medical School, D-30625 Hannover
[4] Trauma Department, University of Saarland, 66421 Homburg, Germany

Abstract. Recurrent carcinomas may infiltrate the bony pelvis. If infiltrating the sacrum it is difficult to resect the tumor cause of the nerve roots that may be damaged during the operation.

In this study three cases of recurrent carcinomas infiltrating the sacrum are presented. All were resected using a navigation system (Surgigate, Medivision, Oberdorf, Switzerland). With this system it was possible to detect the tumor margins on the monitor screen and to perform a resection outside the margins of the tumor using navigated chissels.

Further developments such as CT and MRI fusion may help to improve such surgical procedures and may allow extend indications for computer aided surgery also in tumor cases.

1 Objective

The bony pelvis, especially the sacrum can be infiltrated by recurrent carcinomas of the rectum or the genitourinary system. The danger of a wide resection with an increased rate of nerval complications may be implyed by scar tissues from previous operations or radiation. Computer assisted surgery (CAS) could be a solution to increase the accuracy of tumor resections. Currently, navigation systems use the precise Computed tomography data allowing procedures like navigated pedicle screw applications, cup placement in hip arthroplasty and other procedures [1,2].

Navigated chisels or drilling machines may allow to extend the indications for CAS besides the commercially available applications. This study reports on CAS supported resection of recurrent carcinomas within the pelvis in three patients.

2 Methods

The CAS system Surgigate®, Module "Spine" was used with navigated chissels from the PAO-Module (Medivision, Oberdorf, Switzerland) in all cases because no specific application are available to support the resection of tumors.

Patient 1. A 37 y old male with a recurrent chondrosarcoma located presacral on the left side of S 2 (Fig. 1). Because the recurrent tumor was small and located next to the sacral cortex a tumor resection including the anterior cortex of S2 preserving the nerval roots of S2 were performed.

W. Niessen and M. Viergever (Eds.): MICCAI 2001, LNCS 2208, pp. 1245-1247, 2001.

For registration four titanium K-wires placed into the iliac chrest in local anesthesia and the most convex part of the promontorium were used as landmarks.

The operation was done in supine position using a median distal laparotomy with a transperitoneal approach. The DRB was placed on the left iliac crest. The tumor was localized according to the MRI presacral on the left side in height of S 2 with the navigated pointer, the ventral cortex of the sacrum was osteotomized preserving the sacral channel with the navigated chisel (Fig. 2) and the tumor could be removed in one block.

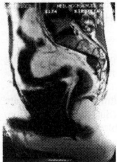
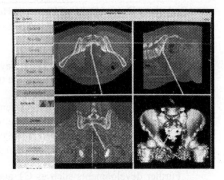

Fig. 1: The MRI showing the chondrosarcoma directly in front of the sacrum.

Fig. 2: Screenshot during the navigated resection of the chondrosarcoma.

Patient 2. A 52 y old female with a recurrent chordoma of the sacrum. CT scans showed an infiltration of the sacrum up to S2 bilateral and an infiltration of the left SI-joint (Fig. 3). The operation was done in prone position. After preparation of the soft tissues the DRB was attached to the sacral body, registration was done using anatomical landmarks for paired point registration: the processus spinosus of S 1 and S 2, the processus transversus bilateral of S1. Surface matching was done using the bony surface of the destructed sacrum. The operation was done using navigated chisels (Fig. 4). The sacrum was removed partially on the levels S1 and S2 including the nerval roots, furthermore the left SI-joint was removed.

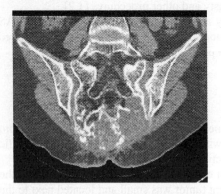
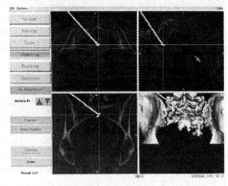

Fig. 3: A CT reformation of the recurrent chordoma showing the infiltration of the sacrum.

Fig. 4: The monitor view during the navigated procedure showing the navigated chissel (green) while resecting the tumor.

Patient 3. A 39 y old female with a recurrent cervix carcinoma infiltrating the body S 1 on the left side (Fig. 5). An exenteration operation with a partial resection of the sacrum was done. Preoperatively 2 titanium pins (1.6 mm diameter) were inserted on the iliac crest bilaterally and a CT was obtained. The operation was done in 3 steps:
1. The patient in prone position doing a CAS supported lumbosacral stabilization to prevent an instability of the posterior pelvic ring due to the partial resection of the sacrum. CAS was used for the placement of the pedicle and the iliac screws. Additionally a hemilaminectomy of S 1 and S 2 and a posterior dissection of the sacroiliac ligaments was performed conventionally.
2. The patient was turned in supine position. The rectum and both ureters were mobilized. The tumor was infiltrating the left common iliac vein and the left obturator nerve, furthermore the left roots of L5 and S 1. The DRB was attached to the left iliac crest after dissection of the vessels and partial replacement with Gore-Tex was done. Paired point registration was done using the fiducials, the SIAS bilateral and the convexity of the promontorium, surface registration on both iliac bones. With navigated chisels an osteotomy of L5 and S 1 paramedian on the right side was performed (Fig. 6). The infiltrated S 1 was identified on the screen and the left S 2 body was resected as well. The tumor could be removed en bloc.
3. A corticospongous bone transplant of the left iliac crest was done for stabilization and the defect between L5 and the left ilium was covered. A Wolter plate was placed additionally for stabilization and the patient was mobilized with full weight bearing.

3 Discussion and Conclusion

Although existing navigation systems support specific steps as pedicle screw placement in the field of orthopaedic surgery, the provided tools allow an extension of indications.
Our experience is limited to three patients, yet, however we found the identification and the resection in critical regions like those close to the sacrum can be done with a high accuracy, if CAS supported. Further developments as CT- and MRI fusion or an intraoperative integration of imaging techniques like ultrasound could lead to improved results and a more extended spectrum of indications.

References

1. Langlotz U, Langlotz F, Hiogne D, et al. *A Novel System for Complete THR Planning and Intraoperative Free-Hand Navigation.* in *CAOS Computer Assisted Orthopaedic Surgery.* 2000. Davos, Switzerland.
2. Lavallee, S, P Sautot, J Troccaz, et al.: *Computer-assisted spine surgery: A technique for accurate transpedicular screw fixation using CT data and a 3-D optical localizer.* J Image Guid Surg, 1(1): 65-73,1995.

Remote Analysis for Brain Shift Compensation

P. Hastreiter[1], K. Engel[2], G. Soza[3], M. Bauer[3], M. Wolf[4], O. Ganslandt[1],
R. Fahlbusch[1], G. Greiner[3], T. Ertl[2], Ch. Nimsky[1]

[1] Neurocenter, Dept. of Neurosurgery, University of Erlangen-Nuremberg, Germany
hastreiter@nch.imed.uni-erlangen.de
[2] Visualization and Interactive Systems Group, University of Stuttgart, Germany
[3] Computer Graphics Group, University of Erlangen-Nuremberg, Germany
[4] Knowledge Processing Group, Bavarian Research Center for Knowledge-Based Systems

Abstract. The compensation for brain shift is assisted by intraoperative imaging. For the purpose of fast registration and interactive visualization, a framework is presented based on local desktop computers and remote high-end computers with a maximum of compute power and graphics capacity. In this context, functional markers resulting from preoperative measurements (MEG, fMRI) are mapped to the intraoperative situation. Overall, results from 5 cases demonstrate the value of the suggested environment.

Keywords: Brain Shift, Registration, Visualization

Introduction Preoperative planning and navigation in neurosurgery are assisted by information from different imaging modalities. As a drawback, preoperative data invalidates during surgery due to the brain shift phenomenon. Therefore, intraoperative imaging is applied for compensation providing anatomical data. However, functional information resulting form magnetoencephalography *(MEG)* or functional MRI *(fMRI)* is exclusively based on preoperative imaging [1]. Therefore, alternative approaches try to predict the occurring deformation or calculate the transformation based on pre- and intraoperative anatomical images. These approaches are based on mathematical models using registration or simulations strategies.

Methods The framework of the presented work aiming at the compensation for brain shift is based on an environment introduced in [2] allowing for access maximal compute power and graphics capacity. For the rigid registration of pre- and intraoperative MR data a hardware accelerated approach suggested in [3] was integrated operating on the remote graphics server. It is based on mutual information and applies 3D texture mapping hardware for all interpolation operations. The subsequent analysis of the image data has been performed with 3D texture mapping on the remote computer applying direct volume rendering which is interactively controlled on the local computer. For the comparative analysis of pre- and intraoperative data synchronized 3D representations are used applying communicating Java viewers. For the transformation of markers indicating functional areas, the brain volume is segmented in the registered datasets using a volume growing strategy. Then, a newly developed approach automatically detects and evaluates corresponding sulci within the registered data. This reference information is consecutively applied to determine the position of preoperatively obtained functional markers within the intraoperative image data. As a result the obtained image data can then be used for an intraoperative functional update of the neuronavigation system.

W. Niessen and M. Viergever (Eds.): MICCAI 2001, LNCS 2208, pp. 1248–1249, 2001.

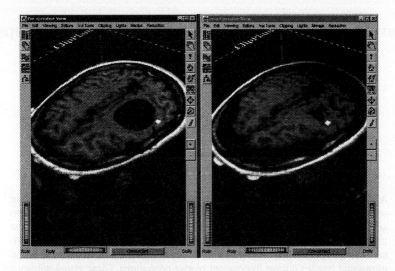

Fig. 1. Communication windows on local client computer: The synchronized 3D representations show preoperative MR *(left)* with a marker from MEG (white square) and intraoperative MR *(right)* including the correct intraoperative location of the MEG marker after transfer.

Results The presented prototype framework was applied in 5 cases with functional markers identifying eloquent brain areas. For an example see Fig. 1. All computation was remotely performed with a SGI Octane ($2 \times$R12000, 300MHz) with 128 Mbytes of graphics memory. The client was located at the operating room providing only low-end graphics capabilities. The connection to the remote server was established via Internet with a communication rate of 10 Mbits/sec. For the visualization a view-port of 600x600 pixels led to a frame rate of 3 fps which is increased to 9 fps reducing the size of the transferred images by a factor of 4. Considering the voxel based registration (about 45 sec) and the mapping of the functional markers an overall processing time of about 10 min was achieved including the transfer of the data to the remote computer. The reduction by a factor of 3.5 compared to a purely local setup enables intraoperative application of the presented approach.

Acknowledgment: This project was partly funded by the Deutsche Forschungsgemeinschaft (DFG) in the context of the project Gr 796/2-1.

References

1. C. Nimsky, O. Ganslandt, H. Kober, M. Möller, S. Ulmer, B. Tomandl, and R. Fahlbusch. Integration of Functional Magnetic Resonance Imaging Supported by Magnetoencephalography in Functional Neuronavigation. *Neurosurgery*, 44:1249–1256, 1999.
2. K. Engel, O. Sommer, and T. Ertl. A Framework for Interactive Hardware Accelerated Remote 3D-Visualization. In *Proc. VisSym*, pages 167–177. Joint Eurographics - IEEE TCVG Symposium on Visualization, 2000.
3. P. Hastreiter and T. Ertl. Integrated Registration and Visualization of Medical Image Data. In *Proc. CGI*, pages 78–85, Hannover, Germany, 1998.

Development of a New Image-Guided Prostate Biopsy System

Jianchao Zeng[1], Ariela Sofer[2], and Seong K. Mun[1]

[1] ISIS Center, Department of Radiology
Georgetown University Medical Center, Washington, DC, USA
zeng@georgetown.edu, http://www.simulation.georgetown.edu
[2] Department of Systems Engineering and Operations Research
George Mason University, Fairfax, VA, USA

Abstract. This paper presents a new image-guided prostate biopsy system under development. The system features a 3-D prostate cancer distribution atlas and new biopsy protocols optimized based on the cancer atlas using a nonlinear integer programming approach. Both the cancer atlas and the optimal protocols are being dynamically registered and superimposed onto the trans-rectal ultrasound images during live-patient biopsy procedures. Clear visual guidance will be provided to the physicians by color-coded spots on top of the ultrasound images, which represent best possible targets for biopsy. Clinical test will be performed to evaluate the system.

1 Introduction

Prostate cancer is usually detected clinically using trans-rectal ultrasound (TRUS) guided needle biopsy. Current ultrasound imaging systems, however, cannot provide enough information to the physicians for the best possible outcome of cancer detection. In this work, we are developing a new image-guided prostate biopsy system for significant improvement of prostate cancer detection.

2 System Development

2.1 Overview of the System

The system configuration is shown in Fig. 1. Built on top of the current TRUS imaging system, the new system will be likely to significantly improve the performance of cancer detection through the introduction of the following new features:

a. *A 3-D atlas of prostate cancer distribution.* The 3-D prostate cancer distribution atlas was developed by first reconstructing over 300 individual 3-D prostate models from real specimens with clinically localized cancers [1]; then dividing each individual prostate model into tiny fine zones, and checking cancer presence in each fine zone for all the models [2].

b. *Optimized biopsy protocols.* Optimal biopsy protocols were developed by making use of the 3-D prostate cancer distribution atlas and a physician needle insertion model [3]. A nonlinear integer program was used to determine optimal biopsy protocols on a 48-zone division of the prostate. For the same number of biopsy needles, these protocols have substantially higher detection rates than the protocols currently used by physicians.

W. Niessen and M. Viergever (Eds.): MICCAI 2001, LNCS 2208, pp. 1250-1252, 2001.

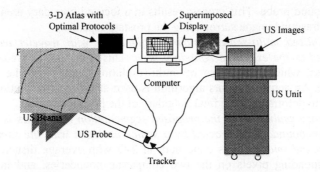

Fig. 1. Image-guided prostate biopsy system with 3-D cancer distribution atlas

c. *Dynamic registration of the 3-D atlas and optimal protocols with ultrasound images.* In order to dynamically register the 3-D cancer distribution atlas with highlighted optimal protocols onto the ultrasound images during the needle core biopsy, we attach a small tracking device Polhemus 3SPACE FASTRAK to the ultrasound probe to track its position and motion during biopsy. Since the developed 3-D cancer atlas is embedded in a bounding box with a number of grids, which represent the corresponding zones in the prostate gland, the registration process can be conveniently converted to the task of finding the bounding box of the individual prostate of the patient based on the ultrasound images, and aligning the two bounding boxes together in real-time.

2.2   Segmentation of the Ultrasound Images

In order to calculate the bounding box of the patient's prostate, we are developing an image segmentation technique to acquire the boundary of a series of transverse ultrasound images (with a few mms interval each) of the prostate. The series of transverse prostate boundaries are used to reconstruct a 3-D prostate surface model of the patient under biopsy procedure. The intersection of the ultrasound beam with the reconstructed 3-D model enables us to extract the corresponding cancer distribution information and optimized biopsy protocols from the cancer distribution atlas, and to superimpose the information on the ultrasound image as color-coded or highlighted grids.

a. *Acquisition of texture statistics around the boundary of prostate capsule using a large set of transverse ultrasound image samples.* For each sample image, we characterize intensity distribution around the prostate boundary. Different scales of neighborhoods of a number of selected boundary points are used to obtain simple local and regional texture information such as mean and standard deviation with Gabor filter. More texture features will also be evaluated for their applicability to the prostate ultrasound images using Gray Level Co-occurrence Matrices.

b. *Boundary area extraction of the individual prostate ultrasound image with texture matching.* The texture matching is guided by prior knowledge of the prostate anatomy and relative position between the prostate and the ultrasound probe. This process results in a focused boundary area (a belt) of the ultrasound image surrounding the prostate capsule.

c. *A localized multi-scale contouring algorithm with wavelet transform is applied to the extracted boundary area.* This algorithm is a coarse-to-fine process, which makes use of multi-resolution features of the ultrasound image. An active contours algorithm is used at different resolution levels in order to deform onto the final boundary of the prostate capsule.

d. *Accuracy evaluation of the proposed segmentation techniques is performed against boundaries extracted by a senior urologist with the same prostate ultrasound images.* It is done both in 2-D with average distance between corresponding pixels on the two comparing boundaries, and in 3-D with volume difference between the two corresponding surface models reconstructed from the boundaries of prostate ultrasound images of the same patient. Refinement of the algorithms is to be performed to the steps a through c until the accuracy reaches a satisfactory level.

3   Summary

A new image-guided prostate biopsy system is now being developed. By using this system, the physicians will be able to make use of a global road map of the patient's prostate (the 3-D overlay display) and/or a 2-D ultrasound image display overlaid with a guidance grid color-coded with the optimized protocols. This combination of both 2-D and 3-D information will significantly enhance the physicians' situation awareness and thus lead to a substantial improved performance of cancer detection.

Acknowledgements

This research was supported in part by The Biomedical Engineering Research Grant RG-99-0115 of The Whitaker Foundation. Ariela Sofer was supported in part by NSF grant DMI-9800544. We thank Dinggang Shen for his valuable comments.

References

1. Zeng, J., Kaplan, C., Bauer, J., Sesterhenn, I., Moul, J. And Mun, S. K.: Visualization and evaluation of prostate needle biopsy. Proceedings of the Medical Image Computing and Computer Assisted Intervention Conference (1998) 285-292
2. Zeng, J., Bauer, J., Sofer, A., Yao, X., Opell, B., Zhang, W., Sestrehenn, I. A., Moul, J. W., Lynch, J., Mun, S. K.: Distribution of Prostate Cancer for Optimized Biopsy Protocols. Proceedings of the Medical Image Computing and Computer Assisted Intervention Conference (2000) 287-296
3. Sofer, A., Zeng, J., Opell, B., Bauer, J., Mun, S.K.: Optimal Biopsy Protocols for Prostate Cancer. In revision for publication in Interfaces (2001)

Intraoperative Tracking of Anatomical Structures Using Fluoroscopy and a Vascular Balloon Catheter

Michael Rosenthal[1], Susan Weeks[2], Stephen Aylward[1],
Elizabeth Bullitt[3], and Henry Fuchs[1]

University of North Carolina at Chapel Hill
[1]Department of Computer Science, CB 3175, [2]Department of Radiology, CB 7510,
[3]Department of Neurosurgery, CB 7060,
Chapel Hill, NC 27599 USA

Abstract. We present preliminary work on a novel technique for tracking anatomical structures during medical procedures. A vascular balloon catheter is placed within a vessel in the structure of interest and is inflated using a radio-opaque contrast material. The balloon catheter is tracked over time using a fluoroscopy system, and three parameters of motion are determined (two of translation, one of rotation) for each view via analysis of the balloon image. These methods are applied to three patient data sets to estimate liver motion during a respiratory cycle.

1 Introduction

We propose the use of a stable intravascular fiducial, in the form of a contrast-filled balloon catheter, to track the motion of soft tissue structures during image-guided procedures. This fiducial produces a consistent image and can be tracked through a series of frames. The fiducial can also be used to correlate images or other data from different stages of a procedure, such as pre-intervention angiography. We have analyzed three series of abdominal patient images containing such fiducials and report the results below.

2 Materials and Methods

Image Acquisition. The images for this study were acquired at North Carolina Memorial Hospital (Chapel Hill, North Carolina, USA) using a Siemens Neurostar biplane fluoroscopy suite. Dr. Weeks captured the images as part of two TIPS procedures in two different patients. A balloon catheter (Meditech Occlusion Balloon, Boston Scientific) was placed in each patient's hepatic vein in the liver as part of the customary procedure for imaging the portal vein. The balloon catheter was inflated using iodinated contrast and a series of fluoroscopic images was captured over a full respiratory cycle. The Institutional Review Board for the School of Medicine has approved the use of these images for research purposes.

W. Niessen and M. Viergever (Eds.): MICCAI 2001, LNCS 2208, pp. 1253-1254, 2001.

Image Analysis. Simple thresholding is performed to create a binary map of the radio-opaque objects in the scene. Connected components analysis is then used to label each distinct region in the binary image. Each region is analyzed to determine its centroid, area, major and minor axis lengths for the best-fitting ellipse, and angular displacement of the major axis relative to the x-axis. The selection of the correct balloon region is performed using a weighted least-squares approach on position and area. Estimated parameters are provided for the first image in the series, while the remaining iterations use the results from the previous step as parameter estimates.

3 Results

The three series of images were analyzed to determine the 2D position, balloon orientation, major and minor axis lengths for the best-fitting ellipse, and the balloon area for each frame. All results are given in Table 1. Image scale varies by series.

Table 1. Results from analysis of fiducial balloon in three series of fluoroscopic images

Results given as mean ± standard deviation	Series Liv01 (n=21)	Series Liv02 (n=11)	Series Liv03 (n=11)
Balloon area (pixels^2)	932.3 ± 33.2	1580.6 ± 36.5	3173.3 ± 75.6
Major axis length (pixels)	44.49 ± 0.74	59.83 ± 0.99	92.08 ± 1.33
Minor axis length (pixels)	28.65 ± 0.46	36.04 ± 0.39	46.23 ± 0.77
Orientation (degrees)	22.27 ± 1.53	24.36 ± 0.67	15.71 ± 0.46
Craniocaudal position (pixels)	636.5 ± 16.0	567.7 ± 8.9	606.0 ± 13.9
Transverse position (pixels)	132.4 ± 2.8	325.6 ± 3.6	324.3 ± 3.8

4 Conclusions

The small variances of the axes lengths and area measures suggest that our methods yield stable estimates of the balloon parameters. As expected, the liver showed very little rotation over the image sequences. The dominant motion was craniocaudal translation, which is consistent with the motion of the attached respiratory diaphragm. These preliminary results suggest that our proposed methods can yield reasonable measurements of the orientation and position of a contrast-filled balloon catheter placed in the liver. Additional studies will be needed to determine the accuracy and precision of these methods across a spectrum of patients and imaging circumstances.

We plan to perform several new studies in the coming months to improve the characterization of our methods. First, we will measure the intrinsic uncertainty of our methods by imaging our fiducial on a precision motion stage and comparing our calculated trajectories to the actual trajectories on the stage. We will then extend our methods to 3D tracking from biplane views and test them using fluoroscopic images from a diverse set of patients. Finally, we plan to investigate the use of Kalman filtering to predict balloon motion and reduce our search space within each image.

Clinical Use of a Mutual Information-Based Automated Image Registration System for Conformal Radiotherapy Treatment Planning

Marc Kessler, PhD[1], Janelle Solock[1], Paul Archer[1], and Charles Meyer, PhD[2]

Department of [1]Radiation Oncology and [2]Radiology
The University of Michigan Medical School, Ann Arbor, Michigan, USA 48109
{MKessler, Jsolack, PGArcher, CMeyer}@umich.edu

Abstract. In this paper we describe the clinical use of an in-house mutual information-based image registration system for improving target volume definition in conformal radiotherapy treatment planning. This system enables a clinician to delineate clinical and anatomic structures on magnetic resonance and nuclear medicine imaging studies and have these structures geometrically mapped to the x-ray CT study used for treatment planning. This system requires very little user interaction and can accommodate a wide range of anatomic sites. These factors combined with consistent accuracy at the sub-voxel to voxel level have improved the overall quality and physician confidence in the delineation of target volumes and surrounding healthy tissues.

1 Introduction

In conformal radiation therapy, accurate delineation of the target volume and surrounding healthy tissues is essential. Modern treatment machines are now capable of delivering highly shaped doses of radiation to a prescribed region while minimizing doses to adjacent tissues. Although x-ray CT is still the primary modality for planning these radiation treatments, other modalities such as magnetic resonance imaging and nuclear medicine studies can provide important data for improving target volume localization. While the practice of incorporating information from multiple modalities into the treatment planning process is by no means new and while most commercial treatment planning systems now offer tools to support this, routine clinical use of these tools is still limited to a few anatomic sites and imaging situations. Requirements placed on the input image data extent, amount of pre-processing involved and the lack of appropriate geometric transforms have confounded broader use of these tools. In order to exploit a wider range of anatomic and functional imaging studies for radiotherapy treatment planning, we have implemented a mutual information-based image registration system. This system requires very little user interaction, is robust to limited and missing data and supports both affine and thin-plate spline geometric transformations [1]. The details of this system and the underlying algorithms are reported elsewhere [2]. In this paper we demonstrate the use of this system using two clinical examples.

W. Niessen and M. Viergever (Eds.): MICCAI 2001, LNCS 2208, pp. 1255-1257, 2001.

2   Clinical Examples

Two clinical cases are described to illustrate the use of the registration system for radiotherapy treatment planning.   One case involves a benign menengioma that enhances well on MR but is difficult to delineate on the treatment planning CT.   The other case involves the use of functional image data from PET to help resolve uncertainties in a CT-based lung tumor target volume.

2.1   MR – CT Case

This case involves the registration of a diagnostic MR with a planning CT for a patient with a benign meningioma located near the base of the skull (Fig. 1). As is often the case, the orientation of the patient's head in the two imaging studies was different.   As is often the case, the patient was imaged wearing a custom-made immobilization mask during the CT procedure but not during the MR because of the space constraints of the head coil.   Although the MR data adequately covered the involved region it did not include the entire cranium. While this situation might have limited the accuracy of a surface-based registration, the MI-based registration behaved properly and was judged to be accurate to within one pixel (1mm).   In addition to the value of the *both* the axial and coronal MR data for delineating the target volume, the coronal MR was essential for accurate localization of the optic nerves and chiasm.

2.2   PET – CT Case

This case involves a large tumor in the upper portion of the right lung (Fig. 2). Using only the CT data, the clinician defined the target volume.   The clinician expressed uncertainty about the detailed extent of parts of the tumor, especially in regions containing CT streak artifacts caused by nearby bones. PET data was acquired to help resolve these uncertainties. A PET-only target volume was delineated and mapped to the CT dataset using a transformation computed using mutual information. A comparison of these volumes is shown in Figure 2. The PET defined target volume not only helped to clarify the superior shape of the tumor (Fig 2-B) but also revealed a portion of the tumor missed in the CT-only target volume (Fig 2-A).

3   Summary

A mutual information-based automatic multimodality image registration system has implemented and applied across a broad spectrum of volumetric data sets of various modalities and anatomies. A practical advantage of this system is the minimal user interaction and data pre-processing required. The major strength, however, is the robustness of the mutual information-based registration metric to sparse or missing data and the ability to register anatomic data with functional data where the precise locations of anatomic features are often difficult to define. These benefits, combined with option of using geometric warping in addition to affine transformations to model certain tissue deformation and machine distortions greatly expands the range of imaging studies that the clinical can quantitatively use to improve the accuracy of target volume and normal tissue delineation for radiotherapy treatment planning.

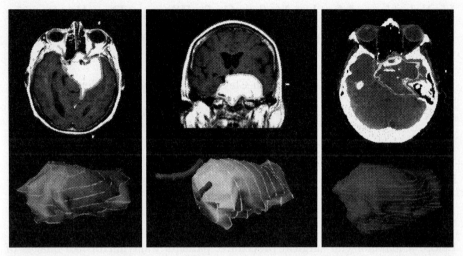

Fig 1. Delineation of target volume and normal tissues using axial (left) and coronal (center) MR imaging series. For this case, the CT target volume (right) was constructed from the logical combination of the mapped structures from the coronal and axial MR data.

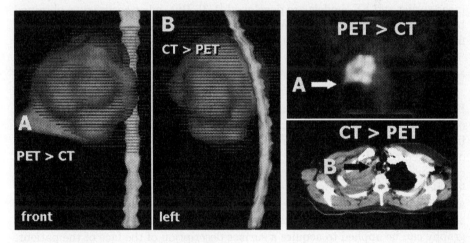

Fig 2. Target volume definition from CT only (contours) and PET only (surface). The long vertical structure is the CT-based spinal cord.

References

1. Bookstein F L 1991. Morphometric tools for landmark data: geometry and biology. Cambridge Univ. Press: New York. 435 pp.

2. Meyer C R, Boes JL, Kim B, Bland B H, et al. 1997, Demonstration of accuracy and clinical versatility of mutual information for automatic multimodality image fusion using affine and thin plate spline warped geometric deformations. *Medical Image Analysis* **1**(3):195-206.

Validation Methods for Soft Tissue Prediction in Maxillofacial Planning Environments

Filip Schutyser, Johan Van Cleynenbreugel, and Paul Suetens

Medical Image Computing (Radiology - ESAT/PSI), Faculties of Medicine and
Engineering, UZ Gasthuisberg, Herestraat 49, B-3000 Leuven, Belgium
Filip.Schutyser@uz.kuleuven.ac.be

Keywords   Soft tissue modelling, maxillofacial surgery simulation

1   Introduction

Before a maxillofacial surgical procedure, patients want mirror-like images of
the probable outcome. Important research activities try to predict 3D soft tissue changes based on the skeletal changes. Major attention was paid on the
biomechanical properties of soft tissues at a certain time instance. (Non-)linear
mass-spring and FE models are developed [1-3]. But, what accuracy is obtained
by a current soft tissue model? What improvements are needed? Some validation
methods for soft tissue deformation prediction are investigated.

2   Methods

From preop CT imaging, a surface description of the face and the skeleton is
obtained. With planning software [4-5], new positions of bone fragments, defining the boundary conditions for soft tissue simulation, are determined. Based
on segmented CT images, a tetrahedral mesh of the soft tissues is automatically constructed. As a simplification, all facial soft tissues are assumed to be
identical linear elastic isotropic materials. With FEM, the constitutive equations
are solved [5]. From the deformed volumetric mesh, predictions of the new skin
surface and the postop CT are derived. After surgery, three dimensional photography can be applied to acquire a surface description of the face of the patient.
Or, from postop CT, the skin surface can easily be extracted. We compare post-
operative outcome and preoperative prediction in two ways.
Surface based validation This validation method compares predicted and
postop skin surfaces. After surface-to-surface registration (ICP, error is a combination of euclidean distance and differences between normals), color-coding
visualises the distances between the surfaces. If the registration fails, matching
based on user-indicated points is a fall-back option.
Volumetric validation This validation method compares predicted and postop
CT volumes. If an unaltered region can be defined in the pre- and postop image
data sets, rigid registration can be applied. The postop data set is resampled
over the grid of the preop dataset (= same grid as predicted CT). The postop
CT and predicted outcome are compared.

W. Niessen and M. Viergever (Eds.): MICCAI 2001, LNCS 2208, pp. 1258–1260, 2001.
© Springer-Verlag Berlin Heidelberg 2001

3   Discussion and Conclusion

As a case study, a hemifacial microsomia patient treated with mandibular unilateral distraction osteogenesis is presented. After preop CT, the optimal surgical procedure is selected with our planning environment [4-5] and the soft tissue deformations were predicted. 64 days after removal of the distractor, the patient was CT-scanned.

Surface based validation (fig 1:a-b). Errors resulting from registration and from prediction can not be separated. A matching algorithm tries to minimise the distance between surfaces. Large soft tissue modelling errors at e.g. the chin can be reduced by the matching algorithm and may result in e.g. a shift of the tip of the nose. But, the same result can be explained as follows: the chin is well-predicted by the simulation, but there is an prediction error at the nose. The surface-based validation method comes up with an average error. Improving the soft tissue model based on these results is very hard.

Volumetric validation (fig 1:c-e). The accuracy of the registration is evaluated on the bony parts. With a good match of postop and planned skull, soft tissues should be the same. For this case, we notice accuracy differences at the left and right side of the patient. Whereas the fit at the left side of the patient is satisfactory, large errors are seen at the right side. With volumetric validation, sources of errors are localised and modelling failures are identified.

Conclusion Surface-based validation, gives a qualitative image of the average error. Localizing sources of error remains difficult. With volumetric validation, identifying sources of error can be done in more detail.

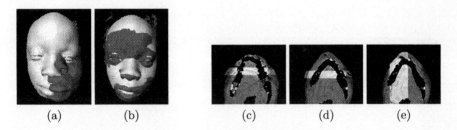

(a)   (b)   (c)   (d)   (e)

Fig. 1. (a-b) *Surface based validation.* The predicted (dark) and postop (bright) skin surfaces are depicted before (a) and after (b) surface based registration. (c-e) *Volumetric validation.* Slices (only soft tissues) from the predicted CT and parts of the registered postop CT in overlay windows (bright parts), are shown.

Acknowledgments
Thanks to Dr. P.A. Diner (Hôpital d'Enfants Armand-Trousseau, Paris, France) for the CT-datasets. The work discussed here belongs, partly to the EU-funded Brite Euram III PISA project, and to a grant for research specialization from the Flemish Institute for stimulation of the scientific-technological research in the industry (IWT) to Filip Schutyser.

References

1. M. Teschner, S. Girod, B. Girod: Optimization Approaches for Soft-Tissue Prediction in Craniofacial Surgery Simulation. MICCAI'99, p. 1183–1190, September 19-22, 1999
2. R.M. Koch, M.H. Gross, F.R. Carls, D.F. von Büren, G. Fankhauser, Y. Parish: Simulating Facial Surgery Using Finite Element Methods. SIGGRAPH 96 Conf. Proc., 1996, p. 421–428
3. S. Zachow, E. Gladiline, H.-C. Hege, P. Deuflhard: Finite-Element Simulation of Soft Tissue Deformation. Proc. CARS 2000, p. 899–904, June 28 - July 1, 2000, San Francisco, USA
4. F. Schutyser, J. Van Cleynenbreugel, N. Nadjmi, J. Schoenaers, P. Suetens: 3D image-based planning for unilateral mandibular distraction. Proc. CARS 2000, p. 899–904, June 28 - July 1 2000, San Francisco, USA
5. F. Schutyser, J. Van Cleynenbreugel, M. Ferrant, J. Schoenaers, P. Suetens: Image-based 3D planning of maxillofacial distraction procedures including soft tissue implications. MICCAI2000, pp. 999-1007, October 11-14, 2000, Pittsburgh, Pennsylvania, USA

Dental Implant Planning in EasyVision

Steven Lobregt, Ted Vuurberg and Joost J. Schillings

Philips Medical Systems Nederland B.V.,
Advanced Development EasyVision Modules,
P.O.Box 10.000, 5680 DA Best, The Netherlands
steven.lobregt@philips.com

Introduction

This work is part of the EC funded PISA project which aims at the development of tools for design and manufacturing of Personalized Implants and Surgical Aids. Sub-optimal implant positioning is a major reason for implant failure and (too) early revision. Although planning is possible to various extends on currently available systems, there is in general no means to transfer the planning to the patient. The PISA project covers the transfer to the patient as well as the planning. Within this project, PMS focused on dental implant planning and design of appropriate drill guides to transfer the planning to the patient. A prototype application was developed on our EasyVision clinical workstation, which includes the following steps:

Segmentation

Various semi-automatic tools are available to obtain a desired segmentation result including thresholding, region growing and watershed separation. If required, the result of these semi-automatic tools can be manually edited and refined in a user friendly and interactive way. Editing can be performed in 2D as well as in 3D.

Curved Path Definition

The first step is to define a suitable cross-sectional plane through the dataset, such that the relevant part of the mandible or maxilla is clearly visible (see figure 1). This base plane can have any orientation with respect to the original slices. Next, a smooth polybezier path, which passes approximately through the center of the bone, is created by a few mouse clicks. This results in the generation of a panoramic view on a curved plane through the created path and perpendicular to the selected base plane, as well as a number of cross-sections perpendicular to this base plane and also locally perpendicular to the curved panoramic plane.

Nerve Canal Modeling and Implant Positioning

If required, the lower alveolar nerve canal in the mandibula can be modeled and visualized, which is helpful to keep implants at a save distance from this nerve canal. Implants can be selected from a list of available models, for instance provided by a preferred supplier. An implant model is placed in initial position by a single mouse

W. Niessen and M. Viergever (Eds.): MICCAI 2001, LNCS 2208, pp. 1261-1262, 2001.
© Springer-Verlag Berlin Heidelberg 2001

click and can be manipulated to optimize the position. The various images give direct feedback to the user by showing cross-sections of CT data and implants, as well as 3D renderings of anatomy with implants (figure 1).

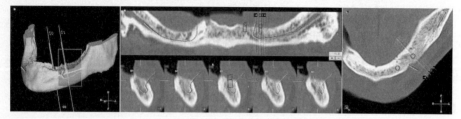

Fig. 1. The UI shows all relevant information: cross-sections of the implant models are shown together with Hounsfield values, 3D renderings and modeled mandibular nerve.

Drill Guide Generation and Interface to Manufacturer

When the implants are positioned optimally with respect to the anatomy and to each other, a drill guide can be generated (figure 2). This is an automatic procedure, which generates a complete CAD compatible description of a suitable drill guide shape, based on the planned positions and sizes of implants and an area of contact between bone and drill guide. The drill guide shape can be exported in STL format to any manufacturer.

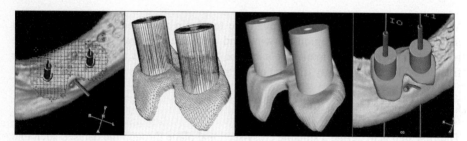

Fig. 2. From left to right: User-modifiable contact area, triangulated surface of automatically generated drill guide shape, same but shaded display, simulation of drill guide shape fitted on mandibula for inspection before manufacturing.

Conclusion

We have developed a prototype application for planning of dental implant placement, which can serve as a basis for surgical planning in a more general sense. The software was fully integrated in the EasyVision clinical workstation environment. Many of the tools, which were developed as part of this work, can be applied in a broader context within future EasyVision products. Examples of these are the functionality to visualize and manipulate triangulated surfaces in combination with voxel-based data, and the functionality for data exchange with CAD/CAM based environments.

Real-Time Simulation of Minimally-Invasive Surgery with Cutting Based on Boundary Element Methods

Ullrich Meier[1,2], Carlos Monserrat[1], Nils-Christian Parr[1,2],
Francisco Javier García[1], José Antonio Gil[1]

[1] MedICLab, ETSIA, DEGI, Universidad Politécnica de Valencia, Camino de Vera s/n,
E-46022 Valencia, Spain
ulme@doctor.upv.es, cmonserr@dsic.upv.es
[2] Institut für Angewandte Mechanik und Bauinformatik,
Technische Universität Braunschweig, Spielmannstraße 11,
D-38106 Braunschweig, Germany

Abstract. Most deformable models for surgery simulation are quite straight-forward to achieve the computational speed required for real time simulation. However, they typically are more adjusted to merely graphical representation needs, i.e. surface-oriented (e.g. mass-spring type models), and neglect mechanical realism, although the simulation of cutting in real time is feasible. Finite element (FEM) based models, in turn, depart from continuum mechanics principles, and therefore are more realistic in many cases. But their volumetric structure is not optimal for graphical representation and in this sense produces excessive data, eventually impeding a real-time simulation of incisions. While parting from the same hypotheses as FEM models, a boundary element (BEM) based algorithm passes the influence of an organ's interior to its surface. Thus, it yields comparable simulation results as the prior, but with less data to process. This enables the consideration in real time of local modifications of the underlying boundary element mesh produced when cutting. Actually, the presented algorithm has been successfully tested to simulate incisions in real time.

A deformable model based on boundary element methods (BEM) departs from the same continuum mechanical hypothesis as those derived from finite element methods (FEM) [2]. However, it only requires the discretization of the organ's surface into 2-D elements and the definition of N nodes on their outline, coinciding with the typical graphical representation of 3-D objects by means of polygons joined at vertices. The resulting system of equations of order $3N$ is of the form

$$\mathbf{H} \cdot U = \mathbf{G} \cdot P + B, \tag{1}$$

where $\mathbf{H}$ and $\mathbf{G}$ are square influence matrices, B the body force vector (gravity), and U and P the nodal displacement and traction vectors. At some nodes, the displacement is prescribed by the virtual tool with which the node is in contact, and the resulting traction determines the respective force fed back. The majority of nodes will be free, though, i.e. have a prescribed zero traction. Thus, by exchanging some few columns of $\mathbf{H}$ and $\mathbf{G}$, all unknowns are on the left, while on the right hand side most matrix columns can be neglected, as they are multiplied with zeros.

W. Niessen and M. Viergever (Eds.): MICCAI 2001, LNCS 2208, pp. 1263-1264, 2001.
© Springer-Verlag Berlin Heidelberg 2001

1264   U. Meier et al.

In order to significantly accelerate the solving time, even more as **H** and **G** are fully populated and not symmetric, (1) is multiplied with the inverse of the modified system matrix **H′**, which is obtained during the preparation phase when time is not yet the ruling factor. Thus, the vector of unknowns is isolated on the left hand side, and the solving of the system is immediate for different tool positions. Nevertheless, whenever it comes to a new contact, or an already existing one is lost, the composition of **H′** and with it its inverse change. But the toggling of some nodes between the two states of "free" and "constrained" only affects a few columns of **H′**. Hence, by resorting to the *Woodbury formula* [3] for the corresponding modification of $\mathbf{H}^{-1}$, the required computations are of the order $O(N^2)$ instead of $O(N^3)$ only.

Cutting, in turn, requires the partitioning of some surface elements and the addition of new elements along the created notch, together with the introduction of the corresponding new nodes. This local re-modeling of the underlying boundary element mesh once more produces changes in a few columns of **H′**, and further leads to some new columns and rows. Again, the Woodbury formula can be employed to modify $\mathbf{H}^{-1}$ correspondingly, and the required modifications do not exceed the order $O(N^2)$.

The result is a deformable model that is comparable to FEM-based models as far as its robustness or high velocity and accuracy when simulating quasi-linear deformations are concerned. In contrast to the other, though, the BEM-based model here proposed permits the inclusion of gravity and the simulation of cutting in real time. However, as with the FEM-based models, the results are less satisfying for large deformations and for tissue properties with important non-linear portions.

The BEM-based deformable model has been tested for organs modeled with several hundred nodes on MedICLab's surgery simulator [1]. Being based on a standard PC with Pentium III processor with 450MHz / 128Mbyte RAM and Windows NT 4.0 (service pack 6), this simulator represents a low cost approach to surgery simulation. For standard deformations, the computational cost was of the order of a millisecond. When creating new contacts with virtual tools or loosing existing ones, the cost was of the order of tens of milliseconds, and of a hundred milliseconds when simulating shear cuts. Resuming, the here exposed algorithm represents an important advance with respect to other deformable models, as it combines the accuracy of a continuum mechanics based model with the possibility to perform cuts. Our future work will therefore be centered in parallelizing the algorithm to further accelerate it and extending the model to include more complex, non-linear tissue properties and large deformations.

References

1. Meier, U., García, F.J., Parr, N.-C., Monserrat, C., Gil, J.A., Grau, V., Juan, M.C., Alcañiz, M.: 3D Surgery Trainer with Force Feedback in Minimally Invasive Surgery. To appear in: Proc. CARS 15, Berlin (2001)
2. Monserrat, C., Meier, U., Alcañiz, M., Chinesta, F., Juan, M.C.: A new approach for the real-time simulation of tissue deformations in surgery simulation. Computer Methods and Programs in Biomedicine, 64(2), 77□85 (2001)
3. Press, W.H. et al.: Numerical Recipes in C. 2nd ed. Cambridge University Press, Cambridge (1992)

3-D Reconstruction and Functional Analysis of the Temporomandibular Joint

Reza Arbab Chirani[1,2], Jean-José Jacq[2,3], Christian Roux[2,3], Philippe Meriot[4]

[1] Université de Bretagne Occidentale, U.F.R. d'Odontologie, Brest, France
[2] Laboratoire de Traitement de l'Information Médicale, INSERM ERM 0102, Brest, France
[3] Ecole Nationale Supérieure des Télécommunications de Bretagne, Brest, France
[4] Centre Hospitalier Universitaire, service de radiologie, Brest, France
{Reza.Arbab-Chirani,Philippe.Meriot}@univ-brest.fr,
{JJ.Jacq,Christian.Roux}@enst-bretagne.fr

Abstract. The 3-D representation of temporomandibular joints can be performed using magnetic resonance imaging. We carried out a MRI on an asymptomatic volunteer subject. Images were reconstructed in three dimensions. This reconstruction allowed the description of the principal anatomical elements of this joint : articular disc, condyle, bilaminar region and temporal bone. A preliminary study of articular function, in the sagittal plane was also carried out with measurement of real movements of the disc.

Extended Summary

Usual 3-D reconstructions of the Temporo Mandibular Joint (TMJ) make use of two medical imaging modalities, MRI and CT scan. 2-D MRI images are used routinely to study TMJ since the eighties. Recently, some attempts have been made to access the 3-D morphology and kinematics of TMJ [2, 3]. In order to study articular dynamics, these representations were often associated to an extra oral movement tracking system [1]. Aims of this work is 1) to propose a 3-D reconstruction methodology of the temporomandibular joint based on MRI slices and 2) to study the function of this joint with measurement of real movements of the articular disc (translation and rotation) in the sagittal plane, during the oral opening movement.

Images of the right and left TMJ - coming from a healthy volunteer - were obtained from a 1.0 Tesla MR system, using a spin-echo sequence. The total number of slice was 90 (15 sagittal slices from each TMJ in three positions: closed jaw, half-open jaw and completely open jaw). The 2D images were segmented through semi-interactive editing of the contours - the 3-D reconstruction being performed by contours stacking. Applications of such a 3-D reconstruction are numerous: representation of anatomical features, representation of articular surfaces and measurement of displacement of movable structures. From these reconstructions, the articular discs were segmented and their principal axes of inertia were computed. These axes allow an approximative measurement of real movements of the articular disc in the sagittal plane, in both translation and rotation, during jaw opening.

Three-dimensional representations, accounting for clinical reality, were obtained for the two right and left TMJ in 3 positions. Figure 1. depicts the 3-D reconstruction of the right TMJ images, in closed position.

W. Niessen and M. Viergever (Eds.): MICCAI 2001, LNCS 2208, pp. 1265-1266, 2001.
© Springer-Verlag Berlin Heidelberg 2001

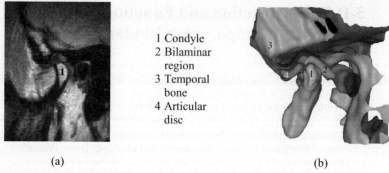

1 Condyle
2 Bilaminar region
3 Temporal bone
4 Articular disc

(a)   (b)

Fig. 1. Right TMJ in closed position. (a) MRI acquisition. (b) 3D reconstruction.

On the 3D representations, the inertia axes of the articular disc are represented in two different positions (Fig. 2.).

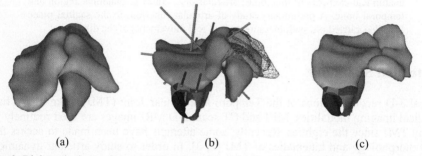

(a)   (b)   (c)

Fig. 2. Right articular surfaces. (a) Closed position. (b) Superimposition of both positions with inertia axes of the disc. (c) opened position.

The real movements for this subject has been measured. We found, for right TMJ, the following values : rotation 47°, translation 2.9 mm (X) and 1.6 mm (Y), which compare favorably to the literature [4]. 3-D reconstruction of the temporomandibular joint images based on MRI allows a precise anatomical description of majority of the components of this joint and constitutes a very promising way in order to study its kinematics.

References

1. Krebs M, Gallo LM, Airoldi RL. A new method for three-dimensional reconstruction and animation of the TMJ. Ann. Acad. Med. Singapore 24 (1995) 11-16

2. Motoyoshi M., Sadowsky PL. Three-dimensional reconstruction system for imaging of the temporomandibular joint using magnetic resonance imaging. J. Oral Sci. 41 (1999) 5-8

3. Price C, Connell DG, MacKay A, Tobias DL. Three-dimensional reconstruction of MRI of the temporomandibular joint by I-DEAS. Dentomaxillofac. Radiol. 21 (1992) 148-153

4. Gerber A, Steinhardt G. Dental Occlusion and the TMJ. Quintessence Publishing (1990)

Methods for Modeling and Predicting Mechanical Deformations of the Breast Under External Perturbations

Fred S. Azar[1], Dimitris N. Metaxas[2], Mitchell D. Schnall[3]

[1]Dept. of BioEngineering, University of Pennsylvania (fredazar@seas.upenn.edu)
[2]Dept. of Computer Science, University of Pennsylvania
(dnm@graphics.cis.upenn.edu)
[3]Dept of Radiology, University of Pennsylvania (schnall@oasis.rad.upenn.edu)

Abstract. Currently, High Field (1.5T) Superconducting MR imaging does not allow live guidance during needle breast procedures, which allow only to calculate approximately the location of a cancerous tumor in the patient breast before inserting the needle. It can then become relatively uncertain that the tissue specimen removed during the biopsy actually belongs to the lesion of interest. A new method for guiding clinical breast biopsy is presented, based on a deformable finite element model of the breast. The geometry of the model is constructed from MR data, and its mechanical properties are modeled using a non-linear material model. This method allows imaging the breast without or with mild compression before the procedure, then compressing the breast and using the finite element model to predict the tumor's position during the procedure in a total time of less than a half-hour.

1 Introduction

The ability to identify a mass in the breast requires the mass to have a different appearance (or a different contrast) from normal tissue. With high-field MRI, the contrast between soft tissues in the breast is 10 to 100 times greater than that obtained with x-rays [1]. A MR image-guided breast localization and biopsy system allows the differentiation between the benign enhancing lesions, and carcinomas [1]. However, the appearance, size and shape of the potential cancer lesion greatly depend on dynamics of the contrast-enhancing agent. Furthermore, the needle is not a very sharp object, and cannot be inserted smoothly in the breast, causing unwanted deformations. The breast could be compressed so as to minimize internal deformations, however that would cause blood to be squeezed out and could dramatically alter the appearance and shape of the lesion on the MR image.

The above limitations coupled with the deformable structure of the breast make needle procedures very sensitive to the initial placement of the needle, and to the amount of breast compression. It thus becomes relatively uncertain that the tissue specimen removed during the biopsy procedure actually belongs to the lesion of interest, due to the added difficulty of accurately locating the tumor's boundaries inside the breast.

We present a virtual deformable breast model of the patient, based on MR data, and using non-linear material models. This model can be used effectively in a *new method for guiding clinical breast biopsy*. This method involves imaging the patient's breast without any or little compression before a needle procedure, then compressing the breast, and its virtual finite element model (by applying the same pressure to

W. Niessen and M. Viergever (Eds.): MICCAI 2001, LNCS 2208, pp. 1267-1270, 2001.

both), and using the displacement of the virtual tumor model to predict the displacement of the real cancer tumor. Other possible applications include registration of data sets from different imaging modalities, diagnosis, measurements, surgery planning, simulations of deformation due to inserting a needle, and further away, virtual surgery, and tele-surgery.

2 Methods

We had presented in [2] an initial attempt to model a patient breast by developing a preliminary FE model of the breast. We extend that methodology to allow clinical use of the model by :

1. Improving the technique. A new meshing algorithm is used to allow variable meshing density in the model, in which the mesh density is increased around the point of interest, and decreased away from it. A new material model for fatty tissue is introduced following the rationale presented in [2]. The non-linear elastic modulus of fatty tissue E_{fat} is a function of the strain ε_{fat} :

$$E_{fat}(\varepsilon_{fat}) = A \cdot \varepsilon_{fat}^2 + B \cdot \varepsilon_{fat} + C \tag{1}$$

where A, B and C are determined based on the boundary conditions. A detailed description of the derivation of this equation can be found in [3]. Finally, a faster time-convergence algorithm employing an Euler method with adaptive step sizing is used. The improvements can reduce the computation time to less than ten minutes.

2. Validating the method. A deformable silicon gel phantom was built to study the movement of a stiff inclusion inside a deformable environment under plate compression [4]. The geometry of the deformable phantom consists of a rectangular box (84x82x70mm) containing a rectangular inclusion (20x23x20mm), which is 4.3 times stiffer than the surrounding silicone. The phantom was imaged undeformed, then compressed 14% (9.8mm). The performance of our software algorithm was compared to that of a commercial FEM software package ABAQUS, by measuring the displacement vectors of the 8 corners of the stiff inclusion and its center.

3. Testing the model and its performance on a patient. A patient's breast was imaged uncompressed and then compressed 26%. The corresponding deformable model was built, and was virtually compressed to match the real compression amount. We tracked the displacement of a small cyst and of two vitamin E pills taped to the superior and inferior parts of the breast. We also tested the model through a convergence analysis and a sensitivity analysis (in which the material parameters were varied over a physiologically relevant range, within two standard deviations of their experimentally derived average value) [3].

3 Results and Discussion

3.1   Silicone Phantom Experiment

The results (Fig. 1) show that all of the average displacement errors per node between the two simulations are under 1mm, and that using a small strain approximation [2] instead of the Lagrangian finite strain expression, in our finite element algorithm does *not* introduce a significant error in simulations of large deformation.

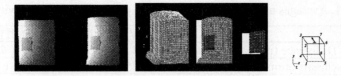

Fig. 1. Uncompressed and compressed axial MR slice of phantom (*left*), 3D view of model including axial slice through center of inclusion and axial view of inclusion center, before and after compression (*center*)

3.2   Patient Breast Compression Experiment

The MR images containing the landmarks and the corresponding model slices are shown in Fig.2. The arrows in the figure indicate the location of the landmarks.

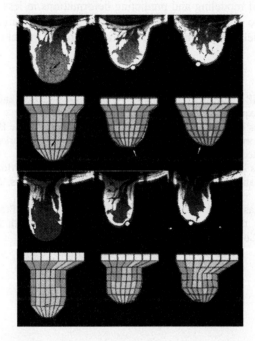

Fig. 2. Uncompressed MR images (*upper left*), uncompressed model slices (*upper right*), compressed MR slices (*lower left*), and corresponding virtually compressed model slices (*lower right*) after virtual compression

All of the simulations in the variational studies were done on a SGI Octane Workstation with 2 195MHz IP30 processors (MIPS R10000 processors), and 256 Megabytes of memory (RAM). The model contains 512 nodes, 343 3D hexahedral elements, and 294 2D triangular elements. Table 1 shows the displacement differences (Model-Real) of the landmarks' center of gravity, and the %Misclassification which compares the number of misclassified pixels in the model with the compressed MRI.

1270   F.S. Azar, D.N. Metaxas, and M.D. Schnall

Table 1. Averages and standard deviations (in parentheses) of sensitivity analysis

	Cyst	Vit. E pill (INF)	Vit. E pill (SUP)
Disp. Difference (mm)	1.3 (*0.1*)	3.5 (*0.1*)	4.6 (*0.1*)
%Misclassification	11.8 (*1.0*)	25.1 (*1.2*)	31.4 (*0.5*)

The convergence analysis shows that the simulation indeed converges to the solution, as the model mesh is refined. The material properties sensitivity analysis (Table 1) shows that large variations in material properties parameters do not significantly affect the parameter results.

4 Conclusion

The final results show that it is possible to create a non-linear deformable model of the breast capable of modeling and predicting deformations in less than a half-hour : the average times to completion were 12 minutes for segmentation of MR data, 3 minutes for the model mesh creation, and 14 minutes for the model simulation.

References

1. Orel SG, Schnall MD *et al.*: MR Imaging-guided Localization and Biopsy of Breast Lesions: Initial Experience. Radiology, Vol. 193 (1994) 97-102
2. Azar FS, Metaxas DN, Schnall MD: A Finite Element Model of the Breast for Predicting Mechanical Deformations during Biopsy Procedures. IEEE Workshop, Mathematical Methods in Biomedical Image Analysis (2000) 38-45
3. Azar FS, Metaxas DN, Schnall MD: A Deformable Finite Element Model of the Breast for Predicting Mechanical Deformations under External Perturbations. J. Acad. Radiology (2001)
4. Azar FS, Metaxas DN, Miller RT, Schnall MD: Methods for Predicting Mechanical Deformations in the Breast during Clinical Breast Biopsy. 26th IEEE Annual N.E. BioEngineering Conference (2000)

Non-linear Soft Tissue Deformations for the Simulation of Percutaneous Surgeries

Jean-Marc Schwartz[1], Ève Langelier[2], Christian Moisan[3], and Denis Laurendeau[1]

[1] Computer Vision and Systems Laboratory, Univ. Laval, Québec (Qc) G1K 7P4, Canada
[2] Biomechanics Laboratory, Univ. Laval, Québec (Qc) G1K 7P4, Canada
[3] iMRI Unit, Quebec City University Hospital, Québec (Qc) G1L 3L5, Canada

Abstract. We introduce a non-linear extension of the tensor-mass method for real-time computation of biological soft tissue deformations. We aim at developing a simulation tool for the planning of cryogenic surgical treatment of liver cancer. This therapy requires careful planning, therefore accurate modeling of the mechanical behavior of organs is required. Our method presently allows real-time computation of non-linear elastic tissue deformations, and further extension towards viscoelasticity modeling is planned.

1 Introduction

The development of surgery simulation systems requires fast algorithms to allow real-time computation of tissue deformations, as well as accurate modeling of soft tissue mechanical properties. We are currently developing a simulation tool for the planning of percutaneous image-guided cryosurgical treatment of liver cancer. This therapy consists in destroying tumor cells through successive application of freezing and passive thawing cycles [3]. Careful planning is required to optimize the destruction of tumor cells vs. damage to healthy cells. In particular accurate modeling of the geometric, thermal, and mechanical behavior of organs is required.

Several methods have been reported for rapid calculation of linear elastic mechanical deformations, from relatively simple physical models such as the spring-mass model to models based of continuum mechanics such as the Finite Element Method [1]. However experimental characterizations suggest that linear elasticity is only a coarse approximation of real properties of biological soft tissues. Among other studies, Miller et al. [2] identified a viscoelastic constitutive model as accurate for modeling brain tissue deformations.

2 Non-linear Modeling

The most promising approach towards real-time computation of non-linear viscoelasticity appeared to be the tensor-mass model introduced by Cotin et al. [1], as it is both time-efficient and physically accurate. It additionally allows local topological changes on mesh elements so that simulation of cutting or perforation is possible. As a first step we show that adequate real-time correction of linear elasticity parameters allows to model different types of non-linear elastic deformations. In our model, expression of force $F_{T_i(j)}$ applied on vertex $P_{T_i(j)}$ within a tetrahedral mesh element T_i is:

W. Niessen and M. Viergever (Eds.): MICCAI 2001, LNCS 2208, pp. 1271-1272, 2001.
© Springer-Verlag Berlin Heidelberg 2001

$$F_{T_i(j)} = \sum_{k=0}^{3} \left([K_{jk}^{T_i}] + \delta\lambda_i[A_{jk}^{T_i}] + \delta\mu_i[B_{jk}^{T_i}] \right) P_{T_i(k)}^0 P_{T_i(k)} \ , \tag{1}$$

where $[K_{jk}^{T_i}]$, $[A_{jk}^{T_i}]$ and $[B_{jk}^{T_i}]$ are 3×3 tensors, λ_i and μ_i are the Lamé coefficients of the material, and $\delta\lambda_i$ and $\delta\mu_i$ are non-linear corrections. Tensors only depend on the geometry at rest so that precomputation is possible.

Fig. 1a shows two examples of simulated non-linear tissue constitutive laws. Both tissues have stiffness increasing with compression, as it typically occurs with biological samples. Stiffness increases linearly for tissue 1 and stepwise for tissue 2. Fig. 1b shows forces calculated in a simulated perforation of these tissues: in both cases, simulation on a macroscopic mesh correctly follows the non-linear constitutive law.

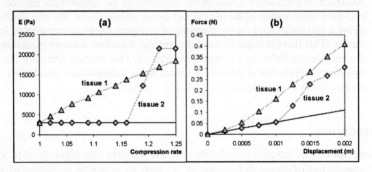

Fig. 1. Two examples of non-linear deformation laws. **(a)** Young's modulus as a function of the rate of compression. **(b)** Corresponding force as a function of displacement in simulated perforation. Dark lines represent the linear elastic case for $E = 3000$ Pa. For all simulations $v = 0.4$.

The linear tensor-mass method can typically deal with meshes of a few thousand nodes in real-time. The non-linear extension increases computing time by a factor 4. However the method remains suitable for real-time applications, provided that the non-linear computational overhead is restricted to a limited number of mesh elements where the highest deformation rates occur.

SEQFurther plans include taking into account viscous effects to allow accurate modeling of biological soft tissues. In addition an experimental setup is under construction to derive experimental data from biological samples in order to assess the accuracy of the model.

References

1. Cotin, S., Delingette, H., Ayache, N.: A Hybrid Elastic Model for Real-Time Cutting, Deformations, and Force Feedback for Surgery Training and Simulation. Visual Computer 16 (2000) 437-452
2. Miller, K., Chinzei, K., Orssengo, G., Bednarz, P.: Mechanical Properties of Brain Tissue in-vivo: Experiment and Computer Simulation. J. Biomech. 33 (2000) 1369-1376
3. Morin, J., Dionne, G., Dumont, M., Fouquet, B., Dufour, M., Cloutier, S., Moisan, C.: MR Guided Percutaneous Cryosurgery of Breast Carcinoma: Technique and Early Clinical Results, Proc. Int. Soc. Mag. Res. in Med. (2000) 71

The Continuous Tabu Search as an Optimizer for 2D-to-3D Biomedical Image Registration

Mark P. Wachowiak and Adel S. Elmaghraby

Department of Computer Engineering and Computer Science
University of Louisville, Louisville, KY 40292, USA
{mpwach01, aselma01}@athena.louisville.edu

Abstract. Both stochastic and direct optimization of similarity metrics have been used in biomedical image registration. This paper proposes an adapted tabu search for registration of 2D ultrasound scans to 3D volumes. Accuracy and efficiency compare favorably with other methods.

1 Continuous Tabu Search

Stochastic global optimizers and stochastic-direct hybrids, which include genetic algorithms and simulated annealing, are used to locate the global optima of complicated and multiextremal functions. These methods have proven effective for biomedical image registration [1], [2]. In this paper, another global optimizer, the continuous tabu search (CTS) (described in [3]), is adapted to image registration.

In the adapted method, after the CTS has identified a number of "promising points" where the optimum may lie, the "affine shaker" (AS) algorithm [4] is applied to locate the best point in each promising area. The shape of the promising area is thus adapted to include areas of the search space that may have been missed during diversification. Finally, an intensified search is conducted around the most promising point using the Nelder-Mead simplex algorithm.

2 Methods and Results

The maximum value of the overlap-invariant normalized mutual information [5] functional was sought. Two 100×100- and one 64×64-pixel images (three experiments) were obtained from a $148\times160\times141$-voxel US volume of a heart (courtesy of TomTec, Inc., Germany). Each experiment consisted of 4 trials for each of 10 initial points at varying distances from a reference ("true" point).

Optimizers were then used to register the 2D slices within the original 3D volume: (1) ASA(0) - Adaptive simulated annealing with slow cooling schedule [6]; (2) ASA(1) - fast cooling; (3) ASA(2) - "medium" cooling; (4) A modified Nelder-Mead simplex algorithm: All reflections of the initial solution in 6D space are examined to prevent finding a local optimum; (5) Tabu / AS, using discretization of the search space [7], AS, and the simplex algorithm for intensification; (6) Tabu' / AS, as (5) above, but restarting the search with a reflected point

W. Niessen and M. Viergever (Eds.): MICCAI 2001, LNCS 2208, pp. 1273–1274, 2001.
© Springer-Verlag Berlin Heidelberg 2001

Experiment		ASA(0)	ASA(1)	ASA(2)	Amoeba	Tabu/AS	Tabu'/AS
% Correct	1	7.50	27.50	7.50	30	40	37.50
Reg.	2	2.50	15	5	0	5	10
	3	5	30	5	10	42.5	52.5
Average		4.17	24.17	5.83	13.33	**29.17**	**33.33**
Mean Func.	1	6.19 ± 0.09	6.17 ± 0.05	6.34 ± 0.07	9.03 ± 0.27	4.68 ± 0.46	4.75 ± 0.25
Evals.	2	6.41 ± 0.00	6.13 ± 0.03	6.22 ± 0.06	N/A	4.30 ± 0.18	4.34 ± 0.51
	3	6.23 ± 0.99	6.18 ± 0.08	6.33 ± 0.12	9.18 ± 0.00	4.98 ± 0.28	5.00 ± 0.25
Average		6.28	6.16	6.30	9.11	**4.66**	**4.70**

Table 1. Percentage of correct registrations and mean number of function evaluation for correct 2D-3D registration ($\times$ 1000).

after 20 iterations without improvement. The number of correct registrations and mean number of function evaluations are shown in Table 1.

The absence of feature extraction and pre-processing, no user interaction, and the large search space contributed to the low percentage of correct registration for all methods. The two CTS techniques correctly registered a larger percentage of trials. ASA(1) also performed very well. CTS outperformed ASA or the simplex in function evaluations for correct registrations. The maximum number of ASA iterations without the simplex stage (here, 4000) was often reached, indicating that CTS may explore the search space in fewer iterations (maximum 200).

Although existing direct and stochastic methods are often effective in image registration, the continuous tabu search can also be used as an optimizer for 2D-to-3D registration, and further work on this technique is warranted.

References

1. Matsopoulos, G. K., Mouravliansky, N. A., Delibasis, K. L., Konstantina, S. N.: Automatic Retinal Image Registration Scheme Using Global Optimization Techniques. IEEE Trans. Info. Tech. in Biomed. **3** (1999) 47–60.
2. Rouet, J.-M., Jacq, J.-J., Roux, C.: Genetic Algorithms for a Robust 3-D MR-CT Registration. IEEE Trans. Info. Tech. in Biomed. **4** (2000) 126–136.
3. Chelouah, R., Siarry, P.: Tabu Search Applied to Global Optimization. Euro. J. of Op. Res. **123** (2000) 256–270.
4. Battiti, R., Tecchiolli, G.: The Continuous Reactive Tabu Search: Blending Combinatorial Optimization And Stochastic Search For Global Optimization. Ann. of Op. Res. **63** (1996) 153–188.
5. Studholme, C., Hill, D. L. G., Hawkes, D. J.: An Overlap Invariant Entropy Measure of 3D Medical Image Alignment. Patt. Recog., **32** (1999) 71–86.
6. Ingber, L., Rosen, B.: Genetic Algorithms and Very Fast Simulated Reannealing: A Comparison. Math. and Computer Model. **16** (1992) 87–100.
7. Siarry, P., Berthiau, G.: Fitting of Tabu Search To Optimize Functions of Continuous Variables. Int. J. for Num. Methods in Eng. **40** (1997) 2449–2457.

Modally Controlled Free Form Deformation for Non-rigid Registration in Image-Guided Liver Surgery

Yoshitaka Masutani and Fumihiko Kimura

The University of Tokyo Graduate School
7 3 1 Hongo Bunkyo ku, Tokyo 113 8656 Japan
{masutani, kimura}@cim.pe.u-tokyo.ac.jp

1. Introduction

One of the difficulties in surgical navigation based on preoperative image information is intra-operative deformation of the organs consisting of soft tissues. In liver surgery, liver shape is deformed dynamically due to patient respiration, posture change and surgical operations. Such intra-operative liver deformation includes so-called large displacement, which requires much computation cost for numerical simulation based on non-linear FEM. Herline [Herline99] reported rigid liver surface registration for such purpose. In this study, we propose a new method of modal representation of liver deformation applied for intra-operative non-rigid registration in image-guided liver surgery. Several experiments with synthetic range data were performed based on error factor analysis.

2. Materials and Methods

We developed a new method for deformation description, *modally-controlled free form deformation*, based on a combination of modal representation and free form deformation (FFD). The FFD [Sederberg86] is a technique for shape manipulation in computer-aided design. By moving control points interactively, object shape is edited. In our method, the, the grid control points surrounding liver shape model are moved in several modes to provide volumetric deformation so that the inner structures such as blood vessels are also deformed. For non-rigid object tracking, Pentland and Scraroff [Sclaroff96] developed a technique of a modal representation of deformation for non-rigid object tracking, based on modal analysis of shape models. In the method, displacement of each vertex is represented by linear combinations of orthogonal eigen-modes. In our study, instead of physically based analysis, artificial and reusable modes, called *generalized geometric modes*, were designed by using several non-linear functions, including bending and twisting of shapes [Barr84]. The modes are: (1) rigid motion (rotation and translation), (2) bending, and (3) twisting (Fig.1) [Masutani01]. The number of parameters is 21, which consists of 6 for rigid motion, 6 for bending 3 axes in 2 directions, and 9 for twisting along 3 axes.

W. Niessen and M. Viergever (Eds.): MICCAI 2001, LNCS 2208, pp. 1275-1278, 2001.
© Springer-Verlag Berlin Heidelberg 2001

We assume that the partial surface of the liver is obtained intra-operatively as range data of unstructured surface point coordinates. For the deformable liver surface matching, the optimization process of the parameter set is performed to minimize the root mean square (RMS) of the distances between range data points and model vertex points. A simple iterative search algorithm in the maximum gradient direction was employed. Based on our preliminary experiments, after a rigid registration with only 6 rigid parameters, registration by using all parameters was performed for faster convergence. The depth information of the range data was employed for the registration for two reasons.

3.   Results, Discussion, and Summary

In this study, we performed preliminary experiments for registration with modal parameter optimization. The 9 types range data (3 types of deformation and 3 view directions) were synthesized by using deformed models and their depth-cueing images. Gaussian noise ($\sigma=2.0$mm) was added to the synthetic range data in the depth direction for simulation of the range sensor errors. The registration errors were evaluated by using root mean square (RMS) of the vertex distances of the two liver models (target and registered). Table 1 shows the RMS errors for the entire liver surface. The errors were generally larger for the larger displacement and non-rigid deformation. As shown in Figure 2, however, the surface matching errors were not uniform on the entire surface. Obviously, the errors were larger outside the range data acquisition area. The RMS errors inside the area were about 4-7 mm. These results naturally showed that the registration is guaranteed only around the range data acquisition area. The registration was about 30 seconds by using a PC workstation with a Pentium III 800 MHz processor.

One of the important properties of our method is that not only the surface but also the inner structures are also deformed according to the same deformation patterns. Though the patterns are based on an approximation of modal deformation theory, we must investigate the errors inside the registered surface before clinical study. Studies by using phantoms made of silicon rubber are currently in progress. For the purpose of analyzing the errors based on the limitation of deformation description, measurement of intra-operative liver deformation and statistical analysis are in progress. Based on the results of the analysis, it might be possible to remove redundant parameters without increasing errors.

Our final purposes of development for intra-operative registration include guidance of surgical robots. One of the potential advantages of such robotic surgery is that surgical operations can be performed with minimal deformation of organs. Therefore, robotic surgery with navigational information based on our registration method is expected to realize more precise and minimally invasive surgeries.

Acknowledgements

This work is a part of the research project: *development of robotic surgery system* in *Research for the Future Program* of Japan Society for Promotion of Science (JSPS) and is financially supported by JSPS.

RMS (mm)	Rest Shape	Registered in View (A)	Registered in View (B)	Registered in View (C)
Deformed #1	24.5	4.3	4.1	5.2
Deformed #2	21.0	5.9	9.7	8.5
Deformed #3	38.8	12.3	12.7	14.5

Table 1. RMS errors of the overall liver surface in registration results

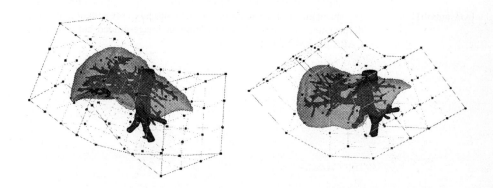

Fig. 1 Liver model deformation by modally controlled FFD
generalized geometric modes of twisting (left), and bending (right)

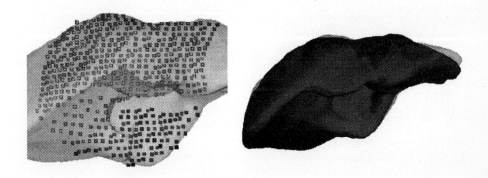

Fig. 2 Registration error analysis by using synthetic range data
synthetic range data (left), and registration result in the view (right)
The given deformed shape is semi-transparent and the registered are opaque.

References

[Herline99]   A. J. Herline, et al., Surface Registration for Use in Interactive Image-
                     Guided Liver Surgery, Proc. MICCAI'99, pp892-899, 1999
[Sclaroff96]   S. Sclaroff, et al., Modal Matching for Correspondence and
                     Recognition, Boston U. tech. rep. TR95-008, 1996
[Sederberg86]   T. W. Sederberg, et al., Free-Form Deformation of Solid Geometric
                     Models, Computer Graphics (Proc. SIGGRAPH), vol.20 no.4 pp151-
                     160, 1986
[Barr84]   A. H. Barr, Global and Local Deformations of Solid Primitives,
                     Computer Graphics (Proc.SIGGRAPH) vol.18 no.3, pp151-160, 1984
[Masutani01]   Y. Masutani, and F. Kimura, A new modal representation of liver
                     deformation for non-rigid registration in image-guided surgery, Proc.
                     CARS'01, pp19-24, 2001

Two-Step Registration of Subacute to Hyperacute Stroke MRIs

P. Anbeek[1], K.L. Vincken[1], M.J.P. van Osch[1], J.P.W. Pluim[1], J. van der Grond[1], M.A. Viergever[1]

[1]Department of Radiology, Image Sciences Institute, University Medical Center, Heidelberglaan 100, rm E01.334, Utrecht, The Netherlands
{nelly, koen, thijs, josien, jeroen, max}@isi.uu.nl

Introduction

In the use of MRI in acute stroke patients, determination of the perfusion-diffusion (PWI-DWI) mismatch is highly important, since it indicates possible enlargement of the ischemic lesion or deterioration of the patient. When quantitative measures are used such as the ADC of CBF to predict ischemic damage, accurate registration of the ischemic lesion on follow-up MRI to the results obtained in the first MRI is essential. Problems in the registration of stroke images include differences in patient orientation and/or low cooperativeness of the patient in the hyperacute stage of stroke. The aim of the present study is to develop a robust method of stroke image registration.

Methods

Registration was performed by Mirit (1), which is based on mutual information. Mirit provides rigid body registration, including rotation, translation and scaling. The image that is modified is the floating image, whereas the image to which the registration is performed is the reference image. We used the MRI data sets of 6 stroke patients, in whom the hyperacute dataset was obtained within 3 hours after the onset of stroke (t0) and at 1 week (t1). Two ways of image registration were compared:
1. One-step: Direct registration of a floating image at t1 (FLAIR, T2-w or PD) to the reference image of different type at t0 (DWI or ADC-map).
2. Two-step: First performing a registration of an image at t1 (FLAIR, T2-w or PD) to an image of the same type at t0. The parameters for translation, rotation and scaling resulting from this registration are used as starting position for the second registration: Registration of the floating image at t1 to a reference image of different type at t0 (DWI or ADC-map).

An example (FLAIR to DWI) of both image registration methods is shown in figure 1. The left side of the picture shows the registration by the one-step method. The right side shows registration by the two-step method. The white line in the picture denotes the contours of the cortex in the DWI scan, which is the reference image. These pictures indicate that for these images the registration and in particular scaling is performed better by the two-step method.

W. Niessen and M. Viergever (Eds.): MICCAI 2001, LNCS 2208, pp. 1279-1280, 2001.

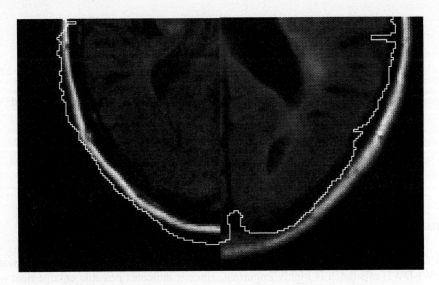

Figure 1: one-step versus two-step registration FLAIR to DWI

Results

In total we compared 72 registrations, 36 registrations by the one-step method with 36 corresponding registrations by the two-step method. Overall, the two-step method yielded in 72% a better registration (p<0.001, Fisher's exact test) when the DWI scan was used as reference image and in 39% (p<0.01) when the ADC-map was used as reference image, compared with the one-step method.

Discussion

The most important finding of the present study is that the two-step registration method is superior to direct registration of follow-up MRI stroke scans to hyperacute stroke scans. Our study has one major limitation. For practical reasons we applied registration by rotation, translation and scaling. It is well known that the current echo planar imaging (EPI) scans may distort the geometry of the brain. Elastic registration, in which is corrected for these image distortions, is the preferred way of registration. However, such a way of image registration is significantly more time consuming.

References

1.   F. Maes et al., IEEE TMI 1997, 16, 187-198.

The Effect of Organ Motion and Image Artifacts on Monomodal Volume Registration

M van Herk, JC de Munck, MTJG Groenewegen, AR Peters and A Touw

Radiotherapy Department, The Netherlands Cancer Institute/Antoni van Leeuwenhoek Huis
Plesmanlaan 121, 1066 CX Amsterdam, the Netherlands
portal@nki.nl

Abstract. Volume registration, by means of minimizing rms pixel value differences, was tested on pairs of pelvic CT scans in a perturbation experiment to determine its robustness. The tests included registration of 9 scans to themselves and registration of 17 clinical image pairs. Local image artifacts have no influence on performance, but global distortions and organ movement severely degraded the reproducibility. By limiting the algorithm to the gray value range of bone the accuracy is improved at the cost of reliability.

1 Introduction

Image registration plays an increasingly important role in many medical procedures. The aim of this study is to evaluate the performance of a "standard" automatic volume registration technique for registering pairs of CT scans and to test the sensitivity of the registration algorithm for image artifacts that might occur in clinical practice.

2 Material and Methods

We used 17 CT scan pairs from eight prostate cancer patients. The rms difference of pixel values between the two scans was minimized by rigid 3-D translation and rotation. Pixels outside the region of overlap of both scans were ignored. Matching was started from random transformations, and the average displacement of pixels in a region of interest compared to a ground truth match was used to measure the performance. Displacements larger than 5 mm are counted as failures. The accuracy is defined as the average displacement of all non-failed matches. In the first, identical data experiments, several image artifacts (e.g., holes, noise, cropping, and distortions) were introduced into copies of the same scan that were then matched. In the second, different data experiments, the planning CT of all eight patients was edited manually using a simple paintbrush program to delete selected structures on all slices. The edited scans were registered with unmodified follow up scans. The ground truth was derived using the same registration technique, i.e., only the reproducibility is measured.

W. Niessen and M. Viergever (Eds.): MICCAI 2001, LNCS 2208, pp. 1281-1282, 2001.
© Springer-Verlag Berlin Heidelberg 2001

3 Results

In the identical data experiments, the match reliability was typically 95% or more, and the introduced artifacts had little influence. The reliability seemed to increase slightly by blurring or adding noise. Cropping of the data if feet-head direction to 1/3 reduced the reliability to 85%. A reduced accuracy was observed by introducing geometrical distortions or simulating patient movement.

In the different data experiments, the match results were consistently different from the ground truth match, i.e., there existed a significant systematic error component. An accuracy of better than 1 mm and a visually correct result is obtained only when registration is limited to pixels that contain bone tissue. However, this procedure results in an extremely poor reliability of 13-15%. The small width of the bony structures and associated small overlap for starting positions more than a few mm away from the correct match may be the cause of this problem. The next best performance (2mm reproducibility and 94% reliability) is obtained when excluding air pixels and removing the table. The influence of the air pixels is probably due to the significant distortions of the skin surface due to normal day to day differences in bladder filling. Removing bowel contrast or the (mobile) femurs had no effect (Fig. 1). Better results were obtained using surface registration of the segmented pelvis.

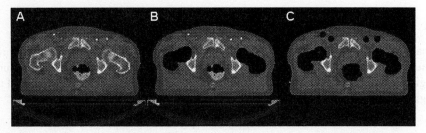

Figure 1. Example of the manual editing process applied in the tests with different data to 17 scan pairs. A) Original slice. B) Femurs removed. The painted region is excluded from the cost function evaluation. C) Bowel (middle) and lymph node (top) contrast removed. Also the table (bottom) was removed. These adaptations hardly improve rms volume registration.

4 Conclusions

Volume registration by minimizing rms pixel value differences is highly robust for local image artifacts. However, the accuracy decreases in the presence of global distortions and organ motion. For this reason, volume registration is not very well suited for accurate rigid registration of pelvic CT. The best results in terms of accuracy, but with a poor reliability, are obtained when limiting the registration to bone pixels only. The next best results (about 2 mm accuracy and 90% reliability) are obtained when excluding air pixels and the table structure. Bowel contrast and the presence of femur movement are not responsible for the poor performance.

A Maximum Likelihood Approach for 2-D to 3-D Registration

Jay B. West, Rasool Khadem, Shao Chin, and Ramin Shahidi

Cbyon Inc., 2275 E. Bayshore Road #101, Palo Alto, CA 94303

Abstract. In this paper, we examine the problem of point-based registration in which a pair of two-dimensional projective views of an object is used to reconstruct the three-dimensional position of given points within the object. The particular application we consider is that of integrating preoperative, three-dimensional information, for example that provided by a CT scan, with the two-dimensional information given by intraoperative fluoroscopy. To facilitate registration, before the preoperative scan we embed small, removable spheres in the patient's anatomy proximal to the site of proposed surgery; the spheres remain in place until the image-guided phase of the operation is complete.

1 Introduction

Once the three dimensional position of the fiducial spheres in physical space has been calculated, the image-to-physical registration step is treated as a simple rigid-body, point-based problem. There is a well-known closed-form solution [1] that gives the rotation and translation which minimizes the sum of squared distances between corresponding points in image and physical space.

We present here a refinement to the traditional method of reconstructing the three-dimensional physical positions of the spheres from the two projective views. Using a maximum likelihood approach linked to a statistical error model for localizing the projections of the spheres in the fluoroscope images, we show how to derive the most likely configuration of the spheres in physical space.

2 Methods

Fluoroscopic images are formed when X-rays are emitted from a source, pass through an object, and are captured by an image intensifier on the other side of the object. By localizing the projection of one of the fiducial spheres in a fluoroscope image, we infer that the physical location of the sphere is at some point on the line joining the source to the point on the image intensifier corresponding to the sphere's projection. If there were no distortion in the images, and if we could localize the projections of the spheres with perfect accuracy, the physical space localization problem would be reduced to that of taking two fluoroscope images at different orientations and finding the intersections of the spheres' projection lines.

W. Niessen and M. Viergever (Eds.): MICCAI 2001, LNCS 2208, pp. 1283–1284, 2001.

We use a calibration jig containing spheres in a known configuration in order to correct for the "pincushion" and ambient magnetic field related distortion common in fluoroscope images. However, because of the finite pixel size and digital nature of the images, it is not possible to localize perfectly the projections of the fiducial spheres. We assume that, for each of the spheres in each of the projections, the distances of the localized positions from the true positions are drawn from a Gaussian distribution with zero mean and standard deviation σ.

Assuming that the X-ray source is at a distance f from the image intensifier, and letting z represent the distance of a fiducial sphere from the source, we have that the localized position of a sphere at this distance from the source is distributed about the true position with a Gaussian distribution having zero mean and standard deviation $\sigma z/f$. If we denote by L_1 and L_2 the derived lines between the projections of the spheres in each view and the source, the traditional approach is to write the three dimensional position of the sphere as the center point of the line P perpendicular to, and joining, L_1 and L_2. Instead, we choose the point that maximizes the product of the probability density functions. From intuitive geometry, it is clear that the optimal choice of point will lie on P. We let z_1 be the distance from the source of the intersection of P with L_1, and z_2 the same for L_2. We write D as length of the line P. Then we wish to choose a point on P at distance d from the intersection of P and L_1 to minimize

$$exp(-d^2 f^2/2\sigma^2 z_1^2)exp(-(D-d)^2 f^2/2\sigma^2 z_2^2). \tag{1}$$

Simple calculus reveals that the optimal choice of d is

$$d = z_1^2/(z_1^2 + z_2^2). \tag{2}$$

3 Conclusion

We have introduced a refinement to the traditional method of reconstructing three dimensional information from a pair of projective views. We have shown that this method may be used to give the most likely spatial positions of fiducial spheres, thus allowing a potential improvement in the registration of three dimensional preoperative images to the physical space of the operating room when intraoperative fluoroscopy is used. In practice, this refinement may give an improvement of the order of 2 mm in localization accuracy.

References

1. P. H. Schönemann, "A generalized solution of the orthogonal Procrustes problem", *Psychometrika*, vol. 31, pp. 1–10, 1966.

How to Trade Off between Regularization and Image Similarity in Non-rigid Registration ?

Pascal Cachier

Projet Epidaure, INRIA, Sophia-Antipolis, France
Pascal.Cachier@inria.fr

1 Introduction

In this work, we propose a new subdivision of intensity-based non-rigid registration algorithms composed of two classes:

Standard Intensity Based (SIB) algorithms. In these algorithms, the same transformation is used to compute the intensity similarity measure while being constrained to remain smooth.

Pair-and-Smooth (P&S) algorithms. These algorithms proceed in two steps, which may alternate or not. In the first step, they look for corresponding points, using the intensity similarity measure. In the second step, they approximate these pairings using a smooth non-rigid transformation. Block-matching, optical flow based and ICP based algorithms belong to this class.

The underlying fundamental difference with SIB registration is that the smoothness of the estimated transformation is balanced with a *geometric* measure (i.e. a distance with the corresponding features found during the first step) instead of an *intensity* measure. This has a strong impact on the smoothness of the registration, which we study in the case of competitive registration.

2 Comparison of Competitive SIB and P&S Algorithms

Competitive algorithms, as defined in [1], use an additional energy E_{reg} (e.g. the linear elastic energy) to regularize the estimation problem on top of the intensity similarity energy E_{sim}. In the case of competitive SIB algorithms, the registration is done by minimizing the weighted sum $E(I, J, T) = E_{sim}(I, J, T) + \lambda E_{reg}(T)$: a trade-off is made between two quantities with different physical dimensions, a geometric measure (E_{reg}) and an intensity measure (E_{sim}). The intensity similarity is related to the amount of *change in the intensity* necessary to go from one image to the other, which is not uniformly proportional to the amount of *motion* necessary to deform one image to the other. Consequently, smoothness largely depends on the local variation of the similarity measure, and so on the local contrast of the image.

On the other hand, competitive P&S algorithms alternate between finding corresponding features (generally points) using the intensity similarity, and smoothing these pairings. The trade-off here is done during the second step, between geometric quantities : this explains why in practice the smoothness of the solutions found by P&S algorithms are much more uniform and controllable.

W. Niessen and M. Viergever (Eds.): MICCAI 2001, LNCS 2208, pp. 1285–1286, 2001.

2.1   Experiment

We have registered a synthetically deformed image with Asym and PASHA algorithms. Asym is a SIB algorithm that minimizes the following classical energy using a gradient descent: $E(I, J, T, \lambda) = \int (I - J \circ T)^2 + \lambda \int ||dT||^2$. PASHA is a P&S algorithm that minimizes the following hybrid energy, introduced in [1] for P&S registration: $E(I, J, C, T) = \int (I - J \circ T)^2 + \sigma \int ||C - T||^2 + \sigma\lambda \int ||dT||^2$. We have run the experiment with a large range of parameters, and kept the result minimizing the average error for both algorithms (fig. 1).

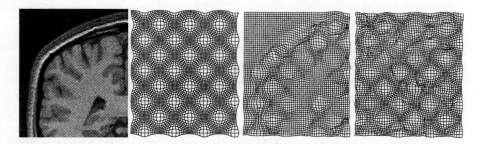

Fig. 1. Left to right: the test image , the synthetic deformation applied to it, and the best result achievable with Asym and PASHA.

With Asym the smoothness of the transformation is non-uniform because of the inhomogeneity of the trade-off: the transformation is almost not estimated on plain areas of the image, while still irregular on the edges in the image. Its average distance to the original transformation is only 1.27 pixel. With PASHA, the quality of the estimation is very uniform, which enables a 35% smaller average distance of 0.83 pixel.

2.2   Two Priors for Non-rigid Registration

PASHA has two parameters σ and λ, corresponding to two separate priors: the level of noise in the image and the smoothness of the transformation. In the classical approach there is only one regularization parameter, which theoretically accounts only for an image noise prior. Unfortunately, in practice it is hardly so: for example, in the previous experiment, best results are obtained for moderate regularization strengths while the images are virtually noiseless. Using two priors enable to separate image reliability and transformation smoothness. We show in [1] that this enables quantitatively better results, whatever the level of noise in the images or the smoothness of the transformation.

References

1. P. Cachier and N. Ayache. Regularization in Image Non-Rigid Registration: I. Trade-Off between Smoothness and Similarity. Technical Report RR-4188, INRIA, 2001. http://www.inria.fr/rrrt/index.en.html.

A Virtual Exploring Robot for Adaptive Left Ventricle Contour Detection in Cardiac MR Images

F. Behloul, B.P.F. Lelieveldt, R.J. van der Geest, J.H.C. Reiber

Div. of Image Processing, Dept of Radiology, C2S, Leiden University Medical Center,
P.O. Box 9600, 2300 RC, Leiden, The Netherlands
F.Behloul@lumc.nl

Abstract. This paper presents an original knowledge driven automatic contour detection approach based on neuro-fuzzy techniques. The method simulates a trained virtual autonomous mobile robot that delineates the organ outlines by combining local image information and global a-priori shape knowledge. In a pilot validation study into left ventricular delineation in cardiac MR images, our novel method demonstrated a high robustness, and a clinically acceptable border localization performance.

1   Introduction

Automatic Left Ventricle (LV) contour detection methods encounter two major problems: (i) Manual expert contours do not always coincide with the location of the strongest local image features (the LV ENDO border is a convex hull around the blood pool), somewhat 'outside' of the strongest edge. (ii) Due to noise and image artifacts in routinely acquired clinical images, a-priori knowledge about the shape *and* image appearance of the LV is essential to achieve robust localization performance.

   We incorporate a-priori shape and appearance knowledge and local information in the simulation and training of a virtual autonomous mobile robot that delineates fully automatically the LV.

2   General Outline of the Method

Our virtual robot is a tri-cycle with a steering front wheel (see Figure 1.a). The robot is subject to non-holonomic kinematic constraints: it can move only along a direction perpendicular to its rear wheel axis (continuous tangent direction) and its turning radius is lower bounded (maximum curvature). The car has a maximum curvature constraint; this provides us with an easy means to go around the papillary muscles (see figure 1.b).

   The robot is provided with range sensors, mounted on its front, left and right sides. They are simulated by rays of limited length, launched from the robot in different directions. The range sensors enable the robot to estimate the distance to the myocardium borders.

   The robot has to navigate around the LV cavity. To isolate the cavities from the background, a fuzzy clustering algorithm is used followed by a region growing. The gray levels are automatically grouped into 3 clusters: very bright (cavities), bright (myocardium) and dark (background). By setting the initial position of the robot outside the LV cavity and the target point inside the LV, the robot navigates around the LV cavity in a wall tracking-mode looking for an opening. Since the cavity is closed, the robot will accomplish a complete loop and stop.

W. Niessen and M. Viergever (Eds.): MICCAI 2001, LNCS 2208, pp. 1287-1288, 2001.

While navigating, the robot delineates the LV contours and distinguishes the septal wall (between left and right ventricular cavities) from the lateral wall. The recognition of septal and lateral wall segments is realized by sampling local image patches of the robot's environment as a grid of 3x3 regions. Each region is characterized by 3 membership degrees to the fuzzy sets: background, myocardium and cavity. The robot uses a trained fuzzy neural network to classify its local patch of image into septum or lateral. The neural network was trained on image data from 21 normal subjects.

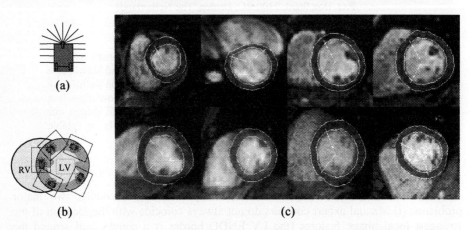

(a)

(b)   (c)

Fig. 1. (a) Tric-cycle model with range sensors (b) Navigation environment in short axis images of the heart. (c) LV contour delineation by the exploring robot. The septum is automatically delimited by the 2 lines going from the cavity to the myocardium.

3   Results and Discussion

The three end-diastolic mid-ventricular slices of 16 normal subjects and 7 infarct patients were considered. An expert observer was asked to draw the LV contours.

The average signed (AS) and root mean square (RMS) border positioning errors were calculated for the ENDO and EPI borders by measuring the distances between corresponding border points along 100 rays perpendicular to the centerline between the manual and the automatic contour. In addition, two clinically important area measures were calculated: ENDO area (cm^2) and EPI area (cm^2).

The automatic detected borders agreed very closely with the manually identified contours (see Figure 1.c). For the endocardium, the AS error was -0.56 ± 1.78 mm and the RMS error was 1.77 ± 0.6 mm. For the epicardium, the AS error was -0.2 ± 2.1 mm and the RMS error was 1.93 ± 0.84 mm. A good correlation was found between the observer's and the robot's LV ENDO and EPI areas (y=1.08*x-0.63, r = 0.89 and y=1.02 *x–0.99, r=0.89). Average paired difference in area measures amounted to – 1.1 ± 1.84 cm^2 and 0.36 ± 2.8 cm^2 for ENDO and EPI contours, respectively, indicating a very slight, but clinically acceptable, overestimation of the LV ENDO area. Our approach has been easily generalized to the image time-series from end-diastole to end-systole. It showed very high robustness to LV shape variation and deformation.

A Mesh-Based Shape Analysis Framework

Jean-José Jacq[1,2] and Christian Roux[1,2]

[1] Département Image et Traitement de l'Information
ENST Bretagne, Technopôle de Brest-Iroise, B.P. 832 - 29285 Brest - France
[2] Laboratoire de Traitement de l'Information Médicale (ERM 0102 INSERM)
CHU Morvan, 5 Avenue Foch, 29200 Brest - France
{JJ.Jacq, Christian.Roux}@enst-bretagne.fr

Abstract. We propose an efficient and non-parametric hierarchical partitioning approach that operates on a general 3D shape. The method suggested makes it possible to process an arbitrary shape provided that it can be described as a triangle mesh. The basic idea is to extend the use of the basin districts concept on curved spaces - such a partitioning process being applied on valuation issued from the computation of main curvatures over a polyhedral support. Hierarchical construction of basin districts is obtained from a Watershed Transform. In our working case, an efficient use of this well known transformation implies to be able to manage front propagations on a polyhedral surface with speed controled by the local characteristics of surface geometry. Moreover, the ability to provide an intrinsic shape partition from any triangle mesh lead us to propose a robust extension to usual mesh simplification algorithms.

Extended Summary

The aim of this work is to provide an interactive, time efficient, flexible and unified set of cooperative shape partitioning tools. As the ultimate goal is to make it possible to an expert (physician, scientist, ...) to separate semi-interactively the major components of a shape, this work also refers to it as a *shape dissection* process. As a result, the common characteristic of the overall process we retained, is to work *directly* on triangle mesh without any global reparameterization. Although involving additional complexity, this generic approach offers two main advantages. On the one hand, as a triangle mesh is a shape representation commonly handled by any infographic system, the interactive use of the algorithms is guaranteed. On the other hand, processing without an intermediate reparameterization makes it possible to process complex biological shapes exhibiting an arbitrary topology.

Although innovating [1, 2, 3], the main idea developed in this work is rather simple. If a Watershed Transform can be defined on a polyhedral support, then a *global* and *hierarchical* partition of the support can be performed. If these valuations are defined as functions of the local curvatures, the partition can be made *intrinsic* to the shape. Another key aspect of this shape partition approach is that it does not imply a very noise sensitive analysis through third order derivatives. Accordingly, it does not require the knowledge of the directions of the principal curvatures. So, the heart of this approach is mainly related to the extension of the immersion simulation [4] on unstructured meshes and involves, in particular, the ability to manage front propagations while solving the Eikonal equation on triangulated domains [5].

W. Niessen and M. Viergever (Eds.): MICCAI 2001, LNCS 2208, pp. 1289-1290, 2001.
© Springer-Verlag Berlin Heidelberg 2001

In order to get an operational framework, this working scheme requires a set of *coprocessing tools* operating directly on a triangulated domain. These tools are also studied here. The main requirement is to be able to manage common signal or image processing tasks (resampling, filtering, computing second order derivatives and geodesic distances) on a polyhedral support while presenting an optimal trade-off between accuracy and efficiency. This analysis framework is embedded in a standard 3-D infographic environment (OpenGL). Figure 1 depicts the full interactive framework when applied to analysis of articular surfaces of a fossil talus bone – this dissection case is based on torsion energy. The whole of the processing steps results depicted by Fig. 1, were obtained interactively from an Apple PowerBook G3.

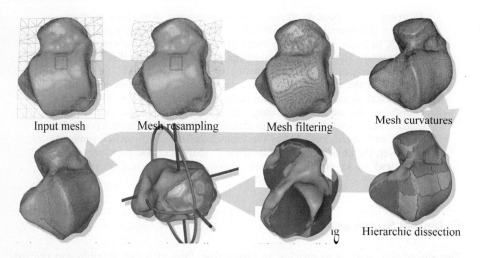

Fig. 1. A mesh-processing framework focusing on hierarchical dissection of anatomical shapes.

References

1. Jacq, J.J.: Partitionnement de Surfaces par Morphologie Géodésique. Application à la morphométrie Interactive du Complexe Péri-talien. In: *Attelier Traitement et Analyse des Images, Méthodes et Applications, TAIMA'99*, 23-26 Mars. 1999, Hammamet, Tunisie.
2. Jacq, J.J., Roux, C., Couture, C.: Segmentation morphologique géodésique de surfaces. Application à la morphométrie interactive des surfaces articulaires en anthropologie. In: *17 ième colloque GRETSI sur le Traitement du Signal et des Images*, 13-17 Sept. 1999, Vannes., 39-42
3. Jacq, J.J., Roux, C.: Hierarchical Shape Dissection Through Front Propagation on Triangle Mesh with Applications. 2001 (*Submitted*)
4. Vincent, L., Soille, P.: Watersheds in Digital Spaces: an Efficient Algorithm Based on Immersion Simulations. *IEEE Trans. on Pattern Analysis and Machine Intelligence*, Vol. 13, No. 6, Jun. 1991, 583-598
5. Sethian, J.A.: *Level Set Methods and Fast Marching Methods*. Cambridge University Press, Aug. 1999, 378p

Acknowledgement. This work has been supported by a grant (99B406) from the French Administration of Research and Technology.

Clinical MRI Based Volumetry: The Cerebral Ventricles

Horst K. Hahn[1], Markus G. Lentschig[2], Burckhard Terwey[2], and Heinz-Otto Peitgen[1]

[1] MeVis – Center for Medical Diagnostic Systems and Visualization,
Universitaetsallee 29, 28359 Bremen, Germany, Email: hahn@mevis.de
[2] Institut für Magnetresonanz-Diagnostik, ZKH St.-Jürgen-Straße, Bremen, Germany

Keywords: Neuroimaging, MRI, volumetry, CSF, ventricles, three-dimensional segmentation, histogram analysis, partial volume effects

1 Introduction

Cerebral ventricular volume is an important factor in quantifying various neurological diseases and in neurosurgical therapy monitoring. We describe a method to efficiently segment and visualize the intracerebral fluid spaces based on MRI and to reproducibly quantify their volumes. At present, no system is available for routine clinical use which is (1) *fast* (less than 10 min for image analysis), (2) *flexible* (robust for normal and pathological anatomy), and (3) *reproducible* (less than 5 % relative variation).

2 Methods

The method presented combines acquisition of thin slices, fast 3D marker-based segmentation, and automatic histogram analysis. T1-weighted anatomic data is acquired on a 1.5 T Siemens Magnetom Vision (Figure 1): MPRAGE, TR 9.7 ms, TE 4.0 ms, flip angle 20 deg, sagittal, FOV 256 mm, matrix 256×256, 160 slices, slice thickness 1.0 mm, acquisition time approx. 8 min. The segmentation algorithm is based on a fast watershed transformation as described in [1]. Additionally, five different marker types are used for ventricle labeling (R, L, 3, and 4) and region exclusion, thereby imposing watersheds at respective borders. The watershed transformation takes approx. 1 sec on a standard PC for a typical region of interest (1 million voxels). It automatically tracks the ventricular boundaries in 3D, taking the marker positions into account. In a standard case, 10 markers suffice to define the ventricular anatomy accurately. The complete segmentation procedure, including user interactions, takes an average of 2 min for all slices.

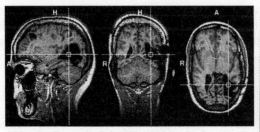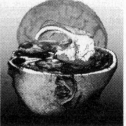

Fig. 1. Patient (F, 29 yrs), postoperative data. **left.** Original data. **right.** Ventricular segmentation result fused with segmented brain and original data. Total ventricular volume: 54.6±0.6 ml.

W. Niessen and M. Viergever (Eds.): MICCAI 2001, LNCS 2208, pp. 1291-1292, 2001.
© Springer-Verlag Berlin Heidelberg 2001

Table 1. Evaluation of total reproducibility on a healthy volunteer (M, 38 yrs) who underwent five separate MRI scans with 30 min rest between acquisitions (V_1–V_5). Volumes in ml.

	V_1	V_2	V_3	V_4	V_5	mean $\pm$ SD	SD/mean	$V_6^\dagger$
right	17.96	17.83	17.73	18.01	17.83	17.87 $\pm$ 0.11	0.63 %	17.84
left	14.37	14.26	14.06	14.37	14.23	14.26 $\pm$ 0.13	0.88 %	14.59‡
3rd	2.22	1.99	2.07	2.17	2.00	2.09 $\pm$ 0.10	4.80 %	2.01
4th	2.64	2.75	2.60	2.74	2.78	2.70 $\pm$ 0.08	2.82 %	2.84
total	37.16	36.95	36.42	37.25	36.98	36.95 $\pm$ 0.32	0.87 %	37.33
lateral	32.33	32.12	31.79	32.39	32.12	32.15 $\pm$ 0.24	0.74 %	32.48

† acquired 2 months later   ‡ significantly enlarged left ventricle

A model based histogram analysis robustly accounts for image noise, non-uniformity, and partial volume effects. The volumes of each of the four segmented ventricles are computed automatically from corresponding over-inclusive regional image histograms. Assuming symmetric, equally distributed partial voluming, we introduce a set of mixed Gaussians to extend the trimodal normal distribution model. Least squared error minimization is used to fit the model. The expected volumetric uncertainties are calculated individually, based on image quality.

3   Results and Discussion

We thoroughly evaluated inter- and intraobserver variance as well as reproducibility for the complete system. Mean values and standard deviations have been recorded. The variance between raters for lateral ventricular volumes is less than 0.5 %. With independently repeated acquisitions on patients and healthy volunteers, reproducibility has been excellent, with relative deviations less than 1 % (Table 1). Larger variations are observed for 3rd and 4th ventricles due to small object sizes and the frequently imprecise delineations in MRI. Repeated acquisitions on a ventricle shaped paraffin phantom yielded a relative standard deviation of 0.4 % for the total volume (Mean $\pm$ SD: 60.89 $\pm$ 0.22 ml).

We present a new semiautomatic approach which speeds up image analysis while improving reproducibility and accuracy compared to manual or semiautomatic slice-based evaluation [2]. User-induced errors are minimized by placing markers inside the objects instead of tracing object borders interactively. The 3D segmentation procedure is equally applicable to normal and pathological anatomy (Figure 1), since it does not require an anatomical model. Furthermore, contralateral differences are directly quantified.

Accurate measurements are achieved on commonly available high-resolution T1-weighted MR images. Image fusion and higher dimensional histogram analysis were avoided. Combining short interaction times, applicability to pathological anatomy, and high reproducibility, the presented method meets the requirements posed by imaging and workflow conditions in a clinical setting.

References

1. H. K. Hahn and H.-O. Peitgen. The Skull Stripping Problem In MRI Solved By A Single 3D Watershed Transform. *MICCAI* (Pittsburgh, Oct 2000), *LNCS*, Springer, Berlin: 134–143.
2. A. Tsunoda, H. Mitsuoka, K. Sato et al. A Quantitative Index of Intracranial Cerebrospinal Fluid Distribution in Normal Pressure Hydrocephalus. *Neuroradiology* 42: 424–429, 2000.

The Importance of Partial Voluming in Multi-dimensional Medical Image Segmentation

Maja Pokrić, Neil Thacker, Marietta L.J. Scott, and Alan Jackson

Imaging Science and Biomedical Engineering
School of Medicine
University of Manchester
Manchester M13 9PT, UK
maja.pokric@man.ac.uk

Abstract. The presented method addresses the problem of multi-spectral image segmentation through use of a model which takes into account partial volumes of tissues being present in a single voxel at boundaries. The parameters of the multi-dimensional model of pure tissues and their mixtures are iteratively adjusted using an Expectation Maximisation (EM) optimisation technique. Bayes theory is used to generate probability maps for each segmented tissue which estimates the most likely *tissue volume fraction* within each voxel.

A common approach for medical image segmentation involves modelling only pure tissue intensity distributions. However, the accurate interpretation of the data requires that partial volume distributions for a mixture of tissues that can be present in any given voxel must be modelled [1]. Knowledge of the physics of image formation in a wide variety of medical image data allows that partial volume distributions for paired tissue combinations can be modelled as a linear process. Hence, we adopted approach whereby the pure tissues have been modelled using a multi-dimensional Gaussian distribution, while mixtures of tissues take the novel form of a triangular distribution convolved with a Gaussian. A multi-variate Gaussian distribution for multi-dimensional data $\mathbf{g}$ for each pure tissue t is defined as:

$$d_t(\mathbf{g}) \; = \; \alpha_t e^{-(\mathbf{g}-\mathbf{M_t})^T C_t (\mathbf{g}-\mathbf{M_t})}$$

where: (i) $\mathbf{M_t}$ is a mean tissue vector; (ii) C_t is an inverse of covariance matrix; (iii) α_t is a constant which gives unit normalisation. Multi-dimensional partial volume distributions is modelled along the line between two pure tissue means $\mathbf{M_t}$ and $\mathbf{M_s}$:

$$d_{ts}(\mathbf{g}) \; = \; \beta_{ts} T_{ts}(h) e^{-(\mathbf{g}-\mathbf{h}\cdot\mathbf{g}/|\mathbf{h}|)^T C_h (\mathbf{g}-\mathbf{h}\cdot\mathbf{g}/|h|)}$$

where: (i) h is a fractional distance between two centres of distribution $[0 < h < 1]$, $h = (\mathbf{g} - \mathbf{M_s})C_h(\mathbf{M_t} - \mathbf{M_s})/|(\mathbf{M_t} - \mathbf{M_s})C_h(\mathbf{M_t} - \mathbf{M_s})|$; (ii) $T_{ts}(h)$ is the 1D partial volume distribution for tissue t generated by partial voluming process

W. Niessen and M. Viergever (Eds.): MICCAI 2001, LNCS 2208, pp. 1293–1294, 2001.

1294   M. Pokrić et al.

with tissue s (iii) C_h is an inverse covariance matrix, $C_h = C_t h + C_s(1-h)$; (iv) β_{ts} is a constant which gives unit normalisation.

Parameters of the model can be iteratively estimated using the Expectation Maximisation (EM) approach [2,3]. EM is used to estimate the parameters by maximising the likelihood of the data distribution. This involves first getting from the likelihood distributions defined above to a probability of a given tissue proportion given the data $P(t|\mathbf{g_v})$. The conditional probability of a grey level being due to a certain mechanism n (either a pure or mixture tissue component) can be calculated using Bayes theory, as follows:

$$P(n|\mathbf{g}) = \frac{d_n(\mathbf{g})f_n}{f_0 + \sum_t d_t(\mathbf{g})f_t + \sum_t \sum_s d_{ts}(\mathbf{g})f_{ts}}$$

where f_n, f_0, f_t and f_{ts} are effectively "priors", expressed here as frequencies (i.e. number of voxels) which belong to a particular tissue type, pure tissues or partial volumes. Unknown tissues are accounted for in the Bayesian formulation by including a fixed extra term f_o for infrequently occuring outlier data in total probability which enables separation of pathological tissues. The EM approach has been applied for the estimation of model parameters for pure and mixture tissues:

$$f_t' = \sum_v^V P(t|\mathbf{g}_v) \qquad and \qquad f_{ts}' = f_{st}' = \frac{1}{2}\sum_v^V P(ts|\mathbf{g}_v) + P(st|\mathbf{g}_v)$$

$$M_t' = \frac{1}{V}\sum_v^V P(t|\mathbf{g}_v)\mathbf{g}_v \qquad and \qquad C_t'^{-1} = \frac{1}{V}\sum_v^V P(t|\mathbf{g}_v)(\mathbf{g}_v-\mathbf{G_t})\otimes(\mathbf{g}_v-\mathbf{G_t})^T$$

The **E**-step recalculates multi-dimensional probability densities, while the **M**-step involves re-estimation of model parameters. Multi-spectral segmentation was performed for six different tissue classes on four co-registred MRI images by applying E- and M-steps in turns. It has been found that the algorithm converges within 10 iterations and that a partial volume model accounts for almost half of data present. This highlighs the importance of inclusion of that part of a model. Inclusion of a partial volume model leads to better visual appearance of segmented tissues as voxels are not simply classified as a single tissue, which causes artifacts at tissue boundaries. This in turn enables creation of better geometric models to be used in simulation and visualisation. This method can be applied on any sequence of images for which the linearity assumption holds.

References

1. Laidlaw, D.H., Fleischer, K.W., Barr, A.H.: Partial-volume Bayesian Classification of Material Mixtures in MR Volume Data Using Voxel Histograms. IEEE Trans. Med. Imag. **17**(1) (1998) 74–86
2. Dempster, A.P.,Laird, N.M., Rubin, D.B.: Maximum Likelihood from Incomplete Data via EM Algorithm. Journal of the Royal Society **39** (1977) 1–38
3. Guillemaud, R., Brady, J.M.: Estimating the bias Field of MR Images. IEEE TRANS. on Medical Imaging **16**(3) (1997) 238–251

Volume Definition Tools for Medical Imaging Applications

Grigoris Karangelis[1], Stelios Zimeras[2], Evelyn Firle[1],
Min Wang[1] , Georgios Sakas[1]

[1] Institut für Graphische Daten Verarbeitung-IGD, Fraunhofer, Darmstadt, Germany
{karangel, efirle, mwang, gsakas}@igd.fhg.de
[2] MedCom GmbH, Darmstadt, Germany.
szimeras@medcom-online.de

Abstract. Central focus of this work, are techniques used to improve time and interaction needed for a user when defining one or more structures. These techniques involve interpolation methods for the manual volume definition and methods for the semi-automatic organ shape extraction.

1   Introduction

In this work we will present a number of methods that improve the time and interaction one needs to define one or more structures. These techniques involve interpolation methods for the manual volume definition and methods for the semi-automatic organ shape extraction. In the next section the interpolation techniques for the manual volume definition would be described. The methods for the automatic shape extraction of structures are located in section 3, and their comparison in section 4. The work concludes with the discussion section.

2   Manual Volume Definition

The manual volume definition is the most common and traditional way to define contours. Usually the user has the possibility to create a contour line using discrete or continuous points. In most systems, the volume definition tools can be applied only on the original, usually axial direction, although images on orthogonal reconstructed planes are provided as well.

Linear Interpolation: Linear interpolation between contours is the first approach used to provide an acceleration tool for the manual contouring. The mechanism of the linear interpolation is applied when between the key contours at least one slice exists. To perform the linear interpolation we create triangles between the contour points of the key contours as described in [1]. For this operation both contour's points must be rotated towards the same rotation direction. The interpolated contour points are created after calculating the intersection of each triangle side with the intermediate slice.

Orthogonal Contour Interpolation: The orthogonal contour interpolation serves to create a volume combining and interpolating orthogonal drawn contours. Principally the algorithm needs at least 2 orthogonal contours to work. The perpendicular plane to these two contours creates intersection points that are the key points to create the new

W. Niessen and M. Viergever (Eds.): MICCAI 2001, LNCS 2208, pp. 1295-1297, 2001.

interpolated contour. In this approach we use the cubic Spine interpolation. In case the lines are completely equal in size and their centres match or have very small distance then the result of the interpolation will be a circle. In any other case that the two vertical lines are unequal the result will be an ellipse.

3 Automatic Contouring

Regarding segmentation techniques, several contour and region approaches have been proposed [3]. The former, are often less robust and more sensitive to noise and variability of data. Hence we will describe and compare in the following section different tools for semi-automatic contouring. For the visual comparison of the semi-automatic techniques, the EXOMIO[1] virtual simulation package was used.

Boundary tracking technique: Boundary tracking techniques is a segmentation method, that given one point along a region's boundary follows the boundary around the region until it returns to the original point. The advantage is that no assumptions need be made a priori about the boundary shape. The algorithm starts with an initial point. Different starting directions are defined until a sharp edge was found. The tracking procedure stops only when passing through the starting point in the original contour direction.

Active Contour Model: Active Contour Models (ACMs) are adaptive contour representations, also known as snakes or deformable models. They are able to recover and represent physical contours of an image, and hence can be used as a model to determine object boundaries in static images as well as for tracking in image sequences. Grosskopf et al. [4] uses the Euler Time Integration to solve the optimisation problem. After initialisation by a user sketch, the contour is deformed to fit the actual object by simulating physical properties of an elastic material or fluid. This method is very reliable to overcome local minima and very fast due to its deterministic character.

4 Comparison of the Semi-automatic Methods

Materials and Measures: The two proposed contouring methods have been applied for a CT tomographic sequence of 8 bit gray scale images of a size 512x512 in which change the shape, and the orientation of the objects.   In this work, segmentation results would be presented for three different regional objects: (a) concave (lungs), (b) convex (lungs), (c) large (skin), (d) small (marrow of the spinal canal). To assess the effectiveness of the methods and its sensitivity, the following object measures are considered: (1) area of a contour, and (2) periphery of a contour.

Segmentation results: The visual comparison of the segmented areas between the boundary tracking (green line-2) and the active contour (red line-1) methods are given in Figure 1 for all the different regions. It is clear that for large segmented areas (Figure 1c) and convex regions (Figure 1b) both methods gives satisfactory results. The contour edges are defined approximate correctly with few false alarm for the active contour technique due to the edge over-smoothness of the process. Different results was found in cases where the areas are concave (Figure 1a) or small and open

---

[1] http://www.medcom-online.de/

(Figure 1d). For the first case, the segmentation using the active contour method is unsatisfactory compared with the boundary tracking method. The regions, where sharp edges were appeared, were over-smoothed or disappeared. For the second case, segmentation results suggest that when the areas are small and open the boundary tracking technique was unable to find the appropriate region with false identification of the areas. Alternatively, the active contour technique gives satisfactory results, where the shape of the region was defined correctly.

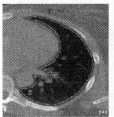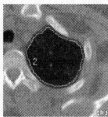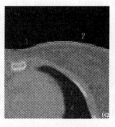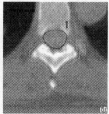

Fig. 1. Visual comparison for different regions; Red line (1): Active contour method, Green line (2): Boundary tracking method. (a) concave (lungs), (b) convex (lungs), (c) large (skin), (d) small (spinal canal marrow).

5   Discussion

In this work different volume definition techniques has been presented. In the first part we present interpolation techniques aim to accelerate the manual contouring process. That includes the well-known linear interpolation technique implemented for simple bisection organ shapes. In addition we introduce a new interpolation method, the orthogonal interpolation, which enables the user to define a volume. At the second part, two contour tracking techniques has been analysed; a boundary tracking and an active contour method. The algorithms have been tested on different regions. For large and convex regions both methods work satisfactory. For concave regions, boundary tracking technique works better compared to the active contour technique. Areas with discontinuities and sharp edges are defined successfully for the boundary tracking method where for the active contour a few false edges are presented. Finally, for small and open regions, active contour method was able to segment the areas, where the boundary tracking method fails.

6   References

1. Ekoule A, Peyrin F.: A Traingulation Algorithm from Arbitrary Shaped Multiple Planar Contours, ACM Trans. On Graphics, Vol. 10, 1991.
2. Haralick R. M. and Shapiro L. G.: Image segmentation techniques, *Comput. Vis. Graph. Im. Proc.*, 29:100-132, 1985.
3. Großkopf S, Park SY, and Kim MH: An improved Active Contour Model for Segmentation of Medical Images, Proc. *3rd Korea-Germany Joint Conference on Advanced Medical Image Processing*, Seoul, Korea, 1998.

Automated Hippocampal Segmentation by Regional Fluid Registration of Serial MRI: Validation and Application in Alzheimer's Disease

Rachael I. Scahill, William R. Crum, Nick C. Fox

Dementia Research Group, Institute of Neurology, 8-11 Queen Square, London, WC1N
3BG United Kingdom
rscahill@dementia.ion.ucl.ac.uk

Voxel-level three-dimensional fluid registration was used to propagate hippocampal segmentation from baseline MR scans onto follow-up scans. In this way automated measurements of hippocampal volume and volume changes were derived. The objective was to compare this technique with the current gold standard of manual segmentation. Serial measurements were performed on 15 normal controls and 12 Alzheimer's disease (AD) subjects. Hippocampal regions on the rigidly-registered repeat scans were generated both by manual segmentation and fluid registration. There was no significant difference between the repeat volumes generated by the two methods (p<0.001), with the mean absolute volume difference being 4.6%. Fluid registration is fully automated and has the potential to track longitudinal structural changes in the hippocampus with application to clinical trials in which large numbers of subjects require serial MR measurements.

Introduction

The hippocampus has been a particular focus for volumetric MR studies in AD due to its early involvement in the disease process, and cross-sectional studies have shown AD subjects with hippocampal volumes decreased by 20-40%. Longitudinal studies reduce the problem of inter-individual variability and have shown greater rates of atrophy in AD subjects compared to controls[1]. However, the measurement errors produced by manual segmentation on serial scans may be of a similar magnitude to the changes expected within the structure, thereby reducing discriminating ability. The development of an automated technique to propagate a manually-generated baseline region onto a repeat scan could reduce this measurement error.

"Fluid Registration" is a non-linear matching algorithm which models the morphological changes within the brain as a compressible viscous fluid[2-3]. This study uses fluid registration to automate serial segmentation and quantification of volumetric change in the hippocampus. A comparison is made between this technique and manual segmentation by an experienced operator.

W. Niessen and M. Viergever (Eds.): MICCAI 2001, LNCS 2208, pp. 1298-1299, 2001.

Materials and Methods

Fifteen control subjects and 12 patients diagnosed with probable AD, according to the NINCDS-ADRDA criteria, underwent two MRI assessments with a mean (±SD) interval of 536 (±380) days. Imaging was performed on a 1.5T GE Signa Unit (General Electric Medical Systems, Milwaukee, WI) yielding 124 contiguous 1.5mm thick slices, with in-plane resolution of 128*256. All manual segmentation was performed using the MIDAS software package[4]. A rigid-body 9 degrees of freedom registration was performed on all repeat scans. An experienced operator, blind to subject condition, outlined the right hippocampus on the baseline and registered repeat scans. Following this a local fluid registration[3] was applied to the manually-defined hippocampal region on the baseline scan. A repeat region was generated and the volume change calculated using the Jacobian values.

Results

The mean baseline hippocampal volumes were 2751 (±294) mm^3 in the controls and 2329 (±560) mm^3 in the AD subjects. There was close correlation between the repeat regions generated by manual segmentation and the fluid model (r=0.9, p<0.001), with a mean absolute volume difference of 109 (± 84) mm^3, 4.6% of hippocampal volume.

Discussion

Manual segmentation remains the most widely used technique for the assessment of hippocampal volume in the study of AD. However, it is time-consuming and subject to observer error. Fluid registration is a fully-automated and unbiased technique for generating serial measurements which are consistent with manual segmentation. It could prove a useful tool with the growing application of serial imaging to the assessment of disease progression and monitoring of drug efficacy in clinical trials.

References

1. Jack CR, Petersen RC, Xu Y, O'Brien PC, Smith GE, Ivnik RJ, Tangalos EG and Kokmen E. Rate of medial temporal lobe atrophy in typical aging and Alzheimer's disease. *Neurology* 1998;51(4):993-9
2. Christensen GE, Rabbitt RD and Miller MI. Deformable templates using large deformation kinematics. *IEEE Transactions in Image Processing* 1998;5:1435-1447
3. Freeborough PA and Fox NC. Modeling brain deformation in Alzheimer's disease by fluid registration of serial 3D MR images. *JCAT* 1998;22(5):838-843
4. Freeborough PA, Fox NC and Kitney RI. Interactive algorithms for the segmentation and quantitation of 3-D MRI brain scans. *Computer Methods and Programs in Biomedicine* 1997;53:15-25

A 3D Statistical Shape Model for the Left Ventricle of the Heart

Hui Luo[1] and Thomas O'Donnell[2]

[1] Dept. of CS and Engineering, SUNY Buffalo, Amherst, NY 14260
huiluo@cse.buffalo.edu
[2] Siemens Corporate Research, Princeton, NJ 08540
odonnell@scr.siemens.com

Abstract. We propose a method for creating a 3-D statistical shape model of the left ventricle from sets of sparse 2-D contour inputs. Since the input contours may not delineate consistent portions of the underlying organ from subject to subject, we apply a model-based approach to make associations (landmarks) between training examples. Included is a measure of confidence in these created landmarks. Statistics on the model shape are garnered via principal component analysis. The results of applying the technique to a 14 subject database are presented.

In this paper we describe a method for developing a statistical shape model of the left ventricle (LV) of the heart. We assume the existence of a set of segmented LV instances culled from both patient and volunteer Magnetic Resonance (MR) datasets. The LVs were segmented using the Argus™ tool which draws 2-D contours on individual image slices. Each MR dataset typically has six to seven short axis slices as well as at least one long-axis slice. The datasets provide sparse but adequate coverage of the LV. Note that the positions of the image slices with respect to the LV vary from dataset to dataset. Therefore contours may delineate different sections of the LV and cannot be used directly as landmarks.

Given these inputs, there are two major issues in developing a statistical model of the LV. First, employing a user-defined landmark-based approach can be challenging as well as time consuming because there are very few distinct features in the underlying LV on which to specify such points. Second, since the landmarks may not be directly delineated by the contours, the concept in confidence in the landmarks must be incorporated.

To address the first concern, we manufacture a dense set of landmarks in a semi-automatic way. As mentioned, the LV has very few distinct, easily labeled points; however, there are several overall shape similarities expressed as regions of curvature. We use a model-based approach to interpolate between sparse contours and align the models using the overall shape [O'Donnell00]. Following this we create a dense set of new associations (landmarks) between the model *surfaces* based on a distance metric. Addressing the second concern, the landmarks are averaged using a weighted sum based on a landmark's proximity to its contours. Finally we create a statistical shape model by principle component analysis using these landmarks.

W. Niessen and M. Viergever (Eds.): MICCAI 2001, LNCS 2208, pp. 1300-1301, 2001.
© Springer-Verlag Berlin Heidelberg 2001

Work closest to ours focuses on the problem of generating dense set of landmarks semi-automatically [Lorenz00, Fleute98, Brett00, Park95]. We view our contributions as: 1) a model-based alignment for sparse inputs. 2) the weighting of landmarks which appropriately describes the reliability of each landmark's situation.

Briefly, our approach is to create a template model, align the datasets making use of this template, fit models to each of the aligned datasets, make associations (landmarks) between the model surfaces (again using the template model), and average those landmarks to create a Procrustes mean shape.

The proposed method has been used to generate 3D statistical LV model from pool of 14 subjects. Table 1 illustrates the relative contribution of the most influential components. From this we can see that nearly 90% of the shape variation can be captured by the first nine eigenvectors.

Table 1. Relative contributions of eigenvectors.

Index	$(\lambda_i/\lambda_{total})$	Cumulative total
1	41.3769%	41.3769%
2	10.4376%	51.8144%
3	9.0261%	60.8406%
4	7.5134%	68.3540%
5	6.2111%	74.5651%
6	4.0443%	78.6094%
7	3.9312%	82.5406%
8	3.4228%	85.9634%
9	3.0939%	89.0573%

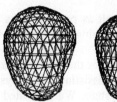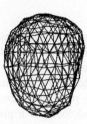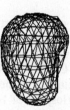

Fig. 1. Leftmost two: The epicardial and endocardial surfaces of the average model. Rightmost two: The result of varying the first mode of variation by three standard deviations.

References

[Fleute98] Fleute M, et. al.,Building a complete surface model from sparse data using statistical shape models: application to computer assisted knee surgery. *MICCAI'98 1998, pp.879-87.*

[Lorenz00] Lorenz C, Krahnstover N. Generation of point-based 3D statistical shape models for anatomical objects. CVIU, *vol.77, no.2, Feb. 2000, pp.175-91.*

[Brett00] Brett AD, Taylor CJ. A method of automated landmark generation for automated 3D PDM construction. *Image & Vision Computing, vol.18, no.9, June 2000, pp.739-48.*

[O'Donnell00] O'Donnell T, et. al., Multi Modality Model-Based Registration. *CVPR00.*

[Park95] Park J, Metaxas D, et. al., Deformable Models with parameter Functions. *CVPR95.*

Robot Assistant for Dental Implantology

R. Boesecke[1], J. Brief[2], J. Raczkowsky[4], O. Schorr[4], S. Daueber[3],
R. Krempien[4], M. Treiber[4], T. Wetter[5] and S. Hassfeld[2]

[1] TaMed GmbH, Hufschmiedstr. ¼, D-69168 Wiesloch, Germany
r.boesecke@praezis.com
[2] Department of Oral and Maxillofacial Surgery, University Hospital Heidelberg
[3] Department of Radiology, University Hospital Heidelberg
[4] Institute of Real-Time Computer Systems & Robotics, University of Karlsruhe
[5] Department of Medical Informatics, University Hospital Heidelberg

Abstract. We introduce a method to apply a preoperative 3D plan for inserting
dental implants with an assisting medical robot. The treatment plan is based on
the 3D visualization of the CT data of the patient's maxilla and mandible, and
supplies the location of the implants in the patient's coordinates. The plan is
then transferred to the surgical robot's coordinate system. The robot guides the
tool, a drill guide. Position, orientation, and depth of the initial drilling is
defined with the tool held by the robot while the surgeon drills. The robot
assists the dentist, and the optimal treatment plan will be applied directly to the
patient.

1 Introduction

The quality of the insertion of dental implants as well as possible risks depend not
only on the surgery planning, but as well on performing the surgery as exact as
possible according to the treatment plan.
Methods of Computer Aided Surgery are used to plan for these parameters. To apply
the so obtained treatment plan, we introduced an assisting robot system at the
University Hospital of Heidelberg as a prototype system. We evaluated the system
accuracy performing 16 operation plans with phantom mandibles.

2 Material and Method

A robot system from Medical Intelligence, Schwabmünchen, Germany, with a reach
of 700 mm was used. The PC based software TomoRob from TaMed, Wiesloch,
Germany, allows for simulation, visualization, and control of the robot. The position
and orientation of the implants was planned based on 3D CT data with TomoRob.
Visualization of the robot, the patient couch, the patient, tools and implants are used
for planning and control of the surgery. The trajectory planning is based on linear
interpolation of start and end point and points between. A collision detection
algorithm is integrated to warn during the computer simulation of the surgery.

W. Niessen and M. Viergever (Eds.): MICCAI 2001, LNCS 2208, pp. 1302-1303, 2001.

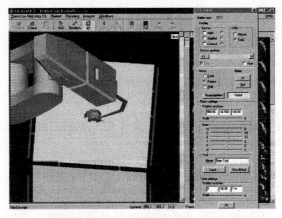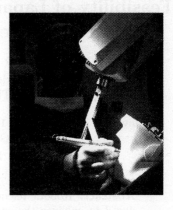

Fig. 1. Simulation before surgery (left). The robot is in surgery position holding the drill guide (right).

After acceptance of the plan by the surgeon, the robot starts to move under control of TomoRob. The communication with the robot controller is based on a standard communication protocol.

With pointing with the robot's pointer to a minimum of three artificial landmarks, the robots coordinate systems, the image coordinate system and the patients coordinate system were referenced. We used the corners of a LEGO block, also visible in the CT data, as landmarks. The fixation of the patients jaws during treatment is still necessary at this stage.

In the current configuration, the robot is mounted on a trolly, which holds the robot, the small robot controller and the laptop computer for TomoRob. The trolly can be connected to a standard operation table with rigid mountings.

Initial drilling was performed by the surgeon. The robot assisted by holding a drill template according to the preoperative determined position data of the implants.

For the 16 performed model operations with altogether 48 drills for implants, post OP CT examinations were performed without the implants in place to avoid artifacts. Then, implant top (bone entrance) positions and implant end positions (implant apex) were compared against the original plan.

3 Results

First and preliminary results show that, after performing the fusion of pre and post OP CT, deviations of about 1 to 2 mm where found for the implant top and implant apex positions. The time saving effect expected from using robots in surgery depends on the effectiveness of the referencing procedure and the optimization and streamlining of the software for practical use.

Feasibility of Laparoscopic Surgery Assisted by a Robotic Telemanipulation System

J.P. Ruurda, I.A.M.J. Broeders, R.K.J. Simmermacher, I.H.M. Borel Rinkes,
and Th.J.M.V. van Vroonhoven

University Medical Center Utrecht, Department of Surgery, P.O. Box 85500,
3508 GA Utrecht, the Netherlands
j.p.ruurda@chir.azu.nl

Abstract. Robotic telemanipulation systems have recently been introduced to enhance the surgeon's dexterity and visualisation in laparoscopic surgery. Technical feasibility of robot-assisted surgery was evaluated in 30 laparoscopic cholecystectomies.

1 Introduction

Where laparoscopic surgery offers the patient clear benefits, it introduces disadvantages to the surgeon as compared to open surgery. Manipulation is compromised by a limitation in degrees of freedom (DOF) of motion, inverted instrument
response and variability in scaling, caused by working with long instruments
through fixed entrypoints.

Visualisation is hampered by the indirect two-dimensional field of view. The
hand-eye co-ordination is further deteriorated by the loss of the eye-hands-target
axis, compromising normal oculovestibular input [1].

In order to cope with these limitations researchers started developing new
tools for laparoscopic surgery, starting with camera guidance systems such as
Aesop and Endoassist [2,3,4]. Finally this resulted in the development of robotic
telemanipulation systems. To demonstrate and evaluate technical feasibility of
robotic assisted surgery, 30 laparoscopic cholecystectomies were performed.

2 Methods

30 robot-assisted laparoscopic cholecystectomies were performed with the Da
Vinci system (Intuitive Surgical, Mountain View, California). The system consists of a master-console, and a 3 armed robotic telemanipulator, located at the
operating table. From the console, the surgeon directly controls the camera-arm
and the two instrument arms with two manipulators. The surgeon's motions are
transposed to the tips of tiny instruments, where the Endowrist system provides
the surgeon with seven DOF. The double optic system provides a 3D image,
integrated in the console. The natural eye-hand-target axis is hereby restored.

Three surgeons were trained to perform laparoscopic cholecystectomies with
the Da Vinci system. Set-up time, OR-time, complications and technical problems were recorded.

W. Niessen and M. Viergever (Eds.): MICCAI 2001, LNCS 2208, pp. 1304–1305, 2001.

3   Results

In 29 cases (29/30; 97%) the cholecystectomy was completed laparoscopically. There was one conversion to an open procedure, caused by the surgeons' incapability to manipulate the gallbladder, due to severe cholecystitis. There were no robot-related complications. In three cases the replaceable blade of the electrocautery instrument detached, but could be removed during the same session.

The time needed to install the robotic system decreased with experience of the OR-crew. Operating time was comparable in robot-assisted cases to the time needed for laparoscopic cholecystectomy in the same clinic.

4   Discussion

Technical feasibility of robot assisted laparoscopic cholecystectomy was repeatedly demonstrated. No significant problems were noted during these procedures, except from the detachment of the electrocautery blade. The introduction of the second-generation blade solved this problem. The system showed to enhance the surgeon's dexterity and visualisation possibilities, providing intuitive control of the instruments.

Time-loss seems eventually to be overcome. Set-up and operating times will further decrease with increasing experience and further development of these robotic systems.

One of the points of criticism towards robotic systems, is the lack of tactile feedback. This is partly compensated for by the 3D visual feedback. Adding tactile feedback is one of the challenging topics in the development of these systems.

Although surgical robotics is considered to be in an early phase of development, the opportunities robotic telemanipulators offer are already distinct. They provide endoscopic surgeons with a dexterity incomparable to the way they used to perform laparoscopic surgery, allowing a precise and intuitive way of performing surgery.

References

1. Satava RM, Ellis SR. Human interface technology. An essential tool for the modern surgeon. Surg Endosc 1994; 8: 817-20
2. Sackier JM, Wang Y. Robotically assisted laparoscopic surgery. From concept to development. Surg Endosc 1994; 8: 63-6
3. Jacobs LK, Shayani V, Sackier JM. Determination of the learning curve of the AESOP robot. Surg Endosc 1997; 11: 54-5
4. Schurr M, Arezzo A, Buess GF. Robotics and systems technology for advanced endoscopic procedures: experiences in general surgery. Eur J Cardiothorac Surg 1999;16 Suppl 2: S97-105

Development of Semi-autonomous Control Modes in Laparoscopic Surgery Using Automatic Visual Servoing

Alexandre Krupa[1], Michel de Mathelin[1], Christophe Doignon[1],
Jacques Gangloff[1], Guillaume Morel[2], Luc Soler[3], and Jacques Marescaux[3]

[1] LSIIT (UPRES-A CNRS 7005), University of Strasbourg I, France
alexandre.krupa|michel.demathelin@ensps.u-strasbg.fr
[2] EDF R&D, Chatou, Paris, France
[3] IRCAD (Institut de Recherche sur le Cancer de l'Appareil Digestif), Strasbourg.

Abstract. This paper presents ongoing research on the development of automatic control modes for robotized laparoscopic surgery. We show how visual feedback can be used in a control scheme to autonomously perform basic surgical subtasks in order to enhance surgeon accuracy and comfort.

1 Objective

Laparoscopic surgical robots have appeared recently. With these systems, robot arms are used to manipulate the instruments and the camera. The surgeon tele-operates the robots through master arms using the visual feedback from the laparoscope. This reduces the surgeon tiredness, and potentially increases accuracy by the use of a high master/slave motion ratio. Our research in this field is aimed at expanding the potentialities of such systems by providing "automatic modes" in which the system autonomously performs simple subtasks. For this purpose, the robot controller uses the visual feedback from the laparoscope to automatically drive instruments, through a visual servo loop, towards their desired location. In cooperation with IRCAD, we particularly focus on liver surgery. This surgery involves a number of repetitive gesture, such as the cleaning-suction process, clamping, cauterization, needle manipulation. It shall be noticed that although these processes are rather simple as compared to critical surgical gestures, it involves repetitive movements for the surgeon who drives master devices.

2 Methodology and Ongoing Experiments

A difficulty in laparoscopic surgery is the lack of depth information due to the monocular vision system. Furthermore, as surgical scenes are poorly structured,

[0] **Acknowledgment:** The experimental part of this work has been made possible thanks to the collaboration of Computer Motion that has graciously provided the medical robot.

W. Niessen and M. Viergever (Eds.): MICCAI 2001, LNCS 2208, pp. 1306–1307, 2001.

it is difficult to extract reliable reference points and visual features to be used in visual servoing techniques. In our approach, we add different structured lightening systems made of laser pointers mounted on a surgical tool-holder. The structured light allows for the robust extraction of visual features that can be used in our image-based control law. The endoscopic camera is mounted on another robot's arm whose relative position is unknown with respect to the other arms holding the surgical tool. This is a major difficulty for visual servoing, that we tackle by robustly identifying part of the Image Jacobian matrix expressing the relationship between visual displacements of the tool in the image around a working position and robot axis rotations. As an example, we can imagine that the surgeon select an area on the monitor screen to indicate a vessel to be reached. By indicating points on the screen, the surgeon specify the target point on the vessel and a desired orientation of the tool with respect to it. Then the projected position and orientation of the tool can be directly controlled with images of the impact laser features as follow (see, e.g., Fig. 1). - Firstly, a rotation around the tool axis is provided for alignment through visual servoing. - Then, laser features are moved onto the projection of the vessel by rotating the tool around the trocard center. - Finally, a simple motion along the tool axis aligns the tool marker with the laser points. We have already successfully tested this vision control with a 6 DOF robot, constrained to 4 DOF (using force feedback), on a laparoscopic trainer (see [1]). An automatic cleaning task has been implemented on a 4 DOF medical robot (Computer Motion) and tests on living animal have been performed.

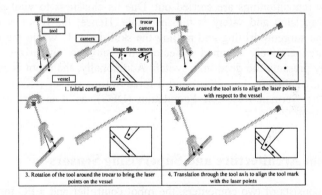

Fig. 1. Example of visual servoing using laser markers.

References

1. A. Krupa, C. Doignon, J. Gangloff, M. de Mathelin, L. Soler, G. Morel. Towards semi-autonomy in laparoscopic surgery through vision and force feedback control. *Proc. of the Seventh International Symposium on Experimental Robotics (ISER)*, Hawaii, December, 2000.

A Supervising System for Robot Application in Surgery

Dirk Engel, Joerg Raczkowsky, Heinz Woern

Institute for Process Control and Robotics, Universität Karlsruhe (TH)
Kaiserstraße 12 , 76128 Karlsruhe, Germany
dEngel@ira.uka.de | rkowsky@ira.uka.de | woern@ira.uka.de

Abstract. In this paper a supervising system for robot application in surgery is described. Since a robot in surgery has to meet special safety requirements the robot application has to be controlled not only by the responsible surgeon but also by redundant sensors. Therefore our robot system for bone repositionings in craniofacial surgery is equipped with internal and external sensors. This paper discusses the use of an infrared navigation system and a force-torque-sensor as supervising sensors.

1. Introduction

The fundamental issue of robots in surgery is the safety of the involved persons: patient, physicians and nurses, for example. Therefore a robust and redundant controlling system is required, in order to be resistant against failure. In craniofacial surgery bone repositionings are carried out. Due its closeness to vital parts, i.e. the brain, high precision and safety is indispensable. Hence, the robot is intended for supporting the surgeon drilling and milling the skull bone 1. While the robot moves along the preoperatively planned trajectory the surgeon authorizes every robot movement by pressing the dead-man switch. Additionally, the robot is supervised by an infrared navigation system (INS) and a force-/torque sensor (FTS). This work is funded by the German Research Foundation (DFG), as it is part of the special research program SFB 414.

2. System Architecture and Supervising Sensors

The system consists of two computers, the robot controller and a PC for sensor data acquisition and processing. Both computers are connected via a RS232 serial line. Further, the PC accesses a digital input signal and the emergency-stop-circuit of the robot controller via a relais card. The digital signal provides the possibility of a so-called soft interrupt; switching logical high to logical low signal causes the robot to move its tool 25 millimeter back from the current location. Such a way the capability of moving the milling cutter out of the bone in the event of failure is retained. Accessing the emergency-circuit, so-called hard interrupt, causes an immediate robot stop.

A rigid body equipped with IR-LEDs which can be tracked by the INS is mounted to the robot tool and is also fixed to the patients head. The INS supervises the

W. Niessen and M. Viergever (Eds.): MICCAI 2001, LNCS 2208, pp. 1308-1309, 2001.

movements of the robot rigid body relative to the patient rigid body. Such a way the INS is able to detect shortcomings of the patient fixation and wrong robot movements, additionally. Computing the relative position brings in the measuring errors of both rigid bodies. Further, the tracked positions do not coincide with the origin of the planning data and robot tool tip position, respectively. Therefore the measured positions have to be transformed into these locations. Transforming the tracked robot tool position into the tool tip position causes an intensification of the measured orientation inaccuracies. An orientation error of $\varphi = 1°$ yields a presumable tool tip positioning error of about d = 3.5 mm, if the distance between rigid body and tool tip is l = 20 cm: $d = l * \tan \varphi$. For that reason not only the measured absolute positioning error is supervised, but two types of errors are distinguished. First, the computed distance d_z between tool tip and trajectory measured along the tool axis (z-axis) and, second, d_y whereby $y = z \times x$ and x is the direction of the trajectory. An error is detected on considering both errors.

The FTS controls the forces and torques affected to the robot tool. It can be used to detect collisions of the robot tool with obstacles during service and approaching movements. Furthermore it is used to control the forces and torques during the milling/drilling process. Since this sensor provides a high data acquisition rate RTLinux 2 is used as real time operating system of the PC. The FTS software client program supervises the forces and torques regarding to the adjusted thresholds. In detail the real time kernel module monitors: the amount of each force/torque direction, the amount of the overall forces and torques, and the force/torque gradients. In case of exceeding an adjusted threshold, the client accesses the digital signal line or the robot emergency-stop-circuit. Fig. 1 depicts the recorded monitoring data of a trajectory milled out in four steps.

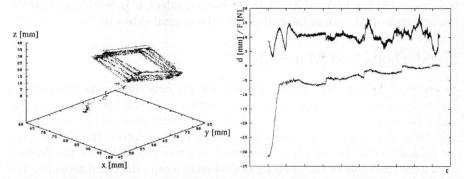

Fig. 1. Left: Trajectory supervised by INS. Right: detected distance d_z to maximal cutting depth (gray) and corresponding overall force (black).

References

1. Engel, D., Raczkowsky, J., Woern, H.: "A Safe Robot System for Craniofacial Surgery", IEEE Inter. Conf. On Robotics and Automation, Seoul, Korea, 2001.

2. RTLinux: http://www.rtlinux.org, March 2001.

A New Diagnostic Method for Alzheimer's Disease Using Pupillary Light Reflex

Xuemin Shi[1], Yi Guo[1], Shogo Fukushima[2], Kenshi Suzuki[2],
Hisashi Uchiyama[1], and Ichiro Fukumoto[1]

[1] Institute of Biomedical Engineering , Nagaoka University of Technology
Kamitomioka 1603 , Nagaoka , Niigata , Japan
shi@stn.nagaokaut.ac.jp
http://bio.nagaokaut.ac.jp/~fukumoto/
[2] Advanced Technology Research Laboratory, Matsushita Electric Works, Ltd., Japan

Abstract. We has developed a lightweight glass-shaped measurement apparatus composed of two CCDs to capture eye images and four white LEDs for light stimulus to diagnose Alzheimer's disease (AD). The AD patients showed significantly smaller miotic rate and longer miotic time than the normal elderly controls for miotic reflex in our clinical experiment.

1 Introduction

Alzheimer's disease (AD) is a neurodegenerative disorder of the central nervous system. As acetylcoline (Ach), a main neural transmitter activating miotic reflex is decreased in the brain of AD than the normal elders, it is considered that the miotic-reflex of AD would be weaker than the normal elders [1].

2 Methods and Materials

In order to lighten the burden imposed on subjects during measurement, a lightweight glass-shaped apparatus for measuring pupil size has been developed, which includes two CCD cameras for both eyes to capture both eye images. The apparatus also includes four controllable white LEDs placed in front of each eye for light stimulus. In the experiment, each eye was stimulated by the flashing light for 0.1 seconds at the intensity of 0.64 cd in a semi-darkened room [2]. The pupil images are transmitted to image processor (60 images/s) and the data are kept with computer. We studied 19 AD patients (mean age 79.4 years, S.D. 8.5 years), 13 Vascular Dementia (VD) patients (mean age 78.9 years, S.D. 8.9 years) and 19 normal elder controls (mean age 80.9 years, S.D. 7.6 years).

3 Results

AD patients showed significantly poor pupillary light reflex on parameters Initial pupil diameter (D_0, $p < 0.05$), Maximum miotic ratio ($p < 0.05$), 10%-50% recovery time ($p < 0.05$), 10%-50% recovery velocity (RV, $p < 0.05$) and Time interval

W. Niessen and M. Viergever (Eds.): MICCAI 2001, LNCS 2208, pp. 1310–1311, 2001.

from 90% miosis to 10% recovery than the controls. VD patients showed significantly smaller D_0 (p<0.01) and RV (p<0.05) than the controls also. Specially, on the parameter RV/MV (MV=10%-90% miotic velocity), the AD patients showed significantly smaller than not only the controls but also the VD patients, suggested that the AD patients owned poor recovery phase more than miotic phase.

4   Discussions

In the experiment AD patients showed significantly poor pupillary light reflex than the controls. It is presumably because the neurotransmitters Ach, effecting miotic phase and norepinephrine (NE), effecting recovery phase of miotic reflex are clearly decreased in AD patients' brains comparing to the controls. VD patients showed significantly smaller D_0 and RV than the controls also. Future investigations are expected to study the amount of ACh in the VD patients. On the parameter RV/MV, the AD patients showed significantly smaller than not only the controls but also the VD patients, suggested that the AD patients owned poor recovery phase more than miotic phase.

5   Conclusions

As the new method (miotic-reflex) is not only simple but also harmless, it may be a new objective method to diagnose and to evaluate senile dementia in the clinical routine in the near future. Matsushita Electric Works is now producing a commercial system of this type.

Acknowledgement

We would like to thank Nagaoka Tamiya Hospital, Syunkouen and Keiseien of Shinseikai of Gunma prefecture for their cooperation.

References

1. X. Shi, H. Uchiyama , I. Fukumoto., A study for objective measurement of the senile dementia by light reflex, JJME Biomedical Engineering, Vol. 12 No. 9, 210/214 (1998).
2. S. Fukushima, X. Shi, et al., A New Objective Approach to Diagnose Dementia by Pupillary Light Reflex Method, Asia-Pacific Congress on Biomedical Engineering IEEE-EMBS Asia-Pasific Conference on Biomedical Engineering, HangZhou, China (2000)

Reduction of Insertion Resistance by Means of Vibration for Catheters and Endoscopes

Kiyoshi Yoshinaka, Ryo Sakamoto, and Ken Ikeuchi

Institute for Frontier Medical Sciences Kyoto University, Kawaharacho 53,
Shogoin,sakyo-ku, Kyoto, 6068507, Japan
{yosinaka,ikeuchi}@frontier.kyoto-u.ac.jp

Abstract. We present a new method to reduce insertion resistance for internal medical instruments by means of vibration. We investigated the relation between frequency of the vibration and the insertion resistance with a pin on flat test system in vitro. And we made a prototype of internal medical probe for in vivo. As a result, vibration is effective to reduce the friction and it is possible to keep a smooth insertion by vibration.

1 Introduction

It is not always easy to insert medical instruments into a human body without injuring tissues. One of the reasons of difficulty to insert these instruments is friction between organic tissue surface and instruments. Then we present a new method to reduce insertion resistance for internal medical instruments by means of vibration. The decrease of the insertion resistance is necessary for no-invasive and rapid insertion into a human body. If friction controled, a novel high quality medical treatment will be realized and this system will greatly lighten doctors burden.

Therefore this paper shows relationship between insertion resistance and vibration, and presents insertion property of a prototype internal probe with vibration in vivo.

2 In Vitro and in Vivo Experiments

We investigated the relation between frequency of the vibration and the insertion resistance with a pin on flat test system in vitro. This experiment system is composed of a linear slider, a vibrating unit, a sensor to measure the insertion resistance and a computer. The computer controls frequency and amplitude of the vibrating unit. Porcine small intestine was used as the test specimen in this experiment.

Next, we made a prototype of internal medical probe shown by Figure.1. This probe is assembled with a vibrating unit, a catheter made of super elastic wire and a capsule. This probe is inserted into a large intestine of a rabbit automatically by the linear actuator and this automated insertion system can measure insertion resistance by the sensor that is installed at the end of catheter. Then we compare the resistance at static insertion with the vibrated insertion.

W. Niessen and M. Viergever (Eds.): MICCAI 2001, LNCS 2208, pp. 1312–1313, 2001.

3   Results

Figure.2 shows that insertion resistance depends on frequency of the vibrating unit, and 90 Hz of vibration is high enough for effective reduction of resistance.

The result of in vivo experiment shows that when insertion resistance is increased, vibration is effective to reduce the friction, and a smooth insertion is kept with vibration. A 70 percent of insertion resistance is decreased by vibration.

These studies indicate the possibility of friction control of the internal medical instrument by vibration.

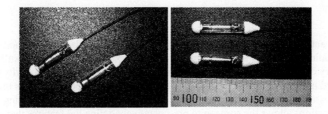

Fig. 1. Apparatus of probes

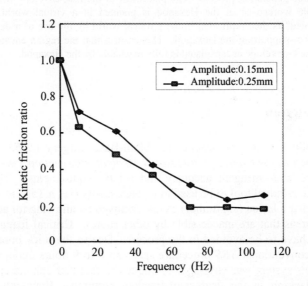

Fig. 2. Effect of vibration amplitude on friction ratio

Hexapod Intervention Planning for a Robotic Skull-Base Surgery System

Charlie Sim[1], Ming-Yeong Teo[1], Wan-Sing Ng[1], Carl Yap[1], Yong-Chong Loh[1],
Tseng-Tsai Yeo[2], Shao-Ping Bai[1], Charles Lo[1]

[1]School of Mechanical & Production Engineering, Nanyang Technological University,
Computer Integrated Medical Intervention Lab, 50, Nanyang Avenue, Singapore 639798
[2] National Neuroscience Institute, Jalan Tan Tock Seng, Singapore 308433

Abstract. This paper introduces a novel intervention planning methodology
facilitating the use of a parallel manipulator (Hexapod) in a robotic skull-base
surgery ("**SBS**") system. This safety intensive procedure requires a cavity to be
created in the skull-base so as to allow access to deep-seated brain areas that are
inaccessible by other routes. An image-guided system (presenting 3-D
information) allows the surgeon to pre-operatively define the features that are to
be avoided. Although the Hexapod used has good positioning accuracy and
high stiffness, its workspace suffers from some undesirable characteristics. A
novel technique has been developed to alleviate this problem by means of
segregating the task-envelope (i.e. the cavity in the skull-base) and Hexapod
workspace generation process. The placement of the task-envelope within the
reachable workspace of the Hexapod is planned in a virtual world. This
"placement" is then replicated in the physical world by the use of a dexterous
base robot supporting the Hexapod. This ensures that the region encapsulated
by the task-envelope encapsulated is fully reachable by the Hexapod.

1.   Introduction

A novel robotic system "*NeuRobot*" for Skull-Base Surgery ("*SBS*") is currently
being developed at *the Computer Integrated Medical Intervention Laboratory*. *SBS*
is a procedure with stringent accuracy and safety requirements. This procedure
requires a bone removal tool to be used to create a cavity (i.e. a Task-Envelope) in the
skull-base so that a lesion (e.g. tumor) can be removed by allowing for access to deep-
seated brain areas that are inaccessible by other routes. Critical features (e.g. vein,
blood vessel) have to be avoided in the process. Due to the thick bone ridge of the
skull-base, a conventional *SBS* procedure spans an 8 to 9 hours duration. The main
reason why this system was envisaged is due to the fact that commercially available
systems are lacking in the degrees-of-freedom required. Eminently, the robotic
manipulator used in other systems possess a large workspace leading to unconstrained
motion that pose danger to both the patient and surgeon alike. One of the main
challenges in developing this system is the use of a parallel manipulator (i.e. the
Hexapod) over a conventional serial robot. The Hexapod has good positioning
accuracy, high stiffness and small workspace acting as a mechanical limit to constrain
the motion available to the end-effector. On the contrary, it suffers not only from a

W. Niessen and M. Viergever (Eds.): MICCAI 2001, LNCS 2208, pp. 1314-1315, 2001.
© Springer-Verlag Berlin Heidelberg 2001

small and oddly distributed workspace, but also a change in the workspace's shape, size and distribution when its orientation is varied. A novel technique has been developed to alleviate this problem by means of segregating the task-envelope (i.e. the cavity in the skull-base) and Hexapod workspace generation process.

2.   Method

Initially, the required image modalities (e.g. CT, MRI) are obtained. The images are fed into an image-guided surgical planning system that will present the images in both 2-D and 3-D to the surgeon, allowing for the topographical assessment of the tumor, skull-base bony structure and the features to be avoided. On each 2-D slice, the surgeon identifies the regions to be avoided. These are called the "no-go" sites (**Fig. 1a.**). Given the "no-go" sites (or a group of sites identifying a "no-go" region) on any given image slice, the largest "go" cavity on each slice is generated by the use of a Voronoi Map. A projection line based algorithm "smooths" the cavities from one slice to another, so as to produce a task-envelope (**Fig. 1b.**) achievable by a surgical bone-removal tool with a straight shank. The algorithm further takes into account the geometrical limitations of the Hexapod.

Next, the workspace is generated in accordance to the end-effector orientation range required by the Hexapod to produce the pre-generated task-envelope (**Fig. 1c.**). This is achieved by the use of a workspace discretisation method. Essentially in robotic *SBS*, the cavity to be created is volume-based, and not just a straight line requiring only a single end-effector orientation. It will be an impossible task for "path-planning" to be performed using the current "state-of-the-art" as most methodologies strictly advocate pure trajectory verification without rectification.

With both the task-envelope and the workspace obtained, the virtual task of placing the task-envelope within the workspace can be easily achieved. This ensures the whole region within the generated task-envelope can be fully reached by the Hexapod carrying the bone removal tool.

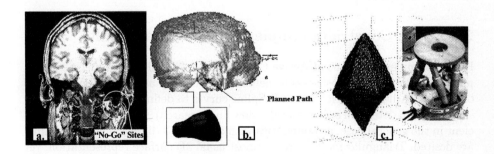

Fig. 1. (a.) Identifying "No-Go" Sites on 2-D Slices; **(b.)** Cavity Produced after "Virtual" Bone-Removal; (inset) Generated Path; **(c.)** Workspace Generated by Discretisation (-5° to 5° orientation range for all axes); (inset) The Hexapod (from Physik Instrumente)

Advances in Active Constraints and Their Application to Minimally Invasive Surgery

Stephen J. Starkie and Brian L. Davies

Imperial College of Science, Technology and Medicine, London SW7 2BX, UK,
s.starkie@ic.ac.uk

Abstract. This paper discusses advances in Active Constraints technology, which is designed to complement the surgeon's skill and improve safety in minimally invasive procedures. These advances include the support for true 3-dimensional constraints, independence of mechanical architecture, distributed constraint auditing, real-time deformation tracking and distributed user interface.

1 Introduction

In minimally invasive neurosurgery the endoscope has to pass through a burr-hole in the skull, causing tool motions to be reversed in an occluded operating field. Active Constraints are intended to improve the safety of such reduced dexterity procedures, by implementing a virtual boundary which encloses the safe regions of the environment. To implement the constraint, an active robotic manipulator holds the tools and is guided under force-feedback control by the surgeon[1].

An important step in improving safety has been to split the control and interface of the system; VxWorks (x86) is used to control the manipulator, and Windows 2000 Pro(x86, accelerated graphics hardware) hosts the distributed user interface. Integration between the controller and the graphical interface is achieved using a proprietary C++ CORBA implementation.

2 Active Constraints Implementation and Results

Previous implementations of Active Constraints [1,2] utilised the specific multi-planar design of knee prostheses to define the boundary as sets of line segments on planes (earlier research [2] used B-Spline curves to define the planar geometry - but collision detection still involved a slow linear search). This method is insufficient in the general case, as boundaries with arbitrary 3-dimensional topography are desired. Triangular meshes are the most usual 3D surface representation, yet this is inelegant for two reasons; it presents a destabilising discontinuous gradients to the underlying force control structures, and accurate search methods[3] for collisions of triangular meshes are too slow for real-time control. If more than two bodies are defined, Bounding Box techniques can be used to cull well seperated bodies, regardless of the underlying representation.

W. Niessen and M. Viergever (Eds.): MICCAI 2001, LNCS 2208, pp. 1316–1317, 2001.

Similarly, volumetric representations suffer from problems of discontinuity and slow search methods, despite allowing the possibility of directly mapping voxel intensities to physical properties, and easy implementation of cutting and tearing of bodies[4].

Parametric surfaces can be specified to be continuous to any order by simply specifying the order of the base polynomials, ensuring reasonable spacing of knots and providing enough control points. In this research, cubic B-Splines are used, as they include the property of local support (provided by the underlying B-Spline polynomials and which is lacking from Bezier surfaces). A B-Spline is a specialization of the more general class of curves called NURBS - Non-Uniform Rational B-Splines [5]. By specifying the knot vectors appropriately (ie; knot vectors are uniform) and the order as 3, they can be guaranteed continuous up to second order.

The boundary search has been implemented as a non-terminating Newton Raphson minimisation of the closest approach vector (CAV) between two surfaces. The method has been implemented on a Neuro-Endoscopic Manipulator, and results have shown that although the iteration is not terminated (in order to continuously track the CAV) it converges after six iterations.

Forces are fed back to the manipulator control by implementing standard mechanical models; the boundary is modelled as a very hard spring, behind a low stiffness membrane and low viscosity damper.

3   Conclusion

This paper has described advances made in Active Constraint technology including the generalisation to 3D using cubic B-Spline boundaries. An extremely fast accurate collision detection algorithm has been developed which can operate in real-time. The technology has been implemented successfully in the control of an active Neuro-Endoscopic Manipulator.

References

1. S J Harris, M Jakopec, R D Hibberd, J Cobb, and B L Davies. Interactive pre-operative selection of cutting constraints, and interactive force controlled knee surgery by a surgical robot. *1st Int. Conf. Medical Image Computing and Computer Assisted Intervention*, pages 996–1006, 1998.
2. S C Ho, R D Hibberd, J Cobb, and B L Davies. Force control for robotic surgery. *Proc. 7th Int. Conf. Advanced Robotics*, 1:21–31, 1995.
3. M Lin. *Efficient Collision Detection for Animation and Robotics*. PhD thesis, University of California at Berkeley, 1993.
4. Sarah F Frisken-Gibson. Using linked volumes to model object collisions, deformation, cutting, carving, and joining. *IEEE Transactions on Visualisation and Computer Graphics*, 5(4), 1999.
5. Les Piegl and Wayne Tiller. *The NURBS Book*. Monographs in Visual Communication. Springer-Verlag, Berlin, 2 edition, 1997.

Motion Correction of MRI from Orthogonal k-Space Phase Difference

Edward Brian Welch[1], Armando Manduca[2]

[1] MRI Research Lab, Dept. of Diagnostic Radiology, Mayo Clinic, Rochester, MN 55905
[2] Biomathematics Resource, Mayo Clinic, Rochester, MN 55905

Abstract. Correction of artifacts in MRI from in-plane 2-D rigid body translational motion is possible using only the raw data of two standard 2DFT images acquired of the same object with phase encode direction swapped. Previous techniques simply use multiple or orthogonal images to reduce artifacts through interference or geometric averaging. The orthogonal k-space phase difference (ORKPHAD) provides an overdetermined system of linear equations which can be solved directly to find the phase errors caused by the motion, and thus correct for arbitrary translations in both image.

1   Introduction

It is well known that rigid body translations of an object in MRI will create image artifacts along the phase encode (PE) direction in standard 2DFT imaging (1). Methods have been proposed to take advantage of the directionality of the artifacts to improve image quality by combining images with dissimiliar artifact patterns. Two such methods are ghost interference techniques (2) and the orthogonal correlation algorithm (ORCA) (3). Neither technique attempts to deduce the motion record or to correct the k-space phase errors caused by the motion. Acquiring two images with swapped PE direction, as in ORCA, makes it possible to determine and correct for the motion directly using the orthogonal k-space phase difference (ORKPHAD).

2   Theory

If one assumes 2-D in-plane translational interview motion, $4N$ unknown motions may corrupt the two NxN images. The phase difference at each point in k-space yields N^2 equations involving only $4N$ unknowns. Equation 1 shows how the motion relates to the phase difference at the (n_1,n_2) position in the k-space phase difference array. The vector $\mathbf{k}$ holds the frequency coefficients across one row or column of k-space. The vectors $\mathbf{P_A}$ and $\mathbf{F_A}$ are the motions in pixels for the first image in the phase and frequency encode directions respectively. Similarly, $\mathbf{P_B}$ and $\mathbf{F_B}$ are the motions for the second image. After the phase difference is properly unwrapped, the motion records can be found by a weighted least squares inversion of the system of equations.

W. Niessen and M. Viergever (Eds.): MICCAI 2001, LNCS 2208, pp. 1318-1319, 2001.

$$\Phi_A - \Phi_B = \frac{2\pi}{N}\left(\mathbf{k}[n_1]\mathbf{P}_A[n_1] + \mathbf{k}[n_2]\mathbf{F}_A[n_1] - \mathbf{k}[n_2]\mathbf{P}_B[n_2] - \mathbf{k}[n_1]\mathbf{F}_B[n_2]\right) \quad [1]$$

3   Methods

Separate volumes of 2-D spin echo images of a volunteer's moving wrist were acquired with orthogonal phase encode directions. The corrupted images were then corrected with the ORKPHAD technique.

4   Results

ORKPHAD successfully improved both corruptions. The results in Fig. 1 show results for slice 6 of the 12 slice volume. All slices showed similar improvement.

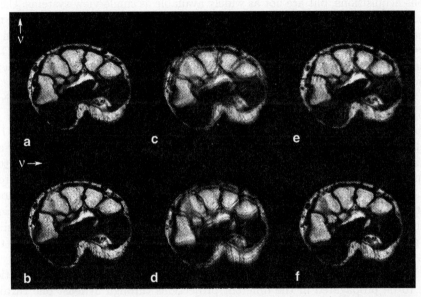

Fig. 1. ORKPHAD results for slice 6: static (**a,b**), corrupted (**c,d**), and corrected (**e,f**).

References

1. Wood ML, Henkelman MR. MR Image Artifacts from Periodic Motion. Medical Physics 1985;12(2):143-151.
2. Xiang QS, Bronskill MJ, Henkelman MR. Two-Point Interference Method for Supression of Ghost Artifacts Due to Motion. J of Magn Reson Imaging 1993;3:900-906.
3. Kruger DG, Slavin GS, Muthupillai R, Grimm RC, Riederer SJ. An Orthogonal Correlation Algorithm for Ghost Reduction in MRI. Magn Reson Med 1997;38:678-686.

3D+t Modeling of Coronary Artery Tree from Standard Non Simultaneous Angiograms[*]

Fabien Mourgues, Frédéric Devernay, Grégoire Malandain, and
Ève Coste-Manière

CHIR Team, www.inria.fr/chir
INRIA, 2004 route des lucioles, 06902 Sophia-Antipolis Cedex, France

1 Method

X-ray angiography provides two-dimensional projections of opacified arteries. Utilizing temporally synchronized projections, from different angles, a 3D model can be reconstructed. Biplane angiography [1] systems can provide two simultaneous acquisitions, but are not as widely available as single-view systems. Using the latter systems, the different projections are acquired sequentially. During the time required to change the position of the imaging system, patient motion or breathing motion may be introduced. We propose a method to construct a 3D+t model of the coronary tree from non-simultaneous sequences, synchronized with the electrocardiogram and acquired on single-view angiography systems.

The first step is extraction and labeling of the coronary tree in the different projections. We chose to address this computationally expensive problem [2, 1] by using a semi-automatic method. All the images are preprocessed with a multi-scale model-based algorithm [3]. Then, the arteries to be reconstructed are selected and labeled by the cardiologist in one image of each sequence with a tool inspired by the intelligent scissors [4], relying on the multi-scale magnitude: from a user-defined seed point, the artery centerline is captured in the neighborhood of the mouse with a shortest path algorithm to the current mouse position. Only the n last pixels are constantly optimized and the correction is possible by guiding the optimized segment using an alternative orientation. Finally, the hierarchical structure of the coronary tree is automatically constructed.

In the second stage of this method, segmentation and labeling information has to be propagated in the different projections through at least one cardiac cycle. Our approach relies on the hierarchical description of the coronary tree, and the modeling of the arteries by B-snakes with an internal energy derived from the multi-scale model-based preprocessing. A two-step optimization - a global transformation followed by a local optimization of the control points - reduces the effects of large displacements, crossings and overlapping arteries.

Then, in the third stage, 3D modeling of the coronary artery tree is performed from two segmented projections corresponding roughly to the same cardiac phase. Since they are extracted from two different sequences, heart motion

---

[*] Thanks to R. Vaillant from GE Medical Systems and to Dr Blanchard, Prof. Carpentier and the Cardiac Surgery team at Hôpital Européen Georges Pompidou, Paris

W. Niessen and M. Viergever (Eds.): MICCAI 2001, LNCS 2208, pp. 1320–1322, 2001.
© Springer-Verlag Berlin Heidelberg 2001

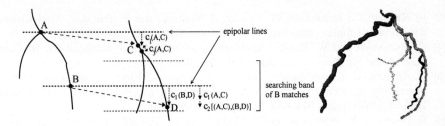

Fig. 1. Left: the penalties of the matching criteria: c_1 penalizes matches which do not respect epipolar geometry, c_2 ensures the deviation continuity from epipolar geometry and c_3 encourages the matching of A and C bifurcations. Right: the final reconstructed tree with sections.

may have occured due to patient's motion or breathing (in the latter, about 10 mm for the inferior-superior translation of the Left Anterior Descending artery). We overcome this difficulty by creating a coherent 3D model by alternately matching the artery pixel strings - as illustrated on figure 1 - and optimizing the sensor parameters by a classical bundle-adjustment method, accomplished on the whole tree. Finally, the 3D skeleton is enriched with sections estimated from the acquisition geometry and the detection scale from the multi-scale preprocessing.

2   Discussion

coronary tree from standard non-simultaneous angiograms has been successfully applied to angiograms acquired on both single-view and biplane angiography systems.

We hope to improve the robustness of the tracking by directly deforming the 3D model obtained at one cardiac phase rather than independently computing the 3D reconstructions. Using its back-projections in all the available sequences would eliminate the artery overlap and crossing problems. Moreover, the measure of sections in all the projections will enable a better quantification of the shape and size of the 3D sections.

After clinical validation, this model could be used to help diagnose cardio-vascular diseases. It can also be integrated in a planning and simulation system for robotically assisted surgery [5] and used in the operating theater to guide the surgeon by augmented reality [6].

References

[1] P. Windiga, M. Garreau, and J.L. Coatrieux. Estimation of search-space in 3D coronary artery reconstruction using biplane images. *Pattern Recognition Letters*, 19:1325–1330, September 1998.

[2] Y. Sato, T. Araki, M. Hanayama, H. Naito, and S. Tamura. A viewpoint deter-mination system for stenosis diagnosis and quantification in coronary angiographic image acquisition. *IEEE Transactions on Medical Imaging*, 17(1), 1998.

1322   F. Mourgues et al.

[3] K. Krissian, G. Malandain, N. Ayache, R. Vaillant, and Y. Trousset. Model-based detection of tubular structures in 3D images. *CVIU*, 80:130–171, 2000.
[4] E. Mortensen and W. Barett. Intelligent scissors for image composition. In *Computer Graphics Proceedings*, pages 191–198, 1995.
[5] L. Adhami, E. Coste-Manière, and JD. Boissonnat. Planning and simulation of robotically assisted minimal invasive surgery. In *Proceedings MICCAI*, volume 1935 of *LNCS*, pages 624–633. Springer, October 2000.
[6] F. Devernay, F. Mourgues, and E. Coste-Manière. Towards endoscopic augmented reality for robotically assisted minimally invasive cardiac surgery. In *Proceedings of Medical Imaging and Augmented Reality*, 2001.

New Tools for Visualization and Quantification in Dynamic Processes: Application to the Nuclear Envelope Dynamics During Mitosis

J. Mattes[1], J. Fieres[1], J. Beaudouin[2], D. Gerlich[1], J. Ellenberg[2], and R. Eils[1]

[1] iBioS, DKFZ Heidelberg, 69 120 Heidelberg, Germany
J.Mattes@dkfz.de
[2] EMBL, Heidelberg, Germany

Abstract. The aim of this paper is to present new tools for visualization and quantification in dynamic processes. We concentrate on the concise description of local quantitative values and on a easy-to-apprehend way to visualize them. Our approach is based on registration in order to obtain a transformation for the whole image space. This transformation permits us to obtain local values such as bending or velocity in each pixel. We define a density function using this values and apply confinement tree analysis on them. We present an application in cell biology where we can obtain new insight into the elasticity properties of the nuclear lamina.

1 Introduction

Modern imaging devices make it possible to study *in vivo* the mechanism of dynamics in living systems. Intra-operative MRI devices producing several images per second, offer nowadays the possibility to follow the heart-cycle in realtime. Tumor growth can be supervised by imaging systems guiding the focus of a radiation source. At a lower scale, fluorescent confocal microscopy permits to observe marked cellular structures such as chromatin or the nuclear envelope over time.

In order to quantitatively analyze and to visualize the movements of objects in the image time series in an easy-to-apprehend way sophisticated computer algorithms are required [1]. A difficulty is a concise quantitative description permitting the comparision of observed motion in different images going beyond the estimation of the velocity vector field. In this paper, we focus on the description and quantification of local deformation and we let aside considerations about the fit of the observed movement with global reference dynamics [3].

2 Methods

Our approach to analyze deformation in the local spatial domain is based on registration in the image time series and on a statistical analysis, namely the confinement tree analysis (CTA) [4], of the local parameters obtained as a result of the registration step. In a first preprocessing step (i), we extract points describing representative structures of the image, eventually after the application

W. Niessen and M. Viergever (Eds.): MICCAI 2001, LNCS 2208, pp. 1323–1325, 2001.

of a filtering operator. In the second step (ii), we register consecutive images based on the extracted point sets. The registration algorithm comprises an error functional, an optimization strategy and a motion model and is detailed in [2]. The error functional is defined using the extracted image structures. The motion model is necessary as the optimization problem is ill posed in order to restrict the solution space and to model the *allowed* volume transformations. It is determined by the initial position of several freely adjustable control points, by the use of thin plate splines to interpolate between them, and by an additional regularization term in the error functional. The obtained transformation permits us, in the third step (iii), to calculate local quantitative values for each pixel such as velocity, strain, or bending. We represent the absolute values obtained for each pixel as an intensity value and produce a new image. Finally, in the fourth step (iv), we apply CTA on the new image as a statistical method to describe the deformation concisely. Given an intensity function $f : \mathbb{R}^d \to \mathbb{R}_{\geq 0}, d = 2, 3$, the *confiners* are defined as the maximal connected subsets (i.e., *components*) C_l of the level sets $\mathcal{L}_l = \{x \in \mathbb{R}^d | f(x) \geq l\}, l \in \mathbb{R}_{\geq 0}$. Considering them taken on several levels $l_k, k = 1, ..., r$ including the 0 level, they define obviously a tree (by "set inclusion") which we will call *confinement tree* [4]. Movements in different images can be compared by comparing corresponding confiners. The area of the confiners indicates to what degree the movement is (homogeneously) directed.

3   Application, Conclusions, and Further Work

We present an application in cell biology where the dynamics of the nuclear envelope during mitosis is investigated. A 4D sequence of fluorescently labeled (by GFP fusion proteins) lamina is acquired with a confocal laser scanning microscop. We obtain one 3D image every 10-30 seconds. We will focus on the formation of holes in the nuclear envelope during its breakdown taking place in prometaphase. To determine deformation in the upper surface of the lamina, artificial landmarks were introduced by photobleaching of a grid.

The upper row in Figure 1 shows the slice representing at best the upper side of the nuclear envelope and the evolution of the bleached grid during time. The confiner contours of the corresponding velocity intensity images shown in the lower row are superimposed. Interestingly, the black area in the middle of image f coincides perfectly with the hole emerging between images b and c. Thus, there is no movement at the emerging hole itself but a strong and homogeneous movement adjacent to it and directed away from it. If we imagine the lamina in this situation as an elastic polymer under tension it appears normal that an emerging hole *causes* this kind of dynamics. The precise coincidence illustrates also how reliable our algorithm estimates the underlying motion. We observe a movement *towards* the hole of the upper confiner in image g and for the confiner in the lower right corner. It seems to represent a back coupling of the movements before and to illustrate vaccilation properties of the lamina. The average area of the selected confiners assesses the movement in image h as highly undirected. This could correspond to the end of a vaccilation-relaxation process.

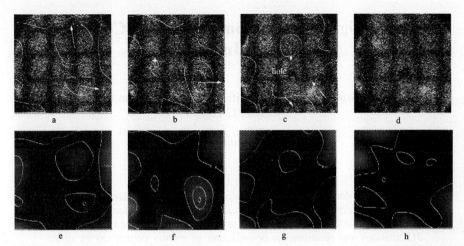

Fig. 1. *Formation of a hole (images c and d, indicated in c) in the lamina and velocity analysis: images a-d show the evolution of the photobleached grid during time with the superimposed confiner contours of the corresponding velocity intensity image depicted in e-h (image e corresponds to images a and b, image f to the images b and c, etc.; image h corresponds to d and the following image in the time sequence which is not shown). The arrows show the average direction of the movement inside a confiner.*

We described, characterized and visualized complex local dynamics by a few image clusters of homogeneous motion connected by a tree structure allowing new ways to analyze them quantitatively. In the presented cell biological application we thus obtained new insight into the physical properties of the lamina and could establish a correlation between surface movement and the formation of a hole in it. In further work we will investigate the possibility to compare local dynamics with reference dynamics, for instance with membrane vaccilations. In long term, we will design a model reproducing the movements of a polymer during the formation of a hole consistently with the imaged data.

References

1. Ferrant, M., Nabavi, A., Kikinis, R., Warfield, S.K.: Real-time simulation and visualization of volumetric brain deformation for image-guided neurosurgery. SPIE Medical Imaging 2001 (in press)
2. Fieres, J., Mattes, J., Eils, R.: A point set registration algorithm using a motion model based on thin-plate splines and point clustering. DAGM 2001, LNCS, Springer Verlag (accepted)
3. Germain, F., Doisy, A., Ronot, X., Tracqui, P.: Characterization of cell deformation and migration using a parametric estimation of image motion IEEE Trans. Biomed. Engineering **46** (1999) 584–600
4. Mattes, J., Demongeot, J.: Tree representation and implicit tree matching for a coarse to fine image matching algorithm. In: MICCAI'99, C. Taylor, A. Clochester (Eds.). LNCS. Springer-Verlag (1999) 646–655

Full 3D Rigid Body Automatic Motion Correction of MRI Images

Yi Su, Armando Manduca, Clifford R. Jack, E. Brian Welch, and
Richard L. Ehman

Mayo Clinic, Rochester, MN 55905 USA

Abstract. We demonstrate the first successful automatic motion correction of
3D MRI data with rigid body motion in all six degrees of freedom. An existing
2D retrospective technique is extended to 3D with a shear-based factorization of
3D rotations and simultaneous optimization of motion corrections in all six
degrees of freedom. Tests on motion corrupted 3D brain images from elderly
research subjects show dramatic improvements in image quality.

1 Introduction

In several ongoing research studies here, high resolution 3D MRI brain scans are
required of elderly, often cognitively impaired individuals. This population is
predisposed to motion and many subjects are simply unable to hold sufficiently still
for the length of the exam. Some form of motion correction is thus imperative.
Recently, automatic methods based on iterative optimization of an image quality cost
function have been proven effective for 2D rigid body motions [1,2]. However, such
schemes require inverse FFTs of the entire data set at each iteration, as well as
regridding in k-space for each trial rotation, making them computationally intensive.
They are also susceptible to local minima, being essentially optimization techniques
in a very high dimensional space. Extrapolation of these techniques to 3D data sets
and motions has not been attempted until now due to the computational requirements
and the increased dimensionality of the search space.

2 Methods

The data obtained in our studies are 3D SPGR acquisitions with TR/TE = 23/9 msec.
The k-space dimensions are 256x144x124 (22x16.5x19.8cm FOV), acquired in xzy
order. We assume no motion during the acquisition of each xz slab (2.85 sec),
reducing the dimensionality of the correction process to six degrees of freedom that
specify the subject's position at each of 144 points in time. The xz slabs are
considered in blocks, with the block size initially 72 slabs and progressively halved
until slabs are considered individually. At a given block size, blocks are optimized
individually, working outward from DC. These six-dimensional optimizations are
performed with a simplex algorithm; at each iteration with a trial set of motion

W. Niessen and M. Viergever (Eds.): MICCAI 2001, LNCS 2208, pp. 1326-1327, 2001.
© Springer-Verlag Berlin Heidelberg 2001

parameters the corresponding corrections are applied to the block under consideration, the entire data set is reconstructed, and the image quality is evaluated. Blocks not currently under consideration have their parameters fixed at the last values found. The cost function is the entropy of the image gradient [2], and 3D rotations are efficiently performed by a factorization into 4 shear operations [3].

3 Results

It is clear that the automatic motion correction dramatically improves the quality of the images (Fig. 1). While further improvement may be possible, the data is now usable for research purposes and would even be suitable for diagnosis. This represents the first successful automatic motion correction of 3D MRI data with rigid body motion in all six degrees of freedom.

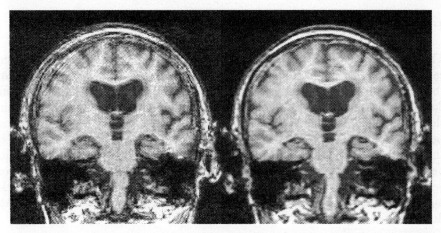

Fig. 1. A typical central slice of a data set with significant motion corruption before (left) and after (right) automatic motion correction.

References

Atkinson, D., Hill, D.L.G., Stoyle, P.N.R., Summers, P.E., Clare, S., Botwell, R., Keevil, S.F.: Automatic Compensation of Motion Artifacts in MRI. Mag. Res. Med. 41 (2000) 163-170

Manduca, A., McGee, K.P., Welch, E.B., Felmlee, J.P., Grimm, R.C. and Ehman, R.L.: Autocorrection in MR Imaging: Adaptive Motion Correction Without Navigator Echoes. Radiology 215 (2000) 904-909

Chen, B., Kaufman, A.: 3D Volume Rotation Using Shear Transformations. Graphical Models 62 (2000) 308-322

Estimating the Motion of the LAD:
A Simulation-Based Study

I.A. Kakadiaris[1*], A. Pednekar[1], G. Zouridakis[2], and K. Grigoriadis[3]

[1] Dept. of Computer Science, Univ. of Houston, Houston TX 77204-3010, USA
[2] Dept. of Neuroscience, Univ. of Texas-Medical School, Houston TX 77030, USA
[3] Dept. of Mechanical Engineering, Univ. of Houston, Houston TX 77204-4792, USA

Abstract. In this paper, we present a simulation-based study of a motion analysis technique designed to intra-operatively estimate the motion parameters of the LAD coronary artery from endoscopic images.

1 Introduction

The epicardial coronary arteries exhibit substantial phasic motion during the cardiac cycle. Our goal is to explore the feasibility of intra-operatively tracking the motion of the Left Anterior Descending (LAD) coronary artery using IR endoscopic images and patient-specific pre-operative data. Reconstruction of the three-dimensional geometry of the coronary arteries (e.g., from biplane projection data [1]) has received extensive attention. However, no parametric model of the arterial lumen that captures both the global and local shape characteristics has been presented. Similarly, although there is a substantial body of work on vessel tracking [2,5], most of the methods are limited to two-dimensional tracking in an image and there is no parametric model of the motion of the LAD during the cardiac cycle.

2 Methods

Modeling the arterial lumen: In our simulation-based study, we start with a triangular mesh of the inner lumen of the LDA. Our first objective is to obtain a parametric model of this mesh. To that end we employ the deformable model framework [4,3] to fit the model to the data. As a geometric model of the LAD we use a deformable model $\mathbf{s}(u,v)$ with a curved axis $\mathbf{e}(u) = (e_1(u), e_2, (u), e_3(u))^\top$

as follows:
$$\mathbf{s}(u,v) = \begin{pmatrix} s_1(u,v) \\ s_2(u,v) \\ s_3(u,v) \end{pmatrix} = \begin{pmatrix} e_1(u) + a_1(u)\ cos(v) \\ e_2(u) + a_2(u)\ sin(v) \\ e_3(u) \end{pmatrix}, \text{ where}$$

$-\frac{\pi}{2} \leq u \leq \frac{\pi}{2}$, $-\pi \leq v \leq \pi$, and $a_1, a_2 \geq 0$ are the parameters that define the superquadric size in the x and y directions, respectively. To capture local deformations we use the finite element method and we represent the deformable model

---

* This material is based in part upon work supported by the Texas Advanced Research Program under Grant No. 003652-0010-1999.

W. Niessen and M. Viergever (Eds.): MICCAI 2001, LNCS 2208, pp. 1328–1331, 2001.

in the form of weighted sums of local polynomial basis functions [4]. Once fitting is accomplished, the estimated values are the parameters of a (pre-operatively obtained) parametric deformable model of the LAD.

Modeling LAD's motion: Our second objective is to describe parametrically the movement of the LAD during the cardiac cycle. For this purpose we obtained, from our colleagues at the Texas Heart Institute, surface meshes of the LAD during five steps of the cardiac cycle. We model the movement of the LAD (due to the heart movement) as a systole/diastole and twist around the major axis of the heart (in this paper, we will not consider the respiratory motion). Let $\mathbf{m}(u, v, t) = (m_1, m_2, m_3)^\top$ be the position of the LAD over time obtained by applying a systole/diastole transformation along with a twist transformation to the initial LAD shape, as described below. Also, let the initial shape $\mathbf{m}(u, v, 0) = \mathbf{s}(u, v)$. The systole/diastole deformation can be parameterized as follows: $\mathbf{o}(u, v, t) = \begin{pmatrix} d^1(u, t) \\ d^2(u, t) \\ d^3(u, t) \end{pmatrix} \mathbf{s}(u, v)$. Given the above primitive $\mathbf{o} = (o_1, o_2, o_3)^\top$, the parameterized twisting results in a new position for the LAD given by:

$$\mathbf{m}(u, v, t) = \begin{pmatrix} o_1 cos(w(u, t)) - o_2 sin(w(u, t)) \\ o_1 sin(w(u, t)) + o_2 cos(w(u, t)) \\ o_3 \end{pmatrix}, \text{ where } w(u, t) \text{ is the time-vary-}$$

ing twisting parameter function along the axis of the heart model.

Model-Based Tracking: Our third objective is to track the motion of the LAD using IR endoscopic images. In this paper, we employ simulated IR endoscopic images. We have developed a model-based tracking technique to estimate the motion of the LAD from IR endoscopic images. The central idea of a model-based tracking approach is the following [3]: Using a previously acquired model of the object that you want to track, for each timestep find the position and orientation of the object such that it produces data like the ones acquired. We use as input the 2D coordinates of the silhouette of the LAD as computed by segmenting the IR images. The output is the functions: $d^1(u, t)$, $d^2(u, t)$, $d^3(u, t)$, and $w(u, t)$.

3   Results

Concerning modeling the shape of the LAD, Fig. 1(a) depicts the estimated deformable model, Fig. 1(b) depicts the estimated axis $\mathbf{e}(u)$, and Fig. 1(c) depicts the variation of the radius of the arterial lumen $a_1(u)$. Concerning our tracking technique, the input to our algorithm was the two-dimensional data of the silhouette of the LAD during a cardiac cycle obtained from simulated IR endoscopic images. Figs. 1(d,e) depict five samples of the estimated position of the LAD over time. The view chosen for Fig. 1(d) clearly shows the systole/diastole of the heart and the view chosen for Fig. 1(e) demonstrates the recovered twisting motion. Figs. 1(f-h) depict the values of the estimated motion parameters.

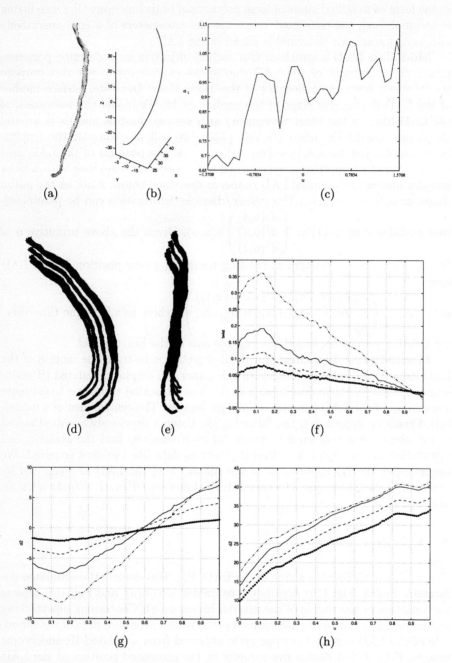

Fig. 1. (a) Deformable model of the LAD, (b) estimated axis, and (c) estimated radius $a_1(u)$. (d,e) Views of the estimated position of the LAD over time, (f-h) Estimated motion parameters $w(u,t)$, $d^1(u,t)$ and $d^2(u,t)$.

References

1. S.-Y.J. Chen and J.D. Carroll. Computer-assisted coronary intervention by use of on-line 3D reconstruction and optimal view strategy. In *Medical Image Computing and Computer-Assisted Intervention*, 1496, pp. 377–385, Cambridge, MA, 1998.
2. Z. Ding and M.H. Friedman. Dynamics of human coronary arterial motion and its potential role in coronary atherogenesis. *J. of Biomech. Engr.*, 122(5):488, 2000.
3. I.A. Kakadiaris and D. Metaxas. Model-based estimation of 3D human motion. *IEEE Transactions on PAMI*, 22(12):1453–1459, 2000.
4. D. Metaxas and D. Terzopoulos. Shape and nonrigid motion estimation through physics-based synthesis. *IEEE Transactions on PAMI*, 15(6):580 – 591, June 1993.
5. M.S. Sussman, A.B. Kerry, J.M. Pauly, N. Merchant, and G.A. Wright. Tracking the motion of the coronary arteries with the correlation coefficient. In *Proceedings of the 7th Scientific Meeting & Exhibition of the International Society for Magnetic Resonance in Medicine*, Philadelphia, Pennsylvania, 24-28 May 1999.

Phase-Driven Finite Element Model for Spatio-temporal Tracking in Cardiac Tagged MRI

Idith Haber[1], Ron Kikinis[2], and Carl-Fredrik Westin[2]

[1] Children's Hospital, Harvard Medical School, Boston MA, USA
[2] Brigham and Women's Hospital, Harvard Medical School, Boston MA, USA
idith.haber@tch.harvard.edu

1 Introduction

MRI tissue tagging[1] of the heart produces noninvasive markers within the muscle wall that can be used to measure motion and deformation (Fig. 1a). However, the widespread use of tissue tagging has been limited by time-consuming image post-processing. This paper outlines a method for automatic 3D tracking of LV motion from 2D MRI images acquired from multiple views. Since the tags form a repetitive pattern in the images, the local phase can serve as a material property that can be tracked. We first derive displacement from local image phase, a quantity previously used for estimating disparity between two 2D images in stereo vision [2, 8] or to measure relative deformation, or strain [7]. Displacement estimates have also been used for least square fitting of a 2D affine motion model to angiography images [5].

In the current work, we use phase-based displacement estimates to drive a 3D finite element deformable model of the left ventricle (LV). Our model enables reconstruction of 3D motion from 2D images and stabilization of the phase-derived displacement estimates, which are susceptible to noise and image artifacts. The basic framework for this model has been previously applied to 3D motion reconstruction of the right ventricles from user tracked tags [4, 3]. We here describe the geometry and constraints that enable phase-based displacement estimates to be used for automatically recovering 3D motion from tagged MR images.

2 Methods

1) Local Phase Estimation: Given an ideal sinusoidal signal, the phase is the argument of the analytic signal. For real signals, we use separable quadrature filters to estimate the analytic signal [6]. In a quadrature filter the real and imaginary parts form a Hilbert pair which makes the filter magnitude response phase invariant. For each coordinate direction u in the frequency domain, the filter is:

$$F(\mathbf{u}) = R(\rho)D(\hat{\mathbf{u}}), \tag{1}$$

where ρ is the magnitude and $\hat{\mathbf{u}}$ is the unit direction u. The directional function $D(\hat{\mathbf{u}})$ is oriented along the initial direction of the tags. The radial frequency function $R(\rho)$ is a Gaussian function on a logarithmic scale, and defines the frequency characteristics of the quadrature filter.

W. Niessen and M. Viergever (Eds.): MICCAI 2001, LNCS 2208, pp. 1332–1335, 2001.

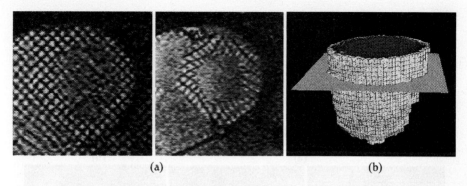

(a)   (b)

Fig. 1. (a) 2D tagged MR images of the left ventricle at beginning systole (relaxed) and end-systole (contracted). Dark bands represent tags that are tracked using local phase. (b) 3D finite element model used for simultaneously tracking in multiple images. A plane is drawn to show the location of the short-axis images.

In the spatial domain, we convolve the complex filter f with each pair of consecutive images $I_t, t = 1, 2$ to obtain $q_t = f(\mathbf{u}) * I_t$. The phase difference $\Delta\phi = arg(q_1 * q_2)$ is calculated with certainty $|q_1 * q_2|$. We estimate the displacement to be $z = \frac{\Delta\phi}{2\pi/\lambda}$, where λ is the tag pattern wavelength. By applying quadrature filters to three mutually perpendicular tagging patterns, we can obtain a field of 3D displacement vectors, $\mathbf{z}$.

2) 3D FEM Deformable Model: Fitting a solid finite element model to the phase-based displacement data ensures smoothness and enables 3D motion estimation. The model geometry is defined using contours traced in the initial, end-diastolic images (Fig. 1b). The finite element formulation and equations governing the model dynamics are derived from the Lagrangian equations of motion [4, 9]:

$$\dot{\mathbf{d}} = \mathbf{K}\mathbf{d} + \mathbf{f} \qquad (2)$$

where $\mathbf{d}$ is the nodal displacement and $\mathbf{K}$ is the finite element stiffness matrix.

The external force $\mathbf{f}$ is a spring-like force designed to approximate the phase-derived displacement: $\mathbf{f} = \mathbf{z} - \mathbf{d}$. The model is iteratively fit between successive image frames using adaptive Euler integration until all forces are minimized.

3 Results and Discussion

Convolution of the quadrature filters with the images resulted in images of the spatial distribution of local phase (Fig. 2a). These two images were then used to estimate the displacement, shown in Fig. 2b.

In order to assess the accuracy of the fitting, we applied the technique to synthetic image data. This data was generated by prescribing a complicated displacement field for a 3D superquadric geometry and calculating the intersection of this model with simulated image planes. We found that the difference between reconstructed and prescribed nodal displacement was less than one third of the voxel dimension.

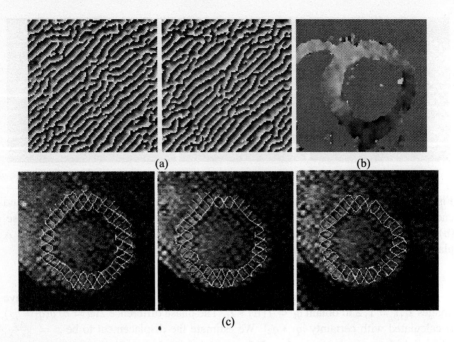

Fig. 2. Results: a) Phase calculated from consecutive images (Grayscale: -2π to 2π) b) Displacement derived from these two (Grayscale is -2.5:2.5mm). c) Representative results of fitting to image data from a normal volunteer. Intersection of model with image planes is shown along with images from consecutive short-axis slices.

The fitting technique was applied to images from several normal subject. We show a representative results Fig. 2c. By viewing intersection points of the model with the original image planes are drawn over the original images, we can see a close agreement.

In conclusion, we describe a phase-based method for fitting a 3D model to tagged MRI. The model allows for the regularization of the phase estimates and integration of motion information from multiple image planes. We found good results when applying the method to MR images of normal hearts.

4   Acknowledgements

This work is funded in part by Boston Children's Heart Foundation, NIH HL63095 (IH), CIMIT and NIH P41-RR13218 (RK,CFW).

References

[1] L. Axel and L. Dougherty. Heart wall motion: Improved method of spatial modulation of magnetization for MR imaging. *Radiology*, 172(2):349–50, Aug 1989.

[2] D.J. Fleet, A.D. Jepson, and M. Jenkin. Phase-based disparity measurement. *CVGIP: Image Understanding*, 53(2):198–210, 1991.

[3] I. Haber. *Three-Dimensional Motion Reconstruction and Analysis of the Right Ventricle From Planar Tagged MRI*. PhD thesis, University of Pennsylvania, Philadelphia, May 2000.

[4] I. Haber, D.N. Metaxas, and L. Axel. Three-dimensional motion reconstruction and analysis of the right ventricle using tagged MRI. *Med Image Analysis*, 4(4):335–355, 2000.

[5] M. Hemmendorff, H. Knutsson, M. T. Andersson, and T. Kronander. Motion compensated digital subraction angiography. In *Proceedings of SPIE's International Symposium on Medical Imaging*, volume 3661, San Diego, USA, February 1999. SPIE.

[6] H. Knutsson. Representing local structure using tensors. In *6th Scandinavian Conf. Image Analysis*, pages 244–51, Oulu, Finland, June 1989.

[7] N. F. Osman, E.R. McVeigh, and J.L. Prince. Imaging heart motion using harmonic phase MRI. *IEEE Trans on Med Imaging*, 19(3).186–201, Mar 2000.

[8] T. Sanger. Stereo disparity computation using gabor filters. *Biol Cybern*, 59:405–418, 1988.

[9] O.C. Zienkiewicz and R.L. Taylor. *The Finite Element Method*. McGraw-Hill, New York, fourth edition, 1989.

JULIUS - An Extendable Software Framework for Surgical Planning and Image-Guided Navigation

Erwin Keeve[1], Thomas Jansen[1], Zdzislaw Krol[1], Lutz Ritter[1],
Bartosz von Rymon-Lipinski[1], Robert Sader[2], Hans-Florian Zeilhofer[2] and
Peter Zerfass[1]

[1] Surgical Simulation and Navigation Group
research center c a e s a r
Friedensplatz 16, 53111 Bonn, Germany
keeve@caesar.de
http://www.caesar.de/ssn
[2] Dept. of Cranio- and Maxillofacial Surgery
Technical University of Munich, Germany

Abstract. In this paper we introduce the extendable and cross-platform software framework JULIUS, which will become public available by the end of this year. JULIUS consists of three conceptual layers and provides diverse assistance for medical visualization, surgical planning and image-guided navigation. The system features a modular and portable design and combines both pre-operative planning and intra-operative assistance within one single environment.

1. Introduction

In image-guided surgery the vision of reality is enhanced using information from CT, MR and other medical imaging data. Certain instruments can be guided by these patient specific images if the patient's position on the operating table is aligned to this data [1, 2, 3, 4]. In order to bring the actual computer-aided pre-operative planning scheme into the OR, it is best to use one single software environment for both the pre-operative planning process and the intra-operative intervention. Since image-guided surgery is a relatively new field, advanced algorithms and techniques should easily be integrated into this environment. To reach this goal, we developed the extendable and cross-platform software framework JULIUS, which can be used as a general software framework for rapid application development as well as a front-end for image-guided surgery.

2. Methods

We developed JULIUS on top of the OpenGL graphics library using the Visualization Toolkit vtk for all visualization tasks and the Qt library for the user interface. JULIUS consists of three conceptual layers - see Figure 1: The *Julius Software Development Kit* (JSDK) builds the core application and controls the data processing pipeline. The *Julius Graphical User Interface* (JGUI) acts like a front-end to the JSDK and offers easy handling combined with time-saving functionalities to increase performance and

W. Niessen and M. Viergever (Eds.): MICCAI 2001, LNCS 2208, pp. 1336-1337, 2001.

productivity. The *Julius Inter-Module Communication* (JIMC) provides information exchange schemes and communication interfaces.

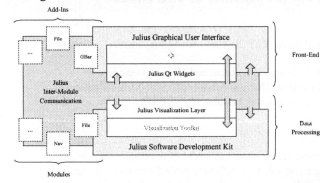

Fig. 1. The three conceptual layers of JULIUS, and the overall system architecture. Future developments can easily be integrated as modules or add-ins.

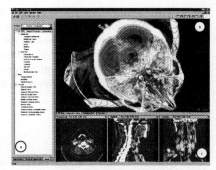

Fig. 2. The JULIUS graphical user interface: a.) The Global Bar window b.) The main window with 3D volume and/or surface visualization c.) The corresponding slice views

3. Results and Conclusions

With JULIUS we have created one single software environment for both pre-operative planning and intra-operative navigation achieving best results in routine surgical cases as well as in new computer-aided intervention methods. Modules for semi-automatic segmentation and registration, 3D reconstruction and visualization have been implemented. Interfaces to external devices like navigation and haptic systems are provided. The software framework has been tested in first surgical trials. We found that the separation between JSDK and JGUI enables on the one hand rapid software development for the scientific developer and on the other hand an intuitive handling for the surgeon. Application areas range from cranio- and maxillofacial surgery, to neurosurgery and orthopaedics. The clinical evaluation of the system in these areas will start within the next months.

References

1. ANALYZE, http://www.mayo.edu/bir/Analyze_Pages/Analyze_Main_TOC.htm
2. Gering D.T., "*A System for Surgical Planning and Guidance using Image Fusion and Interventional MR,*" Master's Thesis, Massachusetts Institute of Technology, 1999.
3. Golland P., Kikinis R., Umans C., Halle M., Shenton M.E., Richolt J.A., "*AnatomyBrowser: A Framework for Integration of Medical Information,*" In Proc. First International Conference on Medical Image Computing and Computer-Assisted Intervention; MICCAI'98, Cambridge, MA, pp. 720-731, 1998.
4. Leventon M.E., "*A Registration, Tracking, and Visualization System for Image-Guided Surgery,*" Master's Thesis, Massachusetts Institute of Technology, 1997.

A Statistical Model of Respiratory Motion and Deformation of the Liver

J.M. Blackall, A.P. King, G.P. Penney, A. Adam, and D.J. Hawkes

Division of Radiological Sciences and Medical Engineering
The Guy's King's and St. Thomas' Schools of Medicine and Dentistry
Guy's Hospital, London SE1 9RT, UK

Abstract. This paper presents a statistical model of the respiratory motion and deformation of the liver. Individual models were made for seven volunteers using a series of MR images taken throughout the breathing cycle. One image was selected as a template and the others were registered to this using an intensity-based non-rigid registration algorithm. The resulting free-form transformations allowed us to map landmarks defined on the template image into their correct positions throughout the breathing cycle. Principal component analysis of these landmarks was used to produce a statistical model of motion and deformation. Results showing typical motion and deformation for a single volunteer are presented.

1   Introduction

Much of the motion and deformation of abdominal structures during interventional procedures may be attributed to respiration and so will be approximately periodic and potentially predictable over the breathing cycle. A number of studies have been carried out into the motion of the liver and other abdominal organs during respiration [1,2]. This paper describes a statistical approach to modelling breathing motion and deformation of abdominal structures.

2   Method

We construct volunteer-specific statistical models of the liver by using a voxel-based non-rigid registration technique [3] to coregister a number of MR images acquired throughout the breathing cycle. The resulting free-form transformations are used to propagate landmarks derived from a segmented liver surface of a template image to the other images [4]. The statistical analysis is performed using these corresponding surface landmarks to form a Point Distribution Model (PDM) as described in [5].

3   Results

Statistical models were constructed using the technique described above for a total of seven volunteers. In this section we present results from one of these which was selected as a representative example.

W. Niessen and M. Viergever (Eds.): MICCAI 2001, LNCS 2208, pp. 1338–1340, 2001.
© Springer-Verlag Berlin Heidelberg 2001

Figure 1 illustrates the first mode of variation for the representative volunteer liver model. These renderings were produced by varying the weight for the first eigenmode only, whilst setting the others to zero. It can be seen that this mode of variation consists primarily of a rigid-body translation in the cranio-caudal direction. The magnitude of this translation, computed over all seven volunteers, is equal to 19 ± 8mm for shallow breathing, and 37 ± 8mm for deep breathing.

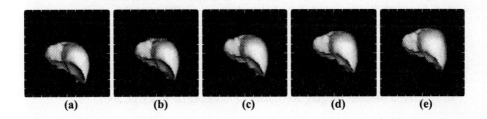

    (a)   (b)   (c)   (d)   (e)

Fig. 1. Renderings illustrating the first mode of variation for a single volunteer. Animations of this and other modes of variation for all seven volunteers can be viewed at http://www-ipg.umds.ac.uk/MICCAI2001/liverModels.html

The other modes of variation typically capture deformation. The maximum magnitude of this deformation was approximately 15mm for deep breathing and 10mm for shallow breathing. A few areas seem more prone to large deformations, particularly the superior surface of the liver, which is in direct contact with the diaphragm, and the inferior surface of the liver, which is in contact with the back of the body cavity and is compressed against this surface as the diaphragm descends.

For all seven individuals the first eigenmode accounted for a large percentage of the total variation. For the volunteer shown in figure 1 the first five modes of variation accounted for 81%, 9.1%, 4%, 3.2% and 2.5% of the total variation respectively.

4   Discussion

This paper has presented work which applies a statistical approach to the analysis of respiratory motion and deformation in abdominal structures.

Previous work [4] has used binary segmented images to compute the non-rigid registrations. Our registrations were computed using the segmented grey level images, which allows the intensities of internal liver structures to contribute to the similarity measure, and may well lead to a more accurate registration. In [6] the entire MR images were coregistered, without segmentation of the liver. This approach will cause difficulties when there is a large relative motion between the liver and surrounding tissue.

Models of respiratory motion have the potential to widen the applicability of image guidance in the abdominal and thoracic region and could prove useful for treatment planning in other applications such as radiotherapy.

References

1. S. C. Davies, A. L. Hill, R. B. Holmes *et al.* Ultrasound Quantitation of Respiratory Organ Motion in the Upper Abdomen. *Br. J. Radiol.*, 67:1096–1102, 1994.
2. I. Suramo, M. Paivansalo, and V. Myllya. Cranio-caudal Movements of the Liver, Pancreas and Kidneys in Respiration. *Acta Radiologica Diagnosis*, 25(2):129–131, 1984.
3. D. Rueckert, C. Hayes, C. Studholme *et al.* Non-rigid Registration of Breast MR Images Using Mutual Information. *Proc. MICCAI'98, Springer*, 1144–1152, 1998.
4. A. F. Frangi, D. Rueckert, J. A. Schnabel *et al.* Automatic 3D ASM Construction via Atlas-Based Landmarking and Volumetric Elastic Registration. *In Proc. IPMI'01, Springer, 2001.*
5. T. F. Cootes, C. J. Taylor, D. H. Cooper *et al.* Active Shape Models - Their Training and Application. *Computer Vision and Image Understanding*, 61(1):38–59, 1995.
6. T. Rohlfing, C. R. Maurer, Jr., W. G. O'Dell *et al.* Modeling Liver Motion and Deformation During the Respiratory Cycle using Intensity-Based Free-Form Registration of Gated MR Images. *Proc. Medical Imaging 2000: Image Processing (SPIE 4322)*, 2001.

Evaluation of Soft–Tissue Model Parameters

Matthias Teschner, Sabine Girod, and Kevin Montgomery

National Biocomputation Center
Stanford University, Palo Alto, CA 94304, USA
teschner@stanford.edu

Abstract. Computer–based techniques for the simulation of craniofacial surgical procedures and for the prediction of the surgical outcome have been shown to be very useful. However, the assessment of the accuracy of the simulated surgical outcome is difficult. In this paper, a robust registration technique is described which allows to compare the simulated surgical outcome and the actual surgical result.

1 Methods

In order to simulate craniofacial surgical procedures an existing system is used which is based on a preoperative CT scan of the patient's head and on a preoperative surface scan of the patient's face. The simulated postoperative patient's appearance is compared to a second surface scan which is obtained postoperatively. To enable the comparison, the pre– and postoperative surface scan have to be registered. Registration is required due to the fact, that the pre– and the postoperative scan are most probably obtained with different positions of the patient's head relative to the scanner.

In contrast to the Iterative Closest Point algorithm, which minimizes the mean of the Euclidean distances between corresponding points, a robust registration method is employed, which minimizes the median of the Euclidean distances of corresponding points. This is due to the fact, that the pre– and the postoperative facial scan differ in certain areas, i. e., corresponding points in these areas will still have comparative large Euclidean distances. In case of minimizing the median error instead of the mean error, these points do not falsify the transformation computed by the registration process.

If both scans are registered, the surgery simulation is performed using the preoperative scan of the patient's face and the simulation result is compared to the actual postoperative appearance by assessing the differences of corresponding points. Parameters of the soft–tissue model, such as number of soft–tissue layers or spring constants, are adapted with respect to minimized differences of corresponding points of the simulated and the actual surface of a patient's face.

2 Results

Registration of pre– and postoperative surface scans provides the opportunity to assess the accuracy of the simulation result by comparing the simulated and

W. Niessen and M. Viergever (Eds.): MICCAI 2001, LNCS 2208, pp. 1341–1342, 2001.

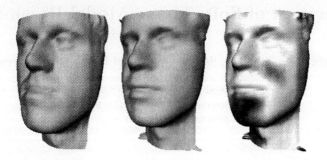

Fig. 1. Left: Praeoperative surface scan. Middle: Postoperative surface scan. Right: Registration error mapped onto the postoperative surface scan. Dark areas represent a large Hausdorff–distance up to 6*mm*. Bright areas are regions with no significant registration error.

the actual postoperative patient's appearance. Differences between both scans can be minimized by the adaption of model parameters. Fig. 1 shows a pre– and postoperative surface scan of a patient's face. Both scans are registered and the registration error is visualized in the right–hand image. Dark colors represent large errors (Hausdorff distances up to 6*mm*). Areas influenced by the surgery show large registration errors. However, these areas do not falsify the registration of the entire scan. Fig. 2 shows two scans with and without swelling. This swelling can be seen in the right–hand image which visualizes the registration error of these two scans. It can be seen that the registration approach is not influenced by areas which are different in both scans. The registration shown in Fig. 1 can be used to compare the simulated postoperative patient's appearance and his actual postoperative appearance. The registration shown in Fig. 2 can be employed to objectively assess the swelling, e. g. by measuring the volume of the swelling.

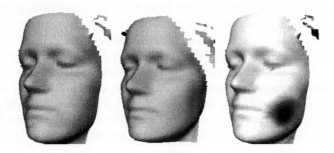

Fig. 2. Left: Surface scan with swelling. Middle: Surface scan without swelling. Right: Registration error mapped onto the surface scan with swelling. Dark areas represent a large Hausdorff–distance up to 4*mm*. Bright areas are regions with no significant registration error.

Bag-of-Particles Model for Simulating Tissue, Organs, and Flow

David J. Stahl, Jr. and Norberto Ezquerra

Georgia Institue of Technology, College of Computing, Atlanta GA, 30332-0280
{stahl, norberto}@cc.gatech.edu

Abstract. We present a physically-based, elastically deformable particle system model that combines the oriented particles used in surface-only models, and the unoriented particles used in volume-only simulations into a *bag of particles*. Multiple species of particles and predefined interspecies parameters determine elastic material properties. Model dynamic behavior and global shape are determined by the response of its particle ensemble to (i) volume forces and surface forces and torques, and (ii) orienting and shaping forces and torques derived from a distance map.

1 Particle Dynamics

Our system employs four potential functions of particle position and orientation that govern particle behavior: one potential that gathers particles into a shapeless, space-filling conglomeration, two potentials that arrange particles into locally planar surface configurations, and one potential that arranges these planar sections into a global object shape. Since the interior of an object does not intrinsically define its shape but is simply a volume filled with material, for our object interiors we use a form of the potential function frequently used in molecular dynamics simulations [1], the Lennard-Jones (LJ) potential, which models condensed matter as an aggregate collection of particles. This potential reasonably models gases and viscous fluids. Particles subject to only a LJ potential will form close-packed, space-filling aggregates in their minimum energy state, but not surfaces. To form surfaces, additional potentials are needed. For this purpose we use the approach of [2], which defines co-normal (CN) and coplanar (CP) potentials that act to arrange oriented particles into locally planar surface sections. To form non-planar surfaces, we add forces to arrange locally planar regions into the desired global object shape, and torques to orient surface particles to the object's surface normal. These forces and torques are obtained from a distance map [3], which defines the distance from a point to the closest point on a surface. The distance map is computed from a voxel bitmap representation of an object, which, in turn, can be obtained from a variety of representations such as polygonal models, implicit functions, or acquired image data.

W. Niessen and M. Viergever (Eds.): MICCAI 2001, LNCS 2208, pp. 1343–1344, 2001.

2   Bags of Particles

The simplest model requires two different particle types: space-filling unoriented volume particles that aggregate due to LJ forces, and oriented surface particles forming an enclosing surface, which are subject to LJ, CN, CP, and distance map forces and torques. The distance map force acts to keep surface particles in surface voxels, and the distance map torque maintains surface particles oriented to the surface normal. To model multiple elastic materials as bags within bags, particles are assigned a species attribute, and a set of inter-species coefficients are used to weight interparticle forces and torques, establishing different elastic behaviors as a function of particle species. Volume particles are free to move within an enclosing structure, such as blood flow within a vessel.

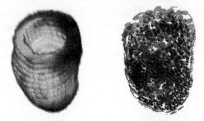

Fig. 1. Left ventricle acquired by PET: volume visualization and bag of particles model.

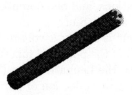

Fig. 2. Bag of particles model of blood flow in a vessel.

References

1. Rapaport, D.C.: The Art of Molecular Dynamics Simulation. Cambridge University Press, Cambridge, United Kingdom, 1995.
2. Szeliski, Richard and Tonnessen, David.: Surface Modeling with Oriented Particle Systems. Computer Graphics **26** (1992) 185–194
3. Danielsson, Per-Erik: Euclidean Distance Mapping. Computer Graphics and Image Processing. **14** (1980) 227–248

Simulated Animal Dissection

Cynthia Bruyns [1,2], Simon Wildermuth [1,2], Kevin Montgomery [1]

1. National Biocomputation Center, Stanford - USA
2. Center for Bioinformatics, NASA Ames Research Center – USA
{bruyns, wis, kevin}@biocomp.stanford.edu

Introduction

We have developed a flexible, multi-user, remote-capable virtual environment system that can be used to simulate rat dissection training. This paper will discuss the technologies required to create a virtual environment for the simulation of a rat dissection procedure incorporating haptic feedback.

Data Acquisition, Segmentation, and Soft-Tissue Deformation

A multidetector computer tomography was performed under 'in vivo' conditions in two anesthetized rats (2x0,5mm collimation, rotation time 0.8s, FOV 11x11cm, 512x512matrix). Using iodinated intravenous contrast material allowed the segmentation and reconstruction of the small internal organs, and to create corresponding high resolution polygon surface models. The reconstructed anatomy of the rat is represented within physically- based modeling simulation system. Bones are modeled as rigid objects that are used primarily for constraining the deformable geometry in space. Solution of the deformation equations is done using a localized semi-static solver, which is a simplification that ignores inertial and damping forces but provides a significant increase in performance. In order to speed up the simulation further, we can solve the deformation equations asynchronously, using a multithreaded model on multi-processor Sun (Mountain View, CA) E3500 8x400 MHz UltraSparc workstation. The simulation system is written in C++ using the OpenGL, GLUT, and POSIX libraries.

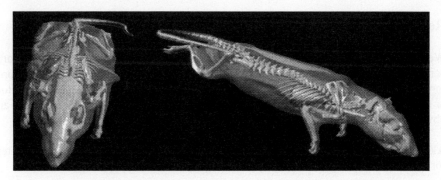

Fig. 1. 3D Surface Model based on high resolution multidetector CT datas

W. Niessen and M. Viergever (Eds.): MICCAI 2001, LNCS 2208, pp. 1345-1346, 2001.
© Springer-Verlag Berlin Heidelberg 2001

Interaction

In order to allow the user to interact with the environment using actual dissection tools, an Ascension Technologies (Burlington, VT) Flock-of-Birds electromagnetic tracker is attached to real surgical forceps, scalpels and scissors. By mapping the actual three-dimensional position and orientation of the tools to their counterpart in the virtual space, the user can easily interact with the tissue of the virtual rat. Probing the virtual rat can be used to extend the grasping or cutting procedures by adding force-feedback in order to give an impression of the compliance of each tissue. The haptic interface is achieved by a device connected to an embedded processor (Intel Pentium-based dedicated PC) and communicating via 100Mbps Ethernet to the Sun server running the simulation. In this way, we can reduce the computation load on the machine controlling the stability of the haptics device.

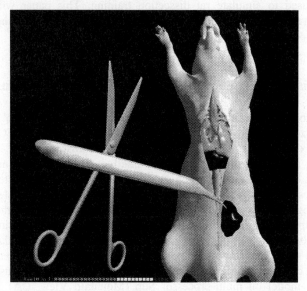

Fig. 2. Demonstrates removing the heart during a virtual animal dissection

Results / Discussion

We have assembled a preliminary environment for simulating tasks that are performed in animal dissection. This system provides for interaction with both non-force-feedback and haptic devices and for display with a stereo workstation monitor or tracked head-mounted display. As features are added to the system, there will be an obvious need to evaluate the effectiveness of the environment as a learning tool.

Aknowledgements: This work was supported by grants to the NASA Ames Center for Bioinformatics. Special thanks to Richard Boyle and Marlyn Vasques.

Virtual Polypectomy

Simon Wildermuth[1,2], Cynthia Bruyns[1,2], Kevin Montgomery[1], Borut Marincek[3]

1. National Biocomputation Center, Stanford - USA
{wis, bruyns, kevin}@biocomp.stanford.edu
2. Center for Bioinformatics, NASA Ames Research Center - USA
3. Institute for Diagnostic Radiology, Univ. Hospital Zurich - Switzerland

1 Introduction

Colorectal cancer is the second leading cause of cancer-related death in the United States and in Europe. If benign adenomas are removed prior to the development of malignancy, colon cancer is essentially preventable [1]. With the introduction of multidetector CT and advanced strategies for fast 3D MR imaging, the concept of virtual colonoscopy has become realistic. Promoting colon polyp screening programs, even more polyps will be found and therefore more polyp extractions are requested. Colonoscopy and endoscopic interventions are already procedures for experienced professionals and for difficult tasks, years of experience is needed [2]. To address a professional learning experience, we have assembled a preliminary environment for simulating tasks that are performed in colonoscopy. Different commercial prototype endoscopy simulators exist and provide realistic interfaces using the same hardware as used for conventional colonoscopy, but none of these products are able to simulate realistic soft tissue deformations using patient specific preoperative CT or MRI colon datasets. This paper presents a virtual environment for the simulation of colonoscopy procedures incorporating patient specific data providing an interactive, semi-immersive, haptic interface to the user.

2 Data Acquisition / Virtual Colonoscopy

Virtual endoscopy (VE) examinations and virtual polyp extractions were performed on clinical cases, using both, multidetector CT as well as MRI. The CTC and MRC techniques require proper patient preparation prior to scanning and instillation of colonic contrast (air for CTC or dilute gadolinium solution for MRC). The segmentation for virtual endoscopy was performed using Amira 2.0 (TGS Inc., San Diego, CA). Amira provides a component for 3D-image segmentation with several special-purpose features, ranging from purely manual to fully automatic methods. Once the lumina of the bowel have been segmented, a corresponding polygonal surface model by using the Generalized Marching Cubes module was created. The high-resolution mesh consisting over 1.4 million triangles was then simplified resulting in a mesh of under 200,000 polygons, which is more reasonable for interactive simulations, yet still provides sufficient fidelity for simulation.

W. Niessen and M. Viergever (Eds.): MICCAI 2001, LNCS 2208, pp. 1347-1348, 2001.
© Springer-Verlag Berlin Heidelberg 2001

3 Soft-Tissue Deformation and Polyp Extraction

In order to provide real-time, haptic-compatible update rates (>1000 Hz) of truly arbitrary deformations, a simplified mass-spring system was used to represent objects within the physically- based modeling simulation system. Solution of the deformation equations is done using a semi-static solver, which ignores inertial and damping forces but provides a significant increase in performance. In order to speed up the simulation further, we track the regions of deformation and only solve those that are currently undergoing interaction or distortion. Finally, we solve the deformation equations asynchronously, using a multithreaded model on multi-processor workstation. The simulation system is written in C++ using the OpenGL, GLUT, and POSIX libraries. The custom haptic handle is achieved by using a prototype device. For probing and tissue extraction, different endoscopic tools were developed and integrated. The score tip of the colonoscope with instrument channel, irrigation, lens and light are modeled and the working channel allows interactions with different instruments (biopsy forceps, snare) for polyp extraction.

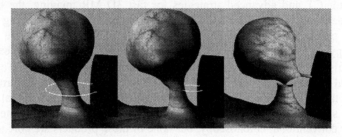

Fig.1. (a) Colonoscope reaching the polyp with the lasso tool. **(b)** Lasso ensnares the base of the polyp, deforming the tissue. **(c)** Cutting the polyp

4 Conclusions

We can import patient specific high-resolution meshes into a system that models colon polyps with different physical properties for interaction with both non-force-feedback and haptic devices. This virtual reality system for simulating virtual colonoscopy and polyp extraction can be used to simulate diverse procedures on a variety of pathologies in a novel physical environment and hopefully can shorten training periods and reduce complications.

References

1. Toribara, N.W. and M.H. Sleisenger, *Screening for colorectal cancer [see comments].* N Engl J Med, Vol. 332 (1995) 861-7
2. Tassios PS, et al. Acquisition of competence in colonoscopy: the learning curve of trainees. Endoscopy. Vol. 3 (1999) 702-6

Real-Time Interactions Using Virtual Tools

Cynthia Bruyns[1,2], Steven Senger[3], Simon Wildermuth[1,2], Kevin
Montgomery[2], and Richard Boyle[1]

[1] Center for Bioinformatics, NASA Ames Research Center
{cbruyns, rboyle}@mail.arc.nasa.gov
[2] National Biocomputation Center, Stanford University
{bruyns, wis, kevin}@biocomp.stanford.edu
[3] University of Wisconsin - La Crosse, Department of Computer Science
senger@csfac.uwlax.edu

Abstract. We extend the current collision response methods to allow
a user to interactively manipulate surface and volumetric meshes with
virtual tools and expand the idea of interaction directions to allow the
same tool to perform multiple tasks.

1 Introduction

We have developed a method to model complex tool and tissue interaction that
can be used to model manipulations such as pushing, pulling, and cutting at
multiple points of contact; and allows for several optimizations to be made within
the collision detection and response schemes.

2 Methods

2.1 Active Objects

Modeled objects have well-defined borders as outlined by the geometric primitives used to represent the volume. These borders can be assigned actions and
can switch which one is implemented depending on the object's state. When
modeling a simple tool, such as a scalpel, one can choose a single edge to be
considered sharp. Figure 1 demonstrates the two states of the sharp edge shown
in green. In the first frame, the surface deforms until the force within the springs
becomes larger than the yield force of the deformable tissue being simulated. In
the second frame, the sharp edge cuts as the user moves the scalpel. A series of
edges can also be specified as sharp in order to model more complex virtual tools
such as scissors. Figure 2 demonstrates the use of multiple edges. The first frame
demonstrates the tissue deformation as the scissors pinch the surface followed,
in the second frame, by surface relaxation as the scissors are opened.

The selection of sharp edges automatically defines allowable cutting directions. Motion along the cut direction allows the cutting action to be implemented, while motion out of the allowed direction causes the object to perform

W. Niessen and M. Viergever (Eds.): MICCAI 2001, LNCS 2208, pp. 1349–1351, 2001.

the pushing action. Figure 3 demonstrates the application of this concept on a simple model. In the first frame, the user has moved the scalpel out of the cutting plane, which does not produce a cut, instead, in the second frame, we see the surface deform as the scalpel pushes the surface to the side.

2.2 Collision Detection

Each object within the virtual environment has a tree of hierarchical bounding spheres [1]. We can choose to speed up the collision detection by pruning the trees to capture only the important aspects of the object interactions. We can also improve performance by leveraging spatial coherence since we typically move through an object by passing over adjacent faces when manipulating a surface, and adjacent tetrahedral when manipulating a volume. We have also developed schemes for adding and removing bounding sphere leafs to the tree as a cut is being created so that entire destruction and recreation of the tree is not necessary.

2.3 Collision Response

Cutting occurs on each intersected element as described in [2]. Because we deal with element states and not an object-wide state, it is possible to cut complex surfaces with folds and multiple layers. Figure 4 demonstrates the ability to interact with these complex objects. In the first frame the scalpel intersects multiple layers forming multiple cut paths. In the second frame, the surfaces relax as the free edges are formed. Using the same face- based cases, we can compose overall tetrahedral cases similar to [3] using only the minimal number of new tetrahedra for each cut. Figure 5 demonstrates the ability to cut a volumetric object composed of tetrahedra.

3 Conclusions

We have demonstrated the ability to model different behaviors within the same virtual object by assigning actions to object borders and report initial results with this system.

Acknowledgements: This work was supported by grants to the NASA Ames Center for Bioinformatics and the National Biocomputation Center. Special thanks to Joel Brown, Fredric Mazzella, and Anil Menon.

References

1. Sorkin, S., Distance Computing Between Deformable Objects. Honors Thesis, Computer Science Department, Stanford University, (2000)
2. Bruyns, C., Senger. S., Interactive Cutting of 3D Surface Meshes. *Computer and Graphics*, **25** (2001) *In Press*
3. Mor, A., Kanade, T., Modifying Soft Tissue Models: Progressive Cutting With Minimal New Element Creation. Lecture Notes in Computer Science, Vol. 1935. Springer-Verlag, Berlin Heidelberg New York (2000) 598-607

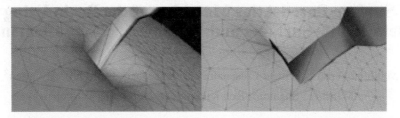

Fig. 1. Object states (a) Tool in pushing mode (b) Tool in cutting mode

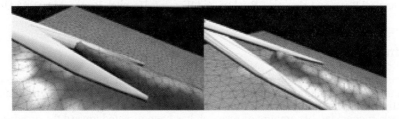

Fig. 2. Use of multiple cutting edges (a) Edges pinching surface (b) Surface relaxing

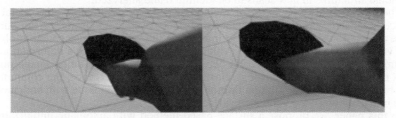

Fig. 3. Action directions a) Tool motion out of plane (b) Pushes aside surface

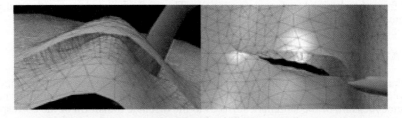

Fig. 4. Cutting multiple layers (a) Side-view (b) Top-view

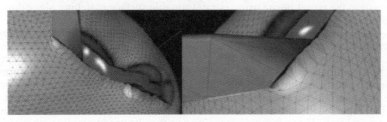

Fig. 5. Cutting a volumetric object

Surface Based Atlas Matching of the Brain Using Deformable Surfaces and Volumetric Finite Elements

Matthieu Ferrant[1], Olivier Cuisenaire[2], Benoît Macq, Jean-Philippe Thiran[2],

Martha E. Shenton[3], Ron Kikinis[3], and Simon K. Warfield[3]

[1] Université catholique de Louvain (UCL/TELE), B-1348 Louvain-la-Neuve, Belgium.
[2] Swiss Federal Institute of Technology (EPFL/LTS), CH-1015 Lausanne, Switzerland.
[3] Surgical Planning Laboratory, Brigham and Women's Hospital, Boston, MA02115 USA.

1 Introduction

The automatic identification and localization of structures in magnetic resonance (MR) brain images are a major part of the processing work for the neuroradiologist in numerous clinical applications, such as functional mapping and surgical planning. To aid in this task, a considerable amount of research has been directed toward the development of 3D standardized atlases of the human brain (e.g. [5]). These provide an invariant reference system and the possibility of template matching, allowing anatomical and functional structures in new scans to be identified and analyzed.

There are mainly two types of methods for doing deformable atlas matching : surface-based and volume based methods. Surface based methods deform key surfaces of the atlas onto the target image and interpolate the surface displacement to obtain a fully volumetric mapping (e.g. [3]). Volumetric methods compute a deformation field that minimizes a similarity criterion between the atlas and the target image under a given regularization constraint (e.g. elastic). To reach convergence, the computations must be done in a multi-resolution fashion (e.g. [1]). The main issue with both methods is the initialization of the volume or surfaces.

In this paper, we propose a surface based method with automatic initialization of the deformable surfaces using a global parametric transformation. We use an elastic volumetric finite element (FE) deformation model to infer a volumetric deformation field from the obtained surface deformations. The method provides us with a fully automated volumetric mapping of the atlas onto a target image.

2 Atlas Matching Algorithm

The landmark deformable surfaces of the atlas (cortical surface and ventricles) are initialized on the target image using a 2nd degree polynomial transform that minimizes a distance measure of the landmark surfaces to the distance transform of the corresponding objects in the target image [2]. The objects are segmented out of the target image using a directional watershed algorithm [2]. We then match the initialized landmark surfaces onto the target image using our deformable surface matching algorithm [4], as illustrated in Figure 1.

We infer a volumetric deformation field from the surface deformations by applying the surface displacements obtained after global registration and active surface deformation as a boundary condition to a volumetric FE tetrahedral mesh we have extracted from the atlas image [4]. After the atlas's volumetric FE mesh has been deformed by the boundary surfaces, the obtained deformation field can be interpolated back onto the image grid to produce a volumetric mapping from the atlas space onto the target image space [4]. Figure 2 illustrates the different volumetric deformation stages of atlas brain onto a target brain. The volumetric mapping can then be used to outline other objects in the target image.

W. Niessen and M. Viergever (Eds.): MICCAI 2001, LNCS 2208, pp. 1352–1353, 2001.
© Springer-Verlag Berlin Heidelberg 2001

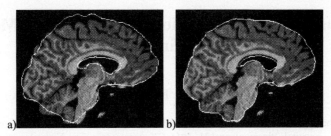

Fig. 1. a) cut through deformable surfaces after 2nd degree polynomial transform overlayed on corresponding cuts through target image. b) Same cut but after active surface deformation.

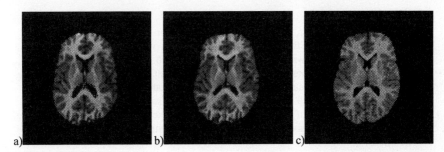

Fig. 2. Volumetric deformations of the atlas MR image illustrating the transformation steps of the algorithm. a) Slice of deformed volume after 2nd degree registration of ventricles and brain surface. b) Same slice after active surface deformation. c) Same slice of target image.

3   Conclusion

We have presented a surface based deformable atlas matching algorithm that automatically initializes the deformable surfaces. An arbitrary number of surfaces can be matched to drive the volumetric warp of the atlas onto a target image, and the finite element formulation of the volumetric match allows for variable elastic deformations of the atlas's objects. Our preliminary experiments show very good correlation of the deformed atlas with the target image.

References

1. G.E. Christensen, S.C. Joshi, and M.I. Miller. Volumetric Transformation of Brain Anatomy. *IEEE Trans. Med. Imag.*, 16(6):864–877, December 1997.
2. O. Cuisenaire. *Distance Transformations : Fast Algorithms and Applications to Medical Image Processing*. PhD thesis, Telecommunications Laboratory, Université catholique de Louvain, B-1348 Belgium, 1999.
3. C. Davatzikos. Spatial Transformation and Registration of Brain Images Using Elastically Deformable Models. *Computer Vision and Image Understanding*, 66(2):207–222, May 1997.
4. M. Ferrant, S.K. Warfield, A. Nabavi, B. Macq, F. Jolesz, and R. Kikinis. Registration of 3D Intraoperative MR Images of the Brain Using a Finite Element Biomechanical Model. In Anthony M. DiGioia and Scott Delp, editors, *MICCAI 2000: Third International Conference on Medical Robotics, Imaging And Computer Assisted Surgery; 2000 Oct 11–14; Pittsburgh, USA*, pages 19–28. Springer, 2000.
5. R. Kikinis, M.E. Shenton, D.V. Iosifescu, R.W. McCarley, P. Saiviroonporn, H.H. Hokama, A. Robatino, D. Metcalf, C.G. Wible, C.M. Portas, R. Donnino, and F.A. Jolesz. A Digital Brain Atlas for Surgical Planning, Model Driven Segmentation and Teaching. *IEEE Trans. on Visualization and Computer Graphics*, 2(3):232–241, 1996.

Evaluation of Cost Functions for Gray Value Matching of 2D Images in Radiotherapy

Niels Dekker, Lennert S. Ploeger, and Marcel van Herk

Radiotherapy Department, The Netherlands Cancer Institute / Antoni van Leeuwenhoek
hospital, Plesmanlaan 121, 1066 CX Amsterdam, The Netherlands
{ndekker, lennert, portal}@nki.nl

Abstract. In this paper, cost functions are tested for 2D registration of portal
and reference images for treatment verification in radiotherapy. Tests were
performed with and without pre-processing for 96 image pairs of various
treatment sites. The best results were obtained when the images were pre-
processed by unsharp masking and histogram equalization. This led to a success
rate of about 88% and a difference with clinical registration of 1.2 mm SD and
1 degree SD for most of the tested cost functions. The number of local minima
with mutual information is much larger than with the other tested cost
functions.

1 Introduction

External beam radiotherapy is often verified by electronic portal imaging, imaging the
patient with the treatment beam. As part of the image analysis to determine the setup
error, the anatomy in a portal image is matched with the anatomy in a reference
image. As reference images, often diagnostic x-ray images or digitally reconstructed
radiographs are used. Because of the complexity of 3D-2D matching, 2D image
analysis is still used on a wide scale. Most automatic matching algorithms for portal
images are based on segmented anatomy. These methods are especially successful for
images of the pelvic region. The purpose of this study is to find a cost function that is
applicable for anatomy matching on a wide range of treatment sites.

2 Material and Methods

In this study 96 pairs of portal and reference images are used. The images were
selected at random from rectum, salivary gland, whole brain, prostate and lung
treatments. For each tumor site, 9 or 10 anterior-posterior and 9 or 10 lateral image
pairs were used. Each of the portal images was matched previously in the clinic.
These clinical matches are considered "ground truth".

It appeared that the result of the cost functions could be improved by applying two
pre-processing steps to both the portal and the reference image: unsharp masking
followed by histogram equalization of the region within the field edge mask.

W. Niessen and M. Viergever (Eds.): MICCAI 2001, LNCS 2208, pp. 1354-1355, 2001.
© Springer-Verlag Berlin Heidelberg 2001

The investigated cost functions are computed from a cross-histogram of pixel values of both images. The following cost functions were tested: 1. Mutual information (MI); 2. The root mean square of the pixelwise differences (RMS); 3. The negated mean pixelwise product (PROD), which is similar to image correlation; and 4. The mean absolute pixelwise difference (DIFF).

For each matched pair of portal and reference images the cost function values were calculated for more than 20,000 transformations; these transformations were generated by varying the translation up to ± 1 cm in horizontal and vertical direction from the clinical match and by varying the rotation up to ± 10 degrees. This search range corresponds with the range of expected setup errors in clinical practice. The step size is 0.7 mm for translation and 1 degree for rotation. The transformation that corresponds to the global minimum of the cost function values is determined. If this transformation lies within a sphere around the clinical match of 4 mm translation and 4 degrees rotation, the match is considered successful. For each cost function the number of successes is counted, and the average and the standard deviation of the results of the successful matches is computed to determine the accuracy compared with the ground truth.

3 Results

Table 1 gives an overview of the successful matches of the tested cost functions. MI had 470 local minima; the other cost functions had 13 to 17 local minima on average.

Table 1. Overview of the performance of the cost functions. The success rate and the mean (standard deviation) of the difference with the clinical match are presented. In all cases, unsharp masking followed by histogram equalization was used as preprocessing.

	MI	RMS	PROD	DIFF
Success rate	78%	89%	88%	89%
Horizontal translation (cm)	0.01 (0.10)	0.01 (0.10)	-0.01 (0.10)	0.01 (0.10)
Vertical translation (cm)	0.00 (0.11)	-0.02 (0.12)	-0.02 (0.12)	-0.02 (0.12)
Rotation (degrees)	-0.05 (0.93)	0.02 (1.02)	-0.18 (1.01)	-0.01 (0.98)

4 Discussion and Conclusions

The success rate is reasonable, if one considers that the existing registration method has a poor success rate for difficult cases like the lung and lateral pelvis images. Good results were obtained for most treatment sites. The largest number of failures occurred for small brain fields, where little anatomical detail is visible. The difference in success rate between the different costs functions is small when pre-processing is applied. In conclusion, gray value matching of portal and reference images is feasible and forms a useful alternative for methods based on segmented anatomy.

Mutual Scale

C.P. Behrenbruch, T. Kadir, M. Brady

Medical Vision Laboratory (Robotics), Department of Engineering Science,
Oxford University, OX1 3PJ, United Kingdom
{cpb,jmb}@robots.ox.ac.uk

Abstract. Intensity-based registration of dynamic imaging data (for example for motion correction of contrast-enhanced MRI) or multi-modal fusion requires the use of a correlation measure that has good photometric invariance properties. We suggest that scale-localized image reconstruction prior to registration (based on the feature saliency of the images to be registered) often produces a better first estimation of a transformation, particularly if intensity conservation is assumed.

Introduction

The motion correction of dynamic soft-tissue imaging (e.g. breast MRI with Gd chelate) and multi-modal fusion (e.g. US-MRI, CT-PET) has lead to the development of registration techniques based on various forms of optical flow or correlated block matching algorithms [1-4]. Many of these algorithms are based on the fundamental assumption that intensities are conserved (in some suitable sense) in order to calculate a displacement field, although in practice, many model-based correction and regularization techniques are used to improve displacement field estimation.

The Mutual Scale Concept

Our hypothesis is that when computing a displacement or motion field between images, significant advantages accrue from using mutually scale-salient representations of the images to be registered. By this, we mean that the images to be registered should first be decomposed into a multi-scale representation and then reconstructed using:

- Scales which best reflect the information content of the images to be registered
- "Mutual Scales" in which *both* images to be registered are well represented.

A demonstration of the concept of image reconstruction at mutual scales is illustrated in Figure 1. In this figure, a breast MRI proton density image (TE=4.2ms, TR=8.9ms, $\alpha=3°$) is compared with a T1-weighted ($\alpha=10°$) image of the same slice. In this case, the intensity transformation is highly non-linear although a number of features remain visually consistent. We illustrate the reconstruction of the image pair at 3 different levels of scale (for example, using a wavelet-based approach, though the precise mechanism for computing the scale space is not the main point of this article). It is evident that most of the intensity transformation is localized at coarse scales (B,F), whilst at finer scales, it is possible to reconstruct a visually similar image via a suitable mutual scale.

W. Niessen and M. Viergever (Eds.): MICCAI 2001, LNCS 2208, pp. 1356-1357, 2001.

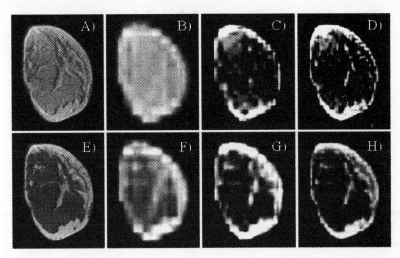

Fig. 1. A) and E) are the original images for which there is a non-linear intensity transformation. B) and F) are "coarse" scale examples which illustrate that the major component of the intensity transformation is localized to a low level of scale. C),G) and D),H) are reconstructions at successively finer scales. The pair D) & H) are a good example of reconstruction at a mutually salient scale.

The concept presented in this short paper is preliminary, however we feel that it demonstrates an inherently intuitive concept that appears not to have been noted before; but which forms the basis of many "workarounds" in image registration. One might argue that the notion of a mutual scale for image registration is simply a form of adaptive denoising or intensity correction. Our hypothesis is that an arbitrary registration approach is more meaningful when the feature scale for matching is appropriately addressed.

Acknowledgements

The Authors wish to acknowledge the Association of Commonwealth Universities (C.B.) Motorola University Partners in Research (T.K.), EPSRC GR/M54995 (M.B.).

References

1. Guimond, A., Roche, A., Ayache, N., Meunier, J.: Multimodal Brain Warping Using the Demons Algorithm and Adaptive Intensity Corrections. IEEE Transactions on Medical Imaging, 20(1), (2001)
2. Hayton, P., Brady, J.M., Tarassenko, L., Moore, N.: Analysis of dynamic MR breast images using a model of contrast enhancement. Medical Image Analysis, 1(3), Oxford University Press (1997) 207-224
3. Roche, A., Guimond, A., Ayache, N., Meunier, J.: Multimodal Elastic Matching of Brain Images. In Computer Vision - ECCV 2000, volume 1843 of LNCS, Dublin, Ireland, Springer Verlag (2000) 511-527
4. Thirion, J-P.: Image matching as a diffusion process: an analogy with Maxwell's demons. Medical Image Analysis, Oxford University Press (1998) 243-260

Fast Linear Elastic Matching Without Landmarks

Samson J. Timoner[1], W. Eric L. Grimson[1], Ron Kikinis[2], and
William M. Wells III[1,2]

[1] MIT AI Laboratory, Cambridge MA 02139, USA
samson@ai.mit.edu
[2] Brigham and Women's Hospital, Harvard Medical School, Boston MA, USA

Introduction: Non-rigid matchers generally constrain estimated displacement fields in uniform intensity regions of medical data. Elastic models are popular regularizers since they are easy to understand and simulate, and their smoothness properties may be as likely as other constraints.

Unfortunately, using an elastic energy function with image driving forces leads to ill-conditioned equations. To better constrain these equations, other authors have added landmarks or otherwise changed the boundary conditions of the problem[1]. However, reliable landmarks are difficult to find in medical images and we therefore avoid them. Our main contribution in this paper is to develop a fast nonrigid registration method using the ill-conditioned equations.

Methods: The matching process starts by meshing one volume with tetrahedra. We have written a tetrahedral mesher that accurately and compactly represents often irregular medical shapes without creating skewed tetrahedra. We use a probabilistic framework to match the mesh to the other volume by maximizing the log probability of the deformation field given the data, $\log P(r|\text{data})$. Equivalently, we maximize $\log P(\text{data}|r) + \log P(r)$.

Our image agreement term, $P(\text{data}|r)$, is based on the joint probability $P(I_2, I_1)$ that the volumes have joint intensities (I_2, I_1) when registered. Many authors assume the intensity distribution of each voxel is independent. A continuous version of this idea is more suitable to volumetric representations. Using this assumption, $\log P(\text{data}|r) = \sum_{\text{Tetrahedra}} \int_{tet} \log P(I_2, I_1) dV$, where I_2 changes depending on the warp.

The probability of a deformation, $P(r)$, can be estimated using statistical physics where the probability that a system is in a configuration is $e^{-E/T}$ where T is a temperature and we choose E as the linear elastic energy of the mesh. That energy can be locally written as is $\frac{1}{2} r^T K r$ where K is an elasticity matrix[2].

We use a modified Newton based solver to find the zeros in the gradient of the maximization function. Given the guess r_k in the kth iteration, the change in the deformation field, δr, in the $k + 1^{th}$ iteration solves

$$[\frac{K}{T} + \epsilon I]\delta r = \frac{-Kr_k}{T} + \sum_{\text{Tetrahedra}} \frac{d(\int_{tet} \log P(I_2, I_1) dV)}{dr}.$$

W. Niessen and M. Viergever (Eds.): MICCAI 2001, LNCS 2208, pp. 1358–1360, 2001.
© Springer-Verlag Berlin Heidelberg 2001

Because K is ill conditioned [1], we use a standard method to improve the matrix conditioning by adding a small ϵ to the diagonal of the matrix.

After the addition of this term, the elasticity matrix is still poorly-conditioned. Solving a poorly-conditioned linear system is possible using standard Krylov subspace based solvers, though may require many iterations. One common method in a Newton solve is to find an approximate solution to the matrix equation, using only a few iterations of the iterative matrix solve. Using this technique, the matrix solve time can be improved by more that a factor of 100. And, because there may be no exact solution, little is lost in solving the system approximately.

Experiments: We tested our matcher applied to a the manually segmented, left hippocampus-amygdala complex from a data set of 30 patients. One complex from a randomly chosen patient was meshed and matched with the rest of the patients. These data sets represent an interesting challenge because of the need of the bulbous head of one amygdala to be captured by the other (Figure 1).

For 1000 node meshes the matcher converged in under 50 iterations in less than 1 minute on a 450 Mhz Pentium III. Tests on larger meshes showed that 50 iterations were still sufficient and, as expected, the iteration time scaled linearly with the number of nodes. Figure 1 shows the error in the match. In the cases with highest error, we found the segmentations to have unphysical protrusions or minimal resemblance to the other data sets. The matcher tended to smooth these features leading to errors.

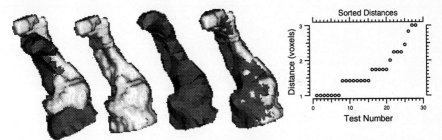

Fig. 1. The left image shows the initial alignment of the mesh (dark) with a triangulated surface of a labeled amygdala (light). The remaining images shows the surfaces after warping. The plot shows the distance between the two surfaces for each match in voxels, calculated as the upper quantile of the undirected Hausdorff metric.

Conclusions: We presented a fast, elastic volumetric matcher that does not use landmarks. We tested the matcher using label maps and showed good results.

Acknowledgements: S.J. Timoner is supported by the Fannie and John Hertz Foundation and NSF ERC grant, J.H.U Agreement #8810274. W. Wells was supported by the same NSF grant. Dr. Martha Shenton provided segmented images for the matching experiments. Her work was supported by NIMH grants R01 50740 and K02 01110, and a Veterans Administration Merit Award.

1360   S.J. Timoner et al.

References

1. Y. Wang and L. H. Staib. Elastic model based non-rigid registration incorporating statistical shape information. In *MICCAI 98*, pages 1162–1173, Cambridge, MA, Oct. 1998.
2. O.C. Zenkiewicz and R.L. Taylor. *The Finite Element Method*, volume 1. McGraw-Hill, Berkshire, England, fourth edition, 1989.

Endoscope Calibration and Accuracy Testing
for 3D/2D Image Registration

Rasool Khadem[1], Michael R. Bax[2], Jeremy A. Johnson[2], Eric P. Wilkinson[2]
and Ramin Shahidi[2]

[1] CBYON, 2275 East Bayshore Road #101, Palo Alto, CA 94303, USA
rasool@cbyon.com
[2] Image Guidance Laboratories, 300 Pasteur Drive #S-012, Stanford, CA 94305-5327, USA
http://igl.stanford.edu

Abstract. New surgical navigation techniques incorporate the use of live surgical endoscope video with 3D reconstructed MRI or CT images of a patient's anatomy. This image-enhanced endoscopy requires calibration of the endoscope to accurately the register the real endoscope video to the virtual image. The calibration and accuracy testing of such a system and a simple yet effective linear method for lens-distortion compensation are described.

1 Background and Theory

Today lightweight endoscopes are used in small body cavities, but they display only visible surfaces and are unable to view the interior of opaque tissue. Combining endoscopic video with overlaid volumetrically-reconstructed CT or MRI patient images permits surgeons to look beyond visible surfaces and provides "on-the-fly" 2D and 3D information for planning and navigation [1]. Precise endoscope calibration and exhaustive accuracy testing are necessary to ensure surgical quality.

Following calibration, tracking the position and rotation of the endoscope enables the rendering of virtual images to match the endoscope video. A ray from the center of projection (the optical origin) to a point in physical space passes through the image projection plane (the CCD). Errors such as residual lens distortion or tracking error cause this intersection to be some distance e from the image point, as in Fig. 1(a).

Adding full non-linear radial lens-distortion compensation to the rendering engine causes a drop in performance; an alternative method, here named "constant-radius linear compensation", is to linearly scale the virtual image such that the radii of the predefined region of interest in each image are made equal.

2 Method

A STORZ Tricam endoscope with a 50200A telescope, Traxtal universal passive trackers, and an NDI Polaris hybrid optical tracking system were used.

Tsai's calibration algorithm [2] was used. The calibration target was a planar grid pattern of black dots 1 and 2 mm in diameter, with the grid rows and columns spaced

W. Niessen and M. Viergever (Eds.): MICCAI 2001, LNCS 2208, pp. 1361-1362, 2001.

3 mm apart. This was mounted in a jig with an attached tracker such that the telescope of the endoscope in calibration is positioned 15 mm away from the center of the
target and angled 30° from the normal of the target plane.

The physical target for accuracy testing was a version of the calibration target large
enough to fill the field of view (FOV) of the endoscope at a distance of 65 mm, and
mounted on a tracked moveable plate. The grid position was localized relative to the
tracker. The grid was stepped through a set of distances from 5 to 65 mm from the tip
of the endoscope's telescope. At each position the image error e was found for each
dot in the endoscope video image. This was repeated for 20 separate calibrations.

3   Results

Fig. 1(b) shows the mean error between the rendered location of the dots in the virtual
image and the corresponding dots in the endoscope video image, normalized to the
diameter of the FOV, as a function of distance from the center of the image. Fig. 1(c)
shows the normalized error as a function of distance of the target plane from the endoscope tip. It can be seen that constant-radius linear compensation is an effective
scheme for overcoming lens distortion without a rendering performance loss.

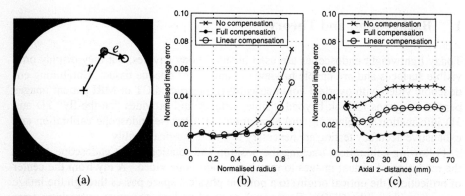

(a)   (b)   (c)

Fig. 1. (a) Image space error: a point in the video image (*gray dot*) and the projection ray
intersection with the image plane (*white dot*). (b) Mean image error versus image radius and
(c) mean image error versus target plane distance, normalized to the FOV diameter.

References

1. D.J. Vining, Virtual Endoscopy: Is It Reality? Radiology **200** (1996) 30–31
2. Tsai, R.Y.: An Efficient and Accurate Camera Calibration Technique for 3D Machine Vision. Proc. of the IEEE Conference on Computer Vision and Pattern Recognition (1986)
   364–374
3. Khadem, R., Yeh, C., Sadeghi-Tehrani, M., Bax, M.R., Johnson, J.A., Welch, J.N., Wilkinson, E.P., Shahidi, R.: Comparative Tracking Error Analysis of Five Different Optical
   Tracking Systems. Computer Aided Surgery **5** (2000) 98–107

Fast Non-rigid Multimodal Image Registration Using Local Frequency Maps

B.C. Vemuri and J. Liu

Department of Computer and Information Science and Engineering
University of Florida
vemuri|jliu@cise.ufl.edu

Abstract. In this paper, we present a novel and computationally efficient multimodal image registration scheme that is capable of handling non-rigidly misaligned multi-modal data sets. The algorithm is based on a level-set based image registration algorithm applied to local frequency representations of the input images. The algorithm has been tested on several data sets and we present one of these examples.

1 Introduction

In this paper, we present a novel method for non-rigidly registering multi-modal images. Our method involves first deriving a brightness "invariant" representation of the image and then using the level-set curve evolution technique for image registration introduced in Vemuri et.al., [1] on these "invariant" representations of the input images.

2 Local Frequency Representation & Matching

The *Gabor Filter* is a well-known quadrature filter. *It achieves the theoretical lower bound of the uncertainty principle.* Local frequency computation can be achieved by Gabor filtering the input data and then computing the gradient of local phase followed by summing the squared magnitude of local frequency maps over a discrete set of orientations for a fixed frequency [2]. We present and example local frequency representation in figure 2 which depicts a pair of T1 & T2 MR slices and their corresponding local frequency maps.

Given two local frequency maps $F_1(X)$ and $F_2(X)$, we want to find the non-rigid transformation between them. This can be achieved by decomposing the non-rigid deformation into incremental rigid transformation and using a moving grid implementation of the following evolution equation:

$$V_t = [F_2(X) - F_1(V(X))]\frac{\nabla F_1(V(X))}{\|\nabla F_1(V(X))\|} \ \ with \ \ V(X,0) = \mathbf{0} \qquad (1)$$

where $V = (u,v,w)^T$ is the displacement vector at X and the operation $V(X) = (x-u, y-v, z-w)$. For an efficient implementation of this equation, see [1].

W. Niessen and M. Viergever (Eds.): MICCAI 2001, LNCS 2208, pp. 1363–1365, 2001.
© Springer-Verlag Berlin Heidelberg 2001

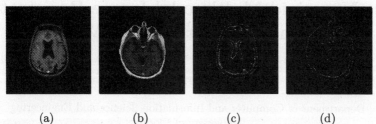

(a)   (b)   (c)   (d)

Fig. 1. (a) T1-weighted MR, (b) T2-weighted MR slices, (c) and (d), corresponding slices of local frequency maps.

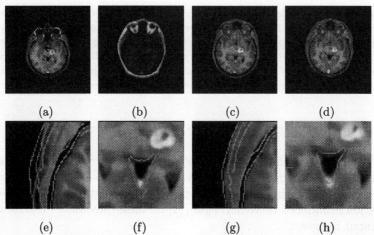

(a)   (b)   (c)   (d)

(e)   (f)   (g)   (h)

Fig. 2. Non-Rigid Registration Example: (a) source image, (b) target image,
(c) globally transformed source image with superimposed target edge map, (d)
non-rigidly transformed source with superimposed target edge map. The second
row is the zoom-in version of (c) and (d): (e) left upper and (f) central parts of
(c); (g) left upper (h) central parts of (d).

3   Implementation Results

We report a registration experiment with a pair of MR images obtained using
a T1 and T2 weighted imaging protocols respectively. Each image was obtained
from different subjects making it apt for the application of a non-rigid deformation. Figure 2 shows the registration results for the T1 and T2 weighted
MR brain scans being registered. Fig. 2(a) and (b) depict the source and target
images to be registered. Prior to application of the non-rigid registration, we
rigidly align the data sets. Figure 2(c) depicts the globally transformed source
and the locally transformed source image is shown in fig. 2(d). 2(c) and 2(d)
have been superimposed with the edge map of target image to visually demonstrate the accuracy of the registration. Figures 2(e) and 2(f) depict the residual
mis-alignment after the application of the global rigid transform to the source

using a close up view at two different locations in the source. Figures 2(g) and 2(h) depict the close up view of the alignment achieved after the application of a non-rigid deformation to the globally transformed source image at the same locations as in 2(e) and 2(f). As is evident, the mis-alignment has been dramatically reduced after the application of the non-rigid deformation. The average CPU time taken for computing the local frequency map from the input image is 366sec. and that for estimating the global rigid motion is 37sec. on an R10000 single CPU of an SGI Onyx. The time taken to compute non-rigid deformation is 357sec., which is much faster than most of the reported non-rigid registration schemes in literature.

4 Summary

In this paper, we presented a novel and efficient non-rigid multimodal image registration scheme. The algorithm involved constructing local frequency maps of the input data followed by an application of the level-set based non-rigid registration scheme [1]. The algorithm was tested on several data and illustrated via one example.

Acknowledgments

We thank Drs. Bova & Bouchet and Mr. Moore for providing the image data. This research was partially supported by the grants NSF IIS9811042 and NIH RO1-RR13197.

References

1. B. C. Vemuri et.al., [2000], "A Level-set based approach to image registration," *IEEE Workshop on MMBIA*, June 10-12, Hilton Head, SC, pp. 86-93.
2. B. C. Vemuri, J. Liu, J. L. Marroquin, [2001], "Robust Multimodal Image Registration using Local Frequency Representation," *IPMI'01*, June 18-22, Davis, CA, pp. 176-182.

Accuracy Validation of Cone-Beam CT Based Registration

Yoshikazu Nakajima[1], Toshihiko Sasama[1], Yoshinobu Sato[1], Takashi Nishii[2], Nobuhiko Sugano[2], Takashi Ishikawa[4], Kazuo Yonenobu[2], Takahiro Ochi[3], Shinichi Tamura[1]

[1] Division of Interdisciplinary Image Analysis
[2] Department of Orthopaedic Surgery
[3] Division of Computer Integrated Orthopaedic Surgery
Osaka University Graduate School of Medicine
[4] Hitachi Medical Corporation
nakajima@image.med.osaka-u.ac.jp
http://www.image.med.osaka-u.ac.jp/nakajima

Abstract. In this paper, the accuracy of intraoperative registration using cone-beam CT for computer-assisted surgery is preliminarily evaluated. Since cone-beam CT enables whole-surface detection of bone without surgical exposure, highly accurate registration is potentially attainable. In *in vitro* experiments, much higher accuracy could be attained by acquiring the intraoperative bone surface using cone-beam CT (0.56 mm) as compared with that of our routinely used protocol employing a 3-D positional sensor (1.43mm).

1 Introduction

Percutaneous surgical procedures and endoscopic surgeries are being increasingly used because of their minimal invasiveness. However, the surgeon does not have a direct view, or has only a restricted view, of anatomical structures. Hence, computer assistance is useful in these procedures, for which accurate registration between preoperative and intraoperative data without surgical exposure is a key technology.

For registration in computer-assisted bone surgery, the x-ray fluoroscope is suitable for the intraoperative localization of bone without surgical exposure. To improve the accuracy and reliability of registration, combining images from two or more views has been proposed [1]. The cone-beam CT scanner is regarded as an extension of the multiview x-ray fluoroscope, and is compact enough for use in the operating room. While the contrast resolution of the CT value in cone-beam CT is still insufficient for diagnosis involving soft tissues, the spatial resolution is isotropic with respect to all three axes and is thus well-suited to 3-D acquisition. Since bone has inherently high contrast in the CT value, cone-beam CT can be particularly useful for 3-D bone surface scanning. In this paper, we consider the use of cone-beam CT as an intraoperative modality for bone surface detection to attain intraoperative registration with high accuracy without surgical exposure.

W. Niessen and M. Viergever (Eds.): MICCAI 2001, LNCS 2208, pp. 1366–1368, 2001.
© Springer-Verlag Berlin Heidelberg 2001

2   Method

The accuracy of cone-beam CT based registration (CB-REG) was evaluated by comparing it with 3-D positional sensor based registration (PS-REG) using a pelvis specimen. The experimental methods were as follows.

1. **Preoperative surface model generation:** A pelvis surface was generated using preoperative CT images with 3-mm thickness by using a conventional helical CT scanner.

2. **Intraoperative surface point collection:** For PS-REG, 30 surface points in the surgical exposure region were sampled using an Optotrak (Northern Digital Inc.) 3-D positional sensor (Fig. 1(a)). The number of sample points, 30, was determined by considering the trade-off between registration accuracy and the time needed for point collection [2]; this number is routinely used for hip-joint surgical navigation in our hospital. (Note that sampling points on the bone surface is not always easy because it is covered in muscle and other tissues.)

   For CB-REG, a pelvis surface was first generated from cone-beam CT (Hitachi Medical Corp.) images by using the same process as that employed for surface generation from helical CT images. After removing the surfaces of artificial markers (ceramic balls, described below) for accuracy evaluation, intraoperative points on the pelvis surface were collected automatically and randomly. Registration was performed using three protocols. In the first (CB-REG1), 30 surface points were collected in the surgical exposure region on the pelvis surface generated from the cone-beam CT images (Fig. 1(b)) to examine the difference in accuracy between point collection by Optotrak and cone-beam CT. In the other two protocols, which were designed to examine differences arising from the extent of the sample region, 1000 surface points were collected in the surgical exposure region (CB-REG2) or over the whole surface (CB-REG3. Fig. 1(c)).

3. **Registration:** By using the iterative closest point algorithm, registration between the preoperative pelvis surface and the intraoperative sample points was performed.

4. **Accuracy evaluation:** The target registration error (TRE)[3] at the acetabular center was calculated by using the gold-standard of registration, which had been estimated from four micron-accurate ceramic balls fixed to the pelvis surface. The average and standard deviation of the TRE were evaluated using 20 sets of sample points for each protocol.

3   Results and Discussion

As shown in Table 1, by using the same number of sample points (30) and the same sampling area (surgical exposure), the average TRE was improved from 1.43 mm (PS-REG) using Optotrak to 0.80 mm (CB-REG1) using cone-beam CT. By increasing the number of sample points from 30 to 1000, the standard deviation (SD) of the TRE was improved from 0.73 mm (CB-REG1) to 0.13 mm

1368   Y. Nakajima et al.

(CB-REG2), while the average remained almost the same. Further, by expanding the sampling area to the whole surface, the average TRE was improved to 0.56 mm (CB-REG3). In summary, the findings showed that registration with much higher accuracy is potentially attainable by acquiring the intraoperative bone surface using cone-beam CT as compared with our current routinely used protocol (PS-REG).

We consider that 0.56 mm, which was derived from *in vitro* experiments, can be regarded as the upper limit of accuracy attainable using cone-beam CT. In future work, we aim to study how the degree of accuracy using *in vivo* images can be brought close to this upper limit. Furthermore, since cone-beam CT based registration entails radioactive exposure, the overall advantages and disadvantages to the patient will need be sufficiently considered in clinical application.

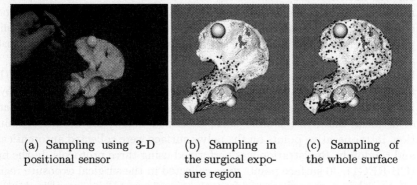

(a) Sampling using 3-D positional sensor

(b) Sampling in the surgical exposure region

(c) Sampling of the whole surface

Fig. 1. Intraoperative point sampling on the pelvis surface

Table 1. Results of accuracy evaluation

	PS-REG	CB-REG1	CB-REG2	CB-REG3
Sample method	Point collection by using 3-D positional sensor	Point collection on the bone surface generated from cone-beam CT images		
Sample number	30	1000		
Sample region	Surgical exposure region			Whole surface
Average TRE (in mm)	1.43	0.80	0.82	0.56
Standard deviation (in mm)	2.06	0.73	0.13	0.24

References

1. S. Lavalée, R. Szelski: Recovering the Position and Orientation of Free-Form Objects from Image Contours Using 3D Distance Maps, *IEEE Trans. on PAMI, 17* (4), 378-390 (1995).
2. T. Sasama, Y. Sato, N. Sugano, *el al.*: Accuracy Evaluation in Computer Assisted Hip Surgery, *Computer Assisted Radiology and Surgery (CARS'99)*, Paris, 772-776 (1999).
3. C.R. Maurer, J.M. Fitzpatrick, M.Y. Wang, *et al.*: Registration of Head Volume Images Using Implantable Fiducial Markers, *IEEE Trans. on Medical Imaging, 16* (4), 447-462 (1997).

Morphogenesis-Based Deformable Models Application to $3D$ Medical Image Segmentation and Analysis

Luis Ibáñez[1], Chafiaâ Hamitouche[2], Martial Boniou[2], and Christian Roux[2]

[1] Computer science department, division of neurosurgery,UNC, USA
[2] Département ITI - LATIM -INSERM 0102, ENST Bretagne, France
chafiaa.hamitouche@onst-bretagne.fr

Abstract. This paper introduces the concept of structured deformable model and presents its application to 3D medical image analysis. A structured deformable model is composed of a group of basic shape elements. A generic model of a biological shape can be build following a growth process controlled by the morphogenesis. This model can be fitted to a specific biological shape by adjusting the parameters of the model based on the information given by a 3D image of the targeted biological structure. An application to bone joint modelling is presented and discussed.

1 Introduction

Since the introduction of Snakes [1], Deformable models have been widely used in applications related with image segmentation of biological shapes [2]. The approach presented in this paper follows the trend of introducing more anatomical information and specific behavior into models. It designs a deformable model by considering the biological process responsible of organ morphogenesis. The hypothesis is that we can better model a form if we take into account the real biological mechanisms that leads to shape formation.

2 Modelling and Segmentation of Osteo-articular Shapes

Morphogenesis Knowledge Biological shape is the result of dynamical systems evolution [3]. Organ shape is, in fact, the spatial distribution of a particular kind of cells and a specific inter-cellular material. Biological shape results from interactions of tissues at cellular level. A tissue finish in space when particular conditions needed to maintain its coherence falls under a certain threshold. These considerations lead to the hypothesis that the families of shapes found in biological organs should belong to the varieties of shapes of zero sets found in implicit functions. In the case of bone modelling, the model is designed by considering the relative positions and sizes of chondrification centers and the geometric configurations of tendons and muscles insertions, using implicit surfaces to emulate the local morphology as described in osteology, arthrology and myology.

W. Niessen and M. Viergever (Eds.): MICCAI 2001, LNCS 2208, pp. 1369–1370, 2001.

Building Generic Shapes. Application to the Elbow Joint Metaballs paradigm was chosen here to build our model by making a gaussian sum of implicit functions that represent our ossification centers like local morphogenetic fields controlled by a few parameters.The articulation to model is composed of three bones epiphyses : the distal region of *humerus*, the *radius* head, and the *ulna*. An homotopy process [4] for mesh constructing implies a progressive modelling from an initial state where each element is collapsed into a simple shape (sphere) with a known mesh for each of the three bone extremities. Then the parameters variations imply a simulated morphogenesis until an adult final stage. The elbow modelling is shown in Figure 1. In order to fit the structured model against the real image, a good rigid transformation is performed to superimpose one over the other in an optimization process.

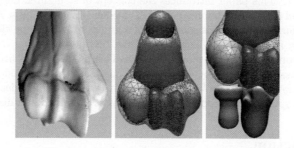

Fig. 1. Humerus distal head (left). Model (center). Complete Elbow Model (right).

3   Conclusion

The structured deformable model presented in this paper is a flexible tool for modelling biological shapes. The main advantage of this method is the possibility of interpreting in biological terms all the elements composing the model. Future work will be directed to the analysis of particular shapes with the aim of determining the appropriated combination of basic metaball elements that should be used to reproduce a good approximation of the shape.

References

1. M. Kass, A. Witkin and D. Terzopoulos, "Snakes: Active contour models", Int. J. Comput. Vision, Vol. **1**, No. 4, 1988, 321-331.
2. T. McInerney, D. Terzopoulos, "Deformable models in medical image analysis", Proc. Workshop on Math. Methods in Biomed. Image Anal., June 1996, 171 - 180.
3. R. Thom, *Stabilité Structurelle et Morphogénèse*, Essai d'une thoèrie générale des modèles. ed. InterEditions, 2nd Ed. 1977.
4. H. Lamure, D. Michelucci, Solving Geometric Constraints By Homotopy, IEEE TVCG, Vol **2**, N. 1, Mar. 1996, 28-35.

Grey-Level Morphology Based Segmentation of T1-MRI of the Human Cortex

Roger Hult[1,2] and Ewert Bengtsson[1]

[1] Centre for Image Analysis, Uppsala University, SE-752 37 Uppsala, Sweden,
[2] Dept. Clinical Neuroscience, Human Brain Informatics
Karolinska Institute, SE-171 76 Stockholm, Sweden,
{rogerh, ewert}@cb.uu.se
http://www.cb.uu.se

Abstract. In this paper an algorithm for fully automatic segmentation of the cortex from T1-weighted transversal, coronal or sagittal MRI data is presented. A histogram-based method is used to find accurate threshold values. Four initial masks are generated, containing background, brain tissue, 3D grey-level eroded brain tissue and 3D grey-level dilated surrounding fat. Information from previous slices are used to avoid leaking from non-brain tissue.

1 Overview of the Method

A histogram-based method is used to select the threshold intervals. The different kinds of tissues that are found are brain matter (white and grey matter), dark tissue types (fluids, bone, background) and bright tissue types (fat). The thresholding is performed on kernel density estimates (continuous histogram (KDE)). From this KDE the four greatest maxima of the second derivative are chosen and sorted. The interval from the lowest to the second maximum correspond to CSF and bone, and below the first threshold is air. Grey matter is approximately the second to third threshold and white matter is the third to fourth threshold. Surrounding tissues (and sometimes some internal structures in the brain) are above the fourth threshold. The histogram from the start slice has been used.

Two additional volumes are calculated. The original volume , called **OrgImage**, is grey-level-eroded using a $3 \times 3 \times 3$ structure element; this new volume is given the descriptive name **MinImage**. The original volume is also grey-level-dilated using a $3 \times 3 \times 3$ structure element; called **MaxImage**. These images are used to eliminate false connectivities to surrounding tissues. In the grey-level eroded volume the background is below the second max found from the second derivate of the continuous histogram. In the grey-level dilated volume the surrounding tissue is above the third max.

In the transaxial case a slice in the middle of a brain is selected as the start slice, see Fig. 1a). Objects large enough are decided to be brain tissue. The segmented slice is used as a mask on following slices. In the sagittal case, two slices are determined, one in the left and one in the right hemisphere, see

W. Niessen and M. Viergever (Eds.): MICCAI 2001, LNCS 2208, pp. 1371–1372, 2001.

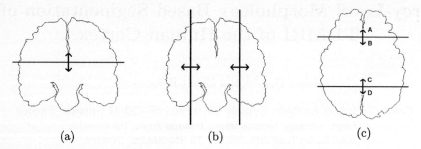

Fig. 1. How the algorithm advances on: a) A transaxial volume. b) A sagittal volume. c) A coronal volume.

Fig. 1b). As in the transaxial case, the information from previously segmented slices is used. In the coronal case, two starting positions are selected, see Fig. 1c). Here the same algorithm that is used to determine the start slices in the two other algorithms is used for all slices from position B to C in conjunction with propagating information from previous slices. For the slices from position A and position D, outwards, the same criterias that were used in the sagittal case are used. The information from previously segmented slices are also used.

2   Results

The segmentation algorithm generates reproducible results and has been visually evaluated on 30 patient data sets in transaxial, sagittal and coronal cases. A frequent problem is when cranial nerves that link brain tissues to non-brain tissue cause bridges that the binary morphology doesn't break. When involving both grey-level dilations and erosions these bridges are almost always broken. Another problem is that the algorithm does not handle volumes that are severely shaded very well. The main reason for this is our using the mid-slice only as a base for the automatic thresholding. This can be compensated for and more slices can be used in the thresholding. The method is improved from earlier work [2], [1].

References

[1] R. Hult. Grey-level Morphology Based Segmentation of MRI of the Human Cortex. Accepted for publication, September 2001.
[2] R. Hult, E. Bengtsson, and L. Thurfjell. Segmentation of the Brain in MRI Using Grey Level Morphology and Propagation of Information. In *Proceedings of 11th Scandinavian Conference on Image Analysis, Kangerlussuaq, Greenland*, volume I, pages 367–373, 1999.

An Active Contour Model for Segmentation Based on Cubic B-splines and Gradient Vector Flow

Matthias Gebhard, Julian Mattes, and Roland Eils

IBioS, German Cancer Research Center, D-69120 Heidelberg, Germany
m.gebhard@dkfz-heidelberg.de
http://www.dkfz-heidelberg.de/ibios

Abstract. The aim of this paper is to present advances in segmentation for visualization and quantitative analysis in bioimaging. Here, we combine two existing approaches for segmentation with snakes. Firstly, we use cubic B-splines to represent the snake using coarse-to-fine control point insertion; this allows to smooth adaptively the resulting contour while reducing the risk to get attracted from misdetected edges. Secondly, we put the snake in a gradient vector flow (GVF) field. This enables the snake to evolve into concavities of the shape. Further, sensitive parameters drop out in our setting and the attraction range with respect to initialization of the snake is enlarged.

1 Introduction

Imaging of cell biological objects *in vivo* leads often to a low signal to noise ratio as—because of their movement—a small capture time must be chosen in relation to the movement of objects [6]. For quantitative analysis of volume changes or surface deformation we need a robust and meaningful segmentation method which works semi-automatically by user interaction [4].

2 Definitions and Notations

To represent snake splines we use uniform B-splines where the basis functions are equidistantly located in the parameter space. A parameterized curve can be defined as $\mathbf{M}(u) = [x(u), y(u)], u \in [0, k]$, (here, $k \in \mathbb{N}$). The construction of a closed B-spline curve $\mathbf{M}(u)$ starts with the determination of k control points $\mathbf{P_i}, i = 1, ...k, \mathbf{P_i} \in \mathbb{R}^2$ (this also determines the range of the parameter interval).

We define $P = (\mathbf{P_i})^T$ built up from the control points $\mathbf{P_i}$, $P \in \mathbb{R}^{k \times 2}$. For cubic B-splines the basis functions are of order three and differ only by translation [1]:

$$\mathbf{M}(u) = \sum_{i=1}^{k} B(u, i)\mathbf{P_i}$$

One of the basic ideas of the primary snakes is the evolution of a contour over the image in search of minimizing a specific energy functional [2], traditionally defined by

W. Niessen and M. Viergever (Eds.): MICCAI 2001, LNCS 2208, pp. 1373–1375, 2001.
© Springer-Verlag Berlin Heidelberg 2001

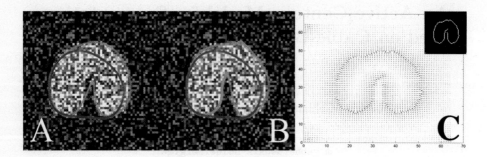

Fig. 1. Comparison between result obtained with the initial number of control points (CP) (A) and after CP insertion where the number of CP's are doubled (B). The blue line correspondes to the initial curve generated by the blue CP's, the red curve representing the *polygon snake* and the green shows the *snake spline* curve respective with its CP's (green). The GVF field corresponding to the Canny edge (C) image

$$E = \int_0^k \frac{1}{2}(\alpha|\mathbf{M}'(u)|^2 + \beta|\mathbf{M}''(u)|^2) + \gamma E_{ext}(x(u))du \qquad (1)$$

where α and β are weighting parameters for the internal energy representing the stretching and bending, $\mathbf{M}'(u), \mathbf{M}''(u)$ denotes $(\frac{\partial x(u)}{\partial u}, \frac{\partial y(u)}{\partial u})^T, (\frac{\partial^2 x(u)}{\partial u^2}, \frac{\partial^2 y(u)}{\partial u^2})^T$, respectively, and γ is the weight for the external energy E_{ext}.

The second term defines an important property of the snake, the smoothness of the contour. As smoothness is therefore contained in the definition of the spline [1], the functional for minimization can be rewritten as

$$E = \int_0^k E_{ext}(\mathbf{M}(u))du \qquad (2)$$

This approach shows some advantages to the classical description of snakes described in [1],[3],[7].

3   Evolution of the Snake

We construct the snake spline based on a manual initialization of the control points P and let them evolute over time in a given strength field, where we used the GVF field. To find the solution of equation 2, the parametrized variable $\mathbf{M}(u)$ must be treated as a function of time $\mathbf{M}(u(t), t)$. The evolution of the control points under time can be described as [3]:

$$\frac{dP(t)}{dt} = B^+ \frac{dM(t)}{dt} = B^+ F_{ext} = -B^+ \nabla I(M) =$$

$$-B^+ \nabla I(BP(t)) = B^+ V(BP(t)) \qquad (3)$$

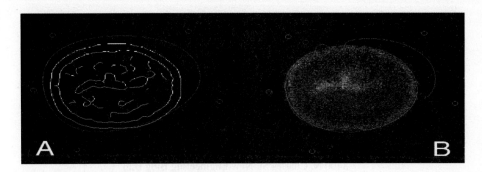

Fig. 2. Segmentation of nuclear membrane. (A) Initial snake spline defined by a set of five control points (blue). (B) The red curve representing the *polygon snake* and the green curve shows the *snake spline* respective with its control points (green)

$V(BP(t))$ are the contour points of the snake under the influence of the GVF vector field V. This ordinary differential equation can be solved by Runge and Kutta [5].

Acknowledgements

The authors want to thank D. Gerlich from the DKFZ Heidelberg and J. Ellenberg, EMBL Heidelberg for providing the nuclear envelope image shown in Fig. 2. We also thank B. Jähne for generously supporting this work.

References

1. Patrick Brigger, Jeff Hoeg, Michael Unser, B-Spline Snake: A Flexible Tool for Parametric Contour Detection, IEEE transaction on image processing, vol. **9**, no. 9, 1484-1496, 2000
2. M. Kass, A. Witkin and D. Terzopoulos, Snakes: Active contour models, Int. J. Comput. Vis., pp. 321-331, 1987
3. Leitner F., Marque I., Lavallee P. and Cinquin P.: Dynamic segmentation: Finding edge with snake splines, Curves and Surfaces, pp. 279-284, Chamonix, France, 1990, 1991
4. Leitner F., Paillasson S., Ronot X., Demongeot J.: Dynamic functional and structural analysis of living cells: new tools for vital staining of nuclear DNA and for characterisation of cell motion, Acta Biotheor., **43(4)**, pp. 299-317, Dec. 1995
5. Press, Teukolsky, Vetterling, Flannery: Numerical Recipes in C, Second Edition, Cambridge University Press, 1999
6. Tvaruskó W., Bentele M., Misteli T., Rudolf R., Kaether C., Spector D.L., Gerdes H.H., Eils R.: Time-resolved analysis and visualization of dynamic processes in living cells, Proc. Natl. Acad. Sci. USA, Vol. **96**, pp. 7950-7955, July 1999
7. Xenyang Xu and Jerry L. Prince, Snakes, Shapes and Gradient Vector Flow, IEEE Transaction on Image Processing, pp. 66-71, 1997

Approximate Volumetric Reconstruction from Projected Images

Gabor Fichtinger[1], Sheng Xu[1], Attila Tanacs[1], Kieran Murphy[2], Lee Myers[3], Jeffery Williams[4,]

[1]Center for Computer Integrated Surgical Systems and Technologies,
Johns Hopkins University, Baltimore, MD, 21218
3400 N. Charles St, New Engineering Bldg B26
contact: gabor@cs.jhu.edu
[2]Department of Radiology, Johns Hopkins University Hospital, Baltimore, MD
[3]Department of Radiation Oncology, Johns Hopkins University Hospital, Baltimore, MD
[4]Department of Neurosurgery, Johns Hopkins University Hospital, Baltimore, MD

Abstract A significant problem in planning of volumetrically prescribed localized treatments is the mathematical impossibility to determine the exact three dimensional shape and volume of a target object from its projected images. Reconstruction accuracy also varies with viewing angle, depending on the convexity and aspect ratios of the target object. In response to this problem, we are developing a robust and efficient technique for approximate volumetric reconstruction, which (A) uses no prior information of the shape and volume of the target, (B) does not require exact silhouettes, (C) accepts arbitrary number of images, (D) produces solid object and measure of its volume, (E) provides confidence measure of the reconstruction and drawing of silhouettes, (F) is robust, fast and easy to implement. Preliminary tests suggest that fairly convex objects can be reconstructed from four views, and typically six views with table rotation allow us to reconstruct fine details as small as 1 mm. The method is applicable for any X-ray guided volumetric treatment. Pilot applications will be planning of radiosurgery of arterioveneous malformations (AVMs) and radio-frequency ablation of soft tissue lesions.

1 Introduction

Contrast-enhanced angiography is the primary imaging modality in AVM radiosurgery and it has assumed significant role in minimally invasive local therapies. A fundamental obstacle in planning such therapies is the lack of reliable volumetric appreciation of the target. The problem has not been researched during the last half decade since fusion of angiography to CT/MRI had become available for AVM radiosurgery planning. At the same time, even state-of-the-art radiosurgery systems, like BrainLAB or Leibinger, merely back-project the silhouettes to reconstructed CT/MRI planes, without giving volumetric appreciation of the target. In general, it is impossible to reconstruct an object exactly in 3D from its projective images. Worse yet, in angiography images the target does not present well defined boundaries and the doctor must depend on subjective clinical judgment when outlining the target

W. Niessen and M. Viergever (Eds.): MICCAI 2001, LNCS 2208, pp. 1376-1378, 2001.

object (Figure 1.) Current methods fail to address the fact that contours, as subjectively drawn by the physician, do not necessarily correspond to a three-dimensional object. Several prior volumetric reconstruction methods exist that also place limitations on the number of projections and the rotational freedom of the X-ray source [1,3]. In 1996, during the peak of interest in mono-modal angiographic planning of AVM radiosurgery, Yeung et al. [2] proposed a method based on pure back-projection from contours. The paper, to-date perhaps the most general and robust method,

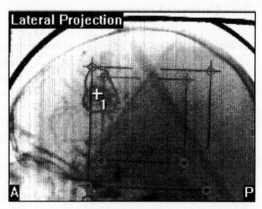

Figure 1: Stereotactic angiogram of an AVM for radiosurgery planning. The target is contoured by the physician around the + marker.

underestimated the problem that back-projection alone produces only a cloud of disjoint voxels that has to be solidified later, in order to receive a solid 3D object. The paper also did not address directional robustness and consistency of contours. Parallel to medical applications, a family of shape recovery methods have also emerged in the fields of pattern recognition and computer vision [3,4,5,6]. These algorithms, besides being rather complex and difficult to implement, deal with solid physical objects with well defined boundaries, therefore, are not suitable for our purpose.

2   Methods

We propose a combination of forward- and back-projections for reconstruction that begins after the surgeon draws the silhouettes of the target in each 2D image. From back-projections of the silhouettes, we determine a closest fitting regular shape that is guaranteed to cover the object in 3D. Then using primarily forward projection, all excess parts are carved off the encompassing shape, till we receive the reconstructed object. In the most conservatively approach, the object must fit inside all silhouettes. Multiple methods were developed to carry out this phase. A fast algorithm takes advantage of occasional convexity of silhouettes, while a voxel-by-voxel method works for all shapes of silhouettes. Finally, the obtained object is projected forward on to each image plane, where the shadow of the reconstructed object is compared to the silhouettes drawn by the surgeon, so that confidence and consistency of silhouette lines could be calculated and visually interpreted. Objects with large aspect ratio inevitably have preferential directions allowing significantly more accurate reconstruction than other projection angles. Part of our robustness analysis is quantitative prediction for the inaccuracy of reconstruction caused by sub-optimal projection angles.

3   Current Status

Currently we are experimenting with synthetic data generated by forward-projection of various objects onto the planes of a hypothetic imager. Objects that are convex in the center of gravity and that have no large aspect ratio can be reconstructed with high accuracy from three or four images. According to expectations, objects with large aspect ratio were reconstructed significantly more accurately from perpendicular directions than from parallel directions, with respect to their long axis. Figure 2 shows a highly complex synthesized tree-branch phantom, similar to the one reported by Yeung [2]. When the object was projected in preferential directions, the relative error was 4.3%, 3.6%, and 0.8% from 3,5, and 7 shots, respectively. When the same object was projected in random directions, the mean relative error was 11.3% in 20 random experiments, from seven projections in each. Based on visual inspection, our results appear to be at least as accurate as Yeung's who did not report numbers. Imperfect silhouettes with known measures of inconsistency have been also synthesized, numerical evaluation of these is in progress. While still more phantom and synthetic studies will be carried out, clinical robustness will also be examined in post-operative analysis of fluoroscopic images of liver lesions and intracranial AVMs.

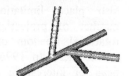

Figure 2: Synthetic tree-branch phantom

Acknowledgements

The project is supported by the National Science Foundation under the Engineering Research Center grant #EEC9731478.

References

[1] Foroni, R.; Gerosa, M. Shape recovery and volume calculation from biplane of atreriovenous malformations. Rad. Onc. Biol. Phys., Vol. 35, No.3, pp. 565-577
[2] Yeung D; Chen N; Ferguson RD; Lee LI; Kun LE Three-dimensional reconstruction of arteriovenous malformations from multiple stereotactic angiograms. Med Phys 1996 Oct;23(10):1797-1804
[3] Chang, S.K.; Wang, Y. R. Three dimensional object reconstruction from orthogonal projections. Patt. Recongnit. 7:167-176; 1975
[4] Xu, G.; Tsuji, S. Recovering surface shape from boundary. Int. Conf. Art. Intel. 2:731-733; 1987
[5] Ulupinar, F.; Nevatia, R. Shape from contours: SHGCs. In: Proc. IEEE Int. Conf. Computer Vision 582; 1990
[6] Ulupinar, F.; Nevatia, R. Inferring shape from contours for curved surfaces. Atlantic City: Proceeding International Conference Pattern Recognition. 1990: 147-154.

Implicit Snakes: Active Constrained Implicit Models

T.S. Yoo[1] and K.R. Subramanian[2]

[1] National Library of Medicine, Natl. Inst. of Health, Bethesda, MD, 20894, USA
yoo@nlm.nih.gov
[2] Dept. of Computer Science, Univ. of North Carolina, Charlotte, NC, 28223, USA
krs@cs.uncc.edu

Extended Abstract: We are exploring new techniques for active contour models (popularly known as "snakes"[1]) by combining active segmentation models with the constrained implicit surface model introduced by Savchenko, et al.[4] and reintroduced under the name of variational implicit surfaces as a modeling and shape morphing tool by Turk and O'Brien[5]. In related work, we pursued more efficient numerical methods for these techniques. For a more complete description of our modeling methods, see Morse[2]. Here we show that an active surface model can be created by combining constrained implicit surfaces with a solver that minimizes an appropriate functional. In these examples, our energy minimization techniques are relatively simple; new work in combing the active implicit modeling techniques with aggressive energy functionals is in progress. By extracting implicit models from discrete volume data, we are diverging from similar modeling methods described by Yngve and Turk[6].

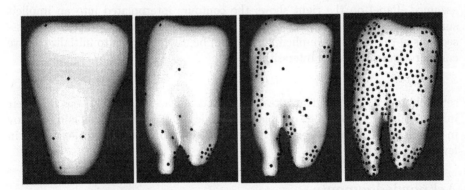

Fig. 1. Active interpolating implicit surfaces applied to a $256 \times 256 \times 163$ CT scan of a tooth. The algorithm was run for 21 iterations, incrementally adding constraints. The implicit model naturally suppresses sampling artifact, guaranteeing smoothness by the underlying radial basis interpolants. Constraints are indicated by small spheres on the surface boundary.

Figure 1 shows our method applied to an X-ray CT scan of a tooth. The first frame shows the first iteration of the progressive interpolating implicit surface

W. Niessen and M. Viergever (Eds.): MICCAI 2001, LNCS 2208, pp. 1379–1381, 2001.
© Springer-Verlag Berlin Heidelberg 2001

algorithm. An initial set of constraints was actively moved toward areas of high boundary strength, and an interpolating implicit function was generated. The remaining frames show progressive refinement through 21 iterations, introducing additional constraints. Unlike a polygonal model, the final implicit surface can be sampled with arbitrary resolution. Figure 2 shows this process applied through a hybrid approach to intravascular ultrasound data (IVUS) of a canine aorta. The method correctly creates the partially occluded blood vessel from the slice data. The arterial vessel is segmented through a combination of 2D active contours and 3D interpolation. By definition, implicit surfaces are closely related to level

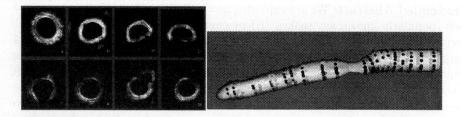

Fig. 2. Active constrained implicit surfaces generalized to active contours. The left panel shows ultrasound data collected using an endovascular transducer on a catheter. The data are slices, sampled at arbitrary angles along the vessel. Active interpolating surfaces were adapted to active interpolating contours to segment the individual slices. Particularly difficult slices due to poor signal can be avoided and the gaps interpolated if smoothness and connectedness can be assumed. Panel on the right shows the contours interpolated into an implicit surface, successfully mapping the 2.5 D problem into the 3D domain. Cross-sections of the resulting implicit surface can be used as priors to initialize active contour segmentation on interstitial slices

set techniques[3]. The advantages of implicit surfaces and level sets are their inherent ability to adapt to complex topologies. Our current focus is to employ in our methods improved partial differential equations similar to those used in level set algorithms.

Acknowledgements

We are indebted to Greg Turk, James O'Brien, and Gary Yngve for their insights and inspiration in implicit surfaces and to Bryan Morse, David Chen, and Penny Rheingans for their continued contributions to this and related work.

References

[1] M. Kass, A. Witkin, and D Terzopolous. Snakes: active contour models. *Int. Journal of Computer Vision*, 1:321–331, 1987.

[2] B.S. Morse, T.S. Yoo, P. Rheingans, D.T. Chen, and K.R. Subramanian. Interpolating implicit surfaces from scattered surface data using compactly supported radial basis functions. In *Proceedings of Shape Modeling International (SMI) 2001*, pages 89–98, May 7-11, Genova, Italy, 2001.

[3] S. Osher and J. A. Sethian. Fronts propogating with curvature dependent speed: Algorithms based on hamilton-jacobi formulation. *Journal of Computational Physics*, 79:12–49, 1988.

[4] V. Savchenko, A. Pasko, G. Okunev, and T.L. Kunii. Fronts propogating with curvature dependent speed: Algorithms based on hamilton-jacobi formulation. *Computer Graphics Forum*, 14(4):181–188, 1995.

[5] G. Turk and J.F. O'Brien. Shape transformation using variational implicit functions. *Computer Graphics Forum*, 14(4):181–188, 1995.

[6] G. Yngve and G. Turk. Creating smooth implicit surfaces from polygonal meshes. *Technical Report GIT-GVU-99-42, Graphics, Visualization and Usability Center, Georgia Institute of Technology*, 1999.

Towards a Robust Path Growing Algorithm for Semi-automatic MRI Segmentation

Casper F. Nielsen and Peter J. Passmore

School of Computing Science, Middlesex University, Bounds Green Road
London, N11 2NQ, United Kingdom
{c.nielsen, p.passmore}@mdx.ac.uk

Abstract. Segmentation of MRI volumes is complicated by RF inhomogeneity, noise and partial volume artifacts. Fully automatic methods often do not cope well with a combination of these problems. Semi-automatic methods are generally too simplistic or require a large amount of user interaction to work. Adaptable Class-Specific Representation (ACSR), implemented by the Path Growing Algorithm (PGA), is a semi-automatic segmentation framework, which has previously been demonstrated to produce accurate and robust segmentation of colour cryo section volumes with a minimal requirement for user interaction. This paper presents an evaluation of three different PGAs to implement ACSR for the MRI modality. Results are based on simulated data from the BrainWeb image database. Future work towards a robust solution is discussed.

1   Introduction

ACSR [1,2] allows the user to define the goal of a segmentation visually by selecting representative class templates. The standard PGA, combined with Learning Vector Quantization (LVQ), has previously been used to implement robust ACSR segmentation of colour cryo section volumes [2] from the Visible Human Project. This study aims to bring the benefits of ACSR segmentation to the MRI modality.

2   Evolving the PGA for MRI Segmentation

A path in the PGA is a connected, acyclic chain of points where no point is repeated twice. All possible paths with distinct point sets are grown from a seed point via a $2n$-connected expansion in n-dimensional space. All points in an image successively become the seed point and a path hierarchy *for each class* at every point is created by calculating the distance of each path to each class template and the path spread. Class-specific sampling windows are built from the winning paths and compete for the final classification. Boundary artefacts are eliminated or significantly reduced. To speed up ACSR segmentation the PGA may be combined with a preliminary crude segmentation step using LVQ, in which the PGA is applied only at boundary points (partial ACSR). See [1,2,4] for a complete description and notation of the PGA.

W. Niessen and M. Viergever (Eds.): MICCAI 2001, LNCS 2208, pp. 1382-1383, 2001.
© Springer-Verlag Berlin Heidelberg 2001

Due to less rich point descriptors in MRI compared to colour cryo section data we introduce *path descriptors*, constituted by the path median and the path average intensity difference between the seed point and all other points in the path. We consider three variations of the PGA with path descriptors: Sampling window built from a single path (PGA-SPD); sampling window built from a single path with the seed point shifted one point in the direction of growth for the calculation of path average intensity difference (PGA-SPDS) to achieve greater tolerance to noise; sampling window built from two full paths with shifted seed point (PGA-DPDS). In partial ACSR the LVQ segmented boundaries are dilated by a small factor and the PGA is applied at the boundary points. The three new algorithms were tested with dilation factors of 1, 3 and ∞ (full ACSR) on simulated T1 MRI volumes from the BrainWeb database (http://www.bic.mni.mcgill.ca/brainweb) with varying levels of RF inhomogeneity and noise (3% noise, 20% inhomogeneity; 3% noise, 40% inhomogeneity; 7% noise, 20% inhomogeneity). Template selection was based on a simulated user in the form of the BrainWeb ground truth for the classes CSF, white matter and grey matter in eight slices per volume. Results were compared to previously published results by Dzung and Prince [3], where MRF segmentation was based on a standard Expectation Maximization (EM) algorithm and the Adaptive Generalized EM algorithm (AGEM).

Best results were found for PGA-SPDS with a dilation factor of 3, which was consistently better than the standard EM algorithm for all volumes and comparable to AGEM at the highest level of inhomogeneity and noise. Error rates (the ratio of misclassified pixels to the total number of pixels in the three segment classes) for this volume were 8.858% for PGA-SPDS, 10.699% for EM and 8.414% for AGEM.

3 Conclusion

We conclude that the single path representation with seed point shifting for path average intensity difference produced consistently better results. Partial ACSR not only speeded up the segmentation process but improved results, which were however affected by the lack of explicitly templated inhomogeneities. Future work will seek to reduce error rates through automated template creation at slice level from the initial LVQ segmentation. The work described in this paper is discussed in detail in [4].

References

1. Nielsen, C. F., Passmore, P. J: A Solution to the Problem of Segmentation Near Edges Using Adaptable Class-Specific Representation, Proc. 15th IEEE ICPR, (2000) 436-440
2. Nielsen, C. F., Passmore, P. J.: Achieving Accurate Colour Image Segmentation in 2D and 3D with LVQ Classifiers and Partial ACSR, Proc. Fifth IEEE WACV, (2000) 72-78
3. Dzung, L. P., Prince, J. L.: A Generalized EM Algorithm for Robust Segmentation of Magnetic Resonance Images, Proc. 33rd Ann. Conf. Inf. Sciences and Systems, (1999) 558-563
4. Nielsen, C. F., Passmore, P. J.: Towards a Robust Path Growing Algorithm for Semi-Automatic MRI Segmentation, Middlesex Uni. CS Tech. Report no. CS-01-01, (2001)

Integrated System for Objective Assessment of Global and Regional Lung Structure

J.M. Reinhardt[1], J. Guo[2], L. Zhang[1], D. Bilgen[1], S. Hu[1,5], R. Uppaluri[3,5], R.M. Long[3], O.I. Saba[1], G. McLennan[4], M. Sonka[3], and E.A. Hoffman[2,1]

[1] Department of Biomedical Engineering
[2] Department of Radiology
[3] Department of Electrical and Computer Engineering
[4] Department of Internal Medicine
University of Iowa, Iowa City, IA 52242
[5] G.E. Medical Systems, Milwaukee, WI 53201

Abstract. Sub-second multi-slice CT scanners can now provide detailed pulmonary structural and functional information. We describe an integrated software system to facilitate quantitative analysis of pulmonary anatomy and physiology. This system includes tools for lung, airway, lung lobe segmentation, parenchymal tissue characterization, as well as regional pulmonary ventilation and perfusion.

We have developed an integrated system for objective assessment of the lung from volumetric CT images. The system includes analysis tools to study lung structure via image segmentation and analysis applications that analyze the structure and function depicted in the images. The overall system architecture is shown in Figure 1. The inputs to the system are volumetric X-ray CT data (three or four dimensional) of the thorax. Processing is started by lung segmentation, followed by airway tree and lung lobe segmentation. Following segmentation, measurements are made for regions of interest, which can be automatically defined using anatomic landmarks. Lung and lobar volumes are computed. The airway tree topology is described by the branchpoints; additional measurements for the tree branches include cross-sectional area along branch; branch diameters and wall thicknesses as a function of branch generation; wall thickness uniformity along a branch and across branches of the same generation; volume of air and wall tissue along individual airway branches expressed per branch, per lobe, and per lung. The segmentation processing provides a structural decomposition that can be used for regional reporting of image-based measurements of lung anatomy or physiology (ventilation, perfusion, airway reactivity, etc.). A database is used to store intermediate and final results, patient information, and anatomic information. Reports and summary statistics can be extracted from the database and formatted into an HTML document.

Acknowledgements: This work was supported in part by HL64368-01 and HL60158-02 from the National Institutes of Health, by an NSF CAREER award, and by a Biomedical Engineering Research Grant from the Whitaker Foundation.

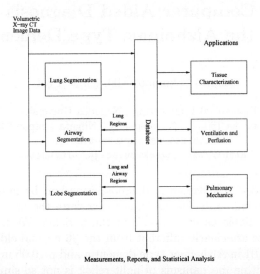

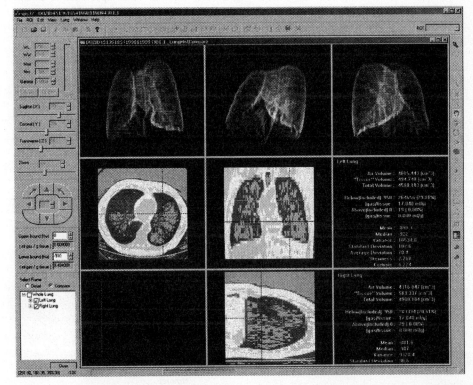

Fig. 1. Top: System architecture. Bottom: One view of analysis system showing volume-rendered views, cross-sections highlighting suspected pathology in green, pixel histograms, and textual summary statistics.

Computer Aided Diagnosis
for the Alzheimer Type Dementia

Ichiro Fukumoto MD. Ph.D. Prof.

Institute of Biomedical Engineering , Nagaoka University of Technology
Kamitomioka 1603-1 , Nagaoka-city , Niigata , Japan 940-2188
ichiro@vos.nagaokaut.ac.jp
http://bio.nagaokaut.ac.jp/~fukumoto/

We have proposed a new dementia diagnostic method by human eye light reflexes, which demands only few seconds to measure the miotic responses and
which is highly reliable as well as safe to the patients. We found that the 35
demented patients are clearly different from the 36 normal elders in the miotic
parameters ($p<0.01$ in Alzheimer type dementia and $p<0.05$ in vascular dementia.) But the eliciting mechanisms of light reflex is not so simple and it is nor
easy to understand the measured results in the clinical settings. In this study an
attempt is studied to elucidate the neuro-physiological mechanism of the light
reflexes with mathematical modeling and computer simulations.

The subject's eye is lightened by visible light from a small lamp in 5 seconds.
The pupil images are recorded by an infrared video camera and the change of
pupil diameter is analyzed by a personal computer to calculate the miotic parameters such as constriction time(s) & constriction rate(%). The subjects are
composed of 26 normal elders, 24 Alzheimer patients (AD), 13 vascular dementia (VD) and 9 other types of dementia. The age of the 4 subject groups are
all in 70s. The time courses of the pupil diameter in the dementia patients are
clearly different from the one of the normal people as is shown in Fig.1. We have
especially noticed the minimal point of the curve and have extracted the two representing parameters, namely the constriction rate and the constriction time of
the minimal point. A theoretical model based on the neuro physiological knowl-

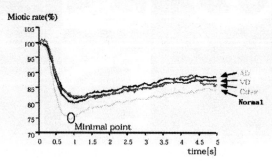

Fig. 1. The time courses of the pupil diameter in the normal and the demented people.

edge is constructed and the computer simulations using the model are executed
in order to analyze the differences between the normal and the demented elders

W. Niessen and M. Viergever (Eds.): MICCAI 2001, LNCS 2208, pp. 1386–1387, 2001.
© Springer-Verlag Berlin Heidelberg 2001

numerically. The model is divided into four sub-models (the primary miotic process, the secondary mydriatic process, the balancing model, modifying miotic parameter model) which reflect the neuro-physiology of the light reflex in the demented patients. In these sub-models, the decreasing activity of acetylcholine or increasing activity of adrenaline in the demented brain is considered to affect the pupil constriction and dilating force parameters namely dP,kP,dS,kS. The mathematical model based on the theoretical model is expressed into the three simple equations described below.

1. The activity level of the parasympathicus nerve:P(t)
   (a) The delay time of the P(t) :dP
   (b) The time constant of the P(t) : kp
   (c) The initial value of the P(t) : P0
   (d) $P(t) = P0^* \exp(-kp(t-dP))$
2. The activity level of the sympathicus nerve:S(t)
   (a) The delay time of the S(t): dS
   (b) The time constant of the S(t) : kS
   (c) The initial value of the S(t) : S0
   (d) $S(t) = S0^*(1-\exp(-kS(t-dS)))$
3. A function of pupil area: $R(t) =P(t)+S(t)$

Figure 2 shows an example of the simulation result (lines) as well as the measured data (circles). The results of the simulation suggest that the demented patients have the decreased activity of parasympathetic system as well as the increased activity of sympathetic system.

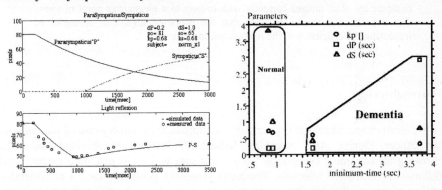

Fig. 2. The simulation result of the demented elder's light reflex.

Fig. 3. The parameter analysis of the miotic parameters.

The miotic parameter analyses of the model using kp, dP, dS show that the demented patients can be clearly discriminated from the normal subjects as is shown in Fig.3. It may be more easy to detect the neuro physiological changes of the demented brain, if one could adopt the neurological parameters obtained from the computer simulations on the dementia screenings, as well as the measured data from the light reflexes. The another computer simulation has been executed with good coincidences to the light reflexes too, in which the atrophic level of patients' hippocampus can be detected by MRI brain images.

CAD System for the Assistance of Comparative Reading for Lung Cancer Using Serial Helical CT Images

M. Kubo [1], T. Yamamoto [1], Y. Kawata [1], N. Niki [1], K. Eguchi [2], H. Ohmatsu [3], R. Kakinuma [3], M. Kaneko [4], M. Kusumoto [4], N. Moriyama [4], K. Mori [5], and H. Nishiyama [6]

[1] University of Tokushima, Tokushima, Japan,
[2] National Shikoku Cancer Center Hospital, Ehime, Japan,
[3] National Cancer Center Hospital East, Chiba, Japan,
[4] National Cancer Center Hospital, Tokyo, Japan,
[5] National Tochigi Cancer Center Hospital, Tochigi, Japan,
[6] Social Health Insurance Medical Center, Tokyo, Japan

Abstract. The objective of this study is to develop a computer-aided diagnosis (CAD) system to support comparative reading of sequential helical CT images for lung cancer screening without using film displays. The placement of pulmonary shadows between sequential helical CT images sometimes differs due to the changes in lung size and shape caused by inspiration. The proposed algorithm consists of two sections; identification of region of interest and the comparison of sequential CT images. We validated the effectiveness of the algorithm by its application to images from 60 subjects. The algorithm could compare the slice images correctly with respect to a physician's point of view. The experimental results indicate that the proposed algorithm is useful in increasing the efficiency of the mass screening process.

1 Introduction

Early detection and treatment is necessary to improve the recovery rate of patient with lung cancer. During mass screening, helical CT images are obtained under the following measurement conditions: 10.0 mm beam width; 50 mA tube current; and 10.0-mm reconstructed intervals. The mass screening generates such a considerable number of images that are time-consuming to assess, it can be difficult for clinicians to make use of them in clinical setting. In particular, comparative reading of sequential helical CT images burden to be registration in lung size and shape caused by inspiration. In this paper, we analyze the motion of the pulmonary structure using the serial images taken at early diagnosis that differ with regard to the extent of inspiration. We then present a new algorithm that matches the slice position of each image in the scan sequence based on the motion of the lung.

W. Niessen and M. Viergever (Eds.): MICCAI 2001, LNCS 2208, pp. 1388-1390, 2001.
© Springer-Verlag Berlin Heidelberg 2001

2 Algorithm for Comparison of Each Slice of Serial Cases

Expert physicians make the comparative reading of the lung based on the position of the pulmonary blood vessels in each image. We analyzed the motion of the pulmonary structure using 17 pairs of sequential images. The comparison results between each sequential image were confirmed the motion of the superior surface of diaphragm and the lung base, while the apexes of the lung and the aortic arch essentially did not moved.

We present an algorithm for each part; the upper lung and lower lung. This algorithm consists of two processes, the region detection process and the comparison process between each slice of serial cases.

In the region detection algorithm, the left and right lung regions are automatically identified in the CT image using the lung extraction method of a conventional CAD system [1]. In the comparison process, the current case is used us the reference and the retrospective case is used as the candidate. An image is selected, which is similar to the present case. This process consists of five stages as follows;

(Stage-1) Corrections of coarse difference in the scan positions using the position of the apex of lung and the backbone as reference points
(Stage-2) Matching of each image of the upper lung using lung shape [2]
(Stage-3) Matching of each sequential image of the lower lung using the pattern of the pulmonary blood vessels
(Stage-4) Evaluation of continuity between upper and lower lung results
(Stage-5) Amendment of discontinuities between results

3 Experiment

The proposed algorithm was tested using 3,502 images (136 pairs) from 60 subjects. The same data was visually analyzed to provide ground truth data. Table 1 shows the results of the tests, where judgment I defines the difference between ground truth and result of test is not any, judgment II defines the difference is one slice, judgment III defines the difference is two slices, and judgment IV defines the difference is more than three slices. Cumulative rate within one slice difference is 3,481 images and 99.4% in all of judgment I and II, and one within two slice difference is 3,490 images and 99.7% in all of judgment I through III.

The cases of judgment IV show three characteristics such as the shrunk lung, the expansion heart and the whitish lung's background. The proposed method using the lung shape and heart shape is difficult to apply in case of no enough inspired air.

4 Conclusion

We present a new CAD system to support effectually the comparative reading using the serial helical CT images for lung cancer screening without using the film display. Cumulative rate within one slice difference was 3,481 images and 99.4% in all of judgment I and II. The experimental results of the proposed algorithm indicate that our CAD system without using the film display is useful to increase the efficiency of the mass screening process. In future work, we will examine the proposed algorithm using many cases.

Table 1. Result of the proposed method

judgment	slice difference	No. of slices	rate (%)
I	0.0-0.5	3227	92.1
II	0.5-1.0	254	7.3
III	1.0-2.0	9	0.3
IV	2.0-	12	0.3

References

1. K. Kanazawa, Y. Kawata, N. Niki, et al., "Computer-aided diagnosis for pulmonary nodules based on helical CT images," Comput. Med. Imag. Graph., 22, pp.157-167, 1998.
2. Y. Ukai, N. Niki, H. Satoh, K. Eguchi et al., "Computer aided diagnosis system for lung cancer based on retrospective helical CT image," in Image Processing, Kenneth M, Hanson, ed, Proc. SPIE 3979, pp. 1028-1039, 2000.

Classification of Breast Tumors on Digital Mammograms Using Laws' Texture Features

Celia Varela[1], Nico Karssemeijer[2], and Pablo G. Tahoces[3]

[1] Department of Radiology, University of Santiago de Compostela,
15782 Santiago de Compostela, Spain
mrcuca@usc.es
[2] University Hospital Nijmegen, Department of Radiology,
PO Box 9101, Nijmegen, 6500 HB, The Netherlands
nico@radiology.azn.nl
[3] Department of Electronic and Computer Science,
University of Santiago de Compostela,
15782 Santiago de Compostela, Spain

1 Introduction

Mammographic screening is widely used for early detection of breast cancer. Despite the success of screening programs, negative effects should not be underestimated. In many countries, only 15%-40% of detected lesions which are biopsied are subsequently determined malignant. Radiologists might improve their performance, when they could use objective computer-aided diagnosis programs developed with the aim of reducing false positives.

Spiculated margins and irregularly shaped masses are two of the main diagnostic features used by radiologists for identifying potentially malignant lesions. In this study we present a digital image processing algorithm to classify breast lesions based on quantitative measures of tumor shape, contrast, and spiculation.

2 Material and Methods

The data set for this study included 131 regions of interest (ROIs). The number of malignant and benign images were 65 and 64 respectively, corresponding to 39 patients for both type of lesions. The ROIs had a pixel size of 100 microns and a depth resolution of 12 bits. Cases were taken from the Galician screening program and from the Digital Database for Screening Mammography (DDSM)[1].

Our study consisted in two main steps:1) Mass segmentation and transformation of its border, 2) Feature extraction and its implementation in a classifier to discriminate between malignant and benign mass.

2.1 Mass Segmentation and Border Transformation

The algorithm used for segmentation was an adaptive region growing algorithm[2] . The border region surrounding the mass was transformed into a rectangular band[3]. By this transformation spicules were transformed into vertical lines perpendicular to the mass contour.

W. Niessen and M. Viergever (Eds.): MICCAI 2001, LNCS 2208, pp. 1391–1392, 2001.

Two low resolution images were obtained by resampling the image by a given factor (0.7 and 0.5). In this way, features were extracted at two different resolutions.

2.2 Feature Extraction and Classification

Different types of features were extracted from the segmented mass region itself and from its corresponding rectangular band. From the segmented mass region a peak-related and a contrast measure were calculated.

Features based in Laws' texture energy features were extracted from the straighten border region. Three Laws' filters (vertical, horizontal, and symmetrical) were applied to the transformed image. Vertical filter was intended to enhance spiculation, where horizontal filter would suppress them.

From each Laws' image two different features were calculated from the distribution of the gray level values of the pixels in the image: the standard deviation and the skewness. Besides, the ratio of the vertical and horizontal features was also calculated. The filters were applied to the original transformed border region and also to its low-resolution versions. Thus, 24 features were extracted from the rectangular region. Therefore, a total of 26 features were extracted for each ROI.

The classifier used in this study was a three layered feed-forward network using backpropagation as learning algorithm. A leave-one-case-out method was used to train and test the generalization capability of the classifier. The classifier performance was evaluated with receiver operating characteristic (ROC) analysis.

3 Results

The best results corresponded to an area under the ROC curve of 0.87. The classifier used as input features extracted from the highest resolution image joined with the peak-related and the contrast feature. Future work is planned to develop new features and also to enlarge the database.

References

1. Heath, M., Bowyer, K.W., Kopans, D., et al.: Current status of the Digital Database for Screening Mammography. In: Karsseimeijer, N., Thijssen, M., Hendriks, J.,van Erning, L. (eds). Digital Mammography, Kluwer Academic Publishers (1998) 457-460.
2. Tahoces, P.G., Varela, C., Méndez, A.J., Souto, M., Vidal, J.J.: An automatic algorithm for segmentation of mammographic masses on a computerized detection scheme. In: Lemke, H.U., Vannier, M.W., Inamura, K., Farman, A.G., Doi, K. (eds.): Cars 2000. Computer Assisted Radiology and Surgery. Elsevier Science, Amsterdam (2000) 1038.
3. Sahiner, B., Chan, H.P., Petrick, N., Helvie, M.A., Goodsitt, M.M.: Computerized characterization of masses on mammograms: The rubber band straightening transform and texture analysis. Med Phys 25 (1998) 516-526.

Computer-Aided Diagnosis of Pulmonary Nodules Using Three-Dimensional Thoracic CT Images

Y. Kawata[1], N. Niki[1], H. Ohmatsu[2], M. Kusumoto[3], R. Kakinuma[2],
K. Mori[4], H. Nishiyama[5], K. Eguchi[6], M. Kaneko[3], N. Moriyama[3]

[1]Dept. of Optical Science, Univ. of Tokushima, [2]National Cancer Center East,
[3]National Cancer Center, [4]Tochigi Cancer Center,
[5]The Social Health Medical Center, [6]National Shikoku Cancer Center
{kawata, niki}@opt.tokushima-u.ac.jp

Abstract. We are developing computerized feature extraction and classification methods to analyze malignant and benign pulmonary nodules in three-dimensional (3-D) thoracic CT images. Internal structure features were derived from CT density and 3-D curvatures to characterize the inhomogeneous of CT density distribution inside the nodule. In the classification step, we combined an unsupervised k-means clustering (KMC) procedure and a supervised linear discriminate (LD) classifier. The KMC procedure classified the sample nodules into two classes by using the mean CT density values for two different regions such as a core region and a complement of the core region in 3-D nodule image. The LD classifier was designed for each class by using internal structure features. The stepwise procedure was used to select the best feature subset from multi-dimensional feature spaces. The discriminant scores output from the classifier were analyzed by receiver operating characteristic (ROC) method and the classification accuracy was quantified by the area, Az, under the ROC curve. We analyzed a data set of pulmonary nodules in this study. The results of this study indicate the potential of combining the KMC procedure and the LD classifier for computer-aided classification of pulmonary nodules.

1. Introduction

We are developing computerized feature extraction and classification methods to analyze malignant and benign pulmonary nodules in three-dimensional (3-D) thoracic images. The purpose of this research is to design a hybrid classifier combining an unsupervised and a supervised model to improve the classification performance.

2. Method and Result

3-D thoracic images were reconstructed from thin-section CT images obtained by the helical CT scanner. In the 3-D thoracic image, pulmonary nodules were segmented by a deformable surface model. From the resulting nodule region, curvature indexes (shape index and curvedness) and CT density were computed and then a set of

W. Niessen and M. Viergever (Eds.): MICCAI 2001, LNCS 2208, pp. 1393-1394, 2001.

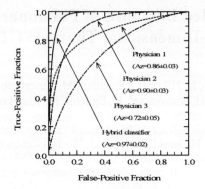

Fig. 1. Comparison of ROC curves of the hybrid classifier and physicians.

histogram features was measured from the distribution of the curvature indexes and CT density over the nodule region. The histogram features measure the amount of voxel which has a particular shape category and CT value in the nodule. Additionally, we introduced the topological and shape distribution features to characterize the internal structure of the nodule. We divided the inside of the nodule into four shape categories by using the shape index value and then, computed the topological features of each 3-D cluster which constructed from a set of voxels with the same shape category. The topological features used here were the Euler number, the number of connected components, cavities, and holes of each 3-D cluster. The shape distribution feature quantified how each shape category distributes inside the nodule by using a technique computing 3-D Euclidean distance transform. In the classification step, we designed a hybrid classifier that combined an unsupervised k-means clustering (KMC) procedure and a supervised linear discriminate (LD) classifier. The KMC procedure classified the sample nodules into two classes by using the mean CT density values for two different regions such as a core region and a complement of the core region in 3-D nodule image. The LD classifier was designed for each class. The discriminate scores output from the classifier were analyzed by receiver operating characteristic (ROC) methodology. The ROC curves using two experienced physicians and one inexperienced physician were shown in Fig.1. The data set included 141 pulmonary nodules (34 benign and 107 malignant cases. The ROC curve of the hybrid classifier was also plotted. The physicians 1, 2, and 3 respectively have 15 years, 12 years, and one year of experience in the chest radiology. This result highlights the promise of the hybrid classifier in the classification between benign and malignant nodules.

3. Conclusion

The application results of our method to the 3D thoracic images have demonstrated that the hybrid classifier is a promising approach for improving the accuracy of classifiers for CAD applications.

Ophthalmic Slitlamp-Based Computer-Aided Diagnosis: Image Processing Foundations

Luca Bogoni[1], Jane C. Asmuth[1], David Hirvonen[1], Bojidar D. Madjarov[2], and Jeffrey W. Berger[2]

[1] Medical Imaging Group,Sarnoff Corporation,
{lbogoni}@sarnoff.com
[2] Department of Ophthalmology, Scheie Eye Institute

Abstract. Computer aided diagnosis and treatment of retinal disorders is enabled through an ophthalmic augmented reality environment being developed around the standard slitlamp biomicroscope. This system will allow the physician to view superimposed fundus photographic and angiographic data on the real-time slitlamp biomicroscopic image. The overlay capability requires real-time image acquisition, processing, mosaicking and comparison. Non-real time capabilities include the co-registration of similar or differing sources such as slitlamp biomicroscope, fundus photograph, or angiograms. Mosaicking enables the creation of montages from a collection of images and provides a context for robust registration and comparison. This paper outlines the image-processing architecture and controls to provide these functionalities.

1 Introduction

Diagnosis and treatment of retinal disorders is enabled through an ophthalmic augmented reality (OAR) environment being developed around the standard slitlamp biomicroscope. This concept was first proposed in [3] and will allow the physician to view superimposed fundus photographic and angiographic data on the real-time slitlamp biomicroscopic image. This "augmented" slitlamp image will enable more precise laser treatment for diseases such as diabetic retinopathy and age-related macular degeneration [4]. Figure 1 shows a conceptual overview of the augmented reality system. The slitlamp image is sent, through a beam-splitter, to the CCD camera and then connects to the video-capture board on the local PC. The enlargement of the screen shows a snapshot of the current application tracking the slitlamp image onto a fundus image. Once the slitlamp image has been aligned, a portion of the corresponding area of the angiogram image is extracted. The extracted image is then viewed on a miniature display which interfaces with one of the oculars of the biomicroscope. Effectively, the physician will merge these two image sources (live and overlay) and see a floating picture of the angiogram positioned directly onto the section of the retina currently being examined via the biomicroscope.

The augmented reality system contains three major design components: *registration,* presentation,*control.* The registration is the process that aligns a *floating*

W. Niessen and M. Viergever (Eds.): MICCAI 2001, LNCS 2208, pp. 1395–1397, 2001.

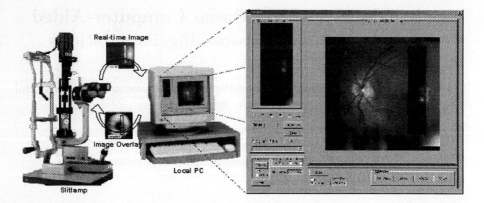

Fig. 1. Overview of the closed loop augmented-reality system connected to the slitlamp biomicroscope.

image to the coordinate frame of another *reference* image, [1], [5], and [2]. The presentation provides a meaningful view of the data to the physician [3]. The control strategy ties the system together and enables real-time registration and presentation. It directs the process of registration and dictates what portions of the images are to be displayed.

2   From Slitlamp Images to Angiograms

In order to relate the registration between the type of images sources, it is necessary to establish a cycle of transformations. Clinically establishing the relation between fundus and angiogram provides a means of relating visual/functional cues of the angiogram with particular loci on the fundus. Thus, the ability to establish this transformation cycle fullfils a procedural requirement for registration as well as a clinical role of providing context and functional interpretation.

These transformations are: *slitlamp image to mosaic* (f2M), *mosaic to fundus image* (M2F) *fundus to angiogram* (F2A) and *angiogram to slitlamp image* (A2f). This alignment is obtained by composing the various transformations $T_{f2A} = F2A \circ M2F \circ f2M$ and then by taking the inverse, T'_{f2A}. In this manner, the angiogram is expressed in the coordinate frame of the slitlamp and the appropriate portion of the angiogram may be extracted.

3   Results

Figure 2 shows the overlaid results from applying the cycle of transformations discussed earlier. Currently, f2M is running on a 300 MHz Pentium II as part of a multi-threaded non-optimized application at approximately 7 frames/second. Improvements in the computational speedup are expected once the Acadia [6], a new vision processing board, will be integrated as part of the augmented reality system.

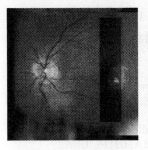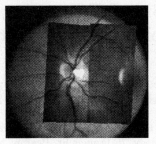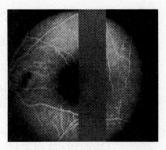

Fig. 2. Registration examples of images warped to the coordinate frame of another. Left: slitlamp image to slitlamp mosaic (f2M); Center: slitlamp mosaic to fundus image (M2F); Right: Fundus to angiogram (F2A). For emphasis, only a small portion of the angiogram is displayed.

We have introduced the image processing architecture and controls to express and recover the sequence of transformation which lead from a slitlamp image acquisition to the extraction of the corresponding angiogram. While this process is being developed as part of an ophthalmic augmented reality system, the ability to perform the intermediate registration will enable to relate multiple image modalities. For instance, once slitlamp mosaics can be constructed and registered to fundus images, it will be possible to compare current images with previously acquired images and both qualify and quantify the change that have taken place. Therefore, registration will facilitate computer-aided diagnosis.

The process of clinical evaluation is also part of the next step in the development and evaluation of the effectiveness of the system and the accuracy of the registration process.

References

1. Asmuth,J.C.,Madjarov, B.D., Sajda, P.,Berger, J.W.: Mosaicking and Enhancement of Slitlamp Biomocroscopic Fundus Images. British Journal of Ophthalmology - Accepted for publication, 2001.
2. Bergen,J.R., Anandan, P., Hanna, K., Hingorani, R.: Hierarchical model-based motion estimation. Proc. of ECCV, (1992) 5-10.
3. Berger,J.W., Leventon, M.E., Hata, N., Wells, WM.III, Kikinis, R.: Design considerations for a computer-vision-enabled ophthalmic augmented reality environment, Vol. 1205. Lecture Notes in Computer Science, Springer-Verlag (1997) 399-408.
4. Berger,J.W., Shin, D.S.: Image-guided macular laser therapy: Design consideration and progress toward implementation, Vol. 3591. Proc. SPIE: Opthalmic Technologies (1999) 241-247.
5. Can, A., Stewart, C.V., Roysam, B., Tanenbaum, H.L.: A Feature-based technique for joing, linear estimation of high-order image to mosaic transformations: application to moaicing the curved human retina. In: Proc. of IEEE Conf. CVPR (2000) 415–438.
6. van der Wal,G.,Hansen, M., Piacentino,M.: The Acadia Vision Processor. In: Proc. of the IEEE Intl. Workshop on CAMP, (2000).

Multiresolution Signal Processing on Meshes for Automatic Pathological Shape Characterization

Sylvain Jaume[1], Matthieu Ferrant[2], Andreas Schreyer[1], Lennox Hoyte[1], Benoît Macq[2], Julia Fielding[1], Ron Kikinis[1], and Simon K. Warfield[1]

[1] Brigham and Women's Hospital and Harvard Medical School, Thorn 329, Department of Radiology, 75 Francis St, Boston, MA, 02115, USA,
[2] Université catholique de Louvain, Telecommunications Laboratory, Place du Levant 2, 1348 Louvain-la-Neuve, Belgium

Abstract. We present a method based on multiresolution signal processing on meshes to create a thickness atlas. We applied this method to construct an atlas of bladder wall thickness. Bladder cancer is associated with increased bladder wall thickness. A thickness atlas helps to detect abnormal thickening in the bladder wall. Extracting inner and outer surface meshes from segmented images, we compute the thickness on the inner surface and map it to a sphere. We average the thickness at each position on the sphere to create a thickness atlas. We then compute Z-score values on the configuration of the patient's bladder to show regions of unusual thickness.

1 Introduction

Anatomical structures such as bladder wall, prostate wall, heart and cortical gray matter, have a varying thickness. A local thickening of the inner surface can be the first sign of an abnormality and is difficult to be distinguished from the normal variation in thickness. Aligning many surfaces and averaging their thickness values would create a thickness atlas. Areas where thickness is both large and highly different from the atlas would mean a high likelihood of abnormality. While Angenent et al. [1] formulate a conformal mapping with minimal area distortion, we use the wavelets on meshes introduced by Guskov et al. [3] to align surfaces onto a sphere. The benefits are a progressive alignment of the shape from large scale to finer details and a small distortion of the surface parameterization.

2 Algorithm

Inner and outer surface meshes are extracted by Marching Cubes [5] from manually segmented and coherently oriented scans. Each vertex of the inner surface gets a thickness value which is the distance to the closest vertex on the outer surface. We then create a *Progressive Mesh* [4] for each subject model.

W. Niessen and M. Viergever (Eds.): MICCAI 2001, LNCS 2208, pp. 1398–1400, 2001.

When traversing this representation from coarse to fine, we minimize the curvature of the vertices involved in a *vertex split* by divided differences [2] and project them to a sphere. Since any position on one sphere can be mapped to another sphere with 2 angles, we can average the thickness at this position on all models to create an atlas. For each subject, a Z-score, $Z(v) = |thickness(v) - atlas\ thickness(v)|/atlas\ standard\ deviation(v)$, estimates the likelihood of pathological thickness at the vertex v.

3   Results

We implemented our method in the Visualization Toolkit [6] and applied it on 24 bladder cases to increase the specificity of tumor detection. Figure 1 illustrates our results. Each value of the spherical thickness atlas is an average over all 24 inner surfaces mapped to a sphere. Center images depict one case where a high thickness value matches a high Z-score (white areas). This suspicious area correlates with the abnormality detected by an expert on the CT images (arrow on the right image).

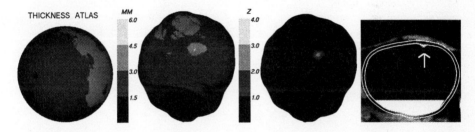

Fig. 1. Thickness atlas from 24 subjects *(left)*, inner surface of one bladder where gray scale codes the thickness *(center left)* and the Z score *(center right)*, CT slice overlayed with cuts through the inner and outer meshes in white *(right)*, the arrow shows an abnormality detected by an expert.

4   Discussion and Conclusion

We presented an algorithm to automatically create a thickness atlas from segmented 3D images of the inner and outer volumes of an anatomical structure. Our method is based on multiresolution signal processing on meshes and introduces small parameterization distortion. The difference between the local thickness in a new scan and the atlas thickness improves the detection of abnormalities. Results on 24 bladder CT scans showed the potentiality of the method for further applications such as designing a thickness atlas of the cortical gray matter.

Acknowledgements: Special thanks to Igor Guskov for many helpful discussions. Sylvain Jaume is working towards a Ph.D. degree with a grant from the Belgian FRIA. This investigation was supported by NIH P41 RR13218, NIH P01 CA67165 and NIH R01 RR11747.

References

[1] S. Angenent, S. Haker, A. Tannenbaum, and R. Kikinis. *System Theory, Modeling, Analysis, and Control*, chapter 20 On area preserving maps of minimal distortion, pages 275–287. Kluwer Academic Publishers, 2000.

[2] I. Guskov. Multivariate subdivision schemes and divided differences. Technical report, Department of Mathematics, Princeton University, 1998.

[3] I. Guskov, W. Sweldens, and P. Schröder. Multiresolution signal processing for meshes. In *Computer Graphics (SIGGRAPH 97 Proceedings)*, pages 325–334, 1997.

[4] Hoppe H. Progressive meshes. In *Computer Graphics (SIGGRAPH 96 Proceedings)*, pages 99–108, 1996.

[5] W.E. Lorensen and H.E. Cline. Marching cubes: a high resolution 3D surface construction algorithm. In *Computer Graphics (SIGGRAPH 87 Proceedings)*, pages 163–169, 1987.

[6] W. Schroeder, K. Martin, and B. Lorensen. *The Vizualisation Toolkit: An Object-Oriented Approach to 3D Graphics*. Prentice Hall PTR, New Jersey, second edition, 1998.

Interactive Visualisation of MRI Vector and Tensor Fields

Abhir Bhalerao[1] and Paul Summers[2]

[1] Department of Computer Science
University of Warwick, UK
abhir@dcs.warwick.ac.uk
[2] Clinical Neurosciences
Kings College Medical School, UK
p.summers@iop.kcl.ac.uk

Methods for visualising and analysing MR phase images that depict motional properties of blood or molecular diffusion in a way that meets the needs of the expert users has been a topic of intense study in recent years e.g., [2, 3]. The clinical attraction of phase contrast imaging has been its ability to depict flowing blood whereas diffusion imaging is associated both with delineating strokes and identifying patterns or pathways of connectivity within the brain. There are similarities in the pre and post-operative questions asked by experts for these two types of MR images, e.g. does a particular vessel feed or drain a given region or what are the terminal connections of a neuronal tract, and what is the flow pattern in a given region or what is the connectivity of a cortical region.

We have developed a graphical tool, **Angiotool** [1], that attempts to meet some of the requirements of clinical experts by providing a set of *low-level* and semi-automated visualisation and analysis tools – low-level in this context meaning they are accountable and their effects transparent to the user. The tools are also consistent in the data navigation and interaction interfaces, to some extent, across MR image types.

The **orthogonal views** can show both slice data and MIPs (Figure 1). Point-and-click cursor navigation in the slice data *continues* to operate on the MIP image allowing any image feature, such as a vessel, to be manually tracked in the other two views which are automatically centred on the cursor position. The **render window** maintains a depth buffer of the current projection from which the cursor position can readily be mapped. Also, a *limited* MIP, where image voxels between a pair of depth planes either side of the cursor position, can be used to prevent depth ambiguity errors which may result from the projection of brightest pixels. The **3D analysis window** is linked to the the render window and displays results of analyses on the volume data. An examples of such an analyses iis tracking, either as flow stream generation or as the derivation of neuronal tract orientation. Flow tracking experiments involve setting one or more particles (or seeds) into the velocity field (Figure 1(a)-(c),(e)). The tracking process is local and relies solely on the velocity data at each point using a physical space, point tracking algorithm. Tracking in diffusion data is performed on a derived vector field such as the principal eigenvector which represents the

W. Niessen and M. Viergever (Eds.): MICCAI 2001, LNCS 2208, pp. 1401–1403, 2001.

local anisotropy modulated by a scalar or the fractional anisotropy index which measures the eccentricity of the tensor. Simulation results, such as flow streams, are buffered by Angiotool which can be recorded or replayed.

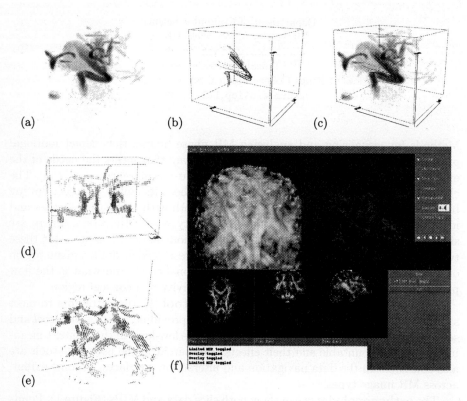

(a)   (b)   (c)

(d)

(f)

(e)

Fig. 1. Flow tracking experiments to determine the neck of a giant cerebral aneurysm: (a) User selects starting point(s) in MIP view. (b) By reversing the direction of flow from the seed point, blood flow is followed from within the aneurysm back through the neck and into the feeding artery. (c) Overlay of MIP with flow experiment precisely locates the neck. (d) Example of velocity data depicted as a field of vectors. (e) Plot of principal eigenvectors across a slice from an example diffusion image. (f) Overview of diffusion tensor image analysis: all tracks from a central slice across the brain. The MIP and orthogonal views show a scalar (derived) image of fractional-anisotropy using a magnitude image for the tensor tracking.

The current implementation is built upon open standards technologies: GUI toolkits using X and Motif and 3D graphics using OpenGL. While not as extensible or general purpose as comparative surgical planning and analysis tools, we believe that the presented GUI model could usefully form the basis of other clinical applications of this type.

References

[1] A. Bhalerao and P. Summers. Angiotool: A Tool for Interactive Visualization of MRI Vector and Tensor Fields. Research Report CS-RR-382, Department of Computer Science, University of Warwick, Coventry, UK, May 2001.

[2] T. M. Koller. *From Data to Information: Segmentation, Description and Analysis of the Cerebral Vascularity.* PhD thesis, Swiss Federal Instititute of Technology, Zurich, 1995.

[3] C-F. Westin, S. E. Maier, B. Khidhir, P. Everet, and F. A. Jolesz nd R. Kikinis. Image Processing for Diffusion Tensor Magnetic Resonance Imaging. In *Proc. of MICCAI'99*, pages 441–452, 1999.

Tracking Methods for Medical Augmented Reality

Abhilash Pandya, M.S.[1], Mohamad Siadat, M.S.[1], Lucia Zamorano, M.D. Dr. Med.[1], Jainxing Gong, Ph.D.[1], Qinghang Li.[1], M.D. Ph.D, James Maida, M.S.[2], Ioannis Kakadiaris, Ph.D[3]

1. Neurosurgery Department suite 930, 4160 John R, Detroit, Mi. 48201
2. NASA, Johnson Space Center, Houston , Tx.
3. University of Houston, Houston, Tx.
This work is partially funded by NASA grant 99-HEDS-01-079
apandya@neurosurgery.wayne.edu

Introduction

Recently, the capabilities of real-time PC-based video image processing and computer graphic systems converged to make possible the display of a virtual graphical image correctly registered with a view of the 3D environment of the user's object of interest. The generation of an Augment Reality scene can now be done with a PC computer graphics system. An Augmented Reality (AR) system generates a composite view for the user. It is a combination of the real scene viewed by the user and a virtual scene generated by the computer (a 3D model) that augments the scene with additional information. Fig. 1 displays one possible AR scene where a phantom is overlaid with graphics models of tumors. One of the most important issues to consider for a very accurate AR application is the method for tracking the various elements of the environment such as the video camera.

Methods

For the camera tracking there are at least three different methods: 1) tracking using an infrared camera tracking system, 2) tracking using a precise robot arm and 3) a camera calibration method using pattern recognition techniques. Note that for the two former methods we need to estimate the camera parameters (calibrate the camera) to generate an accurate AR scene. An infrared stereo-camera with its LEDs is considered enough hardware for both camera calibration and camera tracking. Tracking can be achieved by a robot in which the geometrical information (position and orientation of the mounted camera) is calculated through forward kinematics. A robot also provides enough information for the camera calibration procedure. The third method for camera tracking uses the captured frames in which several well-known patterns are tracked. This method works based on image processing techniques [1] and needs minimum hardware requirements. In the third method the information needed for camera calibration procedure [2] has to be provided either by a special geometrical instrument or through the two former methods. So the camera calibration method is used for camera tracking as well as camera parameter estimation (camera calibration).

W. Niessen and M. Viergever (Eds.): MICCAI 2001, LNCS 2208, pp. 1404-1405, 2001.

Results/Conclusions

There are some limitations and strengths for using each of the systems outlined for camera tracking. Line-of-site and lighting condition issues exist for both the pattern recognition and infrared tracking. The virtual objects will only appear when the tracking marks are in view and the lighting conditions are properly adjusted. A robotics-based camera overcomes both of these problems. There are also range issues. For the pattern recognition system, the larger the physical pattern the further away the pattern can be detected and so the greater the tracking volume. The infrared camera distance to the phantom limits the IR tracking (typically the range is 1 meter). The robotic solution is dependent on the robotic kinematics and the range of motion of each of the joints. For the restricted volume needed for neurosurgery applications, all the mentioned methods could be potentially used [4,5]. For redundancy, a solution that relies on more than one modality would be advantageous. For instance, using infrared guided tracking with image processing would provide continuous tracking during non-optimal scenarios. This paper represents work in progress.

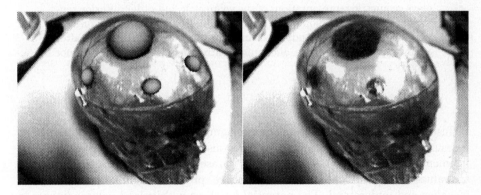

Fig. 1. An AR scene: A see-through phantom is overlaid with graphics models of the "tumors".

References

1. ArtoolKit http://www.hitl.washington.edu/resarch/shared_space/download/

2. Weng J., Cohen P., Herniou M., "Camera Calibration with Distortion Model and Accuracy Evaluation," IEEE Trans. PAMI, vol. 14, no. 10, 1992.

3. Pandya A., Siadat M., Gong J., Li Q, Zamorano L., Maida J., "Towards Using Augmented Reality for Neurosurgery", Medicine Meets Virtual Reality, Jan 2001.

4. Pandya A., Zamorano L., Siadat M., Gong J., Li. Q, Maida J., "Advanced Surgical Image Environments", The 5th Annual Neurosurgery Detroit Symposium—Neurosurgery in the 21st Century, Nov. 3-5th 2000

Toward Application of Virtual Reality to Visualization of DT-MRI Volumes

S. Zhang[1], Ç. Demiralp[1], M. DaSilva[1], D. Keefe[1], D. Laidlaw[1],
B.D. Greenberg[1], P.J. Basser[2], C. Pierpaoli[2], E.A. Chiocca[3], and
T.S. Deisboeck[3]

[1] Brown University, Providence, RI 02912, USA
[2] STBB, NICHD, National Institutes of Health, Bethesda, MD 20892, USA
[3] Neurosurgical Service and Brain Tumor Center, Mass. General Hospital, Harvard
Medical School, Boston, MA 02114, USA

Abstract. We describe a virtual reality application for visualizing tensor-
valued volume data acquired with diffusion tensor magnetic resonance
imaging (DT-MRI). We have prototyped a virtual environment that displays geometric representations of the volumetric 2nd-order diffusion tensor data and are developing interaction and visualization techniques for
two application areas: studying changes in white-matter structures after
gamma-knife capsulotomy and pre-operative planning for brain tumor
surgery.

1 Introduction

Diffusion Tensor Magnetic Resonance Imaging (DT-MRI) has the potential to
measure fiber-tract trajectories in soft fibrous tissues, such as nerves, muscles,
ligaments, and tendons [1]. However, the datasets produced are volumetric with
six values at each spatial location and, hence, present a significant challenge to
visualize and understand. The potential for these multivalued volume images is
likely to be great but is, as yet, not well explored.

A number of methods have been developed that display the data as 3D
models [2,3]. Some methods, including ours, track the fiber-tract trajectories in
DT-MRIs [1,2,4]. We generate a large set of streamtubes and streamsurfaces to
represent, respectively, linear structures like fiber tracts and planar structures.
With traditional monocular single-screen displays, it is difficult to interpret these
complex geometric models. The situation is exacerbated when the complexity of
the models is increased to meet user requirements for more detail. An immersive
virtual environment such as the Cave [5] has the advantages of head-tracked
stereo display, a large display surface, and interactivity [10]. For some tasks, users
can improve performance on similar complex models in such an environment by
200% over working with a static image [9]. Virtual environments have already
been used in some surgical applications [11].

This short paper describes our efforts to use the Cave for DT-MRI visualization. Our targeted applications include studying changes in white matter
structures before and after gamma-knife capsulotomy and pre-operative planning
for brain tumor surgery.

W. Niessen and M. Viergever (Eds.): MICCAI 2001, LNCS 2208, pp. 1406–1408, 2001.
© Springer-Verlag Berlin Heidelberg 2001

2   Method

Virtual Reality Setup Our Cave is an $8 \times 8 \times 8$ foot cube with rear-projected front and side walls and a front-projected floor. A user wears a pair of LCD shutter glasses that support stereo viewing. The glasses have an attached tracker that relays their position and orientation to the computer. In our application, the virtual environment consists of a room the size of the Cave itself and a table under the visualization of the DT-MRI data. The user can walk around, bend over, and move his/her head to observe the visualization from different perspectives.

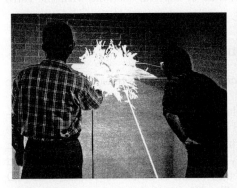 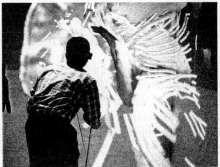

Fig. 1. Two users observe the DT-MRI **Fig. 2.** A user takes a closer look by visualization in the Cave.   moving toward the virtual brain.

DT-MRI Visualization We have displayed DT-MRI and T2-weighted images of a human brain (courtesy Dr. Susumu Mori, Johns Hopkins University). Both of the datasets are registered in a $256 \times 256 \times 40$ volume. Each voxel is $0.89 \times 0.89 \times 3.2mm$.

We use three kinds of geometric models, streamtubes, streamsurfaces, and isosurfaces, to present different types of structures in the brain. Fibrous structures in the brain, like white-matter tracts, yield diffusion tensors with linear anisotropy. Streamtubes are thin tubes that follow the direction of fastest diffusion in regions of linear anisotropy. Analogously, streamsurfaces follow planar structures in regions of planar anisotropy. Colors are mapped on the geometric models to display the magnitude of linear or planar anisotropy. Initially we generate the geometric models from a dense set of seed points in the volume. We then use a culling algorithm to pick a representative subset for display [4,6]. We also generated isosurfaces of the ventricles from the T2-weighted image to give the user an anatomical context.

The doctors who first used our system suggested that viewing typical 2D T2-weighted sections might help in identifying anatomical features in the 3D models. We provide a 2D slicer that the user can move through a 3D scalar dataset that is co-registered with the DT-MRI data. The user can also change the dataset carried by the slicer. We have displayed the T2-weighted image with the slicer to validate the ventricle models, displayed the linear anisotropy image to validate and understand the streamtube models, and displayed the planar anisotropy image to validate and understand the streamsurface models.

Interaction The current interaction scheme is a simple one. The geometric models and sections appear stationary above the virtual table. The user walks around and changes head position to examine the data from different perspectives. With a three-button wand, the user can point to features of interest using a virtual laser pointer, can change the position of the slicer with two of the buttons, or can choose among axial, coronal, or sagittal sections with the third button.

3   Discussion and Conclusion

We have constructed a virtual environment for visualizing tensor-valued volume data acquired with DT-MRI.

Three of the authors who are MDs have used the system and provided feedback. Two are neurosurgeons from MGH and one an MD/PhD studying obsessive compulsive disorder at Butler Hospital in Providence, RI. Their experience with the system suggests that it is sufficiently easy to use. They had each also viewed static images of the geometric models and found it easier to visualize the 3D structures in the virtual environment. The 2D sections were reported to be a very valuable additional tool within the virtual environment.

Our long-term goal is to provide an efficient and effective visualization of DT-MRI volume data together with other medical imaging modalities. As effectiveness can be measured only in the context of a specific application, we intend to pursue the applications we have described. As a first step, we have constructed a framework in which geometric models are put into a fully immersive virtual environment. Users move in the virtual environment and observe the visualization in the same way they would view a physical object in the real world. The environment shows strong potential for understanding these complicated datasets and the underlying anatomy and pathology that they measure.

References

1. Peter Basser et al., *Magn. Reson. Med.*, 44:625-632 (2000)
2. Rong Xue et al., *Magn. Reson. Med.*, 42:1123-1127 (1999)
3. Gordon Kindlmann et al., *Proc. IEEE Visualization*, 183-189 (1999)
4. Song Zhang et al., *Proc. ISMRM* (2001)
5. Carolina Cruz-Neira et al., *SIGGRAPH*, 135-142 (1993)
6. Song Zhang, *Master's Thesis*, Brown University (2000)
7. Will Schroeder et al., *The Visualization Toolkit*, Prentice Hall (1996)
8. Enrico Gobetti et al., *Proc. IEEE Visualization*, 435-438 (1998)
9. Colin Ware et al., *ACM Transactions on Graphics*, 15(2)121-140 (1996)
10. Andrew Forsberg et al., *Proc. IEEE Visualization*, 457-460 (2000)
11. S. Taylor et al., *Computer-Integrated Surgery*, MIT Press (1996)

Registration and Visualization of Transcranial Magnetic Stimulation on MR Images

O. Cuisenaire[1], M. Ferrant[2], Y. Vandermeeren[3], E. Olivier[3], and B. Macq[2]

[1] Swiss Federal Institute of Technology (EPFL-LTS), Lausanne, Switzerland
[2] Université catholique de Louvain (UCL-TELE), Louvain-la-Neuve, Belgium
[3] Université catholique de Louvain (UCL-NEFY), Brussels, Belgium
Olivier.Cuisenaire@epfl.ch, http://ltswww.epfl.ch/~cuisenai

1 Introduction

Transcranial Magnetic Stimulation (TMS) has been widely used in the mapping of the primary motor cortex, as well as in the study of language, memory, mood, auditory or visual perception [4]. Similarly to EEG or MEG, it provides information - Motor Evoked Potentials (MEP) - located on the surface of the scalp and requires a registration between the physical space (PhS) and a MRI for proper interpretation.

Several methods have been proposed for this registration. Wang [5] and Bastings [1] use a magnetic field (MF) digitizer to acquire points on the scalp surface. Wang attaches the MF transmitter on the patient's head while Basting uses two receivers, one fixed on the patient to track head motion and one mobile to acquire the data. Bastings uses 6 MRI-visible landmarks for registration while Wang uses approx. 400 points for MRI to PhS registration, then landmarks for PhS to PhS registration in repeat experiments on the same patient. Ettinger [3] and Potts [4] use a combination of laser to digitize the head surface and optical tracking using LEDs to follow head motion.

In this paper we propose a registration method based on Bastings' and Wang's, but that improves them both in terms of precision and ease of use.

2 Method

PhS points are acquired using a MF digitizer (Polhemus Isotrak II). One receiver is fixed on the patient's forehead and the other is a hand held stylus. The scalp surface is characterized by acquiring about 150 points following the pattern illustrated in Figure 1.1. The coil location and orientation are determined from 3 measures, one at the coil center and the other two in the coil plane.

Both the head (for registration) and the cortical surface (for visualization) are segmented using a semi-automated algorithm based on interactive threshold and mathematical morphology processing. The registration algorithm finds the rigid transform that minimizes the mean square distance between the PhS digitized points and the MRI head surface. This distance is precomputed using a fast Euclidean distance transform, as explained in details in [2].

W. Niessen and M. Viergever (Eds.): MICCAI 2001, LNCS 2208, pp. 1409–1411, 2001.

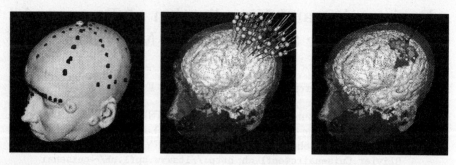

Fig. 1. 1. points used for registration 2. magnet locations 3. interpolated MEPs

Typical results are illustrated at figure 1. The motor cortex was stimulated at points of a regular grid. In Figure 1.2, registered coils centers are represented by spheres and their orientation by lines. The amplitude of the recorded MEP at each location is color coded. In Figure 1.3 the coil locations are projected onto the brain surface and MEP values are interpolated to form a continuous map. For quantitative analysis, the center of gravity (CoG) of the MEPs is also computed.

3   Discussion

The procedure was validated using 4 different methods. Firstly with synthetic PhS points generated from the MRI scalp to which an arbitrary transform was applied. The algorithm converges for all translations and rotation of up to 30°. The mean residual error was $0.17mm$ over a test set of 100 different arbitrary transforms. Secondly 5 sets of PhS points were digitized for the same patient and registrations were performed. In average, the residual mean square distance from registered points to scalp surface was $1mm$. Thirdly, those 5 registrations were used to determine the location of several MRI-visible markers. The mean error was found to be $3.8mm$ while the same test using our implementation of Basting's [1] method lead to an error of $9.7mm$. Finally, the reproducibility of the method was assessed by computing the CoGs of the MEPs on the brain surface using the 5 registrations. The average distance to the mean CoG was approx. $1mm$, 5 times less than using Basting's method.

Ease of use was evaluated in terms of operator time required. Scalp digitization requires between 1 and 3 minutes, while each coil location requires approx. 30 seconds. Both the semi-automatic segmentation and the registration take less than a minute. This is orders of magnitude faster than reported by Wang [5].

References

1. Bastings et al.: Co-registration of cortical magnetic stimulation and functional magnetic resonance imaging. NeuroReport **9** (1998) 1941–1946

2. Cuisenaire O.: Distance transformation, fast algorithms and applications to medical image processing. Ph.D. Thesis, October 1999, Université catholique de Louvain.
3. Ettinger et al.:Experimentation with a Transscranial Magnetic Stimulation System for Functional Brain Mapping. CVRMed/MRCAS'97, Grenoble, France.
4. Potts G.F. et al.: Visual Hemifield Mapping Using Transcranial Magnetic Stimulation Coregistered with Cortical Surfaces Derived from Magnetic Resonance Images. J Clin Neurophysiology, **15** (1998) 344–350
5. Wang et al.: Head surface digitization and registration: a method for mapping positions on the head onto magnetic resonance images. Brain Topography. **6** (1994) 185–192

Automated Image Rectification in Video-Endoscopy

Dan Koppel[1], Yuan-Fang Wang[1], and Hua Lee[2]

[1] Department of Computer Science,
{dkoppel,yfwang}@cs.ucsb.edu
[2] Department of Electrical and Computer Engineering,
University of California, Santa Barbara, CA, 93106, USA
hualee@ece.ucsb.edu

Abstract. Video-Endoscopy has proven to be significantly less invasive to the patient. However, it also creates a more complex and difficult operating environment that requires the surgeon to operate through a video interface. Visual feedback control and image interpretation in this operating environment can be troublesome. **Automated image analysis has tremendous potential in improving the surgeon's visual feedback, resulting in better patient safety, reduced operation time, and savings in health care.** In this paper, we present our design of an image rectification algorithm for maintaining the head-up display in video-endoscopy and report some preliminary results.

Video-endoscopy [1, 2] are minimally invasive surgical procedures where small incisions are made on the patient to accommodate surgical instruments such as scalpels, scissors, staple guns, and a video endoscope. The scope acquires video images of the bodily cavity that are displayed on a monitor to provide visual feedback to the surgeon.

Though video-endoscopy has proven to be tremendously beneficial in shortening the recuperation time and lowering the treatment cost [1, 2], this patient-oriented technology has increased the difficulty of performing the procedures for the surgeon. E.g. in open surgery, though the surgeon may move about the operating table and view the body anatomy from different viewpoints, the surgeon's sense of up and down is maintained. Or in the computer graphics terminology, the "head-up" vector, which indicates one's general perception of the "up" direction in the environment, is unchanged.

But in video-endoscopy, the bodily cavity is not exposed and the surgeon's perception of the "up" direction is established through the understanding of the anatomy. A large, about-the-axis rotation of the scope and the camera will change the orientation of the body anatomy, which often times results in the loss of one's orientation and bearing. Hence, how to compensate for the about-the-axis rotation of the video scope to maintain the right "head-up" display (i.e., a display where the image is rectified and re-oriented in such a way that the view corresponds to that taken with an upright camera) is important.

We propose a new formulation for rotation sensing and compensation based on novel image analysis techniques. The image analysis tasks proposed here can be stated succinctly as follows: Given a video sequence taken during an endoscopy surgery, with large panning and rotation of the scope, deduce the amount of the about-the-axis rotation relative to a specified reference frame. The images are then rectified and displayed in such a way as if the camera is held in an upright orientation.

W. Niessen and M. Viergever (Eds.): MICCAI 2001, LNCS 2208, pp. 1412–1414, 2001.

The essence of our rotation estimation and compensation scheme is to track anatomical features in an endoscopic video sequence and use the tracked features over time to deduce the camera motion parameters. The recovered motion parameters then allow rotation of the camera's head-up vector relative to that of a reference frame computed. Images can then be re-rendered by compensating for the rotation of the head-up vector.

Fig. 1 shows some image segmentation and tracking results. This preliminary result shows our ability to distinguish instrument regions from organ regions (see caption for explanation). Fig. 2 shows 2D and 3D tracking results over a sequence of about 200 frames. Fig. 2 (a) shows typical 2D feature location errors as a function of time, while Fig. 2 (b) shows the absolute error in estimated angle of rotation in 3D camera motion. Both results are quite good.

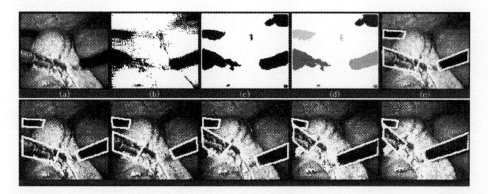

Fig. 1. Upper row: **(a)** Original image. **(b)** Binary image from color classification. Black and white pixels represent surgical instruments and organs, respectively. **(c)** Directional median filters were used to suppress noise. **(d)** Labeled image, different colors represent isolated instrument regions. **(e)** Computed bounding boxes that delineate instrument regions in images. Lower row: Tracking of instrument region.

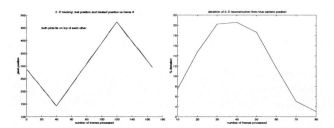

Fig. 2. **(a)** shows the 2D tracking error positions as function of time over about 200 frames. **(b)** shows the 3D tracking error (deviation in estimated angle of rotation from ground truth).

Acknowledgment: This research was supported in part by Karl Storz Imaging, Inc. and the State of California Micro Program.

1414   D. Koppel, Y.-F. Wang, and H. Lee

References

[1] J. F. Hulka and H. Reich. *Textbook of Laparoscopy, 2nd Ed.* W. B. Saunders, Philadelphia, PA, 1994.
[2] J. G. Hunter and J. M. Sackier (eds.). *Minimally Invasive Surgery*. McGraw-Hill, New York, 1993.

Java Internet Viewer: A WWW Tool for Remote 3D Medical Image Data Visualization and Comparison

Chris A. Cocosco and Alan C. Evans

McConnell Brain Imaging Centre, Montreal Neurological Institute,
McGill University, Montreal, Canada
c.cocosco@ieee.org
http://www.bic.mni.mcgill.ca/users/crisco/jiv/

Introduction: There is a growing need in the research and clinical medical imaging community for Internet-capable tools that facilitate remote data dissemination and interaction. 3-dimensional (3D) medical imaging datasets typically require special-purpose, non-portable, software to be installed and maintained on each workstation. Internet technologies have potential for improving this.

We developed JIV: a powerful, robust, portable, extensible, and open-source Java application ("applet") for visualization and side-by-side comparison of multiple 3D image datasets. It is designed to work through the WWW; it only requires a common Web browser, and can cope with slow networks and less capable workstations. Moreover, JIV provides features and a level of performance usually only found in traditional stand-alone workstation applications.

Previously reported projects [1,2,3] only have limited user interface functionality. Furthermore, they download slice images only when and if required; thus, their interactive performance is unsatisfactory when used over common long-distance Internet connections (which cannot guarantee a high transfer rate).

Design & Implementation: A convenient way to visualize 3D medical imaging datasets is by three orthogonal 2D slices through the same location in the volume. When several image volumes are to be compared, it is desirable to visualize their slices side-by-side, all at the same position in the volume.

With respect to how and when to download the 3D image data, the following three operation modes are supported by JIV:

1. *All up-front:* all of the data is downloaded and stored in client's memory before the user can view and interact with any of it.
2. *On demand:* download slice image data only when and if the user wants to view that particular slice.
3. *Hybrid (background download):* first download only the slices required by the initial cursor positions; then continue downloading all of the data in a background thread (as in (1)); if the user requests slice images which are not already downloaded, they will be downloaded with priority (as in (2)).

W. Niessen and M. Viergever (Eds.): MICCAI 2001, LNCS 2208, pp. 1415–1416, 2001.

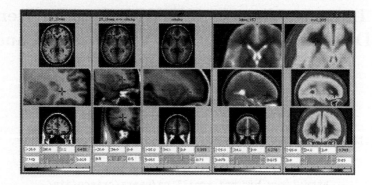

Mode (1) guarantees the best interactive response of the viewer; however, the user has to wait for all the data to download before the JIV interface becomes available – this can take a long time on a slow network link. Mode (2) minimizes the data downloads and the amount of memory required by the applet, but (like in [1,2,3]) its interactive response time is highly dependent on the server and on the network. Mode (3) is the best compromise for most situations. Our implementation does not temporarily freeze while waiting for data to arrive: instead, it displays a discernible pattern for the image areas it does not yet have, and replaces it with the real image as soon as it becomes available. To our knowledge, no other published work provides this background download feature.

The gray-level image data is displayed using a user-controlled color-mapping; an efficient mouse-based user input scheme provides fast roaming through the volume, and continuously adjustable zoom and pan.

Results: JIV was tested and was proved to be robust on a variety of computer platforms: Linux-i386, SGI IRIX, MacOS, and various MS Windows (Win32) versions. The interactive performance, defined as screen update time following user input, is good when JIV is running on recent PC hardware with enough memory (RAM). In conclusion, JIV is a convenient and platform-independent software for the remote visualization of 3D medical image data; for example, it can be used in remote data processing – when data goes to a central, well-equipped, site for image processing and storage. This software proved useful (both remotely and locally, in our lab) for efficient simultaneous visualization and comparison of many 3D image datasets, such as evaluating the performance of registration or segmentation methods.

Acknowledgements: Peter Neelin; Dr. Alex Zijdenbos; Dr. Louis Collins.

References

1. S. Vetsch, et al. A parallel pc-based visible human slice web server. *The Second Visible Human Project Conference*, 1998.
2. P. Golland, et al. *Computer Aided Surgery*, 4(3):129–43, 1999.
3. J. T. Lee, et al. *NeuroImage*, 11(5):S918, 2000.

Applications of Task-Level Augmentation for Cooperative Fine Manipulation Tasks in Surgery[1]

Rajesh Kumar[1,3], Aaron C. Barnes[2,3], Gregory D. Hager[1,3],
Patrick S. Jensen[2,3], Russell H. Taylor[1,3]

[1] The Department of Computer Science,
[2] Wilmer Eye Institute, Johns Hopkins Medical Institutions,
{abarnes,psjensen}@jhu.edu
[3] NSF Engineering Research Center for Computer
Integrated Surgical Systems and Technology,
The Johns Hopkins University, Baltimore, Maryland, USA
{rajesh, hager, rht}@cs.jhu.edu

Abstract. We report on applications of an augmentation system for cooperative fine manipulation using the steady hand manipulation paradigm. Using the "steady hand" robot as the experimental platform we investigate using such a system for creating composite retinal images using a GRIN lens endoscope and for puncturing small blood vessels in the retina.

1 Introduction

Performance of fine and dexterous tasks such as microsurgery is seriously affected due to limitations imposed by physical attributes of the sensory motor, muscular and skeletal systems on manual dexterity, precision and perception. These limitations provide a clear opportunity for augmentation. Using the "steady-hand" approach, we explore applications of a supervisory framework for human augmentation.

The "steady hand" robot used for these experiments was first reported in [1]. The task-level system used here is described in [2]. An explicit task representation is provided by the user for each task that includes planning inputs, safety considerations, and performance parameters. The task-level system generates a representation for the corresponding finite state machine (FSM). Each state of this FSM represents a step in the task, and each transition a termination predicate. The System maintains a basic set of states, and transitions. A detailed description of the task-level system appears in [2].

---

[1] The authors gratefully acknowledge the support of the National Science Foundation under grant #IIS9801684, and the ERC grant #EEC9731478. This work was also supported in part by the Johns Hopkins internal funds. We also thank XACTIX Inc. and Insight Instruments Inc. for some of the equipment used for these experiments.

W. Niessen and M. Viergever (Eds.): MICCAI 2001, LNCS 2208, pp. 1417-1418, 2001.

2 Experiments

We are experimenting with simple microsurgical tasks such as tool guidance and positioning, constrained and guarded tool motions.

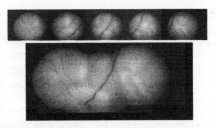

Retinal Mosaics: For these experiments, a porcine eye was positioned naturally in a phantom head, and a port was created in the eye for positioning the GRIN lens endoscope (Insight IE 3000, Insight Instruments Inc.) such that the RCM point is at the port. A task strategy for collecting the images was then executed. The images and the robot position at which they are taken were then used to construct the composite image. An example of a line of 5 images and the corresponding composite image appear in figure 1.

Figure 1: GRIN lens endoscope images and the composite image.

Retinal Vein Cannulation: In these experiments directed at positioning a tool in the occluded vessel, a porcine eye was mounted naturally in a face phantom and a MEMS micro-needle (XACTIX Inc.) was mounted on a 2mm shaft to be used as the probe. The micro-needle mimics a micro-pipette used in experimental vein cannulation treatment. Although they can not deliver anti-coagulants, micro-needles allow us to prototype experiments for evaluating augmentation strategies. The lens of the porcine eye was removed to improve access to the retina. The GRIN lens endoscope was positioned to image the target blood vessel for visual verification.

Lack of blood flow often caused the vessels to be partially collapsed. As a result, our first attempts to cannulate the vessels by approaching them in a perpendicular

 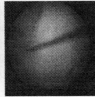

direction were unsuccessful. We modified our approach to be at a small angle to the vessel, and this allowed us to successfully cannulate sub-millimeter vessels. Figure 2(right) shows the micro-needle positioned in a small retinal vessel. Since not all vessels can be reached by approaches with small angles, we are exploring the alternative of mounting the micro-needles at an angle to the shaft. Further experiments are ongoing.

Figure 2: Experimental Setup for retinal cannulation (left), micro-needle positioned in a vessel (right).

References

[1]   R. H. Taylor et al, A Steady-Hand Robotic System for Microsurgical Augmentation, Medical Image Computing and Computer-Assisted Intervention -MICCAI'99, pp1031-1041, Cambridge, UK, 1999.

[2]   R. Kumar et al, An Augmentation System for Fine Manipulation, Medical Image Computing and Computer-Assisted Intervention- MICCAI'2000, pp956-963, Pittsburgh, PA, 2000.

Virtual Fixtures for Robotic Cardiac Surgery

Shinsuk Park[1] Ph.D., Robert D. Howe[1] Ph.D., and David F. Torchiana[2] MD

[1] Harvard University, Division of Engineering and Applied Sciences, Cambridge, Mass., USA
{sspark, howe}@deas.harvard.edu
[2] Massachusetts General Hospital, Division of Cardiac Surgery, Boston, Mass., USA

Abstract We are developing virtual fixtures for the internal mammary artery (IMA) harvest portion of robot-assisted coronary artery bypass graft procedures. A preoperative CT scan will be processed to define the location of the IMA. In surgery, the patient's anatomy will be registered to the image data, then a virtual fixture will constrain the instrument's motions, as commanded by the surgeon, to appropriate paths adjacent to the artery. As a preliminary test, a virtual wall is implemented on a commercial surgical robot system. Results from a dissection task show that execution is faster and more precise than with conventional freehand techniques.

1 Introduction

Traditional methods in cardiothoracic surgery require large incisions such as sternotomies. Recent work has demonstrated that robotic systems enable execution of coronary artery bypass graft (CABG) procedures through small incisions [1]. In practice, these systems have proved cumbersome to use, with shortcomings that include decreased visual and haptic information, motion constraints, and the need for cognitive spatio-motor remapping from the surgeon's hands to the instrument space.

We propose to help alleviate these difficulties through *virtual fixtures* [2]. A virtual fixture is a computer-generated constraint that simplifies task execution by reducing precision requirements or the number of degrees of freedom that must be controlled. On a desktop computer, these fixtures are analogous to computer mouse features such as snap-to-grid that make it simpler to precisely position the cursor. In this study, the validity of the concept of virtual fixtures is tested on the ZEUS surgical robot system (Computer Motion, Inc., Goleta, Calif.). We report the results of *in vitro* testing of a virtual wall fixture for a blunt dissection task that prevents the surgical instrument from entering a specified volume of tissue.

2 Methods

This project focuses on robot-assisted minimally-invasive coronary artery bypass graft (CABG) procedures. In this procedure, the interior mammary artery (IMA) is mobilized from the interior chest wall, and one end is attached to the coronary arteries to provide a new blood supply for the heart. Approximately 10-20 cm are dissected free, using blunt dissection and a harmonic scalpel or electrocautery. In the minimally invasive robotic approach, this is a laborious process that can occupy the majority of the operating time, over an hour in some cases. This study focuses on development of virtual fixtures for the IMA harvest portion of robot-assisted CABG procedures.

W. Niessen and M. Viergever (Eds.): MICCAI 2001, LNCS 2208, pp. 1419-1420, 2001.
© Springer-Verlag Berlin Heidelberg 2001

In the planned procedure, the patient will undergo a CT scan with arterial contrast agent before surgery. In initial animal tests, metal pins will be inserted between the ribs to provide fixed landmarks during imaging and surgery. The resulting image set will be processed to define the location of the artery relative to the registration pins. During the procedure, the surgeon will bring the tip of a robot-mounted instrument into contact with each pin to establish registration; future implementations will use landmark-based registration. A virtual fixture will constrain the instrument's motions, as commanded by the surgeon, to appropriate dissection planes adjacent to the artery. This reduces precision requirements on the surgeon.

We have implemented virtual fixtures on the ZEUS surgical robot system. The complete system comprises two instrument positioner robot arms controlled by the surgeon in manual teleoperation mode, and a third endoscope positioner. The virtual fixture uses a single instrument positioner. To assess the performance benefits of a virtual fixture, we compared blunt dissections with and without the aid of a *virtual wall*. The computer-generated virtual wall confines the slave instrument tip to the region outside a specified plane. The slave instrument is free to follow the master instrument in all three dimensions outside the proscribed region, while it follows only lateral motions on the wall surface if the master controller is moved within the region.

Four subjects (2 surgeons and 2 engineers) were instructed to dissect a 2 x 1.5 x 1 cm segment from a block of soft material simulating tissue, but to avoid penetrating the wall, as marked with lines on the material. The subjects were seated in front of a video monitor providing an image of the operative site, and manipulated the master controller as in the unmodified system. Performance measures include time to completion and number of excursions into the wall beyond a safety margin of 5 mm.

3   Results and Discussion

The effect of the fixture on task performance is summarized in Tables 1 and 2. The virtual wall reduced completion time by over 27% and eliminated excursions beyond the desired region, emphasizing the safety benefits of using the fixture.

Implementation of the image processing, registration, and surgeon interface portions of the system are underway. We are examining issues of registration accuracy, including instrument deflection and tissue movement between imaging and procedure.

Table 1. Time to completion (sec).

Virtual Fixture	Subject				Means
	1	2	3	4	
OFF	211	472	223	321	307
ON	173	345	155	215	222

Table 2. Number of excursions.

Virtual Fixture	Subject				Means
	1	2	3	4	
OFF	25	2	3	3	8
ON	0	0	0	0	0

References

1. Stephenson, E. R. Jr, Sankholkar, S., Ducko, C. T., Damiano, R. J. Jr: Robotically assisted microsurgery for endoscopic coronary artery bypass grafting. *Ann. Thoracic Surg.* 66 (3) (1998) 1064-1067.
2. Rosenberg, L. B.: Virtual fixtures: Perceptual Tools for Telerobotic Manipulation. In: *Proc. IEEE Virtual Reality Annual Intl. Symposium* (1993) 76-82.

The Clinical Use of Multi-modal Resources (2D/3D/Statistics) for Robot Assisted Functional Neurosurgery

Alim-Louis Benabid[1], Dominique Hoffmann[1], Luc Court[1], Vincent Robert[2],
Sébastien Burtin[2], Patrick Pittet[2], Jörg Fischer[3]

[1] Service de NeuroChirurgie, Centre Hospitalier Universitaire, Grenoble, France
[2] Integrated Surgical Systems SA, Bron, France,[3] IVS Solutions AG, Chemnitz, Germany

Abstract. This paper presents specific techniques and their implementation to integrate in the planing of functional neurosurgery all the available resources (3D preoperative examinations, intra-operative 2D radiographic X-rays, statistical database and atlases).
Keywords. Functional Neurosurgery – Image fusion – Co-Registration – Statistical Data – Stereotactic Robot.

1 Introduction

We present in this paper different methods to combine all the available information for planning of stereotactic functional neurosurgery and their implementation within a planning software (VoXim™, IVS Solutions AG) . This software is used to drive a stereotactic robot (NeuroMate™, ISS SA) for an optimal targeting of the planned trajectory[2][3]. [1]

2 Co-registration and Fusion

<u>Co-registration</u> of two modalities consists in the computation of the rigid transformation matrix $^{im2}T_{im1}$ used to convert coordinates expressed in the first image referential in coordinates expressed in the second image referential. After co-registration of two modalities, it is possible to display a point defined on one modality on the other modality and vice-versa. Stereotactic trajectories can also been displayed on both modalities.
<u>Fusion</u> consists in the construction of a new hybrid data set from co-registred exams. Fusion allows a very synthetic management of multi-modalities. **For stereotactic applications, Fusion does not bring any additional information to co-registered modalities.**

---

[1] This work has been granted by the French Government

W. Niessen and M. Viergever (Eds.): MICCAI 2001, LNCS 2208, pp. 1421-1423, 2001.

2.1 Fusion of Tri-dimensional Data Sets

Different methods have been implemented for fusion of 3D reconstructed data sets:

Paired points matching (The most standard method): ISS localizer can be used for high accuracy image fusion (0.3 to 0.5 mm with CT/CT matching) .
Automatic fusion of same modalities (performed with the same patient position) (for instance T1 /T2 MRI exams): co-registration based on imaging system coordinates
Automatic fusion of framebased exams: co-registration based on frame coordinates
Fusion of framebased/frameless exams: co-registration based on robot basis coordinates
Local Matching (in case of image distortions): local paired points or manual matching.

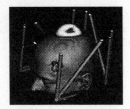 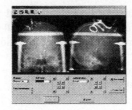 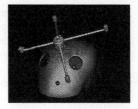

Fig. 1. Framebased 3D exam – Framebased 2D exams – Frameless 3D exam

2.2 Co-registration

2D/3D Co-registration
To co-register two perpendicular X-rays views (framebased), the frame coordinates are used if the 3D exam is performed in framebased mode (automatic co-registration), and the robot basis if the 3D exam is performed in frameless mode.
Integration of statistical data [1][6][7]
Statistical data does not bring a high level of accuracy but they are very useful for target presetting and for trajectory verification. We are currently gathering our functional cases in a statistical database. Each target is validated by microelectrode recording and clinical results evaluation. In order to reduce the effect of patient to patient variations, statistical coordinates of functional targets are defined in an anatomical referential defined by anatomical landmarks (the anterior and posterior commissures and the mid-plane). This orthogonal referential is scaled with the thalamus height and the intercomissure distance. To preset functional targets with their statistical coordinates on images, we co-register the image referential with the described natomical referential. The landmarks are defined on images (2D or 3D data sets) and are introduced in a paired points matching algorithm. The same co-registration technique can also be applied for statistical brain atlases integration (Scaling can be performed by using the Talairach proportional grid).

5   Conclusions

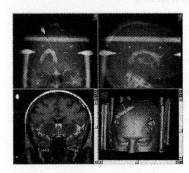

Some very simple, reliable, and useful methods are presented and discussed for integration of different modalities in the functional planning. These methods have been implemented in the VoXim™ software and are currently clinically used. They are helping us to define the optimal planning. Thanks to the NeuroMate™ stereotactic robot, the optimal targeting of the planned trajectory can be performed. This image and robotic guidance simplify dramatically the surgical procedure and leads to a very high level of accuracy.

References

1.Benabid, A.L., Pollak, P., Hoffmann D., Limousin P., Gao, D.M., LeBas, J.F., Benazzouz, A., Segebarth, C., Grand, S.
"Chronic Stimulation for Parkinson's Disease and other Movment Disorders"Textbook of Stereotactic and Functional NeuroSurgery Gildenberg-Tasker Mc Graw Hill 1998, p. 337-349

2. Zamorano, L., Pandya, A., Li, Q.H., Perez-de-laTorre, R., Pittet, P. Badano, F., Robert, V
" The clinical use and accuracy of the NeuroMate Robot for open NeuroSurgery"
Proceedings of the 14th International Congress and Exhibition Computer Assisted Radiology and Surgery (CARS 2000) Elsevier Science B.V. p. 185-190

3. Eldridge, P., Byrne, P., Golash, A., Varma, T., Pittet, P. Badano, F., Nahum, B, Michel, JP
" The clinical use and accuracy of the NeuroMate Robot for open NeuroSurgery"
Proceedings of the 14th International Congress and Exhibition Computer Assisted Radiology and Surgery (CARS 2000) Elsevier Science B.V. p. 980

4. Mösges, R., Lavallée, S.
"Multimodal information for Computer Integrated Surgery"
Computer Integrated Surgery Technology and Clinical Applications, The MIT Press 1996

5. Bucholtz, R.D., Sturm, C.D., Hogan, R.E.,
"The Use of Three Dimensional Images in Stereotactic Neurosuregry"
Textbook of Stereotactic and Functional NeuroSurgery Gildenberg-Tasker Mc Graw Hill 1998, p. 337-349

6. Coffey, R.J.
"Stereotactic Atlases in Printed Format"
Textbook of Stereotactic and Functional NeuroSurgery Gildenberg-Tasker Mc Graw Hill 1998, p. 237-248

7. Finnis, K.W., Starreveld, Y.P., Parrent, A.G., Sadikot, A.F., Peters, T.M.
"3D Functional Database of Subcortical Structures for Surgical Guidance in Image Guided Stereotactic Neurosurgery"   Proceedings of the 2nd International Conference Medical Image Computing and Computer-Assisted Intervention –MICCAI'99. Springer p. 758-757

Application of Compact Pneumatic Actuators to Laparoscopic Manipulator

Kim Daeyoung[1], Ryoichi Nakamura[2], Etsuko Kobayashi[1],
Ichiro Sakuma[1] and Takeyoshi Dohi[1]

[1]Institute of Environment Studies, Graduate School of Frontier Sciences,
[2]Department of Precision Machinery Engineering, Graduate School of Engineering
The University of Tokyo, 7-3-1 Hongo Bunkyo-Ku, Tokyo, 113-8656, Japan
{young, ryoichi, etsuko, sakuma, dohi }@miki.pe.u-tokyo.ac.jp

Abstract. In this study, as an alternative actuator for medical robot, pneumatic actuators are applied to laparoscopic manipulator, and their effectiveness was evaluated. Pneumatic actuators have a strong advantage in application to medical systems that the whole mechanism can be sterilized including actuator. We have developed a new laparoscopic manipulator system. Compared with other types of laparoscopic manipulators, it is small and light. The control system can be placed far from the patient by connecting controlling system and the manipulator with air tubes. In conclusion, we confirmed that the range of view and resolution were very useful and acceptable for clinical use and that this paper provides significant first step toward a clean and small medical robot useful in future.

1. Introduction

There are a growing number of examples of surgical robot systems[1][2]. Repeatable tool position, steady motion, and stability in a fixed position are fundamental advantages of the use of robots. Nevertheless, there are still many problems in motor-driven robot. Generally, it is very difficult to sterilize electric motors as a whole and big. Special mechanisms are used to separate sterilized part and non-sterilized part[2], or the total system is covered by sterilized drapes.

Motivated by the need for providing a *small and clean* robot, we studied the effectiveness of pneumatic actuators to Laparoscopic Manipulator.

2. System

At first, we designed the system that can be fixed on the end of steady holder. At the tip of the holder, 2DOFs' joint. The joint (in the circle) has motions of rolling and pitching, so it is possible to rotate the laparoscope.

W. Niessen and M. Viergever (Eds.): MICCAI 2001, LNCS 2208, pp. 1424-1425, 2001.
© Springer-Verlag Berlin Heidelberg 2001

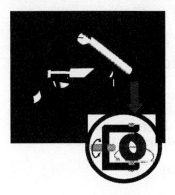 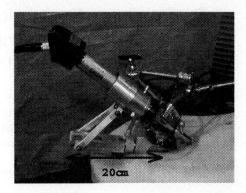

Fig. 1.(a) The concept of the structure (b) Prototype of pneumatic laparoscope system

The cylinder-A controls the horizontal movements, and the cylinder-B controls the vertical movements (Fig.1(a)). By the sliding of the cylinder-A, the laparoscope rotates the y-axis in xz- plane. When the□cylinder-B slides, the laparoscope rotates the x-axis.

3. Discussion and Conclusion

In this study, a small and light laparoscopic manipulator was realized by introducing pneumatic linear actuators.

For the size(20cm×10cm×10cm),it makes possible to reduce the space could be obstruct. About the view range, we knew 38° in horizontal and 18 ° in vertical range that it could see the whole of the liver model when it is far from 20cm from the tip of laparoscope. The resolution less than 0.5mm in cylinder, corresponding to 0.3° in angle of view.

Simple structure and connecting mechanism made it easy to assemble the system after sterilization since the whole mechanism can be sterilized including actuator.

We confirmed the effectiveness of pneumatic actuator in designing clean and compact medical robots.

This study was partly supported by the Research for the Future Program (JSPS-RFTF 99I00904).

References

1. Taylor RH, Funda J, Eldridge B, Gomory S, Gruben K, LaRose D, Talamini M, Kavossi L, Anderson J A   Telerobotic Assistant for Laparoscopic Surgery. Computer Integrated Surgery: The MIT Press, (1995) pp 581-592
2.Etsuko Kobayashi 5-links laparoscope manipulator for minimally invasive operation, 1997

Performance Evaluation of a Cooperative Manipulation Microsurgical Assistant Robot Applied to Stapedotomy

Peter J. Berkelman*, Daniel L. Rothbaum M.D., Jaydeep Roy, Sam Lang,
Louis L. Whitcomb, Greg Hager, Patrick S. Jensen, Eugene de Juan,
Russell H. Taylor, and John K. Niparko M.D.**

Johns Hopkins University

Abstract. This paper reports the development of a full-scale instrumented model of the human ear that permits quantitative evaluation of the utility of a microsurgical assistant robot in the surgical procedure of stapedotomy.

1 Introduction

The need for microsurgical assistants arises from the normal limitations of human dexterity resulting from tremor, jerk, drift, and overshoot [1, 2]. Recently developed robotic assistant devices offer the possibility of extending human performance to permit fine manipulation tasks that are normally considered difficult orimpossible[3, 4, 5, 6, 7, 8, 9]. The "steady-hand" robot employed in these experiments cooperatively assists a surgeon to manipulate microsurgical tools [9]. In this paradigm, both the user and the robot cooperatively hold and manipulate the surgical instrument [8]. This paper reports the development of a full-scale instrumented model of the human ear that permits quantitative evaluation of the utility of the "steady-hand" robot in the surgical procedure of stapedotomy. The model enables direct measurement of intra-operative parameters for two important steps in the stapedotomy operation: (i) fenestration and (ii) prosthesis crimping. Using this instrumented surgical model, we plan to compare performance measures of stapedotomy performed (a) manually and (b) with robotic assistance and, further, to evaluate the effect of expert/novice differences in the comparative performance of human-robotic augmentation.

Otosclerosis, a disorder of the middle ear that causes conductive progressive hearing loss, occurs when bony deposits cause the stapes-the innermost bone of the middle ear-to become immobilized. In consequence, sound vibrations cannot propagate to the inner ear. In stapedotomy, part of the immobilized stapes bone is removed and replaced by a small piston-shaped prosthesis. To achieve contact

---

* Currently at the University of Grenoble
** We gratefully acknowledge the support of the National Science Foundation under grants IIS9801684 and EEC9731478, the Johns Hopkins University, and the National Institutes of Health under Training Grant 5-T32-HL07712.

W. Niessen and M. Viergever (Eds.): MICCAI 2001, LNCS 2208, pp. 1426–1429, 2001.

between the stapes prosthesis and inner ear, the footplate is fenestrated with a micro-pick. After the prosthesis has been placed within the fenestration, it is attached by crimping an integral wire to the long process of the incus, the second of the three bones of the middle ear.

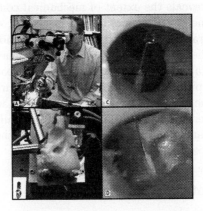

Fig. 1. (A) Dr. Larry Lustig using the stapedotomy surgical station. (B) View of the temporal bone and endoscopes. (C) and (D) View from the endoscopic cameras.

2 Experimental Methodology

Our goal is to compare the performance of otologic surgeons with and without robotic assistance. Using the instrumented model ear, we are able to compare performance variables during both the fenestration and crimping steps of stapedotomy. Performance variables will be measured for skilled operators performing multiple repetitions of a procedure both with and without robotic assistance. To replicate closely actual operative conditions, the procedures reported herein are performed in a prepared human temporal bone. The temporal bone has been drilled to permit 1) visual access to two endoscopic cameras mounted nearly-orthogonal to one another and 2) positioning of an artificial stapes bone mounted on a load cell. To ensure authentic yet repeatable experimental trials, we employ synthetic artificial stapes bone samples exhibiting mechanical properties typical of actual stapes footplates. The experimental setup is pictured in Figure 1.

We measure performance variables for fenestration of the stapes footplate as follows: (i) To measure perforation diameter, we photograph the fenestrated stapes footplate, and analyze the image digitally to measure the actual fenestration diameter. (ii) To measure the perforation placement around a desired point, we employ the same digital imaging technique of the previous step. (iii) To measure force applied to the stapes footplate, we record forces on the load cell upon which the stapes bone is mounted.

We measure performance variables for crimping of the stapes prosthesis to the incus bone as follows: (i) To measure the degree of circumferential contact between the prosthesis wire and incus bone, we employ a sensitive high-impedance op-amp circuit to measure electrical continuity between the each of the electrodes on the artificial incus and the prosthesis wire. The number of incus electrodes exhibiting continuity reveals the extent of mechanical contact between prosthesis wire and incus bone. (ii) To measure crimp quality, experienced otologists judge post-crimping frame-grabbed images from the endoscopic cameras. (iii) To measure force applied to the oval window during crimping, we use the load cell upon which the stapes bone is mounted. (iv) To measure movement of the prosthesis during crimping, we film the crimping procedure with two endoscopic cameras. By moving the robot in a pre-defined trajectory, we are able to calculate the exact angle between the cameras. Thus, after optically tracking the images on each camera, we can reconstruct the movement of the piston prosthesis in three-dimensional space.

Acknowledgements

We gratefully acknowledge the contribution of Professors Dan Stoianovici and Dr. Louis R. Kavoussi M.D., who permitted us to employ the Remote Center of Motion (RCM) surgical robot module, reported in [10], as a component of the steady hand robot; JHU Professor Robert Cammarata; students Ingrid Shao; Han Seo Cho; Matthew Hansen,Jason Wachs, Rajesh Kumar and Aaron Barnes; machinists Terry Shelley and Jay Burns; and Drs. Howard Francis M.D. and Larry Lustig M.D. for their help in various parts of the project.

References

[1] C. N. Riviere, P. S. Rader, and P. K. Khosla, "Characteristics of hand motion of eye surgeons," in *Proc. of the 19th Conf. of the IEEE Engineering in Medicine and Biology Society*, (Chicago), pp. 1690–1693, October 1997.

[2] C. N. Riviere and P. K. Khosla, "Accuracy of positioning in handheld instruments," in *Proc. of the 18th Conf. of the IEEE Engineering in Medicine and Biology Society*, October 1996.

[3] H. Kazerooni, "Human/robot interaction via the transfer of power and information signals — part i: Dynamics and control analysis," in *Proceedings of IEEE International Conference on Robotics and Automation*, vol. 3, pp. 1632–1640, 1989.

[4] H. Kazerooni, "Human/robot interaction via the transfer of power and information signals — part ii: An experimental analysis," in *Proceedings of IEEE International Conference on Robotics and Automation*, vol. 3, pp. 1641–1649, 1989.

[5] H. Kazerooni and J. Guo, "Human extenders," *ASME Journal Dynamic Systems, Measurement, and Control*, vol. 115, pp. 281–290, June 1993.

[6] S. D. Ho, R. Hibberd, and B. Davies, "Robot assisted knee surgery," *IEEE EMBS Magazine Special Issue on Robotics in Surgery*, pp. 292–300, April-May 1995.

[7] J. Troccaz, M. Peshkin, and B. Davies, "The use of localizers, robots, and synergistic devices in CAS," in *Proc. First Joint Conference of CVRMed and MRCAS*, (Grenoble), 1997.

[8] R. H. Taylor, J. Funda, B. Eldridge, K. Gruben, D. LaRose, S. Gomory, and M. Talamini, *A Telerobotic Assistant for Laparoscopic Surgery*, ch. 45, pp. 581–592. MIT Press, 1996.

[9] R. H. Taylor, P. Jensen, L. L. Whitcomb, A. Barnes, R. Kumar, D. Stoianovici, P. Gupta, Z. Wang, E. deJuan, and L. R. Kavoussi, "A steady-hand robotic system for microsurgical augmentation," *International Journal of Robotics Research*, vol. 18, pp. 1201–1210, December 1999.

[10] D. Stoianovici, L. L. Whitcomb, J. H. Anderson, R. H. Taylor, and L. R. Kavoussi, "A modular surgical system for image guided percutaneous procedures," in *Lecture Notes in Computer Science 1496: Medical Imaging and Computer-Assisted Intervention - MICCAI'98* (W. M. Wells, A. Colchester, and S. Delp, eds.), vol. 1496, pp. 404–410, Berlin, Germany: Springer-Verlag, October 1998.

A Modular Robotic System for Ultrasound Image Acquisition

Randal P. Goldberg[1], Mazilu Dumitru [2], Russell H. Taylor[1,3], Dan Stoianovici[1,2]

1 Mechanical Engineering Department, The Johns Hopkins University, Baltimore, MD, USA
2 Brady Urological Institute, Johns Hopkins Hospital, Baltimore, MD, USA
3 Computer Science Department, The Johns Hopkins University, Baltimore, MD, USA

Abstract. This paper reports a modular robotic system currently in development for performing intra-operative 3-D ultrasound scans. The final goal is to be able to utilize ultrasound as a guidance and imaging modality for a variety of computer integrated surgery applications by overcoming the limits it's handheld nature presents. The primary component of the system is a compact 3 DOF robot called the Translational Remote Center of Motion Robot (TRCM). This unit, which can be used standalone or as a dexterity end effector for a larger degree of freedom base robot, can perform the motions necessary to locate and perform force controlled scans of target anatomy quickly and safely. This relatively inexpensive unit, while designed with the ultrasound application in mind, also becomes a useful general purpose robot for any application in which an RCM mechanism is desired.

1 Introduction

Ultrasound is a useful imaging tool for surgeons, capable of providing both 2-D images as well as 3-D models of the anatomy. These scans can be performed intraoperatively to provide real time information to the surgeon both about the target anatomy, as well as the location of surgical tools (such as needles in percutaneous therapy).

A major roadblock to the incorporation of ultrasound imaging in CIS applications is that it utilizes a handheld scanner to acquire the images. It is useful for giving the surgeon qualitative information about the anatomy, such as whether a tumor has grown or shrank, or in general where an instrument is relative to the anatomy is. Unfortunately, the images reflect both movements of the probe by the operator, as well as changes to the anatomy. In addition, there are many other operator dependant variables associated with ultrasound, such as variable scan times and inconsistent image quality due to changes in the applied force. These makes it difficult to perform the quantitative image processing necessary for it to be used as an effective tool to guide computer integrated surgery applications.

Several robotically assisted ultrasound systems have been developed, though not with the express purpose of intra-operative scanning. [1,2] In addition, they rely on large, specialized high degree of freedom robots to manipulate the ultrasound probe.

W. Niessen and M. Viergever (Eds.): MICCAI 2001, LNCS 2208, pp. 1430-1432, 2001.

2 Robot Design

A set of design requirements for the system was developed through conversations with members of the Johns Hopkins Hospital Ultrasonography department.   It was decided that the ability to generate three target motions were desired: rotation and fan type scans, and translation for tracking patient motion and force control. (Figure 1) In addition, the range of motion for each of these degrees of freedom was determined from sonographer requests. Clearly rotation type models require 180° of motion to complete.   For the remaining two degrees of freedom, observation of and discussion with the clinicians led to a target of 120° of motion minimum for the fan type scan, and 50mm minimum of translational motion.

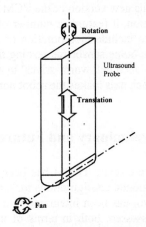

Figure 1: Desired Robot Degrees of Freedom

In   addition,   a   simple   experiment   was performed with an instrumented ultrasound probe, to get a range of values for the forces the robot would encounter during a scan.   Over a variety of scans, the sonographer produced an average of 7 N of force. This value agrees with the more complete evaluation reported in [1], and was used as a starting point for the translation stage design.

The two rotational motions lend themselves to RCM type designs, so a number of these were evaluated. Based on range of motion requirements, and the desire for a compact design, the mini "RCM" configuration was selected. [3] The mini "RCM" uses a chain drive to implement a parallelogram mechanism for it's pitch stage. For the ultrasound application, this degree of freedom actuates the fan type scan, and is adapted directly from the standard robot.

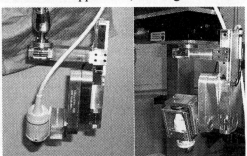

Figure 2: TRCM with US Probe on Passive Arm (left) and on a 3DOF cartesian base robot(right)

The difficulty in using the mini "RCM" for ultrasound arose from the size of the tool and the required range of   motion.   When   the ultrasound probe is mounted on the robot, with it's face centered at the RCM point, it interferes with the pitch degree of freedom, limiting its range of motion. To overcome this, the roll stage of the robot was offset. This allows the ultrasound probe (and other large instruments) to be mounted at the RCM point, while maintaining full 360° motion in both rotation joints.

The adjustable angle joint, which in the mini "RCM" allows tools to be placed at the RCM point, was removed, and in its place a translation stage was inserted. The translation stage uses a miniature ball screw actuator, and runs on a pair of recirculating linear ball bearings.

This new version of the RCM has been dubbed the Translational RCM (TRCM). In addition, it features a number of improvements over previous mini "RCM" versions. These include incorporation of high resolution redundant encoders on all three axes and a home sensor for zeroing the pitch stage. In addition, the TRCM utilizes newly developed ball worm drives[4] in each of the rotation stages. The use of ball type drives on each axis makes the robot non-back drivable and very stiff with zero backlash.

3 Preliminary and Future Work

The prototype TRCM has been constructed, and is shown in Figure 2 in two of its envisioned configurations for intrapoerative ultrasound. Force sensing and basic robot control has been integrated into the robot. In the future, the robot's performance will be assessed, both in terms of its usefulness as a stand alone tool for intraoperative ultrasound, as well as in a variety of cooperative configurations.

Acknowledgments

The authors gratefully acknowledge the support of the National Science Foundation Engineering Research Center Grant #EEC9731478. We also thank Dr. Sheila Sheth and Robert De Jong for supplying ultrasound equipment and assistance. In addition, we thank Louis L. Whitcomb for his input over the course of the project.

References

1) S. E. Salcdean, G. Bell, S Bachmann, W. –H. Zhu, P. Abolmaesumi, and P. D. Lawrence, "Robot-assisted diagnostic ultrasound – design and feasibility experiment," MICCAI '99, UK, 1999

2) E. Degoulange, L. Urbain, P. Caron, S. Boudet, J. Gariepy, J.-L. Megnien, F. Pierrot, and E. Dombre, "HIPPOCRATE: an intrinsically safe robot for medical applications," Proc. IEEE/RSJ Int. Conf. on Intelligent Robots and Systems, IROS'98, Victoria, pp. 959-964,1998

3) Stoianovici, D., Whitcomb, L.L., Anderson, J.H., Taylor, R.H., Kavoussi L.R, "A Modular Surgical Robotic System for Image Guided Percutaneous Procedures," Lecture Notes in Computer Science, Springer-Verlga, Vol. 1496, Pp. 404-410, 1998

4) Stoianovici D, Kavoussi LR: Ball-Worm Transmission, (1999), Regular U.S. utility and PCT application filled by the Johns Hopkins University (#DM-3512)

A Mechatronic System
for the Implantation of the Acetabular Component
in Total Hip Alloarthroplasty

Fridun Kerschbaumer[a], MD; Juergen Wahrburg[b], PhD and Stephan Kuenzler[a]

[a] Department of Arthritis Surgery, University of Frankfurt, Marienburgstr. 2,
60525 Frankfurt (Main), Germany
kerschbaumer@em.uni-frankfurt.de

[b] University of Siegen, Hoelderlinstr. 3, 57068 Siegen, Germany.
wahrburg@zess.uni-siegen.de

Abstract. The paper presents a novel approach to integrate a robot and an optical 3D digitizing system. In a first application, the combined system is used as a sophisticated tool for precise preparation of the acetabulum and for reproducible positioning of the cup implant. A prototype system has been set up and successfully tested in laboratory as well as in cadaver trials. A major advantage of the system is the support of less invasive interventions without loosing accuracy or other drawbacks. Future work will extend its application also to the femoral part of the total hip replacement procedure.

Introduction

Surgical robots are already clinically used in total hip replacement (THR) procedures to prepare the femur by precisely milling the cavity for the stem prosthesis. However, the implantation of the acetabular component is still carried out conventionally by hand. This contribution illustrates the design of a new mechatronic system to support the implantation of the acetabular THR component by improving as well the geometric quality of the reamed bony bed as the placement of the implant in the optimal position and orientation.

System Description

The selected approach is based on the combination of a robot carrying the surgical tools and an optical 3D digitizing system to register the position and the structure of the acetabulum. A control PC connects both systems and coordinates their operation. The combination of a passive digitizing system and an active robotic system exploits the advantages of both systems, that is, easy, fast and safe registration combined with precise, tremor-free guidance of the surgical tools.

A new modular surgical tool system is being developed comprising instruments similar to those used in manually performed operations. The instruments are fixed on a one-degree-of-freedom carriage which is mounted at the wrist of the robot and moved manually by the surgeon. A quick-lock mechanism faciliates fast changes of the tools during surgery. Furthermore it will offer easy adaptation of the tool system for use in other orthopedic procedures, e.g. knee surgery.

W. Niessen and M. Viergever (Eds.): MICCAI 2001, LNCS 2208, pp. 1433-1434, 2001.
© Springer-Verlag Berlin Heidelberg 2001

The intraoperative registration is carried out by scanning the acetabulum and certain bony landmarks using the pointer of the digitizing system. After the alignment of the pre- and intraoperative data sets the robot positions the surgical tool mounted on the carriage in a position close to the operating area. If the surgeon has moved the carriage up to its end position, the reamer and the implant respectively will be exactly in the position and orientation as determined during preoperative planning. Special reamers have been developed to produce a smooth bony surface.

Patient movements that may occur during the intervention are automatically corrected. A reference frame of the optical digitizing system is rigidly fixed close to the acetabulum. Any deviation of position and orientation of this frame are measured by the system and directly transformed into a correcting movement of the robot.

The architecture of the new mechatronic system combing a 3D digitizer and a robot is illustrated in Fig. 1:

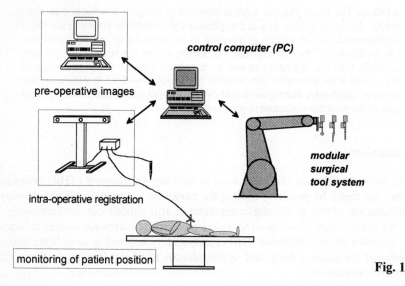

Fig. 1

Conclusion

A prototype of the system has already been used in laboratory and cadaver trials. The results have turned out that it is possible to achieve an overall accuracy of 1 mm or 1° angle deviation with a minimal invasive surgical technique. The robotic system is not expected to prolong the operation time more than 15 minutes in comparison to manual performance, as similar or even more efficient surgical instruments are applied. This compensates for the short additional time needed for registration. The course of the operative procedure is similar to conventional THR surgery, giving the surgeon the possibility to control every step of the operation.

The ongoing research focuses on the extension of the system to also perform the femoral part of the THR procedure. Further methods for intraoperative registration using X-rays are investigated.

Optimal Port Placement in Robot-Assisted Coronary Artery Bypass Grafting

Shaun Selha, B.S.[1], Pierre Dupont, Ph.D.[1], Robert Howe, Ph.D.[2], and
David Torchiana, M.D.[3]

[1] Aerospace and Mechanical Engineering, Boston University, Boston MA, USA
{busds, pierre}@bu.edu
[2] Division of Engineering & Applied Science, Harvard University, Cambridge MA,
USA
howe@deas.harvard.edu
[3] Division of Cardiac Surgery, Massachusetts General Hospital, Boston MA, USA
dtorchiana@partners.org

Abstract. A computer-based algorithm is being developed which, using
preoperative images, provides the surgeon with a list of feasible port
triplets ranked according to tool dexterity and endoscope view quality
at each surgical site involved in a procedure. Computer simulation will
allow the surgeon to select from among the proposed port locations.
The procedure selected for the development of the system consists of
left internal mammary artery (LIMA) take-down and bypass grafting.
Human trials will begin within a month. Data collected from these trials
will be used to validate the system.

1 Introduction

Robotic assistance enables the use of minimally-invasive techniques in coronary
artery bypass grafting by scaling hand motions, decreasing tremor, and enhancing manipulation. In these procedures, endoscopes and instruments are inserted
through small incisions or "ports" to access the surgical site. In initial trials of
this approach, inappropriate port locations have posed a number of difficulties,
including poor dexterity, inability to reach all the required tissue structures, and
collisions between the instruments, both within and outside the patient's body.

A graphical simulation system [1] and an algorithmic approach to port placement [2] have been presented in the literature for the daVinci™ robot system.
Experimental guidelines for the selection of port locations for the ZEUS™ robot
system made by Computer Motion, Inc. appear in [3]. This abstract presents an
algorithm for optimizing port placement for the ZEUS™ system.

The three main issues in defining optimal port placement are tool dexterity,
endoscope viewpoint and workspace limits. Tool dexterity is defined by the relative orientation of the tools with respect to each other and to the surgical site.
Endoscope viewpoint is defined with respect to the tools and with respect to the
surgical site. Workspace limits are reached when a desired tool motion would
cause a tool / endoscope / patient collision or a robot /robot / patient collision.

W. Niessen and M. Viergever (Eds.): MICCAI 2001, LNCS 2208, pp. 1435–1436, 2001.

2 Approach

At this stage, our efforts have focused on tool dexterity and endoscope viewpoint. Aspects of workspace limits are incorporated through selection of feasible port locations as defined below. The algorithm takes as inputs a CT image of the patient's thorax (with artery locations visualized by contrast agent), an array of possible port locations in the intercostal spaces, and a set of surgical sites where tissue is to be manipulated. Its output is a set of feasible port locations ranked according to a cost function. The latter is based on the optimal orientation of the tools and endoscope with respect to each other and with respect to the surgical sites.

Each surgical site is defined by a point in space and surface normal direction at the point. For LIMA takedown, the spatial curve describing artery location is discretized and the resulting set of points is used for site definition. Feasible port triplets correspond to a subset of array triplets that fall within workspace limits, meet minimum dexterity and viewing requirements and satisfy surgeon preferences. Optimal kinematic dexterity and endoscope viewpoint are defined with respect to a surgical site based on clinical experience. These can be modified according to the procedure, tools and surgeon preferences.

A nested search is used to consider feasible port locations and all surgical sites. Due to the constrained relative positioning of the endoscope and tools, the set of feasible triplets is modest. The result is a ranking of feasible port triplets according to a weighted average of their dexterity measure at all surgical sites. The results are displayed graphically, superimposed on the preoperative image, showing the grid of feasible port locations and surgical sites. The user can select port triplets from among those with highest ranking and manipulate a display of the tools and endoscope. Tool color changes to indicate when dexterity or workspace limits are exceeded. Additional two-dimensional views of the feasible port location grid depict through color-coding their relative optimality to assist the user in comparing port locations.

Data collection during upcoming human trials will permit evaluation of the system. Future work will consider robot interference, robot placement and arm posture as well as the placement of additional assist ports.

References

1. L. Adhami, E. Coste-Maniere and J.-D. Boissonnat. Planning and simulation of robitically assisted minimal invasive surgery. *Proc MICCAI '00*. Lecture notes in computer science. Vol. 1935, Springer, October 2000.
2. E. Coste-Maniere, L. Adhami, R. Severac-Bastide, A. Lobontiu, J. Salsibury Jr., J.-D. Boisonnat, N. Swarup, G. Guthart, E. Mousseaux and A. Carpentier. Optimized Port Placement for the totally endoscopic coronary artery bypass grafting using the daVinci robotic system. *Proc Intl Symp Exp Rob*. Springer, December 2000.
3. H. Tabaie, J. Reinbolt, W. Graper, T. Kelly and M. Connor. Endoscopic coronary artery bypass graft (ECABG) procedure with robotic assistance. *Heart Surg Forum* #1999-0552, 2:310-317, 1999.

Author Index

1440   Author Index

Lecture Notes in Computer Science

For information about Vols. 1–2118
please contact your bookseller or Springer-Verlag